Pediatric Psychopharmacology

PEDIATRIC PSYCHOPHARMACOLOGY

Principles and Practice

Edited by

ANDRÉS MARTIN, M.D., M.P.H.
LAWRENCE SCAHILL, M.S.N., PH.D.
DENNIS S. CHARNEY, M.D.
JAMES F. LECKMAN, M.D.

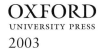
OXFORD
UNIVERSITY PRESS
2003

OXFORD
UNIVERSITY PRESS

Oxford   New York
Auckland   Bangkok   Buenos Aires   Cape Town   Chennai
Dar es Salaam   Delhi   Hong Kong   Istanbul   Karachi   Kolkata
Kuala Lumpur   Madrid   Melbourne   Mexico City   Mumbai   Nairobi
Sâo Paulo   Shanghai   Singapore   Taipei   Tokyo   Toronto

Published by Oxford University Press, Inc.
198 Madison Avenue, New York, New York, 10016
http://www.oup-usa.org

Oxford is a registered trademark of Oxford University Press

Library of Congress Cataloging-in-Publication Data

Pediatric psychopharmacology : principles and practice / edited by Andrés Martin . . . [et al.].
    p. ; cm.   Includes bibliographical references and index.
ISBN 0-19-514173-3
1. Pediatric psychopharmacology. 2. Psychotropic drugs. I. Martin, Andrés.
[DNLM: 1. Mental Disorders—drug therapy—Child. 2. Psychopharmacology—Child. 3. Psychotropic Drugs—therapeutic use—Child. WS 350.2 P371 2003]
RJ504.7 .P397 2003
615'.78—dc21   2002022460

The science of medicine is a rapidly changing field. As new research and clinical experience broaden our
knowledge, changes in treatment and drug therapy do occur. The author and publisher of this work have
checked with sources believed to be reliable in their efforts to provide information that is accurate and complete,
and in accordance with the standards accepted at the time of publication. However, in light of the possibility
of human error or changes in the practice of medicine, neither the author, nor the publisher, nor any other
party who has been involved in the preparation or publication of this work warrants that the information
contained herein is in every respect accurate or complete. Readers are encouraged to confirm the information
contained herein with other reliable sources, and are strongly advised to check the product information sheet
provided by the pharmaceutical company for each drug they plan to administer.

9 8 7 6 5 4

Printed in the United State of America
on acid-free paper

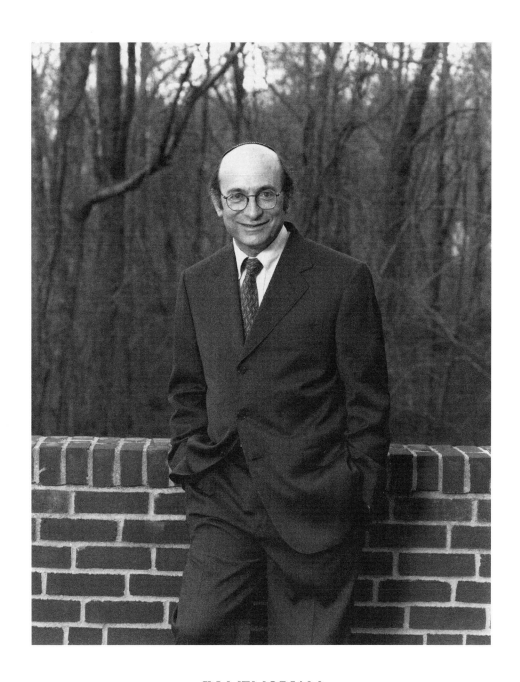

IN MEMORIAM

Donald J. Cohen, M.D.
September 5, 1940–October 2, 2001

Foreword

It is still early in our understanding of the pathogenesis and treatment of psychiatric disorders—the brain is, after all, the most complex object of study in the history of science. Knowledge about the pathogenesis and treatment of pediatric psychiatric disorders has been even harder won than knowledge about adult mental illness because the inherent difficulties of understanding brain and behavior are further complicated by challenges posed by development. Pediatric psychopharmacology has faced additional hurdles, as there are special ethical challenges in the conduct of clinical research, including clinical trials. Moreover, the field of pediatric psychopharmacology developed against the backdrop of entrenched prescientific approaches to childhood psychiatric disorders, approaches that often had strong biases against drug treatment for children that were based entirely in untested theory. Despite these hurdles, the last decade has seen pediatric psychopharmacology emerge as a discipline with a growing knowledge base and an increasingly well-defined set of research goals. The progress in pediatric psychopharmacology evidenced by this volume is particularly important for the sake of the children whom it will benefit. Psychiatric disorders that occur in childhood not only cause suffering, disability, and family distress but may also cast a lifelong shadow. A child with an untreated mood or anxiety disorder, for example, or untreated attention-deficit hyperactivity disorder, may have difficulties learning in school and problems developing healthy family and peer relationships. Over time, such children exhibit elevated risks of developing secondary psychiatric disorders, including substance use disorders, and of school failure and legal difficulties. Early and appropriate diagnosis and treatment can avert such downward spirals.

This volume brings together our best current understandings of relevant neurobiology, pharmacology, and treatment for a broad range of childhood mental disorders and as such, it is both significant and useful. I sincerely hope, however, that the authors of this volume are dedicated to this project for the long haul, because, as significant as the progress of the last decade has been, we are just at the beginning of what we must achieve in basic science, clinical investigation, and treatment recommendations. Emerging approaches to brain and behavior derived from sources as diverse as the genome project and cognitive neuroscience are creating new opportunities for research in pediatric psychopharmacology, but the wise use of these tools will require hard work, new ideas, and ingenuity. For example, genetic approaches to pathogenesis and treatment development, while very promising, have also proven extremely difficult. Perhaps it should have come as no surprise that the genetic contribution to risk of abnormalities in cognition, emotion, and behavioral control are based not on single genetic mutations but on the complex interaction of multiple genetic variants and nongenetic factors. Similarly, deep understandings of human brain development and its relation to behavioral maturation and disease risk will not be easily achieved. It is only in recent years that a basic platform for such knowledge—atlases of human brain anatomy as it changes over the course of development—have begun to emerge. Other critically important areas of science are just beginning to coalesce. One such area that should have an impact on pediatric psychopharmacology is social neuroscience, the attempt to show how the brain supports social behavior, including interpersonal interactions, and to understand how social interactions shape the brain. Even for use of existing medications, much remains to be done in the arena of treatment studies. Well-designed and larger-scale clinical trials for such common childhood and adolescent illnesses as depression and anxiety disorders have either only recently been completed or are still under way. Clinical trials in young children are much in need, but raise daunting ethical questions.

With full recognition that we still have far to travel, the appearance of this volume documents the fact that pediatric psychopharmacology has reached its own important developmental milestone. What is contained in this volume and the implied promise it holds for the future will be of enormous benefit to children and families.

Steven E. Hyman
Provost
Harvard University
Cambridge, MA

Preface

The student who has the capacity to be parented—to appreciate the nurturance and to show this through his own growth—will develop the ability to parent: to be loyal to the values of his teachers by conveying them to his own students.

Donald Cohen (1986)

If we take eternity to mean not infinite temporal duration but timelessness, then eternal life belongs to those who live in the present. Our life has no end in just the way in which our visual field has no limits.

Ludwig Wittgenstein (1922)

Pediatric Psychopharmacology: Principles and Practice first became a concrete idea in the fall of 1999, shortly after the publication of the first edition of *Neurobiology of Mental Illness*. Under the lead editorship of Dennis Charney (together with Eric Nestler and Steven Bunney, when all three were still at Yale), *Neurobiology of Mental Illness* set a new standard for scholarship in the rapidly evolving field of biological psychiatry, and provided a powerful impetus and central model for this book. Like many others, we thought then that a critical mass of knowledge and evidence had accrued in the field of pediatric psychopharmacology, such that the time was ripe for organizing a similarly comprehensive volume that was entirely devoted to the topic. Developing that original idea into the specific project that it has become today has been a challenging task involving difficult choices. Among the many decisions made, however, the easiest and least disputed of all proved in the end to be the most daunting. We agreed from the outset that Donald Cohen would be the optimal person to write the volume's introduction, as we could think of no one better able to contextualize its scope within the broader domain of child and adolescent psychiatry.

Things turned out very differently. Donald J. Cohen, M.D., Sterling Professor of Child Psychiatry, Psychology and Pediatrics, and Director of the Yale Child Study Center since 1983, died at the age of 61 on October 2, 2001. As our friend, mentor, and colleague, Donald followed with interest and excitement the progress of the book, but in the end, his untimely death did not permit him to write what he had gladly agreed to contribute: where there was to be his introduction now stand his photograph and a memorial note instead. Even if our loss is recent as we write these lines, this volume has proven to be an active way of mobilizing our grief, as it has become an effective vehicle for carrying his vision forward. It has, in fact, made Donald present in our lives in unsuspected ways.

Donald Cohen did not see himself as a psychopharmacologist, much as he did not see himself as a therapist, a psychoanalyst, a researcher, or a policy-maker. Not only did he find fault with such traditional demarcations as applied to himself, he also saw them more broadly as shortsighted truncations and pigeonholings of our field and of our professional selves. A master humorist, with tongue in cheek he boasted about having the very same prescription pad that he had received upon graduating from medical school. Donald was the ultimate advocate for children and for child psychiatry, a specialty he saw at the core of pediatrics. He felt an enormous sense of pride on seeing the growth of the field during the decades of his active work, and remained the perennial optimist to the end, hopeful that its major breakthroughs and most effective therapies were near at hand.

As we completed this project, it became clear that Donald's vision was woven into the fabric of the entire volume. For example, we propose an integrated model that places psychopharmacology as but one (albeit a powerful one) among the many tools available for the treatment of psychiatrically ill children and adolescents. Much as he would, we advocate for thoughtfulness and restraint in the prescription of psychotropic drugs, for the judicious use of diagnostic labels, and for the conceptualization of childhood psychiatric disorders within a developmental framework. Instead of a pathway toward the diagnostic and therapeutic minimization of the psychiatrically ill child, we see (and practice on a daily basis) psychopharmacology as another venue toward the deeper understanding and more effective treatment of affected youngsters. These overarching tenets are at the core of the volume. Even while bringing together a large body of knowledge and serving as a benchmark for the advances of the basic and clinical sciences that underlie psychopharmacology, this book is in some ways more than just dedicated to Donald Cohen; it is largely imbued with his vision for this novel and promising discipline. As a reminder of this vision, we have started the preface and each of the part introductions that follow with citations from his extensive body of writings.

The volume is divided into four major sections. The first, *Biological Bases of Pediatric Psychopharmacology*, provides a foundation of neurobiology upon which the rest of the volume is built. The molecular and genetic mechanisms that underlie brain development and drug action are presented as fundamental building blocks for the larger part, *Developmental Psychopathology*, devoted to discrete diagnostic entities. Here one of Donald's central views, concerning the interplay between normal developmental trajectories, their disrupted course under disease states and the individual's adaptation to such dysregulation, is extended further, with particular attention paid to psychotropic drug effects. This first section benefits richly from the genetic and brain imaging findings of the "decade of the brain," and reflects the increasing depth in our understanding of the workings of the brain under normal and pathological states.

The second section, *Somatic Interventions*, reviews the current state of knowledge of the various drug classes routinely used in child psychiatry. It addresses in particular age-specific differences relevant to medication action, including variations in response or side effect profiles, as well as regulatory issues pertaining to children. Other somatic interventions, such as complementary and alternative medicine approaches, as well as electroconvulsive and related treatments, are also discussed. Of note, the chapter devoted to the α agonists is a fitting tribute to the man who first proposed the use of clonidine for the treatment of a child psychiatric condition in the 1970s.

The third and longest section, *Assessment and Treatment*, begins with general approaches and tools that are applicable across disorders. These include paying attention to the whole child, rather than merely to the symptoms; the importance of careful diagnostic assessment and measurement of symptom severity; and a full appreciation of the child's personal experience of being ill and being treated with medication. The section encompasses a broad range of clinical populations, including the vulnerable and traditionally "orphan" ones in research and practice: very young children, and those with comorbid mental retardation, medical illness, or severe substance abuse. Each of the disorder-specific chapters is in turn related back to the underlying developmental psychopathology and drug-specific principles previously presented. Our goal has been to achieve the most integrated flow possible throughout the book. In so doing, we hope to emulate Donald's uncanny ability to move seamlessly between basic research and the care of vulnerable, suffering children.

Even if the shortest, the book's final section, *Epidemiological, Research, and Methodological Considerations*, is quintessential Donald Cohen, in that it highlights the moral and scientific imperative *to know*, which is necessary to be our most clinically effective selves. In Donald's view, every single clinical encounter is, or should be, research. The ethical quandary for him lay not in whether to do research in children, but rather in *not* doing it. As a mover and shaper of policy, he devoted much of his energy to increasing funding to bolster these activities at the local and federal levels, as well as internationally. The volume thus ends appropriately with a chapter on international perspectives on pediatric psychopharmacology.

The success of *Neurobiology of Mental Illness* (the second edition of which is well under way) reflects and contributes to the exciting developments rapidly taking place in the field of biological psychiatry. We appreciate that part of such success can be attributed to the editorial excellence of Oxford University Press. We too are excited about the rapidly paced developments that propel our field each day, grateful to the volume's authors for their engagement and commitment to this work, and indebted to Fiona Stevens at Oxford for her superb and patient editorial support. More than anything, we are profoundly grateful and indebted to Donald Cohen, our mentor and friend. We miss him dearly, and hope in some modest way to celebrate his life and his gifts through this volume, our own posthumous gift back to him.

New Haven, Connecticut   A.M.
New Haven, Connecticut   L.S.
Bethesda, Maryland   D.S.C.
New Haven, Connecticut   J.F.L.

REFERENCES

Cohen, D.J. (1986) Research in child psychiatry: lines of personal, institutional and career development. In: Pincus, H.A. and Pardes, H., eds. *Clinical Research Careers in Child Psychiatry*. Washington, DC. American Psychiatric Association, p. 74.
Wittgenstein, L. (1922) *Tractatus Logico-Philosophicus*, 6.4311. Trans. C.K. Ogden (Routledge and Kegan Paul, 1922); Rev. Trans. By D. Pears and B. McGuiness (London: Routledge, 1961).

Contents

Contributors, xv

SECTION I BIOLOGICAL BASES OF PEDIATRIC PSYCHOPHARMACOLOGY

I-A DEVELOPMENTAL PRINCIPLES OF NEUROBIOLOGY AND PSYCHOPHARMACOLOGY

1. Overview of Brain Development, 3
   Flora M. Vaccarino
   James F. Leckman

2. Synaptic Function and Biochemical Neuroanatomy, 20
   Stephan Heckers
   Christine Konradi

3. Mechanisms of Signal Transduction and Adaptation to Psychotropic Drug Action, 33
   Lara M. Tolbert
   Carrol D'Sa
   Ronald S. Duman

4. Pharmacokinetics I: Developmental Principles, 44
   Alexander A. Vinks
   Philip D. Walson

5. Pharmacokinetics II: Cytochrome P450–Mediated Drug Interactions, 54
   Jessica R. Oesterheld
   David A. Flockhart

I-B GENETIC PRINCIPLES

6. Molecular Genetics, 69
   Surojit Paul
   Paul J. Lombroso

7. Pharmacogenetics, 84
   George M. Anderson
   Jeremy Veenstra-VanderWeele
   Edwin H. Cook

I-C DEVELOPMENTAL PSYCHOPATHOLOGY

8. Neurobiology of Attention Regulation and its Disorders, 99
   Amy F.T. Arnsten
   Francisco X. Castellanos

9. Neurobiology of Early-Life Stress and its Disorders, 110
   Christine Heim
   Charles B. Nemeroff

10. Neurobiology of Early-Onset Mood Disorders, 124
    Joan Kaufman
    Hilary Blumberg

11. Neurobiology of Early-Onset Anxiety Disorders, 138
    Vivian Koda
    Dennis S. Charney
    Daniel Pine

12. Neurobiology of Obsessive-Compulsive Disorder, 150
    Tanya K. Murphy
    Kytja K.S. Voeller
    Pierre Blier

13. Neurobiology of Tic Disorders, Including Tourette's Syndrome, 164
    James F. Leckman
    Chin-Bin Yeh
    Paul J. Lombroso

14. Neurobiology of Immune-Mediated Neuropsychiatric Disorders, 175
    Mary Lynn Dell
    Charlotte S. Hamilton
    Susan E. Swedo

15. Neurobiology of Childhood Schizophrenia and Related Disorders, 184
    Rob Nicolson
    Judith L. Rapoport

16. Neurobiology of Affiliation: Implications for Autism Spectrum Disorders, 195
Sherie Novotny
Martin Evers
Katherine Barboza
Ron Rawitt
Eric Hollander

17. Neurobiology of Aggression, 210
Marcus J.P. Kruesi
Sondra Keller
Mark W. Wagner

18. Neurobiology of Eating Disorders, 224
Walter Kaye
Michael Strober
Kelly L. Klump

19. Neurobiology of Substance Abuse and Dependence Disorders, 238
Leslie K. Jacobsen

SECTION II   SOMATIC INTERVENTIONS

II-A   PSYCHOTROPIC AGENTS

20. Stimulants, 255
Rebecca E. Ford
Laurence Greenhill
Kelly Posner

21. Adrenergic Agonists: Clonidine and Guanfacine, 264
Jeffrey H. Newcorn
Kurt P. Schulz
Jeffrey M. Halperin

22. Antidepressants I: Selective Serotonin Reuptake Inhibitors, 274
Sufen Chiu
Henrietta L. Leonard

23. Antidepressants II: Tricyclic Agents, 284
Karl Gundersen
Barbara Geller

24. Antidepressants III: Other Agents, 295
John T. Walkup
Julia Ritter-Welzant
Elizabeth Kastelic
Nandita Joshi
Emily Frosch

25. Mood Stabilizers: Lithium and Anticonvulsants 309
Pablo Davanzo
James McCracken

26. Antipsychotic Agents: Traditional and Atypical, 328
Robert L. Findling
Nora K. McNamara
Barbara L. Gracious

27. Anxiolytics: Benzodiazepines, Buspirone, and Others, 341
Shannon R. Barnett
Mark A. Riddle

28. Miscellaneous Compounds: Beta-Blockers and Opiate Antagonists 353
Jan K. Buitelaar

II-B   OTHER SOMATIC INTERVENTIONS

29. Complementary and Alternative Medicine in Pediatric Psychopharmacology, 365
Joseph M. Rey
Garry Walter
Joseph P. Horrigan

30. Electroconvulsive Therapy and Transcranial Magnetic Stimulation, 377
Garry Walter
Joseph M. Rey
Neera Ghaziuddin

SECTION III   ASSESSMENT AND TREATMENT

III-A   GENERAL PRINCIPLES

31. Clinical Assessment of Children and Adolescents Treated Pharmacologically, 391
Robert L. Hendren
Stephanie Hamarman

32. Clinical Instruments and Scales in Pediatric Psychopharmacology, 404
L. Eugene Arnold
Michael G. Aman

33. Thinking About Prescribing: The Psychology of Psychopharmacology, 417
Kyle D. Pruett
Andrés Martin

34. Combining Pharmacotherapy and Psychotherapy: An Evidence-Based Approach, 426
John S. March
Karen Wells

III-B   SPECIFIC DISORDERS AND SYNDROMES

35. Attention-Deficit Hyperactivity Disorder, 447
   Thomas Spencer
   Joseph Biederman
   Timothy Wilens
   Ross Greene

36. Depressive Disorders, 466
   Boris Birmaher
   David Brent

37. Bipolar Disorder, 484
   Gabrielle A. Carlson

38. Anxiety Disorders, 497
   Michael Labellarte
   Golda Ginsburg

39. Obsessive-Compulsive Disorder, 511
   Daniel A. Geller
   Thomas Spencer

40. Tourette's Syndrome and Other Tic Disorders, 526
   Robert A. King
   Lawrence Scahill
   Paul Lombroso
   James F. Leckman

41. Early-Onset Schizophrenia, 543
   Helmut Remschmidt
   Johannes Hebebrand

42. Autistic and Other Pervasive Developmental Disorders, 563
   Christopher J. McDougle
   David J. Posey

43. Post-traumatic Stress Disorder, 580
   Craig L. Donnelly

44. Eating Disorders, 592
   Katherine A. Halmi

III-C   SPECIAL CLINICAL POPULATIONS

45. Substance-Abusing Youths, 605
   James G. Waxmonsky
   Timothy Wilens

46. Individuals with Mental Retardation, 617
   Michael G. Aman
   Ronald L. Lindsay
   Patricia L. Nash
   L. Eugene Arnold

47. The Medically Ill Child or Adolescent, 631
   Jonathan A. Slater

48. Psychopharmacology During Pregnancy: Infant Considerations, 642
   Elizabeth A. Walter
   C. Neill Epperson

49. Psychopharmacological Treatment of Preschoolers, 654
   Samuel L. Judice
   Linda C. Mayes

III-D   OTHER AREAS OF CLINICAL CONCERN

50. Agitation and Aggression, 671
   Jean A. Frazier

51. Elimination Disorders: Enuresis and Encopresis, 686
   William Reiner

SECTION IV   EPIDEMIOLOGICAL, RESEARCH, AND METHODOLOGICAL CONSIDERATIONS

52. Pediatric Psychopharmacoepidemiology: Who Is Prescribing? And For Whom, How, and Why?, 701
   Peter S. Jensen
   Aryeh Edelman
   Robin Nemeroff

53. Clinical Trials Methodology and Design Issues, 712
   Benedetto Vitiello

54. Regulatory Issues, 725
   Thomas P. Laughren

55. Ethical Issues in Research, 737
   Kimberly Hoagwood

56. International Perspectives, 746
   Per Hove Thomsen
   Hiroshi Kurita

   Appendix: Pediatric Psychopharmacology at a Glance, 757

   Index, 765

Contributors

MICHAEL G. AMAN, PH.D.
Ohio State University
Columbus, OH

GEORGE M. ANDERSON, PH.D.
Child Study Center
Yale University School of Medicine
New Haven, CT

L. EUGENE ARNOLD, M.D.
Ohio State University
Columbus, OH

AMY F.T. ARNSTEN, PH.D.
Department of Neurobiology
Yale University School of Medicine
New Haven, CT

KATHERINE BARBOZA, B.A.
Mount Sinai School of Medicine
New York, NY

SHANNON R. BARNETT, M.D.
Division of Child and Adolescent Psychiatry
Johns Hopkins Medical Institutions
Baltimore, MD

JOSEPH BIEDERMAN, M.D.
Pediatric Psychopharmacology Unit
Massachusetts General Hospital
Department of Psychiatry
Harvard Medical School
Boston, MA

BORIS BIRMAHER, M.D.
Western Psychiatric Institute and Clinic
University of Pittsburgh Medical Center
Pittsburgh, PA

PIERRE BLIER, M.D.
Department of Psychiatry
University of Florida
Gainesville, FL

HILARY BLUMBERG, M.D.
Department of Psychiatry
Yale University School of Medicine
West Haven, CT

DAVID BRENT, M.D.
Western Psychiatric Institute and Clinic
University of Pittsburgh Medical Center
Pittsburgh, PA

JAN K. BUITELAAR, M.D.
Department of Child and Adolescent Psychiatry
University Hospital Utrecht
Utrecht, The Netherlands

GABRIELLE A. CARLSON, M.D.
Division of Child and Adolescent Psychiatry
State University of New York at Stony Brook
Stony Brook, NY

FRANCISCO X. CASTELLANOS, M.D.
Child Study Center
New York University School of Medicine
New York, NY

DENNIS S. CHARNEY, M.D.
Mood and Anxiety Disorders Program
National Institute of Mental Health
Bethesda, MD

SUFEN CHIU, M.D., PH.D.
McLean Hospital
Department of Psychiatry
Harvard Medical School
Belmont, MA

EDWIN H. COOK, M.D.
University of Chicago
Chicago, IL

PABLO DAVANZO, M.D.
Division of Child and Adolescent Psychiatry
University of California, Los Angeles
Los Angeles, CA

MARY LYNN DELL, M.D., TH.M.
Department of Psychiatry
George Washington University School of Medicine and
Children's National Medical Center
Alexandria, VA

CRAIG L. DONNELLY, M.D.
Pediatric Psychopharmacology
Department of Psychiatry
Dartmouth-Hitchcock Medical Center
Lebanon, NH

CARROL D'SA, PH.D.
Department of Psychiatry
Yale University School of Medicine
New Haven, CT

RONALD DUMAN M.D.
Department of Psychiatry
Yale University School of Medicine
New Haven, CT

ARYEH EDELMAN, B.A.
Center for the Advancement of Children's Mental Health
New York State Psychiatric Institute
Columbia University College of Physicians and Surgeons
New York, NY

C. NEILL EPPERSON, M.D.
Gynecologic Behavioral Health Clinic
Departments of Psychiatry and Obstetrics and Gynecology
Yale University School of Medicine
New Haven, CT

MARTIN EVERS, B.A.
Mount Sinai School of Medicine
New York, NY

ROBERT L. FINDLING, M.D.
Departments of Psychiatry and Pediatrics
University Hospitals of Cleveland
Case Western Reserve University
Cleveland, OH

DAVID A. FLOCKHART, M.D., PH.D.
Pharmacogenetics Core Laboratory
Division of Clinical Pharmacology
Departments of Medicine and Pharmacology
Georgetown University Medical Center
Washington, DC

REBECCA E. FORD, M.A.
New York State Psychiatric Institute
Columbia University College of Physicians and Surgeons
New York, NY

JEAN A. FRAZIER, M.D.
McLean Hospital
Department of Psychiatry
Harvard Medical School
Belmont, MA

EMILY FROSCH, M.D.
Division of Child and Adolescent Psychiatry
Department of Psychiatry and Behavioral Sciences
Johns Hopkins Medical Institutions
Baltimore, MD

BARBARA GELLER, M.D.
Washington University School of Medicine
St. Louis, MO

DANIEL A. GELLER, M.D.
Pediatric Obsessive Compulsive Disorder Clinic
McLean Hospital
Department of Psychiatry
Harvard Medical School
Belmont, MA

NEERA GHAZIUDDIN, M.D., MRCPSYCH (UK)
Division of Child and Adolescent Psychiatry
University of Michigan, Ann Arbor
Ann Arbor, MI

GOLDA GINSBURG, PH.D.
Division of Child and Adolescent Psychiatry
Johns Hopkins Medical Institutions
Baltimore, MD

BARBARA L. GRACIOUS, M.D.
University Hospitals of Cleveland
Case Western Reserve University
Cleveland, OH

ROSS GREENE, PH.D.
Departments of Psychiatry and Psychology
Harvard University
Boston, MA

LAURENCE L. GREENHILL, M.D.
New York State Psychiatric Institute
Division of Child and Adolescent Psychiatry
Columbia University College of Physicians and Surgeons
New York, NY

KARL GUNDERSEN, M.D.
Washington University School of Medicine
St. Louis, MO

KATHERINE A. HALMI, M.D.
New York–Presbyterian Hospital–Westchester Division
Weill Medical College of Cornell University
White Plains, NY

JEFFREY M. HALPERIN, PH.D.
Department of Psychology
Queens College of City University of New York
New York, NY

STEPHANIE HAMARMAN, M.D.
University of Medicine and Dentistry of New Jersey
Newark, NJ

CHARLOTTE S. HAMILTON, M.D.
Pediatrics and Developmental Neuropsychiatry Branch
National Institute of Mental Health
Bethesda, MD

JOHANNES HEBEBRAND, M.D.
Department of Child and Adolescent Psychiatry
Phillips University
Marburg, Germany

STEPHAN HECKERS, M.D.
Massachusetts General Hospital
Department of Psychiatry
Harvard Medical School
Charlestown, MA

CHRISTINE M. HEIM, PH.D.
Department of Psychiatry and Behavioral Sciences
Emory University School of Medicine
Atlanta, GA

ROBERT L. HENDREN, D.O.
Division of Child and Adolescent Psychiatry
Department of Psychiatry
University of California Davis School of Medicine
Sacramento, CA

KIMBERLY HOAGWOOD, PH.D.
Child and Adolescent Services Research
New York State Psychiatric Institute
Columbia University College of Physicians and Surgeons
New York, NY

ERIC HOLLANDER, M.D.
Department of Psychiatry
Mount Sinai School of Medicine
New York, NY

JOSEPH P. HORRIGAN, M.D.
University of North Carolina at Chapel Hill
Chapel Hill, NC

STEVEN HYMAN, M.D.
Harvard University
Cambridge, MA

LESLIE K. JACOBSEN, M.D.
Department of Psychiatry
Yale University School of Medicine
West Haven, CT

PETER S. JENSEN, M.D.
Center for the Advancement of Children's Mental Health
New York State Psychiatric Institute
Department of Psychiatry
Columbia University College of Physicians and Surgeons
New York, NY

NANDITA JOSHI, M.D.
Division of Child and Adolescent Psychiatry
Johns Hopkins Medical Institutions
Baltimore, MD

SAMUEL L. JUDICE, M.D.
Child and Adolescent Psychiatry Clinics
Langley Porter Psychiatric Institute
University of California, San Francisco
San Francisco, CA

ELIZABETH KASTELIC, M.D.
Division of Child and Adolescent Psychiatry
Department of Psychiatry and Behavioral Sciences
Johns Hopkins Medical Institutions
Baltimore, MD

JOAN KAUFMAN, PH.D.
Department of Psychiatry
Yale University School of Medicine
New Haven, CT

WALTER KAYE, M.D.
Western Psychiatric Institute and Clinic
University of Pittsburgh School of Medicine
Pittsburgh, PA

SONDRA KELLER, M.D.
Department of Psychiatry and Behavioral Sciences
Medical University of South Carolina
Charleston, SC

ROBERT A. KING, M.D.
Tic Disorders Clinic
Child Study Center
Yale University School of Medicine
New Haven, CT

KELLY L. KLUMP, PH.D.
Department of Psychology
Michigan State University
East Lansing, MI

VIVIAN H. KODA, PH.D.
Department of Psychiatry
Columbia University College of Physicians and Surgeons
New York, NY

CHRISTINE KONRADI, PH.D.
Laboratory of Molecular and Development Neuroscience
McLean Hospital
Department of Psychiatry
Harvard Medical School
Belmount, MA

MARCUS J.P. KRUESI, M.D.
Youth Division, Department of Psychiatry and Behavioral
Sciences
Medical University of South Carolina
Charleston, SC

HIROSHI KURITA, M.D.
Department of Mental Health
Graduate School of Medicine
The University of Tokyo
Tokyo, Japan

MICHAEL LABELLARTE, M.D.
Division of Child and Adolescent Psychiatry
Johns Hopkins Medical Institutions
Baltimore, MD

THOMAS P. LAUGHREN, M.D.
Division of Neuropharmacological Drug Products
Food and Drug Administration
Rockville, MD

JAMES F. LECKMAN, M.D.
Child Study Center
Yale University School of Medicine
New Haven, CT

HENRIETTA L. LEONARD, M.D.
Brown University School of Medicine
Providence, RI

RONALD L. LINDSAY, M.D.
Ohio State University
Columbus, OH

PAUL J. LOMBROSO, M.D.
Child Study Center
Yale University School of Medicine
New Haven, CT

JOHN S. MARCH, M.D., M.P.H.
Child and Family Study Center
Department of Psychiatry and Behavioral Sciences
Duke University Medical Center
Durham, NC

ANDRÉS MARTIN, M.D., M.P.H.
Child Study Center
Yale University School of Medicine
New Haven, CT

LINDA C. MAYES, M.D.
Child Study Center
Yale University School of Medicine
New Haven, CT

JAMES MCCRACKEN, M.D.
Division of Child and Adolescent Psychiatry
University of California, Los Angeles
Los Angeles, CA

CHRISTOPHER J. MCDOUGLE, M.D.
Indiana University School of Medicine
Indianapolis, IN

NORA K. MCNAMARA, M.D.
University Hospitals of Cleveland
Case Western Reserve University
Cleveland, OH

TANYA K. MURPHY, M.D.
Department of Psychiatry
University of Florida
Gainesville, FL

PATRICIA L. NASH, M.D.
Ohio State University
Columbus, OH

CHARLES B. NEMEROFF, M.D., PH.D.
Department of Psychiatry and Behavioral Sciences
Emory University School of Medicine
Atlanta, GA

ROBIN NEMEROFF, PH.D.
Center for the Advancement of Children's Mental Health
New York State Psychiatric Institute
Columbia University College of Physicians and Surgeons
New York, NY

JEFFREY H. NEWCORN, M.D.
Mount Sinai School of Medicine
New York, NY

ROB NICOLSON, M.D.
Children's Hospital of Western Ontario
London, Ontario, Canada

SHERIE NOVOTNY, M.D.
Mount Sinai School of Medicine
New York, NY

JESSICA R. OESTERHELD, M.D.
The Spurwink School
Bath, ME

SUROJIT PAUL, PH.D.
Yale Child Study Center
Yale University School of Medicine
New Haven, CT

DANIEL S. PINE, M.D.
Section on Development and Affective Neuroscience
National Institute of Mental Health
Bethesda, MD

DAVID J. POSEY, M.D.
Indiana University School of Medicine
Indianapolis, IN

KELLY POSNER, PH.D.
New York State Psychiatric Institute
Columbia University College of Physicians and Surgeons
New York, NY

KYLE D. PRUETT, M.D.
Child Study Center
Yale University School of Medicine
New Heaven, CT

JUDITH L. RAPOPORT, M.D.
Child Psychiatry Branch
National Institute of Mental Health
Bethesda, MD

RON RAWITT, M.D.
Mount Sinai School of Medicine
New York, NY

WILLIAM REINER, M.D.
Johns Hopkins Medical Institutions
Baltimore, MD

HELMUT REMSCHMIDT, M.D.
Department of Child and Adolescent Psychiatry
Philipps University
Marburg, Germany

JOSEPH M. REY, M.D., PH.D.
University of Sydney
North Ryde, N.S.W., Australia

MARK A. RIDDLE, M.D.
Division of Child and Adolescent Psychiatry
Johns Hopkins Medical Institutions
Baltimore, MD

JULIA RITTER-WELZANT, M.D.
Shepard-Pratt Hospital
Baltimore, MD

LAWRENCE SCAHILL, M.S.N., PH.D.
Child Study Center
Yale University School of Medicine
New Haven, CT

KURT P. SCHULZ
The Graduate Center of the City University of New York
Mount Sinai School of Medicine
New York, NY

JONATHAN A. SLATER, M.D.
New York Presbyterian Medical Center
Columbia University College of Physicians and Surgeons
New York, NY

THOMAS SPENCER, M.D.
Pediatric Psychopharmacology Unit
Massachusetts General Hospital
Department of Psychiatry
Harvard Medical School
Boston, MA

MICHAEL STROBER, PH.D.
Neuropsychiatric Institute and Hospital
University of California, Los Angeles
Los Angeles, CA

SUSAN E. SWEDO, M.D.
Pediatrics and Development Neuropsychiatry Branch
National Institute of Mental Health
Bethesda, MD

PER HOVE THOMSEN, M.D.
Borne-Ungdomspsykiatrisk Hospital
Risskov, Denmark

LARA M. TOLBERT, PH.D.
Department of Psychiatry
Yale University School of Medicine
New Haven, CT

FLORA M. VACCARINO, M.D.
Child Study Center
Yale University School of Medicine
New Haven, CT

JEREMY VEENSTRA-VANDERWEELE, PH.D.
Departments of Psychiatry and Pediatrics
University of Chicago
Chicago, IL

ALEXANDER A. VINKS, PHARM. D., PH.D.
Division of Clinical Pharmacology
Children's Hospital Medical Center
Cincinnati, OH

BENEDETTO VITIELLO, M.D.
Child and Adolescent Treatment and Prevention
Intervention Research Branch
National Institute of Mental Health
Bethesda, MD

KYTJA K.S. VOELLER, M.D.
Morris Child Development Center
Department of Psychiatry
University of Florida
Gainesville, FL

MARK W. WAGNER, M.D.
Youth Division, Department of Psychiatry and Behavioral Sciences
Medical University of South Carolina
Charleston, SC

JOHN T. WALKUP, M.D.
Division of Child and Adolescent Psychiatry
Johns Hopkins Medical Institutions
Baltimore, MD

PHILIP D. WALSON, M.D.
Division of Clinical Pharmacology
Children's Hospital Medical Center
Cincinnati, OH

ELIZABETH A. WALTER, M.D.
Mental Health Center
Billings, MT

GARRY WALTER, M.D., FRANZCP
University of Sydney
Concord West, N.S.W., Australia

JAMES G. WAXMOSNSKY, M.D.
Massachusetts General Hospital
Department of Psychiatry
Harvard Medical School
Boston, MA

KAREN WELLS, PH.D.
Child and Family Study Center
Department of Psychiatry and Behavioral Sciences
Duke University Medical Center
Durham, NC

TIMOTHY WILENS, M.D.
Substance Abuse Program in Pediatric Psychopharmacology
Massachusetts General Hospital
Department of Psychiatry
Harvard Medical School
Boston, MA

CHIN-BIN YEH, M.D.
National Defense Medical Center
Taipei, Taiwan, Republic of China

I | BIOLOGICAL BASES OF PEDIATRIC PSYCHOPHARMACOLOGY

. . . a focus on the interplay between normal and atypical development, an interest in diverse domains of functioning, and an emphasis on the utilization of a developmental framework for understanding adaptation across the life course are among those elements that are integral to a developmental psychopathology approach.

> *D. Cicchetti and D. J. Cohen (1995)*
> Developmental Psychopathology, Vol. I—
> Theory and Methods, *p. 3.*

THE book's first section is subdivided into three main parts. The first of these, *Developmental Principles of Neurobiology and Psychopharmacology,* starts with an overview of brain development that highlights molecular mechanisms involved in this life-long process, and their relevance to pediatric pychopharmacology. The two chapters that follow describe molecular mechanisms involved in drug action, starting at the synaptic cleft and moving through multiple messenger cascades into the heart of the cell's genetic machinery. The two last chapters are devoted to pharmacokinetics—the body's handling of alien molecules—with particular and clinically relevant attention paid to drug interactions.

A short intermediary part, *Genetic Principles,* provides an overview of those mechanisms that are set in downstream motion following psychotropic drug engagement and are ultimately responsible for the ensuing end-organ effects. The chapter on pharmacogenetics provides an up-to-date account of progress in this emerging field, and offers a glimpse ahead at one of the most exciting areas of pharmacology, one that may ultimately allow a more rational approach to medication choice for individual patients.

The third part, *Developmental Psychopathology,* delves into detailed disease-specific overviews. Each of the chapters covers issues pertaining to nosology and classification, to genetic determinants, brain systems implicated, environmental influences, and nature–nurture interactions. Neurotransmission and neuromodulation, and hormonal and other developmental influences are addressed and, whenever available, relevant animal models are incorporated into the discussion. The interplay of normative and derailed development is a core concept for these chapters. Of the part's 12 chapters, 9 are devoted to traditionally defined disease categories, and 3 cover the overarching areas of early-life stress, aggression, and affiliative behaviors.

DEVELOPMENTAL PRINCIPLES OF NEUROBIOLOGY AND PSYCHOPHARMACOLOGY

1 | Overview of brain development

FLORA M. VACCARINO AND JAMES F. LECKMAN

What no one could have anticipated, however, are the implications for psychotherapy of the new evidence we have for neurogenesis and plasticity in the brain throughout life (Gross, 2000; Shin et al., 2000). Every day thousands of new neurons are added to the adult brain, some of them in circuits known to be crucial for learning and memory. Their actual number is small in proportion to the total population of neurons, but they may function in learning and memory by permitting the development of new connections as well as modulating older ones. Psychotherapy may literally alter brain structure by altering brain function (Eisenberg, 2000).

Eisenberg (2001, p. 745)

For most species, the nervous system is the most complex part of the organism. In mammalian species, over one-third of the entire set of genes is expressed in the central nervous system (CNS). The reason for this abundance in gene expression (over 30,000 genes are possibly expressed within the CNS) lays in the intrinsic complexity, both structural and functional, of the CNS. It is reasonable to assume that CNS-specific transcripts are necessary to encode the wide variety of molecular components of the mature CNS; moreover, a substantial percent of these transcripts guide CNS morphogenesis and are primarily expressed during its formation. In this chapter, we will introduce the reader to some of the basic rules that control CNS development and discuss how the workings of this genetic machinery are dependent on cell-to-cell communication and variations in the environment. Throughout this chapter, we will draw parallels between CNS development and aspects of the function of the mature brain to illustrate the conservation of mechanisms regulating brain plasticity throughout life. We also explore the ontogenesis of neurotransmitter and neuromodulatory systems that are targets of many of the pharmacological agents used in the pediatric age range. We have deliberately chosen examples to illustrate specific principles of CNS development of particular significance for the understanding of developmental psychopathology. For more complete and systematic accounts, the reader is encouraged to consult one of a growing set of volumes on this topic (Kandel et al., 2000).

GENES THAT SHAPE THE CENTRAL NERVOUS SYSTEM

The ontogenetic development of the central nervous system is driven by hierarchical sets of evolutionary conserved genes. Although the sequence of gene expression that controls neural development is preset and stereotyped, it is also driven to a large extent by local interactions among developing cells. The evolutionary advantage of these interactions is that complex systems are able to reassess cellular identities and make appropriate adjustments to environmental perturbations. This is particularly true at the earliest stages of embryonic development, when there is the need to coordinate reciprocally the layout of different tissues and compartments. Regulatory interactions allow higher organism to use alternative genetic pathways to adjust to environmental fluctuations; the system thus becomes more flexible and less prone to failure. As the genetic blueprint unfolds, cell fates become increasingly autonomous and less sensitive to variations in the environment.

Development involves the proliferation of cells to generate a multicellular organism, differentiation, and sorting of these cells into appropriate patterns. Pattern formation involves a series of cell fate decisions and the proper positioning of the progenitor and differentiated cells. These decisions are arranged in a hierarchy of choices, where the simplest (i.e., axis formation) prefigures and regulates the more complex, such as the location of different neuronal types.

During CNS patterning, cells reciprocally coordinate their replication rate, fate, and relative position. These interactions are mediated by direct cell-to-cell contacts, by the local action of secreted polypeptides called *morphogens*, and by hormonal influences from the macroenvironment.

Morphogens are "form-generating" substances, whose configuration within a tissue "prefigures" the pattern (Meinhardt, 1983). These substances set up an extracellular concentration gradient, which in turns orchestrates a coherent set of cellular behaviors that will eventually result in the proportionate growth of an organ, including the finest details. For example, different scalar concentrations may specify the type of cells and their relative position within the field. Morphogens act by altering the pattern of gene expression in target cells, because different genes whose activation depends on different thresholds will be turned on at different distances from the morphogen's source.

Specific examples can be found from the earliest stages of development. In *Drosophila,* before egg fertilization, localized morphogens present in the egg cytoplasm—the products of "maternal effect genes"—direct early pattern formation. Four maternally derived signals are responsible for the formation of the principal body axes—the anterior–posterior, the dorsoventral, and the terminal. These are established independently and provide a pattern for subsequent development (St Johnston and Nusslein-Volhard, 1992). One of the maternal signals, the *Drosophila*'s homologue of the epidermal growth factor (EGF), establishes the dorsal side of the fertilized egg by binding to its receptor, the EGFR. In mammals, EGFR regulates the development of the cerebral cortex and the proliferation of stem cells in the adult mammalian forebrain (Sibilia et al., 1998). In the absence of EGFR signaling, the cerebral cortex undergoes progressive degeneration, which suggests that this receptor is essential for cortical neuron survival. This example illustrates the striking conservation of molecular signals across development, often used with disparate functional outcomes.

Another maternal signal in the insect is the transcript of a gene called *bicoid,* which is present only at the anterior end of the egg (Fig. 1.1). The bicoid gene product is transcribed in an anterior-to-posterior gradient highest at the anterior pole of the embryo. *Bicoid* is a homeodomain transcription factor that binds the regulatory region of zygotic genes named *gap* genes, turning them on. These genes, in turn, control the development of the head. Since *bicoid* binding sites on different gap genes have different threshold affinities for *bicoid,* the concentration gradient of this morphogen defines different areas of gene expression along the embryo (Fig. 1.1).

Gap genes are activated in discrete blocks that segmentally organize the body plan; as their name suggests, their inactivation results in the creation of a missing part in the developing embryo. For example, orthodenticle (*otd*) and empty spiracles (*ems*) are activated by high concentrations of *bicoid* in partially overlapping regions of the insect head (Finkelstein and Perrimon, 1990). *Otd* and *ems* are required for the specification of the first and the second and third segments of the insect brain. Even though a segmental organization is much less obvious in the vertebrate CNS,

gap genes are evolutionarily conserved and exert a similar function in higher species (Fig. 1.1). The mammalian homologues of *otd* and *ems, Otx1/Otx2* and *Emx1/Emx2,* are expressed in partially overlapping domains of the mammalian forebrain (Simeone et al., 1992; see the next section).

SELECTOR GENES CREATE REGIONAL DIVERSIFICATION

The orderly sequence of gene expression during subsequent development divides the embryo into units called *compartments.* Because cells belonging to one compartment do not mix with cells of other compartments, the founder cells of one compartment share a "genetic address" given by the expression of a unique combination of homeodomain selector genes. *Homeodomain genes* are master regulators of gene transcription present in all eukaryotes (Krumlauf, 1992). By binding to gene promoters through a conserved DNA-binding motif, the homeodomain (Gehring et al., 1994) selector genes give to the cells of one compartment a set of specific instructions that define their identity.

Hox genes are homeodomain selector genes that regulate segmentation in the vertebrate neural tube (Lumsden and Krumlauf, 1996). Loss-of-function mutations of *Hox* genes result in growth abnormalities, deletions of rhombomeres, and alterations in cellular identities leading to cell intermixing and axonal pathfinding defects (Capecchi, 1997). Embryonic defects produced by thalidomide or retinoids toxicity have been attributed to misregulation of homeobox genes in the hindbrain and forebrain. Interesting parallels can be drawn between mouse mutants lacking *Hoxb2* and *Hoxb1,* in which the facial motor neurons fail to be specified, and the autistic features of Moebius syndrome (Gillberg and Steffenburg, 1989; Goddard et al., 1996). Early developmental defects in the rhomboencephalon have been hypothesized to occur in some cases of autism (Gillberg and Steffenburg, 1989; Rodier et al., 1996).

Several families of homeodomain genes expressed in the anterior part of the CNS, the prosencephalon, have now been described (Fig. 1.2). Their function has been determined in the mouse by gene inactivation studies.

The inactivation (knockout) of the *Otx2* gene by homologous recombination results in a failure of development of the whole prosencephalon (Acampora et al., 1995). This is the result of an apparent failure of primary regionalization of the CNS. *Otx1,* a close *Otx2* homologue, is important for development of the cerebral cortex. In the absence of *Otx1,* the cerebral cortex is smaller and has an abnormal lamination; as a result,

DROSOPHILA   MOUSE

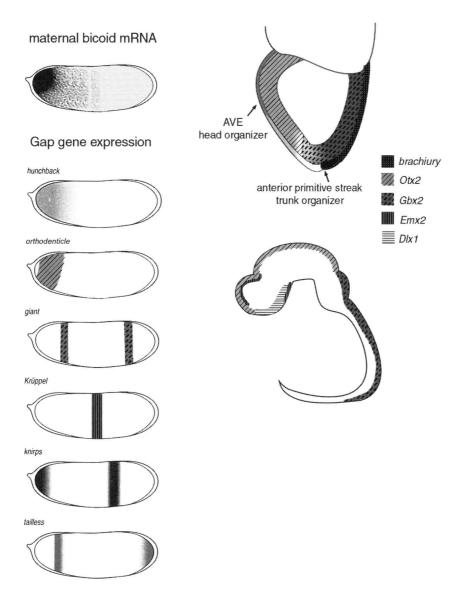

maternal bicoid mRNA

Gap gene expression

hunchback

orthodenticle

giant

Krüppel

knirps

tailless

AVE
head organizer

anterior primitive streak
trunk organizer

brachiury
Otx2
Gbx2
Emx2
Dlx1

FIGURE 1.1 The earliest genes that establish an anteroposterior pattern within the CNS. Drosophila's early development is shown on the left. In *Drosophila*, anteroposterior patterning begins in the egg through maternally expressed genes such as *bicoid*. Gap genes are directly or indirectly the targets of *bicoid* and other maternally expressed morphogens. Anteroposterior patterning in vertebrate development (shown on the right) begins just before gastrulation. At this stage, the mammalian embryo is shaped as a cup. Two signaling centers, the head and the body organizers, are situated in the anterior visceral endoderm (AVE, head organizer) and the anterior primitive streak (anterior primitive streak trunk organizer), respectively. The AVE expresses the homeobox genes *Otx2, Hesx-1, and LIM-1*. The body organizer expresses *LIM-1, goosecoid, brachiury, and HNF-3B*. Genes within the head and body organizers directly or indirectly result in the transcription of *Otx2* and *Gbx2* in the neuroectoderm, which later specify the anterior and posterior CNS, respectively.

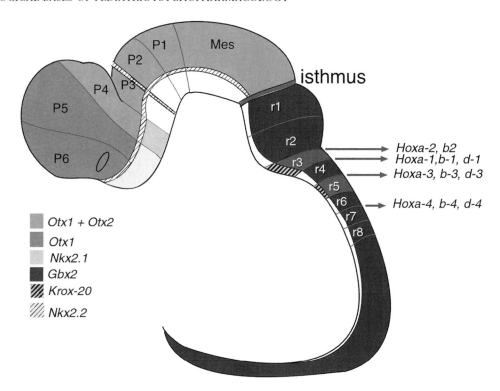

FIGURE 1.2 The prosomeric model of forebrain patterning, defined by gene expression boundaries. Schematic representation of the expression of *Gbx2, Nkx2.1, Nkx2.2, Otx1, Otx2,* and *Krox-20* in the mouse embryonic neural neural tube (embryonic day 11.5). The upper limits of expression of *Hox* genes in the brain stem are indicated by arrows. For more details, see Simeone et al. (1992); Rubenstein et al., (1994) Bulfone et al., (1995); and Shimamura et al., (1995).

mice develop intractable seizures (Acampora et al., 1996). Whereas a complete lack of function of *Otx* genes can result in an anencephalic phenotype, a partial lack of function of these genes causes a lack of midline structures and the partial fusion of the two lateral ventricles, a human malformation called *holoprosencephaly*. While most forms of holoprosencephaly are expected to be lethal, milder forms are compatible with life.

Emx genes are important for the genesis of the hippocampus (Pellegrini et al., 1996) and point mutations of *Emx2* are associated with schizencephaly (Brunelli et al., 1996). Thus, these homologues of early segmentation genes in *Drosophila* serve fundamental functions in the development in the human brain.

ORGANIZER REGIONS ORIGINATE LONG-RANGE MOLECULAR SIGNALS

Organizers are groups of cells that lead to the generation of a new structure in surrounding tissue. These actions at a distance are mediated by the release of diffusible factors (morphogens) by cells within the organizer that induce cascades of gene expression in distant cells.

In the spinal tube, two morphogens acting in a contrasting manner, Sonic hedgehog (*Shh*) and bone morphogenetic protein (BMP), are generated along opposite sides, the ventral and dorsal neural tube. *Shh* diffuses within the ventral tube and specifies as many as five distinct progenitor domains, which in turn will give rise to distinct neuronal groups such as motor neurons; ventral and dorsal interneurons (Briscoe et al., 2000; Fig. 1.3A,B). Conversely, BMP4 is present in the dorsal midline and it induces sensory interneurons in the dorsal spinal cord (Liem et al., 1995).

These diffusible ligands specify the fate of progenitor cells by modifying the expression of specific transcription factors. For example, *Shh* increases the expression of *HNF3* and *Nkx 2.1* and down-regulates *Pax3* and *Msx1*, resulting in a rapid disappearanceof these genes from ventral regions. Once established, these transcrip-

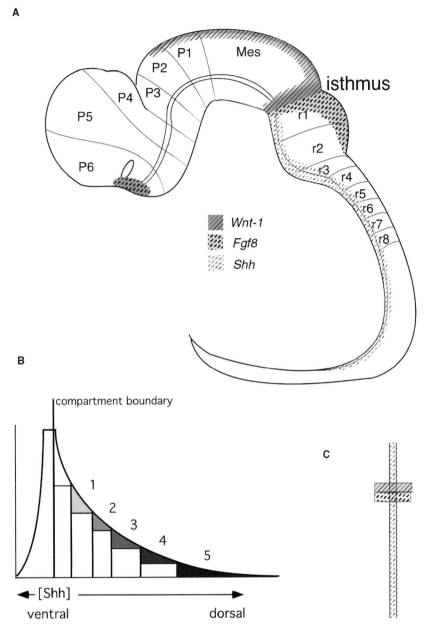

FIGURE 1.3 Morphogens within the CNS. **A:** Schematic view of a mouse embryo at approximately embryonic day 10.5–11.5 showing the distribution of *Wnt-1*, *Fgf8*, and *Sonic hedgehog (Shh)*. These morphogens are involved in the determination of neuronal fates by forming gradients along the anteroposterior and dorsoventral axes. **B:** The shape of Shh gradient from ventral (highest concentrations) to dorsal (lowest concentrations) is related to the determination of different progenitor pools along the dorsoventral axis of the neural tube. Because target genes may respond at different thresholds of *Shh*, progenitor fields will subsequently differentiate into specific neuronal types. Subsequently, reciprocal inhibitory interactions among the genes sharpen the boundaries. **C:** The intersection between two or more morphogens may be needed for the specification of neurons in particular loci within the CNS. For example, the location and number of aminergic progenitors may be specified the intersection of *Shh* with *Fgf8* at precise positions in the CNS.

tional domains stabilize and maintain their expression by reciprocal cross-repressive interactions.

Just above the brain stem, there is the isthmus, a constriction that delimits mesencephalon from rhombencephalon. At this boundary *Otx2* and *Gbx2* expression abuts each other. These genes are involved in the differentiation of the brain and spinal tube, respectively. Several morphogens are also expressed at the isthmus, notably *Wnt-1* and several members of the fibroblast growth factor (FGF) family, including *Fgf8, Fgf17,* and *Fgf18* (Fig. 1.3A). A recent experiment has shown that a localized source of *Fgf8* introduced in the caudal diencephalon (P2) is capable of inducing a second midbrain in this forebrain location, which is in a mirror image orientation with respect to the normal midbrain (Crossley et al., 1996). The second midbrain is flanked by a rudimentary cerebellum; this suggests that the ectopic source of *Fgf8* results in a new, isthmus-like organizing center. This respecification occurs because *Fgf8* induces in the forebrain genes typical of the isthmus and hindbrain, such as *Gbx2*, while repressing forebrain genes such as *Otx2*. Because *Otx2* and *Gbx2* reciprocally antagonize each other, any decrease in *Otx2* expression produces an expansion of the *Gbx2*-positive area and a repositioning of the isthmus (Acampora et al., 1997). The importance of *Fgf8* is confirmed by the fact that caudal midbrain and rostral hindbrain regions are absent when there is a deficient *Fgf8* gene (Meyers et al., 1998).

Thus, there may be signaling centers that regulate forebrain regional identity in a manner similar to that described for the hindbrain and spinal cord (Rubenstein and Shimamura, 1997). Interestingly, *Fgf8* is also expressed within the anterior neural ridge, the leading edge of the anterior neural plate. In this location, *Fgf8*, in conjunction with other FGFs and BMP, influences the development of the olfactory bulbs and dorsal cerebral hemispheres. In addition, *Shh* secreted from cells along the ventral midline of the brain intersects FGF ligands diffusing from the isthmus and anterior neural ridge (Fig. 1.3A,C). Their cooperation apparently induces dopaminergic and serotoninergic cells (Ye et al., 1998). Subtle variations in these interactions among *Shh*, FGFs, and possibly other morphogens may alter the development of these cell types. The dopaminergic and serotoninergic systems are implicated in affective disorders, psychoses, obsessive-compulsive disorders, and autism. Future studies linking gene knockout for these secreted factors with precise aspects of CNS development are eagerly awaited.

DIVERSIFICATION AND EXPANSION OF CEREBRAL CORTEX DURING THE COURSE OF EVOLUTION

After the initial regional specification of the CNS, each region achieves further definition through evolved mechanisms for the control of its overall growth and for the differentiation of appropriate numbers of the indigenous cell types. The cerebral cortex has undergone a considerable expansion in its surface area during phylogenesis. The surface area of the human cortex is 1000-fold larger than that of the mouse and 100-fold larger than that of the monkey. This increase in surface area is not matched by a corresponding increase in thickness (the human cortex is only three-fold thicker than the mouse) (Rakic, 1995). Thus, the fundamental unit of the cortex (i.e., cortical column or radial unit) has remained substantially the same during the evolution of the mammalian species, but the number of these units has increased. Second, there should be a mechanism operative during ontogenesis that leads to an increase in cortical surface area while maintaining the correct proportion of the different neuronal types.

Cortical neurons are generated in a layer of cells situated around the embryonic cerebral ventricles, the *pseudostratified ventricular epithelium* (PVE). Progenitor cells within this layer proliferate and, after their final mitosis, leave the PVE and start migrating toward the primordial cerebral cortex (cortical plate). Although cortical areas differ, the pattern of neurogenesis appears to be similar throughout the cerebral cortex. The mechanisms that control the emergence of diversity within cortical areas may be intrinsic to the progenitors (i.e., there may be a protomap present within the ventricular neuroepithelium). Alternatively, the incoming afferent population may account for the generation of these regional differences while maintaining a fundamental identity in the cellular components of the cortex (Shatz et al., 1990). Recent data suggest that the embryonic cortical plate contains gradients of the homeodomain genes *Emx2* and *PAX6* and growth factor receptors much before the ingrowth of thalamic afferents. Although we do not know whether these early gene gradients are related to the regional characteristics of the mature cerebral cortex, it is now clear that the embryonic cerebral cortex acquires regional characteristics early in development, both in rodents and in the rhesus monkey (Donoghue and Rakic, 1999).

The expansion of founder cells that are originally specified to the cortical field directly affects cerebral cortical size. It has been postulated that founder population expands through symmetric divisions before

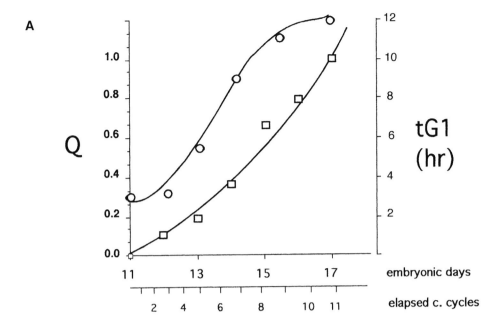

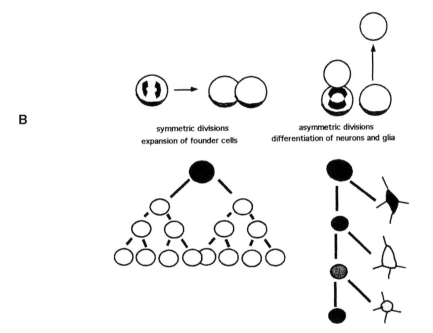

FIGURE 1.4 **A:** The progression of Q through cortical neurogenesis. Schematic time course of the proportion of cells that quit the cell cycle (Q, squares), and of the length of G1 (circles) during cerebral cortical neurogenesis. Q and G1 are plotted as a function of the cell cycle of the neurogenetic interval in the mouse cerebral cortical wall. The pseudostratified ventricular epithelium expands before Q = 0.5 (corresponding to embryonic day 14, as neurons of layer IV are forming) and contracts afterwards. Adapted from Takahashi et al., (1996); Miyama et al. (1997). **B:** Symmetric and asymmetric divisions. Symmetric divisions generating mitotic cells will exponentially increase the progenitor cell population, whereas asymmetric divisions generating a mitotic and a postmitotic daughter will keep the progenitor population at steady-state levels. The progenitor cells exhibit time-dependent changes in fate, giving rise first to neuronal and then to glial progeny (shown as a progressive change in gray shading).

neurogenesis begins (Rakic, 1995), whereas a predominant asymmetric mode of division underlies the generation of neurons (Fig. 1.4B). The molecular mechanisms of asymmetric division are likely to be similar to those controlling the formation of compartments—that is, the differential inheritance of selector genes between the two daughter cells (Jan and Jan, 1995). It is likely that cell death may also regulate the number of cortical founder cells, because mice lacking cell death effector molecules have profound abnormalities in brain anatomy (Roth et al., 2000). The time course of morphogenetic cell death in the developing cortex is the subject of intense investigation (see section "Large Numbers of Neurons Naturally Die During CNS Maturation" later in this chapter).

Cortical progenitor cells undergo a defined number of cell cycles to generate the cerebral cortex—there are 11 cell cycles in the mouse. The cell cycle length increases with the progression of neurogenesis because of a lengthening of the G1 phase (Fig. 1.4A). Takahashi et al. (1996) evaluated the kinetics of growth of the progenitor population by measuring the fraction of progenitor cells that exit the cycle (the Q fraction). Q increases in a nonlinear fashion through mouse neurogenesis, from 0 at the beginning (when all the cells are proliferative) to 1 at the end (when all the progenitor cells exit the cycle) (Fig. 1.4A). After embryonic day 14 ($Q < 0.5$), the rate of cells leaving the proliferative population exponentially increases, resulting in the contraction of the PVE and a massive generation of cortical neurons. Neurons populating the dense upper cortical layers are formed during the last 2 to 3 days of neurogenesis (Takahashi et al., 1996).

The progression of the cell cycle is regulated through a checkpoint in early G1. Exposure to growth factors binding to receptor tyrosine kinases (RTK) during this phase leads to an early commitment of the cell to divide again, whereas growth factor deprivation in G1 leads to the degradation of D cyclins and to a failure to re-enter the cycle (Ross, 1996). Both EGF and basic FGF (Fgf2) are present in the developing cerebral cortex and are candidate mitogenic molecules that may affect the G1 checkpoint (Weiss et al., 1996). Fgf2 acts before and during neurogenesis, much earlier that EGF; EGF-responsive stem cells are the progeny of those that respond to Fgf2 (Vaccarino et al., 1995; Tropepe et al., 1999). The microinjection of Fgf2 in the embryonic cerebral ventricles increases the generation of cortical neurons; conversely, mice lacking a functional Fgf2 gene have a decrease in the number of cortical cells and a decrease in the number of neuronal progenitors early in neurogenesis (Vaccarino et al., 1999; Fig. 1.5). Thus, Fgf2 is required for the attainment of an appropriate

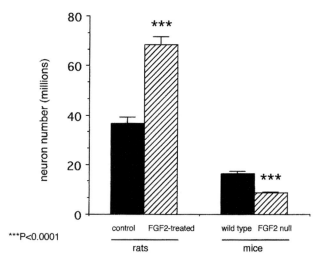

FIGURE 1.5 Fgf2 is both sufficient and necessary for the development of a normal number of neurons in the cerebral cortex. Adult control rats have approximately twice as many cortical neurons compared to wild-type mice. The number of cortical neurons doubled in rats that had received an Fgf2 microinjection during embryogenesis (Fgf2-treated rats). Conversely, mice with a germline disruption of the *Fgf2* gene (*Fgf2* −/− mice) had half the number of cortical neurons compared to wild type mice. Total neuron number was estimated by stereological techniques on cresyl violet–stained sections. Significance was determined by by ANOVA with Sheffe post-hoc test; ***$p < 0.0001$.

cell number in the cortex. Recent data suggest that Fgf2 regulates the expansion of cortical founder cells before neurogenesis begins (Raballo et al., 2000). Interestingly, Fgf2 is not necessary for either the development of the basal ganglia or the generation of cortical interneurons that migrate into the cerebral cortex from the ganglionic eminences (Raballo et al., 2000). It is thus possible that fundamentally different mechanisms regulate the number of glutamatergic cortical pyramidal cells and the γ-aminobutyric acid (GABA) ergic cortical intereneurons (see next section).

In summary, ligands for RTK interact within microdomains of the PVE to regulate the timing of exit from the cell cycle, the number of progenitor cell divisions, and cell differentiation. These interactions occurring in an individual are likely to lead to variations in the number of glutamatergic and GABAergic neurons as well as glia born during this phase of CNS development.

NEURONAL MIGRATION IN THE CEREBRAL CORTEX: RADIAL AND TANGENTIAL

In laminar structures such as the cerebral and cerebellar cortices, glial cells of a specialized nature, which are the Bergmann glia and the radial glia for the cerebellum and cerebral cortex, respectively, are thought to guide young neurons in their radial migratory path. Another set of neurons migrates nonradially through unknown routes, possibly using early axonal tract or other astroglial cells (see below).

In the developing cerebral cortex, cells of the marginal zone (the Cajal-Retzius cells) are the first to be born. Subsequently, neurons pile up underneath the marginal zone to form cortical layers, in the sequence 6-5-4-3-2. The youngest cells always penetrate and migrate past the last ones and occupy the area nearest the marginal zone.

Several human genetic mutations exist that disrupt neuronal migration and cortical layer morphogenesis. These cause an arrest of the migration of cortical neurons, which produces various degrees of mental retardation and seizures (Gleeson and Walsh, 2000).

The analysis of several mouse mutants has given important insights into the complex signaling mechanisms that guide migrating neurons and has emphasized the importance of genetic components in the mechanism of cell migration. The *reeler, scrambler,* and *yotari* mutations in the mouse cause an identical phenotype in which younger migrating neurons are unable to penetrate the layer of older neurons. As a result, there is an inversion of cortical layers and a consequent disorganization of the cerebral cortex and other laminated structures (Caviness, 1982; Sheppard and Pearlman, 1997). The *reeler* gene encodes for reelin, a secreted protein produced by Cajal-Retzius cells and densest in the marginal zone. The *scrambler* and *yotari* mutations disrupt components of the intracellular reelin pathway. Recently, it was found that the double null mutation for the apolipoprotein E (ApoE) receptor 2 and the very low–density lipoprotein receptor (VLDLR) reproduces the reeler phenotype. This is because *reelin* binds to both ApoE2 and VLDLR with high affinity and this binding transduces the *reelin* signal. Signaling through non-receptor tyrosine kinases is critically involved in the regulation of neuronal migration.

A mutation in the *reeler* gene has recently been associated with autism (Keller et al., 2000). Mild abnormalities in cortical neuron migration and in reelin-containing cortical interneurons have been observed in the brains of schizophrenic subjects (Guidotti et al., 2000). Therefore, a mutation in the *reelin* gene has also been implicated in schizophrenia. Changes in reelin have also been reported in the hippocampus in affective disorders (Fatemi et al., 2000).

Glutamatergic pyramidal cells migrate in a radial fashion from the dorsal PVE, and are lineally distinct from GABAergic interneurons, which are tangentially

dispersed. The origin of the tangentially migrating cells was unknown until recently. Many GABA neuron precursor cells reach the developing cortex and hippocampus from the ganglionic eminences, which are located in the ventral part of the telencephalon (Anderson et al., 2001; Fig. 1.6). Progenitor cells of the basal telencephalon are genetically distinct from those located in the dorsal PVE, as they express different sets of homeodomain genes, including *Dlx* and *Nkx* (Figs. 1.1 and 1.2), which are not shared by dorsal cortical progenitors. The exact proportion of cortical interneurons that migrate in the cerebral cortex from the basal telencephalon has not been established.

The common origin of cortical and basal ganglia GABAergic cells and their dependence on a common set of genes necessary for their differentiation and migration pose interesting clinical questions. Deficits in cortical cell migration and in GABAergic interneurons

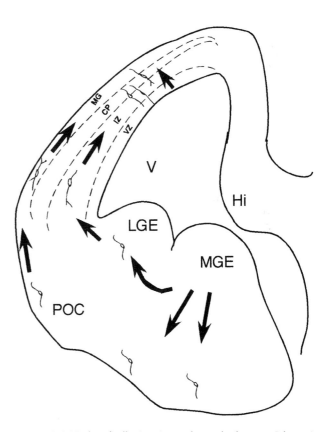

FIGURE 1.6 Modes of cell migration to the cerebral cortex. Schematic drawing of the cerebral cortical wall of the rodent at about embryonic day 13.5. The arrows indicate the main routes of cell migration. Abbreviations: CP, cortical plate; Hi, hippocampal formation; IZ, intermediate zone; LGE, lateral ganglionic eminence; MGE, medial ganglionic eminence; MZ, marginal zone; POC, primary olfactory cortex; V, lateral ventricle; VZ, ventricular zone; Adapted from (de Carlos et al. (1996).

have been observed in schizophrenia (Akbarian et al., 1996; Benes et al., 1996). Similarly, abnormalities in cortical interneurons have been reported in Tourette's syndrome and obsessive-compulsive disorder (Ziemann et al., 1997; Greenberg et al., 2000). These last conditions are thought to be disorders of the basal ganglia. It is now clear that events occurring during the development of the ganglionic eminences may influence the development of the cerebral cortex and the hippocampus as well; conversely, cortical interneurons are disrupted because of gene abnormalities not within the cortex, but within the basal telencephalon.

LARGE NUMBERS OF NEURONS NATURALLY DIE DURING THE EARLY PHASE OF CENTRAL NERVOUS SYSTEM MATURATION

Neurons are produced in excess and are later eliminated by a process of natural cell death called *apoptosis*. The death of a cell is carried out by a program encoded by its own genome and is descriptively characterized by a stereotyped sequence, starting with shrinkage and breakage of the chromatin in the nucleus (Fraser and Evan, 1996). This death program involves a common set of molecules conserved throughout evolution, beginning with primitive unicellular eukaryoriotes (Vaux and Strasser, 1996). The reason for the conservation of cell death programs throughout animal evolution may be that the ability of an organism (or of a colony of cells) to kill part of itself may provide a competitive advantage to the remaining cells. In general, cells eliminated by apoptosis are abnormal and/or potentially dangerous (i.e., cells that fail to follow the appropriate programs of division or differentiation; cancer cells; autoreactive lymphocytes; or virally infected cells). In addition, apoptosis plays a role in selecting neurons that have established unique patterns

of signaling. This will contribute to tissue sculpting during morphogenesis and the maturation of neuronal circuitry in the CNS.

In general, excess cells undergo apoptosis under conditions of scarcity of trophic factors. For example, in sympathetic ganglia, neurons undergo cell death in early embryogenesis unless they are able to connect with their target, a source of nerve growth factor (NGF), for which several neurons compete. In the CNS, growth factors may be delivered to a neuronal cell body not only retrogradely by the target but also anterogradely by the afferents. Furthermore, neuronal activity may regulate the synthesis of growth factors, and patterns of activity in the CNS are not only triggered by afferent stimulation but are often a characteristic of the network (for example, re-entrant circuitry).

Different cell populations die at different times. For example, in rodents, sympathetic neurons are pruned down by mid-gestation, whereas for cranial regions of the neuraxis the phase of cell death extends into the perinatal period. In the mammalian cerebral cortex, it has been estimated that approximately 40% to 50% of neurons die, and this process is completed in rat by the third postnatal week in concomitance to synaptogenesis (Ferrer et al., 1990; Fig. 1.7).

INBORN GENETIC PROGRAMS CONTROL FORMATION OF NEURONAL CONNECTIONS, WHEREAS ACTIVITY REGULATES THEIR REMODELING

One of the most formidable tasks for neurons within the developing CNS is to successfully "find" the appropriate target to establish synaptic connections. In the adult human CNS, over a trillion neurons each connect with, on average, a thousand target cells according to precise patterns essential for proper functioning (Tessier-Lavigne and Goodman, 1996). Rather than es-

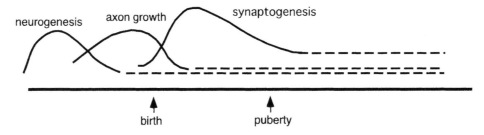

FIGURE 1.7 Time course of neuronal and synaptic remodeling in the rodent cerebral cortex. Neurogenesis and pruning of cells, axon collaterals, and synapses are distinct processes with partially overlapping time courses. Data are compiled from Fraser & Evan (1996); Vaux Strasser, (1996); Ferrer et al. (1990).

tablishing random connections that are later shaped into the normal pattern of connectivity, from the very beginning neurons are endowed with the capability to "choose" appropriate targets. Different mechanisms underlie the directed growth of the axon, the recognition of the target, and the transformation of the growth cone into a synapse; these mechanisms appear to be independent of electrical activity (Goodman and Tessier-Lavigne, 1997). The growth of axons toward the target is orchestrated by homeodomain proteins, which control the transcription of genes that regulate axonal pathfinding, differential cell adhesion, and synapse formation. The resulting pattern of connectivity is largely accurate and can be later refined by mechanisms influenced by electrical activity.

Growing axons "navigate" in the developing neuropil with the help of a sophisticated structure, the growth cone, and make few errors of navigation. The philopodia, dynamic web-like structures at the end of the growth cone of immature neurons, are able to "sense" or explore variations in the surrounding environment. These cues result in either axon growth (attractive cues) or withdrawal and an abrupt turn in a different direction (repulsive cues). Attractive and repulsive cues are either diffusible (long-range) or nondiffusible (short-range) (Tessier-Lavigne and Goodman, 1996). Once the target is finally reached, the growth cone stops and transforms into a synapse.

Short-range cues generally involve contact of axons with cell surface and extracellular matrix proteins. Adhesive substrates, or *cell adhesion molecules* (CAMs), are divided into three families; the cadherins, the integrins, and the immunoglobulin (Ig) superfamily. These transmembrane proteins possess a large extracellular moiety mediating adhesion and an intracellular portion that is linked to the cytoskeleton (Reichardt and Tomaselli, 1991). Members of the Ig superfamily promote adhesions between cells by interactions among different members, such as N-CAMs, L1, and axonin-1, expressed on the surface of adjacent cells. Their reciprocal binding is also influenced by their degree of glycosylation and their sialic acid content.

Diffusible (long-range) factors are soluble attractants or repulsants for growth cones, are distributed in concentration gradients, and aid selective growth in a particular direction. For example, cells at the ventral midline of the CNS express netrins, which attract axons toward the midline in the formation of commissural connections (Serafini et al., 1996). Other long-range cues are provided by ligands for receptor tyrosine kinases (RTKs). For example, axons express RTKs that recognize gradients of ligands secreted by the target.

Retinal axons follow a downward gradient of FGF to enter the tectum (McFarlane et al., 1996), whereas an increasing gradient of NGF or NT3 is required for target recognition in other areas (ElShamy et al., 1996).

After reaching the target area, axons may have to be sorted according to a particular layer, or they must be arranged according to the original topographical information that they carry, such as in maps. A classic example is the arrangement of retinal axons in the tectum, which must reproduce a map of the retina. Experiments have shown that the retinotopic order is preserved even when size disparities are introduced, suggesting that selective affinity for molecular gradients are involved (Patterson and Hall, 1992). Members of the ephrin (Eph) family of RTKs precisely orchestrate these cellular behaviors. Their membrane-anchored ligands are expressed as anterior-to-posterior gradients in the tectum and act as region-specific contact repellents (Tessier-Lavigne and Goodman, 1996).

In a second phase, connections are rendered more precise by elimination of axons and synapses by activity-dependent processes during early postnatal development (Innocenti, 1981). In rodents, this process extends into the first weeks after birth (see Fig. 1.7). In the fetal rhesus monkey, new axons start growing into the two major cerebral commissures (the corpus callosum and the anterior commissure) in the last weeks of gestation, their growth peaking at birth. Axons are subsequently eliminated in the first 2 or 3 postnatal months at a precipitous rate. For example, during the first 3 postnatal weeks, axons are eliminated from the anterior commissure and from the corpus callosum at an average rate of 1 and 50 axons/second, respectively (LaMantia and Rakic, 1994). The processes regulating this wholesale elimination are of interest, because the morphometry of the cerebral commissures correlates with a variety of behavioral differences, including gender, sexual orientation, and handedness (Allen and Gorski, 1991).

Similar to axons, synapses are initially overproduced in the infant primate, reaching their maximum number during infancy (2–4 months of age) (Rakic et al., 1986). Cortical synapses are eventually pruned down to a density of approximately 15 to 20 synapses/100 μm^2 of neuropil. Axons and synapses are eliminated through different time courses (Fig. 1.7). In primates, the adult number of synapses in the primate cerebral cortex is not achieved until near adolescence (Rakic et al., 1986).

Axonal and synapse elimination occurs at the same time as growth of myelin, increase in size of neurons and glia, and other processes; this suggests that the mammalian brain may be considerably more plastic than previously thought. Recent large-scale magnetic resonance imaging (MRI) longitudinal studies of normal human development have revealed that both white matter and gray matter of the cerebral cortex increase in volume during the postnatal period. For the cerebral cortical gray matter, the mean peak volume is reached at age 12 years, only to decrease thereafter. Remarkably, different cortical areas differ with respect to the age of peak growth, with the temporal lobe reaching a peak volume later (age 18 years) than the frontal or parietal lobes. The anterior portion of the corpus callosum increases until adolescence. Hence, increases in cortical volume occur throughout childhood, adolescence, and, sometimes, early adulthood (Giedd et al., 1999; Rapoport et al., 1999; Sowell et al., 1999).

Determination of the cellular and molecular processes that underlie these maturational events is under intense debate. While the anatomical substrate of this growth is still unknown, the magnitude of these phenomena is such that it is likely to involve all components of the CNS, including neurons, glia, and their connections. The prevailing view has been that neurons are generated only during embryogenesis, and that their number decreases during the postnatal period through programmed cell death. More recently, these ideas have been challenged, as experiments in rodents, primates, and humans have shown that new neurons are normally generated in the hippocampus, olfactory bulb, and possibly other areas in adult brains (see section "Pluripotent Cells in Adult Forebrain May Be Involved in Regeneration"). Future research looking into the cellular basis of brain growth and remodeling from infancy into early adulthood is likely to shed light on the pathogenesis of disorders with onset in childhood and adolescence.

EXUBERANT CONNECTIONS ARE PRUNED OFF AS A CONSEQUENCE OF ACTIVITY-RELATED PROCESSES

Critical periods are those in which the synaptic circuitry of a given brain region becomes stabilized in a functionally optimized conformation. The cerebral cortex and other brain structures contain functional maps for the activities characteristic of a species. The best example is the ocular dominance columns and other physical and functional characteristics of the circuitry within the visual cortical system that process information derived from the left and right visual fields, producing a map of the visual world. Other internal maps exist for the body (somatosensory, motor corti-

ces), the external physical environment (hippocampus), and possibly an individual social environment.

The primary visual cortex, like the rest of the cerebral cortex, is organized into vertical assemblies of neurons called *cortical columns*, which are the functional units of cortical information processing (Mountcastle, 1957). The initial formation of these columns is independent of visual experience (Crowley and Kats, 2000). In the primary visual cortex, separate cortical columns receive input from the right or the left eyes (ocular dominance). The maintenance of these connections is critically dependent on patterns of visual activity. If animals are deprived of visual input from one eye during the first 2 to 3 weeks after birth (the critical period), the cortical area occupied by columns for the functional eye enlarges at the expense of that for the deprived eye, which eventually becomes virtually unable to drive cortical activity (Wiesel and Hubel, 1963). This physical and functional "disconnection" of an inactive input occurs only during the critical period, as eye suture after the first weeks of life no longer affects cortical representation; however, the effects are permanent for the life of that individual. One mechanism responsible for these effects is synaptic plasticity; generally connections whose activity is temporally correlated are strengthened, whereas connections that display non-correlated activity tend to be weakened. This phenomenon is apparently consolidated during sleep.

Critical periods may vary depending on the area of the brain and the activity involved. Despite the evidence that patterns of neural activity influence the organization of neuronal circuitry, the mechanisms involved remain elusive. Neuronal activity drives the selective survival and sprouting of branches, accompanied by the local addition of synapses, within appropriate areas; furthermore, the lack of activity promotes the pruning of synaptic connections from inactive areas (Katz and Shatz, 1996). These competitive processes increase the refinement and precision of maps and require the activity of excitatory receptors (Constantine-Paton et al., 1990; Antonini and Stryker, 1993) and locally released growth factors (Thoenen, 1995; Inoue and Sanes, 1997).

Changes in synaptic structure and strength are also thought to underlie learning. Long-term potentiation (LTP) and long-term depression (LTD) consist of increases or decreases in synaptic strength, which depend on previous patterns of activity. N-methyl-D-aspartate (NMDA) receptors and growth factors are also involved in LTP and LTD. Thus, similar or identical mechanisms are used during the development of synaptic connections and the remodeling of these connections during learning (Kandel et al., 2000).

PLURIPOTENT CELLS IN ADULT FOREBRAIN MAY BE INVOLVED IN NEURONAL REGENERATION

Most progenitors are lineage restricted to produce either neurons or glia (Luskin et al., 1988). These progenitors have a limited life span (see Fig. 1.4B). Recent studies have shown that in addition to fate-restricted progenitors, the forebrain contains pluripotent stem cells capable of differentiating into many different cell type, including neurons and glia (Weiss et al., 1996). A small number of these pluripotent cells persist in the subependimal zone of the adult brain in virtually every mammal that has been examined (Reynolds and Weiss, 1992). These cells normally give rise to neurons that migrate in the olfactory bulb (Luskin, 1993). Under normal conditions, neurogenesis does not seem to occur in either the adult striatum or the cerebral cortex, although cortical cell genesis has been observed in the adult primate (Gould et al., 1999). Nevertheless, rodent or human stem cells expanded in vitro in the presence of either Fgf2 and EGF and transplanted in vivo are able to populate various regions of the adult CNS, including the cerebral cortex, striatum, and substantia nigra (Gage et al., 1995; Fricker et al., 1999). Although the efficiency may be low, the new neurons appear to be perfectly integrated in the transplanted regions.

The adult hippocampus also contains progenitors/ stem cells that are capable of differentiating into new hippocampal granule neurons. Hippocampal progenitor cells will give rise to new neurons in adult rodent, primate, and human brains (Eriksson et al., 1998). The new hippocampal granule cells extend axons that are appropriately connected to the pyramidal cells in the CA3 region.

The conditions that promote adult neurogenesis and the functional significance of adding extra neuronal cells to the adult synaptic circuit are presently not clear. For example, increased neurogenesis in rodents has been associated with exposure to an enriched environment, the performance of learning tasks, or simply running in a wheel (Kempermann et al., 2000). In contrast, stress strongly decreases the proliferation of adult progenitor cells in both rodents and primates (Gould et al., 1997). Cell damage or death promotes neurogenesis in the cerebral cortex, where neurogenesis does not normally occur in the adult (Magavi et al., 2000). These finding have generated considerable interest, since the theoretical possibility exists that new neurons could be generated to replace those lost to disease or degeneration (Weiss et al., 1996). For example, in depression and post-traumatic stress disorder there are decreases in hippocampal volume that may reflect cell loss (Bremner et al., 2000; Sheline, 2000). Cell loss has been found in the prefrontal cortex of depressed patients (Rajkowska, 2000). In addition, chronic antidepressant treatment increases neurogenesis in the hippocampus (Malberg et al., 1999).

THE IMPACT OF GONADAL STEROIDS AND DEVELOPMENT OF SEXUALLY DIMORPHIC AREAS

Gonadal steroids act on the developing nervous system to create a variety of gender differences in neural organization. There are also marked gender differences in the incidence of certain neuropsychiatric disorders of childhood and adolescent onset that are likely influenced by these developmental mechanims (female predominance: adolescent onset depression and eating disorders; male predominance: autism, other pervasive developmental disorders [PDDs], Tourette's syndrome, and childhood-onset obsessive-compulsive disorder). Sexually dimorphic behaviors in invertebrate and vertebrate species have been linked to structural differences in the CNS (Goy and McEwen, 1980; Allen and Gorski, 1991). Although some of these effects are likely to be hormone-independent, gonadal steroids (estrogens and androgens) acting during the course of CNS development can influence the number, size, and connectivity of neurons in a variety of brain regions (Arnold and Gorski, 1984; Pilgrim and Hutchinson, 1994; Balan et al., 1996). For example, the increased size of the anteroventral periventricular nucleus of the hypothalamus in male rats appears to depend on the action of testicular hormones during the neonatal period, although the actual structural difference between the sexes is not obvious until puberty (Davis et al., 1996).

Intriguingly, for many areas of the brain, the action of testosterone depends on its conversion to estradiol by aromatase. The emergence of sexually dimorphic regions may depend on the creation of gender-specific networks of estrogen-forming neurons. For example, investigators have measured aromatase activity in two strains of mice selectively bred for behavioral aggression. The animals bred to have short attack latency showed a different developmental pattern of aromatase activity in both the amygdala and the hypothalamus (Hutchinson et al., 1995).

Traditionally, investigators have focused on the role of steroid receptors acting via the nucleus and the binding of the steroid–receptor complex to specific DNA regions to alter the transcription of specific genes (Evans, 1988). More recent studies have indicated that estrogen may also act through effects on the signaling pathway of NGF to induce changes in dendritic arborization and synapse formation. For example, ovariectomized females rats lose dendritic spines in specific hippocampal regions. When treated with estrogen, these animals show a 30% increase in NMDA receptors in the same hippocampal regions (Gazzaley et al., 1996; Wooley et al., 1997).

FUTURE PROSPECTS: ALTERATION OF NEURONAL DEVELOPMENT AND VULNERABILITY TO PSYCHOPATHOLOGY

The past decade has seen unprecedented advances in our understanding of the mechanisms involved in the morphogenesis and activity-mediated sculpting of brain circuitry. The reciprocal interplay of conserved genetic programs and the ever-changing macro- and microenvironment is a recurrent theme. These events set the stage for individual differences and range of phenotypic diversity seen within the human species (Bartley et al., 1997). A deeper understanding of these mechanisms should lead the way to improved treatments and preventive interventions.

Many psychopathological states, such as schizophrenia, autism, or Tourette's syndrome, are fundamentally developmental disorders that likely involve allelic variants that confer vulnerability to specific environmental risk factors (Ciccheti and Cohen, 1995). A developmental perspective is of value in considering childhood-onset disorders and will likely prove to be broadly useful. For example, the ability of estrogens to maintain a rich dendritic arborization in regions of the hippocampus may herald an effective means of maintaining mental function and preventing the toxic effects of substances such as β-amyloid (Tang et al., 1996).

In addition, gene programs that are instructing the development of the CNS may be "reactivated" at later stages, in connection with brain plasticity that characterizes learning (Vaccarino et al., 2001).

REFERENCES

Acampora, D., Avantaggiato, V., Tuorto, F., and Simeone, A. (1997) Genetic control of brain morphogenesis through *Otx* gene dosage requirement. *Development* 124:3639–3650.

Acampora, D., Mazan, S., Avantaggio, V., Barone, P., Tuorto, F., Lallemand, Y., Brulet, P., and Simeone, A. (1996) Epilepsy and brain abnormalities in mice lacking the *Otx1* gene. *Nat Genet* 14:218–222.

Acampora, D., Mazan, S., Lallemand, Y., Avantaggiato, V., Maury, M., Simeone, A., and Brulet, P. (1995) Forebrain and midbrain regions are deleted in Otx2$^{-/-}$ mutants due to a defective anterior neuroectoderm specification during gastrulation. *Development* 121:3279–3290.

Akbarian, S., Kim, J.J., Potkin, S.G., Hetrick, W.P., Bunney, W.E., and Jones, E.G. (1996) Maldistribution of interstitial neurons in prefrontal white matter of the brains of schizophrenic patients. *Arch Gen Psychiatry* 53:425–436.

Allen, L.S., and Gorski, R.A. (1991) Sexual dimorphism of the anterior commisssure and massa intermedia of the human brain. *J Comp Neurol* 312:97–104.

Anderson, S.A., Marin, O., Horn, C., Jennings, K., and Rubenstein, J.L. (2001) Distinct cortical migrations from the medial and lateral ganglionic eminences. *Development* 128:353–363.

Antonini, A., and Stryker, M.P. (1993) Development of individual geniculocortical arbors in cat striate cortex and effects of binocular impulse blockade. *J Neurosci* 13:3549–3573.

Arnold, A.P., and Gorski, R.A. (1984) Gonadal steroid induction of structural sex differences in in the central nervous system. *Ann Rev Neurosci* 7:413–442.

Balan, I.S., Ugrumov, M.V., Borislova, N.A.B.N., Calas, A., Pilgrim, C., Reisert, I., Thibault, J., Calas, A., Pilgrim, C., Reisert, I., and Thibault, J. (1996) Birthdates of the tryosine hydroxylase immunoreactive neurons in the hypothalamus of male and female rats. *Neuroendocrinology* 64:405–411.

Bartley, A.J., Jones, D.W., and Weinberger, D.R. (1997) Genetic variability of human brain size and cortical gyral patterns. *Brain* 120:257–269.

Benes, F.M., Vincent, S.L., Marie, A., and Khan, Y. (1996) Upregulation of GABA$_A$ receptor binding on neurons of the prefrontal cortex in schizophrenic subjects. *Neuroscience* 75:1021–1031.

Bremner, J.D., Narayan, M., Anderson, E.R., Staib, L.H., Miller, H.L., and Charney, D.S. (2000) Hippocampal volume reduction in major depression. *Am J Psychiatry* 157:115–118.

Briscoe, J., Pierani, A., Jessel, T., and Ericson, J. (2000) A homeodomain protein code specifies progenitor cell identity and neuronal fate in the ventral neural tube. *Cell* 101:435–445.

Brunelli, S., Faiella, A., Capra, V., Nigro, V., Simeone, A., Cama, A., and Boncinelli, E. (1996) Germline mutations in the homeobox gene *EMX2* in patients with severe schizencephaly. *Nat Genet* 12:94–96.

Bulfone, A., Smiga, S.M., Shimamura, K., Peterson, A., Puelles, L., and Rubenstein, J.L.R. (1995) T-brain-1: a homolog of brachyury whose expression defines molecularly distinct domains within the cerebral cortex. *Neuron* 15:63–78.

Capecchi, M.R. (1997) *The Role of Hox Genes in Hindbrain Development, 1st ed.* New York: Oxford University Press.

Caviness, V.S., Jr. (1982) Neocortical histogenesis in normal and reeler mice: a developmental study based upon [³H] thymidine autoradiography. *Dev Brain Res* 4:293–302.

Ciccheti, D., and Cohen, D.J. (1995) *Developmental Psychopathology*. New York: John Wiley and Sons.

Constantine-Paton, M., Cline, H.T., and Debski, E. (1990) Patterned activity., synaptic convergence., and the NMDA receptor in the developing visual pathways. *Ann Rev of Neurosci* 13:129–154.

Crossley, P.H., Martinez, S., and Martin, G.R. (1996) Midbrain development induced by FGF8 in the chick embryo. *Nature* 380:66–68.

Crowley, J.C., and Kats, L.C. (2000) Early development of ocular dominance columns. *Science* 290:1321–1324.

Davis, E.C., Shryne, J.E., and Gorski, R.A. (1996) Structural sexual dimorphisms in the anteroventral periventricular nucleus of the rat hypothalamus are sensitive to gonadal steroids postnatally, but develop peripubertally. *Neuroendocrinology* 63:142–148.

de Carlos, J.A., Lopez-Mascaraque, L., and Valverde, F. (1996) Dynamics of cell migration from the lateral ganglionic eminence in the rat. *J Neurosci* 16:6146–6156.

Donoghue, M.J., and Rakic, P (1999) Molecular evidence for the early specification of presumptive functional domains in the embryonic primate cerebral cortex. *J Neurosci* 19:5967–5979.

Eisenberg, L. (2000) Is psychiatry more mindful or brainier than it was a decade ago? *Br J Psychiatry* 176:1–5.

Eisenberg, L. (2001) The past 50 years of child and adolescent psychiatry: a personal memoir. *J Am Acad Child Adolesc Psychiatry* 40 (7):743–748

ElShamy, W.M., Linnarsson, S., Lee, K.-F., Jaenisch, R., and Enfors, P. (1996) Prenatal and postnatal requirements of NT-3 for sympathetic neuroblast survival and innervation of specific targets. *Development* 122:491–500.

Eriksson, P.S., Perfilieva, E., Bjork-Eriksson, T., Alborn, A.M., Nordborg, C., Peterson, D.A., and Gage, F.H. (1998) Neurogenesis in the adult human hippocampus. *Nat Med* 4:1313–1317.

Evans, R.M. (1988) The steroid and thyroid receptor superfamily. *Science* 240:889–895.

Fatemi, S.H., Earle, J.A., and McMenomy, T. (2000) Reduction in reelin immunoreactivity in hippocampus of subjects with schizophrenia, bipolar disorder and major depression. *Mol Psychiatry* 5:654–653.

Ferrer, I., Bernet, E., Soriano, E., del Rio T., and Fonseca, M. (1990) Naturally occurring cell death in the cerebral cortex of the rat and removal of dead cells by transitory phagocytes. *Neuroscience* 39:451–458.

Finkelstein, R., and Perrimon, N. (1990) The orthodenticle gene is regulated by bicoid and torso and specifies *Drosophila* head development [see comments]. *Nature* 346:485–488.

Fraser, A., and Evan, G. (1996) A license to kill. *Cell* 86:781–784.

Fricker, R.A., Carpenter, M.K., Winkler, C., Greco, C., Gates, M.A., and Bjorklund, A. (1999) Site-specific migration and neuronal differentiation of human neural progenitor cells after transplantation in the adult rat brain. *J Neurosci* 19:5990–6005.

Gage, F.H., Coates, P.W., Palmer, T.D., Kuhn, H.G., Fisher, L.J., Suhonen, J.O., Peterson, D.A., Suhr, S.T., and Ray, J. (1995) Survival and differentiation of adult neuronal progenitor cells transplanted to the adult brain. *Proc Natl Acad Sci USA* 92:11879–11883.

Gazzaley, A.H., Weiland, N.G., McEven, B.S., and Morrison, J.H. (1996) Differential regulation of NMDAR1 mRNA and protein by estradiol in the rat hippocampus. *J Neurosci* 16:6830–6838.

Gehring, W.J., Qian, Y.Q., Billeter, M., Furukubo-Tokunaga, K., Schier, A.S., Resendez-Perez, D., Affolter, M., Otting, G., and Wuthrich, K. (1994) Homeodomain-DNA recognition. *Cell* 78:211–223.

Giedd, J.N., Blumenthal, J., Jeffries, N.O., Castellanos, F.X., Liu, H., Zijdenbos, A., Paus, T., Evans, A.C., and Rapoport, J.L. (1999) Brain development during childhood and adolescence: a longitudinal MRI study. *Nat Neurosci* 2:861–863.

Gillberg, C., and Steffenburg, S. (1989) Autistic behaviour in Moebius syndrome. *Acta Pediatr Scand* 78:314–316.

Gleeson, J.G., and Walsh, C.A. (2000) Neuronal migration disorders: from genetic diseases to developmental mechanisms. *Trends Neurosci* 23:352–359.

Goddard, J.M., Rossel, M., Manley, N.R., and Capecchi, M.R. (1996) Mice with targeted disruption of *Hoxb-1* fail to form the motor nucleus of the VIIth nerve. *Development* 122:3217–3228.

Goodman, C.S., and Tessier-Lavigne, M. (1997) Molecular mechanisms to axin guidance and target recognition. In: (Cowan, W.M., Jessel, T.M., and Zipursky, S.L., eds). Molecular and Cellular Approaches to Neural Development, 1st ed. New York: Oxford University Press, pp. 108–178.

Gould, E., McEwen, B.S., Tanapat, P., Galea, L.A.M., and Fuchs, E.

(1997) Neurogenesis in the dentate gyrus of the adult tree shrew is regulated by psychosocial stress and NMDA receptor activation. *J Neurosci* 17:2492–2498.

Gould, E., Reeves, A.J., Graziano, M.S.A., and Gross, C.G. (1999) Neurogenesis in the neocortex of adult primates. *Science* 286:548–552.

Goy, R.W., and McEwen, B.S. (1980) *Sexual Differentiation of the Brain.* Cambridge, MA: MIT Press.

Greenberg, B.D., Ziemann, U., Cora-Locatelli, G., Harmon, A., Murphy, D.L., Keel, J.C., and Wassermann, E.M. (2000) Altered cortical excitability in obsessive-compulsive disorder. *Neurology* 54:142–147.

Gross, C.G. (2000) Neurogenesis in the adult brain: death of a dogma. *Nat Rev Neurosci* 1:67–73.

Guidotti, A., Auta, J., Davis, J.M., Gerevini, V.D., Dwivedi, Y., Grayson, D.R., Impagnatiello, F., Pandey, G., Pesold, C., Sharma, R., Uzunov, D., and Costa, E. (2000) Decrease in reelin and glutamic acid decarboxylase 67 (GAD67) expression in schizophrenia and bipolar disorder: a postmortem brain study. *Arch Gen Psychiatry* 57:1061–1069.

Hutchinson, J.B., Beyer, C., Hutchinson, R.E., and Wozniak, A. (1995) Sexual dimorphism in the developmental regulation of brain aromatase. *J Steroid Biochem Mol Biol* 53:307–313.

Innocenti, G.M. (1981) Growth and reshaping of axons in the establishment of visual callosal connections. *Science* 212:824–827.

Inoue, A., and Sanes, J.R. (1997) Lamina-specific connectivity in the brain: regulation by N-cadherin, neurotrophins, and glycoconjugates. *Science* 276:1428–1431.

Jan, Y.N., and Jan, L.Y. (1995) Maggot's hair and bug's eye: role of cell interactions and intrinsic factors in cell fate specification. *Neuron* 14:1–5.

Kandel, E.R., Schwartz, J.H., and Jessel, T.M. (2000) *Principles of Neural Science, 4 ed.* New York: McGraw-Hill.

Katz, L.C., and Shatz, C.J. (1996) Synaptic activity and the construction of cortical circuits. *Science* 274:1133–1138.

Persico, A.M., D'Agruma, L., Maiorano, N., Totaro, A., Militerni, R., Bravaccio, C., Wassink, T., Schneider, C., Melmed, R., Trillo, S., Montecchi, F., Palermo, M., Pascucci, T., Puglisi-Allegra, S., Reichelt, K.-L., Conciatori, M., Marino, R., Quattrocchi C.C. Baldi, Zelante A., Gasparini P. and Keller F. (2001) *Reelin* gene alleles and haplotypes as a predisposing factor to Molecular Psychiatry 6:150–159 autistic disorder.

Kempermann, G., van Praag H., and Gage, F.H. (2000) Activity-dependent regulation of neuronal plasticity and self repair. *Prog Brain Res* 127:35–48.

Krumlauf, R. (1992) Evolution of the vertebrate *Hox* homeobox genes [review]. *Bioessays* 14:245–252.

LaMantia, A.-S., and Rakic, P. (1994) Axon overproduction and elimination in the anterior commissure of the developing rhesus monkey. *J Comp Neurol* 340:328–336.

Liem, K.F.J., Tremml, G., Roelink, H., and Jessel, T.M. (1995) Dorsal differentiation of neural plate cells induced by BMP-mediated signals from epidermal cells. *Cell* 82:969–979.

Lumsden, A., and Krumlauf, R. (1996) Patterning the vertebrate neuraxis. *Science* 274:1109–1115.

Luskin, M.B. (1993) Restricted proliferation and migration of postnatally generated neurons derived from the forebrain ventricular zone. *Neuron* 11:173–189.

Luskin, M.B., Pearlman, A.L., and Sanes, J.R. (1988) Cell lineage in the cerebral cortex of the mouse studied in vivo and in vitro with a recombinant virus. *Neuron* 1:635–647.

Magavi, S.S., Leavitt, B.R., and Macklis, J.D. (2000) Induction of neurogenesis in the neocortex of adult mice. *Nature* 405:951–955.

Malberg, J.E., Eissch, A.J., Nestler, E.J., and Duman, R.S. (1999) Chronic antidepressant administration increases granule cell neurogenesis. *Soc Neurosci Abstr* 25:1029.

McFarlane, S., Cornel, E., Amaya, E., and Holt, C.E. (1996) Inhibition of FGF receptor activity in retinal ganglion cell axons causes errors in target recognition. *Neuron* 17:245–254.

Meinhardt, H. (1983) Cell determination boundaries as organizing regions for secondary embryonic fields. *Dev Biol* 96:375–385.

Miyama, S., Takahashi and T., Nowakowski, R.S. and Caviness, V.S. (1997) A gradient in the duration of the G1 phase in the murine neocortical proliferative renoepithelium. *Cerebral Cortex* 7:678–689.

Meyers, E.N., Lewandoski, M., and Martin, G.R. (1998) An *Fgf8* mutant allelic series generated by Cre-and Flp-mediated recombination. *Nat Genet* 18:136–141.

Mountcastle, V.B. (1957) Modality and topographic properties of single neurons of cat's somatic sensory cortex. *J Neurophysiol* 20:408–434.

Patterson, P.H., and Hall, Z.W. (1992) *An Introduction to Molecular Neurobiology*. Sunderland, MA:Sinauer Associates.

Pellegrini, M., Mansouri, A., Simeone, A., Boncinelli, E., and Gruss, P. (1996) Dentate gyrus formation requires *Emx2*. *Development* 122:3893–3898.

Pilgrim, C., and Hutchinson, J.B. (1994) Developmental regulation of sex differences in the brain: can the role of gonadal steroids be redefined? *Neuroscience* 60:843–855.

Raballo, R., Rhee, J., Lyn-Cook, R., Leckman, J.F., Schwartz, M.L., and Vaccarino, F.M. (2000) Basic fibroblast growth factor (Fgf2) is necessary for cell proliferation and neurogenesis in the developing cerebral cortex. *J Neurosci* 20:5012–5023.

Rajkowska, G. (2000) Postmortem studies in mood disorders indicate altered numbers of neurons and glial cells. *Biol Psychiatry* 48:766–777.

Rakic, P. (1995) A small step for the cell, a giant leap for mankind: a hypothesis of neocortical expansion during evolution. *Trends Neurosci* 18:383–388.

Rakic, P., Bourgeois, J.-P., Eckenhoff, M.F., Zecevic, N., and Goldman-Rakic, P.S. (1986) Concurrent overproduction of synapses in diverse regions of the primate cerebral cortex. *Science* 232:232–235.

Rapoport, J.L., Giedd, J.N., Blumenthal, J., Hamburger, S., Jeffries, N., Fernandez, T., Nicolson, R., Bedwell, J., Lenane, M., Zijdenbos, A., Paus, T., and Evans, A. (1999) Progressive cortical change during adolescence in childhood-onset schizophrenia. A longitudinal magnetic resonance imaging study. *Arch Gen Psychiatry* 56:649–654.

Reichardt, L.F., and Tomaselli, K.J. (1991) Extracellular matrix molecules and their receptors: functions in neural development. *Ann Rev Neurosci* 14:531–570.

Reynolds, B.A., and Weiss, S. (1992) Generation of neurons and astrocytes from isolated cells of the adult mammalian central nervous system. *Science* 255:1707–1710.

Rodier, P.M., Ingram, J.L., Tisdale, B., Nelson, S., and Romano, J. (1996) Embryological origin for autism:developmental anomalies of the cranial nerve motor nuclei. *J Comp Neurol* 370:247–261.

Ross, E.M. (1996) Cell division and the nervous system: regulating the cycle from neural differentiation to death. *Trends Neurosci* 19:62–68.

Roth, K.A., Kuan, C.-Y., Haydar, T.F., D'Sa-Eipper, C., Shindler, K.S., Zheng, K.S., Kuida, K., Flavell, R.A., and Rakic, P. (2000) Epistatic and independent functions of Caspase-3 and Bcl-X$_L$ in developmental programmed cell death. *Proc Natl Acad Sci USA* 97:466–471.

Rubenstein, J.L.R., Martinez, S., Shimamura, K., and Puelles, L. (1994) The embryonic vertebrate forebrain: the prosomeric model. *Science* 266:576–580.

Rubenstein, J.L.R., and Shimamura, K. (1997) Regulation of patterning and differentiation in the embryonic vertebrate forebrain. In: Cowan, W.M., Jessel, T.M., and Zipursky, S.L., eds. *Molecular and Cellular Approaches to Neural Development, 1st ed.* New York: Oxford University Press, pp. 356–390.

Serafini, T., Colamarino, S.A., Leonardo, E.D., Wang, H., Beddington, R., Skarnes, W.C., and Tessier-Lavigne, M. (1996) Netrin-1 is required for commissural axon guidance in the developing vertebrate nervous system. *Cell* 87:1001–1014.

Shatz, C.J., Ghosh, A., McConnell, S.K., Allendoerfer, K.L., Friauf, E., and Antonini, A. (1990) Pioneer neurons and target selection in cerebral cortical development [review]. *Cold Spring Harb Sympo Quant Biol* 55:469–480.

Sheline, Y.I. (2000) 3D MRI studies of neuroanatomical changes in unipolar major depression: the role of stress and medical comorbidity. *Biol Psychiatry* 48:791–800.

Sheppard, A.M., and Pearlman, A.L. (1997) Abnormal reorganization of preplate neurons and their extracellular matrix: an early manifestation of altered neocortical development in the *reeler* mutant mouse. *J Comp Neurol* 378:173–179.

Shimamura, K., Hartigan, D.J., Martinez, S., Puelles, L., and Rubenstein, J.L.R (1995) Longitudinal organization of the anterior neural plate an d neural tube. *Development* 121:3923–3933.

Shin, J.J., Fricker-Gates, R.A., Perez, F.A., Leavirt, B.R., Zurskowski, D., and Macklis, J.D. (2000) Transplanted neuroblasts differentiate appropriately into projection neurons with correct neurotransuitrer and receptor phenotype in neocortex undergoing targeted project neuron degeneration. *J Neurosci* 20:7404–7416.

Sibilia, M., Steinbach, J.P., Stingl, L., Aguzzi, A., and Wagner, E.F. (1998) A strain-independent postnatal neurodegeneration in mice lacking the EGF receptor. *EMBO J* 17:719–731.

Simeone, A., Acampora, D., Gulisano, M., Stornaiuolo, A., and Boncinelli, E (1992) Nested expression domains of four homeobox genes in developing rostral brain. *Nature* 358:687–690.

Sowell, E.R., Thompson, P.M., Holmes, C.J., Batth, R., Jernigan, T.L., and Toga, A.W. (1999) Localizing age-related changes in brain structure between childhood and adolescence using statistical parametric mapping. *Neuroimage* 9:587–597.

St Johnston, D., and Nusslein-Volhard, C. (1992) The origin of pattern and polarity in the *Drosophila* embryo. *Cell* 68:201–219.

Takahashi, T., Nowakowski, R.S., and Caviness, V.S. (1996) The leaving or Q fraction of the murine cerebral proliferative epithelium: a general model of neocortical neuronogenesis. *J Neurosci* 16:6183–6196.

Tang, M., Jacobs, D., Stern, Y., Marder, K., Schonfeld, P., Gurland, B., Andrews, H., and Mayreux, R. (1996) Effect of oestrogens during menopause on risk and age of onset of Alzheimer's disease. *Lancet* 348:429–432.

Tessier-Lavigne, M., and Goodman, C.S. (1996) The molecular biology of axon guidance. *Science* 274:1123–1133.

Thoenen, H. (1995) Neurotrophins and synaptic plasticity. *Science* 270:593–598.

Tropepe, V., Sibilia, M., Ciruna, B.G., Rossant, J., Wagner, E.F., and van der Kooy, D. (1999) Distinct neural stem cells proliferate in response to EGF and FGF in developing mouse telencephalon. *Dev Biol* 208:166–188.

Vaccarino, F.M., Schwartz, M.L., Hartigan, D., and Leckman, J.F. (1995) Effect of basic fibroblast growth factor on the genesis of excitatory and inhibitory neurons in primary cultures of cells from the mammalian telencephalon. *Cereb Cortex* 1:64–78.

Vaccarino, F.M., Schwartz, M.L., Raballo, R., Nilsen, J., Rhee, J., Zhou, M., Doetschman, T., Coffin, J.D., Wyland, J.J., and Hung, Y.-T.E. (1999) Changes in cerebral cortex size are governed by fibroblast growth factor during embryogenesis. *Nat Neurosci* 2: 246–253.

Vaccarino, F.M., Ganat Y., Zhang Y., Zhang W. (2001) Stem cells in Neurodevelopment and plasticity. *Neuropsychopharmocology* 25:805–815.

Vaux, D.L., and Strasser, A. (1996) The molecular biology of apoptosis. *Proc Natl Acad Sci USA* 93:2239–2244.

Weiss, S., Reynolds, B.A., Vescovi, A.L., Morshead, C., Craig, C.G., and van der Kooy, D. (1996) Is there a neural stem cell in the mammalian forebrain? *Trends Neurosci* 19:387–393.

Wiesel, T.N., and Hubel, D.H. (1963) Single-cell responses in striate cortex of kittens deprived of vision in one eye. *J Neurophysiol* 26:1003–1017.

Wooley, C.S., Weiland, N.G., McEwen, B.S., and Schwartzkroin, P.A. (1997) Estradiol increases sensistivity of hippocampal CA1 pyramidal cells to NMDA receptor–mediated synaptic input: correlation with dendritic spine density. *J Neurosci* 17:1848–1859.

Ye, W., Shimamura, K., Rubenstein, J.L., Hynes, M.A., and Rosenthal, A. (1998) FGF and *Shh* signals control dopaminergic and serotonergic cell fate in the anterior neural plate. *Cell* 93:755–766.

Ziemann, U., Paulus, W., and Rothenberger, A. (1997) Decreased motor inhibition in Tourette's disorder: evidence from transcranial magnetic stimulation. *Am J Psychiatry* 154:1277–1284.

2 | Synaptic function and biochemical neuroanatomy

STEPHAN HECKERS AND CHRISTINE KONRADI

How are the 10^{11} neurons in the central nervous system arranged to process information? How do they communicate through their 10^3–10^4 connections with each other? Most importantly for psychiatrists; how can environmental influences, such as a pharmacological intervention or psychotherapy, influence the way in which the brain processes information?

In this chapter we will focus on two basic principles of neurotransmission that may help to understand normal brain function on the one hand, and the current practice of clinical psychopharmacology on the other. First, the anatomic organization of neurotransmitter systems determines their behavioral affiliation. Second, neurotransmitter receptors modulate the electrical properties (via ion channels) or the biochemical properties (via second messenger systems) of neurons. We will then review these two basic principles for some of the neurotransmitter systems relevant to the practice of neuropsychopharmacology.

NEURAL CIRCUITRY

Neurons are arranged in distributed networks to govern human behavior (Mesulam, 1998). Here we focus on four major anatomical systems: the cortex, the thalamus, the basal ganglia, and the medial temporal lobe (Fig. 2.1).

The thalamus is the gateway to cortical processing of all incoming sensory information, represented in Figure 2.1 by the three major systems: somatosensory (S), auditory (A), and visual (V). Primary sensory cortices (S1, A1, V1) receive information from the appropriate input modules (sensory organ + thalamus). The association cortex integrates information from primary cortices, from subcortical structures, and from brain areas affiliated with memory to create an internal representation of the sensory information. The medial temporal lobe (i.e., hippocampus, amygdala) serves two major functions in the brain: to integrate multimodal sensory information for storage into and retrieval from memory, and to attach limbic valence to sensory information. The basal ganglia are primarily involved in the integration of input from cortical areas. The basal ganglia modulate cortical activity via a cortico-striato-pallido-thalamo-cortical loop. The most prominent projections to the striatum arise from the motor cortex.

These four systems provide the anatomical basis for the three most basic brain functions: the reception of sensory information, the creation of an internal representation, and the creation of a response. Several other systems are involved in information processing in the brain (e.g., the cerebellum and the hypothalamus), but for the purpose of this chapter we will focus on this core set of cerebral structures. The processing of information in this circuitry has to occur extremely fast. For example, how else would the brain process a painful or threatening stimulus and produce an appropriate response to avoid the stimulus? All major pathways in this circuitry are glutamatergic, which, as we will see, allows for fast processing of information. The glutamatergic pathways are under inhibitory control within each of the brain regions by so-called interneurons, which use γ-aminobutyric acid (GABA) as a neurotransmitter.

The function of these four systems is modulated by several groups of neurons that are characterized by their use of a specific neurotransmitter: cholinergic neurons in the basal forebrain and brain stem, dopaminergic neurons in the substantia nigra and ventral tegmental area, noradrenergic neurons in the locus ceruleus, and serotonergic neurons in the raphe nuclei. The broken arrows in Figure 2.1 indicate the four neurotransmitter-specific projection systems. Most of the therapeutic agents used in the current practice of psychopharmacology are aimed at strengthening or inhibiting these modulatory systems.

How do the four major anatomical systems and the

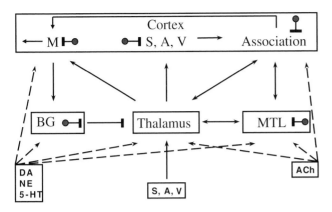

FIGURE 2.1 Neural circuitry. This diagram provides a basic scheme of information processing in the human brain. Excitatory neurons using glutamate as a neurotransmitter are shown as arrows, inhibitory neurons using GABA are shown as circles. The glutamatergic projection neurons are under inhibitory control by GABAergic interneurons. Diffuse-projecting neurotransmitter systems (using acetycholine [Ach], dopamine [DA], norepinephrine [NE], and serotonin [5-HT]) located in the basal forebrain and brainstem are shown as dashed lines. Sensory information of the somatosensory, auditory, and visual realm arrive at the cortex via the thalamus. Primary sensory information is then relayed to association cortex, medial temporal lobe (MTL), and thalamus for further processing. One of the output modules, the motor cortex (M), is fine-tuned via inhibitory neurons in the basal ganglia (BG).

neurotransmitter-specific diffuse projection systems communicate with each other? To answer this question we have to review the basic anatomy of a neuron.

Anatomy of the Neuron

Neurons have three compartments: dendrites, cell body (perikaryon), and axon (Fig. 2.2). *Dendrites* create a network of fibers providing the neuron with input from other cells. The *cell body* integrates the different inputs provided by the dendrites. This integration can occur through a modulation of the membrane potential or at the level of the nucleus (regulation of gene expression). One function of the cell body is the synthesis of all cell-specific receptors and enzymes needed for neurotransmitter production. The *axon* is the output station of the neuron. The axon can be short (local circuit neuron) or long (projection neuron). If a deviation from the resting membrane potential is above a certain threshold, an action potential is created and travels downstream rapidly. The *nerve terminal* is the widened terminal part of the axon. It provides a small area of close contact with dendrites of neighboring cells: a *synapse*. Variations of this typical scheme include synapses between two axons, between two dendrites, and neu-

rotransmitter release in medial parts of the axon (varicosities, boutons).

The Synapse

The presynaptic neuron, which releases the neurotransmitter into the synapse, can express two types of proteins that affect synaptic communication [see (1) and (2) in Fig. 2.2]:

1. Membrane-bound receptors bind the intrinsic neurotransmitter (autoreceptor) or transmitters of neighboring neurons (heteroreceptor) and affect the cell via intracellular messengers. One response, for example, is the modulation of neurotransmitter release (Langer, 1997).

2. Membrane-bound reuptake transporters pump the released neurotransmitter back into the cell (Amara, 1995; Lester et al., 1996).

The neuron receiving the input (postsynaptic cell) can be modulated via two different types of receptors [see (3) and (4) in Fig. 2.2]:

3. Fast-acting, class I (ionotropic) receptors. The neurotransmitter binds to the receptor protein and within milliseconds leads to a change in the permeability of the associated ion channel, allowing the influx of ions such as Ca^{2+}, Na^+, K^+, or Cl^-.

4. Slow-acting, class II (G protein–coupled) receptors. The neurotransmitter binds to the receptor protein and thereby changes the protein conformation. This change is relayed to an associated G protein, which binds guanidine triphosphate (GTP) to be activated. G proteins regulate two major classes of effector molecules: ion channels and second messenger–generating enzymes.

Synaptic communication between neurons does not only involve the classical neurotransmitter systems reviewed in this chapter. Two other classes of neurotransmitters are also known to affect brain function: neuropeptides and atypical neurotransmitters, such as nitric oxide and carbon monoxide. These neurotransmitters are not stored in vesicles, are not released by exocytosis, and do not bind to postsynaptic receptors. We have chosen not to review these neurotransmitters here, since they do not yet have implications for the current practice of neuropsychopharmacology. They are, however, promising targets for the development of new treatment strategies, and the interested reader is referred to other articles for review (Hokfelt, 1991; Snyder and Ferris, 2000).

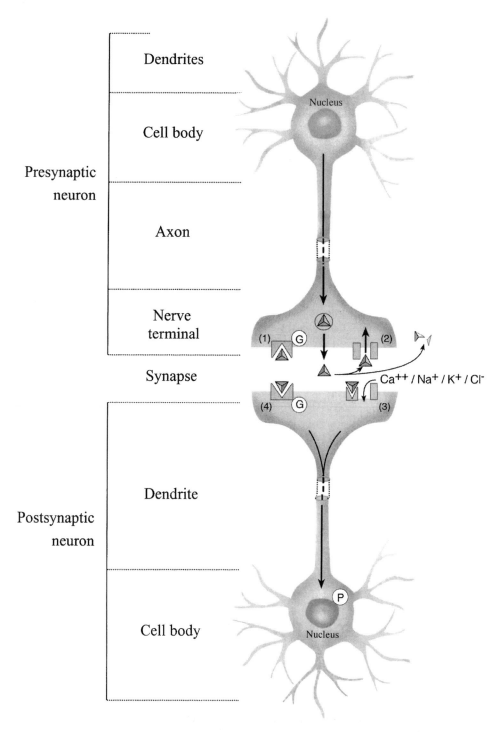

FIGURE 2.2 The anatomy of the neuron. Communication between two neurons occurs at the synapse. The presynaptic neuron produces and releases the neurotransmitter into the synaptic cleft. Four mechanisms (1–4) are important to understand the function of most neurotransmitter systems. The release of neurotransmitter can be modulated via presynaptic receptors (1). The amount of neurotransmitter in the synaptic cleft can be decreased by reuptake into the presynaptic neuron (2) or via enzymatic degradation. Neurotransmitter effects at the target neuron are relayed via fast-acting ion channel–coupled receptors (3) or via slower-acting G protein–coupled receptors (4). Down-stream effects of postsynaptic receptors include the phosphorylation (P) of nuclear proteins.

NEUROTRANSMITTER SYSTEMS

Although there are many more neurotransmitter systems in the brain, in clinical psychopharmacology we are concerned primarily with six systems: the glutamatergic, GABAergic, cholinergic, serotonergic, noradrenergic, and dopaminergic. These six systems can be divided into two groups on the basis of their anatomical characteristics.

The first group includes the glutamatergic and GABAergic systems. These two classes of neurons are by far more prevalent and more widely distributed than any other neurotransmitter system in the human brain. The major functional implication of such widespread distribution is that the modulation of glutamatergic and GABAergic neurotransmission affects many neural systems.

The second group of neurotransmitter systems comprises the cholinergic, serotonergic, noradrenergic, and dopaminergic neurons. These four systems originate from small groups of neurons, densely packed in circumscribed areas of the forebrain or brain stem, which project to their target areas typically via long-ranging projection fibers. Since these neurotransmitter-specific projection systems reach selected neural systems, their modulation leads to more circumscribed effects.

Glutamatergic Neurotransmission

Glutamate (Glu) is the most abundant amino acid in the central nervous system (CNS). It serves many functions as an intermediate in neuronal metabolism, e.g., as a precursor for GABA. About 30% of the total glutamate in the brain functions as the major excitatory neurotransmitter.

Anatomy

Glutamatergic neurons are widely distributed throughout the entire brain. Most glutamatergic neurons are so-called projection neurons: their axon projects into distant brain regions. Prominent glutamatergic pathways are the connections between different regions of the cerebral cortex (cortico-cortical projections), the connections between thalamus and cortex, and the projections from cortex to striatum (extrapyramidal pathway) and from cortex to brain stem/spinal chord (pyramidal pathway).

The hippocampus is characterized by a series of glutamatergic neurons, which can create rhythms of electrical activity necessary for the generation of memory traces in the brain. The cerebellum, a region dedicated to the temporal processing of motor and cognitive in-

formation, is also rich with glutamatergic neurons (Ozawa et al., 1998).

Synaptic organization

Glutamate acts at three different types of ionotropic receptors [see (1) in Fig. 2.3] and at a family of G protein–coupled (metabotropic) receptors [see (2) in Fig. 2.3] (Nakanishi, 1992; Nakanishi et al., 1998; Vandenberg, 1998). Binding of glutamate to the ionotropic receptor opens an ion channel, allowing the influx of Na^+ and Ca^{2+} into the cell. N-methyl-D-aspartate (NMDA) receptors bind glutamate and NMDA. The receptor consists of two different subunits: NMDAR1 (seven variants) and NMDAR2 (four variants). The NMDA receptor is highly regulated at several sites. For example, the receptor is virtually ineffective unless a ligand (such as glycine) binds to the glycine site and it is blocked by binding of ligands (MK-801, ketamine, and phencyclidine [PCP]) to the PCP site inside the channel. α-amino-3-hydroxy-5-methyl-4-isoxazole propionic acid (AMPA) receptors bind glutamate, AMPA, and quisqualic acid, while kainate receptors bind glutamate and kainic acid.

The metabotropic glutamate receptor family includes at least seven different types of G protein–coupled receptors ($mGluR_{1-7}$). These are linked to different second messenger systems and lead to the increase of intracellular Ca^{2+} or the decrease of cyclic AMP (cAMP). The increase of intracellular Ca^{2+} leads to the phosphorylation of target proteins in the cell.

Glutamate is removed from the synapse by high-affinity reuptake; two transporter proteins are expressed in glial cells and one in neurons [see (3) in Fig. 2.3].

Function

The widespread distribution of glutamatergic neurons explains why glutamate is involved in many brain functions. Modulation of glutamatergic activity is therefore most likely to have widespread effects. Excess stimulation of glutamatergic receptors, as seen in seizures or stroke, can lead to unregulated Ca^{2+} influx and neuronal damage (Dingledine et al., 1990; Coyle and PuTtfarcken, 1993; Loscher, 1998).

Several brain functions have been linked to specific glutamate receptor subtypes in selected brain regions. For example, glutamatergic neurons and NMDA receptors in the hippocampus are important for long-term potentiation (LTP), a crucial component in the formation of memory (Wilson and Tonegawa, 1997). Animal models with selective lesioning or strengthening of NMDA receptors in the hippocampus have demonstrated that this glutamate receptor subtype is crucial for normal memory function.

Abnormalities of the glutamate system have also been documented in neuropsychiatric disorders. For example, compounds such as PCP and ketamine, which block the NMDA receptor, can induce psychotic symptoms. By contrast, compounds such as d-cycloserine or glycine, which increase NMDA receptor function via the glycine binding site, can decrease psychotic and/or negative symptoms in schizophrenia (Farber et al., 1999; Goff et al., 1999, Heresco-Levy et al., 1999).

GABAergic Neurotransmission

GABA is an amino acid with high concentrations in the brain and the spinal chord. It acts as the major inhibitory neurotransmitter in the CNS.

Anatomy

GABAergic neurons can be divided into two groups: short-ranging neurons that connect to other neurons in the same brain region and medium/long-ranging neurons that project to distant brain regions. The vast majority of GABAergic neurons are short-ranging neurons (also called *interneurons* or *local circuit neurons*) in the cortex, thalamus, striatum, cerebellum, and spinal chord. Various subtypes of the GABAergic interneurons provide tonic as well as phasic inhibitory control over glutamatergic projection cells. An intricate balance of inhibitory (GABAergic) and excitatory (glutamatergic) tone is essential for normal function (Somogyi et al., 1998).

There are three groups of medium/long-ranging GABAergic neurons with projections into other brain regions. The most important are the projections from caudate/putamen to globus pallidus and from globus pallidus in turn to thalamus and substantia nigra. This pair of GABAergic neurons in the striato-pallido-thalamic pathway is part of a larger cortico-striato-pallido-thalamo-cortical circuit involved in modulating cortical output. Another important group of GABAergic projection neurons connects the septum with the hippocampus and is important in several hippocampal functions, including memory. The third group of long-ranging GABAergic neurons projects from the substantia nigra to thalamus and superior colliculus.

Synaptic organization

GABA acts at two types of receptors [see (1) and (2) in Fig. 2.4]. The GABA$_A$ receptor is a receptor–channel

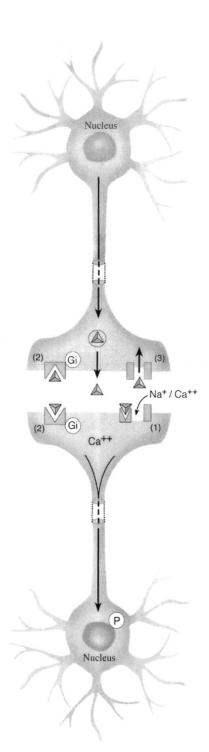

FIGURE 2.3 Glutamatergic synapse. Glutamate binds to ionotropic receptors (1) and metabotropic receptors (2). The glutamate transporter (3) pumps glutamate back into the glutamatergic neuron.

complex comprised of five subunits (Lüddens and Korpi, 1996). Activation leads to the opening of the channel, allowing Cl⁻ to enter the cell, resulting in decreased excitability. Five distinct classes of subunits (six variants of α, four variants of β, three variants of γ, one of δ, and two variants of ρ) are known. Multiple variations in the composition of the GABA$_A$ receptor are known, but the prominent type is created by two α, two β, and one γ or δ subunit. The receptor can be modulated by various compounds that bind to several different sites. Benzodiazepines bind to the α subunit and open the channel if a γ subunit is present and if GABA is bound to the GABA site on the β subunit. Barbiturates and ethanol bind near the Cl⁻ channel and increase channel open time even without GABA present.

The GABA$_B$ receptor is a G protein–coupled receptor with similarity to the metabotropic glutamate receptor (Kaupmann et al., 1997; Bettler et al., 1998). The GABA$_B$ receptor is linked to G$_i$ (decreasing cAMP and opening of K⁺ channels) and G$_o$ (closing Ca²⁺ channels). The net effect is prolonged inhibition of the cell. A well-known agonist is baclofen. The GABA$_B$ receptor is found postsynaptically (causing decreased excitability) and presynaptically (leading to decreased neurotransmitter release).

GABA is removed from the synapse by a sodium dependent GABA uptake transporter [(3) in Fig. 2.4].

Function

GABA is the major inhibitory neurotransmitter in the CNS. Similar to the modulation of glutamatergic receptors, the application of ligands that can strengthen or weaken GABAergic activity has widespread effects.

The cortical, hippocampal, and thalamic GABAergic neurons are crucial for the inhibition of excitatory neurons. Foci of local imbalance, with a subnormal tone of GABAergic inhibition, may spread to distant areas to induce a seizure. GABA$_A$ agonists such as benzodiazepines or barbiturates can decrease the occurrence of seizures or interrupt ongoing seizure activity (Bazil and Pedley, 1998).

Modulation of GABA$_A$ receptors is also beneficial in the treatment of several neuropsychiatric conditions, including anxiety disorders, insomnia, and agitation. The mechanisms are not well understood but may work through a general inhibition of neuronal activity. Benzodiazepines and ethanol use the same mechanism to influence GABA$_A$ receptors. This property is the basis for ethanol detoxification with benzodiazepines (Grobin et al., 1998).

Finally, psychotic disorders, especially schizophrenia

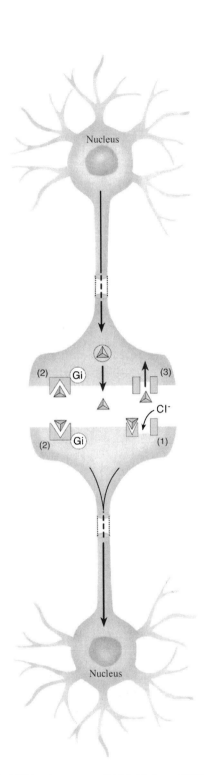

FIGURE 2.4 GABAergic synapse. GABA binds to GABA$_A$ receptors (1) and GABA $_B$ receptors (2). The GABA transporter (3) pumps GABA back into the GABAergic neuron.

and bipolar disorder, are associated with abnormalities of specific subtypes of GABAergic neurons, primarily in the prefrontal cortex and the paralimbic cortex (anterior cingulate gyrus and hippocampus) (Lewis et al., 1999; Benes and Berretta, 2001).

Cholinergic Neurotransmission

Acetylcholine (ACh) has been known as a neurotransmitter since the mid-1920s. In fact, the demonstration that acetylcholine is the *Vagusstoff* ("vagus-substance") released from the vagus nerve to modulate heart function was the first proof for the chemical mediation of nerve impulses (Loewi and Navratil, 1926). In the peripheral nervous system, ACh is found as the neurotransmitter in the autonomic ganglia, the parasympathetic postganglionic synapse, and the neuromuscular endplate.

Anatomy

Cholinergic neurons in the CNS are either wide-ranging projection neurons or short-ranging interneurons. The most prominent group of cholinergic neurons are found in the basal forebrain and include groups in the septum, diagonal band, and nucleus basalis of Meynert. These cholinergic basal forebrain neurons project to many areas of the cerebral cortex, but with regional specificity. The projections are weak in primary sensory and motor areas, become more prominent in association cortex, and are most prominent in paralimbic cortical areas (e.g., cingulate gyrus and hippocampus) (Mesulam, 1996). A smaller group of cholinergic projection neurons are located in the brain stem and project predominantly to the thalamus. The only group of short-ranging cholinergic interneurons are in the striatum and modulate the activity of GABAergic striatal neurons.

Synaptic organization

Acetylcholine acts at two different types of cholinergic receptors [see (1) and (2) in Fig. 2.5]. Muscarinic receptors bind ACh as well as other agonists (muscarine, pilocarpine, bethanechol) and antagonists (atropine, scopolamine). There are at least five different types of muscarinic receptors (M1–M5). All have slow response times. They are coupled to G proteins and a variety of second messenger systems. When activated, the final effect can be to open or close channels for K^+, Ca^{2+}, or Cl^- (Bonner, 1989). Nicotinic receptors are less abundant than the muscarinic type in the CNS. They bind ACh as well as agonists such as nicotine or an-

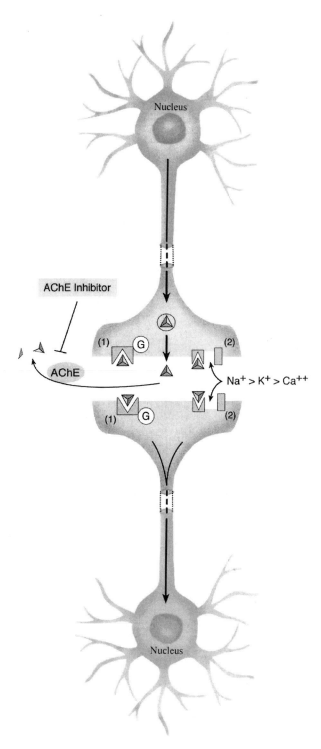

FIGURE 2.5 Cholinergic synapse. Acetylcholine binds to muscarinic receptors (1) and nicotinic receptors (2). Acetylcholinesterase (AchE) cleaves the neurotransmitter acetylcholine into acetylCoA and choline.

tagonists such as d-tubocurarine. The fast-acting, ionotropic nicotinic receptor allows influx of $Na^+ K^+ Ca^{2+}$ into the cell. Presynaptic cholinergic receptors are of the muscarinic or nicotinic type and can modulate the release of several neurotransmitters (Wonnacott, 1997).

Acetylcholine is removed from the synapse through hydrolysis into acetylCoA and choline by the enzyme acetylcholinesterase (AChE). Removing ACh from the synapse can be blocked irreversibly by organophosphorous compounds and in a reversible fashion by drugs such as physostigmine.

Function

The projection patterns of the cholinergic neurons may explain their behavioral affiliations. Cholinergic neurons in the nucleus basalis of Meynert provide tonic and phasic activation of the cerebral cortex to modulate attention and novelty seeking (Detari et al., 1999). The cholinergic neurons of the septum and diagonal band projecting to the hippocampus are essential for normal memory function (Baxter and Chiba, 1999). Alzheimer's disease (AD) and anticholinergic delirium are two examples of a cholinergic-deficit state. Blocking the metabolism of ACh by AChE strengthens cognitive functioning in AD patients and reverses the acute confusional state induced by anticholinergic drugs (Geula, 1998; Giacobini, 1998).

The brain stem cholinergic neurons are essential for the regulation of sleep–wake cycles via projections to the thalamus. The cholinergic interneurons in the striatum modulate striatal GABAergic neurons by opposing the effects of dopamine. Increased cholinergic tone in Parkinson's disease and decreased cholinergic tone in patients treated with neuroleptics are examples of an imbalance of these two systems in the striatum (Calabresi et al., 2000).

Serotonergic Neurotransmission

Serotonin, or 5-hydroxytryptamine (5-HT), is a monoamine widely distributed in many cells of the body, with about 1%–2% of its entire body content present in the CNS.

Anatomy

Serotonergic neurons are found only in midline structures of the brain stem. Most serotonergic cells overlap with the distribution of the raphe nuclei in the brain stem. A rostral group (B6–8 neurons) projects to the thalamus, hypothalamus, amygdala, striatum, and cor-

tex. The remaining two groups (B1–5 neurons) project to other brain stem neurons, the cerebellum, and the spinal chord.

Synaptic organization

Serotonin acts at two different types of receptors: G protein–coupled receptors [see (1) and (2) in Fig. 2.6] and an ion-gated channel [see (3) in Fig. 2.6] (Julius, 1991). With the exception of the $5-HT_3$ receptor, all serotonin receptors are G protein coupled and can be grouped as follows:

1. The $5-HT_1$ receptors ($5-HT_{1A,B,C,D,E,F}$) are coupled to G_i and lead to a decrease in cAMP. The $5-HT_{1A}$ receptor is also directly coupled to a K^+ channel, leading to increased opening of the channel. The $5-HT_1$ receptors are the predominant serotonergic autoreceptors.

2. $5-HT_2$ receptors ($5-HT_{2A-C}$) are coupled to phospholipase C and lead to a variety of intracellular effects (mainly depolarization). Three receptors ($5-HT_{4,6,7}$) are coupled to G_s and activate adenylate cyclase. The function of the $5-HT_{5A}$ and $5-HT_{5B}$ receptors is poorly understood.

3. The $5-H T_3$ receptor is the only monoamine receptor coupled to an ion channel, probably a Ca^{2+} channel. It is found in the cortex, hippocampus, and area postrema. It is typically localized presynaptically and regulates neurotransmitter release. Well-known antagonists are the potent antiemetics ondansetron and granisetron.

Serotonin is removed from the synapse by a high-affinity serotonin uptake site [(4) in Fig. 2.6] that is capable of transporting serotonin in either direction, depending on its concentration. The serotonin transporter is blocked by selective serotonin reuptake inhibitors (SSRIs) as well as by tricyclic antidepressants.

Function

Serotonin has been linked to many brain functions, which is not surprising, considering the widespread serotonergic projections and the heterogeneity of serotonergic receptors (Jacobs and Azmitia, 1992; Lucki, 1998). The modulation of both the serotonergic receptors and the reuptake site is beneficial in the treatment of anxiety, depression, obsessive-compulsive disorder, and schizophrenia (Murphy et al., 1998). Anxiety disorders in particular have been linked to an abnormal serotonergic modulation of the amygdala and the noradrenergic neurons in the locus ceruleus (Gorman et al., 2000). The treatment of psychosis has also benefited from compounds that modulate not only the do-

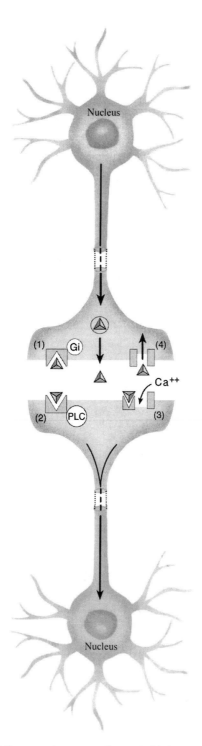

FIGURE 2.6 Serotonergic synapse. Serotonin binds to at least seven different receptors. The most relevant are the 5-HT$_1$ receptors (1), 5-HT$_2$ receptors (2), and 5-HT$_3$ receptors (3). Antagonists of the 5-HT$_2$ receptor include nefazodone and the majority of atypical antipsychotic drugs. The serotonin transporter (4) pumps serotonin back into the serotonergic neuron, which can be blocked by drugs such as venlafaxine, clomipramine, imipramine, and amitriptyline.

paminergic but also the serotonergic system (Meltzer, 1999).

Hallucinogens such as lysergic acid diethylamide (LSD) modulate serotonergic neurons via serotonergic autoreceptors and, by targeting receptors in the visual system, may cause prominent visual hallucinations (Aghajanian and Marek, 1999).

Noradrenergic Neurotransmission

Norepinephrine (NE), a catecholamine, was first identified as a neurotransmitter in 1946. In the peripheral nervous system, it is found as the neurotransmitter in the sympathetic postganglionic synapse.

Anatomy

About half of all noradrenergic neurons, i.e., 12,000 on each side of the brain stem, are located in the locus ceruleus (LC). They provide the extensive noradrenergic innervation of cortex, hippocampus, thalamus, cerebellum, and spinal chord. The remaining neurons are distributed in the tegmental region. They innervate predominantly the hypothalamus, basal forebrain, and spinal chord.

Synaptic organization

Norepinephrine is released into the synapse from vesicles [(1) in Fig. 2.7]; amphetamine facilitates this release. Norepinephrine acts in the CNS at two different types of noradrenergic receptors, the α and the β [see (2a), (2b) and (3) in Fig. 2.7]. α-Adrenergic receptors can be subdivided into α$_1$ receptors (coupled to phospholipase and located postsynaptically) and α$_2$ receptors (coupled to G$_i$ and located primarily presynaptically) (Insel, 1996). β-Adrenergic receptors in the CNS are predominantly of the β$_1$ subtype (3 in Fig. 2.7). β$_1$ receptors are coupled to G$_s$ and lead to an increase in cAMP. Cyclic AMP triggers a variety of events mediated by protein kinases, including phosphorylation of the β receptor itself and regulation of gene expression via phosphorylation of transcription factors.

Norepinephrine is removed from the synapse by means of two mechanisms. In the first, catechol-O-methyl-transferase (COMT) degrades intrasynaptic NE. In the second, the norepinephrine transporter (NET), a Na$^+$/Cl$^-$–dependent neurotransmitter transporter, is the primary way of removing NE from the synapse [(4) in Fig. 2.7]. The NET is blocked selectively by desipramine and nortriptyline. Once internalized,

NE can be degraded by the intracellular enzyme monoamine oxidase (MAO).

Function

Noradrenergic projections are involved in the modulation of sleep cycles, appetite, mood, and cognition by targeting the thalamus, limbic structures, and cortex. An increase in noradrenergic function appears to convey some of the therapeutic effect of antidepressants, although the exact mechanisms remain poorly understood (Charney, 1998; Anand and Charney, 2000; Frazer, 2000).

An important anatomical feature of the LC is the rich innervation by afferents from the sensory systems. This puts the LC in the position to monitor the internal and external environments. The widespread LC efferents in turn then lead to an inhibition of spontaneous discharge in the target neurons. Therefore, the LC is thought to be crucial for fine-tuning the attentional matrix of the cortex and the activity in limbic structures. Anxiety disorders may be due to perturbations of this system.

The LC neurons express a variety of autoreceptors, which allow compounds such as clonidine to decrease, and others such as yohimbine to increase LC firing (Buccafusco, 1992). Clonidine is used in the treatment of opiate withdrawal, since it decreases LC firing during the withdrawal from morphine.

Dopaminergic Neurotransmission

Dopamine (DA) was initially considered merely an intermediate monoamine in the synthesis of NE and epinephrine. However, in the late 1950s, DA was discovered to be a neurotransmitter in its own right.

Anatomy

There are three groups of dopaminergic neurons in the human, which differ in the length of their efferent fiber systems. Wide-ranging projections, functionally the most relevant, are located in two neighboring regions of the brain stem, the substantia nigra (SN) and the ventral tegmental area (VTA) (Fig. 2.8). The SN neurons, also called *A9 neurons,* project primarily to the caudate and putamen. The VTA neurons, also called *A10 neurons,* project to limbic areas such as the nucleus accumbens and amygdala (so-called mesolimbic projections) and the frontal, cingulate, and entorhinal cortex (so-called mesocortical projections).

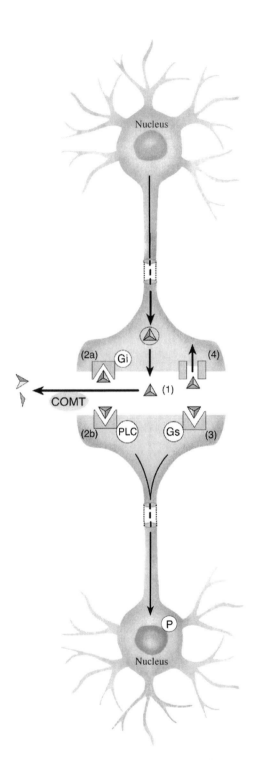

FIGURE 2.7 Noradrenergic synapse. The release of norepinephrine (1) can be enhanced by compounds such as amphetamine. Once released, norepinephrine binds to α2 receptors (2a), α1 receptors (2b), and β1 receptors (3). Norepinephrine is removed from the synapse via cleavage by catechol-O-methyl-transferase (COMT) or via reuptake by the norepinephrine transporter (4).

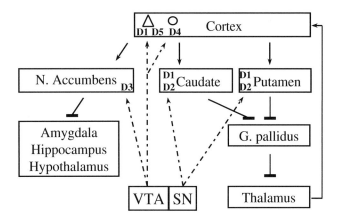

FIGURE 2.8 Dopaminergic neurons. Dopaminergic neurons of the substantia nigra (SN) target GABAergic projection neurons of the caudate and putamen via D_1 and D_2 receptors. Dopaminergic neurons of the ventral tegmental area (VTA) target cortical pyramidal cells via D_1 and D_5 receptors, cortical interneurons via D_4 receptors, and GABAergic projection neurons of the nucleus accumbens via D_3 receptors.

Intermediate-length systems originate in the hypothalamus and project to, among others, the pituitary gland. Finally, ultrashort systems are found in the retina and olfactory bulb.

Synaptic organization

Dopamine is released into the synapse from vesicles [see (1) in Fig. 2.9]; this process is facilitated by stimulant drugs, such as amphetamine and methylphenidate. Dopamine acts at two different classes of DA receptors in the CNS, the D_1 receptor family [see (2) in Fig. 2.9] and the D_2 receptor family [see (3) in Fig. 2.9] (Baldessarini and Tarazi, 1996). The D_1 receptor family includes the D_1 and D_5 receptors. Both are coupled to G_s and lead to an increase in cAMP. The D_2 receptor family includes the D_2, D_3, and D_4 receptors. All are coupled to G_i and lead to a decrease in cAMP. There is a predilection of the different DA receptors for expression in specific brain areas (Fig. 2.8):

D_1: striatum, cortex, SN, olfactory tubercle

D_2: striatum, SN, pituitary gland, retina, olfactory tubercle

D_3: nucleus accumbens

D_4: on GABAergic neurons in cortex, thalamus, hippocampus, SN

D_5: hippocampus, cortex, hypothalamus.

Presynaptic dopaminergic receptors are typically of the D_2 type and found on most portions of the dopaminergic neuron (as autoreceptors). They regulate DA

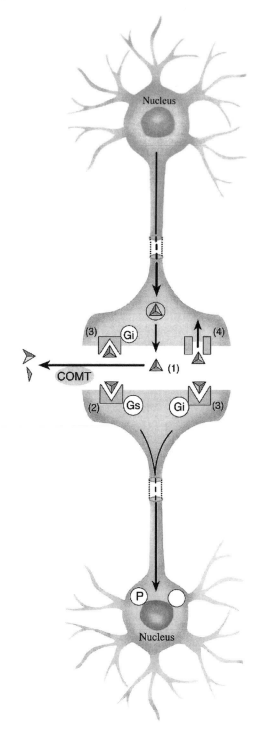

FIGURE 2.9 Dopaminergic synapse. The release of dopamine (1) can be enhanced by compounds such as amphetamine and methylphenidate (1). Once released, dopamine binds to two types of dopamine receptors. The family of D1 receptors includes the D1 and D5 receptor (2) and the family of D2 receptors includes the D2, D3, and D4 receptors (3). Dopamine is removed from the synapse via cleavage by catechol-O-methyl-transferase (COMT) or via reuptake by the dopamine transporter (4).

synthesis and release, as well as the firing rate of DA neurons. Autoreceptors are 5–10 times more sensitive to DA agonists than postsynaptic receptors.

Dopamine is removed from the synapse via two mechanisms. First, COMT degrades intrasynaptic DA. Second, the dopamine transporter (DAT) [see (4) in Fig. 2.9], a Na^+/Cl^-–dependent neurotransmitter transporter, transports DA in either direction, depending on the concentration gradient. The DAT is blocked selectively by drugs such as cocaine, amphetamine, bupropion, and nomifensine.

Function

The effects of DA on brain function are linked to its projection patterns. Furthermore, DA affects brain functions primarily by modulation of other neurotransmitter systems (Missale et al., 1998).

The dopaminergic projections of the SN to the striatum modulate the neuronal excitability of GABAergic neurons in the striatum (Joel and Weiner, 2000; Nicola et al., 2000). By targeting either D_1 or D_2 receptors on different subpopulations of GABAergic projection neurons, they are in the position to specifically alter the flow of information within the cortico-striato-pallido-thalamo-cortical circuit subserving several behaviors, including motor function and cognition. Parkinson's disease and extrapyramidal side effects due to treatment with neuroleptics are examples of a decreased function of this dopaminergic projection.

Dopaminergic projections of the VTA to limbic structures such as the nucleus accumbens are known to be involved in reward behavior and in the development of addiction to drugs such as ethanol, cocaine, nicotine, and opiates (Diana, 1998; Koob, 1998; Spanagel and Weiss, 1999; Berke and Hyman, 2000). Dopaminergic projections of the VTA to the cortex play a role in the fine-tuning of cortical neurons (i.e., better signal-to-noise ratio) (Goldman-Rakic, 1998). It appears that dopaminergic projections to pyramidal neurons act via D_1 receptors, whereas dopaminergic projections to GABAergic interneurons act via D_4 receptors (Goldman-Rakic et al., 2000). This could provide the basis for specific effects of dopaminergic modulation, based on their preference for postsynaptic dopaminergic receptors.

Dopaminergic projections from the hypothalamus to the pituitary gland tonically inhibit the production and release of prolactin via D_2 receptors. The blockade of these receptors leads to hyperprolactinemia, a common side effect of compounds such as typical antipsychotic drugs.

CONCLUSION

Information processing in the human brain via neurochemically defined neuronal systems is complex. Therefore, it remains a challenge to conceptualize psychiatric disorders and their treatment in a reductionistic framework of chemical neuroanatomy. We can nonetheless broadly state that the anatomic organization of neurotransmitter systems determines their behavioral affiliation, and that receptors modulate the electrical or biochemical properties of neurons, with direct relevance to the mechanism of action of psychotropic drugs. Future research will provide more detailed information on the subtypes of neurons and specific neurotransmitters systems that are abnormal in psychiatric disorders, and provide a more rational approach to the development of new treatment interventions.

REFERENCES

Aghajanian, G.K., and Marek, G.J. (1999) Serotonin and hallucinogens. *Neuropsychopharmacology* 21:16S–23S.

Amara, S.G. (1995) Monoamine transporters: basic biology with clinical implications. *Neuroscientist* 1:259–267.

Anand, A. and Charney, D.S. (2000) Norepinephrine dysfunction in depression. *J Clin Psychiatry* 61:16–24.

Baldessarini, R.J. and Tarazi, F.I. (1996) Brain dopamine receptors: a primer on their current status, basic and clinical. *Harv Rev Psychiatry* 3:301–325.

Baxter, M.G. and Chiba, A.A. (1999) Cognitive functions of the basal forebrain. *Curr Opin Neurobiol* 9:178–183.

Bazil, C.W. and Pedley, T.A. (1998) Advances in the medical treatment of epilepsy. *Annu Rev Med* 49:135–162.

Benes, F.M. and Berretta, S. (2001) GABAergic interneurons: implications for understanding schizophrenia and bipolar disorder. *Neuropsychopharmacology* 25:1–27.

Berke, J.D. and Hyman, S.E. (2000) Addiction, dopamine, and the molecular mechanisms of memory. *Neuron* 25:515–532.

Bettler, B., Kaupmann, K., and Bowery, N. (1998) $GABA_B$ receptors: drugs meet clones. *Curr Opin Neurobiol* 8:345–350.

Bonner, T.I. (1989) The molecular basis of muscarinic receptor diversity. *Trends Neurosci* 12:148–151.

Buccafusco, J.J. (1992) Neuropharmacologic and behavioral actions of clonidine: interactions with central neurotransmitters. *Int Rev Neurobiol* 33:55–107.

Calabresi, P., Centonze, D., Gubellini, P., Pisani, A., and Bernardi, G. (2000) Acetylcholine-mediated modulation of striatal function. *Trends Neurosci* 23:120–126.

Charney, D.S. (1998) Monoamine dysfunction and the pathophysiology and treatment of depression. *J Clin Psychiatry* 59 Suppl 14:11–14.

Coyle, J.T. and Putfarcken, P. (1993) Oxidative stress, glutamate, and neurodegenerative disorders. *Science* 262:689–695.

Detari, L., Rasmusson, D.D., and Semba, K. (1999) The role of basal forebrain neurons in tonic and phasic activation of the cerebral cortex. *Prog Neurobiol* 58:249–277.

Diana, M. (1998) Drugs of abuse and dopamine cell activity. *Adv Pharmacol* 42:998–1001.

Dingledine, R., McBain, C.J., and McNamara, J.O. (1990) Excitatory amino acid receptors in epilepsy. *Trends Pharmacol Sci* 11: 334–338.

Farber, N.B., Newcomer, J.W., and Olney, J.W. (1999) Glycine agonists: what can they teach us about schizophrenia? *Arch Gen Psychiatry* 56:13–17.

Frazer, A. (2000) Norepinephrine involvement in antidepressant action. *J Clin Psychiatry* 61:25–30.

Geula, C. (1998) Abnormalities of neural circuitry in Alzheimer's disease: hippocampus and cortical cholinergic innervation. *Neurology* 51:S18–S29; discussion S65–67.

Giacobini, E. (1998) Cholinergic foundations of Alzheimer's disease therapy. *J Physiol Paris* 92:283–287.

Goff, D.C., Tsai, G., Levitt, J., Amico, E., Manoach, D., Schoenfeld, D.A., Hayden, D.L., McCarley, R., and Coyle, J.T. (1999) A placebo-controlled trial of D-cycloserine added to conventional neuroleptics in patients with schizophrenia. *Arch Gen Psychiatry* 56: 21–27.

Goldman-Rakic, P.S. (1998) The cortical dopamine system: role in memory and cognition. *Adv Pharmacol* 42:707–711.

Goldman-Rakic, P.S., Muly, E.C., 3rd, and Williams, G.V. (2000) D(1) receptors in prefrontal cells and circuits. *Brain Res Brain Res Rev* 31:295–301.

Gorman, J.M., Kent, J.M., Sullivan, G.M., and Coplan, J.D. (2000) Neuroanatomical hypothesis of panic disorder, revised. *Am J Psychiatry* 157:493–505.

Grobin, A.C., Matthews, D.B., Devaud, L.L., and Morrow, A.L. (1998) The role of GABA(A) receptors in the acute and chronic effects of ethanol. *Psychopharmacology (Berl)* 139:2–19.

Heresco-Levy, U., Javitt, D.C., Ermilov, M., Mordel, C., Silipo, G., and Lichtenstein, M. (1999) Efficacy of high-dose glycine in the treatment of enduring negative symptoms of schizophrenia. *Arch Gen Psychiatry* 56:29–36.

Hokfelt, T. (1991) Neuropeptides in perspective: the last ten years. *Neuron* 7:867–879.

Insel, P.A. (1996) Adrenergic receptors—evolving concepts and clinical implications. *N Engl J Med* 334:580–585.

Jacobs, B.L., and Azmitia, E.C. (1992) Structure and function of the brain serotonin system. *Physiol Rev* 72:165–229.

Joel, D. and Weiner, I. (2000) The connections of the dopaminergic system with the striatum in rats and primates: an analysis with respect to the functional and compartmental organization of the striatum. *Neuroscience* 96:451–474.

Julius, D. (1991) Molecular biology of serotonin receptors. *Ann Rev Neurosci* 14:335–360.

Kaupmann, K., Huggel, K., Heid, J., Flor, P.J., Bischoff, S., Mickel, S.J., McMaster, G., Angst, C., Bittiger, H., Froestl, W., and Bettler, B. (1997) Expression cloning of GABAb receptors uncovers similarity to metabotropic glutamate receptors. *Nature* 386:239–246.

Koob, G.F. (1998) Circuits, drugs, and drug addiction. *Adv Pharmacol* 42:978–982.

Langer, S.Z. (1997) 25 years since the discovery of presynaptic receptors: present knowledge and future perspectives. *Trends Pharmacol Sci* 18:95–99.

Lester, H.A., Cao, Y., and Mager, S. (1996) Listening to neurotransmitter transporters. *Neuron* 17:807–810.

Lewis, D.A., Pierri, J.N., Volk, D.W., Melchitzky, D.S., and Woo, T.U. (1999) Altered GABA neurotransmission and prefrontal cortical dysfunction in schizophrenia. *Biol Psychiatry* 46:616–626.

Loewi, O. and Navratil, E. (1926) Über humorale Übertragbarkeit der Herznervenwirkung. X. Mitteilung. Über das Schicksal des Vagusstoff. *Pflugers Arch Gesamte Physiol* 214:678–688.

Loscher, W. (1998) Pharmacology of glutamate receptor antagonists in the kindling model of epilepsy. *Prog Neurobiol* 54:721–741.

Lucki, I. (1998) The spectrum of behaviors influenced by serotonin. *Biol Psychiatry* 44:151–162.

Lüddens, H. and Korpi, E.R. (1996) GABAa receptors: pharmacology, behavioral roles, and motor disorders. *Neuroscientist* 2:15–23.

Meltzer, H.Y. (1999) The role of serotonin in antipsychotic drug action. *Neuropsychopharmacology* 21:106S-115S.

Mesulam, M.M. (1996) The systems-level organization of cholinergic innervation in the human cerebral cortex and its alterations in Alzheimer's disease. *Prog Brain Res* 109:285–297.

Mesulam, M.M. (1998) From sensation to cognition. *Brain* 121: 1013–1052.

Missale, C., Nash, S.R., Robinson, S.W., Jaber, M., and Caron, M.G. (1998) Dopamine receptors: from structure to function. *Physiol Rev* 78:189–225.

Murphy, D.L., Andrews, A.M., Wichems, C.H., Li, Q., Tohda, M., and Greenberg, B. (1998) Brain serotonin neurotransmission: an overview and update with an emphasis on serotonin subsystem heterogeneity, multiple receptors, interactions with other neurotransmitter systems, and consequent implications for understanding the actions of serotonergic drugs. *J Clin Psychiatry* 59 Suppl 15:4–12.

Nakanishi, S. (1992) Molecular diversity of glutamate receptors and implications for brain function. *Science* 258:597–603.

Nakanishi, S., Nakajima, Y., Masu, M., Ueda, Y., Nakahara, K., Watanabe, D., Yamaguchi, S., Kawabata, S., and Okada, M. (1998) Glutamate receptors: brain function and signal transduction. *Brain Res Brain Res Rev* 26:230–235.

Nicola, S.M., Surmeier, J., and Malenka, R.C. (2000) Dopaminergic modulation of neuronal excitability in the striatum and nucleus accumbens. *Annu Rev Neurosci* 23:185–215.

Ozawa, S., Kamiya, H., and Tsuzuki, K. (1998) Glutamate receptors in the mammalian central nervous system. *Prog Neurobiol* 54: 581–618.

Snyder, S.H., and Ferris, C.D. (2000) Novel neurotransmitters and their neuropsychiatric relevance. *Am J Psychiatry* 157:1738–1751.

Somogyi, P., Tamas, G., Lujan, R., and Buhl, E.H. (1998) Salient features of synaptic organisation in the cerebral cortex. *Brain Res Brain Res Rev* 26:113–135.

Spanagel, R. and Weiss, F. (1999) The dopamine hypothesis of reward: past and current status. *Trends Neurosci* 22:521–527.

Vandenberg, R.J. (1998) Molecular pharmacology and physiology of glutamate transporters in the central nervous system. *Clin Exp Pharmacol Physiol* 25:393–400.

Wilson, M.A. and Tonegawa, S. (1997) Synaptic plasticity, place cells and spatial memory: study with second generation knockouts. *Trends Neurosci* 20:102–106.

Wonnacott, S. (1997) Presynaptic nicotinic ACh receptors. *Trends Neurosci* 20:92–98.

3 | Mechanisms of signal transduction and adaptation to psychotropic drug action

LARA M. TOLBERT, CARROL D'SA, AND RONALD S. DUMAN

The predominant mechanism by which neurons communicate with and are modulated by one another in the central nervous system (CNS) is through chemical transmission. During this process, molecules released from a presynaptic neuron travel a short distance across the synaptic cleft and interact with receptor proteins located on the plasma membrane of the postsynaptic neuron. The binding of these neurotransmitters, or chemical ligands, to receptors on the postsynaptic neuron initiates a chain of events by which the neuron produces a response to the stimulation. Typically, there are four mechanisms by which a ligand can trigger a response. Monoamine neurotransmitters, as well as amino acid and peptide neurotransmitters, bind to metabotropic receptors, or G protein–coupled receptors, so named because they produce their response via intermediary GTP-binding proteins. Some monoamine and amino acid neurotransmitters can also produce faster responses by directly binding to ion channels in the postsynaptic membrane, altering the membrane potential of the postsynaptic cell by allowing specific ions to flow down their electrochemical gradient. Neurotrophins, growth factors, and some hormones act on membrane-bound receptors which either have intrinsic enzymatic (e.g., kinase) activity or which bind to intracellular proteins with such activity. Finally, lipophilic hormones, such as steroids, can diffuse through the neuronal membrane and activate intracellular receptors that bind to specific sequences on DNA to initiate transcription. This chapter will focus on the first three of these signal transduction mechanisms, which have the most relevance to the actions of currently available psychotropic drugs.

Chemical transmission by neurotransmitters is tightly regulated by a number of distinct mechanisms. As described in the previous chapter, neurotransmitters released from the presynaptic neuron are subject to degradation by enzymes localized on the postsynaptic membrane. For example, acetylcholine released into the synaptic cleft is metabolized by acetylcholinesterases, and catecholamines such as norepinephrine and dopamine are degraded by both catechol-O-methyltransferase and monoamine oxidase. Neurotransmitters are also quickly cleared from the synaptic cleft both actively by reuptake pumps in the membrane of the presynaptic cell and surrounding glia and passively by diffusion. Enzymes involved in neurotransmitter degradation and transporters involved in reuptake are frequently targets of acute psychotropic drug action. Release of neurotransmitter into the synaptic cleft is controlled by feedback mechanisms involving neurotransmitter receptors on the presynaptic membrane. Activation of such autoreceptors serves to decrease the rate of neurotransmitter release, contributing to the regulation of neurotransmitter available to stimulate postsynaptic receptors. In addition to the mechanisms regulating the availability of neurotransmitters at postsynaptic targets, a number of additional mechanisms exist within the postsynaptic neuron to regulate the response of the neuron to a neurotransmitter. Such regulation may involve phosphorylation of the activated receptor, translocation of the receptor away from the membrane, or, over a longer time frame, decreased synthesis of the receptor. These processes will be discussed more thoroughly below.

The cellular consequences of neurotransmission can be both short term (acute) and long term (chronic). Acutely, stimulation of neurotransmitter receptors alters levels of intracellular signaling molecules, which may induce the neuron to fire or alter the responsiveness of the neuron to further stimulation. Over time, the persistent activation of receptors that occurs with chronic drug administration ultimately leads to long-term cellular adaptations that may either serve to counteract the effects of the drug, leading to tolerance, or underlie its therapeutic effects. Mechanisms for such adaptations are also discussed in detail below.

NEUROTRANSMITTER RECEPTORS

Classical neurotransmitters include the monoamines serotonin, epinephrine, norepinephrine, dopamine, acetylcholine, and histamine, and amino acids such as GABA, glutamate, aspartate, and glycine. These compounds exert their effects through one or both of two major classes of receptors: ionotropic receptors, which regulate the flow of ions into and out of the cell, and metabotropic receptors, which direct changes in the levels of intracellular signaling molecules, or second messengers. Signaling through ionotropic receptors is often referred to as *fast synaptic transmission,* because ligand binding results in immediate opening of a channel, allowing ions to flow within a few milliseconds of activation. Signaling through metabotropic receptors, which triggers a cascade of signaling events involving the sequential activation of several tiers of proteins, occurs on a time scale of hundreds of milliseconds to possibly several hours. The actions of psychotropic drugs are mediated predominantly by this second class of receptors.

Ionotropic Receptors

Ionotropic receptors, often referred to as *ligand-gated ion channels,* are large protein complexes composed of five subunits that combine to form a pore through the plasma membrane. In the absence of ligand, the channel remains in a closed position, impermeable to ions. Upon neurotransmitter binding, the channel undergoes a conformational change, opening the pore and allowing specific ions to flow down their electrochemical gradients. The membrane potential of a given cell can be affected by excitatory neurotransmitters, which mediate depolarization and increase the likelihood of firing, and inhibitory neurotransmitters, which induce hyperpolarization and decrease the possibility of firing. In the CNS, the primary excitatory neurotransmitter is glutamate, which can bind to three subtypes of ionotropic glutamate receptors, NMDA, AMPA, and kainate, resulting in an influx of Na^+ into the cell, and also of Ca^{2+} in the case of NMDA receptors and some AMPA receptor subtypes. The predominant inhibitory neurotransmitter in the brain is GABA, which acts on $GABA_A$ receptors to allow Cl^- ions to flow into the

cell. In the brain stem and spinal cord, glycine is the major inhibitory neurotransmitter, also acting on a Cl^- channel. Many psychotropic drugs mediate their effect by binding directly to ion channels. Nicotine, for example, is an agonist at nicotinic acetylcholine receptors, which are permeable to cations, such as Na^+ and Ca^{2+}. Several hallucinogenic drugs, such as phencyclidine, bind to the open conformation of NMDA glutamate receptors, effectively blocking ion flow. Drugs that induce seizures, such as bicuculline and picrotoxin, reduce the activity of $GABA_A$ receptors—bicuculline by blocking ion flow through the channel, and picrotoxin by interfering with GABA binding to the receptor. Conversely, benzodiazepines and barbiturates, while having no activity by themselves, enhance the activation of $GABA_A$ receptors in the presence of GABA (see Deutch and Roth, 1999, and Swank et al., 2000, for further reading).

G Protein–coupled (Metabotropic) Receptors

Most monoamine and peptide neurotransmitters act by binding to G protein–coupled receptors. These receptors are composed of a single polypeptide chain that winds itself through the membrane a total of seven times. The seven transmembrane segments align themselves in the cell membrane in a circular fashion such that a ligand-binding site is formed within the membrane bilayer. Signaling through G protein–coupled receptors takes place in several steps. First, ligand binding induces a conformational change in the receptor that allows for activation of its cognate G protein(s). The activated G protein then goes on to influence the activity of either an effector enzyme, such as adenylyl cyclase or phospholipase C, or of an ion channel. Alterations in the activity level of effector enzymes and ion channels, in turn, result in changes in the concentration of intracellular second messengers, which can lead to both immediate and long-lasting changes within the cell.

The G protein cycle

The G proteins with which G protein–coupled receptors interact are heterotrimeric complexes composed of α, β, and γ subunits. In its inactive state, the G-protein α subunit is bound to GDP and associates with a βγ dimer. Upon receptor activation, the α subunit "opens" its guanine nucleotide binding site and releases its bound GDP, allowing GTP, which is present in higher concentrations in the cell, to bind in its place. The GTP-bound α subunit has a lower affinity for the βγ dimer and dissociates from it, freeing both the α subunit and the βγ dimer to activate downstream targets (See Fig. 3.1). The catalytic activity of the α subunit is limited in duration by its intrinsic GTPase activity, which hydrolyzes GTP into GDP, thus returning it to its inactive conformation. The GDP-bound α subunit then reassociates with the βγ dimer, completing the cycle (see Bourne, 1997, and references therein).

RGS proteins

Recently, it was discovered that G-protein activity is controlled by another class of proteins. These proteins, termed *RGS proteins* (for *r*egulators of *G*-protein *s*ignaling), enhance the rate of GTP hydrolysis. This activity reduces the amount of time the G-protein α subunit spends in its active GTP-bound conformation, in effect limiting the response to receptor activation.

RGS proteins in the brain have a discrete pattern of expression, with RGS4 being the isoform most highly expressed and most widely distributed throughout the brain, including the cerebral cortex, striatum, thalamus, and several brain stem nuclei. In contrast, the distribution of another isoform, RGS9, is primarily restricted to striatal regions. The localization of RGS9 in the striatum, which parallels the distribution of several dopamine receptor subtypes, suggested that this isoform might have a role in regulating G-protein signaling in striatal neurons, particularly via dopamine receptors (Gold et al., 1997; Rahman et al., 1999). In fact, recent studies have demonstrated that over-expression of RGS9-2 in rat striatum decreases behavioral responses to D_2-selective, but not D_1-selective, agonists (Rahman et al., 2000). Interestingly, RGS proteins have been found to act primarily on G_i/G_o, and less frequently on G_q. No RGS proteins have been found for G_s (see Berman and Gilman, 1998, for review).

Second messenger pathways

The nature of the second messenger response to a given neurotransmitter depends on the subtype of receptor to which it binds and the G protein to which the receptor is coupled. Three of the most commonly utilized G proteins include G_s, which stimulates adenylyl cyclase to produce cyclic AMP (cAMP); G_i, which inhibits adenylyl cyclase, resulting in lower intracellullar levels of cAMP; and G_q, which activates phospholipase C to produce the second messengers IP_3 and DAG. In general, these activities refer to the function of the α subunit; however, it should be pointed out that the βγ complex has its own set of activities (on adenylyl cyclase, phospholipase C, K^+ channels, mitogen-activated protein kinase [MAPK]) that are just now becoming better clarified.

Cyclic AMP pathway. The intracellular concentration of the second messenger cAMP can be positively or negatively regulated by receptors that couple to G_s and those that couple to G_i, respectively. These G proteins act on the effector enzyme adenylyl cyclase, which catalyzes the production of cAMP from ATP (Fig. 3.2). The effects of cAMP in the cell are mediated primarily by cAMP-dependent protein kinase (PKA; Schulman and Hyman, 1999). PKA has a wide variety of intracellular substrates whose activation can result in both rapid cellular changes (e.g., both ionotropic and metabotropic receptors) and long-term adaptations (transcription factors). Structural proteins and enzymes that synthesize and degrade neurotransmitters are also targets for phosphorylation by PKA. One particularly well-characterized target for PKA is the transcription factor CREB, or *c*AMP *r*esponse *e*lement–*b*inding protein. CREB binds as a dimer to genes containing an eight-nucleotide sequence (TGACGTCA) known as a *CRE site*, and may mediate low levels of transcription of these genes in the absence of stimulation. Upon phosphorylation by PKA or one of several other kinases at the residue Ser-133, CREB binds to CREB-binding protein (CBP), which in turn activates transcription (Montminy et al., 1990; Meyer and Habener, 1993; Hyman and Nestler, 1999).

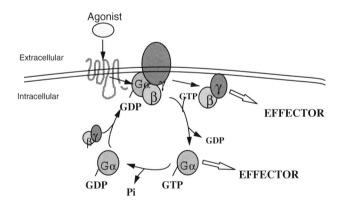

FIGURE 3.1 G-protein activation cycle. Agonist interaction with a G protein–coupled receptor promotes the dissocation of GDP from the α subunit, allowing GTP into the nucleotide binding site. The GTP-activated α subunit dissociates from the βγ complex, and both entities are then able to regulate the activity of effector elements, such as adenylyl cyclase, phospholipase C-β, or ion channels. The intrinsic GTPase activity of the α subunit quickly hydrolyzes the GTP (within milliseconds), serving to turn off G-protein activity by placing the G protein in its GDP-bound, inactive form, which can reassociate with the βγ complex.

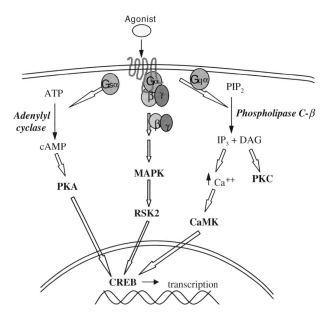

FIGURE 3.2 G_s- and G_q-coupled second messenger pathways. Activation of G_s-linked receptors results in stimulation of adenylyl cyclase activity, leading to an increase in intracellular cyclic AMP (cAMP, a second messenger that leads to activation of protein kinase A (PKA). One target of PKA is the transcription factor cAMP response element binding protein (CREB), resulting in increased expression of genes containing a CRE site. Agonist stimulation of G_q-linked receptors causes activation of phospholipase C-β, which cleaves phosphatidylinositol-4,5-bisphosphate (PIP$_2$), a phospholipid component of the membrane, into the second messengers diacylglycerol (DAG) and inositol-1,4,5-trisphophate (IP$_3$). DAG activates a Ca^{2+}-sensitive kinase, PKC, and IP$_3$ triggers release of Ca^{2+} from intracellular stores. CaMK is activated by increased intracellular Ca^{2+} concentrations, and CREB is also a substrate for phosphorylation by CaMKII and IV. The βγ complex released by receptor activation has its own set of activities, one of which includes the activation of mitogen-activated protein kinase (MAPK), which can mediate CREB phosphorylation via the Rsk family of protein kinases.

Recent studies looking at cellular changes resulting from long-term antidepressant treatment suggest that the activity of several components of the cAMP pathway, including adenylyl cyclase, PKA, and CREB, are up-regulated following chronic antidepressant administration (Duman, 1998). The up-regulation of CREB by antidepressants is of particular interest as the transcription factor may mediate changes in gene transcription that underlie the long-term therapeutic action of these drugs. Interestingly, antidepressants result in increased CREB expression and function exclusively in the hippocampus, cerebral cortex, and amygdala (Nibuya et al., 1996; Thome at al., 2000), while cocaine and morphine affect CREB levels in the nucleus accumbens and locus coeruleus with no detectable effect in the hippocampus (Guitart et al., 1992; Widnell et al., 1994).

Phosphodiesterases

Levels of cAMP are controlled by a group of enzymes called *phosphodiesterases* (PDEs). The PDEs oppose the action of adenylyl cyclases by hydrolyzing cAMP into AMP. These enzymes could be potential targets for therapeutic agents. Theophylline, for example, is a PDE inhibitor used in the treatment of asthma. Inhibitors of PDEs also show promise as antidepressants. Inhibitors of the PDE4 isoform, such as rolipram, have been shown to have antidepressant activity in behavioral models of depression (Wachtel and Schneider, 1986; Griebel O'Donnell, 1993; O'Donnell, and Frith 1999). Furthermore, clinical studies indicate that rolipram has antidepressant efficacy in patients suffering from depression (Bertolino et al., 1988; Bobon, et al., 1988; Eckmann et al., 1988; Hebenstreit et al., 1989; Scott et al., 1991; Fleishchhacker et al., 1992).

Phosphoinositol pathway. Receptors that couple to the G protein G_q result in stimulation of the enzyme phospholipase C-β. This enzyme cleaves phosphotidylinositol-4,5-bisphosphate, a component of the membrane bilayer, into the second messengers diacylglycerol (DAG) and inositol-1,4,5-triphosphate (IP$_3$) (Fig. 3.2). Thus, two major signaling molecules are produced, each with their own unique functions. IP$_3$ is released into the cytosol, and can subsequently bind to IP$_3$ receptors on smooth endoplasmic reticulum (ER) and other organelles, resulting in the release of Ca^{2+} from intracellular stores. DAG, which remains linked to the plasma membrane, together with the released Ca^{2+}, activates protein kinase C (PKC). PKC, like PKA, can activate gene transcription, resulting in long-term cellular changes. One substrate for phosphorylation by PKC is the serum response factor, resulting in the induction of the intermediate early gene, c-*fos*. Fos binds to a member of the Jun family of transcription factors to form the AP-1 DNA binding complex, which activates transcription of genes containing a TRE (tetradecanoyl-phorbol acetate [TPA] response element), or more commonly, AP1, site (see Hyman and Nestler, 1999).

Calcium

In addition to participating in the activation of PKC, calcium released from intracellular organelles has several other effects on cellular processes. Most of these actions are mediated through the protein calmodulin (CaM). Calmodulin has no activity in and of itself, but in the Ca^{2+}-bound state, serves to modulate the activity of several other proteins, including some forms of adenylyl cyclase and phosphodiesterase, calcineurin (a protein phosphatase), and protein kinases known as Ca^{2+}/calmodulin-dependent protein kinases (CaMK). CaMKII is the best-characterized member of the CaMK family, and has been found to be particularly enriched in neurons. Both CaMKII and CaMKIV have been found to phosphorylate CREB at its Ser-133 site, demonstrating a point of convergence between the two major second messenger pathways (Deisseroth et al., 1998).

Ion channels. G proteins are also involved in the coupling of some receptors to ion channels. A classic example is the modulation of inwardly rectifying potassium channels by m2 acetylcholine receptors. Other receptors have been shown to modulate Ca^{2+} and/or K^+ channels by either G protein α or $\beta\gamma$ subunits.

Regulation of signaling

Aside from the regulation of G-protein activity by RGS proteins, signaling through G protein-coupled receptors can also be regulated at the level of the receptor itself (see Deutch and Roth, 1999). Such regulation occurs through several well-characterized mechanisms (Fig. 3.3). Within seconds to minutes of agonist acti-

vation, receptors generally undergo phosphorylation at sites within their third intracellular loop and C tail by at least two families of protein kinases. The second messenger kinases, PKA and PKC, in addition to phosphorylating activated receptors, can also participate in what is termed *heterologous desensitization* of a receptor. These kinases are activated by changes in levels of second messengers rather than by the receptor itself, and thus can phosphorylate unstimulated receptors as well as agonist-occupied receptors. Phosphorylation by these kinases leads to a conformational change in the receptor, such that the receptor is no longer able to interact with G proteins. Another family of protein kinases, the G protein–coupled receptor kinases (GRKs), of which there are six known members (GRK1–6), are involved exclusively in "homologous desensitization" of receptors because they phosphorylate only agonist-stimulated forms of a receptor. Desensitization by GRKs similarly impedes interaction of the receptor with its cognate G protein; however, GRK-mediated phosphorylation itself is not sufficient. Rather, the GRK-phosphorylated carboxy tail of a receptor serves as a docking site for a member of the arrestin family, the binding of which serves to uncouple the receptor from the G protein with which it interacts.

On a slightly longer time scale (several minutes), a second mechanism for receptor regulation becomes evident. Following agonist activation, many receptors undergo redistribution from the plasma membrane into intracellular compartments, or endosomes, in a process referred to as *receptor-mediated endocytosis,* or alternatively, *internalization.* Receptor internalization may be followed by transport of the receptor into lysosomes, where the receptor is degraded, or by recycling of the receptor back to the plasma membrane. Until recently, it was assumed that internalization was another means for desensitizing the receptor to further stimulation. While this appears to be true for some receptors, either by serving to down-regulate the receptors in lysosomes or by simply removing the receptor away from the agonist, it has become clear that for other receptors, internalization serves other functions. The role of internalization has been best characterized for the β_2-adrenergic receptor (reviewed in Lefkowitz, 1998). For this receptor, it was discovered that internalization led to dephosphorylation, and thus reactivation, of the receptor. It was demonstrated that blockade of internalization interfered with resensitization of the receptor, leading to a prolonged desensitization. More recently, it has been found that internalization of the β_2 receptor is not only a means of resensitization but also serves as a means of "switching" coupling of the receptor from G_s to G_i (Daaka et al., 1997). Such a change in G-protein signaling has at least two effects.

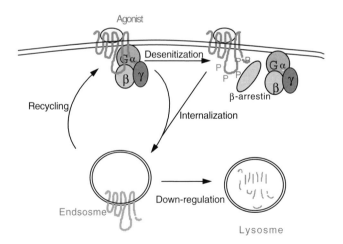

FIGURE 3.3 Mechanisms of G protein–coupled receptor regulation. The agonist-induced activity of G protein–coupled receptors can be regulated by a number of processes, several of which have a direct effect on the receptor itself. These include (*1*) an uncoupling of the receptor from its cognate G protein by receptor phosphorylation in a process termed *desensitization;* (*2*) internalization of the receptor into an intracellular compartment inaccessible to hydrophilic ligands, which may be followed by recycling of the receptor back to the plasma membrane; and (*3*) transport of the receptor protein into lysosomes, where the receptor is degraded. (P represents site of phosphorylation.)

First, it provides another mechanism of desensitization, in that receptors at the cell surface produce an increase in cAMP via G_s, whereas internalized receptors produce a decrease in cAMP levels via G_i. Second, it has been found that $\beta\gamma$ subunits released from activated G_i are capable of stimulating the MAPK cascade. Thus, at least for the β_2 receptor, internalization functions not only to temporarily desensitize the receptor to activation of the cAMP pathway but also to initiate signaling to MAPK. Recently, a number of other G protein–coupled receptors have been found to signal to the MAPK pathway via G_i as well as G_q and G_s, and many of these receptors seem to require internalization for such signaling to take place.

In addition to the above regulatory mechanisms, which take place fairly quickly, continued agonist stimulation of a receptor can ultimately lead to a decrease in total receptor number. Such receptor downregulation can be precipitated by degradation of the receptor in lysosomes, as mentioned above, or, over a longer time frame, by reduced receptor synthesis resulting from decreased gene expression, or by destabilization of the corresponding mRNA transcript.

NEUROTROPHIN RECEPTORS

The *neurotrophins* are a family of peptide factors that contribute to neuronal differentiation, neurite outgrowth, and survival (reviewed in Segal and Greenberg, 1996; Kaplan and Milller, 1997; Friedman and Greene, 1999). This family includes nerve growth factor (NGF), brain-derived neurotrophic factor (BDNF), neurotrophin (NT)-3, and NT-4/5. Signaling via neurotrophins differs somewhat from signaling through conventional neurotransmitters. First, neurotrophins bind to their receptors as dimers—i.e., two neurotrophin molecules associate prior to binding receptors on the cell surface. Second, neurotrophins, while they can be released in a regulated fashion upon depolarization as traditional neurotransmitters are, are often released constitutively, or continuously, by some neurons. A third difference is that neurotrophins can act bidirectionally. Often, a neurotrophic factor is "target-derived," meaning that it is released by the target cell of an innervating neuron. In such a way, a cell can control the number of neurons that connect with it. Neurotrophins can also act anterogradely, i.e., from a neuron to its target cell.

The receptors through which neurotrophins act belong to a third class of membrane-bound receptors, which possess intracellular kinase activity. These receptors, called *receptor tyrosine kinases,* are composed of a single polypeptide chain having an extracellular ligand-binding domain, a single transmembrane domain, and an intracellular kinase domain. The subfamily of receptors to which neurotrophins bind are the Trk receptors, with TrkA being the receptor for NGF, TrkB for BDNF and NT-4/5, and TrkC for NT-3. Signaling by the Trk receptors tends to conform to the general model for signaling by the receptor tyrosine kinase family as a whole. Ligand binding induces receptor dimerization, which leads to intramolecular phosphorylation of tyrosine residues within the kinase domain, and subsequently, cross-phosphorylation of tyrosines outside the kinase domain. Phosphorylated tyrosines serve as docking sites for SH2 domain–containing adaptor proteins and enzymes that initiate a chain of phosphorylation events, ultimately leading to cellular adaptations, often involving alterations in gene expression.

At least three signaling pathways have been described for the Trk receptors (Fig. 3.4). The best characterized of these is the activation of the Ras/MAPK cascade initiated by binding of an adaptor protein, such as Shc, to the activated Trk receptor. Binding of Shc via its SH2 domain to phosphotyrosines on the Trk receptor leads to Shc phosphorylation, which in turn leads to its binding to another SH2-containing adaptor protein, Grb2. Grb2 associates with the guanine nucleotide exchange factor, SOS, via its SH3 domains. SOS, in turn, activates the small G protein, Ras, by catalyzing the exchange of GDP for GTP. GTP-bound Ras goes on to activate a member of the Raf family of serine/threonine kinases, bringing it to the cell membrane, where it phosphorylates, and thus activates, the dual-specificity kinase, MEK. Phosphorylation of MAPK, also called *ERK,* by MEK at both a threonine and a tyrosine residue leads to MAPK activation and its subsequent translocation into the nucleus. MAPK phosphorylates transcription factors, such as Elk, as well as members of another family of kinases, the ribosomal S6 kinases (rsks), whose substrates include another subset of transcription factors, including CREB. Changes in gene expression resulting from activation of transcription factors ultimately contribute to the neuronal differentiation mediated by neurotrophins. This pathway also appears to play a large role in mediating neurite outgrowth.

A second pathway initiated by Trk receptors occurs through the direct binding of the enzyme PLC-γ to an alternative phosphotyrosine residue on the Trk receptor. PLC-γ, like PLC-β activated by G_q, catalyzes the formation of DAG and IP_3 from PIP_2. This pathway also seems to culminate in the activation of MAPK,

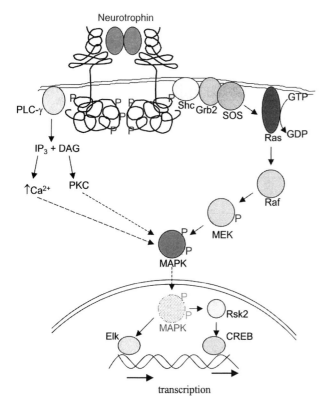

FIGURE 3.4 Signaling cascades activated by neurotrophins. Neutrotropins act on receptor tyrosine kinases, which transduce their signal by sequential activation of protein tyrosine kinases. The major pathway following neurotrophin activation is Ras-dependent activation of MAPK, which involves the recruitment of the adaptor protein Shc, followed by binding of Grb2, which associates with the GTP exchange factor SOS. SOS, in turn, activates Ras, which, in its GTP-bound form, can activate the MAPKKK (or MEKK) Raf. Raf then phosphorylates MEK, whose primary substrate is MAPK. Dually phosphorylated MAPK translocates into the nucleus, where it affects gene transcription by phosphorylating transcription factors directly or indirectly via Rsk kinases. A presumably redundant pathway for MAPK activation occurs via PLC-γ, a pathway that may also be dependent on Ras. Not shown here is the activation of PI3-K, which involves the kinase Akt and may be important for mediating neuronal survival. (P represents site of phosphorylation.)

and may serve as an alternative mechanism for mediating the effects of this kinase.

Activation of the enzyme PI3 kinase (PI3K) constitutes a third pathway of Trk receptor signaling. The precise mechanism by which PI3K activation occurs has not yet been completely elucidated, but appears to involve Trk activation of intermediate proteins, such as insulin receptor substrate (IRS)-1,2 and the IRS-like protein Gab1. Downstream of PI3K activation is stimulation of the kinase Akt, which is largely responsible for the survival effects mediated by this pathway.

MOLECULAR MECHANISMS OF NEURONAL ADAPTATION

Often, the long-term physiological consequences that occur with chronic drug exposure cannot be fully accounted for by a drug's immediate, or acute, pharmacological activity. Rather, such long-lasting effects are mediated by molecular adaptations that occur within cells exposed to the drug over a long period of time (see Nestler and Hyman, 1999). These molecular changes can serve one of two functions: to counteract the acute effects of a drug, or to potentiate the response to the drug. As an example of the former, opiates, which are agonists at δ-, κ-, and/or μ-opioid receptors, act acutely via G_i to reduce intracellular levels of cAMP. Over time, however, the continued presence of these drugs produces an up-regulation of certain components of the cAMP pathway, PKA and AC, which compensate for their inhibitory effect on the cAMP system and restore cAMP to its normal level. This compensatory up-regulation, which occurs in brain regions such as the nucleus accumbens and locus coeruleus involved in drug reinforcement and dependence, respectively, is proposed to be responsible for mediating some of the behavioral aspects of drug addiction (see Nestler, 1999). Simply stated, such up-regulation provides an explanation of how drug tolerance might develop, in that it requires progressively higher doses to overcome the effect of an increasingly active cAMP system. Furthermore, up-regulation of the cAMP system in the locus coeruleus following chronic drug use could account for the withdrawal symptoms following termination of the drug, as removal of inhibition of cAMP would tilt the balance in favor of the acquired overactive cAMP pathway.

Antidepressant drugs, by contrast, require long-term administration for their therapeutic effects to become evident. Thus, it is clear that the acute actions of these drugs, which are most often to enhance synaptic levels of monoamines, are not sufficient in themselves to mediate their therapeutic effects. Neither is the effect of increased monoamines on postsynaptic second messenger systems, which occurs relatively quickly as well, adequate to account for the therapeutic actions of antidepressants. The most obvious explanation, then, is that molecular adaptations in response to chronic exposure to these drugs are what underlie their therapeutic effects. Consistent with this idea, several hypotheses as to the nature of the relevant molecular adaptations have been proposed. Two models focus on adaptations of the 5-HT$_{1A}$ receptor. One theory proposes that desensitization of presynaptic somatodendritic 5-HT$_{1A}$ autoreceptors is responsible for the therapeutic action of antidepressants (Blier and Montigny, 1994; Béïque et al., 2000). Desensitization of these receptors, which control the firing rate of serotonergic neurons, would result in a disinhibition of these neurons, yielding an increase in the release of serotonin into the synaptic cleft. This model would account for the observation that the rate of therapeutic action of selective serotonin reuptake inhibitors (SSRIs) is enhanced when 5-HT_{1A} antagonists are added to the regimen. A related model suggests that the progressive sensitization of postsynaptic 5-HT_{1A} receptors that has been shown to occur with chronic antidepressant treatment is responsible for the therapeutic action (Haddjeri et al., 1998). Yet another potential explanation is that the up-regulation of components of the cAMP system, including PKA and CREB, in limbic brain regions following chronic administration of an antidepressant is what mediates the antidepressant effect (Duman et al., 1997; Duman, 1998). This theory would account for the actions of not only those agents that enhance synaptic levels of serotonin but also those that increase norepinephrine, since up-regulation of the cAMP cascade occurs in response to administration of both norepinephrine- and serotonin-selective reuptake inhibitors.

Regulation of Protein Phosphorylation

The capacity of a cell to respond and adapt to extracellular signals is critically dependent on its ability to regulate the activity of its protein constituents. One of the primary mechanisms by which the activity of proteins in a cell is regulated is by phosphorylation (see Nestler and Hyman, 1999). The addition or removal of a phosphate group to or from the hydroxyl moieties on Ser, Thr, or Tyr residues serves to modulate protein function, and for some proteins, can function as an on/off switch for their activity. The spectrum of proteins influenced by phosphorylation includes both ligand- and voltage-gated ion channels; receptors for neurotransmitters, growth factors, and hormones; neurotransmitter-synthesizing enzymes; and transcription factors; as well as the kinases which catalyze phosphorylation themselves. The effect of phosphorylation on the activity of a particular protein depends on the nature of the protein and the site of the phosphorylated residue. Phosphorylation can modulate protein function in both a positive and negative direction. For example, as mentioned earlier, phosphorylation of G protein–coupled receptors by second messenger–dependent kinases such as PKA serves as a means for desensitizing the receptor toward further agonist stimulation. In contrast, phosphorylation of NMDA and AMPA ionotropic glutamate receptors enhances channel opening. The effect of phosphorylation on the activity of the transcription factor CREB depends on the site at which phosphorylation occurs. Kinases that mediate phosphorylation at Ser-133 increase CREB's transcriptional activity through increased binding to CBP, but phosphorylation at Ser-142 inhibits the transcription factor. Phosphorylation can not only serve to influence protein activity but also enhance or reduce protein–protein interactions. Phosphorylation of a number of G protein–coupled receptors by βARK increases their affinity for the adaptor protein β-arrestin, which has two functions: to block receptor–G protein interaction and to target the receptors to clathrin-coated vesicles for internalization (see Lefkowitz, 1998). Similarly, tyrosine phosphorylation of receptor tyrosine kinases is involved in binding of adaptor proteins, such as Shc, via their SH2 domains, linking the receptors to enzymes further downstream in the signaling cascade.

Regulation of Gene Expression

In addition to changes in protein activity, long-term cellular adaptations can be mediated by changes in the levels of protein expressed in a cell (see Nestler and Hyman, 1999; Schulman and Hyman, 1999). As is evident from the signal transduction pathways described previously, the final targets of most signaling cascades initiated by neurotransmitters, neurotrophins, and other signaling molecules are transcription factors. The activation, or in some cases, inhibition, of transcription factors results in increased or decreased, respectively, expression of genes containing response elements for those transcription factors. Often, the expression of transcription factors themselves is regulated by receptor activity. For example, immediate early genes, such as c-*fos*, a component of the AP-1 transcription factor complex, are not expressed constitutively, but are induced upon neuronal depolarization or activation of signaling cascades. CREB, by contrast, is expressed constitutively, but its transcription rate may be increased or decreased following receptor activation. As mentioned earlier, CREB levels have been shown to be up-regulated in the hippocampus following chronic antidepressant treatment. Such increased expression of this transcription factor implies that increased expression of genes containing a CRE site may mediate the therapeutic effects of long-term antidepressant administration. In fact, two such genes have been identified. It has been shown that similar paradigms of antidepressant administration result in increased expression of the neurotrophin BDNF and its receptor TrkB in the same regions of the hippocampus where induction of

CREB expression occurs (Nibuya et al., 1995, 1996). Brain-derived neurotrophic factor is an attractive candidate for mediating antidepressant action. In addition to its known effects on neuronal survival and differentiation, it also has been shown to play a role in synaptic plasticity. Furthermore, administration of BDNF directly into rat hippocampus has been demonstrated to have antidepressant-like action in several models of depression (Siuciak et al., 1996).

CELLULAR MECHANISMS OF NEURONAL ADAPTATION

The intracellular signaling pathways outlined above modulate neuronal function and underlie the ability of the brain to adapt to pharmacological and environmental stimuli. Besides the adaptations that occur at the biochemical and molecular level, chronic exposure to psychotropic drugs produces structural changes in neurons. These changes, which serve as a form of drug-induced neural plasticity, include alterations in dendritic spine morphology, cytoskeletal proteins, and neuronal number and provide an explanation as to how psychotropic drug exposure produces persistent changes in behavior. Studies to date have focused on these structural changes in anatomically well-defined brain regions that mediate the actions of the drug. Drugs of abuse such as cocaine, morphine, and amphetamine induce cellular changes in the mesolimbic dopamine system, the region associated with craving and drug reinforcement. Morphological adaptations in response to stress, antidepressants, and mood stabilizers by contrast, have mainly been characterized in the hippocampus and prefrontal cortex, which suggests that dysfunction of adaptive plasticity in these regions could be involved in the pathophysiology and treatment of affective disorders. We discuss below the regulation of dendritic spine morphology and neurogenesis by psychotropic drugs.

Regulation of Dendritic Spines and Cellular Morphology

The *dendrite* is a dynamic component of the neuron that receives afferent inputs and responds to its surrounding environment by modifying its apical and basilar spines. These changes in spine density and dendritic spine length can cause alterations in synaptic transmission, and study of these adaptations is a major area of research in understanding the structural basis of drug-induced neural plasticity. Using the Golgi staining method, Robinson and Kolb (1999a,b) have shown

that the psychostimulants cocaine and amphetamine increase dendritic number and apical spine density of neurons in the nucleus accumbens shell and layer V pyrimidal cells of the prefrontal cortex. Cocaine also increases dendritic branching and spine density of basilar dendrites of layer V pyrimidal neurons. The opiate morphine decreases apical dendritic spine density and number in of these processes. These changes might be explained by the alterations in levels of neurofilaments and other cytoskeletal proteins in cell bodies of these neurons in the ventral tegmental area by chronic exposure to drugs of abuse (Beitner-Johnson et al., 1992). As mentioned previously, chronic psychotropic drug exposure alters the levels of trophic factors such as glial-derived neurotrophic factor (GDNF) and BDNF. Changes in levels of these neurotrophins could dramatically affect the synaptic architecture, dendritic morphology, and growth and survival of neurons (Duman et al., 2000; Messer et al., 2000).

A role for plasticity in the actions of antidepressant drugs has been demonstrated in the hippocampus. This region, containing the CA1 and CA3 pyramidal neurons and dentate gyrus granule cells as its primary cell groups, is a remarkable plastic structure. Stress and glucocorticoids decrease the number and length of apical dendrites of CA3 neurons, resulting in atrophy and, in severe cases, death of hippocampal neurons (Sapolsky, 1996; McEwen, 1999). Postmortem studies have indicated that there is also a decease in neuronal size and glial number in the prefrontal cortex and orbitofrontal cortex of depressed patients. In contrast, administration of tianeptine, an atypical antidepressant, blocks the stress-induced atrophy of CA3 pyramidal neurons (Watanabe et al., 1992). Also, repeated electroconvulsive shock theraphy (ECT) induces sprouting of granule cells, with no evidence of cell loss. This effect is long-lasting and attenuated in BDNF heterozygous knockout mice, indicating the importance of this neurotrophin in cell survival and plasticity (Vaidya et al., 1999; 2000). These findings have contributed to the hypothesis that the therapeutic action of antidepressants may involve a reversal of stress-induced cellular atrophy, primarily by increasing the levels of the neurotrophic factor BDNF (Duman, 2000).

Regulation of Neurogenesis

Another level of cellular adaptation to psychotropic drug exposure involves the change in neuronal number through neurogenesis. Recent research has demonstrated that in the adult hippocampus, new cells constantly arise from immature neural precursor cells in the subgranular zone of the dendate gyrus, migrate into the granule cell layer, extend processes to the CA3 pyramidal layer, and make synaptic connections as mature neurons (Gould and Tanapat, 1999). This neurogenic process is dynamically regulated by several environmental and pharmacological factors and could underlie the adaptive function of the brain. Interestingly, changes in hippocampal neurogenesis are observed only after chronic and not acute exposure to psychotropic drugs, consistent with their clinically relevant actions. For example, long-term exposure to the opiates morphine and heroin decreases the proliferation and survival of new hippocampal neurons (Eisch et al., 2000). Also, stress and stress hormones down-regulate neurogenesis and may contribute to the reduction in hippocampal volume seen in patients with post-traumatic stress disorder (PTSD) and depression (Gould and Tanapat). Chronic, but not acute, treatment with different classes of antidepressants, lithium, and electroconvulsive therapy increase cell proliferation and neuronal number. This may be the mechanism, at least in part, through which these drugs exert their therapeutic effects and reverse the stress-induced atrophy of hippocampal neurons (Chen et al., 2000; Malberg et al., 2000). Future research in this field will identify the mechanisms underlying the regulation of neurogenesis and determine if the new neurons formed make a major contribution to brain function in the adult.

REFERENCES

Béïque, J.-C., Blier, P., de Montigny, C., and Debonnel, G. (2000) Potentiation by (-)pindolol of the activation of postsynaptic 5-HT$_{1A}$ receptors induced by venlafaxine. *Neuropsychopharmacology.* 23(3):294–306.

Beitner-Johnson D., Guitart X., and Nestler E.J. (1992) Neurofilament proteins and the mesolimbic dopamine system: common regulation by chronic morphine and chronic cocaine in the rat ventral tegmental area. *J Neurosci* 12(6):2165–2176.

Berman, D.M. and Gilman, A.G. (1998) Mammalian RGS proteins: barbarians at the gate. *J Biol Chem* 273(3):1269.

Bertolino, A., Crippa, D., di Dio, S., Fichte, K., Musmeci, G., Porro, V., Rapisarda, V., Sastre-y-Hernandez, M., and Schratzer, M. (1988) Rolipram versus imipramine in patients with major, "minor," or atypical depressive disorder: a double-blind study, double-dummy study aimed at testing a novel therapeutic approach. *Int Clin Psychopharmacol* 3:245–253.

Blier, P. and de Montigny, C. (1994) Current advances and trends in the treatment of depression. *Trends Pharmacol Sci* 15:220–226.

Bobon, D., Breulet, M., Gerard-Vandenhove, M.A., Guiot-Goffioul, F., Pomteux, G., Sastre-y-Hernandez, M., Schratzer, M., Troisfontaines, B., von Frenckell, R., and Wachtel, H. (1988) Is phosphodiesterase inhibition a new mechanism of antidepressant action? A double blind double-dummy study between rolipram and desipramine in hospitalized major and/or endogenous depressives. *Eur Arch Psychiatry Neurol Sci* 238(1):2–6, 1988.

Bourne, H.R. (1997) How receptors talk to trimeric G proteins. *Curr Opin Cell Biol* 9(2):134.

Chao, M., Casaccia-Bonnefil, P., Carter, B., Chittka, A., Kong, H., and Yoon, S.O. (1998) Neurotrophin receptors: mediators of life and death. *Brain Res Rev* 26:295–301.

Chen G., Rajkowska G., Du F., Seraji-Bozorgzad N., and Manji H.K. (2000) Enhancement of hippocampal neurogenesis by lithium. *J Neurochem* 75(4):1729–1734.

Daaka, Y., Luttrell, L.M., and Lefkowitz, R.J. (1997) Switching of the coupling of the β$_2$-adrenergic receptor to different G proteins by protein kinase A. *Nature* 390:88–91.

Deisseroth, K., Heist, E.K., and Tsien, R.W. (1998). Translocation of calmodulin to the nucleus supports CREB phosphorylation in hippocampal neurons. *Nature* 392(6672):198–202.

Deutch, A.Y. and Roth, R.H. (1999) Neurotransmitters. In: Zigmond, M.J., Bloom, F.E., Landis, S.C., Roberts, J.L., and Squire, L.R., eds. *Fundamental Neuroscience.* San Diego: Academic Press, pp. 193–234.

Duman, R.S. (1998) Novel therapeutic approaches beyond the serotonin receptor. *Biol Psychiatry* 44:324–335.

Duman, R.S. (1999) The neurochemistry of mood disorders: preclinical studies. In: Charney, D.S., Nestler, E.J., and Bunney, B.S., eds. *Neurobiology of Mental Illness*, New York; Oxford University Press, (pp. 333–347).

Duman, R.S., Heninger, G.R., and Nestler, E.J. (1997) A molecular and cellular theory of depression. *Arch Gen Psychiatry* 54:597–606.

Duman, R.S., Malberg, J., Nakagawa, S., and D'Sa, C. (2000) Neuronal plasticity and survival in mood disorders. *Biol Psychiatry* 48:732–739.

Eckmann, F., Fichte, K., Meya, U., and Sastre-y-Hernandez, M. (1988) Rolipram in major depression: results of a double-blind comparative study with amitriptyline. *Curr Ther Res* 43:291–295.

Eisch, A.J., Barrot, M., Schad, C.A., Self, D.W., and Nestler, E.J. (2000) Opiates inhibit neurogenesis in the adult rat hippocampus. *Proc Natl Acad Sci* USA 97(13):7579–7584

Fleischhacker, W.W., Hinterhuber, H., Bauer, H., Pflug, B., Berner, P., Simhandl, C., Wolf, R., Gerlach, W., Jaklitsch, H., Sastre-y-Hernandez, M., Schmeding-Wiegel, H., Sperner-Unterweger, B., Voet, B., and Schubert, H. (1992) A multicenter double-blind study of three different doses of the new cAMP-phosphodiesterase inhibitor rolipram in patients with major depressive disorder. *Neuropsychobiology* 26:59–64.

Friedman, W.J. and Greene, L.A. (1999) Neurotrophin signaling via Trks and p 75. *Exp Cell Res* 253:131–42.

Gold, S.J., Ni, Y.G., Dohlman, H.G., and Nestler, E.J. (1997) Regulators of G-protein signaling (RGS) proteins: region-specific expression of nine subtypes in rat brain. *J Neurosci* 17(20):8024–8037.

Gould E. and Tanapat P. (1999) Stress and hippocampal neurogenesis. *Biol Psychiatry* 2000; 46(11):1472–1479.

Griebel, G., Misslin, R., Vogel, E., and Bourguignon, J.J. (1991) Behavioral effects of rolipram and structurally related compounds in mice: behavioral sedation of cAMP phosphodiesterase inhibitors. *Pharmacol Biochem Behav* 39(2):321–323.

Guitart, X., Thompson, M.A., Mirante, C.K., Greenberg, M.E., and Nestler, E.J. (1992) Regulation of CREB phosphorylation by acute and chronic morphine in the rat locus coeruleus. *J Neurochem* 58:1168–1171.

Haddjeri, N., Blier P., and de Montigny, C. (1998) Long-term antidepressant treatments result in a tonic activation of forebrain 5-HT$_{1A}$ receptors. *J Neurosci* 18:10150–10156.

Hebenstreit, G.F., Fellerer, K., Fichte, K., Fischer, G., Geyer, N., Meya, U., Sastre-y-Hernandez, M., Schony, W., Schratzer, M., and Soukop, W. (1989) Rolipram in major depressive disorder: results of a double-blind comparative study with imipramine. *Psychopharmacology* 22:156–160.

Hyman, S.E. and Nestler, E.J. (1999) Principles of molecular biology. In: Charney, D.S., Nestler, E.J., and Bunney, B.S., eds. *Neurobiology of Mental Illness*. New York: Oxford University Press, pp. 61–72.

Kaplan, D.R. and Miller, F.D. (1997) Signal transduction by the neurotrophin receptors. *Curr Opin Cell Biol* 9:213–21.

Lefkowitz, R.J. (1998) G protein–coupled receptors: new roles for receptor kinases and β-arrestins in receptor signaling and desensitization. *J Biol Chem* 273(30): 18677–18680.

Malberg J.E., Eisch A.J., Nestler E.J., and Duman R.S. (2000) Chronic antidepressant treatment increases neurogenesis in adult rat hippocampus. *J Neurosci* 20(24):9104–9110.

McEwen B.S. (1999) Stress and hippocampal plasticity. *Annu Rev Neurosci* 22:105–22.

Messer, C.J., Eisch, A.J., Carlezon, W.A., Jr., Whisler, K., Shen, L., Wolf, D.H., Westphal, H., Collins, F., Russell, D.S., and Nestler, E.J. (2000) Role for GDNF in biochemical and behavioral adaptations to drugs of abuse. *Neuron* 26:247–257.

Meyer, T.E. and Habener, J.F. (1993) Cyclic adenosine 3',5'-monophosphate response element–binding protein (CREB) and related transcription-activating deoxyribonucleic acid–binding proteins. *Endocr Rev* 14:269–290.

Montminy, M.R., Gonzalez, G.A., and Yamamoto, K.K. (1990) Regulation of cAMP-inducible genes by CREB. *Trends Neurosci* 13: 184–188.

Nestler, E.J. (1999) Cellular and molecular mechanisms of addiction. In: Charney, D.S., Nestler, E.J., and Bunney, B.S., eds. *Neurobiology of Mental Illness*. New York: Oxford University Press, pp. 61–72.

Nibuya, M., Morinobu, S., and Duman, R.S. (1995) Regulation of BDNF and trkB mRNA in rat brain by chronic electroconvulsive seizure and antidepressant drug treatments. *J Neurosci* 15:7539–7547.

Nibuya, M., Nestler, E.J., and Duman, R.S. (1996) Chronic antidepressant administration increases the expression of cAMP response element binding protein (CREB) in rat hippocampus. *J Neurosci* 16:2365–2372.

O'Donnell, J.M. (1993) Antidepressant-like effects of rolipram and other inhibitors of cyclic adenosine monophosphate phosphodiesterase on behavior maintained by differential reinforcement of low response rate. *J Pharmacol Exp Ther* 264(3):1168–1178.

O'Donnell, J.M. and Frith, S. (1999) Behavioral effects of family-selective inhibitors of cyclic nucleotide phosphodiesterases. *Pharmacol Biochem Behav* 63:185–192.

Rahman, Z., Gold, S.J., Potenza, M.N., Cowan, C.W., Ni, Y.G., He, W., Wensel, T.G., and Nestler, E.J. (1999) Cloning and characterization of RGS9-2: a striatal-enriched alternatively spliced product of the *RGS9* gene. *J Neurosci* 19(6):2016–2026.

Rahman, Z., Wein, M., Gold, S.J., Colby, C.R., Chen, C.K., Self, D., Neve, R.L., Simon, M.I., and Nestler, E.J. (2000) Functional role of RGS9-2 in striatum. *Soc Neurosci Abstr* 26:1938.

Robinson T.E. and Kolb B. (1999a) Alterations in the morphology of dendrites and dendritic spines in the nucleus accumbens and prefrontal cortex following repeated treatment with amphetamine or cocaine. *Eur J Neurosci* 11(5):1598–1604.

Robinson T.E. and Kolb B. (1999b) Morphine alters the structure of neurons in the nucleus accumbens and neocortex of rats. *Synapse* 33(2):160–162.

Sapolsky R.M. (1996) Stress, glucocorticoids, and damage to the nervous system: the current state of confusion. *Stress* 1:1–19.

Schulman, H. and Hyman, S.E. (1999) Intracellular signaling. In: Zigmond, M.J., Bloom, F.E., Landis, S.C., Roberts, J.L., and Squire, L.R., eds. *Fundamental Neuroscience*. San Diego: Academic Press, pp. 269–316.

Scott, A.I., Perini, A.F., Shering, P.A., and Whalley, L.J. (1991) Inpatient major depression: is rolipram as effective as amitriptyline? *Eur J Clin Pharmacol* 40:127–129.

Segal, R.A. and Greenberg, M.E. (1996) Intracellular signaling pathways activated by neurotrophic factors. *Annu Rev Neurosci* 19: 463–489.

Siuciak, J.A., Lewis, D.R., Wiegand, S.J., and Lindsay, R.M. (1996) Antidepressant-like effect of brain derived neurotrophic factor (BDNF). *Pharmacol Biochem Behav* 56:131–137.

Swank, R.P., Smith-Swintosky, V.L., and Twyman, R.E. (2000) Monoamine neurotransmitters. In: Sadock, B.J., and Sadock, V.A., eds. *Comprehensive Textbook of Psychiatry 7th ed.* Philadelphia: Lippincott Williams & Wilkins, pp. 50–59.

Thome, J., Impey, S., Storm, D., and Duman, R.S. (2000) cAMP-response element-mediated gene transcription is upregulated by chronic antidepressent treatment. *J Neurosci* 20:4030–4036.

Vaidya V.A., Siuciak J.A., Du F., and Duman R.S. (1999) Hippocampal mossy fiber sprouting induced by chronic electroconvulsive seizures. *Neuroscience* 89:157–166.

Vaidya V.A., Terwilliger R.Z., and Duman R.S. (2000) Alterations in heavy and light neurofilament proteins in hippocampus following chronic ECS administration. *Synapse* 35(2):137–43.

Wachtel, H. and Schneider, H.H. (1986) Rolipram, a novel antidepressant drug, reverses the hypothermia and hypokinesia of monoamine-depleted mice by an action beyond postsynaptic monoamine receptors. *Neuropharmacology* 25(10):1119–1169.

Watanabe Y., Gould E., Daniels D.C., Cameron H., and McEwen B.S. (1992) Tianeptine attenuates stress-induced morphological changes in the hippocampus. *Eur J Pharmacol* 222:157–162.

Widnell, K.L., Russell, D., and Nestler, E.J. (1994) Regulation of cAMP response element binding protein in the locus coeruleus in vivo and in a locus coeruleus-like (CATH.a) cell line in vitro. *Proc Natl Acad Sci USA* 91:10947–10951.

4 | Pharmacokinetics I: developmental principles

ALEXANDER A. VINKS AND PHILIP D. WALSON

Rational pharmacotherapy is dependent upon a basic understanding of the way patients handle drugs (pharmacokinetics) and their response to specific drug effects (pharmacodynamics). Most drugs have been developed and tested in young to middle-aged adults. The evaluation of medications in children has always lagged behind that in adults. In 1964, Dr. Harry Shirkey first called attention to this major public health problem. He coined the term "therapeutic orphans" to describe children as a result of the lack of formal drug studies in children (Shirkey, 1968, 1999).

Important advances in pediatric clinical pharmacology have been made since then, although reluctance to pursue pharmacokinetic and pharmacodynamic studies in children remained (Kauffman and Kearns, 1992). Consequently, even at the present time many drugs that are being routinely used in children have not been adequately tested for safety and efficacy (t Jong et al., 2000). The primary reasons for this situation are the ethical constraints fueled by fears and anxiety about doing studies in children and the fact that drug companies have had little economic incentive to study drugs in the pediatric population. Any pediatric use of a drug not described in the Food and Drug Administration (FDA)–approved labeling is considered "off label." Because the label frequently does not contain pediatric dosing information, doses are derived from the adult dose adjusted for body weight or body surface area. This does not take into account, however, all aspects of pediatric physiology, and can thus put the child or adolescent at risk for failing therapy or for adverse drug reactions.

In 1990, the Institute of Medicine sponsored a workshop to address the lack of pediatric labeling. This workshop produced recommendations that eventually led to the pediatric provisions of the FDA Modernization Act (FDAMA) of 1997, as well as to the 1998 FDA Pediatric Rule (FDAMA, 1999). Stimulated by FDAMA and the 1998 Rule, researchers have developed many more protocols that now include early studies in children with emphasis on pharmacokinetic and pharmacodynamic behaviors that are important to understand and predict developmental differences in drug response.

THE TARGET CONCENTRATION STRATEGY

While imperfect, there is almost always a better relationship between the action of a given drug and its concentration in the blood or at its site(s) of effect than between the dose of the drug given and the effect. *Pharmacokinetics* is the science that can explain and predict the relationship between a dosing regimen and the concentration of a drug in various body compartments. A basic understanding of pharmacokinetic (PK) principles and the effects of development on them are required to better understand and predict drug actions. In Figure 4.1 the interrelationship between drug input (dosage), pharmacokinetics, pharmacodynamics, and clinical effects is schematically conceptualized (Breimer and Danhof, 1997).

There are many practical, physiologic, and pathophysiologic factors that determine how much drug effect will be associated with a drug prescription. Clinicians make a diagnosis and then prescribe a dosing regimen: drug, dose, formulation, route, frequency, and duration. Once a drug is prescribed there are many factors that determine how much effect, either therapeutic or toxic, is seen in the individual patient. Prescriptions must be filled correctly, the prescription filled must contain the correct drug and amount, the dosage regimen must be taken or given, the drug must get into the patient and get to the site(s) of action, and the effects produced will depend on the patient's physiology and on other drugs present. Patients may never fill the prescription, pharmacy or pharmaceutical errors can alter the amount of drug delivered or, in fact, the type of

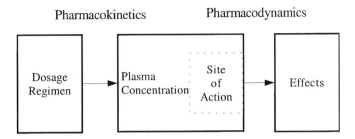

FIGURE 4.1 Schematic representation of the interrelationship between drug input (dosage), pharmacokinetics (concentration), pharmacodynamics, and clinical effects.

drug given, and parents or patients may or may not comply with instructions. All of these pre-dose factors can alter the amount of drug the patient receives. Drug concentration measurements can identify or eliminate the uncertainty about a number of these factors in patients who have unusual or unexpected drug responses. However, patients who actually take or are given the same amount of a drug may also have very different amounts of drug in their body or blood at different times after dosing. The ability to explain or predict the inter- and intraindividual differences in drug concentrations over time requires knowledge of some basic PK principles.

Much of our current knowledge of pediatric pharmacokinetics comes from the ability to measure serum concentrations for drugs, especially those with narrow therapeutic ranges or low safety margins. Therapeutic drug monitoring of drugs has been done for years for compounds such as digoxin, aminoglycosides, and theophylline. Increasingly, measurements of psychoactive drug concentrations have given important insights into the different PK behavior in children and adolescents (Preskorn et al., 1986; Preskorn, 1997).

Unfortunately, incorrect sample collection or analysis, or improper interpretation of results, can diminish the value of therapeutic drug monitoring (TDM) results. In addition, there are financial implications to the usefulness of TDM. There are ample studies showing that, when properly ordered, assayed, and interpreted, psychoactive drug TDM can occasionally be useful in all patients, and always in some clinical situations (Walson, 1994).

For some psychotropic drugs (e.g., lithium and some antidepressants) a good correlation exists between plasma levels and therapeutic or toxic effects. Optimum steady-state levels can now be predicted from single-dose blood level data of some drugs (lithium, nortriptyline, desipramine). Altered PK behavior in children has to be taken into consideration in using psychotropic drugs. With development of suitable drug assays, plasma level control of therapy is becoming an increasing part of a good clinical practice.

The potential of psychoactive TDM to improve therapy has been limited to date because many clinicians lack basic PK training and pharmaceutical marketing departments actively discourage TDM of their drugs. In order to correct this situation, clinicians must appreciate the basic PK principles necessary to correctly order and interpret TDM results, as well as to understand or predict drug actions in their individual patients.

This chapter will give a basic overview of pharmacokinetics and development. The review should allow clinicians to better understand drug disposition issues so as to inform their ordering and interpretation of TDM, as well as help them to understand or design and interpret clinical drug trials.

PHARMACOKINETIC PRINCIPLES

The basic processes that control the concentration of drug at the site(s) of action resulting from a given dosage regimen include: absorption, distribution, metabolism, and excretion. Collectively, these processes are referred to as *ADME* and provide an organized format for describing the pharmacokinetics of a particular drug and its dosage form. Absorption and distribution are primarily responsible for determining the speed of onset of drug effect, while the processes of metabolism and excretion terminate the action of the pharmacologic agent by removing the active form of the drug from the body. Taken together, these four processes determine the duration of drug action (Rowland and Tozer, 1995).

Drug absorption occurs from the site(s) of drug absorption (e.g., gut, lung, nasal epithelium) by either active (e.g., transport mediated) or passive mechanisms. The bioavailability (*F*) of a drug is the fraction that reaches the systemic circulation and is ultimately available to exert a biological effect on target tissues. This percentage is determined by the total amount absorbed and, for an orally administered drug, the metabolic elimination during first passage through the intestine and liver (first-pass effect). Absorption depends heavily on the route of entry, with intravenous administration producing the equivalent of 100% absorption (or $F = 1$). Oral administration is by far the most common route of administration, but also the most unpredictable in terms of final bioavailability. An orally administered drug is absorbed from the gastrointestinal tract and must first enter the portal circulation, where it passes through the liver before reaching the systemic circulation. During this first pass, a considerable portion of the drug is metabolized. Thus, only a fraction of the drug that was absorbed from the gastrointestinal tract enters the systemic circulation.

Most psychotropic medications are given orally and are absorbed after dissolution, primarily in the small intestine. The rate of absorption (expressed as a rate constant Ka [1/h]) is usually passive and obeys first-order principles, meaning that the rate of absorption is dependent on the amount of drug at the site of absorption, with a constant fraction absorbed per unit of time.

An often-misunderstood principle is that concentration in the blood rises until the rate of absorption equals the rate at which drug is being removed from the body (the so-called peak). This peak does not occur when absorption is complete but rather when the rate of absorption equals the rate of elimination. The time to peak is therefore determined by both absorption and elimination rates in the individual patient. Patients with faster elimination will have earlier peaks than will patients with slower elimination, even when the rate of drug absorption is the same (Fig. 4.2). The extent of absorption is usually expressed as the fraction absorbed or bioavailability. This is an important determinant of drug action. While rate and extent of absorption are related, they are different. In general, the onset and magnitude of effects are related to the *rate* of absorption, while the average steady state concentrations are related to the *extent* of absorption.

Once a drug is absorbed or enters the blood by direct injection, it is distributed throughout the body to various extravascular tissues. The PK term most often used to quantify the distribution of a drug throughout the body is the *apparent volume of distribution*. This volume does not necessarily correspond to a physiological space, and therefore, is preceded by the word *apparent*. For most clinical applications, pharmacokinetic analysis can be simplified by representing drug distribution within the body by a single compartment

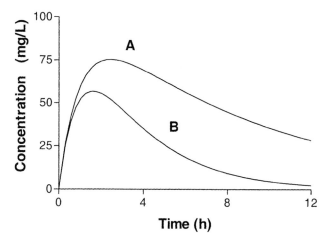

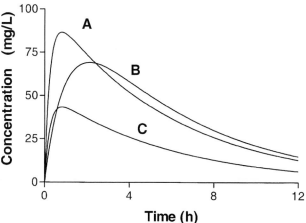

FIGURE 4.2 **A:** Effect of differences in elimination rate ion the maximum concentration (C_{max}) and time to maximum concentration (T_{max}) reached after a single oral dose. The drug absorption rate is the same (Ka = 1 h^{-1}) for curves A and B. The $t_{1/2}$ for curve A is 6 hours ; the $t_{1/2}$ for curve B is 2 hours. **B:** Differences between absorption rates can have a pronounced effect on the time (T_{max}) at which the maximum concentration (C_{max}) is reached. Curve A shows an orally administered drug with an absorption rate 4 times faster than that of curve B. Curve C shows the effect of a 50% decrease in bioavailability of drug A. The half-life (4 hours) is similar for scenarios A–C.

in which drug concentrations are uniform (Rowland and Tozer, 1995).

The relationship between the amount of drug absorbed (D), plasma concentration (C_p), and volume of distribution (V_d) can be summarized by the simple equation: $C_p = D/V_d$. Note that the larger the V_d, the smaller the C_p. The V_d is the constant which when multiplied by the concentration gives the amount of drug in the body. The fact that it is not a true volume is best illustrated by the fact that some drugs have V_ds of many thousands of L/kg of body weight.

The two most important factors affecting distribution are fat stores and the relative proportion of total body water to extracellular water. The V_d of highly lipophilic drugs, including most neuroleptics and antidepressants, is affected substantially by the proportion of body fat.

Most psychotropic drugs follow *first-order elimination*, or *linear kinetics*, in which a constant fraction of drug is eliminated independent of the amount circulating in the bloodstream. First-order kinetics implies that a linear relationship exists between changes in dosage and in plasma concentration. Such a linear association allows for clinically relevant predictions of the impact of a dose change on circulating drug levels.

The pharmacokinetic term *clearance* (CL) best describes the efficiency of the elimination process. Clearance by an elimination organ (e.g., liver, kidney) is defined as the volume of blood, serum, or plasma that is totally 'cleared' of drug per unit time. This term is additive; the total body or systemic clearance of a drug is equal to the sum of the clearances by individual eliminating organs. Usually this is represented as the sum of renal and hepatic clearances: CL = CL renal + CL hepatic. Clearance is constant and independent of serum concentration for drugs that are eliminated by first-order processes, and therefore may be considered proportionally constant between the rate of drug elimination and serum concentration.

However, for some drugs (most notably phenytoin, salicylate, and ethanol) hepatic metabolizing enzymes become saturated even at normal therapeutic concentrations. This is due to the relatively small concentration of hepatic enzymes available to metabolize these drugs (capacity-limited elimination). The elimination of these drugs is described by *zero-order*, or *nonlinear* (Michaelis-Menten), *kinetics*. This process is characterized by the elimination of a constant amount of drug per unit of time, regardless of the plasma level. Certain psychotropic drugs, such as fluoxetine and nefazodone, have been observed to demonstrate zero-order kinetics at clinically relevant doses, making the relationship between dose changes and subsequent plasma levels much less predictable (Janicak et al., 1993). Nonlinear elimination and enzyme saturation resulting in decreased clearance may also occur at very high concentrations of any drug and should always be considered as a potential complication in case of intoxication.

For drugs that follow first-order kinetics, in addition to clearance, the half-life is a useful pharmacokinetic parameter to describe elimination. The elimination half-life ($t_{1/2}$) is the time required for the concentration of drug to decrease by 50%. In clinical practice, this parameter is referred to as the *plasma* (or serum) *half-life* and is usually assessed by measuring the fall of

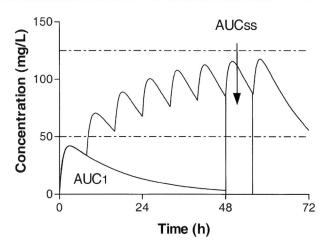

FIGURE 4.3 Plasma concentration time profile of drug with a half-life of 4 hours administered every 8 hours. Steady state is reached after 4–5 times the half-life. The concentration time curve after the first dose shows the area under the curve (AUC_1) after a single oral dose that is equivalent to the AUC at steady state (AUCss). The broken lines represent the therapeutic range (arbitrary).

plasma or serum drug concentration and by graphically plotting the logarithm of the drug concentration versus time. The elimination half-life can be useful when determining frequency of dosing and dosing intervals. When a drug is dosed at regular intervals, it is the plasma half-life that determines the plasma steady-state concentration (C_{ss}). *Steady state* is defined as an equilibrium between the amount of drug ingested and the amount of drug eliminated, resulting in no net change in plasma concentration over time. Steady state (C_{ss}) is reached after approximately 4–5 times the half-life (Fig. 4.3).

A common error is to confuse half-lives with number of doses. Unless given at an interval of a half-life, there is no relationship between number of doses given and steady state. Conversely, if drug intake is stopped, it takes 4–5 half-lives (not doses missed) for drug elimination to be complete (Table 4.1).

TABLE 4.1. *Fraction of Drug Eliminated and Fraction Remaining in the Body as a Function of Half-life*

Half-lives (n)	Fraction Eliminated (%)	Fraction Remaining (%)
1	50	50
2	75	25
3	87.5	12.5
4	93.8	6.25
5	96.9	3.12

Although elimination half-life is usually associated with clearance, it should be noted that this parameter is also influenced by distribution. This concept is important to appreciate when individualizing drug therapy, since it is clearance that determines steady-state concentrations for any given dose absorbed.

Vignette 4.1 Blood Concentration of Phenytoin in Hypoalbuminemia

An 8-year-old child with grand mal seizures experiences nystagmus while on 200 mg/day of long-term phenytoin treatment, given in three divided doses. A steady-state phenytoin concentration of 5.0 mg/L is measured (therapeutic range, 8–20 mg/L). Beside normal laboratory results, it was noted that the child had profound hypoalbuminemia. Free (unbound) phenytoin concentration was 2.4 mg/L (therapeutic range 0.2-2 mg/L).

In this example, the increased unbound phenytoin concentration resulted in a larger volume of distribution (more free drug distributed to the tissues), increased clearance (more free drug available for metabolism), but no change in the drug's half-life. The paradox in this case is that the increased clearance caused the total phenytoin blood concentration to go down, while the free concentration was elevated and led to clinical toxicity. Moreover, the unchanged half-life would not have clarified the cause of the 'subtherapeutic' phenytoin level.

PHARMACOKINETICS IN CHILDREN AND ADOLESCENTS

Children and adolescents display some unique pharmacokinetic properties; they are not "small adults" in the way they handle drugs and they do not necessarily require smaller doses (Kearns and Reed, 1989). Children and adolescents have greater metabolic capacity than adults, if corrected for size, and therefore more rapidly eliminate drugs that utilize hepatic pathways (e.g., neuroleptics, tricyclic antidepressants, pemoline and methylphenidate (Geller, 1991). Because they have relatively more efficient renal elimination, children and adolescents will eliminate drugs that use renal pathways (e.g., lithium) more rapidly than adults. Compared to adults, children have greater body water and relatively less adipose tissue. This can have a pronounced impact on drug distribution and accumulation of lipophilic drugs and metabolites. Therefore, the appropriate dose of a psychotropic medication in the pediatric age group should be empirically determined in combination with therapeutic drug monitoring. Dosing

should not be solely based on adult extrapolations from a proportion of body weight, as such an approach may lead to subtherapeutic concentrations. In addition, infants, children, and adolescents are not a homogenous group in terms of drug distribution patterns (Morselli et al., 1980; Kearns and Reed, 1989). These differences can be especially pronounced around the time of puberty, when hormonal changes can influence drug clearance and plasma drug concentrations achieved (Morselli and Pippinger, 1982).

Although PK data in children and adolescents are limited, clinical observations suggest that children and adolescents require larger, weight-adjusted doses of most drugs than do adults to achieve comparable blood levels and therapeutic effects (Soldin and Steele, 2000). This appears to be mostly the result of increased rate of metabolism and elimination.

DEVELOPMENTAL FACTORS AFFECTING DRUG DISPOSITION AND PHARMACOKINETIC

Absorption and Bioavailability

Drugs are administered by intravenous routes or extravascular routes including oral, sublingual, subcutaneous, intramuscular, rectal (by enema or suppository), and transdermal. Available dosage forms include suspensions, immediate-release capsules or tablets, sustained-release capsules or tablets, and enteric-coated capsules or tablets that resist dissolution in the acidic pH of the stomach.

Drugs may be formulated as their salt forms (i.e., hydrochloride salt for base, sodium salts for acids) that dissociate in the body, or they may be formulated as the free acid or base. The fraction of the drug absorbed can be difficult to predict, as it is influenced by many factors. The extent and rate of absorption are partly determined by the physicochemical properties of the drug. Favorable absorption is related to lipid solubility, nonpolarity, and small molecular size. Reduced absorption is often observed for highly polar, non–lipid-soluble, and large–molecular size drugs.

Other important determinants of drug absorption are the degree of ionization, determined by the pK_a of the drug and the pH of the surrounding milieu. The gastrointestinal epithelium is more permeable to the nonionized form because this portion is usually lipid-soluble and favors absorption. The degree of drug ionization will change as the pH increases from the stomach through the distal portion of the gut. The major factors influencing gastrointestinal absorption are pH-dependent diffusion and gastric emptying time. Slow gastric emptying time may retard drug absorption and can be rate limiting. This is because the major absorption occurs in the proximal bowel, which has the greatest absorptive surface area. A slow transit time or slow intestinal motility may, however, facilitate and prolong the absorption of some drugs. Gastric acid production and intestinal motility undergo substantial changes during the early stages of life but tend to be less different from adult values after the first year of life.

Little information is available regarding the effect of age on the absorption of psychotropic drugs (Prandota, 1985). However, the paucity of drug formulations appropriate for children results in the crushing, mixing, or dissolving of adult formulations in various liquids and solids. This may alter both the rate and extent of drug absorption. Different foods or liquids used as a concomitant vehicle can have different pH values and thus may affect drug stability or absorption. Sustained-release products designed and tested in adults are a special problem. These dosage forms may not work the same in children, regardless of whether they are crushed or not, because of differences in gastrointestinal transit time. A product designed to release drug evenly over 24 hours simply will not work the same in a child with decreased transit time, because only a fraction of the drug would be delivered. If a child is stabilized on a given dose and transit time, toxicity could be seen if the child becomes constipated, or a loss of efficacy seen if diarrhea develops. There are also developmental changes in diet, biliary secretion, and surface area, which could change the rate or extent of drug absorption. Drug concentration "peaks" can occur sooner in children. This is often assumed to be the result of more rapid absorption; perhaps as a result of formulation differences. However, this may be the result of more rapid clearance rather than any difference in absorption rate. Since peak concentrations occur when the rate of absorption equals the rate of elimination (Fig. 4.2), in children with more rapid drug elimination, even when they have identical absorption rates, drug concentration will peak at an earlier time.

Drug Distribution and Protein Binding

After a drug is absorbed, it is distributed into various tissue compartments. The rate at which this occurs is determined by the blood flow to the tissues as well as the rate of transfer of the drug from the blood into the tissues. This transfer depends on the vascular permeability to the drug, the relative binding of the drug to blood versus tissue components, the availability of active transport processes, and the concentration gradient between blood and tissues. Many of these processes are altered during development. Drug distribution never stops; however, eventually the rates of transfer into and out of the tissues become equal. The time period prior to this equilibrium condition is called the *distribution phase*. Drug concentrations measured during the distribution phase will have a different relationship to drug action than will concentrations measured after distribution is complete. This is true for drugs with very slow or rapid elimination. Appreciation of this principle is required to design studies to determine whether a concentration/effect relationship exists. For example, clonazepam studies that failed to find a concentration/effect relationship ignored the fact that clonazepam has an extensive, prolonged distribution phase (Greenblatt et al., 1987). The same patient can have distribution phase concentrations that are 10 times pre-dose concentrations. Concentrations drawn at random times after dosing would not be expected to relate to effects (Walson and Edge, 1996). There is a common misconception that the distribution phase can be ignored for drugs such as clonazepam, which have slow elimination (i.e., long half-lives). Many centrally active drugs have prolonged distribution phases that must be appreciated to both properly interpret concentrations and design studies to investigate concentration/effect relationships (Preskorn et al., 1986).

Two important factors affecting distribution that change substantially during development are the amount of body fat and the relative proportion of total body water. For highly lipophilic drugs, such as most neuroleptics and antidepressants, the volume of distribution is greatly affected by the amount of body fat. The proportion of body fat is highest in the first year of life, followed by a steady decrease until an increase occurs at puberty (Milsap and Szefler, 1986). Children and adolescents at different ages have varying degrees of fat stores, and in general tend to have a proportion of body fat less than that found in adults. Hence, in children one would expect to find a larger plasma concentration with lipophilic drugs than that in adults after being given the same weight-adjusted dose. It has been demonstrated, however, that children actually exhibit a lower plasma concentration than that of adults under these conditions. Therefore, other mechanisms (such as increased metabolism) must explain the lower plasma concentration of lipophilic drugs in children (Fetner and Geller, 1992).

The relative volume of extracellular water is high in children and tends to decrease with development. Extracellular water decreases gradually from about 40%–50% of body weight in the newborn to about 15%–20% by age 10–15 years. Total body water (TBW) decreases rapidly from about 85% of body weight in a small premature infant to about 70% in the full-term newborn to about 60% in the 1-year-old infant, and adult values (55% TBW) are gradually attained by 12 years of age. The percent of intracellular water remains stable form the first months of life through adulthood. Thus, drugs that are primarily distributed in body water (e.g., lithium) can be expected to have a lower plasma concentration in the pediatric population than that in adults because the volume of distribution is higher in children (Fetner and Geller, 1992).

The amount of drug that binds to the receptor at the site of action determines the magnitude of drug effect. This in turn is determined by the amount and strength of drug binding to various proteins in blood and tissues. A major factor that affects distribution of a drug, and differs between pediatric patients and adults, is the extent to which the drug is bound to proteins (Grandison and Boudinot, 2000). The amount of protein available, a drug's binding affinity for protein, and its competition for binding with other endogenous and exogenous binding substrates all can impact the volume of distribution. Only the unbound drug is usually available to pass across membranes, distribute to extravascular tissues, and have pharmacological effects. Albumin is the primary plasma binding protein and at the early stage of life albumin concentration is directly related to gestational age. Albumin levels rapidly increase to adult levels by the end of the first year. Acid and neutral compounds bind primarily to albumin, which has high capacity to bind drugs. Many basic compounds also bind to the low-capacity binding alpha-1-acid glycoprotein (AAG). This protein is of particular importance, as its concentration in serum increases in conditions of stress, inflammation, and malignant disease. In general, changes in protein binding have the largest effects on drugs that are highly bound to blood proteins, or on drugs for which binding can be saturated at therapeutic concentrations (e.g., valproic acid (Herngren et al., 1991). Drug binding depends on the presence of other drugs or drug metabolites (displacement) (MacKichan, 1989) and certain disease states (hepatic impairment, renal disease, malnutrition) (Blaschke, 1977; Krishnaswamy, 1989; Vanholder et al., 1993). For instance, the selective serotonin reuptake inhibitors (SSRIs) fluoxetine, paroxetine, and sertraline are highly protein bound to albumin and AAG. This raises the possibility of displacement interactions with other highly protein-bound drugs. However, SSRIs are weakly bound to AAG. It appears that this is the reason for highly bound SSRIs not increasing the free fraction of other, concomitant highly bound drugs (Preskorn, 1997). Drug protein binding may be reduced in young infants (Notarianni, 1990) and certain disease

states, but overall does not appear to be an important developmental factor in older children and adolescents (Grandison and Boudinot, 2000).

Drug Metabolism and Elimination

Drugs have to exhibit a sufficient degree of lipid solubility (lipophilicity) to be orally absorbed and distributed to receptors, e.g., in the central nervous system. For subsequent effective excretion from the body, conversion to more water-soluble (hydrophilicity) metabolites is required. The enzymes involved in this biotransformation are most highly concentrated in the liver, but are also present in several tissues throughout the body, such as small intestine, lung, kidney, and adrenals. Most psychoactive drugs undergo extensive metabolism in the liver, although some may be excreted unchanged (e.g., lithium, gabapentin). The metabolic processes involved are categorized as either phase I or phase II reactions.

Phase I metabolic reactions involve oxidation, reduction, or hydrolysis of the parent molecule, resulting in the formation of a more polar compound. Phase 1 reactions are mediated by the cytochrome P450 (CYP) family of enzymes. While metabolism used to be thought of as the body's detoxification process, phase I metabolites may be equally or even more pharmacologically active than the parent compound. Drug metabolism in general, and CYP-based mechanisms in particular, are discussed in detail in Chapter 5.

Phase II metabolism involves conjugation with endogenous substrates such as sulfate, acetate, or glucuronic acid. Drugs may be conjugated directly or made more amenable to conjugation following the introduction of a functional group by phase I metabolism (e.g., hydroxylation). It is well recognized that the maturation of drug-metabolizing enzymes is a predominant factor responsible for age-related changes in metabolic drug clearance. For instance, neonates are deficient in many of the enzymes responsible for both phase I and phase II drug metabolism. Unfortunately, when unappreciated these deficiencies have led to a number of adverse reactions, such as the "gray baby" syndrome associated with chloramphenicol use (Weiss et al., 1960). Recent advances in our understanding of the ontogeny of the enzymes responsible for drug metabolism can explain past cases of drug toxicity in the neonate and help prevent such events in the future.

Developmental Aspects of Selected Cytochrome P-450 Isoforms

With increasing knowledge of mammalian drug biotransformation processes, it has become apparent that not only are there developmental differences in expression among drug metabolizing enzyme families (cytochromes P450, glucuronosyl transferases etc.) but individual drug metabolizing enzymes may have unique developmental profiles that influence the therapeutic response to a given drug. Knowledge regarding CYP ontogeny is quite limited, despite our increasing understanding of genetic variation in CYP activity in adults. For instance, CYP2D6 phenotyping data suggest that enzyme activity in the newborn is markedly reduced, with activity gradually increasing during the first month of life to about 20% the adult activity level (Treluyer et al., 1991). In older children CYP2D6 catalytic activity becomes comparable to that of adults around the age of 10 years, but possibly much earlier, around the age of 3–5 years.

Based on available data, CYP3A4 activity is low at birth but increases rapidly during the early stages of life to reach approximately 50% of adult levels at ages 6–12 months. During infancy, CYP3A4 activity appears to be slightly higher than that in adults, with a gradual decline to levels approximating those in the adult occurring around the time of puberty (de Wildt et al., 1999; Lacroix et al., 1997). The implications of these changes depend on the specific CYP involved in a particular drug's clearance and on the number of alternative pathways, as well as on induction or inhibition by other drugs. For instance, maturational changes in CYP3A4 activity are reflected by increased clearance in young children for midazolam and immunosuppressive drugs such as ciclosporine and tacrolimus. As a consequence, higher dosages are required, compared to adults, to reach the desired target blood concentrations.

Therapeutic Drug Monitoring

The developmental changes in pharmacokinetics of psychotropic medications that occur between birth and adolescence to adulthood create challenges for physicians who desire to prescribe medications on a rational, age-appropriate, individual basis. Routine therapeutic drug monitoring of prescribed drugs including active metabolite(s) can be of great help to individualizing dose requirements during long-term treatment (Van Brunt, 1983; Balant-Gorgia and Balant, 1987, 1992; Mitchell, 2000). The ratio of metabolite to parent drug can also give important information on (non)compliance and can reveal unusual metabolic patterns.

Patients with lower or higher effects than expected 3–4 weeks after initiation of therapy or a dose change may benefit from TDM. In the nonresponding patient, concentration measurements will help the clinician in the decision to increase the dose or consider alternate therapy. Generally accepted indications for concentration measurements are summarized in Table 4.2.

Appropriate timing of drug concentration measurements is crucial for the appropriate interpretation of the level and subsequent dose adjustment. Within a dosing interval the pre-dose or trough concentration is usually the most informative sampling time, when steady state is achieved but efficacy is questioned. In case of adverse events or (suspected) toxicity, sampling is preferably done at the time the side effects are experienced. Random sampling often results in not very useful drug monitoring, because of the lack of necessary information, such as the actual time of drug intake, concomitant medications, and time of sampling. Therapeutic drug monitoring laboratories can play an important role in improving the efficient use of TDM by providing up-to-date guidelines and teaching physicians about all the information necessary to interpret a result. This information must either be included in the laboratory requests or obtained by TDM or clinical pharmacokinetic monitoring services, such as those commonly run by clinical pharmacists and pharmacologists (Ensom et al., 1998; Murphy et al., 1996). Ideally, a PK interpretation should be reported back to the clinician along with the results.

For several drug classes, including psychotropic drugs, the use of population models and the application of a Bayesian optimization algorithm has been shown to be clinically useful and cost-effective (Burton et al., 1985; Taright et al., 1994; van Lent-Evers et al., 1999; Rousseau et al., 2000). The method of Bayesian forecasting is derived from Bayes' theorem, and is based on the concept that prior PK knowledge of a drug, in the form of a population model, can be combined with individual patient data, such as drug concentrations (Jelliffe et al., 1998). The idea is to make an individualized model of the behavior of the drug in a particular patient to see how the drug has been handled, and to obtain the necessary information to make

TABLE 4.2 *Indications for Therapeutic Drug Monitoring of Psychotropic Drugs*

Inadequate response

Higher than standard dose required

Serious or persistent side effects

Suspected toxicity

Suspected noncompliance

Suspected drug–drug interactions

New preparation, changing brands

Other illnesses, e.g., hepatic/renal problems, inflammatory diseases rational dose adjustments so as to best achieve the selected target goal(s).

Vignette 4.2 Model-based, Goal-oriented Individualization of Lithium Therapy

A 17-year-old boy with bipolar disorder is started on lithium therapy at 600 mg bid. The initial lithium concentration is 0.8 mmol/L. As the patient's pressured speech and labile mood do not improve with time, the psychiatrist in charge wonders whether the lack of efficacy is due to insufficient coverage or to noncompliance. A repeat trough level is 0.3 mmol/L (Fig. 4.4A).

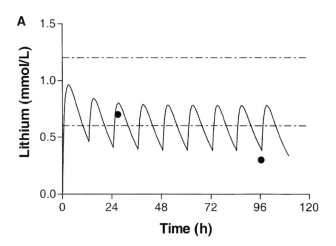

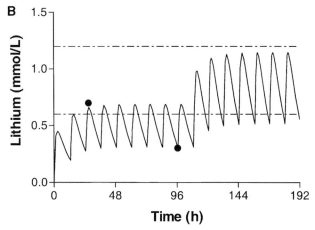

FIGURE 4.4 A: Lithium plasma concentration time profile based on a population pharmacokinetics model (Taright et al., 1994). Closed circles are the actual measured lithium concentrations; broken lines represent the therapeutic range (0.6–1.2 mmol/L). B: Individualized lithium plasma concentration time profile based on the population model with feedback of measured concentrations (Bayesian recalculation). Closed circles are the measured lithium concentrations. The second part of the curve is the predicted lithium concentration profile after increasing the dose to 1000 mg lithium carbonate twice daily, based on a target of 0.6–1.2 mmol/L (broken lines).

In this example, simulation of the lithium serum concentration profile based on population PK data reveals that this patient has a higher than normal clearance. Furthermore, the first level was not a trough level. The model-based profile and subsequent Bayesian individualization process are shown in Figure 4.4B.

Bayesian methods can be more cost-effective than other techniques because they require fewer drug measurements for individual PK parameter estimation and can handle sparse and random samples (Merle and Mentre, 1999). Therapeutic drug monitoring data, when applied appropriately, can also be used to detect and quantify clinically relevant drug–drug interactions (Jerling et al., 1994; Gex-Fabry et al., 1997). However, regardless of which PK dose individualization techniques are used, all are superior to a simple-minded comparison of a result to a therapeutic range. Simply reporting results as below, within, or above a published range is usually uninformative and not cost saving, and can lead to inappropriate actions.

SUMMARY

Development can dramatically alter drug effects. In many cases this is the result of PK changes. Appreciation of developmental PK principles will allow physicians to suspect and evaluate causes of unusual or unexpected drug effects. Often this will require drug concentration measurement and informed interpretation of the drug concentrations. As psychoactive drugs are studied more in children, the clinical and theoretical impact of developmental changes on drug kinetics and effects will be further elucidated. This should improve pediatric psychoactive drug therapy.

REFERENCES

Anonymous. (1999) FDA's FDAMA accomplishments—one year after enactment. *Ann Pharmacother* 33:134.

Balant-Gorgia, A.E. and Balant, L. (1987) Antipsychotic drugs. Clinical pharmacokinetics of potential candidates for plasma concentration monitoring. *Clin Pharmacokinet* 13:65–90.

Balant-Gorgia, A.E. and Balant, L.P. (1992) Milestones in clinical pharmacology. Therapeutic drug monitoring of antidepressants. *Clin Ther* 14:612–614; discussion 611.

Blaschke, T.F. (1977) Protein binding and kinetics of drugs in liver diseases. *Clin Pharmacokinet* 2:32–44.

Breimer, D.D. and Danhof, M. (1997) Relevance of the application of pharmacokinetic–pharmacodynamic modelling concepts in drug development. The "wooden shoe" paradigm. *Clin Pharmacokinet* 32:259–267.

Burton, M.E., Vasko, M.R., and Brater, D.C. (1985) Comparison of drug dosing methods. *Clin Pharmacokinet* 10:1–37.

de Wildt, S.N., Kearns, G.L., Leeder, J.S., and van den Anker, J.N. (1999) Cytochrome P450 3A: ontogeny and drug disposition. *Clin Pharmacokinet* 37:485–505.

Ensom, M.H., Davis, G.A., Cropp, C.D., and Ensom, R.J. (1998) Clinical pharmacokinetics in the 21st century. Does the evidence support definitive outcomes? *Clin Pharmacokinet* 34:265–279.

Fetner, H.H. and Geller, B. (1992) Lithium and tricyclic antidepressants. *Psychiatry Clin North Am* 15:223–224.

Geller, B. (1991) Psychopharmacology of children and adolescents: pharmacokinetics and relationships of plasma/serum levels to response. *Psychopharmacol Bull* 27:401–409.

Gex-Fabry, M., Balant-Gorgia, A.E., and Balant, L.P. (1997) Therapeutic drug monitoring databases for postmarketing surveillance of drug–drug interactions: evaluation of a paired approach for psychotropic medication. *Ther Drug Monit* 19:1–10.

Grandison, M.K. and Boudinot, F.D. (2000) Age-related changes in protein binding of drugs: implications for therapy. *Clin Pharmacokinet* 38:271–290.

Greenblatt, D.J., Miller, L.G., and Shader, R.I. (1987) Clonazepam pharmacokinetics, brain uptake, and receptor interactions. *J Clin Psychiatry* 48 Suppl: 4–11.

Herngren, L., Lundberg, B., and Nergardh, A. (1991) Pharmacokinetics of total and free valproic acid during monotherapy in infants. *J Neurol* 238:315–319.

Janicak, P.G., Davis, J.M., Preskorn, S.H., et al., eds. (1993) Pharmacokinetics. In: *Principles and Practice of Psychopharmacotherapy*. Baltimore: Williams & Wilkins, pp. 59–79.

Jelliffe, R.W., Schumitzky, A., Bayard, D., Milman, M., Van Guilder, M., Wang, X., Jiang, F., Barbaut, X., and Maire, P. (1998) Model-based, goal-oriented, individualised drug therapy. Linkage of population modelling, new 'multiple model' dosage design, bayesian feedback and individualised target goals. *Clin Pharmacokinet* 34:57–77.

Jerling, M., Bertilsson, L., and Sjoqvist, F. (1994) The use of therapeutic drug monitoring data to document kinetic drug interactions: an example with amitriptyline and nortriptyline. *Ther Drug Monit* 16:1–12.

Kauffman, R.E. and Kearns, G.L. (1992) Pharmacokinetic studies in paediatric patients. Clinical and ethical considerations. *Clin Pharmacokinet* 23:10–29.

Kearns, G.L. and Reed, M.D. (1989) Clinical pharmacokinetics in infants and children. A reappraisal. *Clin Pharmacokinet* 17:29–67.

Krishnaswamy, K. (1989) Drug metabolism and pharmacokinetics in malnourished children. *Clin Pharmacokinet* 17:68–88.

Lacroix, D., Sonnier, M., Moncion, A., Cheron, G., and Cresteil, T. (1997) Expression of CYP3A in the human liver—evidence that the shift between CYP3A7 and CYP3A4 occurs immediately after birth. Eur J Biochem 247:625–634.

MacKichan, J.J. (1989) Protein binding drug displacement interactions—fact or fiction? *Clin Pharmacokinet* 16:65–73.

Merle, Y. and Mentre, F. (1999) Optimal sampling times for Bayesian estimation of the pharmacokinetic parameters of nortriptyline during therapeutic drug monitoring. *J Pharmacokinet Biopharm* 27:85–101.

Milsap, R.L. and Szefler, S.J. (1986) Special pharmacokinetic considerations in children. In: Evans, W.E., Schentag, J.J., and Jusko, W.J., eds. *Applied Pharmacokinetics. Principles of Therapeutic Drug Monitoring*. Spokane, WA: Applied Therapeutics, Inc., pp. 294–330.

Mitchell, P.B. (2000) Therapeutic drug monitoring of psychotropic medications. *Br J Clin Pharmacol* 49:303–312.

Morselli, P.L., Franco-Morselli, R., and Bossi, L. (1980) Clinical pharmacokinetics in newborns and infants. Age-related differences and therapeutic implications. *Clin Pharmacokinet* 5:485–527.

Morselli, P.L. and Pippinger, C.E. (1982) Drug disposition during development. In: *Applied Therapeutic Drug Monitoring*. Washington, DC: American Association of Clinical Chemistry, pp. 63–70.

Murphy, J.E., Slack, M.K., and Campbell, S. (1996) National survey of hospital-based pharmacokinetic services. *Am J Health Syst Pharm* 53:2840–2847.

Notarianni, L.J. (1990) Plasma protein binding of drugs in pregnancy and in neonates. *Clin Pharmacokinet* 18:20–36.

Prandota, J. (1985) Clinical pharmacokinetics of changes in drug elimination in children. *Dev Pharmacol Ther* 8:311–328.

Preskorn, S.H. (1997) Clinically relevant pharmacology of selective serotonin reuptake inhibitors. An overview with emphasis on pharmacokinetics and effects on oxidative drug metabolism. *Clin Pharmacokinet* 32:1–21.

Preskorn, S.H., Weller, E., Hughes, C., and Weller, R. (1986) Plasma monitoring of tricyclic antidepressants: defining the therapeutic range for imipramine in depressed children. *Clin Neuropharmacol* 9:265–267.

Rousseau, A., Marquet, P., Debord, J., Sabot, C., and Lachatre, G. (2000) Adaptive control methods for the dose individualisation of anticancer agents. *Clin Pharmacokinet* 38:315–353.

Rowland, M. and Tozer, T.N. (1995) *Clinical Pharmacokinetics. Concepts and Applications, 3rd ed.* Media, PA: Lippincott Williams & Wilkins.

Shirkey, H. (1968) Therapeutic orphans. *J Pediatr* 72:119–120.

Shirkey, H. (1999) Therapeutic orphans. *Pediatrics* 104:583–584.

Soldin, S.J. and Steele, B.W. (2000) Mini-review: therapeutic drug monitoring in pediatrics. *Clin Biochem* 33:333–335.

Taright, N., Mentre, F., Mallet, A., and Jouvent, R. (1994) Nonparametric estimation of population characteristics of the kinetics of lithium from observational and experimental data: individualization of chronic dosing regimen using a new bayesian approach. *Ther Drug Monit* 16:258–269.

t Jong, G.W., Vulto, A.G., de Hoog, M., Schimmel, K.J., Tibboel, D., and van den Anker, J.N. (2000) Unapproved and off-label use of drugs in a children's hospital. N Engl J Med 343:1125.

Treluyer, J.M., Jacqz-Aigrain, E., Alvarez, F., and Cresteil, T. (1991) Expression of CYP2D6 in developing human liver. *Eur J Biochem* 202:583–588.

Van Brunt, N. (1983) The clinical utility of tricyclic antidepressant blood levels: a review of the literature. *Ther Drug Monit* 5:1–10.

Vanholder, R., De Smet, R., and Ringoir, S. (1993) Factors influencing drug protein binding in patients with end-stage renal failure. Eur J Clin Pharmacol 44:S17–S21.

Van Lent-Evers, N.A., Mathot, R.A., Geus, W.P., van Hout, B.A., and Vinks, A.A. (1999) Impact of goal-oriented and model-based clinical pharmacokinetic dosing of aminoglycosides on clinical outcome: a cost-effectiveness analysis. *Ther Drug Monit* 21:63–73.

Walson, P.D. (1994) Role of therapeutic drug monitoring (TDM) in pediatric anti-convulsant drug dosing. *Brain Dev* 16:23–26.

Walson, P.D. and Edge, J.H. (1996) Clonazepam disposition in pediatric patients. *Ther Drug Monit* 18:1–5.

Weiss, C.F., Glazko, A.J., and Weston, J.K. (1960) Chloramphenicol in the newborn infant: a physiologic explanation of its toxicity when given in excessive dose. *N Engl J Med* 262:787–794.

5 | Pharmacokinetics II: cytochrome P450–mediated drug interactions

JESSICA R. OESTERHELD AND DAVID A. FLOCKHART

Fifteen years ago, child psychiatrists' prescribing practices were often quite limited. They were generally free of concerns about possible drug–drug interactions. In the last 10 years, a number of factors have eroded this apparent complacency. Like their adult psychiatry colleagues (Rittmannsberger et al., 1999; Frye et al., 2000). child psychiatrists' prescribing patterns have shifted from monotherapy to co-pharmacy (Safer, 1997). For example, it is commonplace for a hospitalized teen to leave the hospital with an atypical antipsychotic, a mood stabilizer, an acne medication, or an oral contraceptive; or for a depressed latency-aged child who has asthma to be prescribed a selective serotonin reuptake inhibitor (SSRI), a hypnotic, and at least one antiasthmatic. Child psychiatrists have shifted their use of antidepressants to SSRIs, drugs that are likely to produce drug interactions because they cause metabolic drug interactions via inhibition of hepatic cytochrome P450 (CYP) enzymes (Safer, 1997). There has also been an increase in use by children of non-prescription drugs (Adlaf et al., 2000) including drugs of abuse (Weir, 2000), herbals (Walter and Rey, 1999; Chapter 29, this volume), and anabolic steroids (Evans, 1997). Finally, there is a growing list of medications that have been withdrawn from or severely restricted in the U.S. market because of their potential for fatal drug interactions; such drugs include terfenadine, astemizole, and cisapride. Child psychiatrists have even been warned of possible serious drug interactions with drugs that they have used for years, such as pimozide (Friedman, 1994, Horrigan and Barnhill, 1994, Flockhart et al., 2000) and, more recently, thioridazine (Maynard and Soni, 1996, Carrillo et al., 1999).

Any attempt to memorize hundreds of potential drug interactions to prevent dangerous interactions is unproductive. Rather, a child psychiatrist should have a basic understanding of the types and timing of possible drug interactions and then develop prevention strategies in prescribing psychotropics. These may include the *personal formulary approach,* which is designed to enhance awareness of possible drug interactions of particular agents; the use of a *therapeutic alliance* with pharmacists, nurse practitioners, and other professionals to foster mutual cross-checking of drug-prescribing; and continuous review of updated software programs or Web sites each time one uses more than one drug (including nonpsychiatric ones).

The most commonly prescribed psychotropics currently in use in child psychiatry include (1) psychostimulants, (2) SSRIs, (3) central adrenergic agonists, (4) mood stabilizers, (5) tricyclic antidepressants, and (6) antipsychotics (Jensen et al., 1999). Many of the drug interactions affecting SSRIs, tricyclic antidepressants, carbamazepine, and antipsychotics occur during absorption (i.e., in effects on drug transporters, such as P-glycoprotein [P-gp]) or during metabolism (i.e., via interactions with hepatic CYP or enzymes that carry out glucuronidation). If clinicians understand the basics about these processes, they can use up-to-date CYP and P-gp tables that organize a vast amount of drug interaction data into simple groupings that allow a rational approach to prescribing. This chapter will outline such an approach so that child psychiatrists can develop a proactive stance toward possible interactions with drugs they prescribe. Vignettes will be presented to highlight clinically relevant aspects of CYP-based drug interactions. In addition, the authors will focus on central serotonin syndrome (CSS) as an example of the intertwining of CYP-based pharmacokinetic and pharmacodynamic factors that may occur during the use of psychotherapeutics in children.

PHARMACOKINETIC VERSUS PHARMACODYNAMIC INTERACTIONS

Drug interactions are classified as *pharmacokinetic,* i.e., occurring at sites prior to the engagement of drugs with receptors at their sites of action—during absorption, distribution, metabolism, or excretion)—or *pharmacodynamic* i.e., occurring at active sites, as illustrated in Figure 5.1.

An example of a pharmacodynamic drug interaction would be when a child develops a hyperserotonergic state with symptoms of nausea and myoclonus hours after tramadol (an analgesic opioid with pro-serotonergic properties) was added to a regimen of citalopram (another serotonergic agent). An example of a non–cytochrome-mediated pharmacokinetic drug interaction would be when a teenager who has had stable blood levels of lithium develops nausea, tremor, and slurred speech after taking ibuprofen for menstrual cramps, because of diminished renal lithium clearance (Ragheb, 1990). This distinction is obviously artificial, since increases or decreases in drug levels are clinically meaningless unless they cause a pharmacodynamic effect (see Fig. 5.1).

PHASE 1 AND PHASE 2 METABOLISM

Most drugs are absorbed from the small intestine before entering the hepatic vein on their way to the liver. Some drugs are substrates of efflux transporters, such as P-gp (e.g., diltiazem, estradiol; see Table 5.1), which

TABLE 5.1 *Select P-glycoprotein Substrates, Inhibitors, and Inducers*

P-gp Substrates	P-gp Inhibitors	P-gp Inducers
Cimetidine	Chlorpromazine	Amitriptyline
Ciprofloxacin	Clarithromycin[a]	Dexamethasone
Dexamethasone	Cyclosporin	Progesterone
Digoxin	Diltiazem	Rifampin
Diltiazem	Doxepin	St. Johns wort
Enoxacin	Erythromycin[a]	
Erythromycin	Fluphenazine	
Estradiol	Grapefruit juice[a]	
Hydrocortisone	Haloperidol	
Nicardipine	Hydrocortisone	
Quinidine	Imipramine	
Verapamil	Itraconazole[a]	
	Ketoconazole[a]	
	Lidocaine	
	Maprotiline	
	Midazolam	
	Progesterone	
	Propanolol	
	Quinidine	
	Trimipramine	

For additional information, see the following selected references: http://www.aidsinfonyc.org/tag/science/pgp.html; http://www.mhc.com/PGP/index.html. [a]Drugs that are also CYP3A inhibitors

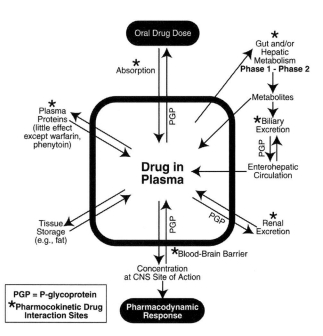

FIGURE 5.1 Pharmacokinetics and pharmacodynamics of a CNS drug. (Adapted from Werry, J.S. and Aman, M.G. (1993) *Practitioner's Guide to Psychoactive Drugs for Children and Adolescents*. New York and London: Plenum Medical Book Company.

act to block absorption from the gut and across the blood–brain barrier (BBB) and facilitate drug elimination in the kidney and bile ducts (see Fig. 5.1). The P-gp-based inhibition of absorption in the small intestine and BBB transport can itself be blocked or induced by other drugs. Only recently has this new category of drug interaction been described (von Moltke and Greenblatt, 2000; Westphal et al., 2000). Loperamide (an over-the-counter antidiarrheal opiate) can cause respiratory depression when the central nervous system (CNS) is exposed to increased levels after BBB P-gp is blocked by quinidine (Sadeque et al., 2000). Not only may other opiates enter the CNS when coadministered with BBB P-gp inhibitors, but other psychiatric and nonpsychiatric drugs can cause CNS toxicity through this mechanism even with "normal" blood concentrations (von Moltke and Greenblatt, 2001). HIV-related dementia may occur when alteration of BBB P-gps allows entry of toxins (Persidsky et al., 2000).

All plants, foods, and most drugs undergo processes that convert them from lipid-soluble to water-soluble agents to be inactivated. Exceptions include drugs that are already water-soluble: lithium (entirely) and gabapentin (mostly) are handled by the kidney. Most psychotropic drugs are metabolized in two steps by two distinct systems (see Fig. 5.2).

Phase 1 metabolic processes involve breaking off a part of the drug and inserting or uncovering a molecule (usually oxygen) to expose a chemical structure that serves as a "functional handle" for further phase 2 processing. The CYP enzymes are those generally responsible for phase 1 actions, and are primarily present in the gut and the liver (as well as in kidney, brain, and other tissues). Other phase 1 hydrolytic enzymes include plasma esterases, which are responsible for initiating metabolism of psychostimulants; microsomal epoxide hydrolases, which form carbamazepine 10,11 epoxide (an active metabolite of carbamazepine); and flavin-containing monooxygenases, which are involved in the metabolism of clozapine and, to a lesser extent, olanzapine (Tugnait et al., 1997; Callaghan et al., 1999).

Phase 2 reactions involve the formation of a link between the functionalized handle of a drug and a conjugate via a transferase. The most abundant conjugate is glucuronic acid, which is "hooked up" to the drug via uridine diphosphate glucuronyl transferases (UGTs). Unlike other phase 2 transferases that are cytosolic, UGTs are microsomal and have close physical proximity to CYPs. A few drugs (e.g., lorazepam, oxazepam, temazepam, lamotrigine, and others) do not undergo phase 1 reactions because they already have "a chemical handle" (a hydroxyl group), and they are directly conjugated. Other phase 2 systems such as N-acetyltransferases are known to acetylate clonazepam, phenelzine, and sulfotransferases, which conjugate acetaminophen. P-glycoproteins and phase 1 and phase 2 reactions are responsible for first pass metabolism, and many psychotropic drugs have a substantial fraction removed prior to entry into the systemic circulation.

CYTOCHROME P450 ENZYMES

Cytochrome P450 enzymes are a superfamily of heme-containing enzymes. Their amino acid sequences have been determined, and a naming system has been developed on the basis of their amino acid similarities. The broadest group is stated first, with increasingly specific groupings designated in the nomenclature. Currently recognized families are named from 1 to 4, and subfamilies from A to E, and specific enzymes are coded by specific genes from 1 on up. For example, CYP2D6 is an enzyme in the CYP2 family and D subfamily and is coded by gene 6. The CYPs that are near each other on the same gene and are related are grouped together (e.g., CYP3A4, CYP3A5, and CYP3A7) and are referred to collectively as *CYP 3A*. Of the 14 families of CYP enzymes identified in humans, one group is located in mitochondria and is involved in synthesis or metabolism of endogenous compounds (e.g., steroids, prostaglandins, and bile acids). The second CYP group is found in endoplasmic reticulum; and these are the phase 1 metabolizers described above.

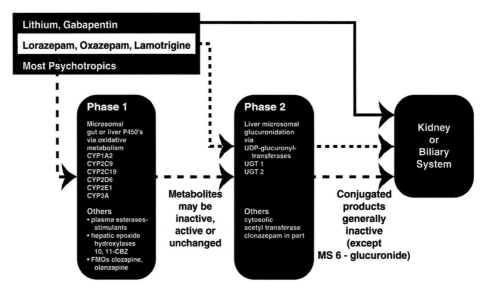

FIGURE 5.2 Phase 1 and phase 2 biotransformation.

At this time, only three families of hepatic CYP enzymes have been shown to be involved in human metabolism of exogenous agents. The responsible hepatic CYPs include CYP1A2, CYP2A6, CYP2B6, CYP2C8, CYP2C9, CYP2C19, CYP2D6, CYP2E1, and CYP3A. The ontogeny, genetics, and abundance of CYP enzymes that are most relevant to child psychiatrist are described in Table 5.2.

CYP3A is by far the single most important hepatic CYP family, since it metabolizes more than 30%–40% of drugs known to be metabolized by human CYP enzymes (de Wildt et al., 1999). Few drugs are substrates of a single CYP (e.g., nefazodone by CYP3A, desipramine by CYP2D6). Most drugs are metabolized by several CYP enzymes. Although there are five CYP enzymes found in the small intestine—CYP1A1, CYP2C19, CYP2D6, CYP3A4, and CYP3A5—CYP3A4 is the lion's share of the total. Drugs or foods may be preferentially metabolized by small intestine or liver CYP3A. Drugs can also inhibit or block a CYP in either the small intestine (e.g., CYP3A by grapefruit juice or St. John's wort) the liver (e.g., CYP3A by nefazodone), or both.

A drug may be a substrate of one or two CYP enzymes and inhibitor of none (e.g., quetiapine is a substrate of CYP3A, and it is not a CYP inhibitor); or a substrate of one and an inhibitor of the same CYP (e.g., nefazodone of CYP3A); or a substrate of one CYP and an inhibitor of another CYP (e.g., quinidine is a substrate of CYP3A and an inhibitor of CYP2D6). All individuals in some classes of drugs are metabolized by the same CYP nonsteroidal anti-inflammatory drugs (e.g., [NSAIDs] and COX-2 inhibitors by CYP2C9), and some members of some classes of drugs are metabolized by different CYPs (e.g., see Table 5.3. for pathways and inhibition of various SSRIs).

A classification system similar to that for the CYPs has been developed to characterize the UGT superfamily. There are two clinically significant hepatic UGT subfamilies (UGT1A and UGT2B) and 10 individual genes found in the liver (Tukey and Strassburg, 2000; http://www.mhc.com//cytochromes//UGT//index.html).

TABLE 5.2 *Hepatic Cytochrome P450 Characteristics*

	CYP1A2	CYP2C9	CYP2C19	CYP2D6	CYP2E1	CYP3A4	CYP3A5	CYP3A7
Chromosome	15	10	10	22	10	7	7	7
Ontogeny	Onset 3 months	Onset after birth	Onset after 1 month	? 3rd term fetus Onset after birth	? 3rd term fetus Onset after birth	? 3rd term fetus Onset 1 week after birth	Present in fetus	Major fetal CYP Decreases after birth
Percentage of adult CYP	50% at 1 year Increases at 3–5 years Decreases past puberty	30% at 1 month Slight decrease at 1 year		25% newborn 50% at 1 month	40% at 7 weeks 40% at 1 year	40% at 1 month 50% at 6–12 months		
Content of total CYPs	15%	20%	5%	<5%	10%	30%	Variable	<1% to variable
Genetics		Polymorphism Absent metabolizer: <% all races	Polymorphism Absent metabolizer: African 4%–7% Asian 12%–22% White 3%–5%	Polymorphism Absent metabolizer: African 7%–10% Asian 1% White 7%–10% Ultrarapid metabolizer: Ethiopian 30% White 1%–3.5%				

CYP, cytochrome P450.

Three extrahepatic UGTs exist, and intestinal UGTs have been shown to conjugate testosterone and some estrogens (Czernik et al., 2000).

Mechanism of Cytochrome P450 Involvement in Drug Interactions

If one drug blocks one or more CYP enzymes and another drug is added that is metabolized only by the blocked CYP, then more of the second drug enters the systemic circulation unmetabolized, and its circulating levels are increased. This effect is amplified with continued dosing of the combination.

Vignette 5.1 Blood Concentration of Substrates Is Increased by Cytochrome P450 Inhibition

A child with Tourette's disorder is treated with a daily dose of 2 mg of pimozide for tics. A family doctor treats a streptococcal pharyngitis with clarithromycin, and 24 hours later the child develops palpitations. An electrocardiogram (ECG) reveals a QTc prolongation to 0.465 milliseconds.

In this example, clarithromycin, a potent CYP3A inhibitor blocks the principal pathway of pimozide metabolism (CYP3A), and plasma concentrations of pimozide increase. A higher pimozide concentration (a pharmacokinetic effect) is associated with prolongation of QTc in EKG readings and potentially fatal torsades de pointes (via potassium channel blockade, a pharmacodynamic effect; see Flockhart et al., 2000, Mayhew et al., 2000). As exemplified by this vignette, the

pharmacokinetic effect of inhibition occurs relatively quickly, since ongoing metabolic processes are interrupted.

Vignette 5.2 Blood Concentrations of Active Metabolites of Substrate Pro-drugs Are Reduced by Cytochrome P450 Inhibitors

A 17-year-old with major depressive disorder is treated with fluoxetine at 40 mg/d. She has a ligament injury while playing soccer. Fluoxetine is discontinued 5 days before surgery. After surgery, she is given oxycodone and continues to complain of pain.

This vignette illustrates a different aspect of CYP inhibition. Oxycodone, hydrocodone, and codeine are all pro-drugs that are converted to active analgesics by CYP2D6 metabolism. If their conversion is blocked by co-prescribed drugs, less analgesia will result. In this example, although fluoxetine itself had been discontinued, its long-lived metabolite, norfluoxetine, was still present, and it inhibited the conversion of the pro-drug oxycodone to its active metabolite.

Types of Cytochrome P450 Inhibitors

There are three biochemical mechanisms of CYP inhibition: competitive, mechanism-based, and metabolite–intermediate-complex (Fig. 5.3). Each type of inhibitor differs in the nature of CYP binding. Competitive inhibitors are reversibly bound and can be "competed off" of the docking site if another substrate of higher affinity is present at a higher concentration. Therefore,

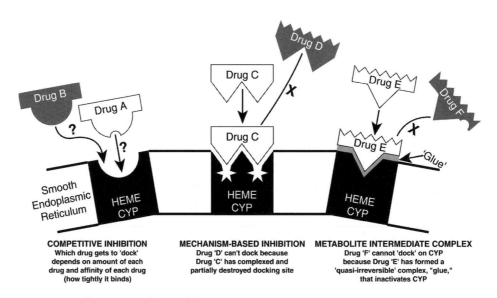

FIGURE 5.3 Different types of CYP inhibitors.

drug interactions are more likely to occur with drugs of the highest affinity (and lowest Kis, e.g., ketoconazole and related compounds are among the most potent competitive inhibitors). Metabolite–intermediate-complex inhibitors bind very tightly to the CYP but do not destroy the docking site, as do mechanism-based inhibitors. Since neither of these latter types of inhibitors can be pushed off the site by other drugs, these types of inhibitors are more likely to cause clinically significant interactions than drugs that are low-affinity competitive inhibitors (e.g., in Vignette 5.1, clarithromycin is a metabolite–intermediate-complex inhibitor).

Intestinal P-glycoprotein and CYP3A as partners in cytochrome P450 inhibition

There is enormous interindividual variation in the amount of both intestinal CYPs and P-gp (Hebert, 1997; Paine et al., 1997). P-glycoprotein acts as a gate-keeper to a drug's contact with intestinal CYP enzymes. Although P-gp and CYP3A4 can function in a complimentar fashion to reduce a drug's entry through the intestine, regulation of their activity is not coordinated (Wacher et al., 1995). It is clear that some drugs are both P-gp inhibitors and CYP3A inhibitors (e.g., erythromycin, ketoconazole, quinidine; see Table 5.1). The blood concentration of vulnerable substrates can be dramatically increased by double inhibitors, and these drug pairs seem more likely to produce clinically significant drug interactions.

Cytochrome P450 inhibition and clearance of drugs metabolized by the liver

Clinicians should note that if a drug has high presystemic clearance (i.e., most of the drug is metabolized before reaching the systemic circulation) and an inhibitor of its metabolism is added, the interaction that results may well be characterized by an immediately elevated plasma drug concentration of the substrate drug (e.g., triazolam is metabolized extensively by CYP3A and ketoconazole has an immediate effect on its concentration; see Greenblatt et al., 1998). An increase in blood concentrations may result in the *immediate* development of symptoms and signs of benzodiazepine toxicity (e.g., increased sedation, impaired psychomotor coordination, confusion). However, if a drug has a low presystemic clearance (i.e., little of the drug is metabolized by CYP3A before reaching the systemic circulation) and an inhibitor of its metabolism is added, little change in plasma drug concentration will occur after the first pass. It is only with repeated drug administration of both drugs that a cumulative effect

will be evident (e.g., alprazolam and ketoconazole will result in little initial benzodiazepine toxicity, but toxicity may develop over a week). This distinction is important for clinicians, as two patterns of drug interaction are evident: those occurring *immediately* after the addition of a second drug, and those occurring *later*, when the second drug has reached steady state.

Cytochrome P450 Induction

Some drugs can also increase the amount of active CYP enzyme via effects on protein stabilization or the transcriptional apparatus. This process is called *induction*.

Vignette 5.3 Blood Concentration of Substrate Is Reduced by Cytochrome P450 Inducer

A 16-year-old-girl who has been using levonorgestrel (Norplant) for contraception without side effects is treated for bipolar affective disorder with gabapentin. Because of inadequate response and weight gain, topiramate is added. Ten days later, the teen complains of breakthrough bleeding.

In this vignette, topiramate (an inducer of CYP3A) has decreased the plasma concentration of levonorgestrel (a CYP3A substrate) by inducing its metabolism. The symptoms of breakthrough bleeding reflect decreased hormonal levels and possible ovulation. Induction takes time to bring about its effect (3–10 days), since it involves the production of additional CYP protein. It also takes time to stop (1–5 days), so an inducer need not be present for induction to continue. In this vignette, a clinician should warn the patient to use barrier contraception for the rest of the cycle, even if topiramate is discontinued. Another vignette illustrates the importance of clinical effects beginning sometime after the introduction of an inducer and lasting well beyond its discontinuation.

Vignette 5.4 Induction of Cytochrome P450 Produces Pharmadynamic Effects after Inducer Is Discontinued

A child with attention-deficit hyperactivity disorder [ADHD] and conduct disorder is treated with 45 mg/d of methylphenidate and 2 mg/d of risperidone. A new diagnosis of complex partial seizures is made and the child is started on carbamazepine. About 10 days after the initiation of carbamazepine, the child develops withdrawal dyskinesias of mouth and tongue. After discontinuation of carbamazepine, the movements last for 1 week.

Typical inducers include the older anticonvulsants, i.e., barbiturates, primidone, phenytoin, and carbamazepine; some newer drugs, e.g., topiramate, felbamate, and oxcarbazepine; and chronic alcohol usage and smoking (see Table 5.3). Foods and herbals such as St. John's wort, brussel sprouts, kale, brocolli and other brassica vegetables, and charbroiled meat may also act as inducers; all induce CYP1A2. It is also now known that P-gp can be induced (see Table 5.1), and some herbals and drugs can be double or triple inducers (e.g., St John's wort induces CYP3A, and P-gp; rifampin is an inducer of CYP2A6, CYP3A, P-gp, and UGT). As a result, both rifampin and St. John's wort can cause very significant reductions in blood concentrations of substrates by increasing metabolism through multiple metabolic pathways.

Hepatic Cytochrome P450 Drug Interaction Table

The Hepatic CYP Drug Interaction Table (Table 5.3) provides a way of anticipating CYP-based interactions. Substrates, inhibitors, and inducers are arranged in vertical columns by CYP. If two drugs are on the same column, the plasma levels of drug can be increased or decreased, depending on whether one drug is an inducer or inhibitor of the substrate of a second drug. This chart can be used to predict the possibility of plasma concentration changes but not the pharmacodynamic consequences of them. Whether, in fact, an interaction will occur depends on host factors, the drugs involved, and the resultant pharmacodynamic changes.

Drug Factors

It has already been stated that the type of inhibitor and whether the second drug has low or high first-pass metabolism are important. Some other important drug factors are (1) how avidly the inhibitor is bound to the CYP, usually measured by an inhibition constant (K_i), with lower values representing tighter avidity; (2) the amount of drug present at the CYP; (3) whether the substrate drug is relatively protected from interaction by virtue of multiple and uninvolved pathways; and (4) whether the substrate drug has a narrow therapeutic index, which may increase the likelihood of toxicity or lack of therapeutic efficacy. Examples of drugs with narrow therapeutic indices that are commonly used in child psychiatry include tricyclics, carbamazepine, thioridazine, and pimozide. Both risperidone and olanzapine shift from atypical to typical antipsychotic profiles when higher doses are used, and higher dosing is associated with increased parkinsonian side effects.

Host Factors

Host factors include the amount of individual CYPs, which may vary as much as 10-to 100-fold between individuals, as well as the efficiency of individual CYPs. The variations are related to (1) food intake (e.g., watercress inhibits CYP2E1; see Leclercq et al., 1998; char-broiled meat induces CYP1A2; see Fontana et al., 1999); (2) cigarette smoking, which potently induces CYP1A2; (3) alcohol intake, which acutely inhibits CYP2E1 and chronically induces it and CYP3A (Fraser, 1997); (4) inflammation and infection (Renton, 2000); (5) gender differences, which may play a role but have not been well characterized; (6) genetic polymorphisms; and (7) youth. Because of the importance of the last two factors, they will be discussed in detail.

Genetic polymorphisms

CYP2C9, CYP2C19, and CYP2D6 have genetic variations that lead to a lack of expression of CYP protein (see Chapter 7). Although the term *slow metabolizer* has been applied, metabolism in these individuals via these routes is not slow, but rather absent (see Table 5.2). This defect leads to increased concentrations of drugs that are substrates of that CYP (the genetic condition analogous to CYP inhibition without an inhibitor).

Vignette 5.5 Increased Blood Concentration of Substrate in Individual Who Is an Absent Metabolizer of Cytochrome P450 Enzymes

A 10-year-old boy has a 4-month history of fears of contamination and of refusing food because "there might be monster drool in it." He is begun on clomipramine (CMI), initially 25 mg at night, and the dosage is gradually increased to three times daily. He complains of mild confusion and dry mouth. A trough blood level of CMI and its demethylated metabolite reveal that CMI is 455 ng/mL and desmethyl CMI is 48 ng/mL.

In this vignette, the child developed central anticholinergic toxicity from the elevated concentration of CMI because he is an "absent metabolizer" of CYP2D6. It is obvious that if an individual is genetically deficient of a given CYP, the addition of an inhibitor of that CYP cannot decrease production any further (e.g., if this child were given paroxetine, blood levels of CMI would not increase, and if the teen in Vignette 5.2 were an absent metabolizer of CYP2D6, she would have had no analgesia from hydrocodone, even without a CYP2D6 inhibitor).

TABLE 5.3 *Cytochrome P450 Drug Interaction Table*

CYP1A2	CYP2C9	CYP2C19	CYP2D6	CYP2E1	CYP3A

Substrates

CYP1A2	CYP2C9	CYP2C19	CYP2D6	CYP2E1	CYP3A
Psychotropics	*Psychotropics*	*Psychotropics*	Psychotropics	Anesthetics	Psychotropics
Clozapine	Fluoxetine	Amitriptyline	*Antidepressants*	Enflurane	*Antidepressants*
Fluvoxamine	Sertraline	Citalopram	Amitriptyline	Halothane	Citalopram
Olanzapine	Valproate	Clomipramine	Citalopram	Isoflurane	Clomipramine
Propranolol		Imipramine	Clomipramine	Sevoflurane	Fluoxetine
	Angiotensin 2	Moclobemide	Desipramine		Imipramine
Others	*blockers*	Sertaline	Fluoxetine	*Others*	Mirtazapine
Caffeine	Irbesartan		Fluvoxamine	Acetaminophen	Sertraline
Ondansetron	Losartan	*Anticonvulsants*	Imipramine	Caffeine	Trazodone
Theophylline		Diazepam	Maprotiline	Ethanol	
Zolmitriptan	*NSAIDs/Cox-2*	Phenytoin	Mirtazapine	Felbamate	*Antipsychotics*
	Blockers	Phenobarbital	Nortriptyline	Isoniazid	(Clozapine)
	Celecoxib	S-mephenytoin	Paroxetine	Theophylline	Haloperidol
	Diclofenac		Sertraline		Quetiapine
	Ibuprofen	*Proton pump*	Trimipramine		Pimozide
	Indomethacin	*blockers*	Venlafaxine		Risperidone
	Meloxicam	Lansoprazole			(Ziprasidone)
	Naproxen	Omeprazole	*Antipsychotics*		
	Piroxicam	Pantaprazole	Chlorpromazine		*Anxiolytics/hypnotics*
			Haloperidol		Alprazolam
	Rofecoxib	*Others*	Perphenazine		Buspirone
	Suprofen	Indomethacin	Risperidone		Clonazepam
		Progesterone	Thioridazine		Diazepam
	Hypoglucemics	Proguanil			Midazolam
	Glipizide		*Psychostimulants*		Triazolam
	Tolbutamide		Amphetamine		Zaleplon
			(Methylphenidates)		Zolpidem
	Others				
	Mestranol		*Others*		Anticonvulsants
	Phenytoin		*Antiarrythmics*		Carbamazepine
	Sulfa drugs		Flecainide		Ethosuximide
	Torsemide		Mexiletine		Tiagabine
	Warfarin				
	Zafirlukast		*Antihistamines*		*Drugs of abuse treatment*
			Mequitazine		Buprenorphine
			Promethazine		Cocaine
					Codeine
			Beta-blockers		Fentanyl
					LAAM
			Cough medicines		Methadone
					PCP
			Drugs of abuse		
			Ecstasy		*Others*
					Calcium channel blockers
			Opiates (pro-drugs)		Cyclosporin
			Codeine		Ethiny lestradiol
			Oxycodone		Erthromycin/macrolides
					HIV antivirals
			Tolterodine		Levonorgestrel
					Nonsedating antihistamines
					Oxybutynin
					Quinidine/quinine
					Steroids
					Tacrolimus
					Tolterodine

(continued)

TABLE 5.3 *Cytochrome P450 Drug Interaction Table (continued)*

CYP1A2	CYP2C9	CYP2C19	CYP2D6	CYP2E1	CYP3A
Inducers					
Brassica Vegetables	Carbamazepine	Carbamazepine	?Dexamethasone	Ethanol (chronic)	Carbamazepine
Carbamazepine	Rifampin	Prednisone	?Rifampin	Isoniazid after	Dexamethasone
Char-broiled meat	Secobarbital	Rifampin		discontinuing	Efavirenz
Cigarette smoke					Ethanol (chronic)
Modafinil					Felbamate
					Modafinil
					Nevirapine
					Oxcarbazepine
					Phenobarbital
					Phenytoin
					Primidone
					Rifampin
					Ritonavir (chronic)
					St. John's wort
					Topiramate
					Troglitazone
Inhibitors					
Amiodarone	Amiodarone	Cimetidine	Amiodarone	Disulfarim	Amiodarone
Caffeine	Fluconazole	Ethinyl	Amitriptyline	Ethanol (acute)	Cimetidine
Cimetidine	Fluoxetine	estradiol	Chlorpheniramine		Diltiazem
Ciprofloxacin	Fluvoxamine	Felbamate	Cimetidine		Erythromycin/macrolides
Enoxacin	Isoniazid	Fluconazole	Clomipramine		Fluconazole
Ethinyl estradiol	Miconazole	Fluoxetine	Cocaine		Gestodene
Fluvoxamine	Phenylbutazone	Fluvoxamine	Desipramine		Grapefruit juice
	Sertraline	Lansoprazole	Dextropropoxyphene		Itraconazole
	Sulfa drugs	Modafinil	Diphenhydramine		Ketoconazole
	Valproate	Omeprazole	Fluoxetine		Nefazodone
	Zafirlukast	Ticlopidine	Haloperidol		Protease inhibitors (acute)
		Topiramate	Imipramine		Zafirlukast
			Methadone		
			Moclobemide		
			Nortriptyline		
			Paroxetine		
			Pimozide		
			Quinidine		
			Ritonavir		
			Sertraline		
			Thioridazine		
			Ticlopidine		

( ) indicate a minor pathway.
CYP, cytochrome P4SO; LAAM, levo-alpha-acetylmethadol ;NSAID, non-steroidal anti-inflammatory drug; PCP, phencyclidine.

CYP2D6 is unique in that there are also genetic variations that lead to a continuum of metabolism, including ultrafast metabolism (the genetic condition analogous to CYP induction without an inducer). Through the mechanism of gene amplification about 30% of Ethiopians (Aklillu et al., 1996) and approximately 1%–3.5% of Caucasians share this trait. At the other end of the continuum, Asians (as a group) have less CYP2D6. As decreased metabolizers of CYP2D6, blood concentrations of CYP 2D6 substrates in some Asians would be somewhat elevated, and the addition of a CYP2D6 inhibitor would further increase levels. One-fifth of Asians are genetically deficient in CYP2C19 (which is involved in some of the demethylation pathways of tricyclic antidepressants). Both factors may be responsible for some Asians having higher plasma levels of tricyclic antidepressants than those of their Caucasian counterparts.

Genotyping has largely replaced the earlier biologic tests used to characterize CYP polymorphisms. Clinically, if a youth has had an adverse outcome from low doses of medications known to be CYP substrates, then a clinician might suspect alterations in metabolic capacity. The history of a child who has not experienced analgesia with codeine (and others) or a child's a bad reaction to cough syrup (because of the accumulation of dextromethorphan) is a clue to the presence of an absent CYP2D6 metabolizer. There are known but less-characterized genetic variations of P-gps and UGTs.

Ontogeny of Cytochrome P450 Enzymes

During fetal life, hepatic drug metabolism is predominantly via CYP3A7 and sulfation (Oesterheld, 1998). Since the UGT enzyme 1A1 is associated with the metabolism of bilirubin and is reduced in newborns, some infants develop icterus. Throughout the 1980s, these vulnerable infants were treated with phenobarbital to induce glucuronidation (Rubaltelli and Griffith, 1992). The rest of the drug-metabolizing CYPs come "online" either during fetal development or during the early months of infancy (see Table 5.2). When these systems reach maximal efficiency is not known, but it is probable that they do so by the toddler years. It is well documented that during latency, children require higher doses of CYP-metabolized drugs. It used to be theorized that this was a consequence of the larger liver and hence larger CYP capacity in children. However, it has been shown that children are better metabolizers, even when considered on a weight-adjusted basis, which suggests that children's CYP enzymes are more efficient. However, a recent attempt to categorize this effect in vitro has *not* shown children's hepatic CYPs to be more efficient than those of adults (Blanco et al., 2000). The efficiency of the CYP enzymes of teens is thought to be comparable to that of adults.

PHARMACOKINETIC/PHARMACODYNAMIC INTERACTIONS AND THE CENTRAL SEROTONIN SYNDROME

Pharmacokinetic changes are clinically important only if they engender pharmacodynamic ones. A dramatic example of this linkage is exemplified by the CSS. Previously thought to be uncommon, more than 125 cases of CSS have been reported (Mills, 1997; Mason et al., 2000, Radomski et al., 2000). Because of the common usage of SSRIs and co-medications, which include St. John's wort, some pro-serotonergic opioids, and ec-

stasy, several authors have warned of the likelihood of both substantial increases in the incidence of CSS and of its current underdiagnosis (Lane and Baldwin 1997; Bowdle 1998; DeBattista et al., 1998, MacKay et al., 1999, Moritz et al., 1999, Sampson and Warner 1999; Beckman et al., 2000; Fugh-Berman, 2000; Perry, 2000). As pediatric clinicians have become more aware of the syndrome, cases have been reported in children and teens (Levy et al., 1996; Pao and Tipnis, 1997; Radomski 1998; Gill et al., 1999; Horowitz and Mullins, 1999; Lee and Lee, 1999; Spirko and Wiley, 1999).

Central Serotonin Syndrome is manifest by autonomic, neuromuscular, and cognitive symptoms. Mild symptoms can include tremor, incoordination, and confusion. Moderate symptoms can manifest as shivering, sweating, hyperreflexia, and agitation, and severe symptoms include fever, myoclonus, and diarrhea. This syndrome is usually associated with two or more drugs that increase central serotonin transmission and affect the 5-HT$_{1A}$ receptor (see Table 5.4).

TABLE 5.4 *Pro-serotonegic Agents Implicated in Central Serotonin Syndrome*

Amitripyline

Amphetamine

Buspirone

Citalopram

Clomipramine

Clonazepam

Cocaine

Dextromethorphan

Fluoxetine

Fluvoxamine

Imipramine

Lithium

Meperidine

Methylenedioxymethamphetamine (MDMA, ecstasy)

Monoamine oxidase inhibitors (MAOIs) and reversible inhibitors of MAO-A

Nefazodone

Paroxetine

St. John's wort

Sertraline

Tramadol

Trazodone

Venlafaxine

Data compiled from Sternbach (1991), Lane et al. (1997), and Gilman (1999).

Symptoms rarely begin after an increase in monotherapy, but more typically, they start immediately or soon after the addition of a second pro-serotonergic agent and then progress rapidly. When SSRIs are one of the causative agents, it is sometimes difficult to diagnose this condition early because the side effects of the SSRIs can overlap with early symptoms of CSS. It is therefore prudent to closely monitor and remove SSRIs if CSS is suspected. When mild, the symptoms usually resolve within 24 hours. More serious symptoms of CSS require vigorous medical support as fatalities have been reported, and agents such as cyproheptadine, a nonselective serotonin receptor antagonist can be used to treat the syndrome (Lane and Baldwin 1997; Graudins et al., 1998).

The most serious cases of CSS have been associated with drugs that block both serotonin exits: reuptake and monamine oxidase routes (e.g., SSRIs or clomipramine and a monoamine oxidase inhibitor [MAOI]). Although child psychiatrists rarely use MAOIs, they should be mindful of serotonergic drugs that they do prescribe and that are more likely to be associated with CSS. Fluvoxamine, fluoxetine, and paroxetine all have nonlinear kinetics and aggressive increases in dosage can result in higher than expected levels of drug at serotonin receptors. Increased levels of serotonin may also occur with *particular combinations* of serotonergic drugs. Fluvoxamine, a potent inhibitor of CYP1A2, CYP2C19, and CYP3A, increases plasma concentrations (up to eight-fold) of the serotonergic tertiary tricyclics (e.g., amitriptyline, clomipramine, and imipramine) since they are substrates of those pathways (Wagner and Vause, 1995). Nefazodone is a potent CYP3A inhibitor and may have similar effects. Since fluoxetine and paroxetine are potent CYP2D6 inhibitors, caution needs to be exercised when they are combined with serotonergic agents that are CYP2D6 substrates (e.g., dextromethorphan in cough syrups, tramadol, and tricyclics). Since St. John's wort is an inducer of CYP3A, it is more likely to cause CSS, in combination with pro-serotonergic agents that are not substrates of this CYP. Central Serotonin Syndrome can also occur when fluoxetine is discontinued and another serotonergic drug is added, since fluoxetine's long-lived metabolite norfluoxetine is present for several weeks after discontinuation (Lane and Baldwin, 1997).

HOW TO USE INFORMATION IN THIS CHAPTER

When reviewing medications of a new patient (including herbal remedies, over-the-counter drugs, anabolic steroids, contraceptives, and recreational drugs) or when a clinician adds a second or third drug to a patient's drug regimen, it is recommended that a proactive stance towards drug interactions be taken. First, one should use a search engine such as PubMed or OVID, entering the names of the drugs in question along with "drug interaction," to ascertain if drug interactions between these drugs have been reported (this search will include pharmacokinetic and pharmacodynamic causes). Even if no drug interactions have been reported, to see if one is possible, a clinician can scan the hepatic CYP Drug Interaction Table (Table 5.3) or a table on the Web at http://www.medicine.iupui.edu/flockhart/ to see if the drugs share CYP pathways. A clinician may also obtain information on the CYP metabolism of specific drugs on Web site: http://www.gentest.com/human_p450_database/index.html. P450+, a commercial database, available at http:www.mhc.com/Cytochrome/ combines CYP-based and glucuronidation-based drug interactions. Epocrates is available for Palm OS handheld devices at http://wwww.epocrates.com/.

Vignette 5.6 How a clinican Deals with a Possible Drug Interaction

A latency-aged child with asthma treated with a new anti-asthma drug, zafirlukast, at 10 mg bid, develops a major depression. Because two relatives with depression have responded to fluoxetine, it is tentatively selected as a possible antidepressant. Fluoxetine is one of the SSRIs in the clinician's personal formulary. Through a check of PubMed no published interaction between these drugs is found. However, a scan of the Hepatic CYP Drug Interaction Table reveals that zafirlukast is an inhibitor of CYP2C9 and CYP3A, pathways of fluoxetine, and norfluoxetine is an inhibitor of CYP2C9, the major pathway of zafirlukast. The clinician decides to be cautious and to start the patient at 5 mg of fluoxetine and to carefully watch for side effects. The clinician alerts the pediatrician to monitor side effects of zafirlukast.

This vignette illustrates several important clinical points. First, there is a variable amount of existing literature available on particular drug interactions. Some drug pairs have undergone in vitro testing, and/or there are relevant case reports and/or clinical studies that detail the extent of the interaction. Since in vivo studies may not show the same results as in vitro studies, a clinician should always give priority to clinical trials or case reports. If a drug is relatively new to the market (as is zafirlukast), there may be few drug interaction studies available. When there are more than two drugs involved, clinicians are usually on their own. Clinicians should expect to anticipate *possible* drug interactions, and they can limit their drug formulary and develop a team approach with colleagues (as illustrated in this vignette).

Second, rarely will clinical studies supply information that allows a clinician to make a "cookbook" translation of the data (e.g., when sertraline is added to desipramine, expect a 25%–40% increase in desipramine in a child who is an extensive metabolizer of CYP2D6; Alderman et al., 1997). If one (or both) of the drugs is a CYP inhibitor and is added to a substrate of that CYP, then the clinician may decide to dose by starting low and going slow or to change one of the medications to a less potent inhibitor or to a drug that is not a substrate. If one of the drugs is an inducer and if an estimation can be made from clinical studies as to the extent of the interaction, then the clinician may decide to use the drug combination and to increase the substrate drug as needed. In either case, the clinician should take into account the drug and host factors as discussed in this chapter and the possible pharmacodynamic effects of co-pharmacy or polypharmacy.

CONCLUSION

In the next few years, advances in genotyping technology will make cytochromal genotyping readily available. Computer drug-interaction programs that detail both *reported* and *predicted* CYP-based, glucuronidation-based, and Pgp-based drug interactions are just emerging to be part of a clinician's armamentarium. To use these "smart" technologies competently, clinicians must still be competent prescribers who understand and use basic information about pharmacokinetics, pharmacodynamics, and drug interactions.

ACKNOWLEDGMENTS
The authors wish to thank Dr. Richard I. Shader for his careful reading of the text, but claim any errors as solely their own. This work was supported in part by a Center for Education and Research in Therapeutics Grant from the Agency for Health Care Research and Quality, Washington, DC, and by R01-GM56898-01 from the National Institute of General Medical Sciences, Bethesda, MD.

REFERENCES

Adlaf, E.M., Paglia, A., Ivis, F.J., and Ialomiteanu. A. (2000) Nonmedical drug use among adolescent students: highlights from the 1999 Ontario Student Drug Use Survey. *CMAJ* 162:1677–1680.

Aklillu, E., Persson, I., Bertilsson, L., Johansson, I., Rodrigues, F., and Ingelman-Sundberg, M. (1996) Frequent distribution of ultrarapid metabolizers of debrisoquine in an ethiopian population carrying duplicated and multiduplicated functional CYP2D6 alleles. *Pharmacol Exp Ther* 278:441–446.

Alderman, J., Preskorn, S.H., Greenblatt, D.J., Harrison, W., Penenberg, D., Allison, J., and Chung, M. (1997) Desipramine pharmacokinetics when coadministered with paroxetine or sertraline in extensive metabolizers. *J Clin Psychopharmacol* 17:284–291.

Beckman, S.E., Sommi, R.W., and Switzer, J. (2000) Consumer use of St. John's wort: a survey on effectiveness, safety, and tolerability. *Pharmacotherapy* 20:568–574.

Blanco, J.G., Harrison, P.L., Evans. W.E., and Relling, M.V. (2000) Human cytochrome P450 maximal activities in pediatric versus adult liver. *Drug Metab Dispos* 28:379–382.

Bowdle, T.A. (1998) Adverse effects of opioid agonists and agonist–antagonists in anaesthesia. *Drug Saf.* 19:173–189.

Callaghan, J.T., Bergstrom, R.F., Ptak, L.R., and Beasley, C.M. (1999) Olanzapine, pharmacokinetic and pharmacodynamic profile. *Clin Pharmacokinet* 37:177–193.

Carrillo, J.A., Ramos, S.I., Herraiz, A.G., Llerena, A., Agundez, J.A., Berecz, R., Duran, M., and Benitez, J. (1999) Pharmacokinetic interaction of fluvoxamine and thioridazine in schizophrenic patients. *J Clin Psychopharmacol* 19:494–499.

Czernik, P.J., Little, J.M., Barone, G.W., Raufman, J.P., and Radominska-Pandya, A. (2000) Glucuronidation of estrogens and retinoic acid and expression of UDP-glucuronosyltransferase 2B7 in human intestinal mucosa. *Drug Metab Dispos* 28:1210–1216.

DeBattista, C., Sofuoglu, M., and Schatzberg, A.F. (1998) Serotonergic synergism: the risks and benefits of combining the selective serotonin reuptake inhibitors with other serotonergic drugs. *Biol Psychiatry* 44:341–347.

de Wildt, S.N., Kearns, G.L., Leeder, J.S., and van den Anker, J.N. (1999) Cytochrome P450 3A: ontogeny and drug disposition. *Clin Pharmacokinet* 37:485–505.

Evans, N.A. (1997) Gym and tonic: a profile of 100 male steroid users. *Br J Sports Med* 31:54–58.

Flockhart, D.A., Drici, M.D., Kerbusch, T., Soukhova, N., Richard, E., Pearle, P.L., Mahal, S.K., and Babb, V.J. (2000) Studies on the mechanism of a fatal clarithromycin–pimozide interaction in a patient with Tourette syndrome. *J Clin Psychopharmacol* 20:317–324.

Fontana, R.J., Lown, K.S., Paine, M.F., Fortlage, L., Santella, R.M., Felton, J.S., Knize, M.G., Greenberg, A., and Watkins, P.B. (1999) Effects of a chargrilled meat diet on expression of CYP3A, CYP1A, and P-glycoprotein levels in healthy volunteers. *Gastroenterology* 117:89–98.

Fraser, A.G. (1997) Pharmacokinetic interactions between alcohol and other drugs. *Clin Pharmacokinet* 33:79–90. Friedman, E.H. (1994) Re: bradycardia and somnolence after adding fluoxetine to pimozide regimen. *Can J Psychiatry* 39:634.

Frye, M.A., Ketter, T.A., Leverich, G.S., Huggins, T., Lantz, C., Denicoff, K.D., and Post, R.M. (2000) The increasing use of polypharmacotherapy for refractory mood disorders: 22 years of study. *J Clin Psychiatry* 61:9–15.

Fugh-Berman, A. (2000) Herb–drug interactions. *Lancet* 8;355:134–138.

Gill, M., LoVecchio, F., and Selden, B. (1999) Serotonin syndrome in a child after a single dose of fluvoxamine. *Ann Emerg Med* 33:457–459.

Gillman, P.K. (1999) The serotonin syndrome and its treatment. *J Psychopharmacol* 13:100–109.

Graudins, A., Stearman, A., and Chan, B. (1998) Treatment of the serotonin syndrome with cyproheptadine. *J Emerg Med* 16:615–619.

Greenblatt, D.J., Wright, C.E., von Moltke, L.L., Harmatz, J.S., Ehrenberg, B.L., Harrel, L.M., Corbett, K., Counihan, M., Tobias, S., and Shader, R.I. (1998) Ketoconazole inhibition of triazolam and alprazolam clearance: differential kinetic and dynamic consequences. *Clin Pharmacol Ther* 64:237–247.

Hebert, M.F. (1997) Contributions of hepatic and intestinal metabolism and P-glycoprotein to cyclosporine and tacrolimus oral drug delivery. *Adv Drug Deliv Rev* 27:201–214.

Horowitz, B.Z. and Mullins, M.E. (1999) Cyproheptadine for serotonin syndrome in an accidental pediatric sertraline ingestion. *Pediatr Emerg Care* 15:325–327.

Horrigan, J.P. and Barnhill, L.J. (1994) Paroxetine-pimozide drug interaction. *J Am Acad Child Adolesc Psychiatry* 33:1060–1061.

Jensen, P.S., Bhatara, V.S., Vitiello, B., Hoagwood, K., Feil, M., and Burke, L.B. (1999) Psychoactive medication prescribing practices for U.S. children: gaps between research and clinical practice. *J Am Acad Child Adolesc Psychiatry* 38:557–565.

Lane, R. and Baldwin, D. (1997) Selective serotonin reuptake inhibitor–induced serotonin syndrome. *J Clin Psychopharmacol* 17:208–221.

Leclercq, I., Desager, J.P., and Horsmans, Y. (1998) Inhibition of chlorzoxazone metabolism, a clinical probe for CYP2E1, by a single ingestion of watercress. *Clin Pharmacol Ther* 64:144–149.

Lee, D.O. and Lee, C.D. (1999) Serotonin syndrome in a child associated with erythromycin and sertraline. *Pharmacotherapy* 19:894–896.

Levy, F., Einfeld, S., and Looi, J. (1996) Combined pharmacotherapy or polypharmacy? *J Paediatr Child Health* 32:265–266.

Mackay, F.J., Dunn, N.R., and Mann, R.D. (1999) Antidepressants and the serotonin syndrome in general practice. *Br J Gen Pract* 49:871–874.

Mason, P.J., Morris, V.A., and Balcezak, T.J. (2000) Serotonin syndrome. Presentation of 2 cases and review of the literature. *Medicine* (Baltimore) 79:201–209.

Mayhew, B.S., Jones, D.R., and Hall, S.D. (2000) An in vitro model for predicting in vivo inhibition of cytochrome P450 3A4 by metabolic intermediate complex formation. *Drug Metab Dispos* 28:1031–1037.

Maynard, G.L. and Soni, P. (1996) Thioridazine interferences with imipramine metabolism and measurement. *Ther Drug Monit* 18:729–731.

Mills, K.C. (1997) Serotonin syndrome. A clinical update. *Crit Care Clin* 13:763–783.

Moritz, F., Goulle, J.P., Girault, C., Clarot, F., Droy, J.M., and Muller, J.M. (1999) Toxicological analysis in agitated patients. *Intensive Care Med* 25:852–854.

Oesterheld, J.R. (1998) A review of developmental aspects of cytochrome P450. *J Child Adolesc Psychopharmacol* 8:161–74.

Paine, M.F., Khalighi, M., Fisher, J.M., Shen, D.D., Kunze, K.L., Marsh, C.L., Perkins, J.D., and Thummel, K.E. (1997) Characterization of interintestinal and intraintestinal variations in human CYP3A-dependent metabolism. *Pharmacol Exp Ther* 283:1552–1562.

Pao, M. and Tipnis, T. (1997) Serotonin syndrome after sertraline overdose in a 5-year-old girl. *Arch Pediatr Adolesc Med* 151:1064–1067.

Perry, N.K. (2000) Venlafaxine-induced serotonin syndrome with relapse following amitriptyline. *Postgrad Med J* 7:54–56.

Persidsky, Y., Rasmussen, J., Suryadevara, R., Poluektova, L., Zelyvianskaya, M., Moran, T., Miller, D., and Gendelman, H. (2000) Impairments of blood-brain barrier function in HIV-1 associated dementia [abstract]. Presented at th 7th Conference on Retroviruses and Opportunistic Infections, Alexandria, VA.

Radomski, J.W. (1998) Serotonin syndrome in a teenager following overdose of dothiepine hydrochloride. *J Child Adolesc Psychopharmacol* 8:201–204.

Radomski, J.W., Dursun, S.M., Reveley, M.A., and Kutcher, S.P. (2000) An exploratory approach to the serotonin syndrome: an update of clinical phenomenology and revised diagnostic criteria. *Med Hypotheses* 55:218–224.

Ragheb, M. (1990) The clinical significance of lithium–nonsteroidal anti-inflammatory drug interactions. *J Clin Psychopharmacol* 10:350–354.

Renton, K.W. (2000) Hepatic drug metabolism and immunostimulation. *Toxicology* 17;142:173–178.

Rittmannsberger, H., Meise, U., Schauflinger, K., Horvath, E., Donat, H., and Hinterhuber, H. (1999) Polypharmacy in psychiatric treatment. Patterns of psychotropic drug use in Austrian psychiatric clinics. *Eur Psychiatry* 14:33–40.

Rubaltelli, F.F. and Griffith, P.F. (1992) Management of neonatal hyperbilirubinaemia and prevention of kernicterus. *Drugs* 43:864–872.

Sadeque, A.J., Wandel, C., He, H., Shah, S., and Wood, A.J. (2000) Increased drug delivery to the brain by P-glycoprotein inhibition. *Clin Pharmacol Ther* 68:231–237.

Safer, D.J. (1997) Changing patterns of psychotropic medications prescribed by child psychiatrists in the 1990s. *J Child Adolesc Psychopharmacol* 7:267–274.

Sampson, E. and Warner, J.P. (1999) Serotonin syndrome: potentially fatal but difficult to recognize. *Br J Gen Pract* 49:867–868.

Spirko, B.A. and Wiley, J.F., 2nd. (1999) Serotonin syndrome: a new pediatric intoxication. *Pediatr Emerg Care* 15:440–443.

Sternbach, H. (1991) The serotonin syndrome. *Am J Psychiatry* 148:705–713.

Tugnait, M., Hawes, E.M., McKay, G., Rettie, A.E., Haining, R.L., and Midha, K.K. (1997) N-oxygenation of clozapine by flavin-containing monooxygenase. *Drug Metab Dispos* 25:524–527.

Tukey, R.H. and Strassburg, C.P. (2000) Human UDP-glucuronosyltransferases: metabolism, expression and disease. *Annu Rev Pharmacol Toxicol* 40:581–616.

von Moltke, L.L. and Greenblatt, D.J. (2000) Drug transporters in psychopharmacology—are they important? *J Clin Psychopharmacol* 20:291–294.

von Moltke, L.L. and Greenblatt, D.J. (2001) Drug transporters revisited. *J Clin Psychopharmacol* 21:1–3.

Wacher, V.J., Wu, C.Y., and Benet, L.Z. (1995) Overlapping substrate specificities and tissue distribution of P450 3A and P-glycoprotein: implications for drug delivery and activity in cancer chemotherapy. *Mol Carcinog* 13:129–134.

Walter, G. and Rey, J.M. (1999) Use of St. John's wort by adolescents with a psychiatric disorder *J Child Adolesc Psychopharmacol* 9:307–311.

Wagner, W. and Vause, E.W. (1995) Fluvoxamine. A review of global drug–drug interaction data. *Clin Pharmacokinet* 29 Suppl 1:26–31.

Weir, E. (2000) Raves: a review of the culture, the drugs and the prevention of harm. *CMAJ* 27:162:1843–1888.

Westphal, K., Weinbrenner, A., Giessmann, T., Stuhr, M., Franke, G., Zschiesche, M., Oertel, R., Terhaag, B., Kroemer, H.K., and Siegmund, W. (2000) Oral bioavailability of digoxin is enhanced by talinolol: evidence for involvement of intestinal P-glycoprotein. *Clin Pharmacol Ther* 68:6–12.

PART

I-B GENETIC PRINCIPLES

6 | Molecular genetics

SUROJIT PAUL AND PAUL J. LOMBROSO

There have been remarkable advances over the last 20 years in our understanding of how genes contribute to both normal and abnormal development. The greatest progress has come from the fields of molecular biology and the neurosciences. Together, these disciplines have deepened our appreciation of the biological and environmental factors that contribute to mental illness. Genes have been implicated in an ever-increasing number of disorders. The sequencing of the human genome will allow researchers to investigate this area with greater ease than was possible before. As a better understanding emerges over the role these genes play, there will be an increasing need to find better techniques to discover psychotropic agents that are capable of interacting with these gene products and modify their actions when necessary. The field of pharmacology has been moving toward an examination of how drugs interact with brain proteins and the regulatory mechanisms that control the synthesis and function of these proteins. This chapter will review the basic concepts of molecular biology as well as summarize some of the most recent discoveries and technical advances.

DNA STRUCTURE

The essential feature of genes as defined by Mendel more than a century ago was that genes were the basic unit of inheritance passed from one generation to the next. The importance of Mendel's discoveries, however, was not fully appreciated until the appearance of the chromosomal theory of inheritance proposed by Sutton and Boveri in the early 1900s. Early cytology showed that a "typical" eukaryotic cell contains a dense nucleus separated by a membrane from the less-dense surrounding cytoplasm. The nucleus consists of a discrete number of thread-like particles, called the *chromosomes*. In human beings, there are 46 chromosomes (22 pairs of homologous chromosomes and two sex chromosomes). Each chromosome forms a continuous structure in which the gene itself has the same linear construction in miniature as the much larger chromosome in which it lies.

Genes are made up of a linear array of deoxyribonucleic acid (DNA) molecules. The total number of nucleotides in the human genome is approximately three billion. Each deoxyribonucleotide is made up of a five-carbon ring sugar (2-deoxyribose), a phosphate group, and one of the following bases: adenine (A) guanine (G), thymine (T) and cytosine (C). The nucleotides are connected to each other by phosphodiester bonds that link the 3'-OH group of one nucleotide with the 5'-OH group of the next nucleotide.

X-ray diffraction studies showed that the high stability of most DNA molecules is maintained by the formation of a double helix (Watson and Creek, 1953). The DNA helix has a diameter of 20 Angstroms and makes a complete turn every 10 nucleotides. It is composed of two polynucleotide chains held together through hydrogen bonding between specific bases (G with C, and A with T). This phenomenon defines one of the most important features of DNA, namely, its complementary base pairing, which predicts that wherever one nucleotide is found the identity of the nucleotide on the other DNA strand is defined. It is this feature that allows for the passage of genetic information from one cell to the next during cell division. In the process of DNA replication, the two strands are separated and act as templates for synthesis of a complementary strand, thereby creating two copies of the original helix.

The sequence of bases in the polynucleotide chain is also important because it determines the exact sequence of amino acids used in the synthesis of a protein. Twenty amino acids are commonly found in proteins, while only four bases are used in the DNA molecule. Thus, more than one base must specify each amino acid. The genetic code is in fact read as triplets and there are 64 possible triplet combinations using 4 nucleotides. Each triplet of nucleotides is termed a *codon*, and given the redundancy, some amino acids are specified by more than one codon.

RNA

The nucleotide sequence on the DNA molecule, however, does not provide a direct template for protein synthesis. Instead, there is an intermediary step required. The DNA is used as a template to synthesize messenger ribonucleic acid (mRNA) through a process known as *transcription*. The primary structure of mRNA is the same as that of DNA: a linear polynucleotide chain with sugar-phosphate bonds. In contrast to double-stranded DNA, RNA generally exists as a single polynucleotide chain and is considerably less stable than DNA. The sugar moiety in the RNA backbone is also different, with ribose being used rather than deoxyribose. Moreover, the base thymine that is found in DNA is replaced by uracil (U). Finally, mRNA molecules are much shorter than genomic DNA, being generally in the order of a thousand to several thousand base pairs long.

Transcription of mRNA from a DNA template involves three distinct stages: initiation, elongation, and termination. Initiation begins with the formation of a complex between an enzyme called *RNA polymerase II* and the DNA near the transcriptional start site. The sequences surrounding this site are part of a regulatory region called the *promoter*. Certain key nucleotide sequences, termed *elements*, are found near the start site and are primarily responsible for the recognition and the binding of the RNA polymerase II to its promoter and initiation of transcription. These elements determine the location of the start point and influence the frequency of transcriptional initiation. In some cases, the transcriptional activity of a gene is greatly stimulated by the presence of sequences termed *enhancers* that are often, but not always, within the promoter region.

Only one of the two DNA strands is transcribed into RNA and is called the *sense strand*. The DNA is unwound in order to make the sense strand available for base pairing. As the transcriptional complex moves along the DNA template extending the RNA chain, a region of local unwinding moves with it. Termination of transcription involves the ability of RNA polymerase II to recognize the sequences that indicate that the end of the gene has arrived and no further bases should be added to the RNA chain.

Transcription of most genes is regulated by several classes of DNA-binding proteins, generally termed *transcription factors*. They recognize specific nucleotide sequences on the DNA molecule and binds tightly to them, forming a complex of regulatory proteins. DNA-binding motifs are present in a large number of regulatory proteins, and include the helix-loop-helix (HLH) motif, leucine zippers, and the zinc fingers. These motifs are present on many different transcription factors that can bind to specific nucleotide sequences and help to determine the precise expression pattern of proteins within different cells (Miller, 1985; Landschulz et al., 1988).

One of the best characterized class of transcription factors are the homeobox (*Hox*) genes (Levine and Hoey, 1988; Gehring, et al., 1994; Burke, 2000). The proteins encoded by these genes contain a highly conserved sequence of 60 amino acids. The conserved domain forms two α-helices that bind within the major groove of the double helix of DNA and, in combination with other proteins, allow RNA polymerase II to gain access to the start site. The evolutionary importance of the *Hox* family of genes is underscored by their presence throughout the phylogenetic tree and their involvement in the early development in insects, worms, and mammals (Murtha et al., 1991). For example, humans and other mammals have four highly conserved clusters of *Hox* genes. These genes and the complex set of intergenic control regions contain the precise instructions for where and when these regulatory genes are expressed in the developing embryo.

Another mechanism that contributes to the regulation of transcription is the fact that chromosomes are tightly packaged into nucleosomes within the nucleus. One group of proteins necessary for compacting DNA within the nuclei of cells is the family of histones. A number of proteins facilitate the binding of histones to DNA and thereby make the underlying genes less accessible to transcriptional activators. In this way, histones function as generalized repressors of transcription. Other proteins can displace histones and thereby permit transcription factors and other regulatory proteins to gain access to the DNA. Disruptions of this regulatory process would be expected to disrupt normal gene expression. Recently, a gene whose product is involved in the binding of histones to DNA was found to be mutated in Rett syndrome, a childhood disorder within the autism spectrum (Amir et al., 1999; Lombroso, 2000)

Gene control is also achieved through the methylation of DNA at specific regulatory sites. The presence of highly methylated regions within a promoter region usually prevents transcription of that gene (Kass et al., 1997). Most of the methyl groups are found on cytosine residues in what are termed CpG "islands" that are high concentrations of the two nucleotides cytosine and guanine. In fact, one of the consequences of the large triplet repeat expansion found in fragile X syndrome is a dramatic increase in these nucleotides and a concomitant increase in methylation immediately adjacent to the transcription start site. Both the trinucleotide expansion and the resulting methylation are thought to lead to the inactivation of the fragile X mental retardation 1 gene (*FMR1*) (Verkerk et al., 1991; Usdin and Woodford, 1995).

Differential methylation of regions on the paternal and maternal chromosomes is also responsible for the genetic mechanism termed *imprinting*. In imprinting, all the genes located within certain critical regions on one of the two chromosomes are not expressed, while genes in the corresponding region of the second chromosome are expressed (Brannen and Bartolomei, 1999). Imprinting is involved in several childhood disorders, including Prader Willi and Angelman syndromes (Cassidy and Schwartz, 1998; Everma and Cassidy, 2000; Greally and State, 2000).

After transcription, the primary RNA transcript undergoes several modifications before the mature mRNA molecule is transported out of the nucleus. This was discovered when a discrepancy was noted between the length of the DNA sequence from which the message was transcribed and the length of the mRNA itself. The sequence on the genomic portion was much longer than the mRNA. It was then discovered that most genes consist of exons that contain the sequence encoding for a protein and the intervening sequences, termed *introns*, that do not encode for protein and must be removed. The process of removing the introns from the primary transcript and joining together the exons is known as *RNA splicing*. Several other modifications occur to the mRNA molecule including the addition of a polyadenyl tail that is believed to provide stability to the mRNA and contribute to how long it will survive in the cytoplasm prior to its own degradation.

PROTEIN SYNTHESIS

The translation of the mRNA into proteins is the final step in the biological flow of information (see Fig. 6.1). Similar to other macromolecular polymerizations, protein synthesis can be divided into initiation, chain elongation, and termination. Critical players in this process are the aminoacyl transfer RNAs (tRNAs). These molecules form the interface between the mRNA and the growing polypeptide. Activation of tRNA involves the addition of an amino acid to its acceptor stem, a reaction catalyzed by an aminoacyl-tRNA synthetase. Each aminoacyl-tRNA synthetase is highly specific for one amino acid and its corresponding tRNA molecule. The anticodon loop of each aminoacyl-tRNA interacts

with a specific codon in the mRNA and transfers the corresponding amino acid to the growing polypeptide chain.

The cytoplasmic organelles that provide the platform for this process are the *ribosomes*. This complex recognizes and binds to a specific region at the 5' end of the mRNA. The signal for initiating a polypeptide chain is a special initiation codon in the mRNA sequence that marks the start of the reading frame. Usually the initiation codon is the triplet AUG, which represents the amino acid methionine, and thus most proteins have this amino acid as the first one in the polypeptide.

The ribosome can carry two aminoacyl-tRNAs simultaneously. In the chain elongation stage, the growing polypeptide is carried on one of these tRNAs. The chain is transferred to the second tRNA, which adds its amino acid to the growing peptide, and displaces the first tRNA. The ribosome then moves one codon along the mRNA to allow the next to be read. Termination of protein synthesis involves the release of the completed polypeptide, expulsion of the last tRNA, and dissociation of the ribosome from the mRNA. This is signaled by specific termination codons (UAA, UAG, or UGA) in the mRNA and requires the participation of various release factors.

Many proteins are modified during or after translation. These modifications include *acetylation*, *methylation*, *disulfide bond formation*, *glycosylation*, and *phosphorylation*. They affect the stability, activity, localization, or function of a protein. Acetylation and methylation result from the addition of an acetyl or methyl group, respectively, to the basic amino acid lysine and less frequently to arginine or histidine. The addition prevents positive charges from forming on the amino group. Another post-translational modification occurs to proteins when a bond is formed between two cysteine residues. This modification most often increases the stability of a protein. A more extensive change in protein structure occurs with glycosylation, which refers to the addition of a carbohydrate side chain to the amino group of asparagine (*N*-linked glycosylation) or to the hydroxyl group of serine, threonine, or hydroxylysine (*O*-linked glycosylation). It is a part of a complex mechanism for transporting proteins through the cell and usually occurs in the endoplasmic reticulum or Golgi apparatus as these proteins are processed for secretion.

The most important modification that occurs to proteins is their phosphorylation. Phosphorylation results in the addition of a phosphate group to the hydroxyl group of a serine or threonine residue and, less frequently, to a tyrosine. The phosphate group intro-

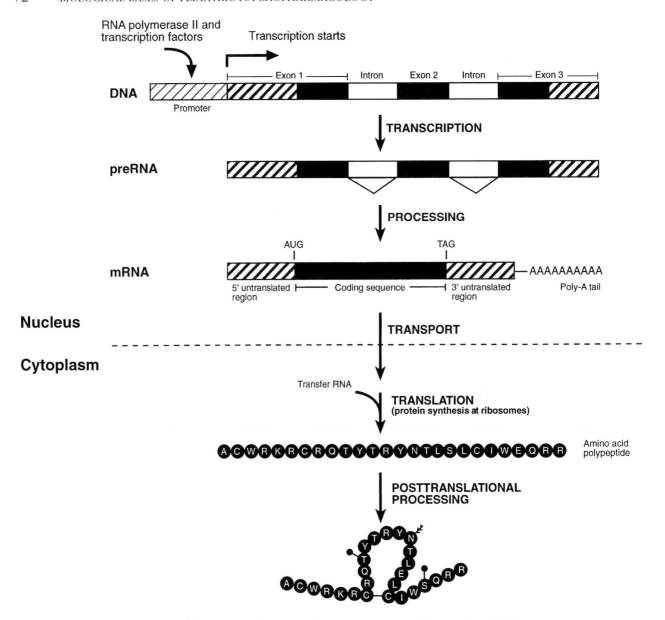

FIGURE 6.1 The different stages of protein synthesis. Transcription and processing of RNA messages occur within the nucleus. The mRNA is then transported into the cytoplasm for translation and post-translational modifications.

duces a large negative charge that has a significant effect on the electrostatic properties of the protein. This leads to a conformational change in the shape of the protein that often changes the activity level of the protein by exposing or hiding specific domains. Many members of the cell signaling cascades, including the mitogen-activated protein (MAP) kinase pathway shown in Figure 6.2, are known to be regulated by phosphorylation.

SIGNAL TRANSDUCTION

The ability of a cell to respond to environmental cues is critical for its survival. Signals arrive from neighboring cells or are transported in the blood and instruct the cell to proliferate, to differentiate into new cell types, or even to die in a normally occurring process termed *apoptosis*. Cells must be able to receive these signals, interpret them correctly, and respond to the sig-

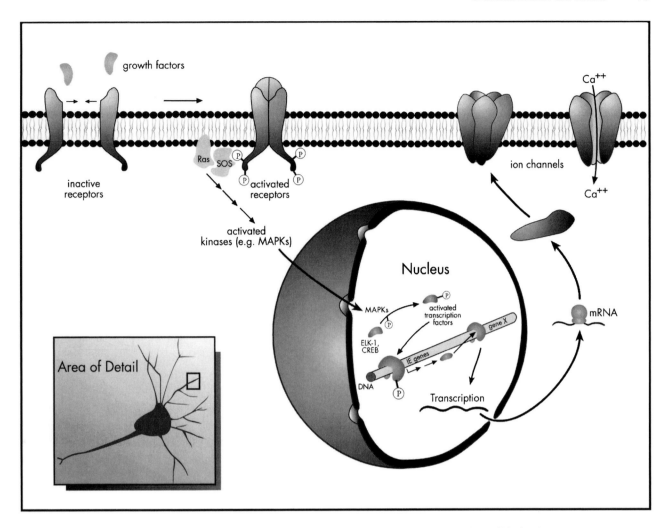

FIGURE 6.2 Signaling pathways. Growth factors activate signaling pathways inside a cell by binding to their specific receptors on the plasma surface. One example of such signaling is shown here, in which the binding of the growth factor to its receptors leads to the assembly of a complex of proteins. A series of phosphorylations occurs that results in the activation of specific transcription factors. These in turn initiate the transcription of messages that are required at that moment. [Adapted from Vaccarino, F. and Lombroso, P.J. (1998) Growth factors. *J Am Acad Child Adolesc Psychiatry* 37:789–790].

nal by initiating the appropriate intracellular response. As might be expected, disruption of these signaling cascades often leads to disease such as diabetes or the uncontrolled cellular growth that occurs in cancer.

One important class of diffusible extracellular signals are *growth factors*. These are molecules used by cells to communicate with each other. There are many different types of growth factors and each is capable of initiating specific intracellular signaling pathways (Fig. 6.2). Each growth factor has a specific receptor on the surface of the cell to which it binds. In the case of nerve growth factor, the binding of the signaling molecule to its receptor leads to the dimerization of

two growth factor receptors. Dimerization in turn activates a kinase domain on both receptors and autophosphorylation occurs at specific tyrosine residues on the intracellular portion of the receptor.

Phosphorylation triggers a second series of events. Phosphorylated amino acids residues act as docking sites for a number of intracellular proteins. These proteins contain their own amino acid motifs that recognize and bind to one or another of the phosphorylated amino acids. Some of these proteins have additional domains that now become activated and bind to other signaling molecules. A complex of proteins is thus assembled at the surface of the cell and specific signaling pathways are activated. In the pathway depicted in Figure 6.2, several kinases are sequentially activated. The end result is phosphorylation of transcription factors either in the cytoplasm or in the nucleus itself. When the phosphorylation occurs in the cytoplasm, the transcription factors are rapidly transported into the nucleus. The transcription factors bind to the promoter region of genes to initiate transcription and produce proteins required at that moment. A signal has moved in this way from the surface of a cell into the nucleus and specific genes are now expressed. The response may be to produce proteins that will initiate cellular division, or the synthesis of cellular structures such as ion channels, as depicted in Figure 6.2.

MUTATIONS

Mutations are any heritable changes that occur to the nucleotide sequence of genes. Changes in this sequence often lead to changes in the amino acid sequence of a given protein, thus altering or abolishing the activity of the protein. However, it is important to note that not all changes to the nucleotide sequence have an effect on protein function. In fact, most mutations are silent in that they either occur outside the coding region or change the sequence in such a way that the amino acid that is altered has no effect on the activity of the protein. In certain instances, of course, mutations may actually benefit the organism and are the underlying basis for evolutionary changes.

We are interested here in those mutations that disturb the function of proteins, as these may lead to specific disorders. In addition, the presence of mutations sometimes allows us to compare the properties of the wild-type (normal) gene with the defective one. By analyzing the changes that occur to the phenotype of the organism, we may gain some insight into the protein's function, as will be discussed further in the section on knockout mice.

All organisms suffer a certain number of mutations as the result of errors in normal cellular operations such as DNA replication. The majority of such mutations are quickly recognized and corrected by specific enzymes that are capable of comparing the two complementary bases on the DNA molecule as replication proceeds. Occasionally, they are not detected and corrected; fortunately, these spontaneous mutations are quite rare. The natural incidence of mutations can be increased by exposure to various environmental factors, and the effectiveness of a mutagen is assessed by the degree to which it increases the rate of mutation.

The most common class of mutation is the *point mutation*, in which the change occurs to a single base pair. There are two types of point mutations. In one, the change results in a stop codon being created where one should not exist. The result of such a mutation is that the protein produced will be truncated at the site of the new stop codon. Such mutations often have dramatic effects by completely inactivating the protein.

The second type of point mutation results in the replacement of one amino acid with another. Such mutations will have more or less of an effect depending on which amino acid is changed. Obviously, if a critical amino acid is replaced by one that is unable to provide the same function, the protein will lose some or all of its activity. Mutations within that *Ras* and *Src* genes are two examples in which point mutations lead to disease. In the case of the Ras protein, substitution of a single amino acid, most commonly at either position 12 or 61, is associated with the occurrence of several human tumors. In the case of the Src protein, a point mutation that occurs in a tyrosine residue leads to the constitutive activation of the protein and is associated once again with several types of tumors.

For a long time, point mutations were thought to be the principal means of disrupting genes. However, we now know that a number of other types of mutations occur. Insertions or deletions within a gene are quite frequent. Mutations of this type may result in the loss of a critical amino acid. More typically, however, they disrupt the downstream amino acid sequence by removing a number of nucleotides that is not a multiple of three and thereby changing the reading frame downstream of the mutation. Duchenne muscular dystrophy (DMD), characterized by progressive muscle degeneration, is an example of a disorder often caused by deletions. The gene that is mutated in DMD patients is located on the X chromosome and encodes a large protein called *dystrophin*. Dystrophin is required inside muscle cells for structural support and is believed to strengthen muscle cells by anchoring the internal cytoskeleton to the surface membrane. Interestingly, there are two forms of muscular dystrophy that differ in the severity of symptoms. Initially, it was thought that the more severe DMD was caused by larger deletions, while the milder Becker muscular dystrophy was caused by smaller deletions. However, it is now thought that the size of the deletion is less important than whether the deletion changes the open reading frame (Monaco et al., 1988). Even small deletions that change the rest of the downstream reading frame are likely to cause more severe illness.

In recent years, a new type of genetic mutation has been discovered. The basis for this mutation is the expansion of a specific series of three nucleotides (Caskey et al., 1992; Warren, 1996; Margolis and Ross, 1999). These trinucleotides are normally found in all humans and do not cause illness until they expand in size. To date, more than 12 human genetic diseases, including fragile X syndrome, Huntington's disease, and myotonic dystrophy, have been associated with expansions of CTG, CGG, or GAA repeats (Fu et al., 1991, 1992; Huntington's Disease Collaborative Research Group, 1993; Jin and Warren, 2000).

Fragile X syndrome is one of the more common forms of mental retardation and the defect is located on the long arm of the X chromosome (Lubs, 1969). In normal individuals, 6 to 50 CGG triplets normally exist within the *FMR1* gene, and are transmitted stably from parents to child. In carriers, there is a mutation in this gene that results in the expansion of the CGG motif to approximately 200 or more. How this occurs remains unclear, but the change is called a *premutation*. In the next generation, there is usually a dramatic expansion to over 1000 repeats and full expression of the syndrome. This huge expansion of CGG triplets leads to a significant increase in DNA methylation and a resultant loss of *FMR1* gene expression (Oberle et al., 1991; Eichler et al., 1993). Although the normal function of FMR1 protein remains unclear, it is known to be a RNA-binding protein and is found associated with ribosomes in the cytoplasm, and it may play a role in the normal translation of mRNA messages into protein (Siomi et al., 1993, 1994).

The progression in severity over several generations is a hallmark of triplet repeat expansions (Fu et al., 1991). This is known as *anticipation* and appears in all of the neuropsychological disorders in which triplet repeat expansions have been found. The extent of anticipation can be quite dramatic. Individuals with myotonic dystrophy, where the expansions are just above the normal threshold, may only develop cataracts late in life. In the next generation, with a slight increase in the expansion, the patient may experience mild muscle weakness. An increase in the next generation results in full-blown myotonic dystrophy in early adulthood. Finally, a still larger expansion results in fatal congenital illness (Fu et al., 1992).

In fragile X syndrome, triplet repeat expansions are responsible for the majority of cases. It should be noted, however, that any mutation that disrupts the functional activity of the FMR1 protein could lead to a similar phenotype. This was in fact established when a patient with severe fragile X syndrome was found who did not have a triplet repeat expansion. Rather, this patient had a point mutation that changed a highly conserved amino acid within the RNA-binding domain of the FMR1 protein (De Boulle et al., 1993; Siomi et al., 1994; Musco et al., 1996). This domain is critical for the proper function of the protein, and mutations in this domain interfere with its ability to bind RNA molecules.

This is one example of *allelic heterogeneity*, in which mutations in different parts of a single gene lead to the identical phenotype. Occasionally, mutations in different parts of a single gene cause very different clinical presentations. For example, several mutations within one of the receptors for fibroblast growth factor have been found that cause distinctly different skeletal abnormalities (Park et al., 1995). By way of contrast, *locus heterogeneity* refers to mutations that occur in different genes, yet affected individuals present with similar clinical features. This can happen, for example, when a mutation occurs in one of several proteins involved in a sequential series of enzymatic reactions. Disruption at any point in the series causes a similar phenotype.

Another type of mutation called a *translocation* involves the inappropriate exchange of genetic material between two chromosomes. A classic example of this is the Philadelphia chromosome, which is formed when the long arms of chromosome 9 and 22 are exchanged. As a consequence of this translocation, a portion of the Abelson (*abl*) gene normally found on chromosome 9 becomes fused to a portion of the breakpoint cluster region (*bcr*) gene on chromosome 22. This fusion results in the production of a chimeric mRNA that encodes for a hybrid protein. As a result, the regulatory region of the abl protein is no longer present and the chimeric protein is constitutively active. As the abl protein is a tyrosine kinase, a number of signaling pathways are activated and, in particular, ones that induce the proliferation of lymphocytes. The Philadelphia chromosome is found in 95% of patients with chronic myelogenous leukemia, 10% to 25% of patients with acute lymphocytic leukemia, and 1% to 2% of patients with acute myelogenous leukemia.

ISOLATION OF GENES

The isolation and characterization of genes may be divided into three epochs. Prior to the 1980s, investigators interested in the molecular basis of a particular disorder had a limited number of tools available. During this classical period, the approach usually consisted of biochemically purifying proteins that were either mutated themselves or directly affected by the mutation of another protein. This approach was severely limited as it required that the protein of interest be overproduced in order to allow for its purification. This is the case for many metabolic disorders in which a specific enzyme in a series of enzymatic steps is mutated and leads to the accumulation of one or more proteins. Once purified, it was possible to determine the amino acid sequence. In the vast majority of illnesses, however, there is no accumulation of protein and this approach proved unfeasible.

The rapid advances in molecular biology during the 1980s and 1990s allowed investigators to use an opposite approach, termed *reverse genetics*. Investigators interested in a particular disorder first accumulated families with affected individuals over several generations. Using linkage analysis techniques, they would determine the approximate chromosomal location of the mutated gene. Advances in cloning techniques allowed for the isolation and sequencing of the gene. The sequence could then be compared to that of the same gene isolated from unaffected individuals in an effort to identify potential mutations. The power of this approach is underscored by the several thousand genes

that have been cloned and implicated in a variety of disorders over the last decade. This compares to the hundreds of proteins that had been purified and implicated in various disorders using the earlier classical approach.

The reverse genetic approach relies on the construction of suitable libraries. The initial step is to homogenize the tissue and isolate the mRNA population. As mRNAs are single stranded and relatively unstable, they are first converted to their complimentary DNA (cDNA) sequence, and then into the more stable double-stranded cDNA molecule. The next step is to find a suitable vector that can carry the cDNA molecule and replicate itself multiple times. This will allow each message to be amplified to the large numbers of copies required for isolation and purification.

A number of different vectors have been used over the years. The one shown in Figure 6.3 is the bacteri-

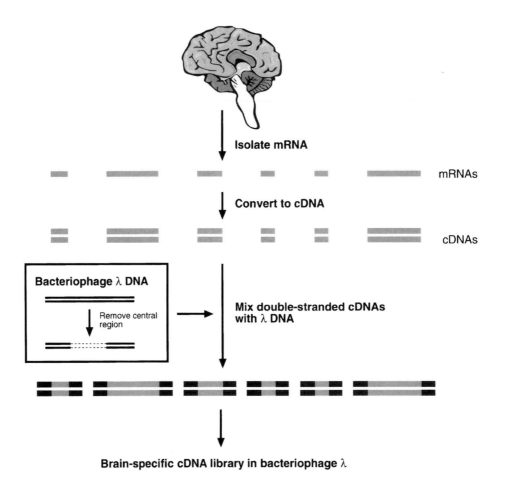

FIGURE 6.3 Construction of a brain-specific cDNA library. Messages (mRNA) are isolated from a tissue of interest. In this case, the target tissue is the brain. The mRNAs are converted to cDNA and each cDNA is inserted into the DNA of the bacteriophage lambda. The end result is a brain-specific cDNA library.

ophage lambda. This minute organism attaches itself to the surface of certain bacteria and injects its DNA into the cell, where approximately 100 copies are made that are repackaged into daughter phages. The phages burst the bacteria, reinfect adjacent bacteria, and repeat the process until all nutrients in the plate are gone.

The DNA of bacteriophage lambda is approximately 50 kilobases in length. It has the interesting property that the central region may be removed or replaced with another DNA sequence, and the bacteriophage is still able to produce progeny. This property allows one to place individual cDNAs into the λ DNA molecule such that each bacteriophage will contain a single cDNA insert. The total population of bacteriophage with their inserts is termed a *cDNA library*.

The next step is to screen the library for the insert of interest (Fig. 6.4). The bacteriophages are mixed with bacteria at the appropriate concentration such that each bacteriophage will infect a single bacteria. The progeny will infect adjacent bacteria and repeat the process of infection, replication and bursting until

millions of copies are produced. As the bacteria are killed, a clear circular area called a *plaque* appears in the bacterial lawn. Placing a filter carefully over the petri dish will allow one to lift the phage off the dish. One now has a faithful copy of the plaques that were produced and one can come back to the master plate at a later time to isolate one or another bacteriophage of interest.

To isolate a specific cDNA clone, one now performs a hybridization with a radiolabeled probe. A *probe* is a piece of DNA made or isolated in the laboratory. The investigator may be interested in isolating the full-length cDNA from which the probe was derived to determine the gene's full sequence. The cDNAs on the membranes represent all the messages from the brain. They are made single stranded and mixed with single-stranded labeled probes. Single-stranded nucleic acids have the property of binding very strongly when complimentary strands are brought together. The probe will therefore bind tightly to the specific cDNA clone that is its complementary strand. It is a relatively easy process to go back to the master plate and isolate the original cDNA clone. In this way, a specific cDNA clone may be isolated and its sequence determined. If one compares the sequence of a gene from individuals affected with a disorder with the sequence from unaffected individuals, potential mutations will be identified. If the same change in nucleotide sequence is found in a number of unrelated individuals with the same disorder, this is now taken as convincing evidence that the mutation is responsible for causing the disorder.

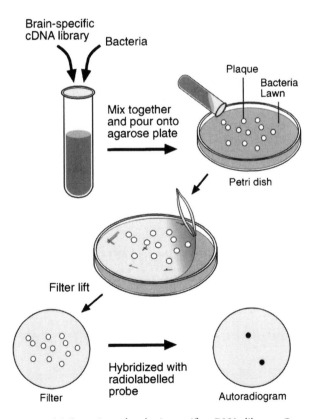

Brain-specific cDNA library

Bacteria

Mix together and pour onto agarose plate

Plaque

Bacteria Lawn

Petri dish

Filter lift

Filter

Hybridized with radiolabelled probe

Autoradiogram

FIGURE 6.4 Screening of a brain-specific cDNA library. Once a cDNA library is available, one can use it to isolate the sequence of any message that is in the library. One must have a portion of the gene to use as a probe. The library may need to be screened several times to isolate the full-length sequence of the gene of interest.

GENE KNOCKOUT

Several approaches are now being taken in an effort to establish the physiological function of a number of genes. One such approach is based on *knockout technology*, which relies on the ability to remove both copies of a gene from an experimental mouse and then examine the mouse for any anatomical, cognitive, or behavioral abnormalities that might appear.

To create a knockout mouse, one starts with a cDNA that encodes the gene of interest. One removes a portion of the gene that renders it inactive, and replaces that portion with a gene that allows one to select out those cells that have replaced a functional copy with the newly constructed mutated version. The new construct is placed into cells termed *embryonic stem* (ES) *cells*, which have the ability to grow into viable offspring when placed into pseudopregnant mothers.

After transfecting the mutated gene construct into the ES cells, an occasional rare homologous recombination event will occur. The mutated gene lines up with one of the two normal copies of the gene. A crossover event occurs in which genetic information is exchanged and one of the genes is replaced with the mutated gene.

As this is a very rare event, it would be difficult to determine which ES cells among the thousands on the petri dish have successfully incorporated the mutated gene. One now takes advantage of having placed a selection gene in the middle of the gene that is being disrupted. In the example in Figure 6.5, the selection gene is the neomycin gene. The protein produced by this gene will protect the cell from being killed by the antibiotic neomycin. Neomycin is added to the ES cells and only those ES cells that have incorporated the mutated gene will survive. Additional selection genes are available to ensure that the incorporation has only occurred by homologous recombination and not by a random insertion elsewhere in the genome, as this

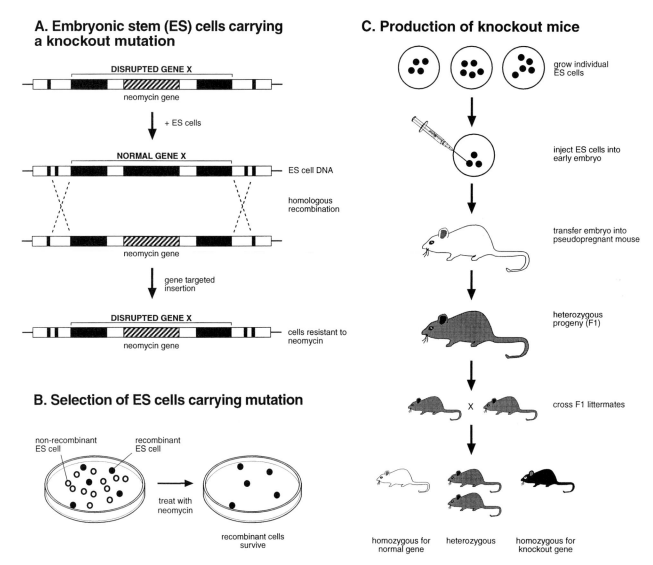

FIGURE 6.5 Knockout technology. **A:** Construction of mutated gene that will be inserted into embryonic stem (ES) cells. These cells are used to produce knockouts as they can be placed into pseudopregnant female mice and will lead to viable offspring. **B:** Selection of ES cells by treatment with neomycin. Neomycin usually kills the ES cells, unless a recombination event has occurred that introduces the neomycin gene into the genome. Those cells will be selected out and can be grown in culture dishes for introduction into pseudopregnant female mice. **C:** Production of knockout mice. The first generation of mice (F1 generation) will have one mutated and one normal copy of the gene of interest. Crosses between the F1 littermates will produce progeny that are homozygous for the mutated gene for behavioral and anatomical studies.

would still maintain the two viable genes as well as the inactive one.

Embryonic stem (ES) cells selected in this manner are placed into a pseudopregnant female. The first generation litter (F1) should have one normal and one mutated copy of the gene. If one then crosses the F1 generation, one-quarter of the next generation will have two copies of the knocked-out gene. These animals can now be examined for any phenotype that results from the absence of that specific gene.

Although some dramatic examples of knockouts exist, several problems are occasionally encountered. One example occurs if the gene is essential for survival: the knockout will be embryonically lethal. Newer techniques have been developed that are termed *conditional knockouts*. In these animals, the gene is normally expressed as long as the animal is given a specific factor, such as the antibiotic tetracycline. When the factor is removed, the gene is repressed and no longer expressed. In this way, it is possible to produce viable offspring in knockouts that would otherwise be lethal. These animals can then be examined later in life to determine if the removal of gene expression now disrupts specific pathways or behaviors.

In a number of cases, the knockout mice have shown a surprising absence of phenotype. For example, this has been seen with knockouts of transcription factors that one would have thought to be critically important. The knockout mice instead show no visible phenotype. It has been proposed that some genes are so critical that a certain amount of redundancy between genes is present, and one gene may be rescued by a close relative.

An example of this is the knockout of a homeodomain-containing transcription factor termed *Distaless* (Dlx-1). Members of the Dlx family are specifically expressed within the central nervous system (CNS) and, in particular, within the basal ganglia (Bulfone et al., 1993). Disruption of Dlx-1 was predicted to disrupt the structure and function of this brain region. The knockout in fact produced very little detectable abnormalities within the basal ganglia. It was only after a second member of the Dlx family was knocked out that a distinct phenotype emerged (Anderson et al., 1997). The double knockout produced dramatic malformations within the basal ganglia.

To summarize, knockouts have proved useful in determining the function of some genes. However, the complexity of gene interactions often leads to the absence of any phenotype, and multiple knockouts are required to tease apart the actual function of a gene or gene family. Moreover, certain genes are absolutely required during early development. Conditional knockout techniques have been developed in attempts to res-cue what otherwise results in embryonic lethal offspring.

FUNCTIONAL GENOMICS

Biomedical research is in the middle of a significant transition. The transition is driven by two primary factors: the massive increase in the amount of DNA sequence information, and the development of technologies to exploit its use. Over the last few years, more than 30 organisms have had their genomes completely sequenced and another 100 or so will follow close behind (see http://www.ncbi.nlm.nih.gov for a list). Within 2002, a 90% draft of the human genome sequence will be at hand, with completion expected by the year 2003.

It is currently estimated that approximately 35,000 genes are present in the human genome. Having the sequence tells us little about the function of these genes and what goes wrong when they are mutated. The challenge thus turns from determining the sequence of genes to understanding their function in a precise and quantitative way. This era is not surprisingly referred to as the period of *functional genomics*.

Among the most powerful and versatile tools devised to provide functional information on genomic sequence are *gene arrays*. High-density DNA arrays allow complex mixtures of RNA and DNA to be tested in a parallel and quantitative fashion (Bowtell, 1999). The analyses of nucleic acid arrays once again involves hybridization of labeled DNA or RNA to DNA fragments attached to specific locations on a solid surface. The attached DNA fragment may vary from 20 nucleotides (for oligonucleotides) up to 1000 base pairs (bp) (for double-stranded cDNAs). Arrays with more than 250,000 different oligonucleotide probes or 10,000 different cDNAs per cm^2 can be produced. The surface on which the probes are directly synthesized or attached may be made of glass, plastic, silicon, gold, a gel or membrane, or beads at the end of fiber-optic bundles (Ferguson et al., 1996; Michael et al., 1998; Walt, 2000). The hybridization sample is usually labeled with a radioactive group or a fluorescent probe. After hybridization, the arrays are scanned to assess the relative abundance of a particular gene in one or more samples.

DNA arrays can be used for many different purposes. The most important application for arrays thus far is the monitoring of gene expression for tens of thousands of genes simultaneously. The basic assumption underlying this approach is that genes that show similar expression patterns (i.e., are either increasing, decreasing, or remaining constant after a specific stimulation) are likely to be functionally related. In this way, genes without previous functional assignments are given tentative biological roles based on the known function of the other genes in the expression cluster. The validity of this approach has been demonstrated for many genes in *Saccharomyces cerevisiae*, an organism for which the functional role of approximately 60% of the genes are known (Cho et al., 1998a,b; Chu et al., 1998; Eisen et al., 1998).

PROTEOMICS

To facilitate our understanding of gene function, large-scale analyses of proteins are also necessary. Proteomics is currently divided into three main areas: (*1*) mass spectrometry for characterization and identification of proteins; (*2*) differential display proteomics for comparison of protein levels; and (*3*) studies of protein–protein interaction by using the yeast two-hybrid system or phage display technology.

The most significant breakthrough in proteomics has been the development and application of mass spectrometry to identify individual proteins. There are two main approaches to mass spectrometric protein identification. In the peptide-mass mapping approach, the mass spectrum of a tryptic peptide mixture is analyzed by matrix-assisted laser desorption/ionization (MALDI) (Henzel et al., 1993). Since trypsin cleaves the protein backbone at the amino acids arginine and lysine, the masses of tryptic peptides can be predicted theoretically for any entry in a protein sequence database. These predicted peptide masses are compared with those obtained experimentally by MALDI analysis. The protein can be identified unambiguously if there is a sufficient number of peptide matches with a protein in the database resulting in a high score. Recent advances in the automation of MALDI identification procedures and the availability of full-length human gene sequences in the databases will allow researchers to analyze hundreds of protein spots and automatically identify them by searching databases.

The second approach is the tandem mass spectrometric method (Wilm et al., 1996; Link et al., 1999; Yates, 2000). This method relies on fragmentation of individual peptides in the tryptic peptide mixture to gain sequence information. Its main advantage is that sequence information derived from several peptides is much more specific for the identification of a protein than a list of peptide masses. The sequence data can be used to search not only protein sequence databases but also nucleotide databases such as expressed sequence tag (EST) databases and, more recently, even raw genomic sequence databases. Biological mass spectrometry is still evolving rapidly owing to continued technological advances in various areas. In the future, this would probably enable researchers to perform the whole proteomic analysis in a single automated experiment without gel separation or enzymatic digestion.

In biomedical study, until recently, differential display proteomics was the most common approach to identify proteins that are up- or down-regulated under diseased condition. In this method, crude protein mixtures obtained from cells or tissues, derived from different conditions, are analyzed by two-dimensional gel electrophoresis and silver staining. Proteins are then subjected to mass spectrometric analysis. Although there are technical challenges to such experiments, the method has been successfully used to identify specific proteins that have been used as diagnostic markers or therapeutic targets (Aicher et al., 1998; Gauss et al., 1999; Ostergaard et al., 1999)

In a more modified approach, differential display proteomics can also be done with no separation of proteins. This is called the *protein chip approach*. In this method, a variety of "bait" proteins such as antibodies, peptides, or protein fragments may be immobilized in an array format on specially treated surfaces. The surface is then probed with the samples of interest. Proteins that bind to the relevant target can then be analyzed by direct MALDI readout of the bound material (Nelson, 1997; Davies et al., 1999). For example, well-characterized antibodies can be used as bait. Protein samples from two different cell states are then labeled by different fluorophores, mixed together, and used as probe. In such a case, the fluorescent color acts as an indicator for any change in the abundance of the protein that remains bound to the chip (Lueking et al., 1999). A number of technical problems would still need to be overcome before applying this technique for large-scale analysis of proteins.

Proteomics can make a key contribution in the identification of interacting protein partners and create a protein–protein interaction map of the cell (Lamond and Mann, 1997; Neubaer et al., 1997; Blackstock and Weir, 1999; Link et al., 1999). This would be of immense value to understanding the biology of the cell and can be further exploited for drug development. The simplest way to study such interaction is to purify the entire multiprotein complex by affinity-based methods. The members of the multiprotein complex can then be identified by mass spectrometry.

However, the most powerful tool to study such protein–protein interactions is the yeast two-hybrid system (Fields and Song, 1989; Allen et al., 1995). In its current form, the system utilizes the efficacy of yeast genetic assays to detect protein–protein interactions via the activation of a reporter gene. Typically, a gene encoding a known protein, termed the *bait,* is fused to the DNA-binding domain of a well-characterized transcription factor (e.g., GAL4, LEXA). A cDNA library is fused to the transcriptional activation domain. The two constructs are then introduced into a yeast strain for translation into proteins. A productive interaction between an unknown protein and the known protein bait results in transcription of an adjacent reporter gene that can be visualized by a color reaction. It is then relatively easy to identify the new gene through DNA sequencing. In this way, many novel protein interactions have been determined.

For large-scale analysis, this strategy has been further modified for use in the array method (Ito et al., 2000; Uetz et al., 2000; Walhout et al., 2000). Such analyses in *Sachromyces cerevisiae* and *Caenorhabditis elegans* have already reported many potential interactions that need to be confirmed by further biological experimentation. Finally, another modification of the yeast two-hybrid system has been recently reported, termed *reverse two-hybrid* (Vidal and Endoh, 1999). This technique is being used to identify compounds and peptides that can disrupt protein–protein interactions and thus have an effect on various signaling pathways.

FUTURE PROSPECTS

Future research efforts in molecular biology, functional genomics, and pharmacogenetics are sure to rapidly expand our understanding of normal development and increase our ability to intervene therapeutically when abnormal development occurs. The new information from the Genome Project will help to unravel the mysteries of evolution as genes are compared throughout the world, and single nucleotide polymorphisms (SNPs) are found that will build a map of humankind's migrations throughout the world. New genes that cause disease will be found and the normal function of these genes will be determined as well as the ways through which they cause illness when mutated. At the same time, ethical dilemmas will emerge as we struggle with issues around the screening of families and children for specific disorders as screening techniques become available.

REFERENCES

Aicher, L., Wahl, D., Arce, A., Grenet, O., and Steiner, S. (1998) New insights into cyclosporine A nephrotoxicity by proteome analysis. *Electrophoresis* 19:1998–2003.

Allen, J.B., Walberg, M.W., Edwards, M.C., and Elledge, S.J. (1995) Finding prospective partners in the library: the two-hybrid system and phage display find a match. *Trends Biochem Sci* 20:511–516.

Amir, R.E., Van den Veyver, I.B., Wan, M., Tran, C.Q., Francke, U., and Zoghbi, H.Y. (1999) Rett syndrome is caused by mutations in X-linked *MECP2*, encoding methyl-CpG-binding protein 2. *Nat Genet* 23:185–188.

Anderson, S.A., Qiu, M., Bulfone, A., Eisenstat, D.D., Meneses, J., Pedersen, R., and Rubenstein, J.L. (1997) Mutations of the homeobox genes *Dlx-1* and *Dlx-2* disrupt the striatal subventricular zone and differentiation of late born striatal neurons. *Neuron* 19: 27–37.

Blackstock, W.P. and Weir, M.P. (1999) Proteomics: quantitative and physical mapping of cellular proteins. *Trends Biotechnol* 17:121–127.

Bowtell, D.D. (1999) Options available—from start to finish—for obtaining expression data by microarray. *Nat Genet* 21:20–24.

Brannen, C.I. and Bartolomei, M.S. (1999) Mechanisms of genomic imprinting. *Curr Opin Genet Dev* 9:164–170.

Bulfone, A., Puelles, L., Porteus, M.H., Frohman, M.A., Martin, G.R., and Rubenstein, J.L. (1993) Spatially restricted expression of Dlx-1, Dlx-2 (Tes-1), Gbx-2, and Wnt-3 in the embryonic day 12.5 mouse forebrain defines potential transverse and longitudinal segmental boundaries. *J Neurosci* 13:3155–172.

Burke, A.C. (2000) *Hox* genes and the global patterning of the somitic mesoderm. *Curr Top Dev Biol* 47:155–181.

Caskey, C.T., Pizzuti, A., Fu, Y-H., Fenwick, R.G. Jr., and Nelson, D.L. (1992) Triplet repeat mutations in human disease. *Science* 256:784–789.

Cassidy, S.B. and Schwartz, S. (1998) Prader-Willi and Angelman syndromes: disorders of genomic imprinting. *Medicine* 77:140–151.

Cho, R.J., Campbell, M.J., Winzeler, E.A., Steinmetz, L., Conway, A., Wodicka, L., Wolfsberg, T.G., Gabrielian, A.E., Landsman, D., Lockhart, D.J., and Davis, R.W. (1998b) A genome-wide transcriptional analysis of the mitotic cell cycle. *Mol Cell* 2:65–73.

Cho, R.J., Fromont-Racine, M., Wodicka, L., Feierbach, B., Stearns, T., Legrain, P., Lockhart, D.J., and Davis, R.W. (1998b) Parallel analysis of genetic selections using whole genome oligonucleotide arrays. *Proc Natl Acad Sci USA* 95:3752–3757.

Chu, S., DeRisi, J., Eisen, M., Mulholland, J., Botstein, D., Brown, P.O., and Herskowitz, I. (1998) The transcriptional program of sporulation in budding yeast. *Science* 282:699–705.

Davies, H., Lomas, L., and Austen, B. (1999) Profiling of amyloid beta-peptide variants using SELDI protein chip arrays. *Biotechniques* 27:1258–1261.

De Boulle, K., Verkerk, A.J., Reymers, E., Vits, L., Hendrickx, J., Van Roy, B., Van den Bos, F., de Graaff, E., Oostra, B.A., and Willems, P.J. (1993) A point mutation in the *FMR-1* gene associated with fragile X mental retardation. *Nat Genet* 3:31–35.

Eichler, E.E., Richards, S., Gibbs, R.A., and Nelson, D.L. (1993) Fine structure of the human *FMR1* gene. *Hum Mol Genet* 2:1147–1153.

Eisen, M.B., Spellman, P.T., Brown, P.O., and Botstein, D. (1998) Cluster analysis and display of genome-wide expression patterns. *Proc Natl Acad Sci USA* 95:14863–14868.

Everman, D.B. and Cassidy, S.B. (2000) Genetics of childhood disorders: XII. Genomic imprinting: breaking the rules. *J Am Acad Child Adolesc Psychiatry* 39:386–389.

Ferguson, J.A., Boles, T.C., Adams, C.P., and Walt, D.R. (1996) A fiber-optic DNA biosensor microarray for the analysis of gene expression. *Nat Biotechnol* 14:1681–1684.

Fields, S. and Song, O.K. (1989) A novel genetic system to detect protein–protein interactions. *Nature* 340:245–246.

Fu, Y.-H., Kuhl, D.P., Pizzuti, A., Pieretti, M., Sutcliffe, J.S., Richards, S., Verkerk, A.J., Holden, J.J., Fenwick, R.G. Jr., and Warren. S.T. (1991) Variation of the CGG repeat at the fragile site results in genetic instability: resolution of the Sherman paradox. *Cell* 67: 1047–1058.

Fu, Y.-H., Pizzuti, A., Fenwick, R.G., Jr., King, J., Rajnarayan, S., Dunne, P.W., Dubel, J., Nasser, G.A., Ashizawa, T., and de Jong, P. (1992) An unstable triplet repeat in a gene related to myotonic dystrophy. *Science* 255:1256–1258.

Gauss, C., Kalkum, M., Lowe, M., Lehrach, H. and Klose, J. (1999) Analysis of the mouse proteome. (I) Brain proteins: separation by two-dimensional electrophoresis and identification by mass spectrometry and genetic variation. *Electrophoresis* 20:575–600.

Gehring, W.J., Qian, Y.Q., Billeter, M., Furukubo-Tokunaga, K., Schier, A.F., Resendez-Perez, D., Affolter, M., Otting, G., and Wuthrich, K. (1994) Homeodomain-DNA recognition. *Cell* 78: 211–223.

Greally, J.M. and State, M.W. (2000) Genetics of childhood disorders: XIII. Genomic imprinting: the indelible mark of the gamete. *J Am Acad Child Adolesc Psychiatry* 39:532–535.

Henzel, W.J., Billeci, T.M., Stults, J.T., and Wong, S.C. (1993) Identifying proteins from two-dimensional gels by molecular mass searching of peptide fragments in protein sequence databases. *Proc Natl Acad Sci USA* 90:5011–5015.

Huntington's Disease Collaborative Research Group. (1993) A novel gene containing a trinucleotide repeat that is expanded and unstable on Huntington's disease chromosomes. *Cell* 72:971–983.

Ito, T., Tashiro, K., Muta, S., Ozawa, R., Chiba, T., Nishizawa, M., Yamamoto, K., Kuhara, S., and Sakaki, Y. (2000) Toward a protein–protein interaction map of the budding yeast: a comprehensive system to examine two-hybrid interactions in all possible combinations between the yeast proteins. *Proc Natl Acad Sci USA* 97:1143–1147.

Jin, P. and Warren, S.T. (2000) Understanding the molecular basis of fragile X syndrome. *Hum Mol Genet* 9:901–908.

Kass, S.U., Pruss, D., and Wolffe, A.P. (1997) How does DNA methylation repress transcription? *Trends Genet* 13:444–440.

Lamond, A.I. and Mann, M. (1997) Cell biology and the genome projects—a concerted strategy for characterizing multi-protein complexes using mass spectrometry. *Trends Cell Biol* 7:139–142.

Landschulz, W.H., Johnson, P.F., and McKnight, S.L. (1988) The leucine zipper: a hypothetical structure common to a new class of DNA binding proteins. *Science* 140:1759–1764.

Levine, M. and Hoey, T. (1988) Homeobox proteins as sequence-specific transcription factors. *Cell* 55:537–540.

Link, A.J., Eng, J., Schieltz, D.M., Carmack, E., Mize, G.J., Morris, D.R., Garvik, B.M., and Yates, J.R., 3rd. (1999) Direct analysis of protein complexes using mass spectrometry. *Nat Biotechnol* 17:676–682.

Lombroso, P.J. (2000) Genetics of childhood disorders: XIV. A gene for Rett syndrome. *J Am Acad Child Adolesc Psychiatry* 38:671–674.

Lubs, H. (1969) A marker X chromosome. *Am J Hum Genet* 21: 231–244.

Lueking, A., Horn, M., Eickhoff, H., Lehrach, H., and Walter, G. (1999) Protein microarrays for gene expression and antibody screening. *Anal Biochem* 270:103–111.

Margolis, R. and Ross, C. (1999) Triplet repeat disorders. *J Am Acad Child Adolesc Psychiatry* 38:1598–1600.

Michael, K.L., Taylor, L.C., Schultz, S.L., and Walt, D.R. (1998) Randomly ordered addressable high-density optical sensor arrays. *Anal Chem* 70:1242–1248.

Miller, J. (1985) Repetitive zinc-binding domains in the protein transcription factor IIIA from *Xenopus oocytes*. *EMBO J* 4:1609–1614.

Monaco, A.P., Bertelson, C.J., Liechti-Gallati, S., Moser, H., and Kunkel, L.M. (1988) An explanation for phenotypic differences between patients bearing partial deletions of DMD locus. *Genomics* 2:90–95.

Murtha, M.T., Leckman, J.F., and Ruddle, F.H. (1991) Detection of homeobox genes in development and evolution. *Proc Natl Acad Sci USA* 88:10711–10715.

Musco, G., Stier, G., Joseph, C., Morelli, M., Nilges, M., Gibson, T. and Pastore, A. (1996) Three-dimensional structure and stability of the KH domain: molecular insights into the fragile X syndrome. *Cell* 85:237–245.

Nelson, R.W. (1997) The use of bioreactive probes in protein characterization. *Mass Spectrom Rev* 16:353–376.

Neubauer, G., Gottschalk, A., Fabrizio, P., Seraphin, B., Luhrmann, R., and Mann, M. (1997) Identification of the proteins of the yeast U1 small nuclear ribonucleoprotein complex by mass spectrometry. *Proc Natl Acad Sci USA* 94:385–390.

Oberle, I., Rousseau, F., Heitz, D., Kretz, C., Devys, D., Hanauer, A., Boue, J., Bertheas, M.F., and Mandel, J.L. (1991) Instability of a 550-base pair DNA segment and abnormal methylation in fragile X syndrome. *Science* 252:1097–1110.

Ostergaard, M., Wolf, H., Orntoft, T.F., and Celis, J.E. (1999) Psoriasin (S100A7): a putative urinary marker for the follow-up of patients with bladder squamous cell carcinomas. *Electrophoresis* 20:349–354.

Park, W.J., Meyers, G.A., Li, X., Theda, C., Day, D., Orlow, S.J., Jones, M.C., and Jabs, E.W. (1995) Novel *FGFR2* mutations in Crouzon and Jackson-Weiss syndromes show allelic heterogeneity and phenotypic variability. *Hum Mol Genet* 4:1229–1233.

Siomi, H., Choi, M., Siomi, M., Nussbaum, R., and Dreyfuss, G. (1994) Essential role for KH domains in RNA binding: impaired RNA binding mutation in the KH domain of FMR1 that causes fragile X syndrome. *Cell* 77:33–39.

Siomi, H., Siomi, M., Nussbaum, R., and Dreyfuss, G. (1993) The protein product of the fragile X gene, *FMR1*, has characteristics of an RNA-binding protein. *Cell* 74:291–298.

Uetz, P., Giot, L., Cagney, G., Mansfield, T.A., Judson, R.S., Knight, J.R., Lockshon, D., Narayan, V., Srinivasan, M., Pochart, P., Qureshi-Emili, A., Li, Y., Godwin, B., Conover, D., Kalbfleisch, T., Vijayadamodar, G., Yang, M., Johnston, M., Fields, S., and Rothberg, J.M. (2000) A comprehensive analysis of protein–protein interactions in *Saccharomyces cerevisiae*. *Nature* 403:623–627.

Usdin, K. and Woodford, K.J. (1995) CGG repeats associated with DNA instability and chromosome fragility form structures that block DNA synthesis in vitro. *Nucl Acids Res* 23:4202–4209.

Verkerk, A., Pieretti, M., Sutcliffe, J., Fu, Y., Kuhl, D., Pizzuti, A., Reiner, O., Richards, S., Victoria, M., Zhang, F., Eussen, B., van Ommen, G., Blonden, L., Riggins, G., Chastain, J., Kunst, C., Galjaard, H., Caskey, C., Nelson, D., Oostra, B., and Warren, S. (1991) Identification of gene (*FMR-1*) containing a CGG repeat coincident with a breakpoint cluster region exhibiting length variation in fragile X syndrome. *Cell* 65:905–914.

Vidal, M. and Endoh, H. (1999) Prospects for drug screening using the reverse two-hybrid system. *Trends Biotechnol* 17:374–381.

Walhout, A.J., Sordella, R., Lu, X., Hartley, J.L., Temple, G.F., Brasch, M.A., Thierry-Mieg, N., and Vidal, M. (2000) Protein interaction mapping in *C. elegans* using proteins involved in vulval development. *Science* 287:116–122.

Walt, D.R. (2000) Bead-based fiber-optic arrays. *Science* 287:451–452.

Warren, S. (1996) The expanding world of trinucleotide repeats. *Science* 271:1374–1375.

Watson, J.D. and Crick, F.H.C. (1953) A structure for DNA. *Nature* 171:737–738.

Wilm, M., Shevchenko, A., Houthaeve, T., Breit, S., Schweigerer, L., Fotsis, T., and Mann, M. (1996) Femtomole sequencing of proteins from polyacrylamide gels by nano electrospray mass spectrometry. *Nature* 379:466–469.

Yates, J.R. (2000) Mass spectrometry: from genomics to proteomics. *Trends Genet* 16:5–8.

7 | Pharmacogenetics

GEORGE M. ANDERSON, JEREMY VEENSTRA-VANDERWEELE, AND EDWIN H. COOK

Pharmacogenetics is usually defined as the study of genetic influences on drug response. *Pharmacogenomics,* a more recently coined and largely interchangeable term, refers to the area of research that employs genetic information in drug design and treatment. Initial pharamacogenetic research dealt with genetic variation in catabolizing enzymes, and examined how this variation influenced the pharmacokinetics of different drugs. More recently, pharmacogenetics has begun to consider pharmacodynamic aspects of drug response. These studies have investigated how genetic variation at the site of drug action can influence drug effects. It is an exciting time for pharmacogenetics/genomics, as recent applications across medical specialties suggest that the approach has great potential. This appears to hold true for neuropsychopharmacology, and for child and adolescent psychopharmacology in particular.

In this chapter, five introductory sections briefly review the range of recent promising clinical applications of pharmacogenetics, the areas of pharmacokinetics and pharmacodynamics, the possible relevance of pharmacogenetics to understanding of disease pathogenesis, and the appropriate genetic methodology to be employed in the investigation of genetic influences in neuropsychiatric illness and in neuropharmacological response. Separate sections then review the evidence supporting roles for dopamine-and serotonin-related alleles in determining risk of neuropsychiatric disorders. These sections are followed by a review of the pharmacogenetic studies examining the role of the corresponding genes in influencing drug response. In coupling the sections on risk and drug response we emphasize the close and reciprocal relationship between disease association studies and pharmacogenetic research. The chapter is written with an eye toward the potential utility of pharmacogenetics in child and adolescent psychopharmacology, and it closes with a look to what the near future may hold in this area.

OVERVIEW OF CLINICAL APPLICATIONS OF PHARMACOGENETICS

The potential clinical utility of pharmacogenetics is great. On the one hand, drug design and development should become more efficient and rapid because of a better understanding of disease mechanism and improved target identification. On the other, drug and dose selection will be more systematic and individualized, shortening an often costly and risky iterative process (Marshall, 1997; Houseman and Ledly, 1998). Exciting clinical applications are already occurring in the fields of cancer chemotherapy, hypertension, asthma, and pain medication requirements.

A number of authors have commented on the hopes raised for pharmacogenetics by the recent clinical advances and by the Human Genome Project (Housman and Ledley, 1998; Evans & Relling, 1999; Coats, 2000; Etkin, 2000; Roses, 2000; Ligett, 2001; Ratain and Relling, 2001. A range of factors has been discussed as possible determinants of when and how pharmacogenetics will affect the practice of medicine, including the rate of advance in understanding the molecular bases of disease, especially for multifactorial disorders (see Risch, 2000); the utility of genetic characterization, categorization, and diagnosis of disease; the success of design efforts using molecularly defined targets; the politics, ethics, and economics of genotyping; and the practical consequences of fragmenting drug markets based on patient genotype. Although it is clear that psychiatry and all of medicine will be affected, the rate and extent of the coming changes are difficult to predict.

PHARMACOKINETIC ASPECTS OF PHARMACOGENETICS

The role of liver microsomal enzymes is discussed extensively in Chapter 5 by Oesterheld and Flockhart in this volume and will be reviewed only briefly here. In phase I drug metabolism, cytochrome P450 (CYP) enzymes oxidize drugs to more readily excreted forms. A substantial amount of the variation in the activity of this family of enzymes (including CYP1A2, CYP2D6, CYP3A4, and CYP3A5) has been attributed to polymorphisms in the corresponding genes. Often, the frequencies of the polymorphisms vary across ethnic groups, contributing to the observed ethnic differences in drug response.

Researchers have also identified genetic variation in the phase II conjugative metabolic enzymes. These enzymes are relevant to the metabolism of almost all psychotherapeutic agents except lithium, and are involved in forming readily excreted conjugates with sulfate, acetyl, and glucuronate moieties. Further clinically relevant application of genetics to pharmacokinetics will require the identification of additional genetic variants contributing to the activity of metabolic enzymes. Many hope that the current cumbersome assays for determination of metabolic status will be replaced in some cases by genotyping of pertinent polymorphisms

PHARMACODYNAMIC ASPECTS OF PHARMACOGENETICS

In contrast to pharmacokinetic studies that investigate genetic influences on drug metabolism and disposition, pharmacodynamic studies focus on genetic variation at the sites of drug action. In neuropsychiatry, as in other fields, these studies have been relatively limited in number. Initial studies have examined neuronal receptors and transporters known to be affected by neuropharmacological agents. This "pharmacodynamic-genetic" approach should complement the pharmacokinetic-based work and lead to a greater understanding of racial, ethnic, and individual differences in drug response. As will be discussed below, an understanding of the genes involved in determining drug response may also contribute to increased understanding of etiology and pathophysiology of the disorders and behaviors under study.

Although genetic influences on the dynamics of drug response have been studied in a wide range of disorders, most of the studies have been carried out in only the past few years. Disorders and behaviors studied include Alzheimer's disease, schizophrenia, depression, suicide, anxiety, obsessive-compulsive disorder (OCD), substance abuse, smoking, and alcoholism. Across these disorders, however, there has been a focus on only a handful of neuroeffector systems. These include apolipoprotein and the cholinergic system (in Alzhei-

mer's disease), the dopaminergic system, and the serotonergic system. Research in Alzheimer's disease has suggested that the APOE-4 allele is associated with greater risk of disease (Blacker et al., 1997), and that patients with the APOE-4 allele have altered lipid transport (Rubinsztein, 1995). Recently, several pharmacogenetic studies have indicated that the E4 allele may influence drug response to anticholinesterase therapy and to cholinomimetics (Poirier, 1999).

Research on dopaminergic and serotonergic agents has the potential for advancing knowledge in a larger range of disorders and behaviors. The wide-ranging clinical utility of agents affecting dopamine receptors and the dopamine transporter, including antipsychotics and stimulants, is clear. The importance of agents affecting serotonin receptors and the serotonin transporter, including the tricyclic antidepressants and the selective serotonin reuptake inhibitors (SSRIs), is also unquestioned. Although the monoamine-related genes have taken a deserved place in the spotlight, genes related to the hypothalamic-pituitary-adrenal axis have been less well studied in neuropsychiatry (see Hinney et al., 1998). Given the important role of stress in the expression of a range of neuropsychiatric phenotypes, this area warrants greater attention.

RELEVENCE OF PHARMACOGENETICS TO UNDERSTANDING PATHOGENESIS

Although it is more traditional to think of drug development as proceeding from an understanding of pathophysiology, knowledge of treatment effects has often been used to generate theories of pathogenesis. In psychiatry, this strategy of selecting candidate genes on the basis of sites of drug action has been attempted with almost all disorders. This approach, however, is often limited by our incomplete understanding of drug action and by the nonspecificity of many agents. A growing area of relevant research concerns the effects of pharmacological agents on gene expression (Nestler, 1997; Paul, 1999). Examination of drug effects on gene expression may help elucidate mechanisms of drug action and pathogenesis.

Genetic studies of pathogenesis without any preconceived notions of pathophysiology (genome-wide screens) may identify completely novel targets for subsequent drug development. Animal models using gene knockout strategies have also provided promising leads for drug development. Advances in combinatorial chemistry and structure-based drug design have dramatically increased the capacity to develop new drugs once targets are identified. Although the polygenic nature of most neuropsychiatric disorders makes it more difficult to identify the genes involved, each gene may provide an option for treatment development. In many cases, the susceptibility genes are predicted to lead to disease only when occurring in combination; this suggests that drugs directed to a target identified by one of these susceptibility genes may be sufficient to ameliorate the syndrome.

GENETIC STUDIES IN NEUROPSYCHIATRY AND PSYCHOPHARMACOLOGY: METHODOLOGY

The first studies of genetic influences on pharmacological response compared drug response in subjects grouped according to genotype. Although statistically efficient, this approach was liable to the same errors that had been noted in case–control studies of disease. As non replicated associations in case–control studies accumulated, genetic epidemiologists identified biases that could contribute to false-positive findings. The most prominent of these was population stratification, in which the cases and controls were drawn from different subpopulations with discrepant gene frequencies (Kang et al., 1999). The risk of admixture artifact was also noted in populations that had undergone nonrandom mating for only a few generations (Spielman and Ewens, 1996). Some investigators have sought to identify rare homogeneous populations to eliminate these biases. However, studies focusing on one ethnic group may not be generalizable to the larger population.

In response to the biases inherent in case–control studies, family-based studies utilizing the transmission/ disequilibrium test (TDT) have become the gold standard in detection of association (Thomson, 1995; Spielman and Ewens, 1996). The family-based studies require analysis of alleles of both parents and the affected individual to determine which of the parental alleles are transmitted to the affected individual. Only data from heterozygous parents are informative and, for a two-allele system, each allele has an expected transmission rate of 50%.

Of special relevance in pharmacogenetics are recently developed TDT analyses for quantitative traits (Allison, 1997; Waldman et al., 1999; Abecasis et al., 2000). This methodology would allow pharmacogenetic studies to focus on gradations of response to a drug, rather than using categorical response and nonresponse groupings. Unfortunately for those trying to apply family-based methods, it can be difficult or impossible to collect DNA from parents of older psychiatric patients.

Given the difficulty and cost of acquiring DNA from parents, investigators have begun looking for ways of controlling for nonindependence within a case–control sample. One of the methods suggested is "genomic control" (GC), in which 20–60 single nucleotide polymorphisms (SNPs) spread throughout the genome are used to estimate the degree of population stratification. The significance level of a candidate gene SNP is then adjusted to reflect true association in the face of population substructure (Bacanu et al., 2000). Pritchard and colleagues (2000) have suggested an alternative method in which subjects are assigned to putative genetic subpopulations on the basis of genotypes at 100 unlinked microsatellite markers throughout the genome. Testing for association within these genetic subpopulations will in theory eliminate the hazards of unknown population substructure. In another alternative to the standard TDT parent–child trio approach, samples of sibling pairs are used to test for association (Spielman and Ewens, 1998).

Review of association studies of psychiatric disorders are restricted to family-based studies. However, all of the existing studies in the neuropsychiatric pharmacogenetic literature have used the case–control design. Although the studies may provide useful leads for follow-up work, this weakness of the pharmacogenetic research performed to date needs to be acknowledged.

ASSOCIATION STUDIES OF DOPAMINE-RELATED ALLELES IN NEUROPSYCHIATRIC DISORDERS

Dopamine-related genes that have been associated with disease by family-based association or linkage methods include the genes for the dopamine D_4 receptor (DRD4), dopamine D_5 receptor (DRD5), dopamine beta-hydroxylase (DBH), and the dopamine transporter (DAT). Replicated findings in attention-deficit/ hyperactivity disorder (ADHD) implicate the DAT, with the 10 copy repeat (of a variable number of tandem repeat [VNTR]) in the 3' untranslated region (3' UTR) of DAT found to be preferentially transmitted from heterozygous parents to children with ADHD in some (Cook et al., 1995; Gill et al., 1997; Waldman et al., 1998; Daly et al., 1999; Curran et al., 2001), but not all (Palmer et al., 1999; Swanson et al., 2000) groups studied. A recent study found linkage and association to the DAT in ADHD only when a haplotype including two additional polymorphisms was considered (Barr et al., 2001). In a meta-analysis, Curran and colleagues (2001) found significant heterogeneity among findings from different TDT studies of the 10-

repeat allele and an overall *p* value of 0.06 (Curran et al., 2001). However, a high level of significance is obtained if heterogeneity is accounted for (E.H. Cook, unpublished results).

Family-based association also has been reported and replicated for the *DRD4* VNTR. The 7-repeat allele, which leads to a longer protein than the 4-copy repeat, was first found to occur at a higher frequency in ADHD using a case–control association design (La-Hoste et al., 1996). Follow-up family-based association studies have now replicated the association (Rowe et al., 1998; Smalley et al., 1998; Swanson et al., 1998). Meta-analysis of the case–control and family-based studies supports the existence of a small, but significant, association with the 7-repeat allele (Faraone et al., 2001). Strong family-based associations have also been reported for *DBH* and *DRD5* in ADHD (Daly et al., 1999). A trend in support of *DRD5* association was observed in a sample of Turkish children with ADHD (Tahir et al., 2000). This association became significant when considering only methylphenidate responders, but was not corrected for multiple tests.

Although the ADHD data represent a relatively strong replication of findings in a complex genetic disorder, the alleles in question explain a relatively small amount of the phenotypic variance. In addition, there may be specific relationships with only certain domains or dimensions of relevant psychopathology. For instance, it has been reported that *DRD4* alleles appear to be more strongly associated with inattention (Rowe et al., 1998) and that *DAT* alleles are more strongly associated with hyperactivity/impulsivity (Waldman et al., 1998). Moreover, the haplotype study of Barr and colleagues (2001) suggests that *DAT* 3' UTR VNTR alleles may actually be linked to an unidentified susceptibility variant.

Dopamine-related alleles have been studied in a range of other disorders as well. Most studies of *DAT* markers in bipolar disorder samples have reported linkage (Kelsoe et al., 1996; Waldman et al., 1997; Bocchetta et al., 1999; Greenwood et al., 2001). In one American TDT study, *DRD4* 7-copy alleles were preferentially transmitted in Tourette's disorder (Grice et al., 1996); however, this latter finding was not replicated in a German follow-up study (Hebebrand et al., 1997). In addition, a single family-based association study of a tetranucleotide repeat polymorphism in the tyrosine hydroxylase gene was negative in Tourette's disorder (Comings et al., 1995). Another finding of interest is the association of novelty- or sensation-seeking behavior and the 7-copy alleles of *DRD4* (Ebstein et al., 1996; Auerbach et al., 1999). The 7-copy findings

in ADHD raise intriguing questions about the relationships between the behaviors being examined.

PHARMACOGENETIC STUDIES OF DOPAMINE-RELATED ALLELES

Compared to the proliferation of case–control and family-based disorder association studies of dopamine-related alleles, there are relatively few pharmacogenetic studies of these genes. The number is substantially increased if studies of dopamine-related genes in alcoholism and addiction are included (Uhl, 1999). Although usually not considered as such, genetic association and linkage studies in these areas can be termed pharmacogenetic, for they deal with genetic effects on drug consumption and response. It should be noted that treatment response in the addiction and alcoholism area can be potentially influenced by the genetics of the drug of abuse as well as by genes related to the effects of any treatment agents employed.

Generating the most interest in the general area of substance abuse has been a possible case–control association between the *Taq*A1 allele of the D$_2$ dopamine receptor (*DRD2*) and alcoholism (Blum et al., 1990; Gelernter et al., 1993), but this association was not supported by family-based studies (Edenberg et al., 1998; Blomqvist et al., 2000). Recent related studies include those examining *DRD2* alleles in cocaine dependence (Gelernter et al., 1999b), *DRD3* alleles in drug abuse in schizophrenia (Krebs et al., 1998), *DRD4* alleles in smoking (Lerman et al., 1998), and *DRD5* alleles in substance abuse (Vanyukov et al., 1998). Also relevant are studies associating specific *DAT* alleles with severity of cocaine-induced psychosis or paranoia (Gelernter et al., 1994) and the report that a specific haplotype at the *DBH* locus, correlated with lower enzyme activity, was associated with cocaine-induced paranoia (Cubells et al., 2000). The highly functional nature of a −1021T/C promoter polymorphism in the *DBH* gene suggests that these alleles may be promising candidates in a range of disorders or behaviors in which dopamine or the enzyme product norepinephrine might play a role (Zabetian et al., 2001).

Before leaving the abuse and addiction area, the exciting work in which animal models are used to map genes for drug abuse, alcoholism, neuroleptic-induced catalepsy, and stimulant response deserves mention (Crabbe et al., 1994; Kanes et al., 1996; Grisel et al., 1997). The application of powerful quantitative trait loci (QTL) approaches to animal models will almost assuredly lead to the identification of genes that are important in human drug abuse and response.

Studies of genetic influences on treatment response to dopaminergic agents are limited, with the neuroleptics receiving most of the attention. Two studies of *DRD3* alleles suggest that neuroleptic and clozapine responses are associated with certain (different) polymorphisms (Shaikh et al., 1996; Krebs et al., 1998). The finding of an association between the functional *DRD3* Ser9Gly polymorphism and clozapine response was not replicated in the study of Malhotra and co-workers (1998). However, a third study did support this finding and an overall meta-analysis is positive (Scharfetter et al., 1999). There have been several negative studies regarding the influence of an exon 3 polymorphism in the *DRD4* gene; an exon 1 polymorphism also appears not to affect clozapine response (Kohn et al., 1997). A study using the *DRD2* agonist bromocriptine to treat alcoholism found the greatest reduction in craving in individuals with one or two copies of the *DRD2* A1 allele (Lawford et al., 1995). A recent report found better acute response (positive symptoms only) to haloperidol in patients with at least one copy of the *DRD2* A1 allele (Schafer et al., 2001). However, the wide disparity in *DRD2* TaqI genotype frequencies in world populations must be considered when evaluating case–control studies involving this polymorphism (Barr and Kidd, 1993).

A number of related studies have focused on the role of dopamine-related alleles in the adverse effects of neuroleptic treatment. The glycine variant of the *DRD3* Ser9Gly polymorphism results in increased ligand binding in transfected cells (Lundstrom and Turpin, 1996) and appears to be associated with the development of tardive dyskinesia (Steen et al., 1997). Two studies have replicated the initial finding (Basile et al., 1999; Segman et al., 1999), and a third study found a significant association with acute akathesia (Eichhammer et al., 2000). One nonreplication of the glycine variant finding has also been reported (Rietschel et al., 2000).

In the first study of a dopamine-related gene's role in pharmacological response in a childhood neuropsychiatric disorder, Winsberg and Comings (1999) examined the influence of *DRD2*, *DRD4*, and *DAT* alleles on methylphenidate response in ADHD. A significantly lower response rate was observed in subjects homozygous for the 10-repeat allele of the *DAT* 3'UTR VNTR, with 5 responders of 17 in the 10/10 group vs. 11 responders of 13 for all other genotypes. Only African-American children were included in this study, and the study was limited by the small number of subjects. Replication is obviously necessary, but interesting questions are raised regarding the relationship of these results to other research findings. Relevant findings include the report of an association between the 10-repeat allele and ADHD risk (see above) and the report of *DRD5* associations in methylphenidate responders (Tahir et al., 2000). Issues raised include possible differences between white and black children, and the question of whether associations might also be seen with response to other stimulants. In general, the area of stimulant response in ADHD appears to offer a fruitful area for applying family-based (TDT) methods, given the number of individuals treated with stimulants and the frequent availability of parental DNA.

ASSOCIATION STUDIES OF SEROTONIN-RELATED ALLELES IN NEUROPSYCHIATRIC DISORDERS

A number of genes encoding proteins within the serotonin system have come under intense scrutiny, including the 5-HT_{2A}, 5-HT_{1B}, serotonin transporter, and tryptophan hydroxylase genes. Many of the disorder association and pharmacogenetic studies have examined a functional polymorphism (5-HTTLPR) in the promoter region of the serotonin transporter gene (*HTT*). The transporter is a critical component of the serotonergic system and it is the principal site of action of the widely prescribed SSRIs. The transporter might also influence the action of other agents with predominant or partial serotonergic effects, such as atypical neuroleptics, hallucinogens, serotonin precursors (tryptophan, 5-hydroxytryptophan), and serotonin-releasing agents such as trazodone and fenfluramine. Importantly, the insertion/deletion polymorphism in the promoter region appears to be functional, with the insertion form (the long, or *l*, allele) leading to higher levels of transporter expression and hence greater transport activity. Initial studies of the functional effects of 5-HTTLPR genotype indicate that the deletion form (short, or *s*, allele) results in lower mRNA levels, transporter protein expression, and uptake rates in transfection systems. Thus, individuals with a short variant on both chromosomes have reduced serotonin transporter expression in lymphoblastoid cell lines (Lesch et al., 1996), reduced whole blood serotonin levels (Hanna et al., 1998), reduced serotonin transporter function in platelets (Greenberg et al., 1999; Anderson et al., 2002) and reduced serotonin transporter expression in brain (Little et al., 1998; Heinz et al., 2000) relative to individuals with two copies of the long variant. In most, but not all (Hanna et al., 1998;

Mann et al., 2000; Willeit et al., 2001), of these studies, the short variant has been dominant for reduced levels, expression, or function.

The initial disease association study of the 5-HTTLPR was reported for the *s* allele and neuroticism in a case–control analysis that was supported by within-family sibling-pairs analysis (Lesch et al., 1996). This association was replicated twice using a similar approach in Israeli and American samples (Hu et al., 2000; Osher et al., 2000), and a Finnish replication study found linkage in a sib-pair sample (Mazzanti et al., 1998). After a mixture of support and nonsupport was found in a number of case–control studies, Gelernter and colleagues (1999a) clearly demonstrated the need for family-based methodology by showing dramatic differences in allele frequencies across populations. The accumulation of family based evidence suggests that variation at this gene does contribute to neuroticism, but analysis of extended haplotypes incorporating additional polymorphisms may help to clarify the picture.

Studies of the 5-HTTLPR extend beyond neuroticism to various other psychiatric phenotypes. In OCD, one family-based study found transmission disequilibrium with the 5-HTTLPR *l* allele (McDougle et al., 1998). Several family-based studies have not found linkage between 5-HTTLPR, or other *HTT* variants, and bipolar disorder (Geller and Cook, 1999; Mundo et al., 2001). In autistic disorder, Cook and colleagues initially reported TDT-based association with a haplotype including the 5-HTTLPR *s* allele (Cook et al., 1997). Three subsequent studies found transmission disequilibrium with the *l* allele in German, Israeli, and French populations (Klauck et al., 1997; Tordjman et al., 2001; Yirmiya et al., 2001), although others have found no significant transmission disequilibrium (Maestrini et al., 1999; Persico et al., 2000). A more extensive study of serotonin transporter gene variants in autism has found that other variants within the serotonin transporter gene show more evidence for linkage disequilibrium with autism risk than the original promoter variant (Kim et al., 2002). When studying a possible allelic influence on severity within domains of autistic behavior, Tordjman et al. (2001) found greater transmission of the *l* allele in less severely socially affected subgroups.

The report of 5-HTTLPR allelic association with severity in specific domains of autistic behavior (Tordjman et al., 2001) raises two general issues. First, the use of overall response as the end point in pharmacogenetic studies may not be sufficiently specific to identify an association between response and genotype. The

recent domain-specific findings regarding DRD4 and DAT alleles in ADHD support this idea. Second, even within domains, there may be greater statistical power in a dimensional rather than a categorical approach. Practically, this will require the development of more quantitative or QTL approaches to estimation of severity of domains affected in neuropsychiatric disorders (e.g., in autism; see Lord et al., 2001).

Genes encoding other proteins within the serotonin system have been studied less extensively than the *HTT*; the next-most studied has been the 5-HT$_{2A}$ receptor. Interest in the 5-HT$_{2A}$ receptor's role in psychiatric disorders and psychopharmacology has been sparked by two key observations. First, agonists at the 5-HT$_{2A}$ receptor, including lysergic acid diethylamide (LSD), have hallucinogenic properties that correspond to their affinities for these receptors (Aghajanian and Marek, 1999). Second, clozapine and other atypical antipsychotic agents act as antagonists at 5-HT$_{2A}$ receptors and this appears to be an important component of their therapeutic action (Meltzer, 1999). Thus, it is not surprising that the role of the 5-HT$_{2A}$ receptor gene (*HTR2A*) in the pathogenesis and treatment of schizophrenia has been extensively studied.

A number of polymorphisms, including several amino acid (AA) variants (nonsynonymous polymorphisms), have been identified within *HTR2A*. The most common of the AA variants is His452Tyr in the C-terminal region of the receptor, with the 452Tyr allele showing a 9% frequency in Caucasian subjects (Ozaki et al., 1997). To date, only a few family-based disorder association studies of *HTR2A* variants have been performed. One family-based study reported significant association in the presence of linkage between schizophrenia and the C allele at a 102-T/C polymorphism in a group of United Kingdom families, most of which were multiplex (Spurlock et al., 1998). This finding is not consistent with a negative TDT in a group of Irish subjects from multiplex families (Hawi et al., 1997). These contradictory results may reflect genetic heterogeneity or, alternatively, they may reflect different patterns of linkage disequilibrium across populations. Family-based association studies using additional markers, perhaps including haplotype analysis, may help resolve these findings.

Interest in the 5-HT$_{2C}$ receptor is based on its possible role in hallucinations and psychosis. As with the 5-HT$_{2A}$ receptor, LSD and clozapine have relatively high affinity for the 5-HT$_{2C}$ receptor. Meltzer (1999) has pointed out a relationship between atypical antipsychotic drug affinity for the 5-HT$_{2C}$ receptor and potential to produce weight gain. Indeed, the *5HT2C* knockout mouse is overweight, with a dimished response to the satiating effects of the 5-HT releaser d-fenfluramine (Vickers et al., 1999). Given that *HTR2C* is located on the X chromosome, one might expect to see gender differences in clozapine response; however, this has not been reported.

Although not yet examined in pharmacogenetic studies, several other 5-HT-related proteins are of special interest in neuropsychiatry. The tryptophan hydroxylase gene, encoding for the rate-limiting enzyme for serotonin synthesis, has been studied primarily in relationship to suicide and alcoholism in adults (Ishiguro et al., 1996; Mann et al., 1997; Tsai et al., 1999). Family-based analyses confirmed earlier case–control associations with suicidal ideation and alcoholism (Nielsen et al., 1998). The apparent involvement of the 5-HT_{1A} receptor in the pathogenesis and treatment of anxiety and depression suggests that family-based studies of *HTR1A* polymorphisms in these disorders are warranted. Interest in the $5\text{-HT}_{1B/1D}$ receptor arises from its possible role in migraine headaches, aggression, substance abuse, alcoholism, and feeding behavior, as well as results of initial association/linkage studies in aggression, alcoholism, and OCD.

PHARMACOGENETIC STUDIES OF SEROTONIN-RELATED ALLELES

From a pharmacogenetic standpoint, the 5-HT_{2A}, 5-HT_{2C}, and serotonin transporter genes are by far the best studied of the serotonin-related genes (Veenstra-VanderWeele et al., 2000). The initial pharmacogenetic studies examining the influence of the variance at the 5-HT_{2A} receptor gene on response to psychopharmacological agents have focused on clozapine (Masellis et al., 2000). Clozapine is used in the treatment of schizophrenia when patients are intolerant or unresponsive to standard treatments. Arranz and colleagues (1998) performed a meta-analysis of the eight studies examining clozapine response and the 102 T/C polymorphism and found significant association. However, this significance disappeared when the original study (Arranz et al., 1995) was excluded. Their meta-analysis of the four studies examining the His452Tyr polymorphism revealed significant association with the 452Tyr allele. A subsequent large, case–control association study in an ethnically diverse United States sample revealed significant association between clozapine response over 6 months and the 452Tyr allele, but not the 102 C allele (Masellis et al., 1998). Analysis of haplotypes did not improve the association with clozapine response (Arranz et al., 1998; Masellis et al., 1998).

Even if the association between clozapine response and the two *HTR2A* polymorphisms is replicated using family-based methods, they appear to make only a modest contribution to determining clozapine response. Using the most generous estimate based on the meta-analysis data, excluding the study of shortest duration, the positive predictive value of the 102 T allele is only 0.57, while the negative predictive value of lacking the T allele (the 102 C/C genotype) is only 0.54 (Arranz et al., 1998). Likewise, the positive predictive value of the 452His/His genotype or one or more copy of the 452Tyr allele was only 0.57 (see Table 7.1). In contrast (although, based on a total of 13 subjects), the negative predictive value of the 452Tyr/Tyr genotype is fairly high (0.85) (Arranz et al., 1998; Masellis et al., 1998). But, with a predicted population frequency for the 452Tyr/Tyr genotype of only 1% (Ozaki et al., 1997), it is difficult to justify screening given the current cost of genetic testing. Although there is some evidence that the 452Tyr allele may have functional significance, this requires further study. A recent extensive review of the pharmacogenetics of clozapine reponse is recommended (Masellis et al., 2000).

The studies focusing on *HTR2C* and clozapine response have used case–control designs to examine a possible association with a nonsynonymous polymorphism in the coding region of the gene (23Ser). Sodhi and colleagues (1995) reported a strong association between the 23Ser allele and good response to clozapine in a population of Western European patients. Rietschel and co-workers (1997) reported a nonsignificant trend toward association between the 23Ser variant and clozapine response in a retrospective analysis of treatment results in German patients. Masellis and colleagues (1998) also reported a nonsignificant trend toward association between the 23Ser allele and good response to 6 months of clozapine treatment in a population of United States Caucasian patients. A nonsignificant trend toward association with the 23Ser allele and retrospectively assessed response to clozapine has been reported for a population of British Caucasian subjects (Arranz et al., 2000b). Malhotra and col-

TABLE 7.1 *Predictive Value of* HTR2A *452His/Tyr Polymorphism in Clozapine Response*

Genotype	Response	Nonresponse	Predictive Value	Confidence Interval
452His/His	402	301	0.57	0.56–0.59
452His/Tyr	65	76	0.54	0.46–0.62
452Tyr/Tyr	2	11	0.85	0.54–0.97
452Tyr	67	87	0.57	0.49–0.64

leagues (1996) found a nonsignificant trend in the opposite direction when they compared subjects' response to 10 weeks of clozapine with their response to 4 weeks of treatment with a typical neuroleptic. Differences in ethnicity may be critical here, given large disparities in 23Ser allele frequency across Caucasian and African-American samples (Masellis et al., 1998).

Given the observed trends toward association between the 23Ser allele and response to clozapine in three of the studies, a preliminary meta-analysis of the four studies that report genotype frequencies in the clozapine response and nonresponse groups is of interest (see Table 7.2). Since *HTR2C* is located on chromosome X and the original association was by allele, rather than genotype, we grouped subjects with one or more copies of the 23Ser allele, including females with both 23Ser/Ser and 23Cys/Ser genotypes. Our simple meta-analysis indicated a significant case–control association across populations ($p = 0.03$, OR = 1.7), suggesting that attempts to replicate the association using family- or genome-based control methods are warranted.

Arranz and colleagues (2000b) reported a positive association between an *HTR2C*-330GT/-244CT repeat polymorphism and retrospectively determined clozapine response. This association exists at the $p = 0.04$ level only when the short allele is considered dominant. Given the need for Bonferroni adjustment in their analysis of 19 polymorphisms in this subject sample, this result must be considered quite tentative. In general, the above meta-analyses point out the benefits of large samples and the need for consistent assessment methodologies.

Initial pharmacogenetic studies of serotonin transporter gene (*HTT*) variants used case–control methods and have generated disparate results in different populations. Positive association of the promoter VNTR polymorphism (5-HTTLPR) with clinical response to fluvoxamine was seen in Italian patients with bipolar or unipolar delusional depression: subjects with one or

more copies of the *l* allele showed significantly greater improvements (Smeraldi et al., 1998). A similar result was obtained in nondelusional unipolar depression patients treated for 4 weeks with paroxetine (Zanardi et al., 2000). An American group studying response to paroxetine in elderly patients with depression observed a more rapid response in subjects with the *l/l* genotype, but found no difference in response rates at the end of 12 weeks (Pollock et al., 2000). This to some extent replicates the Italian finding and indicates that rapidity of response, rather than response itself, may be determined by genotype. However, in a group of Korean patients with unipolar major depression, Kim and colleagues (2000) found that the *s/s* genotype was significantly more frequent among responders than among nonresponders. If the strong associations with opposite alleles persist in family-based studies, it would suggest that these polymorphisms are actually in linkage disequilibrium with the functionally important variant (see Kim et al., 2002).

Although the SSRIs are widely used to treat depression, they have also been found to be useful in the treatment of OCD, social phobia, anxiety, and autism. Genetic effects on SSRI treatment response are thus of interest in a range of psychiatric symptoms and disorders. However, at present, there are only a few studies outside the depression field. Two studies found no association between *HTT* genotypes and SSRI response in OCD (Billett et al., 1997; McDougle et al., 1998), while Whale and colleagues (2000) found significantly higher clomipramine-induced prolactin response in normal control subjects homozygous for the 5-HTTLPR *l* allele.

When speculating about how *HTT* genotype-based differences in transporter expression could mediate differences in SSRI response, several groups have focused on autoreceptor feedback (Kelsoe, 1998; Smeraldi et al., 1998; Whale et al., 2000). Pharmacogenetic studies of the *HTT* may help unravel the complexities of terminal and cell body autoreceptor control of 5-HT neuronal functioning. Because variation in 5-HT transporter expression or function may influence 5-HT levels at all serotonin receptors, *HTT* variants may affect the response to almost any agent affecting the serotonin system (Lesch, 1998; Malhotra et al., 1998). For example, Arranz and colleagues (2000a) found no significant association between response to clozapine in a population of British schizophrenic subjects and any allele of the promoter or intron 2 VNTR polymorphisms. In another study, they found a significant association between the *s/s* genotype and poor response only when no correction for multiple comparisons was employed (Arranz et al., 2000b).

TABLE 7.2 *Meta-analysis of Association Studies on HTR2C Cys23Ser in Clozapine Response*

Association study	Response to Clozapine		Nonresponse to Clozapine	
	Cys only	Ser	Cys only	Ser
Sodhi et al. (1995)	84	19	57	2
Malhotra et al. (1996)	15	3	35	13
Rietschel et al. (1997)	59	19	63	11
Masellis et al. (1998)	55	17	58	9
Total subjects	213	58	213	35

$\chi^2 = 4.68$, 1 df, 2-sided $p = 0.031$.

FUTURE PHARMACOGENETIC APPLICATIONS IN CHILDHOOD AND ADOLESCENT NEUROPSYCHIATRY

Based on existing findings, there are many important hypotheses in pediatric psychopharmacogenetics. Selective serotonin transporter inhibitors have been shown to have efficacy in double-blind studies in children and/or adolescents in the treatment of autism, major depression, OCD, and anxiety disorders. Given the association of the serotonin transporter promoter variant with SSRI treatment response in adult depression (Smeraldi et al., 1998), all of the SSRI-responsive phenotypes should be tested for promoter variant influence on response using family-based or population-based controlled association studies. The report of strong 5-HTTLPR allelic effects on SSRI-induced mania (Mundo et al., 2000) is of special interest given frequent SSRI-induced activation in children.

The hypothesis that the optimal dose of SSRI may be dependent on *HTT* variants is intriguing; it can be speculated that dose–response correlations differ across genotypes; patients with one or two copies of the short variant of the serotonin transporter might respond at lower doses and/or plasma levels of SSRIs than patients with two copies of the long variant. This hypothesis could be tested using flexible-dose placebo-controlled designs coupled with family-based association studies.

It is now feasible to use the TDT approach to test whether *DAT* or *DRD4* genotypes (or both) may affect responsiveness of ADHD to stimulants. The large number of studies examining possible association to risk for ADHD or its component behaviors, as well as the preliminary case–control study of Winsberg and Comings (1999), should serve to stimulate interest in this area. Indeed, the first family-based association study of *DRD4* in ADHD was conducted in patients with a good therapeutic response to stimulants (Swanson et al., 1998); thus, a start has already been made in this direction.

The preliminary findings of a relationship between serotonin 5-HT$_{2A}$ receptor genotype and atypical antipsychotic responsiveness in schizophrenia warrant replication and could be extended to children and adolescents with autism. Investigation along these lines has been included in the (National Institute of Mental Health (NIMH)–sponsored multicenter study of risperidone in autism (Arnold et al., 2000).

Because of the ready availability of parents, pediatric psychopharmacology is in an advantageous position to conduct family-based association studies. The use of standardized assessment instruments and systematic dosing regimens are of obvious importance. The creation of genetic archives would allow subsequent testing of later emerging alleles of interest. Issues of consent and confidentiality need to be carefully addressed to protect the individuals involved while also maximizing the usefulness of the genetic and drug response information.

ACKNOWLEDGMENTS

G.M.A. gratefully acknowledges the support of NIMH (MH30929, MH49351), NICHD (HD03008, HCIDC35482), and the Korczak Foundation for Autism Research; Donald J. Cohen, M.D., is thanked for providing encouragement and, along with David Pauls, Ph.D., helpful insights. E.H.C. acknowledges the generous support of the NIMH (MH52223; MH01389, MH55094), NICHD (HD 35482), the Jean Young and Walden W. Shaw Foundation, and the Brain Research Foundation. Bennett Leventhal, M.D., Catherine Lord, Ph.D., and Nancy Cox, Ph.D., are thanked for encouragement and insights.

REFERENCES

Abecasis, G.R., Cardon, L.R., and Cookson W.O. (2000). A general test of association for quantitative traits in nuclear families. *Am J Hum Genet* 66:279–292.

Aghajanian, G.K. and Marek G.J. (1999) Serotonin and hallucinogens. *Neuropsychopharmacology* 21:16S–23S.

Allison, D.B. (1997). Transmission-disequilibrium tests for quantitative traits. *Am J Hum Genet* 60:676–690.

Anderson, G.M., Gutknecht, L., Cohen, D.J., Brailly-Tabard, S., and Cohen, J.H.M., Ferrari, P., Roubertoux, P.L., and Tordjman, S. (2002) Serotonin transporter promoter variants in autism: functional effects and relationship to platelet hyperserotonemia. *Mol Psychiatry* 2001 in press.

Arnold, L.E., Aman, M.G., Martin, A., Collier-Crespin, A., Vitiello, B., Tierney, E.; Asarnow, R., Bell-Bradshaw, F., Freeman, B.J., Gates-Ulanet, P., Klin, A., McCracken, J.T., McDougle, C.J., McGough, J.J., Posey, D.J., Scahill, L., Swiezy, N.B., Ritz, L., and Volkmar, F. (2000). Assessment in multisite randomized clinical trials of patients with autistic disorder: the Autism RUPP Network. Research Units on Pediatric Psychopharmacology. *J Autism Dev Disord* 30:99–111.

Arranz, M., Collier, D., Sodhi, M., Ball, D., Roberts, G., Price, J., Sham, P., and Kerwin, R. (1995). Association between clozapine response and allelic variation in 5-HT2A receptor gene. *Lancet* 346:281–282.

Arranz, M.J., Bolonna, A.A., Munro, J., Curtis, C.J., Collier, D.A., and Kerwin, R.W. (2000a). The serotonin transporter and clozapine response. *Mol Psychiatry* 5:124–125.

Arranz, M.J., Munro, J., Birkett, J., Bolonna, A., Mancama, D., Sodhi, M., Lesch, K.P., Meyer, J.F., Sham, P., Collier, D.A., Murray, R.M., and Kerwin, R.W. (2000b) Pharmacogenetic prediction of clozapine response. *Lancet* 355:1615–1616.

Arranz, M.J., Munro, J., Sham, P., Kirov, G., Murray, R.M., Collier, D.A., and Kerwin, R.W. (1998) Meta-analysis of studies on genetic variation in 5-HT2A receptors and clozapine response. *Schizophre Res* 32:93–99.

Auerbach, J., Geller, V., Lezer, S., Shinwell, E., Belmaker, R.H., Levine, J., and Ebstein, R. (1999) Dopamine D4 receptor (D4DR) and serotonin transporter promoter (5-HTTLPR) polymorphisms in the determination of temperament in 2-month-old infants. *Mol Psychiatry* 4:369–373.

Bacanu, S.-A., Devlin, B., and Roeder, K. (2000). The power of genomic control. *Am J Hum Genet* 66:1933–1944.

Barr, C.L., and Kidd, K.K. (1993) Population frequencies of the A1 allele at the dopamine D2 receptor locus. *Biol Psychiatry* 34:204–209.

Barr, C.L., Xu, C., Kroft, J., Feng, Y., Wigg, K., Zai, G., Tannock, R., Schachar, R., Malone, M., Roberts, W., Nothen, M.M., Grunhage, F., Vandenbergh, D.J., Uhl, G., Sunohara, G., King, N., and Kennedy, J.L. (2001) Haplotype study of three polymorphisms at the dopamine transporter locus confirm linkage to attention-deficit/hyperactivity disorder. *Biol Psychiatry* 49:333–339.

Basile, V.S., Masellis, M., Badri, F., Paterson, A.D., Meltzer, H.Y., Lieberman, J.A., Potkin, S.G., Macciardi, F., and Kennedy, J.L. (1999). Association of the MscI polymorphism of the dopamine D3 receptor gene with tardive dyskinesia in schizophrenia. *Neuropsychopharmacology* 21:17–27.

Billett, E.A., Richter, M.A., King, N., Heils, A., Lesch, K.P., and Kennedy, J.L. (1997) Obsessive compulsive disorder, response to serotonin reuptake inhibitors and the serotonin transporter gene. *Mol Psychiatry* 2:403–405.

Blacker, D., Haines, J.L., Rodes, L., Terwedow, H., Go, R.C.P., Harrell, L.E, Perry, R.T., Bassett, S.S., Chase, G., Meyers, D., Albert, M.S., and Tanzi, R. (1997) ApoE-4 and age at onset of Alzheimer's disease: the NIMH Genetics Initiative. *Neurology* 48:139–147.

Blomqvist, O., Gelernter, J., and Kranzler, H.R. (2000) Family-based study of *DRD2* alleles in alcohol and drug dependence. *Am J Med Genet* 96:659–664.

Blum, K., Noble, E.P., Sheridan, P.J., Montgomery, A., Ritchie, T., Jagadeeswaran, P., Nogami, H., Briggs, A.H., and Cohn, J.B. (1990) Allelic association of human dopamine D2 receptor gene in alcoholism. *JAMA* 263:2055–2060.

Bocchetta, A., Piccardi, M.P., Palmas, M.A., Chillotti, C., Oi, A., and Del Zompo, M. (1999) Family-based association study between bipolar disorder and *DRD2, DRD4, DAT,* and *SERT* in Sardinia. *Am J Med Genet* 88:522–526.

Coats, A.J.S. (2000) Pharmacogenomics: hope or hype? *Int J Cardiol* 76:1–3.

Comings, D., Gade, R., Muhleman, D., and Sverd, J. (1995) No association of a tyrosine hydroxylase gene tetranucleotide repeat polymorphism in autism, Tourette syndrome, or ADHD. *Biol Psychiatry* 37:484–486.

Cook, E., Courchesne, R., Lord, C., Cox, N., Yan, S., Lincoln, A., Haas, R., Courchesne, E., and Leventhal, B.L. (1997) Evidence of linkage between the serotonin transporter and autistic disorder. *Mol Psychiatry* 2:247–250.

Cook, E., Stein, M., Krasowski, M., Cox, N., Olkon, D., Kieffer, J., and Leventhal, B. (1995) Association of attention deficit disorder and the dopamine transporter gene. *Am J Hum Genet* 56:993–998.

Crabbe, J.C., Belknap, J.K., and Buck, K.J. (1994) Genetic animal models of alcohol and drug abuse. *Science* 264:1715–1726.

Cubells, J.F., Kranzler, H.R., McCance-Katz, E., Anderson, G.M., Malison, R.T., Price, L.H., and Gelernter, J. (2000) A haplotype at the DBH locus, associated with low plasma dopamine beta-hydroxylase activity, also associates with cocaine-induced paranoia. *Mol Psychiatry* 5:56–63.

Curran, S., Mill, J., Tahir, E., Kent, L., Richards, S., Gould, A., Huckett, L., Sharp, J., Batten, C., Fernando, S., Ozbay, F., Yazgan, Y., Simonoff, E., Thompson, M., Taylor, E., and Asherson, P. (2001) Association study of a dopamine transporter polymorphism and attention deficit hyperactivity disorder in UK and Turkish samples. *Mol Psychiatry* 6:425–428.

Daly, G., Hawi, Z., Fitzgerald, M., and Gill, M. (1999) Mapping susceptibility loci in attention deficit hyperactivity disorder: preferential transmission of parental alleles at *DAT1, DBH* and *DRD5* to affected children. *Mol Psychiatry* 4:192–196.

Ebstein, R.P., Novick, O., Umansky, R., Priel, B., Osher, Y., Blaine, D., Bennett, E.R., Nemanov, L., Katz, M., and Belmaker, R.H. (1996) Dopamine D4 receptor (D4DR) exon III polymorphism associated with the human personality trait of novelty seeking. *Nat Genet* 12:78–80.

Edenberg, H.J., Foroud, T., Koller, D.L., Goate, A., Rice, J., Van Eerdewegh, P., Reich, T., Cloninger, C.R., Nurnberger, J.I., Jr., Kowalczuk, M., Wu, B., Li, T.K., Conneally, P.M., Tischfield, J.A., Wu, W., Shears, S., Crowe, R., Hesselbrock, V., Schuckit, M., Porjesz, B., and Begleiter, H. (1998) A family-based analysis of the association of the dopamine D2 receptor (DRD2) with alcoholism. *Alcohol Clin Exp Res* 22:505–512.

Eichhammer, P., Albus, M., Borrmann-Hassenbach, M., Schoeler, A., Putzhammer, A., Frick, U., Klein, H.E., and Rohrmeier, T. (2000) Association of dopamine D3-receptor gene variants with neuroleptic induced akathisia in schizophrenic patients: a generalization of Steen's study on DRD3 and tardive dyskinesia. *Am J Med Genet* 96:187–91.

Etkin, A. (2000) Drugs and therapeutics in the age of the genome. *JAMA* 284:2786–2787.

Evans, W.E. and Relling, M.V. (1999) Pharmacogenomics: translating functional genomics into rational therapies. *Science* 286:487–491.

Faraone, S.V., Doyle, A.E., Mick, E., and Bierderman, J. (2001) Meta-analysis of the association between the 7-repeat allele of the dopamine D4 receptor gene and attention deficit hyperactivity disorder. *Am J Psychiatry* 158:1052–1057.

Gelernter, J., Cubells, J.F., Kidd, J.R., Pakstis, A.J., and Kidd, K.K. (1999a) Population studies of polymorphisms of the serotonin transporter protein gene. *Am J Med Genet* 88:61–66.

Gelernter, J., Goldman, D., and Risch, N. (1993) The A1 allele at the D2 dopamine receptor gene and alcoholism: a reappraisal. *JAMA* 269:1673–1677.

Gelernter, J., Kranzler, H., and Satel, S. (1999b) No association between D2 dopamine receptor (*DRD2*) alleles or haplotypes and cocaine dependence or severity of cocaine dependence in European- and African-Americans. *Biol Psychiatry* 45:340–345.

Gelernter, J., Kranzler, H.R., Satel, and S.L., Rao, P.A. (1994) Genetic association between dopamine transporter protein alleles and cocaine-induced paranoia. *Neuropsychopharmacology* 11:195–200.

Geller, B. and Cook, E. (1999) Serotonin transporter gene (*HTTLPR*) is not in linkage disequilibrium with prepubertal and early adolescent bipolarity. *Biol Psychiatry* 45:1230–1233.

Gill, M., Daly, G., Heron, S., Haw, Z., and Fitzgerald, M. (1997) Confirmation of association between attention deficit hyperactivity disorder and a dopamine transporter polymorphism. *Mol Psychiatry* 2:311–313.

Grant, S.F.A. (2001) Pharmacogenetics and pharmacogenomics: tailored drug therapy for the 21st century. *Trends Pharmacol Sci* 22:3–4.

Greenberg, B.D., Tolliver, T.J., Huang, S.J., Li, Q., Bengel, D., and Murphy, D.L. (1999) Genetic variation in the serotonin transporter promoter region affects serotonin uptake in human blood platelets. *Am J Med Genet* 88:83–87.

Greenwood, T.A., Alexander, M., Keck, P.E., McElroy, S., Sadovnick, A.D., Remick, R.A., and Kelsoe, J.R. (2001) Evidence for linkage disequilibrium between the dopamine transporter and bipolar disorder. *Am J Med Genet* 105:145–51.

Grice, D.E., Leckman J.F., Pauls, D.L., Kurlan, R., Kidd, K.K., Pakstis, A.J., Chang, F.M., Buxbaum, J.D., Cohen, D.J., and Gelernter, J. (1996) Linkage disequilibrium between an allele at the dopamine D4 receptor locus and Tourette syndrome, by the transmission-disequilibrium test. *Am J Hum Genet* 59:644–652.

Grisel, J.E., Belknap, J.K., O'Toole, L.A., Helms, M.L., Wenger, C.D., and Crabbe, J.C. (1997) Quantitative trait loci affecting methamphetamine responses in BXD recombinant inbred mouse strains. *J Neurosci* 17:745–754.

Hanna, G.L., Himle, J.A., Curtis, G.C., Koram, D.Q., Weele, J.V.V., Leventhal, B.L., and Cook, E.H., Jr. (1998) Serotonin transporter and seasonal variation in blood serotonin in families with obsessive-compulsive disorder. *Neuropsychopharmacology* 18:102–111.

Hawi, Z., Myakishev, M.V., Straub, R.E., O'Neill, A., Kendler, K.S., Walsh, D., and Gill, M. (1997) No association or linkage between the 5-HT2a/T102C polymorphism and schizophrenia in Irish families. *Am J Med Genet* 74:370–373.

Hebebrand, J., Nothen, M.M., Ziegler, A., Klug, B., Neidt, H., Eggerman, K., Lehmkuhl, G., Poustka, F., Schmidt, M.H., Propping, P., and Remschmidt, H. (1997) Nonreplication of linkage disequilibrium between the D4 receptor locus and Tourette syndrome. *Am J Hum Genet* 61:238–239.

Heinz, A., Jones, D.W., Mazzanti, C., Goldman, D., Ragan, P., Hommer, D., Linnoila, M., and Weinberger, D.R. (2000) A relationship between serotonin transporter genotype and in vivo protein expression and alcohol neurotoxicity. *Biol Psychiatry* 47:643–649.

Hinney, A., Becker, I., Heibult, O., Nottebom, K., Schmidt, A., Ziegler, A., Mayer, H., Siegfried, W., Blum, W.F., Remschmidt, H., Hebebrand, J. (1998) Systematic mutation screening of the POMC gene. *J Clin Endocrinol and Metab* 83:3737–3741.

Housman, D. and Ledley, F.D. (1998) Why pharmacogenomics? Why now? *Nat Biotechnol* 16:492–493.

Hu, S., Brody, C.L., Fisher, C., Gunzerath, L., Nelson, M.L., Sabol, S.Z., Sirota, L.A., Marcus, S.E., Greenberg, B.D., Murphy, D.L., and Hamer, D.H. (2000) Interaction between the serotonin transporter gene and neuroticism in cigarette smoking behavior. *Mol Psychiatry* 5:181–88.

Ishiguro, H., Saito, T., Shibuya, H., Toru, M., and Arinami, T. (1999) The 5' region of the tryptophan hydroxylase gene: mutation search and association study with alcoholism. *J Neural Transm* 106:1017–1025.

Kanes, S., Dains, K., Cipp, L., Gatley, J., Hitzemann, B., Rasmussen, E., Sanderson, S., Silverman, M., and Hitzemann, R. (1996) Mapping the genes for haloperidol-induced catalepsy. *J Pharmacol Exp Ther* 277:1016–1025.

Kang, A.M., Palmatier, M.A., and Kidd, K. (1999) Global variation of a 40-bp VNTR in the 3'-untranslated region of the dopamine transporter gene (*SLC6A3*). *Biol Psychiatry* 46:151–60.

Kelsoe, J.R. (1998) Promoter prognostication: the serotonin transporter gene and antidepressant response. *Mol Psychiatry* 3:475–476.

Kelsoe, J., Sadovnick, A., Kristbjarnarson, H., Bergesch, P., Mroczkowski-Parker, Z., Drennan, M., Rapaport, M., Flodman, P., Spence, M., and Remick, R. (1996). Possible locus for bipolar disorder near the dopamine transporter on chromosome 5. *Am J Med Genet (Neuropsychiatr Genet)* 67:533–540.

Kim, D.K., Lim, S.W., Lee, S., Sohn, S.E., Kim, S., Hahn, C.G., and Carroll, B.J. (2000) Serotonin transporter gene polymorphism and antidepressant response. *Neuroreport* 11:215–219.

Kim, S.J., Cox, N., Courchesne, R., Lord, C., Corsello, C., Natacha Akshoomoff, N., Guter, S., Leventhal, B.L., Courchesne, E., and Cook, E.H. (2002) Transmission disequilibrium mapping in the serotonin transporter gene (*SLC6A4*) region in autistic disorder. *Amer J Hum Genet* 2002, in press.

Klauck, S.M., Poustka, F., Benner, A., Lesch, K.-P., and Poustka, A. (1997) Serotonin transporter (*5-HTT*) gene variants associated with autism? *Hum Mol Genet* 6:2233–2238.

Kohn, Y., Ebstein, R.P., Heresco-Levy, U., Shapira, B., Nemanov, L., Gritenko, I., Avnon, M., and Lerer, B. (1997) Dopamine D4 receptor gene polymorphisms: relation to ethnicity., no association with schizophrenia and response to clozapine in Israeli subjects. *Eur Neuropsychopharmacol*, 7:39–43.

Krebs, M.O., Sautel, F., Bourdel, M.C., Sokoloff, P., Schwartz, J.C., Olie, J.F., Loo, H., and Poiriet, M.R. (1998) Dopamine D3 receptor gene variant and substance abuse in schizophrenia. *Mol Psychiatry* 3(4):337–341.

LaHoste, G., Swanson, J., Wigal, S., Glabe, C., Wigal, T., King, N., and Kennedy, J. (1996) Dopamine D4 receptor gene polymorphism is associated with attention-deficit hyperactivity disorder. *Mol Psychiatry* 1:128–131.

Lawford, B.R., Young, R.M., Rowell, J.A., Qualichefski, J., Fletcher, B.H., Syndulko, K., Ritchie, T., and Noble, E.P. (1995) Bromocriptine in the treatment of alcoholics with the D2 dopamine receptor Al allele. *Nat Med* 1:337–341.

Lerman, C., Caporaso, N., Main, D., Audrain, J., Boyd, N.R., Bowman, E.D., and Shields, P.G. (1998) Depression and self-medication with nicotine: the modifying influence of the dopamine D4 receptor gene. *Health Psychol* 17:56–62.

Lesch, K.P. (1998) Hallucinations: psychopathology meets functional genomics. *Mol Psychiatry* 3:278–81.

Lesch, K.-P., Bengel, D., Heils, A., Sabol, S.Z., Greenberg, B.D., Petri, S., Benjamin, J., Müller, C.R., Hamer, D.H., and Murphy, D.L. (1996) Association of anxiety-related traits with a polymorphism in the serotonin transporter gene regulatory region. *Science* 274:1527–1531.

Liggett, S.B. (2001) Pharmacogenetic applications of the Human Genome Project. *Nat Med* 7:281–283.

Little, K.Y., McLaughlin, D.P., Zhang, L., Livermore, C.S., Dalack, G.W., McFinton, P.R., DelProposto, Z.S., Hill, E., Cassin, B.J., Watson, S.J., and Cook, E.H. (1998) Cocaine., ethanol., and genotype effects on human midbrain serotonin transporter binding sites and mRNA levels. *Am J Psychiatry* 155:207–213.

Lord, C., Leventhal, B.L., and Cook, E.H. (2001). Quantifying the phenotype in autism spectrum disorders. *Am J Med Genet (Neuropsychiatr Genet)* 105:36–38.

Lundstrom, K. and Turpin, M.P. (1996) Proposed schizophrenia-related gene polymorphism: expression of the Ser9Gly mutant human dopamine D3 receptor with the Semliki Forest virus system. *Biochem Biophys Res Commun* 225:1068–1072.

Maestrini, E., Lai, C., Marlow, A., Matthews, N., Wallace, S., Bailey, A., Cook, E., Weeks, D., Monaco, A., and International Molecular Genetics of Autism Consortium. (1999) Serotonin transporter (*5-HTT*) and gamma-aminobuyric acid receptor subunit beta-3 (*GABRB3*) gene polymorphisms are not associated with autism in the IMGSA families. *Am J Med Genet (Neuropsychiatr Genet)*, 88:492–496.

Malhotra, A.K., Goldman, D., Buchanan, R.W., Rooney, W., Clifton, A., Kosmidis, M.H., Breier, A., and Pickar, D. (1998) The dopamine D3 receptor (DRD3) Ser9Gly polymorphism and schizophrenia: a haplotype relative risk study and association with clozapine response. *Mol Psychiatry* 3:72–75.

Malhotra, A.K., Goldman, D., Ozaki, N., Rooney, W., Clifton, A., Buchanan, R.W., Brier, A., and Pickar D. (1996) Clozapine response and the 5HT2C cys23ser polymorphism. *Neuroreport* 7:2100–2102.

Mann, J.J., Huang, Y.Y., Underwood, M.D., Kassir, S.A., Oppenheim, S., Kelly, T.M., Dwork, A.J., and Arango, V. (2000). A serotonin transporter gene promoter polymorphism (5-HTTLPR) and prefrontal cortical binding in major depression and suicide. *Arch Gen Psychiatry* 57:729–738.

Mann, J.J., Malone, K.M., Nielsen, D.A., Goldman, D., Erdos, J.,

Gelernter, J. (1997) Possible association of a polymorphism of the tryptophan hydroxylase gene with suicidal behavior in depressed patients. *Am J Psychiatry* 154:1451–1453.

Marshall, A. (1997) Laying the foundations for personalized medicines. *Nat Biotechnol* 15:954–957.

Masellis, M., Basile, V., Meltzer, H.Y., Lieberman, J.A., Sevy, S., Macciardi, F.M., Cola, P., Howard, A., Badri, F., Nothen, M.M., Kalow, W., and Kennedy, J.L. (1998) Serotonin subtype 2 receptor genes and clinical response to clozapine in schizophrenia patients. *Neuropsychopharmacology* 19:123–132.

Masellis, M., Basile, V.S., Ozdemir, V., Meltzer, H.Y., Macciardi, F.M., and Kennedy, J.L. (2000). Pharmacogenetics of antipsychotic treatment: lessons learned from clozapine. *Biol Psychiatry* 47:252–266.

Mazzanti, C.M., Lappalainen, J., Long, J.C., Bengel, D., Naukkarinen, H., Eggert, M., Virkkunen, M., Linnoila, M., and Goldman, D. (1998) Role of the serotonin transporter promoter polymorphism in anxiety-related traits. *Arch Gen Psychiatry* 55:936–940.

McDougle, C.J., Epperson, C.N., Price, L.H., and Gelernter, J. (1998) Evidence for linkage disequilibrium between serotonin transporter protein gene (*SLC6A4*) and obsessive compulsive disorder. *Mol Psychiatry* 3:270–273.

Meltzer, H.Y. (1999) The role of serotonin in antipsychotic drug action. *Neuropsychopharmacology* 21:106S–115S.

Mundo, E., Walker, M., Cate, T., Macciardi, F., and Kennedy, J. (2001) The role of the serotonin transporter protein gene in antidepressant-induced mania in bipolar disorder: preliminary findings. *Arch Gen Psychiatry* 58:539–544.

Nestler, E.J. (1997) Molecular mechanisms of opiate and cocaine addiction. *Curr Opin Neurobiol* 7:713–719.

Nielsen, D.A., Virkkunen, M., Lappalainen, J., Eggert, M., Brown, G.L., Long, J.C., Goldman, D., and Linnoila, M. (1998) A tryptophan hydroxylase gene marker for suicidality and alcoholism. *Arch Gen Psychiatry* 55:593–602.

Osher, Y., Hamer, D., and Benjamin, J. (2000). Association and linkage of anxiety-related traits with a functional polymorphism of the serotonin transporter gene regulatory region in Israeli sibling pairs. *Mol Psychiatry* 5:216–219.

Ozaki, N., Manji, H., Lubierman, V., Lu, S.J., Lappalainen, J., Rosenthal, N.E., and Goldman, D. (1997) A naturally occurring amino acid substitution of the human serotonin 5-HT2A receptor influences amplitude and timing of intracellular calcium mobilization. *J Neurochem* 68:2186–2193.

Palmer, C.G., Bailey, J.N., Ramsey, C., Cantwell, D., Sinsheimer, J.S., Del'Homme, M., McGough, J., Woodward, J.A., Asarnow, R., Asarnow, J., Nelson, S., and Smalley, S.L. (1999). No evidence of linkage or linkage disequilibrium between *DAT1* and attention deficit hyperactivity disorder in a large sample. *Psychiatr Genet* 9:157–60.

Paul, S. (1999) CNS drug discovery in the 21st century. From genomics to combinatorial chemistry and back. *Bri J Psychiatry* Suppl 37:23–25.

Persico, A.M., Militerni, R., Bravaccio, C., Schneider, C., Melmed, R., Conciatori, M., Damiani, V., Baldi, A., and Keller, F. (2000) Lack of association between serotonin transporter gene promoter variants and autistic disorder in two ethnically distinct samples. *Am J Med Genet* 96:123–127.

Poirier, J. (1999) Apolipoprotein E4., cholinergic integrity and the pharmacogenetics of Alzheimer's disease. *J Psychiatry Neurosci* 24:147–153.

Pollock, B.G., Ferrell, R.E., Mulsant, B.H., Mazumdar, S., Miller, M., Sweet, R.A., Davis, S., Kirshner, M.A., Houck, P.R., Stack, J.A., Reynolds, C.F., and Kupfer, D.J. (2000) Allelic variation in the serotonin transporter promoter affects onset of paroxetine treatment response in late-life depression. *Neuropsychopharmacology* 23:587–590.

Pritchard, J., Stephens, M., Rosenberg, N., and Donnelly, P. (2000) Association mapping in structured populations. *Am J Hum Genet* 67:170–181.

Ratain, M.J. and Relling M.V. (2001) Gazing into a crystal ball—cancer therapy in the post-genomic era. *Nat Med* 7:283–285.

Rietschel, M., Krauss, H., Muller, D.J., Schulze, T.G., Knapp, M., Marwinski, K., Maroldt, A.O., Paus, S., Grunhage, F., Propping, P., Maier, W., Held, T., and Nothen, M.M. (2000) Dopamine D3 receptor variant and tardive dyskinesia. *Eur Arch Psychiatry Clin Neurosci* 250:31–35.

Rietschel, M., Naber, D., Fimmers, R., Moller, H.J., Propping, P., and Nothen, M.M. (1997) Efficacy and side-effects of clozapine not associated with variation in the 5-HT2C receptor. *Neuroreport* 8:1999–2003.

Risch, N.J. (2000) Searching for genetic determinants in the new millenium. *Nature* 405:847–856.

Roses, A.D. (2000) Pharmacogenetics and the practice of medicine. *Nature* 405:857–865.

Rowe, D., Stever, C., Giedinghagen, L., Gard, J., Cleveland, H., Terris, S., Mohr, J., Sherman, S., Abramowitz, A., and Waldman, I. (1998) Dopamine DRD4 receptor polymorphism and attention-deficit hyperactivity disorder. *Mol Psychiatry* 3:419–426.

Rubinsztein, D.C. (1995) Apolipoprotein E: a review of its role in lipoprotein metabolism., neuronal growth and repair and as a risk factor for Alzheimer's disease. *Psychol Med* 25:223–239.

Schafer, M., Rujescu, D., Giegling, I., Guntermann, A., Erfurth, A., Bondy, B., and Moller, H.J. (2001) Association of short-term response to haloperidol treatment with a polymorphism in the dopamine D(2) receptor gene. *Am J Psychiatry* 158:802–804.

Scharfetter, J., Chaudhry, H.R., Hornik, K., Fuchs, K., Sieghart, W., Kasper, S., and Aschauer, H.N. (1999) Dopamine D3 receptor gene polymorphism and response to clozapine in schizophrenic Pakastani patients. *Eur Neuropsychopharmacol* 10:17–20.

Segman, R., Neeman, T., Heresco-Levy, U., Finkel, B., Karagichev, L., Schlafman, M., Dorevitch, A., Yakir, A., Lerner, A., Shelevoy, A., and Lerer, B. (1999) Genotypic association between the dopamine D3 receptor and tardive dyskinesia in chronic schizophrenia. *Mol Psychiatry* 4:247–253.

Shaikh, S., Collier, D.A., Sham, P.C., Ball, D., Aitchison, K., Vallada, H., Smith, I., Gill, M., Kerwin, R.W. (1996) Allelic association between a Ser-9-Gly polymorphism in the dopamine D3 receptor gene and schizophrenia. *Hum Genet.* 97:714–719.

Smalley, S., Bailey, J., Palmer, C., Cantwell, D., McGough, J., Del'Homme, M., Asarnow, J., Woodward, J., Ramsey, C., (1998) Nelson, S. Evidence that the dopamine D4 receptor is a susceptibility gene in attention-deficit hyperactivity disorder. *Mol Psychiatry* 3:427–430.

Smeraldi, E., Zanardi, R., Benedetti, F., Di Bella, D., Perez, J., and Catalano, M. (1998) Polymorphism within the promoter gene and antidepressant efficacy of fluvoxamine. *Mol Psychiatry* 3:508–511.

Sodhi, M.S., Arranz, M.J., Curtis, D., Ball, D.M., Sham, P., Roberts, G.W., Price, J., Collier, D.A., and Kerwin, R.W. (1995). Association between clozapine response and allelic variation in the 5-HT2C receptor gene. *Neuroreport* 7:169–172.

Spielman, R. and Ewens, W. (1996) The TDT and other family-based tests for linkage disequilibrium and association. *Am J Hum Genet* 59:983–989.

Spielman, R.S. and Ewens, W.J. (1998) A sibship test for linkage in the presence of association: the sib transmission/disequilibrium test. *Am J Hum Genet* 62:450–458.

Spurlock, G., Heils, A., Holmans, P., Williams, J., D'Souza, U.M., Cardno, A., Murphy, K.C., Jones, L., Buckland, P.R., McGuffin, P., Lesch, K.P., and Owen, M.J. (1998) A family-based association study of T102C polymorphism in 5HT2A and schizophrenia plus identification of new polymorphisms in the promoter. *Mol Psychiatry* 3:42–49.

Steen, V.M., Lovlie, R., MacEwan, T., and McCreadie, R.G. (1997) Dopamine D3-receptor gene variant and susceptibility to tardive dyskinesia in schizophrenic patients. *Mol Psychiatry* 2:139–45.

Swanson, J.M., Flodman, P., Kennedy, J., Spence, M.A., Moyzis, R., Schuck, S., Murias, M., Moriarity, J., Barr, C., Smith, M., and Posner, M. (2000) Dopamine genes and ADHD. *Neurosci Biobehav Rev* 24:21–25.

Swanson, J.M., Sunohara, G.A., Kennedy, J.L., Regino, R., Fineberg, E., Wigal, T., Lerner, M., Williams, L., LaHoste, G.J., and Wigal, S. (1998) Association of the dopamine receptor D4 (*DRD4*) gene with a refined phenotype of attention-deficit hyperactivity disorder (ADHD): a family-based approach. *Mol Psychiatry* 3: 38–41.

Tahir, E., Yazgan, Y., Cirakoglu, B., Ozbay, F., Waldman, I., and Asherson, P.J. (2000) Association and linkage of *DRD4* and *DRD5* with attention-deficit hyperactivity disorder (ADHD). *Mol Psychiatry* 5:396–404.

Thomson, G. (1995). Mapping disease genes: family-based association studies. *Am J Hum Genet* 57:487–498.

Tordjman, S., Gutneckt, L., Carlier, M., Spitz, E., Antoine, C., Slama, F., Cohen, D.J., Ferrari, P., Roubertoux, P.L., and Anderson, G.M. (2001) Role of the serotonin transporter in the behavioral expression of autism. *Mol Psychiatry* 6:434–439.

Tsai, S.J., Hong, C.J., and Wang, Y.C. (1999) Tryptophan hydroxylase gene polymorphism (A218C) and suicidal behaviors. *Neuroreport* 10:3773–3775.

Uhl, G.R. (1999) Molecular genetics of substance abuse vulnerability: a current approach. *Neuropsychopharmacology* 20:3–9.

Vanyukov, M.M., Moss, H.B., Gioio, A.E., Hughes, H.B., Kaplan, B.B., and Tarter, R.E. (1998) An association between a microsatellite polymorphism at the DRD5 gene and the liability to substance abuse: pilot study. *Behav Gent* 28:75–82.

Veenstra-VanderWeele, J., Anderson, G.M., and Cook, E.H. (2000) Pharmacogenetics and the serotonin system: initial studies and future directions. *Eur J Pharmacol* 410:165–181.

Vickers, S.P., Clifton, P.G., Dourish, C.T., and Tecott, L.H. (1999) Reduced satiating effect of d-fenfluramine in serotonin 5-HT(2C)

receptor mutant mice. *Psychopharmacology (Berl)* 143:309–314.

Waldman, I.D., Robinson, B.F., and Feigon, S.A. (1997) Linkage disequilibrium between the dopamine transporter gene (*DAT1*) and bipolar disorder: extending the transmission disequilibrium test (TDT) to examine genetic heterogeneity. *Genet Epidemiol* 14(6): 699–704.

Waldman, I.D., Robinson, B.F., and Rowe, D.C. (1999). A logistic regression-based extension of the TDT for continuous and categorical traits. *Ann Hum Genet* 63:329–340.

Waldman, I., Rowe, D., Abramowitz, A., Kozel, S., Mohr, J., Sherman, S., Cleveland, H., Sanders, M., Gard, J., and Stever, C. (1998) Association and linkage of the dopamine transporter gene and attention-deficit hyperactivity disorder in children: heterogeneity owing to diagnostic subtype and severity. *Am J Hum Genet* 63:1767–1776.

Whale, R., Quested, D.J., Laver, D., Harrison, P.J., and Cowen, P.J. (2000). Serotonin transporter (5-HTT) promoter genotype may influence the prolactin response to clomipramine. *Psychopharmacology (Berl)* 150:120–122.

Willeit, M., Stastny, J., Pirker, W., Praschak-Rieder, N., Neumeister, A., Asenbaum, S., Tauscher, J., Fuchs, K., Sieghart, W., Hornik, K., Aschauer, H., Brücke, T., and Kasper, S. (2001) No evidence for in-vivo regulation of midbrain serotonin transporter availability by serotonin transporter promoter gene polymorphism. *Biol Psychiatry* 50:8–12.

Winsberg, B.G. and Comings, D.E. (1999) Association of the dopamine transporter gene (*DAT1*) with poor methylphenidate response. *J Am Acad Child Adolesc Psychiatry* 38:1474–1477.

Yirmiya, N., Pilowsky, T., Nemanov, L., Arbelle, S., Feinsilver, T., Fried, I., Ebstein, R.P. (2001) Evidence for an association with the serotonin transporter promoter region polymorphism and autism. *Am J Med Genet* 105:381–386.

Zabetian, C.P., Anderson, G.M., Buxbaum, S.G., Elston, R.C., Ichinose, H., Nagatsu, T., Kim, K.S., Kim, C.H., Malison, R.T., Gelernter, J., and Cubells, J.F. (2001) A quantitative-trait analysis of human plasma-dopamine beta-hydroxylase activity: evidence for a major functional polymorphism at the DBH locus. *Am J Hum Genet* 68:515–522.

Zanardi, R., Benedetti, F., Di Bella, D., Catalano, M., and Smeraldi, E. (2000) Efficacy of paroxetine in depression is influenced by a functional polymorphism within the promoter of the serotonin transporter gene. *J Clin Psychopharmacol* 20:105–107.

DEVELOPMENTAL PSYCHOPATHOLOGY

8 | Neurobiology of attention regulation and its disorders

AMY F.T. ARNSTEN AND F. XAVIER CASTELLANOS

The word *attention* is an inadequate, singular term for a multitude of interrelated processes. We use a host of adjectives to describe attention—e.g. we say that attention can be divided, oriented, sustained, or focused—and many of these descriptions likely reflect underlying, dissociable neural processes. Complicating matters, attentional resources can be allocated to either external stimuli or to internal stimuli such as memories. Furthermore, we often confuse the regulation of attention (a covert behavior) with the regulation of movement (an overt behavior) when discussing an "attentional" disorder. This may be for good reason: the cortical mechanisms regulating movement are tightly tied to those regulating attention, as discussed below. Attentional processes are also intimately linked to motivation, salience, arousal, and stress, which may enhance or erode aspects of attention in complex ways. This chapter aims to illuminate some of these issues by reviewing what is currently known about brain networks underlying attentional processes, and then relating these mechanisms to attention disorders in children.

BRAIN SYSTEMS MEDIATING ATTENTION

As illustrated in Figure 8.1, different cortical areas make distinct contributions to our attentional experience: The higher order sensory cortices, such as the inferior temporal cortex (ITC), process sensory features and can focus resources on a particular detail, e.g., the color red; the posterior parietal association cortex (PAC) "pays attention," allowing us to orient attention in time and space, and perhaps binding features to allow perception itself; while the prefrontal cortex (PFC) regulates attention, inhibiting processing of irrelevant stimuli, sustaining attention over long delays, and dividing and coordinating attention. The PFC, PAC, and ITC areas are intricately interconnected, creating both feed-forward and feedback loops that work together to provide a unified attentional experience. The following is a brief introduction to the roles these areas play in mediating attention.

Sensory Association Cortices: Inferior Temporal Cortex

Incoming information is processed by parallel yet interconnecting sensory circuits. Electrophysiological studies in monkeys and imaging studies in humans indicate that attention usually has little effect on processing very early in the processing streams, but plays an increasing role as one moves higher up these cortical pathways. For reviews of this field, see Desimone (1996) and Kastner et al. (1998).

The ITC is specialized for processing visual features such as color (in area V4). Processing of a visual stimulus can either be diminished or enhanced, depending upon sensory conditions and internal directions. The activity of ITC neurons is captured by salient stimuli (e.g., high contrasts), but they readily "lose interest" in stimuli—e.g., repeated experience with the same visual stimulus leads to decreased neuronal responding known as *repetition suppression*. This may account for the boredom of repetition in a school setting. Processing of visual stimuli is also diminished by competition from nearby stimuli in the same visual field. Both of these suppressive effects result from intrinsic properties of ITC neurons. (In contrast, processing can be inhibited more thoughtfully by extrinsic projections from the PFC which serve to gate irrelevant stimuli, as will be discussed below.) "Top-down" inputs from the PFC and PAC can also enhance stimulus processing in the ITC. For example, directing attention to a region of space reduces the suppressive interactions between multiple stimuli, particularly for low contrast stimuli. Responses can also be enhanced through learned relevance; for example, attending to a color (e.g., red vs. green) that signals reward increases firing of V4 cells, while the irrelevant color reduces firing. The ITC neu-

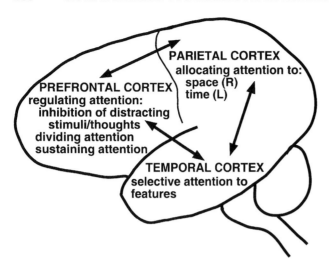

FIGURE 8.1 The prefrontal, parietal, and temporal association cortices form interconnected networks that play complementary roles in attentional processing.

rons can also hold information "on-line" over a short delay if there are no distracters. These enhancing abilities may be conferred by the PFC, which sustains attention during otherwise boring tasks (see below). Thus, top-down projection from the PFC and PAC allows for selective attention in visual cortex.

Posterior Parietal Cortex

The PAC plays a critical role in "paying attention." This cortex is specialized for the analysis of movement and spatial relationships, for analyzing quantity and constructing spatial maps, and for orienting attention in time and space. Indeed, some researchers have proposed that the PAC is responsible for binding features with spatial position to allow perception itself. For reviews of this field, see Coull and Nobre (1998) and Mesulam (2000).

Much of the research on the neural bases of attention has been sparked by interest in the phenomenon of *contralateral neglect*, or the loss of perception for the left side of visual space in patients with right-sided PAC brain lesions (with large lesions, neglect can extend to extravisual modalities as well). The PAC also controls the covert movement of attention, i.e., the orienting of attention without overt movement. Attentional orienting is frequently tested using the Posner paradigm, in which attention is captured by a valid or invalid cue. Patients with PAC lesions, but not those with PFC lesions, are impaired on this task. Imaging studies in humans have since confirmed the importance of the right PAC in the performance of this task. In-

terestingly, recent imaging research in humans has shown that *left* PAC is activated when attention is oriented to an interval in *time* rather than space, while PAC activates bilaterally when one attends to both time and space.

The link between PAC and visuospatial attention has been confirmed by recordings in monkeys (Robinson et al., 1995). Neurons in PAC area 7a increased their firing, depending on whether the animal attended to the region of space where the stimulus occurred. Parietal neurons exhibit a variety of complex, attention-related responses in monkeys performing the Posner task. Neurons in area 7a also appear to create world-referenced maps of visual space, and they project this information to the dorsolateral PFC, which uses this information to effectively guide behavior.

Prefrontal Cortex

The PFC uses representational knowledge, i.e., working memory, to guide overt responses (movement) as well as covert responses (attention), allowing us to inhibit inappropriate behaviors and to attenuate the processing of irrelevant stimuli (for reviews, see Godefroy and Rousseaux, 1996; Goldman-Rakic, 1996; Robbins, 1996; Knight et al., 1999). Patients with PFC lesions are easily distracted, have poor concentration and organization, are more vulnerable to disruption from proactive interference, and can be impulsive, especially when the lesions involve the right hemisphere. Lesions of the PFC impair the ability to sustain attention, particularly over a delay, and reduce the ability to gate sensory input. Such lesions impair divided and focused attention, and these attentional deficits have been associated with lesions in the left, superior PFC. Lesions of the PFC similarly impair attentional function in monkeys and rats, rendering animals more vulnerable to distraction or other types of interference, and impairing attentional regulation on set-shifting tasks.

Electrophysiological studies in monkeys have shown that PFC neurons are able to hold modality-specific information on-line over a delay and use this information to guide behavior in the absence of environmental cues. In contrast to inferior temporal neurons, which stop firing when distracted by a new visual stimulus, PFC neurons can maintain delay-related activity in the presence of distracting stimuli. These studies have also suggested that working memory serves as the basis for behavioral inhibition, as delay-related firing correlates with appropriate behavioral responses in an antisaccade task in which monkeys must look away from a remembered visual stimulus (Funahashi et al., 1993).

Set-shifting is another attentional process linked with PFC function, for example, as assessed in the Wisconsin Card Sorting Task. An animal analog of this task has more precisely examined the PFC mechanisms underlying the ability to switch attentional sets (Robbins, 1996). Lesions to the dorsolateral PFC impaired performance on extradimensional shifting, e.g., when the animal had to switch attention from lines to shapes. In contrast, lesions to the ventromedial PFC impaired performance on intradimensional shifts when the animal had to discriminate between two stimuli within a dimension to learn which was paired with food reward. It has been appreciated for many years that the orbital/ventral surface of the PFC is important for flexible regulation of stimulus–reward responding, i.e., reversal learning. Lesion studies have been corroborated by electrophysiological studies of orbital cortex neurons in the monkey, which rapidly modify their firing in response to changes in reward contingencies (Rolls, 1996). Thus the orbital and medial PFC enables us to inhibit inappropriate affective responses, permitting us to use socially appropriate behavior.

Subcortical Pathways

The PFC, PAC, and ITC all project to the caudate nucleus as part of the cognitive circuit through the basal ganglia, which projects via the thalamus back to PFC (Fig. 8.2). In contrast, the motor circuit involves cortical projections to the putamen, which in turn projects back onto the premotor cortices (Fig. 8.2). This pathway is important for the planning, selection, initiation, and execution of movements. The entire cortical mantle also projects indirectly to the cerebellar cortex (not shown), which ultimately projects back to the primary motor cortex. This pathway serves as a "biological gyroscope," providing on-line correction of movements.

The role of these subcortical structures in the regulation of attention is less clear. The cerebellum is activated during many types of cognitive tasks, but its role in attention is not understood. It is likely that the caudate makes important contributions, but what these are and the ways in which they may be distinct from cortical contributions are currently under investigation (e.g., Crofts et al., 2001).

MODULATION OF CORTICAL CIRCUITS BY THE ASCENDING "AROUSAL" SYSTEMS

Effects of Altering Arousal on Attention

Early studies of the effects of arousal on attention often likened attention to a spotlight that could be widened or focused, moved or stabilized. For example, Hockey (1970) concluded that during conditions of low arousal (drowsiness), the attentional spotlight was diffuse and sluggish; under optimal arousal conditions the spotlight could be focused and moved appropriately, while during overarousal (stress/anxiety), the spotlight became very narrowed and labile. While attention research has become more sophisticated, and we recognize that attention is not a singular spotlight but rather a distributed and complex series of processes, there remains an essential truthfulness to this early research, replicated in recent findings. The following section will review how the ascending "arousal" systems appear to modulate the cortical circuits subserving attention, and thus how changes in arousal, stress, and motivation may alter attentional processing.

The Ascending Arousal Systems

There are a variety of monoaminergic and cholinergic systems that project from the brain stem and basal forebrain to the thalamus and cortex. Acetylcholine (ACh) cells in the pons project to the thalamus, those from the basal forebrain innervate the cortex, and those in the medial septum and diagonal band innervate the hippocampus. There are a variety of ascending monoamine systems as well: the norepinephrine (NE) cells of the locus coeruleus (LC), the dopamine (DA) cells of the ventral tegmental area and substantia nigra, the serotonin (5-HT) cells of the raphe nuclei, and the histamine cells of the posterior hypothalamus (the former two are illustrated in Fig. 8.2). In general, these neuromodulators excite cortical and thalamic cells, switching them from a burst mode that is unresponsive to incoming information to a single spike mode that is capable of processing information (McCormick and Bal, 1997). Very high levels of arousal (anxiety, stress) produce supranormal release of these compounds, particularly DA (reviewed in Birnbaum et al., 1999a). Interestingly, DA innervation of layer III in the PFC peaks around puberty, which may render adolescents more vulnerable to the onset of disorders such as schizophrenia (Lewis, 2001).

Recordings from awake, behaving monkeys suggest that although the NE, DA, and ACh cells all increase their tonic activity during waking, their phasic activity to stimuli occurs in subtly different ways. Both the ACh and DA cells fire in relationship to reward—ACh cells to the reward itself (Richardson and DeLong, 1986) and DA cells to stimuli that signal reward (Schultz et al., 1993). Thus both likely contribute to enhanced attention relative to motivation. In contrast, NE cells appear to fire to stimuli that capture the animal's interest

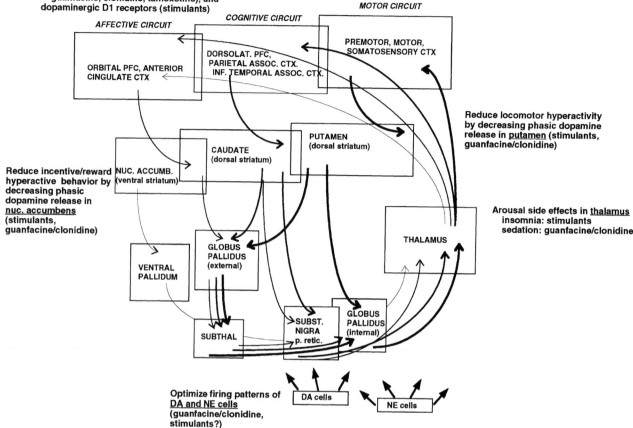

Improve inhibitory control of behavior and attention in both the cognitive and affective realms by optimizing neurochemical influences in <u>prefrontal cortex</u> via: alpha-2A noradrenergic receptors (stimulants, guanfacine, clonidine, tamoxetine); and dopaminergic D1 receptors (stimulants)

Enhance attentional resources in <u>parietal or inferior temporal cortex</u> via: beta and alpha-1 noradrenergic receptors (stimulants,tamoxetine); and dopaminergic receptors (stimulants)

Reduce locomotor hyperactivity by altering catecholamines in <u>motor cortices</u>?

MOTOR CIRCUIT

COGNITIVE CIRCUIT

AFFECTIVE CIRCUIT

PREMOTOR, MOTOR, SOMATOSENSORY CTX

DORSOLAT. PFC, PARIETAL ASSOC. CTX. INF. TEMPORAL ASSOC. CTX.

ORBITAL PFC, ANTERIOR CINGULATE CTX

PUTAMEN (dorsal striatum)

Reduce locomotor hyperactivity by decreasing phasic dopamine release in <u>putamen</u> (stimulants, guanfacine/clonidine)

CAUDATE (dorsal striatum)

Reduce incentive/reward hyperactive behavior by decreasing phasic dopamine release in <u>nuc. accumbens</u> (stimulants, guanfacine/clonidine)

NUC. ACCUMB. (ventral striatum)

THALAMUS

Arousal side effects in <u>thalamus</u> insomnia: stimulants sedation: guanfacine/clonidine

VENTRAL PALLIDUM

GLOBUS PALLIDUS (external)

SUBTHAL

SUBST. NIGRA p. retic.

GLOBUS PALLIDUS (internal)

Optimize firing patterns of <u>DA and NE cells</u> (guanfacine/clonidine, stimulants?)

DA cells

NE cells

FIGURE 8.2 Possible mechanisms by which treatments for ADHD may have their beneficial effects on circuits mediating attention and the regulation of behavior. Parallel corticostriatal loops have been proposed that regulate motor, cognitive, and affective behaviors (Alexander et al., 1986). All of these regions are modulated by norepinephrine (NE) and/or dopamine (DA), and thus may be altered by medications (e.g., stimulants, guanfacine, tamoxetine) that alter catecholamine transmission and are commonly used to treat attention disorders. Note that all of these mechanisms are hypothetical and based on research in animals. Medications may strengthen impulse control and regulation of attention by optimizing catecholamine regulation of prefrontal cortex (PFC) at noradrenergic α_{2A} and dopaminergic D_1 receptors. Posterior cortical attentional processes may also be aided by these medications, but the receptor pharmacology of these mechanisms is more poorly understood. Grace (2001) has proposed that stimulants may reduce locomotor hyperactivity by in-

creasing tonic and decreasing phasic DA release in the striatum. There is also a dense DA innervation of the premotor and motor cortices, but it is not known how this innervation modulates motor cortical function. Medications may optimize the firing of noradrenergic and dopaminergic cells, either through direct actions or indirectly by promoting PFC regulation of these cell groups (the projection from the PFC to the noradrenergic and dopaminergic cell bodies is not shown). Many of the side effects of these medications may also result from actions on these circuits. For example, the insomnia induced by stimulants and the sedation induced by guanfacine may result from drug actions in thalamus, as well as more widespread effects in cortex and excessive actions on catecholamine cells. Abbreviations: ASSOC., association; CTX, cortex; DORSOLAT, dorsolateral; INF., inferior; NUC. ACCUMB., nucleus accumbens; SUBST. NIGRA p. retic., substantia nigra pars reticulata; SUBTHAL., subthalamic nucleus.

102

but not to food per se. In monkeys performing a continuous performance task, LC neurons fired to targets but not distracters (Aston-Jones et al., 1999), perhaps because of PFC regulation of firing. However, when the monkey was drowsy (low tonic activity) or anxious (high tonic activity) this pattern reversed: the salient distracters, but not the subtler targets, engaged phasic LC neuronal firing (Aston-Jones et al., 1999). These may be conditions when there is little PFC regulation of NE cell activity.

NEUROMODULATION OF CORTICAL ATTENTION SYSTEMS

Modulation of Sensory Association Cortices

It has long been appreciated that NE enhances the "signal-to-noise" processing of stimuli in sensory cortex. Waterhouse and colleagues have scrutinized the receptor mechanisms underlying these effects and have found that β-adrenergic receptor stimulation can enhance inhibitory responses, while α_1 adrenergic receptor stimulation can enhance excitatory responses (Mouradian et al., 1991). These effects have been observed in a variety of brain regions, including the auditory and somatosensory cortices, as well as the cerebellum and hippocampus. Norepinephrine and ACh have also been shown to modulate plasticity during development in sensory cortices (e.g., Bear and Singer, 1986). Norepinephrine continues to modulate plasticity of visual receptive fields in the adult brain, enhancing via α_1 adrenoreceptors and decreasing plasticity via α_2 adrenoceptor mechanisms (Kirkwood et al., 1999). There have been few studies of ITC modulation at the behavioral level, although 5-HT antagonists and 5-HT depletion have been shown to *enhance* discrimination responding (Altman and Normile, 1988).

Modulation of Posterior Parietal Association Cortex

Several studies of both human and non-human primates have used the Posner covert attentional orienting paradigm to examine global cholinergic or catecholaminergic manipulations effecting PAC function. Spatial attentional orienting appears particularly sensitive to cholinergic inputs, as lesions of the basal forebrain in monkeys impaired performance of the Posner task, but had no effect on any other test of memory or attention (Voytko et al., 1994). In human patients with Alzheimer's disease, administration of the cholinergic antagonist scopolamine was found to reduce arousal and widen the spatial focus of attentional orienting on a variant of the Posner task (Levy et al., 2000).

Catecholamines also appear to modulate this cortex (reviewed in Coull et al., 2001). Studies in both monkeys and humans have found that clonidine, but not guanfacine, can impair alerting abilities in the Posner task, likely because of reducing NE release. Dopamine receptor blockade also impairs performance.

Modulation of Prefrontal Association Cortex

The neurochemical needs of the PFC have been studied more intensively than other cortical areas because of the immediate relevance of this cortical area to neuropsychiatry and the pioneering work of Brozoski et al. (1979), who found dramatic effects of catecholamine depletion in PFC. The following represents a brief summary of this field. For more detailed reviews of this topic, see Arnsten (1998), Robbins et al. (1998), Sarter and Bruno (2000), and Arnsten and Robbins (2002).

Dopamine

Dopamine modulates PFC functions through actions at both D_1/D_5 and D_4 receptors, and both produce an inverted *U*-shaped dose–response influence on the working memory and attention regulation processes of the PFC. While modest levels of DA are essential to PFC function, high levels of DA release occur during exposure to stress and impair working memory via cAMP/protein kinase A intracellular signaling mechanisms. A similar inverted *U* has been described at the cellular level, where high levels of DA reduce signal transfer and memory-related firing. Limited studies have been done in humans because of the lack of selective D_1/D_5 or D_4 compounds for human use. Human experiments also note an inverted *U*, with the more D_1-like compounds being most effective in improving working memory.

Norepinephrine

Norepinephrine improves PFC function through actions at postsynaptic, α_{2A} receptors at both the cognitive and cellular levels. Thus, α_{2A} agonists enhance, while antagonists erode, memory-related cell firing. The α_{2A} agonist guanfacine improves working memory, attention regulation, behavioral inhibition and planning in rats, monkeys, and humans. Guanfacine is currently used for treating attention-deficit hyperactivity disorder (ADHD), especially in patients who cannot take stimulants, e.g., those with tics (see Chapter 21). It is likely that its therapeutic actions involve strengthening PFC control of behavior (Fig. 8.2).

In contrast, high levels of NE release (e.g., during

stress) impair PFC function through actions at α_1 receptors coupled to protein kinase C. Interestingly, most effective antipsychotic medications, including the atypical neuroleptics, have potent α_1 blocking properties. To date, little effect has been found with β-adrenergic compounds in PFC. This profile contrasts sharply with that of posterior cortical and subcortical areas, which are improved by β and α_1 receptor stimulation, and are impaired or unaffected by α_2 receptor stimulation (reviewed in Arnsten, 2000).

Stimulants

Drugs such as amphetamine and methylphenidate act to enhance the release and/or inhibit the reuptake of both DA and NE. An extensive review of stimulant actions and their relevance to ADHD can be found in Solanto et al. (2001). Methylphenidate can improve PFC working memory function in healthy adult humans and animals (Mehta et al., 2000). It is likely that these improvements are due to both DA and NE beneficial actions in PFC, as well as stimulation of posterior association cortices. Some of the ideas regarding the sites of stimulant therapeutic actions in the brain are illustrated in Figure 8.2.

Acetylcholine

Acetylcholine also has a dramatic influence on PFC function and may be particularly important for the behavioral flexibility supported by medial/orbital PFC and for vigilance during attention tasks. For example, infusion of scopolamine directly into the PFC in rats impairs working memory or sustained attention. These results are consistent with dialysis studies showing ACh release during sustained attention tasks in which rats are working for rewards (Sarter and Bruno, 2000). Conversely, depletion of ACh from the rat PFC reduces PFC neuronal activity, especially activity correlated with the task, such as increased firing to the distracters (Gill et al., 2000). Performance of a sustained attention task in rats can be improved by nicotinic agonists, but less so by cholinergic compounds such as physostigmine. Nicotinic compounds can also improve sustained attention and working memory in humans (Sahakian et al., 1989). However, as stimulation of nicotine receptors increases DA and NE release, this cholinergic effect may actually result via catecholamine mechanisms.

Serotonin

Relatively few studies have examined the role of 5-HT on PFC cognitive functioning. This is partly because of the extraordinary complexity of 5-HT receptor pharmacology, and in part due to early negative results, which dissuaded future experimentation (Brozoski et al., 1979). Studies in humans have found only subtle effects of serotonin depletion on the cognitive and attention functions of the PFC. However, recent studies with selective 5-HT$_{2A}$ receptor compounds have begun to show alterations of function at both the behavioral and cellular levels (Marek and Aghajanian, 1999; Koskinen et al., 2000).

Relation of Neurochemistry to Arousal, Motivation, and Stress

In summary, we have learned that neuromodulators have a critical influence on attentional circuits. When we are drowsy or unmotivated, levels of NE, DA, and ACh release are low in cortex, diminishing the function of all attentional circuits. At optimal levels of arousal and motivation, moderate levels are released which enhance the functioning of both prefrontal and posterior attentional circuits. However, during very high levels of arousal, i.e., during stress when subjects perceive themselves as out of control, very high levels of modulators are released that impair the attentional functions of the PFC, but likely enhance the processing of the PAC and sensory association cortices. Under these conditions, attention would become narrowed on salient signals, and easily captured by parietal mechanisms. However, attention would not be inhibited or regulated by the PFC, thus leaving one more susceptible to environmental factors.

ATTENTION-DEFICIT HYPERACTIVITY DISORDER

The *Diagnostic and Statistical Manual of Mental Disorders, 4th ed.* (DSM-IV) criteria for ADHD include symptoms of inattention and hyperactivity or/impulsivity; patients can have either combined type, or predominantly inattentive (see below) or predominantly hyperactive/impulsive types (American Psychiatric Association, 1994). Many of the symptoms of inattention relate to attentional abilities of the PFC—for example, difficulty sustaining attention, difficulty organizing, easily distracted, and forgetful. However, other symptoms described by DSM-IV could result from either PFC or posterior cortical attentional dysfunction—e.g., does not seem to listen, reluctance or difficulty engaging in tasks that require mental effort, poor attention to details. Thus, these symptoms could arise either due to poor attention regulation by the PFC or due to poor attentional allocation by the posterior cortices. Similarly, many of the symptoms of hyperactivity/

impulsivity describe PFC deficits—e.g., difficulty await-ing turn. But other symptoms in this category could result from dysfunction of either PFC and/or motor cortices and striatum—e.g. acts as if "driven by a mo-tor". Thus, as DSM-IV criteria stand, dysfunction of a variety of corticostriatal circuits may contribute to the ADHD syndrome. Neuroimaging and genetic studies have begun to provide a picture of the biological bases of ADHD. Most of these studies have been performed on patients with the combined profile; studies of inat-tentive types will also be needed (e.g., they may have more posterior cortical problems).

Neuroimaging

The following is a brief review of imaging studies in ADHD. A more comprehensive review can be found in Castellanos and Swanson (2001).

Stuctural imaging

Imaging studies of ADHD have focused on the PFC, basal ganglia, and cerebellum. Volumetric measures have detected smaller right-sided prefrontal regions measured en bloc (Castellanos et al., 1996; Filipek et al., 1997) in boys with ADHD. These reductions cor-related with performance on tasks that required re-sponse inhibition (Casey et al., 1997). In the only pub-lished study to date to report gray–white segmentation, right anterior white matter was also reduced in boys with ADHD (Filipek et al., 1997). Abnormalities of caudate nucleus volume or assymmetry have been re-ported, although the pattern of differences remains complex (Castellanos et al., 1996; Filipek et al., 1997). Girls with ADHD had smaller left and total caudate volumes (Castellanos et al., 2001). A consistent finding in ADHD has been reduced volume of the posterior–inferior cerebellar vermis (reviewed in Castellanos et al., 2001), the only cerebellar region that exhibits DA transporter immunoreactivity (Melchitzky and Lewis, 2000). The function and origin of these DA fibers are not known, but they may form the afferent portion of a cerebellar circuit that influences the ventral tegmental area and the LC (Snider et al., 1976; Dempesy et al., 1983), supporting the speculation that the vermis ex-erts important regulatory influences on PFC-striatal cir-cuitry via the ventral tegmental area and LC.

Functional imaging

Although it would seem that functional imaging studies would be ideal to investigate ADHD, it has been dif-ficult to obtain a consistent picture, perhaps because of interactions between imaging technology and the dis-order itself (e.g., subjects must remain absolutely still and are often surrounded by supervisory adults; the tasks are usually brief and thus do not require sus-tained attention). Despite these limitations, positron emission tomography (PET) was used to demonstrate decreased frontal cerebral metabolism in adults with ADHD (Zametkin et al., 1990). Other investigators have measured local cerebral blood flow, which is linked to neuronal activity and tissue metabolism, with a variety of techniques including[133] Xenon inhalation and single photon emission tomography. Decreased blood flow has been reported in ADHD subjects in the striatum (Lou et al., 1990) and in prefrontal regions (Amen et al., 1993). However, these results remain ten-tative because ethical constraints make it difficult to obtain truly independent observations from normal control children.

By contrast, functional magnetic resonance imaging obviates the need to use ionizing radiation. Early re-sults have been intriguing (Vaidya et al., 1998; Rubia et al., 1999); but important confounds such as medi-cation exposure, first-dose effects, and small sample size require replication.

Neuroreceptor imaging

Positron emission tomographic imaging has been used to examine the neuropharmacology of ADHD. For ex-ample, [18F]F-DOPA uptake was significantly dimin-ished in the left and medial PFC of 17 adults with ADHD compared to that in 23 controls (Ernst et al., 1998), with no differences in striatum or midbrain regions. By contrast, in 10 adolescents with ADHD, [18F]F-DOPA uptake in right midbrain was significantly elevated compared to that in 10 controls ($p = 0.04$, uncorrected for multiple comparisons) (Ernst et al., 1999). If replicated, these preliminary results support the notion that catecholamine dysregulation is central to the pathophysiology of ADHD, and not just to its treatment.

Single photon computed emission tomography (SPECT) with the highly selective DA transporter li-gand [123I] altropane was used to compare 6 adults with ADHD with a database of 30 healthy controls (Dougherty et al., 1999). Striatal binding potential (Bi_{max} / K_d) was elevated in all six ADHD patients. However, this report was questioned because 4 of the 6 patients had been previously treated with stimulants, even though they were all medication-free for at least 1 month.

A second study appears to support the Dougherty study. Ten stimulant-naive adults with ADHD were studied before and after 4 weeks of daily treatment with methylphenidate by SPECT with [Tc-99m]-

TRODAT-1, a SPECT ligand that binds to the DA transporter. Specific binding of [Tc-99m]-TRODAT-1 to the DA transporter was significantly elevated in the patients, compared to age- and sex-matched controls (Krause et al., 2000). Treatment with three doses per day of 5 mg methylphenidate for 1 month significantly decreased specific [Tc-99m]-TRODAT-1 binding in all patients by a mean of 29%. This study shows that even modest therapeutic doses of methylphenidate have robust effects on DA transporter availability. However, a third study of stimulant-naive ADHD adults found no change in striatal DA transporter numbers using [^{123}.I]β-CIT SPECT (van Dyck et al., 2000). Eight of the nine patients in this study were stimulant naive; one had received methylphenidate intermittently between ages 9 and 11 years but had received no stimulants in 14 years. There was no difference between the ADHD adults and the control subjects. The difference in these findings from those of Krause and Doherty suggests that the relationship between prior stimulant use (even in the distant past) and elevated levels of DA transporter in ADHD remains an open question. Alternatively, there may be heterogeneous etiologies underlying ADHD, reflected in the differing outcomes.

Genetics of Attention-Deficit Hyperactivity Disorder

Attention-deficit hyperactivity disorder, like all psychiatric disorders, is not likely to be a single gene disorder. Rather, ADHD falls into the category of complex genetic disorders, which do not follow classic Mendelian inheritance patterns and are believed to result from the combined effects of several genes and interactions with the environment (see Solanto, 2001, for review). A number of dopaminergic candidate genes have been proposed for ADHD because of the consensus that dopaminergic dysregulation is likely to be central to the disorder. The first allelic variation associated with ADHD is in the untranscribed portion of the DA transporter gene (DAT1; see Cook et al., 1995; Waldman et al., 1998; Daly et al., 1999).

Another dopaminergic gene that has aroused interest is the dopamine 4 receptor (DRD4). Some animal studies suggest that DRD4 is involved in the modulation of PFC function (see above). The gene for the DRD4 is particularly interesting, as a large number of allelic variations have been discovered, many of which are determined by the number of 48 base pair repeats in exon 3As noted in a recent meta-analysis (Faraone et al., 2001); most, though not all, studies have found a significant, if modest, association between DRD4 and ADHD.

Finally, one study has found an additive relationship

between alterations in three NE genes, the α_{2A}- and α_{2C}-adrenergic receptors, and the gene for DA β hydroxylase, the synthetic enzyme for NE (Comings et al., 1999). However, this study requires replication before determining the relative roles of DA and NE alterations in this disorder.

In summary, there is surprising consensus that two dopaminergic genes, DAT1 and DRD4, may be associated with susceptibility to ADHD. However, the effects of these genes are modest at best, and the possibility that these findings represent false positives must still be considered. It is also possible that genes involved in NE modulation are affected in some patients. Given the importance of these catecholamines for the modulation of attentional circuits, it would be logical that alterations in these systems would result in impaired attention regulation. However, it is likely that the genetic contributors to the etiology of ADHD will be solidly established as the Human Genome Project approaches its goal of providing the complete sequencing of human DNA.

PHARMACOLOGICAL TREATMENT FOR ATTENTION-DEFICIT HYPERACTIVITY DISORDER: RELEVANCE TO MODULATORY PROCESSES

The most common treatments for ADHD are the stimulant medications methylphenidate and amphetamines. Secondary medications include dopaminergic or noradrenergic reuptake blockers (e.g., a tamoxetine) and α_2-adrenergic agonists. These treatments are reviewed in this volume (see Chapters 20, 21, 24, and 35). Thus, only brief reference will be made here to the possible effects these compounds may have vis-a-vis modulation of attentional circuits. These ideas are summarized in Figure 8.2.

All of these agents serve to facilitate catecholamine transmission; the above discussion has emphasized the importance of proper catecholamine modulation to the integrity of PFC cognitive functioning. Thus it is presumed that stimulants would serve to enhance both DA D_1 and NE α_{2A} receptor stimulation in the PFC. If ADHD involves reduced catecholamine tone in the PFC, as indicated by Ernst and colleagues (1998), stimulant-induced increases would serve to correct this imbalance. More selective DA or NE reuptake blockers would accomplish much the same mission, while α_{2A} agonists would enhance processing by mimicking NE actions at postsynaptic α_{2A} receptors. It is assumed that α_{2A} agonists would not be helpful in patients with posterior cortical dysfunction, as α_{2A} receptor stimulation impairs or has little effect on PAC and ITC function.

However, the posterior cortical areas may be aided by β and α_1-adrenergic receptor stimulation and by dopaminergic stimulation, and thus stimulants may promote the attentional processing abilities of these areas. It is important to note that there has been no direct animal research on catecholamine modulation of posterior cortical function; thus this idea remains speculative.

Stimulants also may reduce hyperactivity through actions in striatum. Grace (2001) has hypothesized that orally administered stimulants may actually reduce phasic DA release by enhancing tonic DA tone, resulting in reduced locomotor activity. This same mechanism could apply to the motor and premotor cortices, which also have relatively high levels of DA innervation. Reduction in phasic DA release in the nucleus accumbens may be particularly important for reducing impulsive actions related to reward (Taylor and Jentsch, 2001).

ANIMAL MODELS OF ATTENTION-DEFICIT HYPERACTIVITY DISORDER

There is no comprehensive animal model of ADHD. The spontaneously hyperactive rat is frequently used as an animal model (Sagvolden, 2001), but rats have limited value because of their small cortex, particularly vis-a-vis the very association cortices thought to be most involved in ADHD. Genetically altered mice with hyperactive phenotypes have been suggested as an animal model, but these animals often do not show the cognitive/attention changes nor pharmacological profiles consistent with ADHD (Gainetdinov et al., 1999). A recent review of rodent models can be found in Ferguson (2001). It is likely that mouse models will be helpful in the future, particularly as animals are identified with impaired PFC function and juvenile hyperactivity that responds to stimulant medication. To date, monkey studies have been more helpful in delineating the cortical mechanisms contributing to attention than as models of ADHD per se.

ATTENTION DYSFUNCTION IN OTHER NEUROPSYCHIATRIC DISORDERS OF CHILDHOOD

Problems with attention are a component of most neuropsychiatric disorders. For example, poor concentration is a major symptom of depression, which may relate to insufficient monoamine stimulation in the PFC. Conversely, the concentration deficits and impulsivity in mania may be associated with a hyper-NE state, and

bipolar disorder in adults has been associated with overactivity of protein kinase C (Manji and Lenox, 1999), and this overactivity impairs PFC function (Birnbaum et al., 1999b). Schizophrenia involves prominent deficits in gating and filtering of inappropriate thoughts and stimulus processing that may contribute to psychotic symptoms. Similarly, post-traumatic stress disorder (PTSD) is thought to involve impaired gating of memories and emotions that the individual would wish to be suppressed. Thus, PFC dysfunction is a factor in many illnesses, but may arise from a variety of differing etiologies. Both genetic factors (e.g., mutations in receptors or transporters) and environmental factors (stress changing the neurochemical environment, trauma during birth, altering developmental processes) likely contribute to these symptoms.

In conclusion, the prefrontal, parietal, and temporal association cortices, and their projections to the striatum, make distinct contributions to attentional experience. These cortical and subcortical areas are profoundly affected by their neurochemical environment. Attention disorders in children involve problems in these circuits that are just beginning to be understood through functional and structural imaging studies. Genetic contributions are likely to be understood in much greater detail in the future with the publication of the Human Genome Project. The development of pharmacological treatments for attentional disorders depends upon our understanding of the corticostriatal circuits underlying these problems, and a sophisticated appreciation of their individual neurochemical requirements.

REFERENCES

Alexander, G.E., Alexander, G.E., DeLong, M.R., and Strick, P.L. (1986) Parallel organization of functionally segregated circuits linking basal ganglia and cortex. *Annu Rev Neurosci* 9:357–381.

Altman, H.J. and Normile, H.J. (1988) What is the nature of the role of the serotonergic nervous system in the learning and memory: prospects for development and effective treatment strategy for senile dementia. *Neurobiol Aging* 9:627–638.

Amen, D.G., Paldi, J.H., and Thisted, R.A. (1993) Brain SPECT imaging. *J Am Acad Child Adoles Psychiatry* 32:1080–1081.

American Psychiatric Association (1994) *Diagnostic and Statistical Manual of Mental Disorders*. Washington, DC: American Psychiatric Association Press.

Arnsten, A.F.T. (1998) Catecholamine modulation of prefrontal cortical cognitive function. *Trends Cogn Sci* 2:436–447.

Arnsten, A.F.T. (2000) Through the looking glass: differential noradrenergic modulation of prefrontal cortical function. *Neural Plasticity* 7:133–146.

Arnsten, A.F.T. and Robbins, T.W. (2001) Neurochemical modulation of prefrontal cortical function in humans and animals. In: Stuss, D. and Knight, R.T., eds. *The Frontal Lobes*, New York: Oxford University Press, pp. 51–84.

Aston-Jones, G., Rajkowski, J., and Cohen, J. (1999) Role of locus coeruleus in attention and behavioral flexibility. *Biol Psychiatry* 46:1309–1320.

Bear, M.F. and Singer, W. (1986) Modulation of visual cortical plasticity by acteylcholine and noradrenaline. *Nature* 320:172–176.

Birnbaum, S.G., Gobeske, K.T., Auerbach, J., Taylor, J.R., and Arnsten, A.F.T. (1999a) A role for norepinephrine in stress-induced cognitive deficits: alpha-1-adrenoceptor mediation in prefrontal cortex. *Biol Psychiatry* 46:1266–1274.

Birnbaum, S.G., Gobeske, K.T., Auerbach, J., Taylor, J.R., and Arnsten, A.F.T. (1999b) The role of alpha-1-adrenoceptor and PKC activation mediating stress-induced cognitive deficits. *Soc Neurosci Abstr* 25:608.

Brozoski, T., Brown, R.M., Rosvold, H.E., and Goldman, P.S. (1979) Cognitive deficit caused by regional depletion of dopamine in prefrontal cortex of rhesus monkey. *Science* 205:929–931.

Casey, B.J., Castellanos, F.X., Giedd, J.N., Marsh, W.L., Hamburger, S.D., et al. (1997) Implication of right frontostriatal circuitry in response inhibition and attention-deficit/hyperactivity disorder. *J Am Acad Child Adolesc Psychiatry* 36:374–383.

Castellanos, F.X., Giedd, J.N., Berquin, P.C., Walter, J.M., Sharp, W., et al. (2001) Quantitative brain magnetic resonance imaging in girls with attention-deficit/hyperactivity disorder. *Arch Gen Psychiatry*, 58:289–295.

Castellanos, F.X., Giedd, J.N., Marsh, W.L., Hamburger, S.D., Vaituzis, A.C., et al. (1996) Quantitative brain magnetic resonance imaging in attention deficit/hyperactivity disorder. *Arch Gen Psychiatry* 53:607–616.

Castellanos, F.X. and Swanson, J. (2002) Biological underpinnings of ADHD. In: Sandberg, S., ed. *Hyperactivity and Attention Disorders of Childhood:Cambridge Monographs in Child and Adolescent Psychiatry*. Cambridge UK: Cambridge University Press, in press.

Comings, D.E., Gade-Andavolu, R., Gonzalez, N., and MacMurray, J.P. (1999) Additive effect of three noradrenergic genes (ADRA2A, ADRA2C, DBH) on attention-deficit hyperactivity disorder and learning disabilities in Tourette syndrome subjects. *Clin Genet* 55:160–172.

Cook, E.H., Jr., Stein, M.A., Krasowski, M.D., Cox, N.J., Olkon, D.M., Kieffer, J.E., and Leventhal, B.L. (1995) Association of attention deficit disorder and the dopamine transporter gene. *Am J Hum Genet* 56:993–998.

Coull, J.T. and Nobre, A.C. (1998) Where and when to pay attention: the neural systems for directing attention to spatial locations and to time intervals as revealed by both PET and fMRI. *J Neurosci* 18:7426–7435.

Coull, J.T., Nobre, A.C., and Frith, C.D. (2001) The noradrenergic alpha2 agonist clonidine modulates behavioural and neuroanatomical correlates of human attentional orienting and alerting. *Cereb Cortex* 11:73–84.

Crofts, H.S., Dalley, J.W., Collins, P., van Denderen, J.C.M., Everitt, B.J., Robbins, T.W., and Roberts, A.C. (2001) Differential effects of 6-OHDA lesions of the prefrontal cortex and caudate nucleus on the ability to acquire an attentional set. *Cereb Cortex*, 11:1015–1026.

Daly, G., Hawi, Z., Fitzgerald, M., and Gill, M. (1999) Mapping susceptibility loci in attention deficit hyperactivity disorder:preferential transmission of parental alleles at DAT1, DBH and DRD5 to affected children. *Mol Psychiatry* 4:192–196.

Dempesy, C.W., Tootle, D.M., Fontana, C.J., Fitzjarrell, A.T., Garey, R.E., and Heath, R.G. (1983) Stimulation of the paleocerebellar cortex of the cat:increased rate of synthesis and release of catecholamines at limbic sites. *Biol Psychiatry* 18:127–132.

Desimone, R. (1996) Neural mechanisms for visual memory and their role in attention. *Proc Nat Acad Sci USA* 93:13494–13499.

Dougherty, D.D., Bonab, A.A., Spencer, T.J., Rauch, S.L., Madras, B.K., and Fischman, A.J. (1999) Dopamine transporter density is elevated in patients with attention deficit hyperactivity disorder. *Lancet* 354:2132–2133.

Ernst, M., Zametkin, A.J., Matochik, J.A., Jons, P.H., and Cohen, R.M. (1998) DOPA decarboxylase activity in attention deficit disorder adults. A [fluorine-18]fluorodopa positron emission tomographic study. *J Neurosci* 18:5901–5907.

Faraone, S.V., Doyle, A.E., Mick, E., and Biederman, J. (2001) Meta-analysis of the association between the dopamine D4 gene 7-repeat allele and attention deficit hyperactivity disorder. *Am J Psychiatry*, 158:1052–1057.

Ferguson, S.A. (2001) A review of rodent models of ADHD. In: Solanto, M.V., Arnsten, A.F.T., and Castellanos, F.X., eds. *Stimulant Drugs and ADHD:Basic and Clinical Neuroscience*. New York: Oxford University Press, pp. 209–220.

Filipek, P.A., Semrud-Clikeman, M., Steingard, R.J., Renshaw, P.F., Kennedy, D.N., and Biederman, J. (1997) Volumetric MRI analysis comparing subjects having attention-deficit hyperactivity disorder with normal controls. *Neurology* 48:589–601.

Funahashi, S., Chafee, M.V., and Goldman-Rakic, P.S. (1993) Prefrontal neuronal activity in rhesus monkeys performing a delayed anti-saccade task. *Nature* 365:753–756.

Gainetdinov, R.R., Wetsel, W.C., Jones, S.R., Levin, E.D., Jaber, M., and Caron, M.G. (1999) Role of serotonin in the paradoxical calming effect of psychostimulants on hyperactivity. *Science* 283:397–401.

Gill, T.M., Sarter, M., and Givens, B. (2000) Sustained visual attention performance-associated prefrontal neuronal activity: evidence for cholinergic modulation. *J Neurosci* 20:4745–4757.

Godefroy, O. and Rousseaux, M. (1996) Divided and focused attention in patients with lesion of the prefrontal cortex. *Brain Cogn* 30:155–174.

Goldman-Rakic, P.S. (1996) The prefrontal landscape: implications of functional architecture for understanding human mentation and the central executive. *Phil Trans R Soc Lond* 351:1445–1453.

Grace, A.A. (2001) Psychostimulant actions on dopamine and limbic system function:relevance to the pathophysiology and treatment of ADHD. In: Solanto, M.V., Arnsten, A.F.T., and Castellanos, F.X., eds. *Stimulant Drugs and ADHD: Basic and Clinical Neuroscience*. New York:Oxford University Press, pp. 134–158.

Hockey, G.R.J. (1970) Effect of loud noise on attentional selectivity. *Q J Exp Psychol* 22:28–36.

Kastner, S., De Weerd, P., Desimone, R., and Ungerleider, L.G. (1998) Mechanisms of directed attention in the human extrastriate cortex as revealed by functional MRI. *Science* 282:108–111.

Kirkwood, A., Rozas, C., Kirkwood, J., Perez, F., and Bear, M.F. (1999) Modulation of long-term synaptic depression in visual cortex by acetylcholine and norepinephrine. *J Neurosci* 19:1599–1609.

Knight, R.T., Staines, W.R., Swick, D., and Chao, L.L. (1999) Prefrontal cortex regulates inhibition and excitation in distributed neural networks. *Acta Psychol* 101:159–178.

Koskinen, T., Ruotsalainen, S., Puumala, T., Lappalainen, R., Koivisto, E., et al. (2000) Activation of 5-HT2A receptors impairs response control of rats in a five-choice serial reaction time task. *Neuropharmacology* 39:471–481.

Krause, K.H., Dresel, S.H., Krause, J., Kung, H.F., and Tatsch, K. (2000) Increased striatal dopamine transporter in adult patients with attention deficit hyperactivity disorder:effects of methylphenidate as measured by single photon emission computed to-mography. *Neurosci Lett* 285:107–110.

Levy, J.A., Parasuraman, R., Greenwood, P.M., Dukoff, R., and Sunderland, T. (2000) Acetylcholine affects the spatial scale of attention:evidence from Alzheimer's disease. *Neuropsychology* 14: 288–298.

Lewis, D.A. (2001) The catecholamine innervation of primate cerebral cortex. In: Solanto, M.V., Arnsten, A.F.T., and Castellanos, F.X., eds. *Stimulant Drugs and ADHD: Basic and Clinical Neuroscience*. New York: Oxford University Press, pp. 77–103.

Lou, H.C., Henriksen, L., and Bruhn, P. (1990) Focal cerebral dysfunction in developmental learning disabilities. *Lancet* 335:8–11.

Manji, H.K. and Lenox, R.H. (1999) Protein kinase C signaling in the brain: molecular transduction of mood stabilization in the treatment of manic-depressive illness. *Biol Psychiatry* 46:1328–1351.

Marek, G.J. and Aghajanian, G.K. (1999) 5-HT2A receptor or alpha1-adrenoceptor activation induces EPSCs in layer V pyramidal cells of the medial prefrontal cortex. *Eur J Pharmacol* 367: 197–206.

McCormick, D.A. and Bal, T. (1997) Sleep and arousal:thalamocortical mechanisms. *Annu Rev Neurosci* 20:185–215.

Mehta, M.A., Owen, A.M., Sahakian, B.J., Mavaddat, N., Pickard, J.D., and Robbins, T.W. (2000) Methylphenidate enhances working memory by modulating discrete frontal and parietal lobe regions in the human brain. *J Neurosci* 20:RC651–RC656.

Melchitzky, D.S. and Lewis, D.A. (2000) Tyrosine hydroxylase– and dopamine transporter–immunoreactive axons in the primate cerebellum. Evidence for a lobular- and laminar-specific dopamine innervation. *Neuropsychopharmacology* 22:466–472.

Mesulam, M.-M. (2000) *Principles of Behavioral and Cognitive Neurology*. New York: Oxford University Press.

Mouradian, R.D., Seller, F.M., and Waterhouse, B.D. (1991) Noradrenergic potentiation of excitatory transmitter action in cerebrocortical slices:evidence of mediation by an alpha$_1$-receptor-linked second messenger pathway. *Brain Res* 546:83–95.

Richardson, R.T. and DeLong, M.R. (1986) Nucleus basalis of Meynert neuronal activity during a delayed response task in a monkey. *Brain Res* 399:364–368.

Robbins, T.W. (1996) Dissociating executive functions of the prefrontal cortex. *Phil Trans R Soc Lond* 351:1463–1471.

Robbins, T.W., Granon, S., Muir, J.L., Durantou, F., Harrison, A., and Everitt, B.J. (1998) Neural systems underlying arousal and attention: implications for drug abuse. *Ann N Y Acad Sci* 846: 222–237.

Robinson, D.L., Bowman, E.M., and Kertzman, C. (1995) Covert orienting of attention in macaques. II. Contributions of parietal cortex. *J Neurophysiol* 74:698–712.

Rolls, E.T. (1996) The orbitofrontal cortex. *Phil Trans R Soc Lond* 351:1433–1444.

Rubia, K., Overmeyer, S., Taylor, E., Brammer, M., Williams, S.C.R., et al. (1999) Hypofrontality in attention deficit hyperactivity dis-order during higher-order motor control: a study with functional MRI. *Am J Psychiatry* 156:891–896.

Sagvolden, T. (2001) The spontaneously hypertensive rat as a model of ADHD. In: Solanto, M.V., Arnsten, A.F.T., and Castellanos, F.X., eds. *Stimulant Drugs and ADHD: Basic and Clinical Neuroscience*. New York:Oxford University Press, pp. 221–238.

Sahakian, B.J., Jones, G., Levy, R., Gray, J.G., and Warburton, D. (1989) The effects of nicotine on attention, information processing and short term memory in patients with dementia of the Alzheimer-type. *Br J Psychiatry* 154:797–800.

Sarter, M. and Bruno, J.P. (2000) Cortical cholinergic inputs mediating arousal, attentional processing and dreaming:differential afferent regulation of the basal forebrain by telencephalic and brainstem afferents. *Neuroscience* 95:933–952.

Schultz, W., Apicella, P., and Ljungberg, T. (1993) Responses of monkey dopamine neurons to reward and conditioned stimuli during successive steps of learning a delayed response task. *J Neurosci* 13:900–913.

Snider, R.S., Maiti, A., and Snider, S.R. (1976) Cerebellar pathways to ventral midbrain and nigra. *Exp Neurol* 53:714–728.

Solanto, M.V. (2001) Attention-deficit/hyperactivity disorder:clinical features. In: Solanto, M.V., Arnsten, A.F.T., and Castellanos, F.X., *Stimulant Drugs and ADHD:Basic and Clinical Neuroscience*. New York:Oxford University Press, pp. 3–30.

Solanto, M.V., Arnsten, A.F.T., and Castellanos, F.X., eds. (2001) *Stimulant Drugs and ADHD: Basic and Clinical Neuroscience*. New York: Oxford University Press.

Taylor, J.R. and Jentsch, J.D. (2001) Stimulant effects on striatal and cortical dopamine systems involved in reward-related behavior and impulsivity. In: Solanto, M.V., Arnsten, A.F.T., and Castellanos, F.X., eds. *Stimulant Drugs and ADHD:Basic and Clinical Neuroscience*. New York:Oxford University Press, pp. 104–133.

Vaidya, C.J., Austin, G., Kirkorian, G., Ridlehuber, H.W., Desmond, J.E., et al. (1998) Selective effects of methylphenidate in attention deficit hyperactivity disorder: a functional magnetic resonance study. *Proc Nat Acad Sci USA* 95:14494–14499.

van Dyck, C.H., Quinlan, D.M., Cretella, L., Staley, J.K., Malison, R.T., et al. (2002) Striatal dopamine transporter availability with [123I]β-CIT SPECT is unaltered in adult attention deficit hyperactivity disorder. *Am J Psychiatry*, 159:309–312.

Voytko, M.L., Olton, D.S., Richardson, R.T., Gorman, L.K., Tobin, J.T., and Price, D.L. (1994) Basal forebrain lesions in monkeys disrupt attention but not learning and memory. *J Neurosci* 14: 167–186.

Waldman, I.D., Rowe, D.C., Abramowitz, A., Kozel, S.T., Mohr, J.H., et al. (1998) Association and linkage of the dopamine transporter gene and attention-deficit hyperactivity disorder in children:heterogeneity owing to diagnostic subtype and severity. *Am J Hum Genet* 63:1767–1776.

Zametkin, A.J., Nordahl, T.E., Gross, M., King, A.C., Semple, W.E., et al. (1990) Cerebral glucose metabolism in adults with hyperactivity of childhood onset. *N Engl J Med* 323:1361–1366.

9 | Neurobiology of early-life stress and its disorders

CHRISTINE M. HEIM AND CHARLES B. NEMEROFF

The relative contribution of disposition and experience to the pathogenesis of mental disorders has been explored in numerous studies. Evidence from these studies suggests a strong genetic contribution to the development of the major psychiatric disorders. In addition, a preeminent role of stressful life events has been documented for several disorders, especially mood and anxiety disorders, but schizophrenia as well. Along with growing societal recognition of the existence and high incidence of child maltreatment and other adverse experiences in children, a large number of studies have evaluated the impact of early untoward life events on the development of mental disorders. Given the accumulating evidence for a strong impact of early adverse experience on the development of mental disorders, considerable attention has recently been directed towards the exploration of the neurobiological mechanisms by which stressful experiences early in life may be translated into mental disease persisting into adulthood. The present chapter summarizes available findings on the relationship between early adversities and mental disease and its neurobiological underpinnings, with a focus on mood and anxiety disorders.

EARLY-LIFE STRESS

Definition

According to prevailing concepts, stress is being experienced when an individual is confronted with a situation that is appraised as personally threatening and for which adequate coping resources are unavailable (Lazarus, 1985). Biological stress reactions are particularly elicited during novel, uncertain, and unpredictable situations (Mason, 1968). These concepts emphasize that individual perception and behavioral adaptations to an event are critical to the experience of stress. In addition, physical stimuli, such as injury, may represent threats to homeostasis and elicit stress responses. Any such situation occurring during development may be classified as early-life stress in humans.

Of obvious importance are incidents of child maltreatment, including sexual or physical abuse, emotional abuse, and neglect. *Sexual abuse* may best be defined as exposure of a child to sexual situations, the passive use of children as sexual stimuli for adults, and sexual contacts between children and older people. *Physical abuse* involves intentional harm to the child's body through excessive force. *Emotional abuse* has been defined as coercive, demeaning, or overly distant behavior by a parent or caretaker that interferes with the child's development. *Neglect* is defined as failure of a caretaker to provide basic shelter, supervision, medical care, or support (Wissow, 1995). Although the need for a uniform definition of child maltreatment has been recognized, there is a large variation of definitions evident in the literature. Other incidents of early-life stress involve the loss of a parent due to death or separation and living with a mentally ill parent, as well as natural disaster, accidents, physical illness, family violence, and war among other difficult experiences. Furthermore, a stressful prenatal or perinatal environment, such as maternal stress during pregnancy or birth complications, may be subsumed to early-life stress.

Prevalence

According to the U.S. Department of Health and Human Services, 1.4 million cases of child maltreatment are reported annually, with 160,000 children suffering serious injuries and 2000 children dying each year as a consequence of maltreatment. Prevalence rates have been evaluated for different types of abuse in clinical, community, and national samples. Prevalence rates of sexual abuse range from 7%–62% in women (McCauley et al., 1997). A reanalysis of 166 studies on the prevalence of sexual abuse in boys revealed rates from

4% to 76%, suggesting that sexual abuse in men is largely underestimated (Holmes and Slap, 1998). Prevalence rates of physical abuse range from 10% to 30% in women and are generally higher in men. The apparent variation across studies is likely due to different case definitions, sample characteristics, and assessment methods. Regarding the prevalence of parental loss, the U.S. Bureau of Census reported that 27% of children lived with only one parent and 4% lived with neither parent in 1995. A vast number of children are exposed to parental psychopathology. For example, 12%–50% of women with young children suffer from depressive episodes. There are also reports that 5%–16% of women are abused during pregnancy, suggesting that a significant number of children experience prenatal stress (see Heim and Nemeroff, 2001).

Relationship to Psychopathology

Approximately two-thirds of sexually abused children exhibit symptoms of anxiety, fear, sleep disturbance, and intrusive thoughts as well as internalizing and externalizing behavioral problems, including crying, irritability, withdrawal, and depression, together with disturbed expressions of anger or aggression. As they grow older, poor academic performance, substance abuse, and delinquency are frequent. Physical abuse and neglect are associated with similar disturbances, suggesting that there is no specific syndrome related to sexual abuse. Increased rates of syndromal major depression, post-traumatic stress disorder (PTSD), attention deficit-hyperactivity disorder (ADHD), and other disorders have been reported for maltreated children and adolescents (e.g., Kendall-Tackett et al., 1993). Likewise, adolescents who experience the separation from parents express more psychiatric symptoms than adolescents of intact families and children of mentally ill or overprotective parents exhibit more mental disorders than children of healthy parents. Thus, it appears that different types of early-life stress have profound and similar immediate effects on mental health in children and adolescents.

Numerous studies found that childhood sexual, physical, and emotional abuse also predisposes victims of such abuse to the development of depression in adulthood (e.g., McCauley et al., 1997). The risk for depression increases with early onset and severity of the abuse as well as with the experience of multiple types of abuse. In addition, child abuse is related to an array of anxiety disorders, including generalized anxiety disorder and PTSD (e.g., Kendler et al., 2000). Other disorders related to childhood abuse include substance abuse, eating disorders, dissociation, and so-

matoform disorders, among others. Depression and anxiety disorders, but other psychiatric disorders as well, often coincide in victims of child abuse, while there is little specificity regarding the long-term consequences of different types of abuse. Other types of early stress, such as parental loss or mental illness of parents, also increase the risk for depression and anxiety disorders, as well as bipolar disorder and schizophrenia, in adulthood (Kessler and Magee, 1993; Agid et al., 2000). Prenatal stress also results in an increased risk for adult depression.

NEUROBIOLOGICAL SYSTEMS INVOLVED IN THE MEDIATION OF STRESS RESPONSES

Corticotropin-Releasing Factor Systems

The relationship between early-life stress and the development of depression and anxiety disorders as well as other mental disorders is hypothesized to be mediated by persistent changes in neurobiological systems that are implicated in the regulation of the stress responses, i.e., corticotropin-releasing factor (CRF) and other neurotransmitter systems. High densities of CRF-containing cell bodies are found in the hypothalamic paraventricular nucleus (PVN), which form the central component of the hypothalamic–pituitary–adrenal (HPA) axis. During stress, CRF is released into the portal circulation and subsequently binds to receptors of the adenohypophyseal corticotropes to stimulate the release of adrenocorticotropin hormone (ACTH), which, in turn, stimulates the secretion of glucocorticoids from the adrenal cortex (Fig. 9.1). Glucocorticoids exert metabolic and immune-modulating effects and inhibit the neuroendocrine stress response via negative feedback, which is mediated by two types of receptors, the mineralocorticoid receptors (MR) in the hippocampus and the widely distributed glucocorticoid receptors (GR). While these effects are critical to the adaptation of an organism to stress, excessive glucocorticoid exposure may be harmful.

Outside of the hypothalamus, an abundant presence of CRF neurons is found in the neocortex, likely influencing cognitive appraisals and behavioral reactions to stress. High densities of CRF neurons are also found in the central nucleus of the amygdala (CeA), which is the key structure in the mediation of emotion (LeDoux, 2000). These CRF neurons likely modulate affective stress responses. The CRF neurons originating from the CeA project directly and indirectly, via the bed nucleus of the stria terminalis (BNST), to the hypothalamic PVN and influence endocrine responses to stress. Fur-

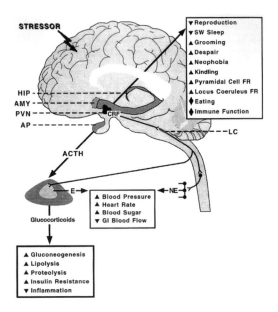

FIGURE 9.1 Endocrine, autonomic, behavioral, and immunological effects of corticotropin-releasing factor (CRF). ▲ increase; ▼ decrease; ♦, both increase and decrease. AMY, amygdala; AP, anterior pituitary; E, epinephrine; FR, firing rate; GI, gastrointestinal; HIP, hippocampus; LC, locus coeruleus; NE, norepinephrine; PVN, paraventricular nucleus; SW, slow wave. Reprinted from Arborelius et al. (1999).

thermore, amygdaloid CRF neurons send projections to brain stem nuclei, including the locus coeruleus (LC), which regulates autonomic outflow and contains the bulk of the noradrenergic projections to the forebrain, and the nuclei raphé (NR), which are the major source of serotonergic projections to the forebrain. These monoaminergic neurotransmitter systems have long been implicated in the pathophysiology of mood and anxiety disorders (Owens and Nemeroff, 1991). An equally widespread distribution of two subtypes of CRF receptors throughout the central nervous system (CNS) suggests that CRF, in fact, serves as a neurotransmitter in these brain regions. Thus, microinjection studies have shown that CRF increases neuronal firing rates in the LC and, at low doses, inhibits neuronal firing rates in the NR, whereas high doses of CRF enhance NR neuronal firing rates (Valentino et al., 1983; Kirby et al., 2000). Monoaminergic neurons themselves send projections to various brain regions that contain CRF neurons or are involved in the stress response. Noradrenergic neurons serve as the major stimulus for CRF release from the PVN. Serotonergic neurons modulate stress responses through projections to the PVN, amygdala, the hippocampus, and the prefrontal cortex. Gamma-aminobutyric acid (GABA)-

containing neurons located in these brain structures exert inhibitory influences on central CRF neurons and stress responsiveness. The strategic distribution of CRF neurons and its receptors throughout the CNS infers a role of CRF as a neuroendocrine releasing factor and a neurotransmitter, which, in concert with other neurotransmitter systems, integrates endocrine, autonomic, and behavioral responses to stress.

Consistent with its neuroanatomical distribution, central administration of CRF to laboratory animals produces physiological and behavioral changes that are reminiscent of stress, depression, and anxiety (Owens and Nemeroff, 1991; Fig. 9.1). Microinjection studies have shown that CRF induces many of the anxiety-like behaviors through actions in neural circuits connecting the amygdala with the noradrenergic neurons of the LC. The effects of CRF are reversed by CRF antagonists and, moreover, CRF antagonists attenuate many anxiety-like responses to stress. Evidence from studies using antisense oligonucleotides against CRF_1 and CRF_2 receptors suggest that the anxiogenic effects of CRF are mediated via binding to the CRF_1 receptor, whereas CRF_2 receptors, which bind with higher affinity to urocortin than to CRF, may mediate stress coping. Accordingly, transgenic mice lacking the CRF_1 receptor are less fearful and show decreased pituitary-adrenal stress responses, whereas transgenic mice lacking the CRF_2 receptor display increased anxiety-like behavior and stress sensitization (see Heim and Nemeroff 2001). Taken together, the depressogenic and anxiogenic properties of CRF are consistent with its neuroanatomical distribution and its mutual interactions with other neurotransmitter circuits involved in the regulation of emotion, and suggest that CRF hyperactivity may constitute the neurobiological substrate of the relationship between early-life stress and mood or anxiety disorders.

Ontogeny of the Neurobiological Stress Response System

It may be assumed that early-life stress induces long-term alterations in this neurobiological stress response system through interference with its ontogeny. It is known that CRF and CRF receptors are evident after 16 days of gestation in rat fetuses and after 12–13 weeks of gestation in human fetuses. In rats, the density and distribution of CRF receptors are subject to substantial modifications throughout the prenatal and postnatal phase, reaching adult status at postnatal day (pnd) 14. Similarly, aminergic innervations of the PVN as well as the hippocampus and the portal vessel system are not fully established at birth and develop until pnd 14 in the rat. Consistent with this lack of development, a stress–hyporesponsive period has been described in rats from pnd 4–14, in which the HPA axis does not respond to a variety of stressors, most likely reflecting a protective mechanism, which prevents adverse glucocorticoid effects on neurodevelopment. The stage of CNS development during pnd 4–14 in rats corresponds to the developmental stage of human fetuses at 24 weeks of gestation. After birth, human infants are capable of mounting significant cortisol responses, which reach adult levels after 3 months (see Graham et al., 1999). Thus, it is plausible that stress during early development interferes with neurodevelopment, thereby inducing long-term maladaptations, which increase the risk for psychopathology.

NEUROBIOLOGICAL CONSEQUENCES OF EARLY-LIFE STRESS

Studies in Rodents

Among animal models of early-life stress are separations of rat pups from their dams, the caregiving adult female rats, during the neonatal period (for detailed description see Animal Models for Psychopharmacological Research, below). Despite the stress–hyporesponsive period, infant rats have been shown to mount pronounced corticosterone responses to maternal separation. One recent study reported that 12-day-old rats exposed to maternal deprivation exhibited increased ACTH responses to restraint stress as compared to nondeprived rats. While CRF mRNA expression in the PVN increased during restraint in both groups, only the maternally deprived rats exhibited increased AVP mRNA expression, which suggests that increased stress responsiveness is due to synergy effects of CRF and AVP (Dent et al., 2000). Interestingly, maternal separation at pnd 3–4 produced increased ACTH responses to stress, whereas maternal separation at pnd 11–12 produced blunted ACTH responses to stress in rats at pnd 20 (van Oers et al., 1998). These findings suggest that there are critical developmental "windows," in which early-life stress may have differential effects on neurobiological function.

A considerable body of literature has focused on the long-term consequences of maternal separation in rats (Table 9.1). Adult rats separated from their dams for 180 minutes/day on pnd 2–14 demonstrate increased CRF concentrations in the median eminence, portal blood, and CSF, as well as increased CRF mRNA expression in the PVN and decreased GR binding in the hippocampus as compared to rats reared under normal conditions. These rats also exhibited increased ACTH and corticosterone responses to a variety of stressors (Plotsky and Meaney 1993). Adult rats removed from their dams for 240 minutes/day on pnd 2–21 exhibited increased median eminence CRF concentrations and decreased pituitary CRF receptor binding as well as increased ACTH, but normal corticosterone responses to foot shock (Ladd et al., 1996). These results suggest that more severe or extended postnatal stress may promote dissociation of pituitary and adrenal reactivity. Rats exposed to maternal separation also developed marked behavioral abnormalities reminiscent of depression and anxiety (Caldji et al., 2000), consistent with increased CRF activity in corticolimbic and brain stem circuits. Accordingly, maternally separated adult rats demonstrated increased CRF mRNA expression in the CeA and BNST as well as increased CRF concentrations and increased CRF receptor binding in the LC (Plotsky et al., in press).

Consistent with the evidence that the LC-noradrenergic neurons project to the hypothalamus, increased PVN norepinephrine (NE) concentrations were measured in maternally separated rats (Liu et al., 2000). Moreover, increased CRF receptor binding has been measured in the NR in maternally separated rats (Ladd et al., 1996), which may be associated with altered neural firing rates. Another recent study found decreased levels of $GABA_A$ and central benzodiazepine receptors (CBZ) in maternally separated rats. Ligand binding to the CBZ enhanced the affinity of the $GABA_A$ receptor for GABA, resulting in reduced anxiety. Decreased levels of these receptors were thus associated with increased behaviors of anxiety in maternally separated rats (Caldji et al., 2000).

In contrast to the long-term consequences of maternal separation, brief handling of rat pups for 15 minutes/day on pnd 2–14 results in a phenotype that is less sensitive to stress and less fearful than that of rats left undisturbed. Remarkably, it has been shown that brief removals of pups result in increased maternal caregiving behavior. Naturally occurring variation in maternal care is strongly associated with neuroendocrine and behavioral stress responsiveness as well as with alterations in neurocircuits implicated in anxiety (Liu et al., 1997; Caldji et al., 1998). Like maternal separation or decreased caregiving behavior, prenatal stress also induces marked increases in fear-related behaviors and ACTH responses to stress along with increases of CRF peptide and CRF receptor binding in the amygdala (e.g., Ward et al., 2000).

TABLE 9.1 *Long-term Neurobiological Changes in Selected Models of Early-Life Stress*

Model	Species	Timing	Neurobiological Changes	
Maternal separation	Rats	180 minutes/day pnd 2–14	ACTH after stress	↑
			CORT after stress	↑
			CRF in CSF, ME, LC	↑
			CRF receptor binding in LC	↑
			CRF mRNA in PVN, CeA, BNST	↑
			NE in PVN	↓
			GABA$_A$ in LC and NTS	↓
			GABA$_A$ γ2 mRNA CeA, LnA, LC, NTS, FC	↓
			CBZ in CeA, LnA, LC, NTS	↓
			GR in hippocampus	↓
	Rats	4–6 hours day pnd 2–14	ACTH basal and after stress	↑
			CORT basal and after stress	↑
			ME CRF	↑
			Pituitary CRF receptor binding	↓
			CRF receptor binding in NR	↑
	Non-human primates	Separated after birth and peer-reared	ACTH after stress	↑
			CORT after stress	↑
Variable foraging demand	Non-human primates	12 weeks beginning at ~17 weeks of age	CSF CRF	↑
			CSF CORT	↓
			Behavioral response to yohimbine	↑
			GH response to clonidine	↓
			Behavioral response to m-CPP	↑
Childhood abuse	Adult humans	Before puberty	24-hour urinary cortisol	↑[a]
			ACTH after psychosocial stress	↓
			CORT after psychosocial stress	↑[b], ↑[c]
			ACTH after CRF challenge	↑[b], ↓[c]
			CORT after ACTH$_{1-24}$ challenge	↓[b], →[c]
			CORT after dexamethasone	↓
			24-hour urinary NE	↑[a]
			Autonomic response to stress/imagery	↑[a,b]
			Prolactin response to m-CPP	↓
			Hippocampus size	↓[a]

ACTH, adrenocorticotropic hormone; BNST, bed nucleus of the stria terminalis; CBZ, central benzodiazepine receptor; CeA, central nucleus of the amygdala; CORT, corticosterone or cortisol; CRF, corticotropin-releasing factor; CSF, cerebrospinal fluid; FC, frontal cortex; GABA, gamma-aminobutyric acid A receptor; GH, growth hormone; GR, glucocorticoid receptor; LC, locus coeruleus; LnA, lateral nucleus of the amygdala; NTS, nucleus tractus solitarius; m-CPP, meta-chlorophenylpiperazine; ME, median eminence; mRNA, messenger ribonucleic acid; NR, nucleus raphé; pnd, postnatal day; PVN, paraventricular nucleus; ↑, increased; ↓, decreased; →, unaltered.

[a]With current major depression. [b]Without current major depression. [c]With current post-traumatic stress disorder.

Studies in Non-Human Primates

Several studies evaluating the consequence of early-life stress in non-human primates have provided findings similar to those in rodents. For example, 6-month-old rhesus monkeys reared without their mothers, but with peers, showed increased cortisol responses to social separation as compared to mother-reared rhesus monkeys, with cortisol increases predicting alcohol preference of these monkeys in young adulthood (Fahlke et al., 2000). Maternally deprived adult non-human primates also exhibited increased pituitary-adrenal activation and distress vocalizations when separated from peers as compared to mother-reared primates (Suomi, 1991). Interestingly, a magnetic resonance imaging (MRI) study found decreased volumes of the posterior corpus callosum, but not of the hippocampus, in prepubescent non-human primates reared under social isolation from 2 to 12 months of age as compared to primates reared in a social environment (Sanchez et al., 1998), paralleling findings in maltreated children (see below).

A series of studies in non-human primates have focused on variations in maternal behavior during infancy (Table 9.1). Mothers of infant bonnet macaques are confronted with low (LFD), high (HFD), or variable foraging demand (VFD), resulting in differential perception of security and maternal care in the infants (for detailed description see Animal Models for Psychopharmacological Research, below). As adults, VFD-reared bonnet macaques demonstrated stable traits of anxiety and significantly elevated cerebrospinal fluid (CSF) CRF concentrations when compared to LFD- or HFD-reared non-human primates (Coplan et al., 1996). The CSF cortisol levels were actually lower in animals exposed to VFD, which suggests dissociation between increased CRF and decreased adrenal activity. The VFD-reared non-human primates further exhibited exaggerated behavioral responses to the administration of the selective α_2-receptor antagonist yohimbine, and reduced growth hormone responses to the α_2 agonist clonidine, reflecting sensitization of the nordrenergic system after early-life stress (Coplan et al., 2000). The VFD reared non-human primates also exhibited decreased behavioral responses to the serotonin (5-HT) agonist meta-chlorophenylpiperazine (m-CPP), which suggests a 5-HT dysfunction (Rosenblum et al., 1994).

Clinical Studies

A number of clinical studies are now available that evaluate neurobiological alterations as a consequence of early-life stress in children or adult humans.

Studies in Children

Several studies recruiting children of different ages who experienced different types of early-life stress at different developmental stages report decreased salivary cortisol concentrations in the morning and/or a lack of decline of cortisol towards the evening, suggesting a disturbed circadian rhythm of the HPA axis (see Heim and Nemeroff, 2001). The absent decline of cortisol in these children may be due to higher numbers of stressful events during the day and/or increased HPA responses to daily stress. Thus, the total 24-hour urinary cortisol excretion is unaltered or increased in maltreated children, depending on the duration of the abuse and the severity of psychopathology (DeBellis et al., 1994a, 1999a). In response to a CRF stimulation test, sexually abused girls, most of whom suffered from dysthymia, demonstrated a markedly blunted ACTH response as compared to controls in one study (De-Bellis et al., 1994a), likely reflecting in part pituitary CRF receptor down-regulation due to hypothalamic CRF hypersecretion. Another study using the CRF stimulation test found enhanced ACTH and normal cortisol responses in abused children with current depression, compared to those in non-abused depressed children and controls (Kaufman et al., 1997). About half of these children were emotionally abused at the time of the study. In a naturalistic stress study, maltreated children did not show an increase of cortisol in a social conflict situation, whereas controls showed increases (Hart et al., 1995), but these results may reflect lack of novelty to such situations in maltreated children, rather than decreased stress sensitivity. Two studies using the dexamethasone suppression test in children with acute parental death (Weller et al., 1990) and children who were in an earthquake 5 years prior to the study (Goenjian et al., 1996) yielded opposite results. While bereaved children were depressed and did not adequately suppress cortisol, the children exposed to the earthquake showed symptoms of PTSD and enhanced suppression of cortisol, similar to some findings in adult patients with PTSD. Taken together, it is evident that neuroendocrine dysfunction in children with early-life stress is highly variable and likely influenced by multiple factors—i.e., type, age at onset and duration of the stressful event, the time elapsed since the event, concomitant stress, and psychopathology.

Similar to findings in animal models of early-life stress, elevated 24-hour urinary NE, epinephrine (E), and dopamine (DA) excretion as well as decreased platelet adrenergic receptors have been measured in abused children with PTSD (Perry, 1994; DeBellis et al., 1999a). Abused children with PTSD also exhibit increased heart rate and blood pressure levels at rest and after orthostatic challenge (Perry, 1994). Elevated catecholamine levels were also found in abused girls without PTSD (DeBellis et al., 1994b) and children whose parents had marital problems (Gottman and Katz, 1989). Notably, decreased levels of NE and DA-β-hydroxylase (DβH), the rate limiting factor in the synthesis of NE, were observed in children who were neglected in infancy (Rogeness and McClure, 1996). These findings suggest that different types or timing of early-life stress may result in differential biological changes, which may in turn be related to differential psychopathology.

Indicative of serotonergic dysfunction, abused children with depression were shown to exhibit increased prolactin, but normal cortisol responses to the injection of L-5-hydroxytryptophan, a precursor of 5-HT, as compared to nonabused depressed children and controls (Kaufman et al., 1998). Likewise, increased prolactin responses to fenfluramine were observed in boys with adverse rearing environment (Pine et al., 1997). Since prolactin, but not cortisol release, is mediated via 5-HT$_{1A}$ receptors, these findings suggest sensitization of these receptors due to early-life stress. Another study recently reported that children with traumatic brain injury (TBI) who had experienced abuse have dramatic increases in CSF concentrations of glutamate, compared to nonabused TBI children (Ruppel et al., 2001).

In a neuroimaging study, maltreated children with PTSD exhibited decreased volumes of the corpus callosum (similar to findings in prepubescent primates with early-life stress), whereas hippocampal volumes were normal in these children (DeBellis et al., 1999b). Furthermore, a proton magnetic resonance spectroscopy study found smaller ratios of N-acetylasparate to creatine in the anterior cingulate of abused children with PTSD than those in controls (DeBellis et al., 2000), which is thought to reflect decreased neural integrity in this brain region.

Studies in adults

A limited number of studies have evaluated the consequences of early-life stress in adults (Table 9.1). Although there is evidence for increased 24-hour urinary cortisol excretion in abused women with PTSD (Lemieux and Coe, 1995), findings on basal plasma or salivary cortisol levels in women with a history of childhood abuse are conflicting, likely because of methodological differences (Heim and Nemeroff, 2001). There is evidence for increased HPA feedback sensitivity in abused women with PTSD (Stein et al., 1997a). Given the preclinical evidence for a sensitization of the

stress responses after early-life stress, it appears important to evaluate stress responsiveness in adults exposed to early-life stress. We found that abused women with or without current depression exhibited markedly increased plasma ACTH responses to psychosocial laboratory stress relative to controls and depressed women without early-life stress (Heim et al., 2000). Abused women with depression also exhibited increased cortisol responses to stress as compared to all other groups. Similar findings were reported for adults with parental loss (Lücken, 1998). While these findings are remarkably consistent with findings from animal studies, they also suggest that there are subgroups of depression with differential pathophysiology depending on early trauma experience. Interestingly, in a standard CRF stimulation test, in which pituitary CRF receptors are selectively stimulated, women abused in childhood who were without depression also exhibited increased ACTH responses, whereas abused women with current depression, like depressed women without childhood abuse experiences, exhibited blunted ACTH responses (Heim et al., 2001). It is plausible that early-life stress is related to sensitization of the CRF neuronal circuits, resulting in high CRF secretion whenever these women are stressed, which at the pituitary eventually leads to CRF receptor down-regulation and, because of CRF actions at extrahypothalamic sites, to symptoms of depression and anxiety. We further reported that abused women without depression released less cortisol during a standard ACTH$_{1-24}$ stimulation test (250 μg) (Heim et al., 2001); this finding suggests peripheral adaptation to CNS hyperactivity.

Parallel to findings in abused children with PTSD, elevated 24-hour urinary NE excretion was reported in abused women with PTSD (Lemieux and Coe, 1995). In addition, increased heart rate or blood pressure responses have been observed during stress induction in adults with early parental loss and in abused women with depression (Lücken, 1998; Heim et al., 2000) as well during mental imaging of abuse experiences in abused women with PTSD (Orr et al., 1998); these findings suggest increased autonomic reactivity. With respect to serotonergic function, a history of severe childhood abuse was found to be highly correlated with blunted prolactin responses to m-CPP in adult women who suffered from borderline personality disorder (Rinne et al., 2000). As this finding is opposite those in maltreated children but comparable to findings in VFD-reared adult non-human primates, these authors suggest that the 5-HT system may undergo a developmental "switch" after early stress.

Neuroimaging studies showing decreased hippocampal volumes have been described in adults with perinatal trauma and in adult women with child abuse and PTSD (Bremner et al., 1997; Stein et al., 1997b; (McNeil et al., 2000). As hippocampal atrophy is not observed in abused children with PTSD (DeBellis et al., 1999b), it may be hypothesized that repeatedly increased cortisol secretion over the course of time induces hippocampal cell loss and impaired neurogenesis in the dentate gyrus, which may further disinhibit cortisol secretion, eventually resulting in measurably smaller hippocampi. Two positron emission tomography (PET) studies reported decreased activation of the anterior cingulate during script-driven guided mental imagery of personal abuse experiences in abused women with PTSD, compared to such activation in abused women without PTSD (see Newport and Nemeroff, 2000); this structure is also abnormally developed in maltreated children with PTSD. These studies also found altered activation of several areas of the frontal cortex that are involved in the processing of emotion.

THE ROLE OF GENES

Family, twin, or adoption studies have provided convincing evidence for a robust genetic basis of most psychiatric disorders, including the mood and anxiety disorders. Although linkage to specific genes has yet to be established, it is assumed that multiple genes act in concert with nongenetic factors, i.e., early environment and adulthood stress, to produce a risk for mental disorders (Hyman 2000). In addition, there appears to be genetic variation with respect to perceived stress (Thapar et al., 1998). Genes may also affect stress reactivity. Thus, findings from animal studies suggest that Fischer 344 rats exhibit higher pituitary-adrenal responses to stress than those of other rat strains (Dhabhar et al., 1997). Remarkably, when chronically stressed, Lewis rats develop a relative adrenocortical hyporesponsiveness to ACTH as compared to other rat strains, whereas hypothalamic CRF mRNA expression is increased (Gómez et al., 1996). Identical-twin studies revealed a medium-sized heritability of cortisol concentrations [h(2)= 0.40 to h(2)= 0.48] (Wüst et al., 2000; Young et al., 2000a). These observations give rise to the hypothesis that there is genetic variation with respect to the neurobiological consequences of early-life stress. Thus, exposure of BALB/cByJ mice, which exhibit greater HPA reactivity to stress than C57BL/6ByJ mice, to early handling results in attenuation of HPA hyperreactivity. While fostering of BALB/cByJ mice by C57BL/6ByJ dams also attenuates HPA hyperreactivity, cross-fostering of the genetically less reactive C57BL/

6ByJ mice to BALB/cByJ dams does not induce any changes (Anisman et al., 1998). Likewise, rhesus monkeys, which carry an allele associated with "reactive temperament," are more vulnerable to maternal separation in terms of neuroendocrine and behavioral maladaptations than monkeys not carrying the allele (Suomi, 1997). Taken together, it appears that early adverse experiences "shape" a preexisting genetic vulnerability to stress and disease, resulting in a stable phenotype with a certain risk to develop disease in response to further stress exposure.

NEUROBIOLOGY OF DISORDERS RELATED TO EARLY-LIFE STRESS

Here we shall summarize the neurobiology of adult depression and anxiety disorders and compare these findings to the consequences of early-life stress. For information on the neurobiology of childhood mental disorders, we refer to Part I-C in this book. Notably, there are marked differences in the neurobiology of childhood depression, as compared to adulthood depression, and there appears to exist a subtype of childhood depression that is related to early trauma and has a distinct neurobiology.

Depression

A number of studies have repeatedly measured increased CRF-like immunoreactivity in the CSF of untreated patients with major depression (e.g., Nemeroff et al., 1984). A recent study using serial CSF sampling over 30 hours has provided evidence for inadequately high CRF activity in major depression in the face of sustained hypercortisolism (Wong et al., 2000). Postmortem studies have further provided evidence for increased CRF concentrations and CRF mRNA expression in hypothalamic tissue of depressed patients as well as decreased CRF receptor binding, likely due to chronic CRF hypersecretion, in the frontal cortex of suicide victims (Nemeroff et al., 1988; Raadsheer et al., 1994, 1995). These findings are consistent with indices of increased CRF activity in the hypothalamus and other structures in animals models of early-life stress. Direct measures of central CRF release in humans with early-life stress are still unavailable.

Indirect evidence for hypothalamic CRF hypersecretion comes from CRF stimulation test studies in which patients with depression typically show blunted ACTH responses, likely reflecting, in part, down-regulation of pituitary CRF receptors. These findings are similar to the reduction of pituitary CRF receptors in maternally deprived rats and compare to blunted ACTH responses to CRF in abused women with depression. Major depression has further been associated with increased cortisol responses to $ACTH_{1-24}$. However, the available findings are inconsistent and likely confounded by lack of control of early-life stress in depressed patients and controls, given the profound effects of early-life stress on adrenal function.

As a possible consequence of direct neurotoxic effects of sustained hypercortisolism, hippocampal atrophy has now repeatedly been reported for depressed patients (Sheline et al., 1996; Bremner et al., 2000a). Hippocampal atrophy may be associated with disinhibition of CRF secretion and further increases in cortisol secretion, which in turn may further damage the hippocampus. Impaired inhibition of the HPA axis is also evidenced by nonsuppression of cortisol by dexamethasone and decreased GR numbers in depressed patients; both findings parallel those in maternally separated rats.

Consistent with feed-forward actions between central CRF and NE systems, sustained increases in CSF NE concentrations of depressed patients have been measured (Wong et al., 2000). Serotonergic systems, which are believed to modulate the stress response, are also altered in depression (Owens and Nemeroff, 1994). Functional imaging studies further revealed decreased cortical GABA concentrations in depressed patients. Many of these findings are similar to reports of noradrenergic, serotonergic, and GABAergic dysfunction in animal models of early-life stress. Findings of structural or functional changes in the prefrontal cortex as well as structural changes in the amygdala are further compatible with an abnormal stress response system in depression (Sheline et al., 1998; Drevets, 1999). However, despite the evidence for increased activation of the stress response system, reduced β-endorphin and normal cortisol responses to psychosocial stress have been reported for depressed patients (Young et al., 2000b). These findings are in contrast to findings in animal models of early-life stress and our findings in adult survivors of child abuse with depression as well as depressed women without abuse, suggesting that there may be different subgroups of depression with distinct neurobiology.

Anxiety Disorders

Increased CRF-like immunoreactivity has also been measured in the CSF of patients with several anxiety disorders, including PTSD and obsessive-compulsive disorder, plausibly accounting for the frequent comorbidity among depression and anxiety disorders related to early-life stress. Consistent with hypothalamic CRF hypersecretion, blunted ACTH responses to CRF stimulation have been reported for PTSD and in panic disorder (see Heim and Nemeroff, 2001). In another study, however, increased ACTH responses to CRF were observed in patients with panic disorder (Curtis et al., 1997). One possible explanation for these findings may be that initial sensitization evolves into CRF receptor down-regulation upon long-term CRF hypersecretion. By and large, these findings parallel our findings in abused women who show pituitary sensitization when not depressed, evolving into blunted responsiveness in the presence of depression.

Interestingly, while peripheral neuroendocrine function appears normal in patients with panic disorder, decreased basal cortisol concentrations have been reported in most studies in PTSD patients. This relative hypocortisolism occurs in the context of increased feedback inhibition of the HPA axis (see Yehuda, 2000). However, a dissociation between central and adrenocortical (re)activity has been found in animal models of severe early-life stress as well as in abused children and women, suggesting that adrenal dysfunction may, at least in part, contribute to hypocortisolism in PTSD. In the face of hypocortisolism, it seems surprising that hippocampal atrophy is one of the most prominent findings in patients with PTSD, including adult survivors of childhood abuse with PTSD (see Newport and Nemeroff, 2000). While increased glucocorticoid sensitivity of hippocampal cells may play a role in the development of hippocampal atrophy, another potential mechanism may involve toxic effects of markedly increased cortisol responses to everyday stress in patients with PTSD.

There is evidence from peripheral catecholamine measures and pharmacological provocation studies suggesting that increased noradrenergic activity may be involved in the pathogenesis of several anxiety disorders, including panic disorder and PTSD. Thus, exaggerated behavioral responses to yohimbine are observed in patients with panic disorder and PTSD, a finding similar to those in VFD reared non-human primates (Coplan et al., 2000). With respect to other neurotransmitter systems, the beneficial effects of serotonergic drugs on symptoms of anxiety suggest serotonergic dysfunction in several anxiety disorders. Thus, several peripheral indices of serotonergic dysfunction have been measured in patients with PTSD (Newport and Nemeroff, 2000). Functional imaging studies further revealed decreased CBZ binding in the CNS of patients with panic disorder or PTSD (Bremner et al., 2000b,c). Taken together, these findings support the claim that that anxiety disorders are associated with alterations in neurotransmitter systems responsive to early-life stress.

IMPLICATIONS FOR PSYCHOPHARMACOLOGICAL RESEARCH

Pharmacological Prevention or Reversal of the Consequences of Early-Life Stress

The tremendous progress in identifying the neurobiological substrates mediating the relationship between early-life stress and psychopathology opens a new area of major interest for psychopharmacology. The evaluation of the potential utility of pharmacological agents targeting CRF and associated neurotransmitter systems in the prevention or reversal of the long-term consequences of early-life stress is of paramount clinical importance.

A number of studies provide evidence that different classes of antidepressants decrease CRF neuronal or HPA axis activity in rodents and primates, including humans (see Heim and Nemeroff, 2001). Many of the above effects were produced by drugs that affect the central serotonergic neurons, including the selective serotonin reuptake inhibitors (SSRIs). The SSRIs have been shown to be effective in the treatment of several psychiatric disorders associated with early-life stress, as well as in early-onset depression in children (Hidalgo and Davidson, 2000; Martin et al., 2000). Interestingly in this regard, in a rodent model it was shown that treatment of maternally deprived rats as adults with the SSRI paroxetine reverses the neurobiological consequences of early-life stress, resulting in unaltered vulnerability to stress, depression, and anxiety (P.M. Plotsky et al., unpublished report). It appears that several available drugs, but namely the SSRIs, may be beneficial in the treatment of children and adults exposed to early-life stress. Future preclinical studies will have to evaluate the efficacy of these drugs in the prevention or reversal of the effects of early-life stress during development. Furthermore, the efficacy of other classes of available drugs known to decrease CRF activity, including the 5-HT/NE reuptake inhibitor venlafaxine and benzodiazepines (Owens et al., 1996; Skelton et al., 2000), in the prevention or reversal of the effects of early-life stress should be studied.

There are also promising novel drugs that may be efficient in the treatment of disorders related to early-life stress. Thus, considerable attention has been directed towards the development and evaluation of CRF receptor antagonists. Given the integral role of CRF and its receptors in the mediation of stress and emotion, the CRF_1 receptor antagonists are being discussed as novel antidepressants and anxiolytics as well as potentially preventive treatments for PTSD (Martin et al., 2000). Oral administration of the CRF_1 receptor antagonist antalarmin significantly decreased CSF CRF, pituitary-adrenal, and autonomic responses to stress and inhibited behaviors indicative of fear and anxiety in adult primates (Habib et al., 2000). The antidepressant and anxiolytic properties of the selective CRF_1 receptor antagonist R121919 was recently demonstrated in a clinical trial of depressed patients (Zobel et al., 2000). Interestingly, treatment of rats exposed to pre- or postnatal stress with CRF receptor antagonists reverses increases of fearful behavior (Kehne et al., 2000; Ward et al., 2000). Given the fact that early-life stress is related to substantial alterations in central CRF systems, it is plausible that CRF_1 receptor antagonists, once they are available, will represent the most direct treatment of symptoms related to early-life stress in children and adults.

Animal Models for Psychopharmacological Research

While there are many possible means of inducing neonatal stress in animals, i.e., pain, cold, and restraint stress, among others, it will be crucial to systematically explore the utility of pharmacological agents in preventing or reversing the consequences of early-life stress using those animal models that have been proven to induce a vulnerable phenotype, including maternal separation in rodents and VFD in non-human primates.

In the frequently used rodent model of maternal separation (Plotsky and Meaney, 1993), time-pregnant Long Evans rats are used. On pnd 2, pups are randomly grouped into 8–10 male pups per dam and then subjected to different rearing conditions from pnd 2 to 14. In the animal facility rearing condition, cages are changed twice per week, beginning at pnd 5, which is associated with brief handling of the pups. In the handling-maternal separation (HMS) 15 condition, pups are removed from the cage daily for 15 minutes, mimicking separation patterns in the wild. In the HMS 180 condition, pups are removed from the home cage daily for 180 minutes. Sometimes a condition of leaving the rat pups completely undisturbed is also included. After pnd 14, pups are subjected to routine care and the long-term consequences are studied after pnd 60. Pharmacological intervention may be started at pnd 60, although the evaluation of the effects of earlier intervention may also be of major interest.

In the VFD paradigm, infant bonnet macaques are differentially reared over 12 weeks, beginning at 17 weeks of age (Coplan et al., 1996). Infants are allowed to habituate to the nursery, which is enclosed by contact-permissive mesh within their mother's pen. Thereafter, rearing conditions are varied: mothers with LFD may easily pick up food without any effort, while mothers with HFD have to dig for their food in wood chip bedding. In the VFD condition, mothers are alternately exposed to LFD/HFD conditions in 2-week blocks. During HFD, these mothers may either dig for food or perform a joystick task to earn food. Water is available for all mothers. Food and water are ad libitum for the infants. After the 12 weeks, bonnet macaques grow up under normal conditions and are studied after 2–4 years.

Considerations on Clinical Research Methods

Placebo-controlled clinical studies on the potential of antidepressants, benzodiazepines, and selective CRF_1 receptor antagonists to prevent or reverse the neurobiological and behavioral consequences of early-life stress are strongly warranted. When planning such clinical trials, one needs to consider that it is difficult to assess neurobiological stress responsiveness before and after treatment because of the confounding effects of habituation to a laboratory stress protocol, posing the challenge of developing different stress protocols that preclude cross-habituation. Another general problem in clinical studies on early-life stress is the controversially discussed creditability of retrospective self-reports on child abuse. On the one hand, abuse early in childhood may not be remembered, and, on the other hand, "false memories" may exist on alleged abuse experiences. To complicate the picture, mental health status may be associated with over- or under-reporting of the abuse. To increase the creditability of retrospective self-reports, it is generally recommended that abuse histories be assessed in standardized personal interviews that comprise a large number of specific questions and have been psychometrically validated, such as the Early Trauma Inventory (Bremner et al., 2000d). It is further helpful to obtain independent corroboration from court, social service, or medical records in retrospective studies. In addition, longitudinal studies will be important in the future, not only for solving the problem of retrospective self-reports but also for the identification of developmental stages that are sensitive to treatment effects. Here the evaluation of the combined effects of psychological and pharmacological treatment may be particularly fruitful.

CONCLUSION

We have summarized findings from preclinical and clinical studies suggesting that early-life stress induces long-lived changes of CNS CRF and adjoined neurotransmitter systems, resulting in enhanced endocrine, autonomic, and behavioral stress responsiveness. With repeated exposure to stress, this vulnerability may evolve in symptoms of depression and anxiety disorders, which are frequently seen in adult survivors of abuse. More studies in humans exposed to early-life stress are needed to evaluate potential alterations in the various central and peripheral components of the stress response system. The development of new techniques allowing for the assessment of central neurotransmitter and receptor changes, particularly the CRF receptors, will considerably advance this field of research in the near future and will increase the comparability of clinical and preclinical findings. Future studies should also identify the roles of predisposition, gender, and critical developmental periods for the effects of stress or treatment, as well as the moderating effects of social buffering in relation to early-life stress. The increasing knowledge on the detrimental effects of early-life stress, along with an increasing understanding of their prevention or reversal, asks for the careful assessment of early adversities in the clinical care of children and adolescents, and for the early application of treatment regimes that target neurobiological systems affected by early-life stress.

REFERENCES

Agid, O., Kohn, Y., and Lerer, B. (2000) Environmental stress and psychiatric illness. *Biomed Pharmacother* 54:135–141.

Anisman, H., Zaharia, M.D., Meaney, M.J., and Merali, Z. (1998) Do early-life events permanently alter behavioral and hormonal responses to stressors? *Int J Dev Neurosci* 16:149–64.

Arborelius. L, Owens, M.J., Plotsky, P.M., and Nemeroff, C.B. (1999). CRF, depression and anxiety. *J Endocrinology* 160:1–12.

Bremner, J.D., Innis, R.B., Southwick, S.M., Staib, L., Zoghbi, S., and Charney, D.S. (2000a) Decreased benzodiazepine receptor binding in prefrontal cortex in combat-related posttraumatic stress disorder. *Am J Psychiatry* 157:1120–1126.

Bremner, J.D., Innis, R.B., White, T., Fujita, M., Silbersweig, D., Goddard, A.W., et al. (2000b) SPECT [I-123]iomazenil measurement of the benzodiazepine receptor in panic disorder. *Biol Psychiatry* 47:96–106.

Bremner, J.D., Narayan, M., Anderson, E.R., Staib, L.H., Miller, H.L., and Charney, D.S. (2000c) Hippocampal volume reduction in major depression. *Am J Psychiatry* 157:115–118.

Bremner, J.D., Randall, P., Vermetten, E., Staib, L., Bronen, R.A., Mazure, C., et al. (1997) Magnetic resonance imaging–based measurement of hippocampal volume in posttraumatic stress disorder related to childhood physical and sexual abuse—a preliminary report. *Biol Psychiatry* 41:23–32.

Bremner, J.D., Vermetten, E., and Mazure, C.M. (2000d) Development and preliminary psychometric properties of an instrument for the measurement of childhood trauma: the early trauma inventory. *Depress Anxiety* 12:1–12.

Caldji, C., Francis, D., Sharma, S., Plotsky, P.M., and Meaney, M.J. (2000) The effects of early rearing environment on the development of GABA$_A$ and central benzodiazepine receptor levels and novelty-induced fearfulness in the rat. *Neuropsychopharmacology* 22:219–229.

Caldji, C., Tannenbaum, B., Sharma, S., Francis, D., Plotsky, P.M., and Meaney, M.J. (1998) Maternal care during infancy regulates the development of neural systems mediating the expression of fearfulness in the rat. *Proc Natl Acad Sci USA* 95: 5335–5340.

Coplan, J.D., Andrews, M.W., Rosenblum, L.A., Owens, M.J., Friedman, S., Gorman, J.M., et al. (1996) Persistent elevations of cerebrospinal fluid concentrations of corticotropin-releasing factor in adult nonhuman primates exposed to early-life stressors: implications for the pathophysiology of mood and anxiety disorders. *Proc Natl Acad Sci, USA* 93:1619–1623.

Coplan, J.D., Smith, E.L., Trost, R.C., Scharf, B.A., Altemus, M., Bjornson, L., et al. (2000) Growth hormone response to clonidine in adversely reared young adult primates: relationship to serial cerebrospinal fluid corticotropin-releasing factor concentrations. *Psychiatry Res* 95:93–102.

Curtis, G.C., Abelson, J.L., and Gold, P.W. (1997) Adrenocorticotropic and hormone and cortisol responses to corticotropin-releasing hormone: changes in panic disorder and effects of alprazolam treatment. *Biol Psychiatry* 41:76–85.

DeBellis, M.D., Baum, A.S., Birmaher, B., Keshavan, M.S., Eccard, C.H., Boring, A.M., et al (1999a) Developmental traumatology. Part I: Biological stress systems. *Biol Psychiatry* 45:1259–1270.

DeBellis, M.D., Chrousos, G.P., Dorn, L.D., Burke, L., Helmers, K., Kling, M.A., et al. (1994a) Hypothalamic-pituitary-adrenal dysregulation in sexually abused girls. *J Clin Endocrinol Metab* 78: 249–255.

DeBellis, M.D., Keshavan, M.S., Clark, D.B., Casey, B.J., Giedd, J.N., Boring, A.M., et al. (1999b) A.E. Bennett Research Award. Developmental traumatology. Part II: Brain development. *Biol Psychiatry* 45:1271–1284.

DeBellis, M.D., Keshavan, M.S., Spencer, S., and Hall, J. (2000) *N*-Acetylaspartate concentration in the anterior cingulate of maltreated children and adolescents with PTSD. *Am J Psychiatry* 157:1175–1177.

DeBellis, M.D., Lefter, L., Trickett, P.K., and Putnam F.W. (1994b) Urinary catecholamine excretion in sexually abused girls. *J Am Acad Child Adolesc Psychiatry* 33:320–327.

Dent, G.W., Okimoto, D.K., Smith, M.A., and Levine, S. (2000) Stress-induced alterations in corticotropin-releasing hormone and vasopressin gene expression in the paraventricular nucleus during ontogeny. *Neuroendocrinology* 71:333–342.

Dhabhar, F.S., McEwen, B.S., and Spencer, R.L. (1997) Adaptation to prolonged or repeated stress—comparison between rat strains showing intrinsic differences in reactivity to acute stress. *Neuroendocrinology* 65:360–368.

Drevets, W.C. (1999) Prefrontal cortical–amygdalar metabolism in major depression. *Ann NY Acad Sci* 877:614–637.

Fahlke, C., Lorenz, J.G., Long, J., Champoux, M., Suomi, S.J., and Higley, J.D. (2000) Rearing experiences and stress-induced plasma cortisol as early risk factors for excessive alcohol consumption in nonhuman primates. *Alcohol Clin Exp Res* 24:644–650.

Goenjian, A.K., Yehuda, R., Pynoos, R.S., Steinberg, A.M., Tashjian, M., Yang, R.K., et al. (1996) Basal cortisol, dexamethasone sup-

pression of cortisol, and MHPG in adolescents after the 1988 earthquake in Armenia. *Am J Psychiatry* 153:929–934.

Gómez, F., Lahmame, A., deKloet, E.R., and Armario, A. (1996) Hypothalamic-pituitary-adrenal response to chronic stress in five inbred rat strains: differential responses are mainly located at the adrenocortical level. *Neuroendocrinology* 63:327–337.

Gottman, J.M. and Katz, L.F. (1989) The effects of marital discord on young children's peer interaction and health. *Dev Psychol* 25: 373–381.

Graham, Y.P., Heim, C., Goodman, S.H., Miller, A.H., and Nemeroff, C.B. (1999) The effects of neonatal stress on brain development: implications for psychopathology. *Dev Psychopathol* 11: 545–565.

Habib, K.E., Weld, K.P., Rice, K.C., Pushkas, J., Champoux, M., Listwak, S., et al. (2000) Oral administration of a corticotropin-releasing hormone receptor antagonist significantly attenuates behavioral, neuroendocrine, and autonomic responses to stress in primates. *Proc Natl Acad Sci USA* 97:6079–6084.

Hart, J., Gunnar, M., and Cicchetti, D. (1995) Salivary cortisol in maltreated children: evidence of relations between neuroendocrine activity and social competence. *Dev Psychopathol* 7:11–26.

Heim, C. and Nemeroff, C.B. (2001) The role of childhood trauma in the neurobiology of mood and anxiety disorders: preclinical and clinical studies *Biol Psychiatry* 49:1023–1039.

Heim, C., Newport, D.J., Heit, S., Graham, Y.P., Wilcox, M., Bonsall, R., et al. (2000) Pituitary-adrenal and autonomic responses to stress in women after sexual and physical abuse in childhood. *JAMA* 284:592–597.

Heim, C., Newport, D.J., Miller, A.H., and Nemeroff, C.B. (2001) Altered pituitary-adrenal axis responses to provocative challenge tests in adult survivors of childhood abuse. *Am J Psychiatry* 158: 575–581.

Hidalgo, R.B. and Davidson, J.R. (2000) Selective serotonin reuptake inhibitors in post-traumatic stress disorder. *J Psychopharmacol* 14:70–76.

Holmes, W.C. and Slap, G.B. (1998) Sexual abuse of boys: definition, prevalence, correlates, sequelae, and management. *JAMA* 280: 1855–1862.

Hyman, S.E. (2000) The genetics of mental illness: implications for practice. *Bull World Health Organ* 78:455–463.

Kaufman, J., Birmaher, B., Perel, J., Dahl, R.E., Moreci, P., Nelson, B., et al. (1997) The corticotropin-releasing hormone challenge in depressed abused, depressed nonabused, an normal control children. *Biol Psychiatry* 42:669–679.

Kaufman, J., Birmaher, B., Perel, J., Dahl, R.E., Stull, S., Brent, D., et al. (1998) Serotonergic functioning in depressed abused children: clinical and familial correlates. *Biol Psychiatry* 44:973–981.

Kehne, J.H., Coverdale, S., McCloskey, T.C., Hoffman, D.C., and Cassella, J.V. (2000) Effects of the CRF(1) receptor antagonist, CP 154,526, in the separation-induced vocalization anxiolytic test in rat pups. *Neuropharmacology* 39:1357–1367.

Kendall-Tackett, K.A., Williams, L.M., and Finkelhor, D. (1993) Impact of sexual abuse on children: a review and synthesis of recent empirical studies. *Psychol Bull* 113:164–80.

Kendler, K.S., Bulik, C.M., Silberg, J., Hettema, J.M., Myers, J., and Prescott C.A. (2000) Childhood sexual abuse and adult psychiatric and substance use disorders in women: an epidemiological and cotwin control analysis. *Arch Gen Psychiatry* 57:953–959.

Kessler RC and Magee WJ. (1993). Childhood adversities and adult depression: basic patterns of association in a US national survey. *Psychol Med* 23:679–690.

Kirby, L.G., Rice, K.C., and Valentino, R.J. (2000) Effects of corticotropin-releasing factor on neuronal activity in the seroto-

122 BIOLOGICAL BASES OF PEDIATRIC PSYCHOPHARMACOLOGY

nergic dorsal raphe nucleus. *Neuropsychopharmacology* 22:148–162.

Ladd, C.O., Owens, M.J., and Nemeroff, C.B. (1996) Persistent changes in corticotropin-releasing factor neuronal systems induced by maternal deprivation. *Endocrinology* 137:1212–1218.

Lazarus, R.S. (1985) The psychology of stress and coping. *Issues Ment Health Nurs* 7:399–418.

LeDoux, J.E. (2000) Emotion circuits in the brain. *Annu Rev Neurosci* 23:155–184.

Lemieux, A.M. and Coe, C.L. (1995) Abuse-related posttraumatic stress disorder: evidence for chronic neuroendocrine activation in women. *Psychosom Med* 57:105–115.

Liu, D., Caldji, C., Sharma, S., Plotsky, P.M., and Meaney, M.J. (2000) Influence of neonatal rearing conditions on stress-induced adrenocorticotropin responses and norepinepherine release in the hypothalamic paraventricular nucleus. *J Neuroendocrinol* 12:5–12.

Liu, D., Diorio, J., Tannenbaum, B., Caldji, C., Francis, D., Freedman, A., et al. (1997) Maternal care, hippocampal glucocorticoid receptors, and hypothalamic-pituitary-adrenal responses to stress. *Science* 12277:1659–1662.

Lücken, L.J. (1998) Childhood attachment and loss experiences affect adult cardiovascular and cortisol function. *Psychosom Med* 60:765–772.

Martin, A., Kaufman, J., and Charney, D.S. (2000) Pharmacotherapy of early-onset depression. Update and new directions. *Child Adolesc Psychiatr Clin North Am* 9:135–157.

Mason, J.W. (1968) The scope of psychoendocrine research. *Psychosom Med* 30:565–575.

McCauley, J., Kern, D.E., Kolodner, K., Dill, L., Schroeder, A.F., DeChant, et al. (1997) Clinical characteristics of women with a history of childhood abuse. *JAMA* 277:1362–1368.

McNeil, T.F., Cantor-Graae, E., and Weinberger, D.R. (2000) Relationship of obstetric complications and differences in size of brain structures in monozygotic twin pairs discordant for schizophrenia. *Am J Psychiatry* 157:203–212.

Nemeroff, C.B., Owens, M.J., Bisette, G., Andorn, A.C., and Stanley, M. (1988) Reduced corticotropin-releasing factor (CRF) binding sites in the frontal cortex of suicide victims. *Arch Gen Psychiatry* 45:577–579.

Nemeroff, C.B., Widerlöv, E., Bisette, G., Walleus, H., Karlsson, L., Eklund, K., et al. (1984) Elevated concentrations of CSF corticotropin releasing factor like immunoreactivity in depressed patients. *Science* 226:1342–1344.

Newport, D.J. and Nemeroff, C.B. (2000) Neurobiology of posttraumatic stress disorder. *Curr Opin Neurobiol* 10:211–218.

Orr SP, Lasko NB, Metzger LJ, Berry NJ, Ahern CE, and Pitman RK (1998). Psychophysiologic assessment of women with posttraumatic stress disorder resulting from childhood sexual abuse. *J Consult Clin Psychol* 66:906–913.

Owens, M.J. and Nemeroff, C.B. (1991) Physiology and pharmacology of corticotropin-releasing factor. *Pharmacol Rev* 43:425–473.

Owens MJ and Nemeroff CB. (1994). Role of serotonin in the pathophysiology of depression: focus on the serotonin transporter. *Clin Chem* 40:288–295.

Owens, M.J., Plotsky, P.M., and Nemeroff, C.B. (1996) Peptides and affective disorders. In: Watson, S.J., ed. *Biology of Schizophrenia and Affective Disorders*. Washington, DC: American Psychiatric Press, pp. 259–293.

Perry, B.D. (1994) Neurobiological sequelea of childhood trauma: PTSD in children. In: Murburg, M., ed. *Catecholamine Function*

in Posttraumatic Stress Disorder: Emerging Concepts. Washington, DC: American Psychiatric Press, pp. 173–189.

Pine, D.S., Coplan, J.D., Wasserman, G.A., Miller, L.S., Fried, J.E., Davies, M., et al. (1997) Neuroendocrine response to fenfluramine challenge in boys. Associations with aggressive behavior and adverse rearing. *Arch Gen Psychiatry* 54:839–846.

Plotsky, P.M. and Meaney, M.J. (1993) Early, postnatal experience alters hypothalamic corticotropin-releasing factor (CRF) mRNA, median eminence CRF content and stress-induced release in adult rats. *Mol Brain Res* 18:195–200.

Plotsky, P.M., Thrivikraman, K.V., Caldji, C., Sharma, S., and Meaney, M.J. (in press) The effects of neonatal rearing environment on CRF mRNA and CRF receptor levels in adult rat brain. *J Neurosci*

Raadsheer, F.C., Hoogendijk, W.J., Stam, F.C., Tilders, F.J., and Swaab, D.F. (1994) Increased numbers of corticotropin-releasing hormone expressing neurons in the hypothalamic paraventricular nucleus of depressed patients. *Neuroendocrinology* 60:436–444.

Raadsheer, F.C., van Heerikhuize, J.J., Lucassen, P.J., Tilders, F.J., and Swaab DF (1995) Corticotropin-releasing hormone mRNA levels in the paraventricular nucleus of patints with Alzheimer's disease and depression. *Am J Psychiatry* 152:1372–1376.

Rinne, T., Westenberg, H.G., den Boer, J.A., and van den Brink, W. (2000) Serotonergic blunting to meta-chlorophenylpiperazine (m-CPP) highly correlates with sustained childhood abuse in impulsive and autoaggressive female borderline patients. *Biol Psychiatry* 47:548–556.

Rogeness, G. and McClure, E. (1996) Development and neurotransmitter interactions. *Dev Psychopathol* 8:183–199.

Rosenblum, L.A., Coplan, J.D., Friedman, S., Gorman, J.M., and Andrews, M.W. (1994) Adverse early experiences affect noradrenergic and serotonergic functioning in adult primates. *Biol Psychiatry* 35:221–227.

Ruppel, R.A., Kochanek, P.M., Adelson, P.D., Rose, M.E., Wisniewski, S.R., Bell, M.J., et al. (2001) Excitatory amino acid concentrations in ventricular cerebrospinal fluid after severe traumatic brain injury in infants and children: the role of child abuse. *J Pediatr* 138:18–25.

Sanchez, M.M., Aguado, F., Sanchez-Toscano, F., and Saphier, D. (1998) Neuroendocrine and immunocytochemical demonstrations of decreased hypothalamo-pituitary-adrenal axis responsiveness to restraint stress after long-term social isolation. *Endocrinology* 139:579–587.

Sheline, Y.I., Gado, M.H., and Price, J.L. (1998) Amygdala core nuclei volumes are decreased in recurrent major depression. *Neuroreport* 9:2023–2028

Sheline, Y.I., Wang, P.W., Gado, M.H., Csernansky, J.G., and Vannier, M.W. (1996) Hippocampal atrophy in recurrent major depression. *Proc Natl Acad Sci USA* 93:3908–3913.

Skelton, K.H., Nemeroff, C.B., Knight, D.L., and Owens, M.J. (2000) Chronic administration of the triazolobenzodiazepine alprazolam produces opposite effects on corticotropin-releasing factor and urocortin neuronal systems. *J Neurosci* 20:1240–1248.

Stein, M.B., Koverola, C., Hanna, C., Torchia, M.G., and McClarty, B. (1997a) Hippocampal volume in women victimized by childhood sexual abuse. *Psychol Med* 27:951–959.

Stein, M.B., Yehuda R., Koverola, C., and Hanna, C. (1997b) Enhanced dexamethasone suppression of plasma cortisol in adult women traumatized by childhood sexual abuse. *Biol Psychiatry* 42:680–686.

Suomi, S.J. (1991) Early stress and adult emotional reactivity in rhesus monkeys. *Ciba Found Symp* 156:171–183.

Suomi, S.J. (1997) Long-term effects of different early rearing experiences on social, emotional and physiologial development in non-human primates. In: Kesheven, M.S. and Murra R.M., eds. *Neurodevelopmental Models of Adult Psychopathology.* Cambridge, UK: Cambridge University Press, pp. 104–116.

Thapar, A., Harold, G., and McGuffin, P. (1998). Life events and depressive symptoms in childhood—shared genes or shared adversity? A research note. *J Child Psychol Psychiatry* 39:1153–1158.

Valentino, R.J., Foote, S.L., and Aston-Jones, G. (1983) Corticotropin-releasing factor activates noradrenergic neurons of the locus coeruleus. *Brain Res* 270:363–367.

van Oers, H.J., DeKloet, E.R., and Levine, S. (1998) Early versus late maternal deprivation differentially alters the endocrine and hypothalamic responses to stress. *Dev Brain Res* 111:245–252.

Ward, H.E., Johnson, E.A., Salm, A.K., and Birkle, D.L. (2000) Effects of prenatal stress on defensive withdrawal behavior and corticotropin releasing factor systems in rat brain. *Physiol Behav* 70:359–366.

Weller, E.B., Weller, R.A., Fristad, M.A., and Bowes, J.M. (1990) Dexamethasone suppression test and depressive symptoms in bereaved children: a preliminary report. *J Neuropsychiatry Clin Neurosci* 2:418–421.

Wissow, L.S. (1995) Child abuse and neglect. *N Engl J Med* 332:1425–1431.

Wong, M.L., Kling, M.A., Munson, P.J., Listwak, S., Licinio, J., Prolo, P., et al. (2000) Pronounced and sustained central hypernoradrenergic function in major depression with melancholic features: relation to hypercortisolism and corticotropin-releasing hormone. *Proc Natl Acad Sci USA* 97:325–330.

Wüst, S., Federenko, I., Hellhammer, D.H., and Kirschbaum, C. (2000) Genetic factors, perceived chronic stress, and the free cortisol response to awakening. *Psychoneuroendocrinology* 25:707–720.

Yehuda, R. (2000) Biology of posttraumatic stress disorder. *J Clin Psychiatry* 61:14–21.

Young, E.A., Aggen, S.H., Prescott, C.A., and Kendler, K.S. (2000a) Similarity in saliva cortisol measures in monozygotic twins and the influence of past major depression. *Biol Psychiatry* 48:70–74.

Young, E.A., Lopez, J.F., Murphy-Weinberg, V., Watson, S.J., and Akil, H. (2000b) Hormonal evidence for altered responsiveness to social stress in major depression. *Neuropsychopharmacology* 23:411–418.

Zobel, A.W., Nickel, T., Kunzel, H.E., Ackl, N., Sonntag, A., Ising, M., et al. (2000) Effects of the high-affinity corticotropin-releasing hormone receptor 1 antagonist R121919 in major depression: the first 20 patients treated. *J Psychiatr Res* 34:171–181.

10 | Neurobiology of early-onset mood disorders

JOAN KAUFMAN AND HILARY BLUMBERG

In this chapter we review extant data on the neurobiology of unipolar and bipolar depressive disorders in children and adolescents. A complement to two recent reviews (Kaufman and Ryan, 1999; Kaufman et al., 2001), this chapter places primary emphasis on those studies in which neuroimaging techniques have been used. Unfortunately, such studies are few and far between. Preclinical models that have guided research on the neurobiology of affective disorders in adults are discussed, and, given the limits in the application of these models to juvenile samples, especially in the case of unipolar disorder, the need for more developmentally focused preclinical work is emphasized.

NEUROBIOLOGY OF MAJOR DEPRESSION IN CHILDREN

The existence of major depressive disorder (MDD) in children and adolescents was controversial prior to the late 1970s (Puig-Antich and Gittleman, 1982). Research over the past two decades, however, has demonstrated clearly that children are capable of experiencing episodes of depression that meet standard *Diagnostic and Statistical Manual of Mental Disorders, 4th ed.* (DSM-IV) criteria for MDD (Ryan et al., 1987; Birmaher et al., 1996b). In addition, MDD in children and adolescents is common, recurrent, and associated with significant morbidity and mortality (Birmaher et al., 1996a). Epidemiological studies estimate the prevalence of depression is 2% in children (Kashani et al., 1983) and 5%–8% in adolescents (Lewinsohn et al., 1994). Within 5 years of the onset of MDD, 70% of clinically referred depressed children and adolescents will experience a recurrence (Kovacs et al., 1984; Rao et al., 1993). Children with depression also have persistent functional impairment even after recovery (Puig-Antich et al., 1993), and as many as 5%–10% of de-

pressed adolescents will complete suicide within 15 years of their initial episode of MDD (Rao et al., 1993; Weissman et al., 1999).

Preclinical Studies of the Effects of Early Stress

Preclinical studies of the effects of stress provide a valuable heuristic in understanding the pathophysiology of depression in adults and organizing findings of the neurobiological correlates of MDD in adult patients. Many of the biological alterations associated with early stress in preclinical studies have been reported in adults with depression and other stress-related disorders. The application of research findings from these preclinical studies to understanding the neurobiology of early-onset affective disorders is more limited, however, for a variety of reasons that will be discussed later in this review.

The neurobiological effects of early stress have been reviewed extensively elsewhere (Francis et al., 1999a; Kaufman et al., 2000). Building on the seminal work of Levine and colleagues (Coe et al., 1978; Wiener et al., 1987; Levine et al., 1993), numerous investigators have demonstrated long-term neurobiological changes in animals subjected to multiple prenatal and postnatal stress paradigms (Takahashi and Kalin, 1991; Graham et al., 1999). Extensive research has been conducted to examine the neurobiological effects of early maternal separation. These experiences are associated in adulthood with increased basal and stress-induced adrenocorticotropin (ACTH) and cortisol secretion; reduced feedback inhibition of the hypothalamic–pituitary–adrenal (HPA) axis, increased central corticotropin-releasing hormone (CRH) and norepinephrine (NE) drive; a decrease in tone of the inhibitory gamma-aminobutyric acid–benzodiazepine (GABA/BZ) system (Francis et al., 1999b; Caldji et al., 2000); altered patterns of dopaminergic and serotonergic innervation to the medial prefrontal cortex (mPFC) (Poeggel et al., 1999; Braun et al., 2000); and exaggerated age-related cell loss in the hippocampus (Meaney et al., 1991; 1993).

Similarities between the Effects of Stress and Neurobiological Correlates of Major Depressive Disorder in Adults

Consistent with this preclinical work is the finding that adults with depression have multiple alterations of the HPA axis, including increased basal cortisol secretion (Schildkraut et al., 1989); reduced negative feedback as evidenced by dexamethasone nonsuppression (Carroll, 1982; American Psychiatric Association, 1987); and blunted ACTH secretion in response to administration of endogenous CRH (Gold et al., 1986; Holsboer et al., 1987; Plotsky et al., 1998). They have also been found to have increased central CRH drive, as evidenced by reports of elevated concentrations of cerebrospinal fluid (CSF) CRH (Nemeroff et al., 1984, 1991) and reduced CRH receptor–binding site number in the frontal cortex of suicide victims (Nemeroff et al., 1988). Depressed adults also have higher CSF NE concentration (Wong et al., 2000) and decreased cortical GABA measured in vivo using proton magnetic resonance spectroscopy (Sanacora et al., 1999). Altered dopamine (DA)/serotonin (S-HT) balance has also been reported in adults with depression (Reddy et al., 1992), with fluoxetine treatment associated with increases in CSF DA/5-HT metabolite concentration ratios (De Bellis et al., 1993).

Studies of adults with depression have reported structural and functional alterations in the mPFC. This region has significant projections to the hypothalamus and other autonomic and subcortical structures that are not only critical in the integration of the stress response but also important in the organization of emotional processing (Nauta, 1971; Devinsky et al., 1995). Alterations reported in this region in adults with depression include reduced gray matter volume in the subgenual PFC (Drevets et al., 1997); changes in regional cerebral blood flow (rCBF) and glucose metabolism in this region (Drevets et al., 1992); and, according to preliminary histopathological studies, a reduction in glia number without a corresponding loss of neurons (Ongur et al., 1998). Alterations in additional regions contained within the mPFC have also been reported in depressed patients, including reductions in glucose metabolism in the ventromedial PFC (Buchsbaum et al., 1997); decreased rCBF in the anterior cingulate (Bench et al., 1992); and changes in rCBF in the rostral anterior cingulate, with the direction of changes in this region preliminarily found to

relate to individual differences in treatment response (Mayberg et al., 1997).

Structural changes in the hippocampus have also been reported in adults with depression in several (Sheline et al., 1996; Shah et al., 1998; (Bremner et al., 2000; Mervaala et al., 2000), but not all, studies of adults with depression (Hauser et al., 1989; Axelson et al., 1993; Vakili et al., 2000). In two of the positive studies, the degree of hippocampal atrophy correlated with total duration of illness (Sheline et al., 1996; Bremner et al., 2000), raising questions as to whether these changes represent primary disturbances associated with the onset of disorder or secondary brain changes related to recurrence and extended glucocorticoid exposure. Adults with depression have also been found to have reduced volume of core amygdala nuclei (Sheline et al., 1998), a critical region involved in the stress response, with abnormalities in resting blood flow and glucose metabolism also reported in this area (Drevets, 1999).

This review of the neurobiological correlates of MDD in adults is not exhaustive, but designed to highlight the value of preclinical models of the effects of stress in generating hypotheses about potential brain changes associated with depression. Reductions in glucose metabolism and/or rCBF have been reported in additional brain regions in depressed adults, including the dorsolateral PFC (Baxter et al., 1989; Bench et al., 1992), parietal lobes (Sackeim et al., 1990), basal ganglia (Buchsbaum et al., 1986; Baxter et al., 1989), and thalamus (Petracca et al., 1995; Nikolaus et al., 2000).

Limitations in the Application of Preclinical Models of Effects of Stress in Organizing Neurobiological Correlates of Major Depressive Disorder in Children and Adolescents

While the preclinical studies examining the neurobiological effects of early stress provide a powerful heuristic for thinking about the pathophysiology of MDD in adults, the application of this literature to understanding the neurobiology of early-onset affective disorders is more limited. Depressed children and adolescents fail to show evidence of hypercortisolemia as is frequently reported in adults (Ryan and Dahl, 1993; Kaufman and Ryan, 1999). To the extent that dysregulation of basal cortisol is found in depressed subjects in this age range, it appears to be more subtle, and is manifest as alterations in the normal diurnal pattern of cortisol secretion. Rather than have increased 24-hour cortisol secretion, depressed youngsters are more likely to only have elevated cortisol output close to the period of sleep onset, a time when the HPA axis is normally quiescent.

This pattern of findings does not usually appear until adolescence in nontraumatized depressed youth, but has been reported in several studies of maltreated preadolescent children with depressive symptomatology (Kaufman, 1991; Putnam et al., 1991; Hart et al., 1996).

In addition to a lack of robust findings in basal cortisol secretion, nontraumatized depressed children and adolescents do not have blunted ACTH response to CRH infusion as is reported in adults (Birmaher et al., 1996b; Dorn et al., 1996). Among depressed children with a history of maltreatment, contradictory findings have been reported in CRH studies. One study reported maltreated children to have blunted ACTH after CRH infusion (De Bellis et al., 1994), whereas another study reported the children to have markedly elevated ACTH secretion after CRH infusion (Kaufman et al., 1997). In the latter study, abnormalities in the HPA axis response to CRH were limited to those maltreated children living in conditions of ongoing chronic adversity (e.g., emotional maltreatment, domestic violence), and most also met criteria for comorbid post-traumatic stress disorder (PTSD). Depressed children with a history of early maltreatment who were living in currently stable and positive environments showed no evidence of HPA axis dysregulation (Kaufman et al., 1997).

To the best of our knowledge, no studies with child and adolescent depressed cohorts have examined hippocampal volume. The one study that examined hippocampal volume in children and adolescents with PTSD ($n = 43$), about half of whom met criteria for comorbid MDD, failed to find evidence of hippocampal atrophy (De Bellis et al., 1999). This finding is not surprising, as most of the children and adolescents in the study had not experienced more than one episode of depression, and hippocampal atrophy was found to be correlated with total lifetime duration of illness in the prior adult studies cited (Sheline et al., 1996; Bremner et al., 2000). Developmental factors may also account for the discrepant findings in child and adult studies. For example, age-dependent changes in sensitivity to some forms of N-methyl-D-aspartate (NMDA) receptor blockade neurotoxicity in corticolimbic regions have been reported in preclinical studies, with cell death minimal or absent prepuberty and reaching peak in early adulthood (Farber et al., 1995).

Instead of hippocampal atrophy, the children and adolescents with PTSD were found to have smaller intracranial and cerebral volumes than matched controls; increased right, left, and total lateral ventricle volume; and decreased volume of the medial and posterior portions of the corpus callosum (CC) (De Bellis et al., 1999). Consistent with this investigation, in a recent abstract, psychiatric inpatients with a history of maltreatment were likewise reported to have a significant reduction in volume of the medial and caudal portions of the CC, compared to psychiatric and healthy controls without a history of early child maltreatment (Teicher et al., 2000).

The medial and caudal portions of the midbody of the CC contain interhemispheric projections from the auditory cortices, posterior cingulate, retrosplenial cortex, and insula, and somatosensory and visual cortices to a lesser extent. It also includes connections from the inferior parietal lobe to the contralateral superior temporal sulcus, cingulate, and parahippocampal gyrus (Pandya and Seltzer, 1986). Several of the regions with interhemispheric projections through the medial and caudal portions of the midbody of the CC are involved in the processing of emotional stimuli and various memory functions—core disturbances frequently observed in children with a history of early trauma.

To the best of our knowledge, there is only one published structural magnetic resonance imaging (MRI) study in prepubescent non-human primates subjected to early stress (Sanchez et al., 1998). Most preclinical studies of early stress have examined the long-term impact of these experiences on brain development in *adult* animals. Interestingly, the study with the young primates also failed to find evidence of hippocampal atrophy. Instead, consistent with the work of De Bellis and colleagues (1999), the investigators reported reductions in the medial and caudal portions of the midbody of the CC in the juvenile, non-human primates subjected to early stress.

As mentioned above, most of the preclinical studies on the effects of early stress have examined the impact of these experiences on adult animals. The preliminary work discussed in this section highlights the need for more developmentally focused preclinical studies of the effects of early stress. In addition, there is a need for more research on the development of the CC, and circadian control of cortisol secretion.

Preliminary Results of Neuroimaging Studies in Children and Adolescents with Depression

Table 10.1 summarizes the results of available pediatric neuroimaging studies in depressed patients. Given the limited amount of available data, published papers and professional presentations are reviewed. Two of the eight studies included seven or fewer depressed subjects, and two had no normal control comparisons. Results from the three largest-scale studies suggest that there are some neuroanatomical correlates of depression that may be evident across the life cycle (e.g., frontal lobe and amygdala volume changes), and others

TABLE 10.1. *Neuroimaging Studies of Children and Adolescents with Major Depression*

Reference	Sample	Ages (years)	Method	Results
Tutus et al., 1998	14 MDD 11 NC	11–15	⁹⁹Tc HMPAO brain SPECT	MDD < NC rCBF left anterofrontal and temporal lobes
Kowatch et al., 1999	7 MDD 7 NC	13–18	⁹⁹Tc HMPAO brain SPECT	MDD > NC rCBF temporal lobe subregions MDD < NC rCBF anterior thalamus, left parietal lobe, right caudate
Dahlstrom et al., 2000	31 DD 10 PC	7–17	[¹²³I]β-CIT SPECT	DD > PC 5-HT transporter availability in hypothalamic/midbrain area DD = PC DA transporter availability in the striatum
Steingard et al., 1996	65 DD 18 PC	6–17	Structural MRI, 5 mm slice thickness	DD < PC frontal lobe volume DD > PC lateral ventricular volume
Botteron et al.,	14 MZ and 22 DZ twins discordant for MDD 12 MZ and 2 DZ NC twins	17–23	Structural MRI, 1 mm slice thickness	Twins with history of MDD < twins no history of MDD = NC subgenual prefrontal cortex volume
Botteron et al., 2000	14 MZ and 22 DZ twins discordant for MDD 12 MZ and 2 DZ NC twin	17–23	Structural MRI, 1 mm slice thickness	Twins with history of MDD = twins with no history of MDD < NC amygdala volume
Thomas et al., 2001	5 MDD 5 NC	8–16	Functional MRI digitized faces with neutral and fearful facial expressions	MDD < NC amygdala response to fearful expressions compared to fixation
De Bellis et al., 1999	44 PTSD 20/44 with comorbid MDD 61 NC	6–17	Structural MRI, 1.5 mm slice thickness	PTSD = PTSD + MDD = NC hippocampal volume PTSD = PTSD + MDD > NC lateral ventricle volume PTSD = PTSD + MDD < NC middle and posterior regions of the corpus callosum

DA, dopamine; DD, depressive disorders (major depression and/or dysthymia); DZ, dizygotic twins; 5-HT, serotonin; [¹²³I] β-CIT, iodine-123-labeled 2β-carbomethoxy-3β(iodophenyl) tropane; MDD, major depressive disorder; MRI, magnetic resonance imaging; MZ, monozygotic twins; NC, normal controls; PC, psychiatric controls; PTSD post-traumatic stress disorder; rCBF, regional cerebral blood flow; SPECT, single photon emission computerized tomography; ⁹⁹Tc HMPAO, technetium-99m hexamethylpropylene amine oxime.

that may only emerge later in development or secondary to biological alterations (e.g., excess cortisol) associated with persistence and recurrence of disorder (e.g., hippocampal atrophy).

Single photon emission computerized tomograph studies

Tutus et al. (1998) and Kowatch et al. (1999) conducted single photon emission computerized tomography (SPECT) studies examining CBF in juvenile samples. The study by Tutus and colleagues included 14 depressed patients and 11 normal controls. Results were consistent with findings reported in adults, with depressed adolescents found to have reduced rCBF in the left anterofrontal and left temporal lobe regions (Tutus et al., 1998). The study by Kowatch and colleagues included only seven depressed and seven normal control subjects. In contrast to studies in adults, and the studies by Tutus, Kowatch, and colleagues reported increased rCBF in the temporal lobe. Consistent with prior studies conducted in adults (Buchsbaum et al., 1986; Baxter et al., 1989; Sackeim et al., 1990; Petracca et al., 1995; Nikolaus et al., 2000), they also reported decreased rCBF in the left parietal lobe, right caudate, and anterior thalamus (Kowatch et al., 1999).

The role of serotonin in the pathophysiology of MDD has long been postulated. Dahlstrom and colleagues (2000) used iodine-123-labeled 2 β-carbomethoxy-3 β (iodophenl) tropane ([123I]β-CIT) as a tracer for monoamine transporters in 31 drug-naive children and adolescents with depressive disorders and 10 psychiatric controls with a range of diagnoses including pervasive developmental, anxiety, and conduct disorders. They reported that depressed patients had significantly higher 5-HT transporter availability in the hypothalamic/midbrain region, and no significant difference in DA transporter availability in the striatum. Without comparable data in normal control children and adolescents and such a mixed cohort of psychiatric controls, it is difficult to speculate on the significance of these findings. Compared to healthy controls, adults with depression have been found to have reduced brain stem 5-HT transporter availability (Malison et al., 1998) and increased striatum DA transporter availability (Laasonen-Balk et al., 1999).

Structural and functional magnetic resonance imaging studies

Steingard and colleagues (1996) conducted the first published report of structural MRI in children and adolescents with depressive disorders (e.g., major depression and dysthymia). Children with depressive disorders were found to have reduced frontal lobe/cerebral volume ratios and increased lateral ventricle/cerebral volume ratios when compared to psychiatric controls. The finding of reduced frontal lobe volume is consistent with results of studies conducted with adults, but lateral ventricle enlargement has not typically been reported in nondelusional mid-life depression (Drevets et al., 1999). These findings need to be replicated and future studies extended to include normal control comparison subjects and the examination of more refined subregions of the frontal lobes. In particular, given replicated positron emission tomography (PET) studies showing reduced rCBF and metabolism in the dorsolateral region of the prefrontal cortex, and human and non-human primate studies suggesting that refinement of inputs in this area continues through adolescence (Alexander and Goldman 1978; Casey et al., 2000), examination of this region is of particular interest in child and adolescent cohorts.

Preliminary yet-to-be published structural MRI work underway at Washington University suggests that subgenual prefrontal cortex/anterior cingulate volume is reduced in early-onset depression, as reported in adult cohorts (Botteron et al., in press). In this study, structural MRI scans were completed in 14 monozygotic (MZ) and 22 dizygotic (DZ) twins who were discordant for a history of MDD, with one of the co-twins having a lifetime history of child- or adolescent-onset depression. Twelve MZ and 2 DZ twins with no lifetime history of psychopathology and no first-degree relatives with a lifetime history of MDD were used as comparison subjects. The volume reduction in the subgenual region appears to represent a "scar" marker (e.g., marker of past episode), and not a putative risk factor, as it was observed in identical twins with a history of MDD, but was not present in co-twins without a history of affective illness

In this study, twins with a history of depression were also found to have reduced amygdala volume (Botteron et al., 2000). The volume reduction in the amygdala appears to represent a potential "risk" marker, and was observed in identical twins with a history of MDD *and* in co-twins without a history of affective illness. Longitudinal follow-up of this cohort will be very informative in determining the predictive significance of this marker over time. Consistent with these structural MRI findings (Botteron et al., 2000), a pilot functional MRI investigation reported depressed children and adolescents to have reduced amygdala activation in processing fearful faces when compared to normal controls (Thomas et al., 2001).

As discussed previously, hippocampal-volume assessments have not been obtained in children and adolescents with primary affective disorders. De Bellis and colleagues (1999) conducted structural MRI assessments in a cohort of 44 children and adolescents with PTSD, about half of whom also met criteria for MDD. Unlike in studies of adults with PTSD or MDD (Bremner et al., 1995; 1997, 2000), no hippocampal volume reductions were found. Given the demonstrated importance of recurrence and total duration of illness on hippocampal-volume measures in adult studies, this finding is not surprising.

Summary

The preliminary results from these studies are promising and demonstrate clearly the feasibility of utilizing neuroimaging methodologies with juvenile samples. The available studies suggest that early-onset depression, like adult depression, is associated with structural and functional changes in frontal and subcortical regions. Some neuroanatomical correlates of depression preliminarily appear to be evident across the life cycle (e.g., frontal lobe and amygdala volume changes), and others seem to emerge later in development or secondary to biological alterations (e.g., excess cortisol) associated with persistence and recurrence of disorder (e.g., hippocampal atrophy). More research needs to be done in this area. Magnetic resonance spectroscopy (MRS) and functional MRI techniques have been little applied in child and adolescent cohorts, and will provide valuable additional data on potential mechanisms involved in the observed structural brain changes associated with early-onset MDD. In addition, more work on MDD in pre-adolescents is needed.

NEUROBIOLOGY OF BIPOLAR DISORDERS IN CHILDREN AND ADOLESCENTS

Adolescent bipolar disorder (BD) was described in the early twentieth century writings of Kraeplin, who noted a significant emergence of BD at puberty (Kraeplin, 1921). It is only within the past decade, however, that adolescent-onset BD has begun to receive significant research attention. Studies estimate the prevalence of bipolar spectrum disorders (e.g., bipolar I, bipolar II, bipolar not otherwise specified) as being 1% in adolescents (Lewinsohn et al., 1995). In addition, it is estimated that 20%–40% of adults with BD experi-

enced their first manic episode in adolescence (Loranger and Levine, 1978; Baron et al., 1983; Joyce, 1984; Lish et al., 1994).

Prepubertal diagnoses of BD are more controversial, and while childhood BD is increasingly accepted as a valid diagnosis, there is no consensus on the appropriate criteria to use to make the diagnosis in preadolescents (see Chapter 37, this volume, and Geller and Luby, 1997; for further discussion). Hyperactivity is frequently the earliest presenting symptom in prepubescent children with BD, and children are often diagnosed first with attention-deficit hyperactivity disorder (ADHD).

The overlap between symptoms of ADHD and BD often makes diagnosis difficult; however, similarities in the clinical picture of both conditions may implicate common neural systems that are important for understanding the neurobiology of these disorders. For example, features of both disorders are abnormalities in impulse control. Prefrontal development is significant in childhood and adolescence, and is related to increased ability to inhibit impulses and refine behavior adaptively to environmental changes. Greater knowledge of the development of the prefrontal cortex is likely to be instrumental in understanding both of these disorders.

There is a paucity of data on the neurobiology of BD in children, adolescents, and adults. Many factors contribute to the dearth of studies in this area, including the lower prevalence of BD, greater difficulty in engaging manic patients in research, and few preclinical models to guide research efforts. Available neurobiological models are reviewed below.

Preclinical Models of Mania and Neurobiological Correlates of Bipolar Disorder in Adults

There are relatively few animal models to inform the study of BD. Available models can approximate some of the symptoms, but cannot mimic the complex nature of mood alterations typical of the disorder. Rodent models of hyperactivity produced by creating right cortical hemispheric lesions mimic some of the symptoms of BD observed during the manic phase of the illness. Lesions in rats that promote hyperactivity/manic-like symptoms are associated with bilateral abnormalities in noradrenergic and dopaminergic function, and ipsilateral abnormalities in serotonergic function (Robinson 1979; Finkelstein et al., 1983). Consistent with these preclinical studies are findings that adults with BD have alterations on peripheral and central indices of noradrenergic, dopaminergic, and serotonergic functioning (Schatzbert and Schildraut, 1995; Willner, 1997; Drevets, 2000).

Brain lesion studies in non-human primates also suggest a potential role for the ventral prefrontal cortex in the pathophysiology of BD. The ventral prefrontal cortex is associated with the ability to rapidly refine behaviors in response to changes in reward contingencies. Animals with ventral prefrontal lesions continue to respond to stimuli that were previously rewarded despite the lack of ongoing positive feedback (Rolls, 1996). Humans with brain lesions in ventral prefrontal regions in the right hemisphere similarly demonstrate disinhibited and perseverative maladaptive behaviors when reward contingencies change (Rolls et al., 1994; Bechara et al., 1997). This behavioral abnormality after right hemisphere brain lesioning is associated with mood elevations (Rolls et al., 1994). Consistent with the results of these preclinical and clinical lesioning studies are findings that adults with mania have decreased regional brain activity in right orbitofrontal cortex, and increased activity in the dorsal anterior cingulate (Blumberg et al., 1999, 2000).

Kindling, however, is probably the most widely investigated preclinical model proposed to understand the pathophysiology of BD (Post and Weiss, 1989). *Kindling* describes the phenomenon that neurons in some areas of the brain, especially in the medial temporal lobes, respond to repeated stimulation by lowering their threshold to firing. Over time, these cells fire to previously subthreshold stimuli and may begin to fire spontaneously. Parallel to the phenomenon of kindling, first episodes of bipolar illness were hypothesized to be frequently associated with significant stressors. Episodes were thought to be more likely to emerge in response to lesser stressors and eventually to occur spontaneously—independent of external stressors (Post et al., 1995). While the relationship between life stressors and the course of bipolar illness appears more complex (Hlastala et al., 2000), preclinical models of kindling have been very useful in the conceptualization of the pathophysiology and treatment of BD (Post and Weiss, 1998). For example, the observations that the repeated stimulation administered in kindling experiments could lead to spontaneous seizures and that kindling phenomemon could be blocked by anticonvulsant agents were instrumental in introducing anticonvulsants as mood-stabilizing agents.

Preclinical studies examining the mechanism of action of mood stabilizers has extended research attention in the neurobiology of BD from a focus on biogenic amines to include study of the second messenger systems. These studies have found that chronic lithium treatment at "therapeutic" levels in adult rats alters activity in the cyclic adenosine monophosphate (cAMP)– and phosphoinositide (PI)–G protein systems (Manji and Lenox, 2000). Other clinically effective mood stabilizers have also been found to affect these signaling pathways, although the various agents have been found to have different effects. Consistent with these studies is the finding that adults with BD have alterations in cerebral and peripheral measures of second messenger systems (Young et al., 1993).

More recently investigation has focused on the effect of mood stabilizers on neuroprotective and neurotrophic factors (Manji et al., 1999; Manji and Lenox, 2000). Lithium and valproic acid have been found to increase neuroprotective protein bcl-2 in the frontal cortex of rats (Manji and Lenox, 2000). These preclinical investigations examining the mechanisms of action of the various mood stabilizers have been critical to generating new hypotheses of the role of neurotrophic factors in the pathogenesis of BD. Consistent with these studies is the finding that lithium increases gray matter volume in adults with BD (Moore et al., 2000a). In addition, in a recent MRS study, chronic lithium administration in adult patients with BD was found to increase brain N-acetylaspartate (NAA), a putative marker for neuronal viability (Moore et al., 2000b).

Utility of Preclinical Models in Organizing Findings of the Neurobiology of Bipolar Disorder in Children and Adolescents

The capacity to evaluate the utility of these various preclinical models in organizing findings on the neurobiological correlates of BD is extremely limited, given the paucity of research in the area. With regard to neurobiological correlates associated with lesioning studies that produce hyperactivity/manic-like symptomatology, peripheral and central indices of noradrenergic, dopaminergic, and serotonergic functioning have been little studied in juvenile BD. To the best of our knowledge there is only one study that examined urinary NE metabolites in a single child with BD (McKnew et al., 1974). The use of kindling models of disorder is supported by studies suggesting the preliminary effectiveness of these agents in juvenile samples (Geller et al., 1998; Kowatch et al., 2000). Also, because younger animals have been found to be more susceptible to kindling, developmentally informed investigations of this phenomenon may help to unravel the causes of rapid cycling in children and adolescents with BD. Whether neurotrophic factors are involved in the pathogenesis of early-onset BD is an area of active research.

Preliminary Results of Neuroimaging Studies in Children and Adolescents with Bipolar Disorder

Structural magnetic resonance imaging

There are few neuroimaging studies in pediatric BD; Table 10.2 delineates the few existing studies. Botteron and colleagues (1995) conducted the first structural MRI study in bipolar children and adolescents. Neuroradiological review of MRI scans from eight children with mania (ages 8 to 16), compared to age-matched healthy controls, suggested that mania was associated with an increased incidence of ventricular abnormalities, especially with temporal horn enlargement or asymmetry, and greater deep white matter hyperintensities. None of these group differences reached statistical significance, however (Botteron et al., 1995).

Friedman, Dasari, and colleagues conducted more recent structural MRI studies of children and adolescents 10 to 18 years of age, including 20 with schizophrenia, 15 with BD, and 16 healthy controls. Decreased thalamic volume (adjusted for total brain volume), decreased intracranial volume, and increased frontal and temporal sulcal size were found in the combined patient group compared to measurements in the healthy control group. However, differences were not detected between the two diagnostic groups (Dasari et al., 1999; Friedman et al., 1999).

The findings above are, for the most part, consistent with those in adults. Volumetric abnormalities have been reported in adults with BD, including increased sulci as well as increases and asymmetries in third and lateral ventricle size, particularly with increases in the left lateral ventricle and temporal horn volumes (Andreasen et al., 1990; Roy et al., 1998; Hauser et al., 2000). There have been conflicting findings about volumes of temporal lobe structures, although recent reports suggest that, in BD, there may be decreased temporal lobe volume and increased amygdala volume, both of which may be more prominent in men with the disorder (Swayze et al., 1992; Strakowski et al., 1999; Altshuler et al., 2000). Deep white matter hyperintensities have been reported (Dupont et al., 1990; McDonald et al., 1999) in BD. Decreased cerebellar vermal volume has also been reported, but this appears to be associated with multiple episodes (DelBello et al., 1999) and may be less likely to be seen in young populations. Adults with BD have also been found to have reduction in the left subgenual prefrontal cortex (Drevets et al., 1997). Study is underway to investigate gray matter abnormalities in this region in juvenile BD samples.

Magnetic resonance spectroscopy

Castillo and colleagues (2000) conducted an MRS study with 10 bipolar and 10 normal control preadolescents 6 to 12 years of age. When compared to controls, bipolar children had increased glutamate/glutamine ratios in the frontal lobe and basal ganglia regions and increased lipid levels in the frontal lobes.

There is an emerging literature in MRS in adults with BD, with reports of decreases in dorsolateral prefrontal cortex of neuronal marker NAA (Winsberg et al., 2000) and abnormalities in phopholipid metabolism (Kato et al., 1995, 1998; Hamakawa et al., 1999). There is preliminary work to suggest that cortical GABA levels and glutamate turnover are decreased in unipolar depression in adults, but these abnormalities may not be present in bipolar depression (Sanacora et al., 1999, Mason et al., 2000).

Summary

Studies with adults implicate frontotemporal regions in the pathophysiology of BD. The few recent neuroimaging studies that have been performed in children highlight the feasibility of applying these new technologies to the study of child and adolescent BD and suggest that frontotemporal structures may also be involved in early-onset cases. Results of preliminary neuroimaging studies in children and adolescents with BD show some continuities with the results of adult studies, with alterations in specific brain regions less likely to be replicated in juvenile samples when the findings are limited in adults to patients with recurrent episodes of illness (e.g., cerebellar vermal volume). This observation highlights the importance of differentiating between primary disturbances associated with the onset of BD and secondary brain changes associated with persistence and/or recurrence of illness.

CONCLUSIONS

Unipolar and bipolar depressive disorders in children and adolescents are serious conditions. The pathophysiology of these disorders is poorly understood. The new tools available through neuroimaging techniques will help to unravel the neuroanatomical systems involved in the onset and recurrence of these disorders. There is a need for more developmentally informed preclinical research and more studies of the normal development of the neural systems implicated in emotional regulation.

TABLE 10.2 *Neuroimaging Studies of Children and Adolescents with Bipolar Disorder*

Reference	Sample	Ages (years)	Method	Results
Botteron et al., 1995	8 BD 5 NC	8–16	Structural MRI	BD ≥ NC deep white matter hyperintensities BD ≥ NC ventricular volume (temporal horn)
Friedman et al., 1999	20 SCHZ 15 BD 16 NC	10–18	Structural MRI	SCHZ = BD < NC intracranial volume SCHZ = BD > NC frontal and temporal lobe sulcal size
Dasari et al., 1999	20 SCHZ 15 BD 16 NC	10–18	Structural MRI	SCHZ = BD < NC thalamic volume
Castillo et al., 2000	10 BD 10 NC	6–12	MRS	BD > NC frontal lobes and basal ganglia GLU/GLN BD > NC frontal lobes lipid levels

BD, bipolar disorder; GLU/GLN, glutamate/glutamine; MRI, magnetic resonance imaging; MRS, magnetic resonance spectros copy; NC, normal control; PFC, prefrontal cortex; SCHZ, schizophrenia.

REFERENCES

Alexander, G.E. and Goldman, P.S. (1978) Functional development of the dorsolateral prefrontal cortex: an analysis utlizing reversible cryogenic depression. *Brain Res* 143:233–249.

Altshuler, L.L., Bartzokis, G., Grieder, T., et al (2000) An MRI study of temporal lobe structures in men with bipolar disorder or schizophrenia. *Biol Psychiatry* 48:147–162.

Andreasen, N.C., Swayze, V.I.I., Flaum, M., Alliger, R., and Cohen, G. (1990) Ventricular abnormalities in affective disorder: clinical and demographic correlates. *Am J Psychiatry* 147:893–900.

American Psychiatric Association (1987) The dexamethasone suppression test: an overview of its current status in psychiatry. The APA Task Force on Laboratory Tests in Psychiatry. *Am J Psychiatry* 144:1253–1262.

Axelson, D.A., Doraiswamy, P.M., McDonald, and W.M., Boyko, O.B., Tupler, L.A., Patterson, L.J., Nemeroff, C.B., Ellinwood, E.H., Jr., and Krishman, K.R. (1993)

Baron, M., Risch, N., and Mendlewicz, J. (1983) Age at onset in bipolar-related major affective illness: clinical and genetic implications. *J Psychiatr Res* 17:5–18.

Baxter, L.R., Phelps, M.E., Mazziotta, J.C., Schwartz, J.M., Gerner, R.H., Selin, C.E., and Sumida, R.M. (1985) Cerebral metabolic rates for glucose in mood disorders. Studies with positron emission tomography and fluorodeoxyglucose F 18. *Arch Gen Psychiatry,* 42:441–447.

Bechara, A., Damasio, H., Tranel, D., and Damasio, A.R. (1997) Deciding advantageously before knowing the advantageous strategy. *Science* 275:1293–1295.

Bench, C., Friston, K., Brown, R., Scott, L., Frackowiak, R., and Dolan, R. (1992) The anatomy of melancholia—focal abnormalities of cerebral blood flow in major depression. *Psychol Med* 22:607–615.

Birmaher, B., Dahl, R.E., Perel, J., et al. (1996a) Corticotropin-releasing hormone challenge in prepubertal major depression. *Biol Psychiatry* 39:267–277.

Birmaher, B., Ryan, N.D., Williamson, D.E., Brent, D.A., and Kaufman, J. (1996b) Childhood and adolescent depression: a review of the past 10 years. Part II. *J Am Acad Child Adolesc Psychiatry* 35:1575–1583.

Blumberg, H., Kaufman, J., Martin, A., and Peterson, B. (2001) Structural and functional MRI studies in children, adolescents, and adults with bipolar disorder. Presented at the *Childhood Depression: A Critical Review Conference.* Banbury Center, NY: Cold Spring Harbor Laboratory.

Blumberg, H.P., Stern, E., Martinez, D., Ricketts, S., de Asis, J., White, T., Epstein, J., McBride, P.A., Eidelberg, D., Kocsis, J.H., and Silbersweig, D.A. (2000) Increased anterior cingulate and caudate activity in bipolar mania. *Biol Psychiatry* 48:1045–1052.

Blumberg, H., Stern, E., Ricketts, S., et al. (1999) Rostral and orbital prefrontal cortex dysfunction in the manic state of bipolar disorder. *Am J Psychiatry* 156:1986–1988.

Botteron, K., Raichle, M., Heath, A., Price, J., Sternhell, K., Singer, T., and Todd, R. (in press) An epidemiological twin study of prefrontal neuromorphometry in early onset depression. *Biol Psychiatry.*

Botteron, K.N., Raichle, M.E., Heath, A.C., and Todd, R.D. (2000) Twin study of brain morphometry in adolescent- or earlier-onset depression. Presented at *Depression in the Twenty-first Century.* Laguna Beach, CA:

Botteron, K.N., Vannier, M.W., Geller, B., Todd, R.D., and Lee, B.C. (1995) Preliminary study of magnetic resonance imaging characteristics in 8- to 16-year-olds with mania. *J Am Acad Child Adolesc Psychiatry* 34:742–749.

Braun, K., Lange, E., Metzger, M., and Poeggel, G. (2000) Maternal separation followed by early social deprivation affects the development of monoaminergic fiber systems in the medial prefrontal cortex of Octodon degus. *Neuroscience* 95:309–318.

Bremner, J.D., Narayan, M., Anderson, E.R., Staib, L.H., Miller, H.L., and Charney, D.S. (2000) Hippocampal volume reduction in major depression. *Am J Psychiatry* 157:115–118.

Bremner, J.D., Randall, P., Scott, T.M., Bronen, R.A., Seibyl, J.P., Southwick, S.M., Delaney, R.C., McCarthy, G., Charney, D.S., and Innis, R.B. (1995) MRI-based measurement of hippocampal volume in patients with combat-related posttraumatic stress disorder. *Am J Psychiatry* 152:973–981.

Bremner, J.D., Randall, P., Vermetten, E., Staib, L., Bronen, R.A., Mazure, C., Capelli, S., McCarthy, G., Innis, R.B., and Charney, D.S. (1997) Magnetic resonance imaging-based measurement of hippocampal volume in posttraumatic stress disorder related to childhood physical and sexual abuse—a preliminary report. *Biol Psychiatry,* 41:23–32.

Buchsbaum, M.S., Wu, J., DeLisi, L.E., Holcomb, H., Kessler, R., Johnson, J., King, A.C., Hazlett, E., Langston, K., and Post, R.M. (1986) Frontal cortex and basal ganglia metabolic rates assessed by positron emission tomography with [8F]2-deoxyglucose in affective illness. *J Affect Disord* 10:137–52.

Buchsbaum, M.S., Wu, J., Siegel, B.V., Hackett, E., Trenary, M., Abel, L., and Reynolds, C. (1997) Effect of sertraline on regional metabolic rate in patients with affective disorder. *Biol Psychiatry* 41:15–22.

Caldji, C., Francis, D., Sharma, S., Plotsky, P.M., and Meaney, M.J. (2000) The effects of early rearing environment on the development of GABA$_A$ and central benzodiazepine receptor levels and novelty-induced fearfulness in the rat. *Neuropsychopharmacology* 22:219–229.

Carroll, B.J. (1982) The dexamethasone suppression test for melancholia. *Br J Psychiatry* 140:292–304.

Casey, B.J., Giedd, J.N., and Thomas, K.M. (2000) Structural and functional brain development and its relation to cognitive development. *Biol Psychol* 54:241–257.

Castillo, M., Kwock, L., Courvoisie, H., and Hooper, S.R. (2000) Proton MR spectroscopy in children with bipolar affective disorder: preliminary observations. *AJNR Am J Neuroradiol* 21:832–838.

Coe, C.L., Mendoza, S.P., Smotherman, W.P., and Levine, S. (1978) Mother–infant attachment in the squirrel monkey: adrenal response to separation. *Behav Biol* 22:256–263.

Dahlstrom, M., Ahonen, A., Ebeling, H., Torniainen, P., Heikkila, J., and Moilanen, I. (2000) Elevated hypothalamic/midbrain serotonin (monoamine) transporter availability in depressive drug–naive children and adolescents. *Mol Psychiatry* 5:514–522.

Dasari, M., Friedman, L., Jesberger, J., Stuve, T.A., Findling, R.L., Swales, T.P., and Schulz, S.C. (1999) A magnetic resonance imaging study of thalamic area in adolescent patients with either schizophrenia or bipolar disorder as compared to healthy controls. *Psychiatry Res* 91:155–162.

De Bellis, M.D., Chrousos, G.P., Dorn, L., Putnam, F.W., and Gold, P. (1994) Hypothalamic pituitary adrenal axis dysregulation in sexually abused girls. *J Clin Endocrinol Metab* 78:249–255.

De Bellis, M.D., Gold, P.W., Geracioti, T.D., Jr., Listwak, S.J., and Kling, M.A. (1993) Association of fluoxetine treatment with reductions in CSF concentrations of corticotropin-releasing hormone and arginine vasopressin in patients with major depression. *Am J Psychiatry* 150:656–657.

De Bellis, M.D., Keshavan, M.S., Clark, D.B., et al. (1999) Developmental traumatology. Part II: Brain development. *Biol Psychiatry* 45:1271–1284.

DelBello, M.P., Strakowski, S.M., Zimmerman, M.E., Hawkins, J.M., and Sax, K.W. (1999) MRI analysis of the cerebellum in bipolar disorder: a pilot study. *Neuropsychopharmacology* 21: 63–68.

Devinsky, O., Morrell, M.J., and Vogt, B.A. (1995) Contributions of the anterior cingulate cortex to behaviour. *Brain,* 118:279–306.

Dorn, L.D., Burgess, E.S., Dichek, H.L., Putnam, F.W., Chrousos, G.P., and Gold, P.W. (1996) Thyroid hormone concentrations in depressed and nondepressed adolescents: group differences and behavioral relations [see comments]. *J Am Acad Child Adolesc Psychiatry* 35:299–306.

Drevets, W.C. (2000) Neuroimaging studies of mood disorders. *Biol Psychiatry* 48:813–829.

Drevets, W.C., Gadde, K., and Krishnan, K. (1999) Neuroimaging studies of mood. In: N Charney, D., Nestler, E., and Bunney, B.S. eds. *Neurobiology of Mental Illness.* New York: Oxford Press, pp. 394–418.

Drevets, W.C., Price, J.L., Simpson, J.R., Jr., Todd, R.D., Reich, T., Vannier, M., and Raichle, M.E. (1997) Subgenual prefrontal cortex abnormalities in mood disorders. *Nature,* 386:824–827.

Drevets, W.C., Videen, T.O., Price, J.L., Preskorn, S.H., Carmichael, S.T., and Raichle, M.E. (1992) A functional anatomical study of unipolar depression. *J Neurosci* 12:3628–3641.

Dupont, R.M., Jernigan, T.L., Butters, N., Delis, D., Hesselink, J.R., Heindel, W., and Gillin, J.C. (1990) Subcortical abnormalities detected in bipolar affective disorder using magnetic resonance imaging. Clinical and neuropsychological significance. *Arch Gen Psychiatry* 47:55–59.

Farber, N.B., Wozniak, D.F., Price, M.T., Labruyere, J., Huss, J., St. Peter, H., and Olney, J.W. (1995) Age-specific neurotoxicity in the rat associated with NMDA receptor blockade: potential relevance to schizophrenia? *Biol Psychiatry* 38:788–796.

Finklestein, S., Campbell, A., Stoll, A.L., Baldessarini, R.J., Stinus, L., Paskevitch, P.A., and Domesick, V.B. (1983) Changes in cortical and subcortical levels of monoamines and their metabolites following unilateral ventrolateral cortical lesions in the rat. *Brain Res,* 271:279–288.

Friedman, L., Findling, R.L., Kenny, J.T., Swales, T.P., Stuve, T.A., Jesberger, J.A., Lewin, J.S., and Schulz, S.C. (1999). An MRI study of adolescent patients with either schizophrenia or bipolar disorder as compared to healthy control subjects. *Biol Psychiatry,* 46:78–88.

Francis, D., Diorio, J., Liu, D., and Meaney, M.J. (1999a) Nongenomic transmission across generations of maternal behavior and stress responses in the rat. *Science* 286:1155–8.

Francis, D.D., Caldji, C., Champagne, F., Plotsky, P.M., and Meaney, M.J. (1999b) The role of corticotropin-releasing factor—norepinephrine systems in mediating the effects of early experience on the development of behavioral and endocrine responses to stress. *Biol Psychiatry* 46:1153–1166.

Geller, B., Cooper, T.B., Zimerman, B., Frazier, J., Williams, M., Heath, J., and Warner, K. (1998) Lithium for prepubertal depressed children with family history predictors of future bipolarity: a double-blind, placebo-controlled study. *J Affect Disord,* 51: 165–175.

Geller, B. and Luby, J. (1997) Child and adolescent bipolar disorder: a review of the past 10 years. *J Am Acad Child Adolesc Psychiatry* 36:1168–1176.

Gold, P.W., Calabrese, J.R., Kling, M.A., Avgerinos, P., Khan, I., Gallucci, W.T., Tomai, T.P., and Chrousos, G.P. (1986) Abnormal ACTH and cortisol responses to ovine corticotropin releasing factor in patients with primary affective disorder. *Prog Neuropsychopharmacol Biol Psychiatry* 10:57–65.

Graham, Y.P., Heim, C., Goodman, S.H., Miller, A.H., and Nemeroff, C.B. (1999) The effects of neonatal stress on brain development: implications for psychopathology. *Dev Psychopathol* 11: 545–565.

Hamakawa, H., Kato, T., Shioiri, T., Inubushi, T., and Kato, N. (1999) Quantitative proton magnetic resonance spectroscopy of the bilateral frontal lobes in patients with bipolar disorder. *Psychol Med* 29:639–644.

Hart, J., Gunner, M., and Cicchetti, D. (1996) Altered neuroendocrine activity in maltreated children related to symptoms of depression. *Dev Psychopathol* 8:201–214.

Hauser, P., Altshuler, L.L., Berrettini, W., Dauphinais, I.D., Gelernter, J., and Post, R.M. (1989) Temporal lobe measurement in primary affective disorder by magnetic resonance imaging. *J Neuropsychiatry Clin Neurosci* 1:128–134.

Hauser, P., Matochik, J., Altshuler, L.L., et al. (2000) MRI-based measurements of temporal lobe and ventricular structures in patients with bipolar I and bipolar II disorders. *J Affect Disord* 60: 25–32.

Hlastala, S.A., Frank, E., Kowalski, J., Sherill, J.T., Tu, X.M., Anderson, B., and Kupfer, D.J. (2000) Stressful life events, bipolar disorder, and the "kindling model." *J Abnorm Psychol* 109:777–786.

Holsboer, F., Gerken, A., Stalla, G.K., and Muller, O.A. (1987) Blunted aldosterone and ACTH release after human CRH administration in depressed patients. *Am J Psychiatry* 144:229–231.

Joyce, P.R. (1984) Age of onset in bipolar affective disorder and misdiagnosis as schizophrenia. *Psychol Med* 14:145–149.

Kashani, J.H., McGee, R.O., Clarkson, S.E., Anderson, J.C., Walton, L.A., Williams, S., Silva, P.A., Robins, A.J., Cytryn, L. and McKnew, D.H. (1983) Depression in a sample of 9-year-old children, Prevalence and associated characteristics. *Arch Gen Psychiatry* 40:1217–1223.

Kato, T., Murashita, J., Kamiya, A., Shioiri, T., Kato, N., and Inubushi, T. (1998) Decreased brain intracellular pH measured by 31P-MRS in bipolar disorder: a confirmation in drug-free patients and correlation with white matter hyperintensity. *Eur Arch Psychiatry Clin Neurosci,* 248:301–306.

Kato, T., Shioiri, T., Murashita, J., Hamakawa, H., Takahashi, Y., Inubushi, T., and Takahashi, S. (1995) Lateralized abnormality of high energy phosphate metabolism in the frontal lobes of patients with bipolar disorder detected by phase-encoded 31P-MRS. *Psychol Med* 25:557–566.

Kaufman, J. (1991) Depressive disorders in maltreated children. *J Am Acad Child Adolesc Psychiatry* 30:257–265.

Kaufman, J., Birmaher, B., Perel, J., Dahl, R.E., Moreci, P., Nelson, B., Wells, W., and Ryan, N.D. (1997). The corticotropin-releasing hormone challenge in depressed abused, depressed nonabused, and normal control children. *Biol Psychiatry* 42:669–679.

Kaufman, J., Martin, A., King, R.A., and Charney, D.S. (2001) Are child-, adolescent- and adult-onset depression one and the same disorder? *Biol Psychiatry* 49:980–1001.

Kaufman, J., and Plotsky, P., Nemeroff, C., and Charney, D. (2000) Effects of early adverse experience on brain structure and function: clinical implications. *Biol Psychiatry* 48:778–790.

Kaufman, J., and Ryan, N. (1999) The neurobiology of child and adolescent depression. In: Charney, D., Nestler, E., and Bunny, B., eds. *The Neurobiological Foundation of Mental Illness.* New York: Oxford University Press, pp. 810–821.

Kovacs, M., Feinberg, T.L., Crouse-Novak, M., Paulauskas, S.L., Pollock, M., and Finkelstein, R. (1984) Depressive disorders in childhood. II. A longitudinal study of the risk for a subsequent major depression. *Arch Gen Psychiatry* 41:643–649.

Kowatch, R.A., Devous, M.D., Sr., Harvey, D.C., Mayes, T.L., Trivedi, M.H., Emslie, G.J., and Weinberg, W.A. (1999) A SPECT HMPAO study of regional cerebral blood flow in depressed adolescents and normal controls. *Prog Neuropsychopharmacol Biol Psychiatry* 23:643–656.

Kowatch, R.A., Suppes, T., Carmody, T.J., Bucci, J.P., Hume, J.H., Kromelis, M., Emslie, G.J., Weinberg, W.A., and Rush, A.J. (2000) Effect size of lithium, divalproex sodium, and carbamazepine in children and adolescents with bipolar disorder. *J Am Acad Child Adolesc Psychiatry* 39:713–720.

Kraeplin, E. (1921) *Manic-Depressive Insanity and Paranoia.* Edinburgh: E & S Livingstone.

Laasonen-Balk, T., Kuikka, J., Viinamaki, H., Husso-Saastamoinen, M., Lehtonen, J., and Tiihonen, J. (1999) Striatal dopamine transporter density in major depression. *Psychopharmacology (Berl)* 144:282–285.

Levine, S., Wiener, S.G., and Coe, C.L. (1993) Temporal and social factors influencing behavioral and hormonal responses to separation in mother and infant squirrel monkeys. *Psychoneuroendocrinology* 18:297–306.

Lewinsohn, P.M., Clarke, G.N., Seeley, J.R., and Rohde, P. (1994) Major depression in community adolescents: age at onset, episode duration, and time to recurrence [see comments]. *J Am Acad Child Adolesc Psychiatry* 33:809–818.

Lewinsohn, P.M., Klein, D.N., and Seeley, J.R. (1995) Bipolar disorder in a community sample of older adolescents: prevalence, phenomenology, comorbidity and course. *J Am Acad Child Adolesc Psychiatry* 34:454–463.

Lish, J.D., Dime-Meenan, S., Whybrow, P.C., Price, R.A., and Hirschfeld, R.M. (1994) The National Depression and Manic-Depressive Association (DMDA) survey of bipolar members. *J Affect Disord* 31:281–294.

Loranger, A. and Levine, P. (1978) Age at onset of bipolar illness. *Arch Gen Psychiatry* 35:1345–1348.

Malison, R.T., Price, L.H., Berman, R., van Dyck, C.H., Pelton, G.H., Carpenter, L., Sanacora, G., Owens, M.J., Nemeroff, C.B., Rajeevan, N., Baldwin, R.M., Seibyl, J.P., Innis, R.B., and Charney, D.S. (1998) Reduced brain serotonin transporter availability in major depression as measured by [123I]-2 beta-carbomethoxy-3 beta-(4-iodophenyl)tropane and single photon emission computed tomography. *Biol Psychiatry* 44:1090–1098.

Manji, H.K., and Lenox, R.H. (2000) The nature of bipolar disorder. *J Clin Psychiatry* 61 Supp 13:42–57.

Manji, H.K., Moore, G.J., and Chen, G. (1999) Lithium at 50: have the neuroprotective effects of this unique cation been overlooked? *Biol Psychiatry* 46:929–940.

Mason, G.F., Sanacora, G., Anand A, et al. (2000) Cortical GABA reduced in unipolar, but not bipolar depression. *Biol Psychiatry* 47:92S.

Mayberg, H.S., Brannan, S.K., Mahurin, R.K., Jerabek, P.A., Brickman, J.S., Tekell, J.L., Silva, J.A., McGinnis, S., Glass, T.G., Martin, C.C., and Fox, P.T. (1997) Cingulate function in depression: a potential predictor of treatment response [see comments]. *Neuroreport* 8:1057–1061.

McDonald, W.M., Tupler, L.A., Marsteller, F.A., Figiel, G.S., DiSouza, S., Nemeroff, C.B., and Krishnan, K.R. (1999) Hyperintense lesions on magnetic resonance images in bipolar disorder. *Biol Psychiatry* 45:965–971.

McKnew, D.H., Jr., Cytryn, L., and White, I. (1974) Clinical and biochemical correlates of hypomania in a child. *J Am Acad Child Psychiatry* 13:576–585.

Meaney, M.J., Aitken, D.H., Bhatnagar, S., and Sapolsky, R.M. (1991) Postnatal handling attenuates certain neuroendocrine, anatomical, and cognitive dysfunctions associated with aging in female rats. *Neurobiol Aging* 12:31–38.

Meaney, M.J., Bhatnagar, S., Diorio, J., Larocque, S., Francis, D., O'Donnell, D., Shanks, N., Sharma, S., Smythe, J., and Viau, V. (1993) Molecular basis for the development of individual differences in the hypothalamic-pituitary-adrenal stress response. *Cell Mol Neurobiol* 13:321–347.

Mervaala, E., Fohr, J., Kononen, M., et al. (2000) Quantitative MRI of the hippocampus and amygdala in severe depression. *Psychol Med* 30:117–125.

Meaney, M.J., Bhatnagar, S., Diorio, J., Larocque, S., Francis, D., O'Donnell, D., Shanks, N., Sharma, S., Smythe, J., and Viau, V. (1993) Molecular basis for the development of individual differences in the hypothalamic-pituitary-adrenal stress response. *Cell Mol Neurobiol* 13:321–347.

Moore, G.J., Bebchuk, J.M., Wilds, I.B., Chen, G., and Manji, H.K. (2000a) Lithium-induced increase in human brain grey matter. *Lancet* 356:1241–1242.

Moore, G.J., Bebchuk, J.M., Hasanat, K., Chen, G., Seraji-Bozorgzad, N., Wilds, I.B., Faulk, M.W., Koch, S., Glitz, D.A., Jolkovsky, L., and Manji, H.K. (2000b) Lithium increases 5N-acetyl-aspartate in the human brain: in vivo evidence in support of bcl-2's neurotrophic effects? *Biol Psychiatry* 48:1–8.

Nauta, W.J. (1971) The problem of the frontal lobe: a reinterpretation. *J Psychiatr Res* 8:167–87.

Nemeroff, C.B., Bissette, G., Akil, H., and Fink, M. (1991) Neuropeptide concentrations in the cerebrospinal fluid of depressed patients treated with electroconvulsive therapy. Corticotrophin-releasing factor, beta-endorphin and somatostatin. *Br J Psychiatry* 158:59–63.

Nemeroff, C.B., Owens, M.J., Bissette, G., Andorn, A.C., and Stanley, M. (1988) Reduced corticotropin releasing factor binding sites in the frontal cortex of suicide victims. *Arch Gen Psychiatry* 45:577–579.

Nemeroff, C.B., Widerlov, E., Bissette, G., Walleus, H., Karlsson, I., Eklund, K., Kilts, C.D., Loosen, P.T., and Vale, W. (1984) Elevated concentrations of CSF corticotropin-releasing factor-like immunoreactivity in depressed patients. *Science* 226:1342–1344.

Nikolaus, S., Larisch, R., Beu, M., Vosberg, H., and Muller-Gartner, H.W. (2000) Diffuse cortical reduction of neuronal activity in unipolar major depression: a retrospective analysis of 337 patients and 321 controls. *Nucl Med Commun* 21:1119–1125.

Ongur, D., Drevets, W.C., and Price, J.L. (1998) Glial reduction in the subgenual prefrontal cortex in mood disorders. *Proc Natl Acad Sci USA* 95:13290–13298.

Pandya, D.N., and Seltzer, B. (1986) The topography of commisural fibers. In: Lepore, F., Ptito, M., and Jasper, H.H., eds. *Two Hemispheres–One Brain: Functions of the Corpus Callosum., Vol 17.* New York: Alan R. Liss, Inc., pp. 47–74.

Petracca, G., Migliorelli, R., Vazquez, S., and Starkstein, S.E. (1995) SPECT findings before and after ECT in a patient with major depression and Cotard's syndrome. *J Neuropsychiatry Clin Neurosci* 7:505–507.

Plotsky, P.M., Owens, M.J., and Nemeroff, C.B. (1998) Psychoneuroendocrinology of depression. Hypothalamic-pituitary-adrenal axis. *Psychiatry Clin North Am* 21:293–307.

Poeggel, G., Lange, E., Hase, C., Metzger, M., Gulyaeva, N., and Braun, K. (1999) Maternal separation and early social deprivation in Octodon degus: quantitative changes of nicotinamide adenine dinucleotide phosphate-diaphorase-reactive neurons in the prefrontal cortex and nucleus accumbens. *Neuroscience* 94:497–504.

Post, R.M., and Weiss, S.R. (1989) Sensitization, kindling, and anticonvulsants in mania. *J Clin Psychiatry* 50 Suppl:23–30.

Post, R.M. and Weiss, S.R. (1998) Sensitization and kindling phenomenon in mood, anxiety, and obsessive compulsive disorders: the role of serotonergic mechanisms in illness progression. *Biol Psychiatry* 44:193–206.

Post, R.M., Weiss, S.R., Smith, M., Rosen, J., and Frye, M. (1995) Stress, conditioning, and the temporal aspects of affective disorders. *Ann NY Acad Sci* 77:677–696.

Puig-Antich, J. and Gittleman, R. (1982) Depression in childhood and adolescence. In: Paykel, E. ed. *Handbook of Affective Disorders.* New York: Guilford Press, pp. 379–392.

Puig-Antich, J., Kaufman, J., Ryan, N.D., Williamson, D.E., Dahl, R.E., Lukens, E., Todak, G., Ambrosini, P., Rabinovich, H., and Nelson, B. (1993) The psychosocial functioning and family environment of depressed adolescents. *J Am Acad Child Adolesc Psychiatry* 32:244–253.

Putnam, F.W., Trickett, P., Helmars, K., Dorn, L., and Everett, B. (1991) Cortisol abnormalities in sexually abused girls. Abstract Annual Meeting of the Washington, DC: American Psychiatric Association Press, pp. 107.

Rao, U., Weissman, M.M., Martin, J.A., and Hammond, R.W. (1993) Childhood depression and risk of suicide: a preliminary report of a longitudinal study. *J Am Acad Child Adolesc Psychiatry* 32:21–27.

Reddy, P.L., Khanna, S., Subhash, M.N., Channabasavanna, S.M., and Rao, B.S. (1992) CSF amine metabolites in depression. *Biol Psychiatry* 31:112–118.

Robinson, R.G. (1979) Differential behavioral and biochemical effects of right and left hemispheric cerebral infarction in the rat. *Science* 205:707–710.

Rolls, E. (1996) The orbitofrontal cortex. *Phil Trans R Soc Lond B* 351:1433–1444.

Rolls, E.T., Hornak, J., Wade, D., and McGrath, J. (1994) Emotion-related learning in patients with social and emotional changes associated with frontal lobe damage. *J Neurol Neurosurg Psychiatry* 57:1518–1524.

Roy, P.D., Zipursky, R.B., Saint-Cyr, J.A., Bury, A., Langevin, R., and Seeman, M.V. (1998) Temporal horn enlargement is present in schizophrenia and bipolar disorder. *Biol Psychiatry* 44:418–22.

Ryan, N., and Dahl, R. (1993) The biology of depression in children and adolescents. In: Mann, J. and Kupfer, D., eds. *The Biology of Depressive Disorders.* New York: Plenum Press, pp. 37–58.

Ryan, N.D., Puig-Antich, J., Ambrosini, P., Rabinovich, H., Robinson, D., Nelson, B., Iyengar, S., and Twomey, J. (1987) The clinical picture of major depression in children and adolescents. *Arch Gen Psychiatry* 44:854–861.

Sackeim, H.A., Prohovnik, I., Moeller, J.R., Brown, R.P., Apter, S., Prudic, J., Devanand, D.P., and Mukherjee, S. (1990) Regional cerebral blood flow in mood disorders. I. Comparison of major depressives and normal controls at rest. *Arch Gen Psychiatry* 47:60–70.

Sanacora, G., Mason, G.F., Rothman, D.L., Behar, K.L., Hyder, F., Petroff, O.A., Berman, R.M., Charney, D.S., and Krystal, J.H. (1999) Reduced cortical gamma-aminobutyric acid levels in depressed patients determined by proton magnetic resonance spectroscopy. *Arch Gen Psychiatry* 56:1043–1047.

Sanchez, M.M., Hearn, E.F., Do, D., Rilling, J.K., and Herndon, J.G. (1998) Differential rearing affects corpus callosum size and cognitive function of rhesus monkeys. *Brain Res* 812:38–49.

Schatzberg, A.F. and Schildraut, J.J. (1995) Recent studies on norepinephrine systems in mood disorders. In: Bloom, F.E. and Kupfer, D.J., eds. *Psychopharmacology: The Fourth Generation of Progress.* New York: Raven Press, pp. 911–920.

Schildkraut, J., Green, A., and Mooney, J. (1989) Mood disorders: biochemical aspects. In: Kaplan, H. and Sadock, B., eds. *Comprehensive Textbook of Psychiatry*, Baltimore: Wilkens & Williams *Vol.* I. pp. 868–879.

Shah, P.J., Ebmeier, K.P., Glabus, M.F., and Goodwin GM (1998) Cortical grey matter reductions associated with treatment-resistant chronic unipolar depression. Controlled magnetic resonance imaging study. *Br J Psychiatry* 172:527–532.

Sheline, Y.I., Gado, M.H., and Price, J.L. (1998) Amygdala core nuclei volumes are decreased in recurrent major depression [published erratum appears in *Neuroreport* (1998) 13;9(10):2436]. *Neuroreport* 9:2023–2028.

Sheline, Y.I., Wang, P.W., Gado, M.H., Csernansky, J.G., and Vannier, M.W. (1996) Hippocampal atrophy in recurrent major depression. *Proc Natl Acad Sci USA* 93:3908–3913.

Steingard, R.J., Renshaw, P.F., Yurgelun-Todd, D., Appelsmans, K.E., Lyoo, I.K., Shorrock, K.L., Bucci, J.P., Cesena, M., Abebe, D., Zurakowski, D., Poussaint, T.Y., and Barnes, P. (1996) Structural abnormalities in brain magnetic resonance images of depressed children. *J Am Acad Child Adolesc Psychiatry* 35:307–311.

Strakowski, S.M., DelBello, M.P., Sax, K.W., et al. (1999) Brain magnetic resonance imaging of structural abnormalities in bipolar disorder. *Arch Gen Psychiatry* 56:254–260.

Swayze, V.W.I.I., Andreasen, N.C., Alliger, R.J., Yuh, W.T.C., and Ehrhardt, J.C. (1992) Subcortical and temporal structures in affective disorders and schizophrenia: a magnetic resonance imaging study. *Biol Psychiatry* 31:221–240.

Takahashi, L.K., and Kalin, N.H. (1991) Early developmental and temporal characteristics of stress-induced secretion of pituitary-adrenal hormones in prenatally stressed rat pups. *Brain Res* 558:75–78.

Teicher, M.H., Anderson, S.L., Dumont, Y., et al. (2000) Childhood neglect attenuates development of the corpus callosum. *Neuroscience* 206:872.

Thomas, K.M., Drevets, W.C., Dahl, R.E., Ryan, N.D., Birmaher, B., Eccard, C.H., Axelson, D., Whalen, P.J., and Casey, B.J. (2001) Amygdala response to fearful faces in anxious and depressed children. *Arch Gen Psychiatry* 58:1057–1063.

Tutus, A., Kibar, M., Sofuoglu, S., Basturk, M., and Gonul, A.S. (1998) A technetium-99m hexamethylpropylene amine oxime brain single-photon emission tomography study in adolescent patients with major depressive disorder. *Eur J Nucl Med* 25:601–606.

Vakili, K., Pillay, S.S., Lafer, B., Fava, M., Renshaw, P.F., Bonello-Cintron, C.M., and Yurgelun-Todd, D.A. (2000). Hippocampal volume in primary unipolar major depression: a magnetic resonance imaging study. *Biol Psychiatry* 47:1087–1090.

Wiener, S.G., Johnson, D.F., and Levine, S. (1987) Influence of postnatal rearing conditions on the response of squirrel monkey infants to brief perturbations in mother-infant relationships. *Physiol Behav* 39:21–26.

Weissman, M.M., Wolk, S., Goldstein, R.B., Moreau, D., Adams, P., Greenwald, S., Klier, C.M., Ryan, N.D., Dahl, R.E., and Wickramaratne, P. (1999) Depressed adolescents grown up. *Jama* 281:1707–1713.

Willner, P. (1997) The mesolimbic dopamine system as a target for rapid antidepressant action. *Int Clin Psychopharmacol* 12 Suppl 3:S7–S14.

Winsberg, M.E., Sachs, N., Tate, D.L., Adalsteinsson, E., Spielman,

D., and Ketter, T.A. (2000) Decreased dorsolateral prefrontal *N*-acetyl aspartate in bipolar disorder. *Biol Psychiatry* 47:475–481.

Wong, M.L., Kling, M.A., Munson, P.J., Listwak, S., Licinio, J., Prolo, P., Karp, B., McCutcheon, I.E., Geracioti, T.D., Jr., DeBellis, M.D., Rice, K.C., Goldstein, D.S., Veldhuis, J.D., Chrousos, G.P., Oldfield, E.H., McCann, S.M., and Gold, P.W. (2000) Pronounced and sustained central hypernoradrenergic function in major depression with melancholic features: relation to hypercortisolism and corticotropin-releasing hormone. *Proc Natl Acad Sci U S A* 97:325–330.

Young, L.T., Li, P.P., Kish, S.J., Siu, K.P., Kamble, A., Hornykiewicz, O., and Warsh, J.J. (1993) Cerebral cortex Gs alpha protein levels and forskolin-stimulated cyclic AMP formation are increased in bipolar affective disorder. *J Neurochem* 61:890–889.

11 | Neurobiology of early-onset anxiety disorders

VIVIAN H. KODA, DENNIS S. CHARNEY, AND DANIEL S. PINE

The past two decades of research on both the longitudinal course and familial distribution of anxiety disorders suggests that many forms of adult anxiety disorders can be conceptualized as developmental conditions. Family studies demonstrate strong associations between anxiety in parents and children (Weissman et al., 1997; Battaglia et al., 1998). Similarly, prospective epidemiological studies find strong associations between anxiety during adolescence and both anxiety as well as major depression during adulthood (Pine et al., 1998). Given this developmental perspective, the expanding knowledge base on the neurobiology of adult anxiety disorder may provide opportunities for enhancing knowledge of childhood anxiety disorders.

Research on clinical characteristics of childhood anxiety disorders outlines the potential utility of a developmental, neurobiological perspective. For example, childhood anxiety disorders exhibit high rates of comorbidity in both community-and clinically based studies (Gurley et al., 1996). Comorbidity appears particularly high for generalized anxiety disorder in children, which shows strong associations with a range of conditions, including social anxiety disorder and major depression (Kessler and Walters, 1998; Pine, 1999). Such high rates of comorbidity raise questions as to the validity of current nosological categories and suggest the need for alternative bodies of knowledge to validate conditions. Recent advances in affective neuroscience generate hope that as understanding of brain function increases, so may the sophistication of approaches to diagnosis and treatment.

A significant challenge in research on anxiety disorders in children is to address the apparent contradiction of the transient nature of many childhood anxiety disorders, juxtaposed against other evidence suggesting that adult mood and anxiety disorders often begin with symptoms of anxiety during childhood. Longitudinal data suggest that this paradox may result from very high rates of childhood anxiety disorders. In most

children, these disorders remit. However, those children who remain anxious may account for a large proportion of adult cases of both mood and anxiety disorders. Given this possibility, there is a pressing need to discover factors that distinguish anxious children at low versus high risk for developing anxiety or depression during adulthood. Available clinical measures provide limited insights on such distinguishing factors. With advances in neurobiological understandings, new avenues for developing such insights may become available.

Work on the neurodevelopmental aspects of many psychiatric disorders remains relatively limited, and research on childhood anxiety represents one of the less developed areas. In two sections, the current chapter reviews the progress that has been made in recent years as well as ongoing efforts to lay the groundwork for future research that may better bridge basic science and clinical research, capitalizing on the considerable recent advances in neuroscience. The initial section reviews phenomenology and introduces data on biological correlates for six childhood anxiety disorders—social phobia, generalized anxiety disorder, separation anxiety disorder, specific phobia, post-traumatic stress disorder, and panic attacks. The subsequent section surveys research on neurobiology in more detail.

PHENOMENOLOGY

Social Phobia

The terms *social phobia* or *social anxiety disorder* refer to a pattern of recurrent fear and apprehension in social situations or scenarios where an individual may be scrutinized. Before modifications in the *Diagnostic and Statistical Manual of Mental Disorders, 4th ed.* (DSM-IV), identification of social phobia in childhood was limited by having the condition closely aligned to both avoidant disorder of childhood and *overanxious disorder*. With changes in DSM-IV that remove these potential problems, available data from epidemiological studies suggest that social phobia represents a relatively common primary diagnosis among adolescents (Pine et al., 1998; Stein et al., 2000; Wittchen et al., 2000; Velting and Albano, 2001).

Early signs of potential risk for social phobia may be manifested in a temperamental profile, such as *behavioral inhibition*, recognizable early in life. This profile refers to a pattern of wariness in novel situations, particularly novel social situations. While children with behavioral inhibition face a high risk for various childhood anxiety disorders, by adolescence this risk is specific for social phobia (Schwartz et al., 1999). Hence, both behavioral inhibition and social phobia may be characterized by an underlying hypersensitivity to social scrutiny. Research on neural aspects of social communication, through face processing, raises questions on the degree to which such hypersensitivity might ultimately be localized in the brain.

As children mature, rates of anxiety in social situations tend to increase. Paralleling this general rise in social anxiety among adolescents, rates of social phobia, a pathological form of social anxiety, tend to peak during adolescence (Pine et al., 1998; Stein et al., 2000). As with other research on developmental changes in fear, this finding raises questions about factors that distinguish adolescents with "normal" as opposed to "pathological" aspects of social anxiety. Specifically, the presence of moderate social anxiety may be viewed as developmentally appropriate and within the range of normal adaptive behavior. For a sizable minority of children and adolescents, however, social anxiety becomes maladaptive, causing significant distress and impairment.

Generalized Anxiety Disorder

Relative to social phobia's adolescent onset and specific longitudinal course, onset for generalized anxiety disorder is not well understood, in part because the conceptualization of this syndrome changed between DSM-III and DSM-IV. In DSM-III/III-R, children who exhibited a pattern of pervasive worries were classified as meeting criteria for overanxious disorder. In DSM-IV, the diagnosis of overanxious disorder was eliminated to facilitate a life-course perspective on the anxiety disorders, and, like adults, children who exhibited a pattern of pervasive worries received the diagnosis of generalized anxiety disorder. Nevertheless, even when one considers data for both generalized anxiety disorder and overanxious disorder, characteristics of chil-

dren with problems in these domains differ from those of children with social phobia. Most importantly, both overanxious disorder and generalized anxiety disorder tend to exhibit very high rates of comorbidity with other anxiety disorders and to predict elevated risk for multiple conditions, including anxiety disorders and major depression (Pine et al., 1998).

High risk for adult psychopathology associated with childhood generalized anxiety disorder has been demonstrated in several studies. Both retrospective and prospective data suggest that adolescent generalized anxiety disorder strongly predicts adult major depression (Kessler and Walters, 1998; Pine et al., 1998). These data are consistent with data from family studies on the associations between childhood generalized anxiety disorder and adult major depression (Pine, 1999). These associations may partially arise through the effects of stress, which is thought to play a prominent role in both anxiety and depression. Consistent with this view, adverse life events during adolescence show the strongest and most consistent association with depression and generalized anxiety disorder (Pine et al., in press). Therefore, neurobiological mechanisms involved in stress mediation may contribute to the strong comorbidity of early-onset generalized anxiety disorder with later adult major depression. As discussed below, investigations of stress-sensitive systems including the hippocampal formation may elucidate mechanisms contributing to such comorbidity.

Separation Anxiety Disorder

Separation anxiety disorder usually develops during middle childhood and must begin before age 18. Rates of the disorder show relatively marked age-related decline, again consistent with age-related changes in the related normal developmental phenomenon of separation anxiety. As with data for social anxiety, these data raise questions about factors that distinguish normal from pathological separation anxiety. Findings from longitudinal studies reveal some specificity in the relationship between separation anxiety disorder and later panic attacks (Pine et al., 1998). Moreover, family studies find that childhood separation anxiety disorder relates to adult panic disorder (Warner et al., 1995; Capps et al., 1996; Weissman et al., 1997; Battaglia et al., 1998). Nevertheless, other data suggest high rates of separation anxiety disorder in children of parents with other psychiatric disorders, such as major depression (Biederman et al., 2001).

Some suggest that childhood separation anxiety disorder and adult panic disorder share a biological substrate, based at least in part on commonalities in respiratory correlates of the two disorders (Pine, 1999). Similarly, both separation anxiety disorder in children and panic disorder in adults are associated with abnormalities within the noradrenergic system that may contribute to risk for the conditions (Sallee et al., 2000).

Panic Disorder

Panic disorder is very rare before adolescence (Costello et al., 1996), exhibiting rates that are generally lower than 1% for lifetime diagnosis (Pine et al., 1998). In general, children tend to exhibit a relatively abrupt increase in rates of panic attacks around puberty (Hayward et al., 1992), though such panic attacks only infrequently progress to full-blown panic disorder (Pine et al., 1998). In these children, panic attacks typically progress to panic disorder over a relatively lengthy period, into early adulthood.

Among both children and adults, panic attacks are associated with a set of respiratory abnormalities (Klein, 1993; Pine et al., 2000). These abnormalities are found not only in panic disorder but also in a range of other conditions, such as separation anxiety disorder and isolated panic attacks, which show strong familial associations with panic disorder. It has been suggested that parents with panic disorder transmit a diathesis for certain forms of anxiety that is apparent in the respiratory system (Pine, 1999), may remain latent (Coryell, 1997), or may vary across development, manifested as separation distress during childhood or as panic attacks after puberty (Klein, 1993; Pine et al., 2000).

Phobic Disorder (Specific Phobia)

Specific phobia refers to unreasonable fear of a specific object or environmental condition that causes impairment in normal functioning, primarily due to avoidance of feared situations or objects. Typical onset occurs during childhood, although it may arise in other developmental periods. Again, data on developmental changes in phobias, as abnormal conditions, show parallels with data on developmental changes in normal specific fears, such as childhood fears of small animals or the dark. Prevalence of specific phobia in children and adolescents has been estimated at approximately 3%–4%, with the highest prevalence generally appearing between 10 and 13 years of age (Fyer et al., 1998; Essau et al., 2000).

Efforts to validate and cluster specific phobias in adults, based on the object to which the phobia is directed, have yielded varying results (Fyer, 1998). Specific phobias in children cluster into three subtypes similar to those found in adults. Children 7 to 19 years of age report animal phobia, blood injection–injury phobia and, environmental-situational phobia (Muris et al., 1999). Of these three subtypes, blood phobia has been shown to result in physiololgical symptomatology consisting of an initial rise in heart rate, followed by vasovagal bradycardia and, frequently, syncope (Marks, 1988). This may indicate a uniquely different neurobiological substrate of phobic responding relative to other specific phobias.

Posttraumatic Stress Disorder

Posttraumatic stress disorder (PTSD) refers to a pattern of anxiety, distress, and avoidance following an event experienced as threatening and/or intensely distressing. This disorder has been reported to have behavioral (Zaidi and Foy, 1994) and neurobiological effects into adulthood (Charney and Bremner, 1999). Much of the developmental research on the condition derives from retrospective studies of adults. The many possible biases inherent in such research preclude the generation of firm conclusions on the developmental course of the condition. An important process in the study of PTSD will be to identify the developmental path of the disorder in the context of the prevalence of anxiety disorders in childhood (Costellot et al., 1996; Pynoos et al., 1999).

Hypothalamic-pituitary-adrenal axis

Recent studies, reviewed below in rodent models, emphasize the impact that trauma exerts on stress system reactivity, particularly reactivity of the hypothalamic–pituitary–adrenal (HPA) axis. Post-traumatic stress responses reported in children following natural disasters (Goenjian et al., 1996; Pynoos et al., 1999) and sexual abuse do suggest resultant dysregulation in the HPA axis (De Bellis et al., 1999). However, unlike relative consistency within adult studies, less clear abnormalities emerge in studies among children (De Bellis et al., 1999). Moreover, data among adults show evidence of reduced hippocampal volumes in PTSD, consistent with evidence both on the role of the hippocampus in HPA axis negative feedback and the possible effects of cortisol on the hippocampus. However, the available data on children, while limited, fail to document evidence of reduced hippocampal volume in PTSD (De Bellis, 1999). Taken together, these data suggest the need for more research on the neuroanatomical and endocrine effects of trauma during development. Overt changes in hippocampal volume and HPA axis regulation seen among formerly traumatized adults may arise over many years (Monk et al., in press).

BRAIN SYSTEMS IN EARLY-ONSET ANXIETY DISORDER

This section reviews three topics relevant to neurobiological research on pediatric anxiety disorders. First, given the wealth of basic science data on fear conditioning, the chapter reviews data on the neuroanatomical and psychiatric correlates of this process. Second, considerable research in clinical anxiety disorders shows evidence of enhanced sensitivity to innately fear-provoking stimuli, in contrast to stimuli that organisms learn to fear through conditioning. The chapter next reviews data in this area. Finally, the chapter reviews in more detail results from the above-noted studies demonstrating developmental plasticity within stress-sensitive systems that regulate the HPA axis.

Considerable research in this area examines fear system function in animals or healthy adults. Nevertheless, as summarized in Table 11.1, considerable research among adults has also begun to examine psychobiological differences between patients with anxiety disorders and various comparison groups. Paralleling each of the forthcoming sections, Table 11.1 summarizes conclusions supported by data on biological correlates of both child and adult anxiety disorders. This includes data for measures of fear conditioning, reactivity to innate fear probes, and regulation of the HPA axis.

Fear Conditioning

In a fear-conditioning experiment, a neutral stimulus, such as a tone or a light, is paired with an aversive stimulus, such as a shock, a loud noise, or an aversive air blast. Following this experience, the formerly neutral stimulus becomes a conditioned stimulus (CS+) and acquires the ability to elicit behaviors and physiological responses formerly only associated with the aversive stimulus, the unconditioned stimulus (UCS). Enthusiasm for this work derives at least partly from the precise delineation of neural circuits, down to the level of the genome, engaged by environmental components that produce fear conditioning (LeDoux,

TABLE 11.1 *Subjective and Physiological Signs of Perturbations in Fear Systems among Adults and Children*[c]

	Magnitude of Association with Clinical Anxiety[a]	Specificity of Findings[b]	Consistency of Findings
Physiologic measures of fear conditioning			
Cue-specific	+/− (+)	+/−	+/−
Contextual	+ (+)	+/−	+
Other (e.g., darkness potentiated)	+ (+)	+/−	+/−
Subjective reactions to innate fear probes			
Social challenges (e.g., Trier social challenge)	++	+/−	+
Respiratory (e.g., CO_2)	++ (+)	++ (+)	++ (+)
Noradrenergic challenge (e.g., yohimbine, clonidine)	++ (+)	++ (+)	++
Serotonergic challenge (e.g., fenfluramine)	+	+/−	+
Perturbation in HPA axis function			
Elevated CSF-CRF	++	+	+
Altered urinary or plasma cortisol	++ (+)	+ (+/−)	+/− (+/−)
Altered ACTH/cortisol response to challenges	++ (+)	+ (+/−)	+/− (+/−)

ACTH, adrenocorticotropin hormone; CRF, corticotropin-releasing factor; (SF, cerebrospinal fluid; HPA, hypothalamic–pituitary–adrenal.
[a]Magnitude of association is indexed from weak (+/−) to strong (++), in terms of effect sizes in studies comparing healthy subjects and patients with anxiety disorders.
[b]Specificity of findings is indexed on the basis of data across multiple diagnoses. Measures receiving +/− ratings show minimal evidence of specificity. Measures receiving ++ or + ratings show specificity, manifest as either consistent abnormalities in a family of conditions (e.g., respiratory/noradrenergic challenges) or distinct abnormalities in distinct conditions (e.g., altered cortisol in PTSD vs. panic disorder).
[c]When available, summary of data in children and adolescents are presented within parentheses.

1998). From a neuroanatomical perspective, the amygdala, a medial temporal lobe structure, plays a central role in mediating fear conditioning, and changes in genes within the amygdala are thought to reflect changes in behavior and physiology associated with this process.

Phenomenology and neuroanatomy

At least two forms of fear or anxiety develop in the classic fear conditioning experiment. First, the conditioned stimulus (CS+) acquires the ability to elicit behavior, such as freezing, typically associated with the unconditioned stimulus (UCS), a process known as *cued conditioning*. Second, the environment in which the CS+ is presented also comes to elicit fear-related behaviors, a process known as *contextual conditioning*. Lesions studies suggest that these are anatomically distinct phenomena (LeDoux, 1998). Lesions of the amygdala impair both cued and contextual fear conditioning. Lesions of other structures, including the hippocampus, interfere with contextual but not cued conditioning.

Other data in animal models suggest that distinct forms of fear can be differentiated on both neuroanatomical and behavioral grounds. For example, Davis (1998) suggests that brain systems involved in conditioning to specific cues are distinguishable from those involved in responses to dangerous environments, such as a well-lit room for a rodent or a dark room for a human. The central nucleus of the amygdala may relate more closely to cue-specific fear, whereas the bed nucleus of the stria terminalis and associated amygdala components may relate more closely to fear of dangerous environments. Recent studies among humans have attempted to identify parallel fear-related behaviors that are distinguishable in terms of their eliciting stimuli. Documenting such phenomenological similarities may facilitate identification of neuroanatomical parallels between fear states in humans and animals.

The amygdaloid complex includes a collection of nuclei and systems, both the basolateral amygdala (lateral, basal and accessory basal nuclei) and surrounding structures, encompassing the central, medial, and cortical nuclei. It has been suggested, however, that these neighboring structures are more similar to each other and other targets of the basolateral amygdala than to the basolateral amygdala itself, and that it may be more useful to view the "basolateral amygdala" and its target areas as parts of a specific network subserving specialized functions (Davis and Whalen, 2001). An extensive animal literature has demonstrated that sensory information from many cortical areas reaches the lateral and basolateral nuclei and that efferents from the lateral and basolateral nuclei project to the central nucleus of the amygdala (Aggelton, 2000). The central nucleus then projects to hypothalamic, motor, and brain stem target areas.

Data from fear conditioning experiments clearly implicate the amygdala and its efferent projections in some forms of fear and anxiety in lower mammals (LeDoux, 1998). Data from lesion studies document parallels in humans, and De Bellis et al. (2000) did find enhanced amygdala volumes in children with generalized anxiety disorder. Moreover, functional imaging studies do reveal amygdala engagement during fear conditioning (Pine et al., 2001).

Studies in anxiety disorders

While lesion and imaging studies provide some evidence to link amygdala function to human fear and anxiety, more evidence of amygdala involvement in human anxiety derives from indirect measures. These measures document behavioral, physiological, and pharmacological similarities between fear states in humans and animals. Similarly, most data examining human amygdala function in clinical anxiety disorders rely on such indirect measures, usually ascertained by assessing physiological changes during fear-conditioning experiments. Conclusions from the available studies are summarized in Table 11.1.

Animal studies using the acoustic startle reflex indicate that explicit cue information (e.g., lights, tone) activates the central nucleus of the amygdala, which in turn activates hypothalamic and brain stem target areas involved in specific signs of fear (Davis, 1998; LeDoux, 1998). It has been further demonstrated that when startle is elicited in rats by dangerous contexts, such as after a bright light has been turned on, there is an increase in the startle reflex. Humans, however, show a significant increase of startle amplitude (eyeblink response) in the dark (Grillon et al., 1998), an effect possibly related to the difference between nocturnal (rats) and diurnal (humans) species. Fear-conditioning studies using these methods in clinical populations show some evidence of abnormal fear conditioning to cues in panic disorder, as well as more consistent evidence of abnormal context conditoning in PTSD (Charney and Bremner, 1999). Fear conditioning studies examining skin conductance responses also document abnormalities in PTSD. Nevertheless, the nature of the findings varies across laboratories, methods, and components of the conditioning experiment, such as during conditioning versus during extinction. These inconsistencies in the clinical literature are reflected in summaries within Table 11.1.

Studies in children and adolescents

Given necessary precautions and prohibitions in extending fear-conditioning studies to clinical developmental populations, few studies investigate affective response to aversive stimuli in children and adolescents. New startle-based methods that may be appropriate for administration in younger populations show promise for extending the investigation of the neurodevelopmental characteristics of fear conditioning.

Children who exhibit a consistent behavioral restraint toward novelty, temperamental sensitivity to negative stimuli, or a reactive "behavioral inhibition system" may exhibit premorbid signs of anxiety disorders (Kagan, 1995; Gray and McNaughton, 2000). Such risk markers may be manifested in laboratory-based measures where there are closer parallels with measures used among other species. For example, parallels between startle regulation in rodents and humans provide a potentially useful index. Positing that startle reflex would be sensitive to differences in emotional reactivity, Grillon et al. (1998) found deficient startle modulation in adolescents with a parental history of anxiety disorder or alcoholism. These researchers also found fear-potentiated startle to discriminate children at high and low risk for anxiety disorders, with different abnormalities for high-risk male and female subjects (Grillon et al., 1998; Merikangas et al., 1999). Overall, startle levels were elevated among high-risk female subjects, whereas high-risk males showed greater magnitude of startle potentiation during aversive anticipation. Importantly, these studies relied on relatively mild UCS, in the form of an air puff to the throat, to elicit fear conditioning. These methods effectively balance ethical constraints in research on children against the need to develop measures of fear conditioning that are suitable for cross-species generalizations.

Important questions remain, however. For one, fear conditioning in these studies tends to show a stronger association with risk for anxiety than with the presence of an anxiety disorder in children. Hence, this raises questions about factors that distinguish between at-risk children with low rates of clinical anxiety and those with high rates, an area where startle data have yet to provide key insights. Secondly, it remains unclear why startle-based measures of fear conditioning may relate to risk for anxiety in some populations, whereas in other populations startle measures less influenced by conditioning, such as baseline startle magnitude, relate to risk for anxiety. Regardless, by demonstrating parallels between startle regulation in human children, adult humans, and other species, Merikangas et al. (1999) generate considerable enthusiasm for further validation of parallels between animal models and paradigms used among human children. Finally, the study of fear conditioning using these methods has been further advanced by the use of functional magnetic reso-

nance imaging (fMRI). Following Merikangas et al. (1999), in a study of adults using air puff as UCS, activation in the right amygdala was found to differ between CS+ and CS− trials (Pine et al., 2001). The specific engagement of the right amygdala is consistent with lateralized effects found in another fMRI study that relied upon shock as a UCS (LaBar et al., 1998). These findings generate considerable enthusiasm for other work comparing the degree of amygdala engagement among children with various levels of anxiety.

Innate Fear-producing Stimuli

As noted above, Davis (1998) suggests that different brain systems may be engaged by innate fear-inducing stimuli, such as bright light exposure in the rodent, as opposed to stimuli that acquire fear-evoking properties through experiences, such as conditioning. Considerable clinical research documents differences in the degree to which patients with anxiety disorders may display selective hypersensitivity to such innately fear-inducing stimuli. As reflected in Table 11.1, research on such hypersensitivity is reviewed by considering three sets of innate fear-inducing stimuli, comprising social, physiological, and pharmacological fear probes.

Face processing: social fear probes

Advances in neuroscience techniques provide unique opportunities for research on innate social fear probes. These techniques have been used to map brain circuitry involved in various aspects of face processing. Features common to all faces, in contrast to non-face objects, engage one set of circuits encompassing portions of the brain's ventral temporal lobe. Aspects of particular faces engage another set of circuits. Some brain regions appear particularly sensitive to the innate emotionally evocative aspects of faces. For example, faces of fearful expressions specifically engage the amygdala, whereas faces evoking angry expressions specifically engage the ventral frontal lobes. Such angry expressions may represent particularly potent, innate elicitors of anxiety in social phobia. These developments, as well as concomitant developments in the field of cognitive neuroscience, make it possible to examine the relationship between amygdala sensitivity for various innate danger cues, as expressed in faces, and developmental changes in various clinical behaviors.

These possibilities generate a series of questions amenable to study with modern neuroscience methods (Pine, 1999). For example, adults with social phobia exhibit hypersensitivity to social situations in which they may be scrutinized. This hypersensitivity may be paralleled by an abnormal sensitivity to facial displays of threat or fear (Ohman, 1986). Evidence from cognitive studies suggests that children with social phobia or other anxiety disorders might also exhibit hypersensitivity for social cues of threat or fear.

Studies in adults, following bilateral amygdala damage, have demonstrated impaired recognition of fear in some, but not all, patients (Adolphs et al., 1995). Neuroimaging studies have demonstrated increased activation in the amygdala during the viewing of fearful facial expressions (Whalen et al., 1998), supporting a hypothesized selective response to facial displays of aversive emotions, particularly fearful faces. Studies in adult social phobia also document enhanced amygdala response to facial displays (see review in Pine, 1999).

Examination of brain circuitry mediating the visual processing of fearful faces has been extended to children and adolescents. Amygdala activation in youth during the viewing of fearful faces compared to control stimuli has been demonstrated in two studies (Baird et al., 1999; Thomas et al., 2001).

Amygdala activation during conscious versus nonconscious visual processing of facial expression has been investigated using emotional faces that are "masked" by neutral faces (Ohman, 1986; Mogg and Bradley, 1998). Viewing consciously, in contrast to unconsciously, perceived emotionally salient faces is hypothesized to engage distinct neural systems (Morris et al., 1998). Neuroimaging in adults has demonstrated that passive viewing of masked fearful faces specifically engages the amygdala and associated subcortical pathways (Whalen et al., 1998). The masked face paradigm developed by Whalen et al. (1998) was used in a neuroimaging study comparing adolescent and adult emotion perception (Pine et al., 2001) to examine possible developmental differences in cortical activation in the ventral temporo-occipital regions involved in face processing. While the study failed to demonstrate hypothesized greater amygdala activation to masked fearful faces in adolescents than in adults, results did reveal cortical brain areas where intensity of activation was stronger in adolescents than in adults. Consistent with neuropsychological findings that face-emotion processing abilities show signs of developmental change during adolescence, this study found differences between adolescents and adults in the degree to which posterior hemisphere brain areas are engaged by viewing masked facial displays of emotion (Pine et al., 2001).

Disturbances in ventilatation: physiological fear probes

Some clinical anxiety disorders in humans may be characterized by specific sensitivities to physiological signs of danger. For example, *panic disorder* is characterized by paroxysms of acute anxiety often accompanied by changes in respiration. This observation has stimulated a series of studies examining respiratory function in panic disorder. Much of this work suggests that panic disorder is characterized by enhanced reactivity to innately dangerous situations that elicit changes in respiration. This includes stimuli such as sodium lactate, doxopram, and CO_2. As reviewed in Table 11.1, studies in this area among adults generate some of the strongest, most consistent evidence of biological correlates of clinical anxiety. Nevertheless, there remains considerable disagreement, fueled partially by the limited understanding of neural regulation of breathing and hypersensitivity to respiratory provocation, on the ultimate origin behind such enhanced reactivity,

Among the various physiological probes that may be used in developmental research, CO_2 possesses considerable advantages, in terms of safety and replicability of associations. In adults, the relationship of ventilatory physiology to anxiety disorders has been demonstrated through research on enhanced sensitivity to CO_2, manifested as both changes in subjective state and physiology, among panic disorder patients (Klein, 1993; Perna et al., 1995). Klein (1993) suggests that these findings reflect an innate sensitivity in panic disorder of the central receptors to signals of possible respiratory compromise. One major question arising in available data concerns inconsistencies in the data for physiological measures. For example, innate hypersensitivity in chemoreceptors should be reflected in physiological responses to stimuli such as CO_2, but the data are more consistent for subjective than for ventilatory indices of CO_2 hypersensitivity. Research in this area has, however, advanced conceptualizations of biological markers in anxiety disorders. Ventilatory measures may be used to refine understandings of *endophenotypes*, categories that refer to more homogenous groups of individuals with a disorder or a latent risk for a disorder.

Ventilatory abnormalities have been identified in first-degree relatives of patients with panic disorder (Perna et al., 1995; Coryell, 1997), as well as in patients with possible precursors for panic disorders, such as separation anxiety disorder (Pine et al., 2000) or isolated panic attacks (Perna et al., 1995). Additionally, studies have found family loading for panic disorder in the relatives of panic patients with respiratory abnormalities (Perna et al., 1996), suggesting that hypersensitivity to CO_2 inhalation may be a trait marker for panic disorder rather than a state marker. These data suggest that parents with panic disorder may transmit a diathesis for certain forms of anxiety (e.g., separation anxiety disorder) that is observable in the respiratory system (Pine, 1999), which may remain latent (Coryell, 1997) or may be variably expressed across development as extreme separation distress during childhood or as panic attacks after puberty (Panksepp, 1998; Pine et al., 1998).

Norepinephrine and serotonin: pharmacological fear probes

There remains a paucity of research on the psychopharmacology of childhood anxiety disorders. However, pediatric psychopharmacology research over the last decade (see Riddle et al., 2001, for review) has begun to generate hypotheses on neurobiological mechanisms underlying childhood anxiety disorders. Such research raises interest in the role for pharmacological probes as precipitants of anxiety.

Most research in the pharmacological precipitants of anxiety among adults examines noradrenergic and serotonergic neurotransmitter systems. The evidence currently indicates a complex dysregulation of norepinephrine (NE) levels and locus coeruleus firing that may lead to increases or decreases in NE release coupled with altered sensitivities of the pre- and postsynaptic receptors (Ressler and Nemeroff, 2000). As summarized in Table 11.1, findings in this area represent a second area of consistency in research on biological correlates of adult anxiety disorders, along with findings for respiratory perturbations. Adults with generalized anxiety disorder, panic disorder, obsessive-compulsive disorder, or social phobia exhibit a blunted growth hormone (GH) response to clonidine challenge, interpreted as a subsensitivity of central α_2-adrenergic postsynaptic receptors (Charney and Bremner, 1999). Adults with panic disorder or PTSD, in contrast, exhibit hypersensitivity to challenges with yohimbine, an α_2-adrenergic antagonist. Such hypersensitivity is manifest most consistently as increases in subjective anxiety, and it appears specific to these two conditions, as opposed to generalized anxiety disorder or major depression. Interestingly, Sallee et al. (1998) reported *enhanced* GH secretion to clonidine challenge in children with anxiety disorders, particularly obsessive-compulsive disorder, findings that run counter to data from adults that document blunted GH response. More consistent with data in adult panic disorder, a subsequent study by Sallee et al. (2000) found enhanced anxiety responses to yohimbine as well as blunted GH response in children with anxiety disorders, particularly among children with separation anxiety disorder.

While considerable research examines serotonergic correlates of adult anxiety disorders, virtually no research in this area has been extended to pediatric populations (Charney and Bremner, 1999; Pine, 1999).

Studies in adults reveal some evidence of serotonergic abnormalities, though the data are less consistent than for noradrenergic measures. Emerging data from therapeutic studies, however, do strongly implicate the serotonergic system in both adult and pediatric anxiety disorders. The selective serotonin reuptake inhibitors (SSRIs) effectively treat virtually all forms of adult anxiety. Until recently, little data have been available on pediatric populations. A mutlicenter study examined the effects of fluvoxamine in children and adolescents with social phobia, separation anxiety disorder, or generalized anxiety disorder. The study showed a robust treatment response (Research Unit on Pediatric Psychopharmacology Anxiety Study Group, 2001).

Stress, Neuroplasticity, and the Hypothalamic–Pituitary–Adrenal Axis

Research on conditioning or innate fear provocation meaningfully extends data on the biology of anxiety from adults to children. Nevertheless, some of the most exciting neurodevelopmental research on anxiety considers associations among neuroplasticity, hippocampal function, stress, and the HPA axis. Conceptually relating the hippocampal formation to emotion, Papez originally proposed that emotional expression was dependent upon the integrative actions of the hypothalamus and the hippocampal formation. More recent conceptualizations have focused on the septohippocampal system (Gray and McNaughton, 2000), which encompasses the hippocampus, dentate gyrus, entorhinal cortex, subicular area, and the posterior cingulate cortex. Both direct and indirect pathways connect the hippocampal formation with thalamic nuclei, the hypothalamus, and the midbrain reticular formation. Noradrenergic innervation of the hippocampal formation arises from cells in the locus coeruleus and projects via the septal region. This long history of research on possible hippocampal contributions to anxiety resonates with more recent work on developmental plasticity in fear.

Early environmental manipulations in animals

Early environmental adversity exerts long-lasting effects on stress responsivity in adulthood. Exposure of rodent pups to handling manipulations results in reduction in fear behaviors, altered regulation of the HPA system, and neurodevelopmental changes within the hippocampus (Meaney et al., 1996). These effects are at least partially a reflection of changes in hippocampal regulation of HPA axis activation.

Extensive investigations using animal models of fear and anxiety have contributed significantly to understanding the effects of early environmental experience on plasticity in hippocampal-based neural circuits (Meaney et al. 1996). Postnatal rearing conditions influence the development of HPA response to stress in rodents. Adult animals exposed to short periods of postnatal handling during the first week of life show a more modest plasma adrenocorticotropin Hormone (ACTH) and corticosterone response to a wide range of stressors, and this handling effect persists throughout the life of the animal (Meaney et al., 1996). Increases in glucocorticoid receptor gene expression in cell fields of the hippocampus have been reported as a result of postnatal handling. The increase in hippocampal glucocorticoid receptor density is suggested to be a critical feature of the handling effect on HPA function, and appears to be mediated by activation of the pituitary-thyroid system that, in turn, leads to an increase in activity within ascending serotonergic systems during the first week of life (Meaney et al., 1996). Earlier studies on the activation of ascending serotonergic systems has shown that chronic handling has a significantly greater effect on serotonin (5-HT) turnover in the hippocampus than does acute handling (Smythe et al., 1994). However, handling has no effect on 5-HT turnover in the amygdala, where there is no effect of handling on glucocorticoid receptor expression (Smythe et al., 1994). In primary hippocampal cell cultures, serotonin increases glucocorticoid receptor expression, and this effect appears to be mediated by increased c-AMP levels (Meaney et al., 2000).

Effects of early environmental adversity on HPA mediation of neurodevelopment have also been demonstrated in non-human primates (Coplan et al., 1995). Corticotropin-releasing hormone (CRH) intracerebroventricular administration in rhesus monkeys that had been separated from their mothers produced behavioral inhibition and increases in ACTH and cortisol. Coplan et al (1995) presented evidence for persistently elevated cerebrospinal fluid concentrations of corticotropin-releasing factor (CRF) in grown macaques that had been reared by mothers in unpredictable environmental conditions. Further studies in adversely reared adult monkeys demonstrated an inverse relationship between mean CRF concentrations and GH response to clonidine (Coplan et al., 2000). In light of evidence that reduced GH response to clonidine has been shown in other anxiety disorders (Charney and Bremner, 1999), Coplan et al. (2000) hypothesize that GH response to clonidine may inversely reflect trait-like increases of central nervous system CRF activity. Data linking childhood anxiety to growth deficits are consistent with this view (Pine et al., 1996). Activity, of the HPA axis, as related to early environmental

manipulations, was also studied over the first 6 months of primate life in stressful housing transitions among mother-reared or peer-reared monkeys (Coplan et al., 1995). Cortisol and ACTH showed increases in both rearing groups in response to separation stress and to housing with unfamiliar mates.

Early adverse environmental conditions in childhood

Adverse early environmental stress has also been investigated in human populations. Observations of the effects of early childhood experience of environmental adversity have led investigators to propose a stress vulnerability mediated by changes in stress-responsive CRF systems implicated in both mood and anxiety disorders (Heim and Nemeroff, 1999). Granger et al. (1996) measured children's adrenocortical reactions to a conflict-oriented mother–child interaction task and found that children's pretask cortisol scores were negatively associated with anxiety symptoms.

Childhood abuse has been associated with a predisposition for the development of anxiety disorders in adulthood, including generalized anxiety disorder and panic disorder (Kaufman and Charney, 1999; Stein et al., 2000), and may increase the risk of developing PTSD in response to extreme stressors such as combat experience in adulthood (Zaidi and Foy, 1994; Bremner, 2001). Parental loss in childhood and negative parenting have also been associated with the development of mood and anxiety disorders, including PTSD (Kendler, 1993).

Hippocampal atrophy

Current theories suggest that hypersecretion of cortisol during stress may damage the hippocampus. Studies have demonstrated reduced hippocampal volume in trauma survivors with PTSD, compared to nontraumatized individuals (Sapolsky, 2000; Bremner, 2001). However, hormonally regulated plasticity in the hippocampus involves multiple influences, and glucocorticoid hormones work in concert with excitatory amino acids and N-methyl-D-aspartate (NMDA) receptors, as well as other neurotransmitters and the GABA-benzodiazepine system (see McEwen, 2000a,b, for review).

Controversy has emerged concerning the association between PTSD and reduced hippocampal volume (Sapolsky, 2000; Yehuda, 2000, 2001; Bremner, 2001), both in terms of the findings and the theoretical perspectives. A study in neurodevelopmental traumatology using MRI has shown that children with a history of abuse did not show reduced hippocampal volume but a smaller overall cerebral volume with larger ventricles and smaller corpus callosum (De Bellis et al. 1999). Selective hippocampal reduction in older subjects may develop after childhood as a result of long-term neural and endocrine activity and the cumulative effects of life experiences (McEwen, 2000a,b).

FUTURE DIRECTIONS

The profile of developmental vulnerability for anxiety disorders presented in this chapter underscores the need for more research on underlying neurobiological mechanisms. As has been shown in research to date, early-onset anxiety disorders have a high comorbidity within anxiety disorders as well as with other disorders, most notably major depressive disorder. Childhood-onset anxiety disorders are often predictors of adult anxiety and mood disorders, and are thought to share common neural substrates and physiological mechanisms. The evolving development of neuroimaging tools and techniques to investigate neural substrates promises to advance this area of research. Advances in the basic neuroscience of anxiety and molecular genetics may offer unique opportunities to understand the transmission of these disorders across generations. Of paramount importance is the need to integrate research efforts in addressing developmental vulnerability. Environmental influences such as early adversity and trauma must be directly investigated in children and adolescents. Longitudinal studies combining neurobiological, neuroimaging, and behavioral measures may move research to the next level of understanding to support early identification, preventive intervention, and effective treatment.

REFERENCES

Aggleton, J.P., ed. (2000) *The Amygdala: A Functional Analysis.* New York: Oxford University Press.

Adolphs, R., Tranel, D., Adolphs, R., Tranel, D., and Damasio, H. (1995) Fear and the human amygdala. *J Neurosci* 15:669–672.

Baird, A.A., Gruber, S.A, Baird, A.A. Gruber, S.A., Fein, D.A., MAAS, L.C., Steingard, R.J., Renshaw, P.F., Cohen, B.M., and Yurgelien Todd, D.A. (1999) Functional magnetic resonance imaging of facial affect recognition in children and adolescents. *J Am Acad Child Adolesc Psychiatry* 38:195–199.

Battaglia, M., Bertella, S., Battaglia, M., Bertrella, S., Bajo, S., Biraghi, F., and Belloo; L. (1998) Anticipation of age at onset in panic disorder. *Am J Psychiatry* 155:590–595.

Biederman, J., Faraone, S.V., Biederman, J., Faraone, S.V., Hirshfield-Becker, D.R., Friedman, D., Rotin, J.A., and Rosenbaum, J.F. (2001) Patterns of psychopathology and dysfunction in high-risk children of parents with panic disorder and major depression. *Am J Psychiatry* 158:49–57.

Bremner, J.D. (2001) Hypotheses and controversies related to effects of stress on the hippocampus: an argument for stress-induced damage to the hippocampus in patients with posttraumatic stress disorder. *Hippocampus* 11:75–81.

Capps, L., Sigman, M., Capps, L., Sigman, M., Sena, R., Henker, B., and Whalen, C. (1996) Fear, anxiety and perceived control in children of agoraphobic parents. *J Child Psychol Psychiatry* 37:445–452.

Charney, D.S. and Bremner, J.D. (1999) The neurobiology of anxiety disorders. In: Charney, D.S., Nestler, E.J., Bunney, B.S., eds. *The Neurobiology of Mental Illness.* New York: Oxford University Press, pp. 494–517.

Coplan, J.D., Rosenblum, L.A., and Gorman, J.M. (1995) Primate models of anxiety. Longitudinal perspectives. *Psychiatry Clin North Am* 18:727–743.

Coplan, J.D, Smith, E.L, Coplan, J.D., Smith, E.L., Trost, R.C., Scharf, B.A., Alternus, M. Bjornson, L., Rosenblum, L.A., Owens, M.J., Nemeroff, C.B., and Gorman, J.M. (2000) Growth hormone response to clonidine in adversely reared young adult primates: relationship to serial cerebrospinal fluid corticotropin-releasing factor concentrations. *Psychiatry Res* 95:93–102.

Coryell, W. (1997) Hypersensitivity to carbon dioxide as a disease-specific trait marker. *Biol Psychiatry* 41:259–263.

Costello, E.J., Angold, A., Costello, E.J., Angold A., Buns, B.J., Stangl, D.K., Tweed, D.L., Erkanli, A., and Worthman, C.M. (1996) The Great Smoky Mountains Study of Youth. Goals, design, methods, and the prevalence of DSM-III-R disorders. *Arch Gen Psychiatry* 53:1129–1136.

Davis, M. (1998) Are there different parts of the amygdala involved in fear versus anxiety? *Biol Psychiarty* 44:1239–1247.

Davis, M. and Whalen, P.J. (2001) The amygdala: vigilance and emotion. *Mol Psychiatry* 6:13–34.

De Bellis, M.D., Casey, B.J., Dahl, R.E., Birmaher, B., Williamson, D.E., Thomas, K.M., Axelson, D.A., Frustaci, K., Boring, A.M., Hall, J., and Ryan, N.D. (2000) A pilot study of amygdala volumes in pediatric generalized anxiety disorder. *Biol Psychiatry* 48:51–57.

De Bellis, M.D., Keshavan, M.S., De Bellis, M.D., Keshavan, M.S., Clark, D.B., Casey, B.J., Giedd, J.N., Boeing, A.M., Frustaci, K., and Ryan, N.D. (1999) A.E. Bennett Research Award. Developmental traumatology. Part II: Brain development. *Biol Psychiatry* 45:1271–1284.

Essau, C.A., Conradt, J., Essau, C.A., Conradt J and Petermann, (2000) Frequency, comorbidity, and psychosocial impairment of specific phobia in adolescents. *J Clin Child Psychol* 29:221–231.

Fyer, A.J. (1998). Current approaches to etiology and pathophysiology of specific phobia. *Biol Psychiatry* 44:1295–1304.

Goenjian, A.K., Yehuda, R., Goenjian, A.K., Yehuda, R., Pynoos, R.S., Steinberg, A.M., Tashjian, M., Yang, R.K., Najarian, L.M. and Fairbanks, L.A. (1996) Basal cortisol, dexamethasone suppression of cortisol, and MHPG in adolescents after the 1988 earthquake in Armenia. *Am J Psychiatry* 153:929–934.

Granger, D.A., Weisz, J.R., Granger, D.A., Weiss, J.R., McCracken, J.T., Ikeda, S.C. and, Douglas, P. (1996). Reciprocal influences among adrenocortical activation, psychosocial processes, and the behavioral adjustment of clinic-referred children. *Child Dev* 69:1503–1513.

Gray, J.A. and McNaughton, N. (2000) *The Neuropsychology of Anxiety: An Enquiry into the Functions of the Septo-Hippocampal System.* New York: Oxford University Press.

Grillon, C., Dierker L., and Merikangas, K.R. (1998) Fear-potentiated startle in adolescent offspring of parents with anxiety disorders. *Biol Psychiatry* 44:990–997.

Gurley, D., Cohen, P., Gurley, D., Cohen, P., Pine, D.S., and Brook,

J. (1996) Discriminating depression and anxiety in youth: a role for diagnostic criteria. *J Affect Disord* 39:191–200.

Hayward, C., Killen, J.D., Hayward, C., Killen, J.D., Hammer, L.D., Litt, J.F., Wilson, D.M., Jimmonds, B., and Taylor, C.B., (1992). Pubertal stage and panic attack history in sixth- and seventh-grade girls. *Am J Psychiatry* 149:1239–1243.

Heim, C. and Nemeroff, C.B. (1999) The impact of early adverse experiences on brain systems involved in the pathophysiology of anxiety and affective disorders. *Biol Psychiatry* 46:1509–1522.

Kagan, J. (1995) *Galen's Prophecy*. New York: Basic Books.

Kaufman, J. and Charney, D.S. (1999) Neurobiological correlates of child abuse. *Biol Psychiatry* 45:1235–1236.

Kendler, K.S. (1993) Twin studies of psychiatric illness. Current status and future directions. *Arch Gen Psychiatry* 50:905–915.

Kessler, R.C. and Walters, E.E. (1998) Epidemiology of DSM-III-R major depression and minor depression among adolescents and young adults in the National Comorbidity Survey. *Depress Anxiety* 7:3–14.

Klein, D.F. (1993) False suffocation alarms, spontaneous panics, and related conditions. An integrative hypothesis. *Arch Gen Psychiatry* 50:306–317.

LaBar, K.S., Gatenby, J.C., LaBar, K.S., Gatenby, J.C., Gore, J.C., LeDoux, J.E., and Phelps, E.A. (1998) Human amydala activation during conditioned fear acquisition and extinction: a mixed-trial fMRI study. *Neuron* 20:937–945.

LeDoux, J.E. (1998) Fear and the brain: where have we been, and where are we going? *Biol Psychiatry* 44:1229–1238.

Marks, I. (1988) Blood-injury phobia: a review. *Am J Psychiatry* 145:1207–1213.

McEwen, B.S. (2000a). Effects of adverse experiences for brain structure and function. *Biol Psychiatry* 48:721–731.

McEwen, B.S. (2000b). The neurobiology of stress: from serendipity to clinical relevance. *Brain Res* 886:172–189.

Meaney, M.J., Diorio, J., Meaney, M.J., Diorio, J., Francis, D., Widdowson, J., LaPlante, P., Caldji, C., Sharma, S. Seckl, J.R., and Plotsky, P.M. (1996). Early environmental regulation of forebrain glucocorticoid receptor gene expression: implications for adrenocortical responses to stress. *Dev Neurosci* 18:49–72.

Meaney, M.J., Diorio, J., Francis, P., Weaver S., Yau, J., Chapman, K., Seckl, J.R., (2000) Postnatal handling increases the expression of cAMP inducible transcription factors in the rat hippocampus effects of thyroid hormone and serotonin *J. Neurosci* 20:3926–3935.

Merikangas, K.R., Avenevoli, S., Merikangas, K.R., Avenevoli, S., Dierker, L., Grillion, C. (1999) Vulnerability factors among children at risk for anxiety disorders. *Biol Psychiatry* 46:1523–1535.

Mogg, K. and Bradley B.P. (1998) A cognitive-motivational analysis of anxiety. *Behav Res Ther* 36:809–848.

Monk, C.S., Pine D.S., Charney, D.S. (in press). A developmental and neurobiological approach to early trauma research. *Semin Clin Neuropsychiatry*

Morris, J.S., Gurley, D., Morris, J.S., Gurley, D., and Dolan, R.J. (1998) Conscious and unconscious emotional learning in the human amygdala. *Nature* 393:467–470.

Muris, P., Schmidt, H., Muris, P., Schmidt, H., and MerCkelbach, H., (1999) The structure of specific phobia symptoms among children and adolescents. *Behav Res Ther* 37:863–868.

Ohman, A. (1986) Face the beast and fear the face: animal and social fears as prototypes for evolutionary analyses of emotion. *Psychophysiology* 23:123–145.

Panksepp, J. (1998) *Affective Neuroscience: The Foundations of Human and Animal Emotions*. New York:

Perna, G., Bertani, A., et al. (1996) Family history of panic disorder and hypersensitivity to CO_2 in patients with panic disorder. *Am J Psychiatry* 153:1060–1064.

Perna, G., Gabriele, A., Perna, G., Bertrani, A., Caldirola, D. and Bellodi L. (1995) Hypersensitivity to inhalation of carbon dioxide and panic attacks. *Psychiatry Res* 57:267–273.

Pine, D.S. (1999). Pathophysiology of childhood anxiety disorders. *Biol Psychiatry* 46:1555–1566.

Pine, D.S., Cohen, P., Pine, D.S., Cohen, P., Gurley, D., Brook, J., and Ma, Y. (1998) The risk for early-adulthood anxiety and depressive disorders in adolescents with anxiety and depressive disorders. *Arch Gen Psychiatry* 55:56–64.

Pine, D.S., Fyer, A., Grun, J., Phelps, E.A., Szeszko, P.R., Koda, V., Li, W., Ardekani, B., Maguire, E.A., Burgess, N., and Bilder, R.M. (2001). Methods for developmental studies of fear conditioning circuitry. *Biol Psychiatry* 50:225–228.

Pine, D.S., Cohen, P., Brook, J. (1996) Emotional problems during youth as predictors of stature during early adulthood: results from a prospective epidemiologic study. *Pediatrics* 97:856–863.

Pine, D.S., Johnson, J., Cohen, P., Brook, J. (in press) Adolescent life events as predictors of adult depression. *J Affect Disord*

Pine, D.S., Klein, R.G., Pine, D.S., Klein, R.G., Coplan, J.D., Papp, L.A., Hoven, C.W., Martinez, J., Kovalenko, P., Mandell, D.J., Moreau, D., Klein, D.F., and Gorman, J.M. (2000) Differential carbon dioxide sensitivity in childhood anxiety disorders and nonill comparison group. *Arch Gen Psychiatry* 57:960–967.

Pynoos, R.S., Steinberg, A.M., Pynoos, R.S., Steinberg, A.M., and Piacenti, J.C. (1999) A developmental psychopathology model of childhood traumatic stress and intersection with anxiety disorders. *Biol Psychiatry* 46:1542–1554.

Research Unit on Pediatric Psychopharmacology (RUH) Anxiety Study Group (2001) Flovoxamine for the treatment of anxiety disorders in children and adolescents. *N Engl J Med* 344:1279–1285.

Ressler, K.J. and Nemeroff, C.B. (2000) Role of serotonergic and noradrenergic systems in the pathophysiology of depression and anxiety disorders. *Depress Anxiety* 12(Suppl 1):2–19.

Riddle, M.A., Kastelic, E.A., Riddle, M.A., Kastelic, E.A., and Frosch, E. (2001) Pediatric psychopharmacology. *J Child Psychol Psychiatry* 42:73–90.

Sallee, F.R., Richman, H., Sallee, F.R., Richman, H., Sethuraman, G. Dougherty, D., Sine, L., and Attman-Hamandzic, S. (1998) Clonidine challenge in childhood anxiety disorder. *J Am Acad Child Adolesc Psychiatry* 37:655–662.

Sallee, F.R., Sethuraman, G., Sallee, F.R., Sethuraman, G., Sine, L., and Lia, H. (2000) Yohimbine challenge in children with anxiety disorders. *Am J Psychiatry* 157:1236–1242.

Sapolsky, R.M. (2000) Glucocorticoids and hippocampal atrophy in neuropsychiatric disorders. *Arch Gen Psychiatry* 57:925–935.

Schwartz, C.E., Snidman, N., Schwartz, C.E., Snidman, N., and Kagan, J. (1999) Adolescent social anxiety as an outcome of inhibited temperament in childhood. *J Am Acad Child Adolesc Psychiatry* 38:1008–1015.

Smythe, J.W, Rowe, W.B., and Meaney, M.J. (1994) Neonatal handling alters serotonin (5-HT) turnover and 5-HT2 receptor binding in selected brain regions: relationship to the handling effect on glucocorticoid receptor expression. *Brain Res Dev Brain Res* 80:183–189.

Stein, M.B., Torgrud, L.J., Stein, M.D., Torgrud, L.J., and Walker, J.R. (2000) Social phobia symptoms, subtypes, and severity: findings from a community survey. *Arch Gen Psychiatry* 57:1046–52.

Thomas, K.M., Drevets, W.C., Thomas, K.M., Drevets, W.C., Whalen, P.J. Eccard, C.H., Darl, R.E., Ryan, N.D., and Casey,

B.J. (2001). Amygdala response to facial expressions in children and adults. *Biol Psychiatry* 49:309–316.

Velting, O.N. and Albano, A.M. (2001) Current trends in the understanding and treatment of social phobia in youth. *J Child Psychol Psychiatry* 42:127–140.

Warner, V., Mufson, L., Warner, V., Mufson, L., and Weissman, M.M. (1995) Offspring at high and low risk for depression and anxiety: mechanisms of psychiatric disorder. *J Am Acad Child Adolesc Psychiatry* 34:786–797.

Weissman, M.M., Warner, V., Wickramaratne, P., Moreau, D., and Olfson, M. (1997) Offspring of depressed parents. 10 years later. *Arch Gen Psychiatry* 54:932–940.

Whalen, P.J., Bush, G., Whalen, P.J., Bush, G., McNally, R.J., Wilhelm, S., McInerney, S.C., Jenike, M.A., and Rauch, S.L. (1998)

The emotional counting Stroop paradigm: a functional magnetic resonance imaging probe of the anterior cingulated affective division. *Biol Psychiatry* 44:1219–1228.

Wittchen, H.U., Fuetsch, M., Wittchen, H.U. Feutsch, M., Sonntag, H., Muller, N., and Liebowitz, M. (2000) Disability and quality of life in pure and comorbid social phobia. Findings from a controlled study. *Eur Psychiatry* 15:46–58.

Yehuda, R. (2000) Biology of posttraumatic stress disorder. *J Clin Psychiatry* 61(Suppl 7): 14–21.

Yehuda, R. (2001) Are glucocortoids responsible for putative hippocampal damage in PTSD? How and when to decide. *Hippocampus* 11:85–89.

Zaidi, L.Y. and Foy, D.W. (1994) Childhood abuse experiences and combat-related PTSD. *J Trauma Stress* 7:33–42.

12 | Neurobiology of obsessive-compulsive disorder

TANYA K. MURPHY, KYTJA K. S. VOELLER, AND PIERRE BLIER

As defined in the Diagnonstic and Statistical Manual of Mental Disorders, 4th (DSM-IV), obsessive-compulsive disorder (OCD) is an anxiety disorder, characterized by obsessions—recurrent, unwanted, and distressing thoughts, images, or impulses—and/or compulsions—complex, repetitive, rule-governed behaviors that the patient feels driven to perform. Patients usually try to actively dismiss obsessions or neutralize them by seeking reassurance, avoiding situational triggers, or by engaging in compulsions. Although compulsions generally serve to alleviate anxiety, they can also engender anxiety if they become too arduous or time-consuming.

The proposed lifetime prevalence of OCD is 2%–3% in adolescents and adults. Approximately half of all OCD patients first present in childhood, before age 15 (Karno et al., 1988). Peak symptom changes often occur around age 10 years (Leonard et al., 1992) and the symptom profile in children can be quite variable. A child with only OCD or tics may develop additional symptoms months or years later. Although there are many similarities between childhood and adult onset OCD, Geller et al. (1998a) propose that there are enough differences between childhood- and adult-onset OCD to view childhood-onset OCD as a developmental subtype of the disorder. The major difference between childhood- and adult-onset OCD is that in children compulsions often precede obsessions and they may lack insight about their symptoms. Childhood-onset OCD is also associated with a poorer treatment response, higher familial risk, and a high rate of comorbid tic, disruptive, and developmental disorders.

One of the challenges of making the diagnosis of OCD in children is to differentiate between the normal self-soothing rituals of childhood and subclinical OCD. In a large survey of children ages 8 to 72 months, Evans et al. (1997) found that 2- to 4-year-olds engage in compulsive-like behaviors more often than younger or older children and that repetitive-oriented behaviors emerge earlier than sensory-perceptual "just right" behaviors. Since sameness and consistency may promote a sense of security at times of transition, many normal children engage in bedtime rituals such as arranging their bedding in a particular way, to ensure that their toes are covered, or checking for "monsters" under the bed. It has been argued that these normal compulsive behaviors of the young child do not constitute a continuum with the pathological OCD behaviors (Leonard et al., 1990). Obsessive-compulsive disorder should be considered when these childhood rituals become persistent and are maladaptive (e.g., time-consuming or distressing).

The clinical course of OCD is often described as chronic and unremitting. That some cases of OCD can show an episodic course is less well recognized (Perugi et al., 1998). In studies on the course of OCD in children and adolescents, the rate of symptom remission is not uncommon but still represents a minority of cases. Although many children (23% to 70%) have a chronic course and continue to meet diagnostic criteria at follow-up (Geller et al., 1998b), the type and severity of symptoms fluctuate and some 12%–50% of children no longer meet diagnostic criteria when re-evaluated 1 to 7 years later (Flament et al., 1990; Leonard et al., 1993; Thomsen, 1995a). This variability in clinical course may be due in part to sampling factors (i.e., some studies are based on clinic referrals, others on epidemiological samples, and samples may differ with regard to age and symptom severity).

Obsessive-compulsive disorder is a brain disorder involving the frontal–subcortical circuits. Environmental, genetic, and clinical factors interact in a complex fashion in the individual patient. This chapter will examine OCD from a neurobiological perspective. The characteristics of OCD that are of specific relevance to this topic are listed in Table 12.1.

TABLE 12.1 *Neurobehavioral Characteristics of Obsessive-Compulsive Disorder*

- Complex repetitive behaviors and cognition
- High incidence of childhood onset
- Changes in symptom content and severity over time
- Anxiety driven
- Improvements with cognitive behavioral therapy
- Improvements with serotonergic, dopaminergic, and opiate therapies
- Worsened by stress
- Worsened by amphetamine or psychostimulants
- Triggered by various etiologic agents
- Increased genetic risk
- With symptom provocation, increased activity of caudate, orbital frontal cortex, anterior cingulate, and thalamus
- Comorbid conditions with other anxiety disorders, attention-deficit hyperactivity disorder, and tic disorders

OBSESSIVE-COMPULSIVE DISORDER BEHAVIORS

Obsessions and compulsions are maladaptive, that is, they impair function. They center on four themes: contamination, sexual/aggressive/checking, ordering and symmetry, and hoarding. Patients with OCD who do not have tics or a family history of tics tend to have more frequent contamination themes (Leckman et al., 1997). Common compulsions include excessive cleaning, checking behaviors, ordering and arranging rituals, counting, repeating routine activities, and hoarding. Compulsions usually involve observable behaviors (e.g., hand washing) but may also consist of covert mental rituals (e.g., counting, or ritualized performance of mental math).

Obsessive-Compulsive Disorder Behaviors from an Evolutionary Perspective

Obsessive-compulsive behaviors can be viewed as evolutionarily conserved normal behaviors, which are disinhibited or overactivated (Swedo et al., 1989a). From a neuroethological perspective, fixed repetitive behavioral routines involving grooming, nesting, reproduction, and avoidance of harm are "hard-wired." In certain breeds of animals, repetitive behavioral sequences occur with great frequency, are inherited, and are typically quite gender-, development-, and environment-specific. Animals manifesting these disordered behaviors are often described as anxious and "high-strung" and may also develop separation anxiety and phobias. In humans, grooming, nesting, and mat-

ing rituals as well as repetitive, intrusive, and time-consuming thoughts and images centering on the loved one can normally be seen. Leckman and Mayes (1998) propose that these behaviors and altered mental states contribute to the development of close pair bonds and parent–infant dyads and contribute to the propagation of our species.

The common pathway is likely due to preservation of neurohormonally mediated behaviors. Certain neuropeptides (melanocortins, orexin, vasopressin, bombesin, arginine vasopressin, somatostatin, and oxytocin) play an important role with regard to memory acquisition, the maintenance and retrieval of certain behavioral sequences such as grooming, or maternal, sexual, and aggressive behaviors. There are also extensive interactions between neuropeptidergic and monoaminergic neuronal systems. Arginine vasopressin is involved in repetitive grooming behaviors and maintaining conditioned responses to aversive stimuli in experimental animals (Leckman et al., 1994).

ETIOLOGICAL FACTORS OF OBSESSIVE-COMPULSIVE DISORDER

It is likely that OCD is the end result of a number of etiologic factors—stress, illness, and genetic predisposition. Early stressful events (disruption of social environment secondary to moves, illnesses, etc.) have been associated with the onset of OCD in some cases. Over 50% of children and adolescents cite a precipitating event (Thomsen, 1995b).

Although most cases of OCD are familial (Riddle et al., 1990), OCD behaviors that closely resemble familial cases have resulted from brain lesions affecting frontal–subcortical structures (tumors, strokes, head injury, carbon monoxide poisoning, manganese intoxication) (Chacko et al., 2000; Weiss and Jenike, 2000). However, in these sporadic acquired cases, symptoms appear late in life, there is no family history of OCD, the standard sensorimotor neurological examination is often abnormal, and neuroimaging studies reveal structural damage (Laplane et al., 1989; Swoboda and Jenike, 1995). In some cases, a specific aspect of OCD spectrum behaviors can occur after a brain injury. For example, Hahm et al. (2001) described a male who compulsively collected toy bullets following a rupture of an anterior communicating artery aneurysm.

Other progressive neurologic disorders that affect components of frontal–subcortical circuits (e.g., postencephalitic Parkinson's disease, neuroacanthocytosis, progressive supranuclear palsy, and Huntington's disease) also can present with OCD symptoms (Cummings and Cunningham, 1992). In chronic, non-postencephalitic Parkinson's disease, patients exhibit symptoms in the OCD spectrum. Although most of these acquired cases are described in adults, head injuries (Max et al., 1995) and a suprasellar germinoma (Mordecai et al., 2000) have resulted in OCD symptoms in children.

In the last few years there has been increased interest in the immune aspects of OCD and related disorders. It has been proposed that some cases of childhood-onset OCD may be related to an infection-triggered autoimmune process similar to that of Sydenham's chorea, a late manifestation of rheumatic fever (Swedo, 1994; Chapter 14, this volume).

GENETIC STUDIES

Twin and family studies have provided strong support for a genetic etiology of OCD. Studies of twins with "obsessional neuroses" have shown consistently higher concordance with monozygotic (MZ) than dizygotic (DZ) twins. In a review, Rasmussen and Tsuang (1984) found a 65% concordance rate in MZ twin pairs. Other studies revealed less striking results with 4.96%–35% of family members of patients with OCD endorsing behaviors in the OCD spectrum (Hanna, 2000; Reddy et al., 2001). Early age of onset correlates with increased familial risk (Geller et al., 1998b; Nestadt et al., 2000) but the risk related to the presence of comorbid tics has had mixed reports (Eapen et al., 1997; Nestadt et al., 2000). Segregation analysis based on symptom factor scores suggested that symmetry and ordering relate to increased genetic risk (Alsobrook et al., 1999). Genetic studies have focused on genes that are related to the catecholaminergic system. Although most candidate gene studies have not uncovered strong associations with any one gene (Frisch et al., 2000), certain alleles showing a sexually dimorphic effect may suggest increased susceptibility in females (Karayiorgou et al., 1999; Enoch et al., 2001).

NEUROPSYCHIATRIC DISORDERS FREQUENTLY COMORBID WITH OBSESSIVE-COMPULSIVE DISORDER

In early-onset OCD, comorbid psychiatric disorders are present in about 80% of the cases. Major depression is seen in approximately 66%; attention-deficit hyperactivity disorder (ADHD), oppositional defiant disorder (ODD), or multiple anxiety disorders in 50%; and enuresis or speech and language disorders in 33%

(Geller et al., 2000). Tics often develop during the course of OCD in childhood, if they are not present at the time of symptom onset. In the presence of tics, obsessions often involve violent or sexual themes, or focus on symmetry. Compulsions involve checking, counting, repeating, touching, or "evening up." Central nervous system (CNS) dysfunction is more evident in early-onset OCD, which suggests that the underlying relationship between OCD and the other disorders is nonspecific or overlapping neurophysiologic dysfunction.

NEUROIMAGING STUDIES

Morphometric magnetic resonance imaging (MRI) studies provide further support for the concept of a subtle developmental brain anomaly. Szeszko et al. (1999) noted that OCD patients had reduced orbitofrontal and amygdala volumes bilaterally, and absence of the normal hemispheric asymmetry of the hippocampus–amygdala complex. Morphometric measurements of the basal ganglia also reveal decreased caudate size (Robinson et al., 1995; Jenike et al., 1996).

Rosenberg et al. (1997b) studied 19 drug-naive children with OCD and found significantly smaller striatal volumes and larger ventricles than in controls, but no differences in volumes of prefrontal cortex, lateral ventricles, or intracranial volume. In a different study Rosenberg et al. (1997a) found that all regions of the corpus callosum, except the isthmus, were significantly larger in OCD patients than in controls. Callosal area correlated significantly with OCD symptom severity but not illness duration. The age-related increase in callosal size seen in the normal subjects was absent in OCD patients. These findings support theories of abnormal development of associational cortex in OCD but also suggest possible abnormalities of other primary cortical regions as well. MacMaster et al. (1999) reported decreased signal intensity in the region of the anterior genu of the corpus callosum in children with OCD compared to controls.

Functional neuroimaging studies provide strong evidence for dysfunction of the cortical-striatal-thalamo-cortical (CSTC) circuitry. Symptoms of OCD are associated with increased activity in orbitofrontal cortex in neutral state (Swedo et al., 1989b; Baxter, 1994; Saxena et al., 1998). Increased activity was also noted in some of these studies in anterior cingulate gyrus, caudate nucleus, and thalamus. Horwitz et al. (1991) found that the pattern of intercorrelations between various brain regions in patients with OCD differed from that of controls.

Studies in which subjects were compared to themselves before and after pharmacological treatment showed a decrease in activity in the caudate, orbitofrontal cortex and/or cingulate cortex (Baxter, 1992; Swedo et al., 1992). Behavior therapy was also employed in some subjects with a finding of decreased activity in the right caudate (Baxter, 1992).

Neuroimaging experiments using provocative measures and circuit-specific cognitive tasks have also been used (Breiter and Rauch, 1996). Increased activity in the right caudate, bilateral orbitofrontal cortex, left anterior cingulate, and left thalamus was reported by Rauch et al. (1994) during a symptom provocation paradigm. Brain activity was measured by functional MRI (fMRI) (Pujol et al., 1999) in patients with OCD during a verbal fluency task and this measurement demonstrated significantly greater activation during word generation and impaired suppression of such activation during the rest period than was observed in controls. Rauch et al. (1997) found that during implicit sequence-learning tasks, OCD patients differed from controls in that they appeared to preferentially activate bilateral medial temporal structures (typically used for conscious, explicit information processing) rather than the striatum, which is used for implicit information processing.

In many of these neuroimaging studies there is a suggestion that right hemisphere structures are more frequently or dramatically involved than those of the left hemisphere. In several studies reporting neurological examination findings, subtle left hemibody signs and synkinesias in both children and adults were detected, suggesting more prominent right than left hemisphere involvement (Denckla, 1989; Hollander et al., 1990).

NEUROPSYCHOLOGIC STUDIES

Neuropsychologic studies have revealed prosodic disturbances and impaired visuospatial processing, deficits that are consistent with right frontal–subcortical dysfunction. In a review, Tallis (1997) identified four broad areas that had been found to be impaired in neuropsychological studies of patients with OCD. In addition to general intellectual function, these patients had an "under-inclusive" cognitive style, manifested impairment on tasks assessing prefrontal-executive function, and had memory deficits. A number of studies have provided support for prefrontal–executive function deficits. Mataix-Cols et al. (1999) demonstrated reduced verbal and design fluency in patients with OCD compared to controls, with evidence of a correlation between severity of OCD symptoms and

design fluency, also pointing to right hemisphere dysfunction. When performing on the Wisconsin Card Sorting Test, patients with OCD required significantly more trials, and made more perseverative and other errors than controls (Lucey et al., 1997). Although the vast majority of such studies have been conducted in adults, when studied, children with OCD have shown similar neurocognitive profiles. However, Beers et al. (1999) found that untreated children with early OCD did not differ from carefully matched controls on an array of neuropsychological tests.

NEUROANATOMICAL FEATURES OF OBSESSIVE-COMPULSIVE DISORDER

The Basal Ganglia

The basal ganglia serve as an important node in a complex system of parallel, segregated, and somatotopically organized CSTC loops that integrate motor and cognitive functions. Inputs flow from the cortex to the basal ganglia through the globus pallidus and substantia nigra to thalamus and, in turn, back to cortex. Research focused on Parkinson's disease (PD) worked out many of the details of the motor system. Projections from a specific region of motor cortex synapse with neurons in the caudate and putamen, which in turn project to the internal segment of the globus pallidus (GP_i) and substantia nigra, pars reticulata (SN_r); from here axons arise and project to the thalamus, and from thalamus back to the same cortical region. Cognitive and emotional processes are handled by CSTC loops that project from associational and limbic areas to the striatum, particularly the ventral striatum or nucleus accumbens (NAc). Although less well studied than its dorsal counterpart, the ventral striatum has a homologous pattern of overall connectivity and histochemistry. It serves as a critical node in the integration of emotional and cognitive behaviors and is thus highly relevant to OCD.

The projections from the cortex are glutamatergic and form synaptic connections with medium-sized spiny neurons in the striatum. These neurons give rise to two pathways that link striatal output (from GP_i) to the thalamus. The direct pathway is GABAergic and inhibitory and projects monosynaptically from putamen to GP_i and from GP_i to SN_r. The indirect pathway is excitatory (GABAergic and inhibitory from putamen to the external segment of the globus pallidus [GP_e] and from GP_e to subthalamic nucleus [STN], but glutamatergic and excitatory from STN to GP_i and SN_r). These pathways are shown in Figure 12.1.

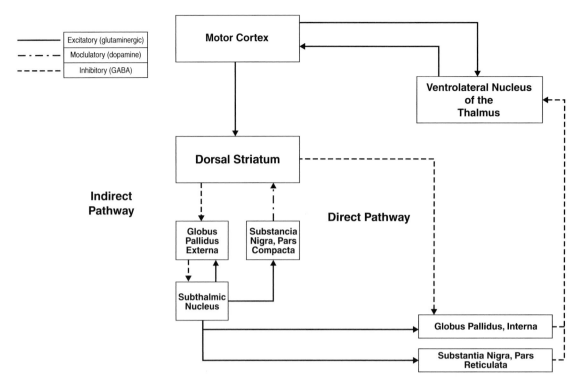

FIGURE 12.1 The classical model of basal ganglia function, based on the motor system. The glutaminergic excitatory projection from the motor cortex impinges on medium spiny neurons in the striatum. Output from the striatum consists of the direct and indirect pathways, which, in the normal nervous system, are balanced. In the direct pathway, the striatum sends an inhibitory (D1) projection on to the globus pallidus interna (Gp$_i$) and the SN$_r$. In the indirect pathway the striatum sends an inhibitory (D2) projection on to the subthalamic nucleus (STN). STN sends excitatory projections to the substantia nigra, pars compacta (SN$_c$) and on to Gp$_i$/SN$_r$. Since the output of Gp$_i$/SN$_r$ on to the ventrolateral nucleus of the thalamus is inhibitory, increased inhibition of STN will diminish its excitatory effect on GP$_i$, with the net result that there is increased inhibition of VL. VL sends an excitatory projection to cortex. With increased inhibition of STN there is increased inhibition of VL, and, as a result, the excitatory projection to motor cortex is damped down, with the resulting motor dysfunction seen in Parkinson's disease. In contrast, in a hyperkinetic movement disorder, there is a decrease in the excitatory input of STN on to GP$_i$/SN$_r$, with a decrease of inhibition of GP$_i$/SN$_r$ resulting in enhanced thalamic activation to motor cortex.

In the classical model of basal ganglia function, neurons in the direct pathway were conceptualized as bearing D$_1$ receptors and co-expressing substance P and dynorphin. Neurons in the indirect pathway had D$_2$ receptors and co-expressed enkephalin. The direct pathway was viewed as releasing movement through disinhibition of the thalamus, whereas enhancing the excitatory activity of the indirect pathway decreased motor activity (Chevalier and Deniau, 1990). This system of checks and balances can be disrupted in several ways. When there is a decrease of normal dopaminergic input, as it is in PD, the excessive output from the basal ganglia results in increased inhibition with the reduction in motor movements. Other alterations in the balance of these two systems results in dyskinesias and stereotypies and the repetitive cognition and motor behaviors associated with OCD.

This classical view of the connectivity of the basal ganglia has been modified to some extent over the last decade by new information relating to the neuroanatomy and physiology of the striatum, and from molecular biology. Although the classical model fits in many ways with neurophysiological studies and clinical observations (i.e., lesioning STN and GP$_i$ improves motor function in both humans with PD as well as experimental animals [Wichmann et al., 1994)]), the circuitry of the basal ganglia is far more complex than originally envisioned (Obeso et al., 2000). First, D_1 and D_2 inputs are confined not just to the neurons in the direct and indirect pathways, respectively, but are found together on the medium spiny neurons in both the direct and indirect pathways (Aizman et al., 2000). Second, rather than acting directly to inhibit striatal neurons, dopamine is now viewed as modulating the interaction of glutamatergic and dopamine receptors and the function of GABAergic and serotonergic neurons. Third, other interneurons have been identified in the striatum that influence striatal activity. For example, cholinergic interneurons have widespread dendritic trees that make it possible to affect neuronal transmission across a large area of the striatum. They likely play an important, albeit currently poorly understood, role in modulating striatal output by interacting with glutamatergic, dopaminergic, and GABAergic neurons (Calabresi et al., 2000).

A fourth modification of the classical model involves nitric oxide (NO), a new form of nonsynaptic interneuronal communication, or volume transmission. Nitric Oxide inhibits the uptake of dopamine, norepinephrine (Lonart and Johnson, 1994), and serotonin (Asano et al., 1997) into neurons and is closely linked to glutamate-mediated neurotransmission. Nitric Oxide synthase is "switched on" only by glutamatergic receptors and appears to enhance the strength of glutamatergic input to monoaminergic neurons without requiring direct synaptic contact (Kiss and Vizi, 2001).

Fifth, the identification of four closed-loop "internal circuits" that are distinct from the CTSC loops has also modified the classical view. These internal circuits are parallel, somatotopically arranged, and highly collateralized projection systems that integrate striatal, thalamic, and cortical activity. If the CTSC loops are considered vertical, the internal circuits are horizontal and appear to modulate the excitability of the basal ganglia and maintain stability in the system (Obeso et al., 2000).

Specific patterns in neuronal pools in the basal ganglia have also been elucidated in the last decade. The firing pattern of neuronal clusters in Gp_i is such that dopamine depletion in PD might be attributed to specific alterations in firing patterns (Obeso et al., 2000). Some neurons fire during movement preparation, whereas others fire while a movement is being performed. Depending on the degree of automatization of a movement, a shift occurs in which neuronal pools are used. When a motor behavior is being learned, associative prefrontal cortex (PFC) and anterior basal

ganglia structures are involved, whereas once the motor sequence has been learned and is relatively automatic, the activation pattern shifts posterior to the premotor and motor areas and posterior basal ganglia (Hikosaka et al., 1999; Jog et al., 1999).

The Striosome and Matrix Compartments

Most relevant to the pathophysiology of OCD are the striosome and matrix compartments, which represent another system integrating specific cortical areas to subcortical circuits (Gerfen, 1989). (Gerfen uses the term *patch*, whereas Graybiel refers to these structures as *striosomes*.) Striosome and matrix differ in connectivity, neurochemical composition, and function. Striosomes stain weakly for acetylcholinesterase and have dense opiate receptor binding, as well as enkephalin- and substance P–like immunoreactivity. They receive input from deep cortical layers V and VI, predominantly from the orbitofrontal, anterior cingulate and posterior medial PFC, amygdala, and hippocampus and project to the substantia nigra, parscompacta and thus influence nigrostrial dopaminergic innervation. Graybiel et al. (2000b) suggest that striosomes are involved in reward-based learning. In contrast, the matrix stains strongly for acetylcholinesterase and manifests somatostatin immunoreactivity. It receives inputs from cortical layers II and III and superficial layer V, predominantly from neocortical parietal and motor areas, and to the nondopaminergic nigrothalamic and nigrotectal system. Thus, there is a relative predominance of allocortical projections to patches and to dopaminergic circuits, and a relative predominance of neocortical sensorimotor projections to matrix (Gerfen, 1989). The striosome–matrix system serves to link cortical influences onto the dopaminergic and GABAergic neurons in the substantia nigra, which in turn modulate thalamocortical activity. The striosome and matrix compartments also follow a topographical organization in that inputs from a given cortical area to striosomes are surrounded by matrix that also receives inputs from the same cortical area. These systems appear to be a way of dispersing cortical inputs and then reintegrating them at the next stage of processing (refer to Fig. 12.2).

Ventral Striatum: Nucleus Accumbens

The ventral striatum, like its dorsal counterpart, is part of a system of CSTC loops. Only recently has it become clear that these loops are as segregated and discrete as those in the dorsal striatum. Glutamatergic inputs, which arise from the orbital and medial prefrontal cor-

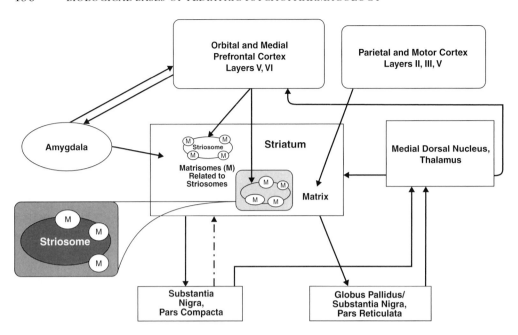

FIGURE 12.2 Details of striosomes and matrisomes in basal ganglia. This diagram presents some of the detail about the OMPFC network pertinent to OCD, based on the research of Graybiel and colleagues (Graybiel 2000a; 2000b; Eblen and Graybiel, 1995). Striosomes, surrounded by a cluster of patchy matrisomes are the target for projections from posterior orbital and mediofrontal (limbic) cortices. This pattern is in contract to projections from other cortical regions, which target matrix. Striosomes have a selective reciprocal projection to dopaminergic SNpc, a system crucial to learning and motivation. Gene induction in the striosomal and matrisomal compartments is relatively balanced in the normal state (represented by gray shading). In the insert, a diagram of the response to dopamine enhancing drugs such as cocaine, amphetamine. These drugs produce stereotypy in experimental animals and may serve as a model for obsessions and compulsions in humans. Here, gene induction (dark gray) is much more striking in the striosome than in the matrix, suggesting an imbalance in the striatal system controlling the integration of thoughts, emotions, and behavior.

tex, hippocampus, and amygdala, converge on single neurons in NAc. The nucleus accumbens projects to the ventral pallidum (VP), which sends an inhibitory projection to the thalamus; this in turn projects back to the cortical areas from which the inputs arose. Prefrontal cortex exerts inhibitory control over the NAc during activation of the amygdala, inhibiting dopamine release from the NAc onto the amygdala (Jackson and Moghaddam, 2001). O'Donnell et al. (1997) suggest that the NAc-reticular thalamic nucleus projection may serve to focus arousal and attention toward stimuli (particularly those that are emotionally charged) and in turn modulate thalamocortical output.

Microstructure of the striatum

Using retrograde horseradish peroxidase, Grofova (1975) demonstrated that medium spiny neurons were

projection neurons, rather than interneurons, as had been previously thought. The medium spiny neurons constitute 90% to 95% of the neuronal population of the striatum and are targets for several different types of neurotransmitters. They receive two types of glutamatergic inputs from the cortex, NMDA and AMPA, as well as both D_1 and D_2 receptors at the synaptic neck.

Because of the complex interactions with the several different neurotransmitters that converge on them, the medium spiny neurons are little models of synaptic plasticity. The immediate-early genes encode proteins that respond rapidly to a variety of inputs, such as environmental stimuli, learning, endogenous anxiety or mood states, or neuropharmacological changes. Berke et al. (1998) demonstrated that following stimulation of striatal D_1 receptors in 6-OHDA–lesioned rats, more than 30 striatal genes were rapidly induced and returned rapidly to baseline. Many of these genes were transcription factors and they may regulate late-response genes that function to maintain the enhanced sensitivity to neurotransmitters. Repeat exposure to the stimulus results in a very rapid response. The ease with which the immediate-early and late-response genes respond to learning, environmental inputs, and pharmacologic changes and store "neuronal memories" may provide a physiological basis for the fluctuating course that is typical of OCD.

THE DOPAMINE SYSTEM

Clear abnormalities of the dopamine system have not been identified in the periphery or the brain of OCD patients. Nevertheless, repetitive stereotypies and OCD-like behaviors can be produced in humans by the administration of exogenous D_2 agonist or stimulants, which suggests that the dopaminergic system may be involved in some way in OCD. Conversely, antipsychotics can be used adjunctively in the treatment of selective serotonin reuptake inhibitor (SSRI)-resistant OCD patients with a definite benefit in a significant proportion of patients.

Dopaminergic neurons arise from two areas—the mesolimbic system, (involved in emotional and cognitive behaviors), which comes from cell bodies in the mesencephalic ventral tegmental area of Tsai (A10), the substantia nigra pars compacta (A9); and the caudo-lateral cell group (A8); and the nigrostriatal system, which is involved in motor function, arises in the substantia nigra pars compacta (SN_c), and projects to the caudate and putamen. The dopamine systems project heavily to associational neocortex—dorsomedial orbital and medial prefronta cortex and inferior parietal cortex—(Lewis et al., 1988), as well as primary motor cortex. Dopaminergic innervation of primary visual, auditory, and somatosensory cortices is relatively sparse (Hokfelt et al., 1986; Foote and Morrison, 1987). Figure 12.3 amply illustrates this.

THE SEROTONIN SYSTEM

Serotonin (5-hydroxytryptamine [5-HT]) has remained the leading target for investigations of the neurochemical underpinnings of OCD, largely because of the remarkable efficacy of SSRIs in the treatment of OCD. More direct measures of neurochemical dysfunction, including paradigms that employ biological markers, pharmacologic challenges, or functional neuroimaging, are needed to confirm a pathophysiol-

ogic role for 5-HT. Acute blockade of 5-HT reuptake appears to be the critical first step in a chain of neural events leading to efficacy in the treatment of OCD. Serotonin-containing terminals are densely scattered throughout the cortex, neostriatum, and hippocampus and neurons of the ventromedial striatum (Molliver, 1987). There are dense projections from ventral PFC to the caudate (Modell et al., 1989). Serotonin serves to modulate other neural networks, and is involved in both tonic and phasic patterns of response. There is also a complex interaction between glutamatergic, dopaminergic, and serotoninergic neurons. Serotonin receptors are localized to the same areas as glutaminergic and dopaminergic terminals and have similar patterns of connectivity. There is a reciprocal relationship between glutamatergic and serotonergic neurons: glutamine strongly inhibits serotonin-containing neurons (Becquet et al., 1990) and, in turn, serotonergic neurons modulate glutamatergic activity. In the caudate 5-HT2$_a$ receptors on GABA interneurons serve to inhibit glutamate projections to the striatum.

Studying peripheral markers of the 5-HT system offers an extremely remote view on the physiology of the central 5-HT system. Despite the fact that the 5-HT reuptake transporters (5-HTT) on platelets appear to be identical to those on 5-HT neurons in the brain, one must take into account that region-specific factors may alter their density and/or function. Similarly, measures of the main metabolite of 5-HT, 5-HIAA, reported to be increased in the CSF of OCD patients and to decline in relation to symptom reduction, also must be interpreted with caution. This pool of 5-HIAA most likely originates from descending 5-HT neurons, which have different characteristics from those giving rise to ascending projections. Furthermore, several factors control the 5-HIAA excretion into the cerebrospinal fluid (CSF). Among them is the access of 5-HT to intracellular monoamine oxidase. Therefore, SRI treatment would be expected to decrease the access of 5-HT to the intracellular enzyme responsible for the production of 5-HIAA.

The pharmacological challenge approach that consists of examining neuroendocrine parameters can be criticized on the basis of the brain region specificity relevance factor; these responses originate from the hypothalamo pituitary complex, whereas OCD has clearly been linked to anomalies in a neurocircuitry comprising a loop from the orbitofrontal cortex to the basal ganglia and the thalamus. The challenge approach consisting of triggering symptoms does bear, considerable face value. Nevertheless, the agonists used in the past made interpretation of the exa-

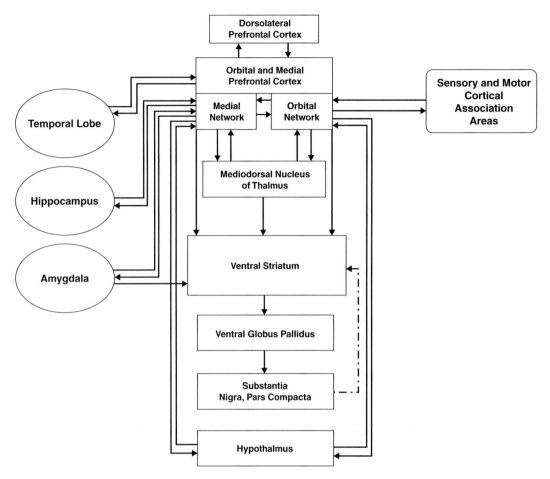

FIGURE 12.3 The CSTC loop relevant to obsessive-compulsive disorder. In the situation involved in OCD, the orbital and medial prefrontal cortex (OMPFC) networks play an important role. OMPFC projects topographically to the medical caudate nucleus, NAc, and ventromedial putamen. It receives projections, which are reciprocal, with minor exception, from numerous cortical association areas, prominently the amygdala, hippocampus, and other temporal lobe regions. There is also one-way glutaminergic projections from anygdala to the nucleus accumbens (Nac). As in the classical CSTC loop, caudate and putamen project topographically to the ventral pallidum, and non-topographically to the substantia nigra, pars compacta (SNpc). The pallidum sends a projection to the mediodorsal nucleus of the thalamus (MD) and the Reticular Thalamic Nucleus (RTN), which in turn project to OMPFC.

cerbations difficult because of their lack of either specificity or brain penetration. Specifically, meta-chlorophenylpipeazin (m-CPP) is a potent 5-HT_{2C} agonist, but an equally effective 5-HT_3 antagonist, a 5-HT_{2A} antagonist, and moderately active 5-HT_{1D} agonist that can decrease 5-HT release, whereas the 5-HT_{1D} agonist sumatriptan exhibits poor penetration of the blood–brain barrier (Hamik and Peroutka, 1989; Sleight et al., 1990). In contrast, 5-HT antago-

nists have been reported to produce a reversal of the beneficial action of SSRIs in OCD. Since the 5-HT_2 antagonist ritanserin and the nonselective $5\text{-HT}_{1/2}$ antagonist metergoline both produced exacerbations, these data tentatively implicate the role of a 5-HT_2 receptor in mediating the anti-OCD effect of SSRIs (Greenberg et al., 1998).

The role of the 5-HT system certainly appears more important in the treatment than in the etiopathology of OCD. Long-term SSRI treatment likely produces its anti-OCD effect by enhancing 5-HT transmission in the orbitofrontal cortex. This would occur as a result of their capacity to desensitize the terminal 5-HT$_{1B}$ autoreceptors in that brain region after an 8-week, but not a 3-week, treatment. This is congruent with the longer delay to obtain an optimal therapeutic effect in OCD than in depression. In brain structures involved in depression, such as the hypothalamus and the hippocampus, a 2- to 3-week SSRI treatment is sufficient to desensitize this autoreceptor normally producing an inhibitory action on 5-HT release (Blier and Bouchard, 1994). In addition, an elevated-dose SSRI regimen is necessary to produce this change, consistent with higher doses generally being required to effectively treat OCD than those for major depression. Also, repeated electroconvulsive shock, which is considered to be devoid of intrinsic anti-OCD efficacy, does not alter 5-HT release nor 5-HT$_{1B}$ autoreceptor function in the orbitofrontal cortex (Bergqvist et al., 1999). Interestingly, this neuronal change produced by SSRIs does not occur in the downstream structure from the orbitofrontal cortex, the head of the caudate nucleus (el Mansari et al., 1995). It is important to emphasize here that 5-HT transmission need not be enhanced in all relays of a loop to dampen the reverberating phenomenon present in this circuitry.

The enhanced 5-HT release would probably act via the activation of postsynaptic 5-HT$_2$ receptors that remain normosensitive after the 8-week SSRI treatment (el Mansari and Blier, 1997). Indeed, the response of orbitofrontal cortex neurons to 5-HT and 5-HT$_2$ agonists is unaltered, whereas that to a 5-HT$_{1A}$ agonist is decreased after such treatment. It has not been conclusively shown that these 5-HT$_2$ receptors are located directly on the glutamatergic pyramidal neurons or on inhibitory GABA interneurons. Wherever their precise localization, the effect of 5-HT on these neurons, which send an excitatory output to the caudate nucleus, is inhibitory in nature, which could account for the dampening of the hyperactivity observed following successful SSRI treatment. These results clearly identify the terminal 5-HT$_{1B}$ autoreceptor and the postsynaptic 5-HT$_2$ receptors as potential novel targets for the treatment of OCD.

THE GLUTAMATE SYSTEM

Pyramidal neurons in the orbitofrontal cortex are glutamatergic in nature and release their excitatory neurotransmitter glutamate in the head of the caudate. The beneficial action of internal capsulotomy (which inter-rupts these glutamatergic fibers) in treatment-refractory patients provides support for their role. More recently, Rosenberg and colleagues (2000) have elegantly shown an elevation of a glutamate signal in the caudate of children with OCD using ^{1}H nuclear magnetic spectroscopy. Furthermore, this elevated signal normalized following effective SSRI treatment. Although there are still some methodological issues to be resolved with this approach (specifically, this signal may not be entirely attributable to glutamate), the results constitute a compelling hypothesis. An important anomaly accounting in part for OCD symptomatology could thus be the hyperactivity of orbitofrontal neurons. These neurons could therefore constitute the effector upon which SSRIs would act to decrease such hyperactivity. This abnormality need not reside only on orbitofrontal cortex neurons. Indeed, the thalamic neurons that project from the thalamus to the orbitofrontal cortex are also glutamatergic. Since SSRIs increase 5-HT transmission in the orbitofrontal cortex but not the head of the caudate nucleus, it is conceivable that if these drugs are also devoid of action in the thalamus, they may not exert a more robust anti-OCD action because of this lack of generalized action on all glutamate neurons of the loop. In contrast, a drug that could directly act on glutamate neurons to decrease release would theoretically be endowed with a rapid onset of action, and potentially exert a more robust action than SSRIs. Agonists of the metabotropic glutamatergic type II receptor do exert such a dampening effect on glutamate release, and strikingly only under excessive release conditions (Schoepp et al., 1999). This preferential action would result from the fact that these glutamate autoreceptors are located extrasynaptically, and thus are not activated under normal physiological conditions. In addition, direct antagonists of the postsynaptic glutamate receptors mediating the excitatory action of this neurotransmitter in the head of the caudate nucleus could be effective anti-OCD agents. These drugs would have to be fairly selective, however, for such neurons to avoid generalized adverse events due to generalized attenuation of glutamate transmission.

CONCLUSIONS

Obsessive-compulsive disorder is a disorder of the frontal–subcortical system. A characteristic of this group of disorders is a complex interaction between the exogenous and endogenous stimuli and the neural systems that link stimuli to cognitive and behavioral responses. Although cortical dysfunction cannot be excluded as a basis for OCD symptoms, there is evidence that basal ganglia dysfunction is likely to play a major role in the pathophysiology of OCD. Graybiel et al. (2000a,b) have suggested that l-DOPA-induced dyskinesias and dopamine-dependent stereotypies, which have similar pathophysiology, serve as a model for the derangement in OCD.

A characteristic feature of striatal neurons is their role in procedural (or habit) learning and memory (as distinct from episodic memory). The synaptic and neurochemical features of the striatum, particularly its richness in neuropeptides and amines, which modulate synaptic transmission along a gradient, make possible a wide range of neuronal responses. Patterns of learned motor behaviors (and presumably patterns of thought) are embedded in the neuronal network of the striatum. This is reflected in the transcriptional genes, which, once induced following even a single exposure to an environmental event or pharmacological manipulation, manifest sensitization to repeated exposures. This would be congruent with the clinical behavior of patients with OCD who present with repetitive thoughts and behaviors following relatively minimal triggering events, which often increase in intensity in response to additional stimuli.

Stereotypies are repetitive motor actions that are similar to each other and represent the inability to initiate normal adaptive responses (Graybiel et al., 2000a, b). An intact nigrostriatal system is required for the production of sterotypic behavior (Ridley, 1994). These stereotypies can be induced in rodents by injecting drugs into the caudate/putamen that activate both D_1 and D_2 receptors. When these drugs are injected into NAc, stereotypic hyperlocomotion occurs. Graybiel et al. (2000a) provided a detailed list of reasons for stereotypies and dyskinesias being likely the same condition: they both require activation of dopamine receptors; they occur in response to chronic intermittent dopamine-receptor agonist treatment; they require activation of glutamate NMDA receptors; they have similar effects on NMDA NR_1 and NR_{2B} receptor subunit phosphorylation and/or increased glutamate transmission, as well as involvement of the C-AMP response element–binding protein (CREB) pathway; and they involve activation of similar transcription factor families, prolonged activation of delta FosB/chronic Fras, and enhanced expression of preprodynorphin/preproenkephalin. These changes are more intense and easily induced in the presence of dopamine depletion or damage to the nigrostriatal system. There is also a tight correlation between the striosome/matrix activation ratio and the amount of stereotypy that an animal manifests. Since striosomes receive input from orbital and medial prefrontal cortex, the relative enhancement of

striosomes over matrix would serve to enhance motivational behaviors (i.e., those triggered by such strong emotions as fear or anxiety). Moreover, because striosomes project to the substantia nigra, they would modulate dopaminergic input to the striatum.

Obsessive-compulsive disorder is a fascinating disorder from a neurobiological point of view because the repetitive behaviors and thoughts associated with OCD have an array of rather unique characteristics: (1) they echo phylogenetically old behaviors that are programmed into vertebrate brains; (2) they can result from genetic predisposition as well as acquired brain lesions that affect frontal–subcortical circuits; (3) they are triggered and exacerbated by anxiety and stress; (4) they can result from disregulation of the dopaminergic system (both hypo- [e.g., PD] and hyperdopaminergic conditions [e.g., stimulants and cocaine]) and diminish in response to SSRIs; and (5) they increase with repetition (practice, a characteristic "striatal" pattern) and decrease with exposure and response prevention in controlled therapeutic settings. Given what we know about frontal–striatal circuitry, it would appear that OCD is not the result of a single specific factor, such as too little serotonin, too much dopamine, or too much anxiety, but rather reflects dysregulation or imbalance of the striatal system. This system serves to integrate "hard-wired" motor and cognitive programs with newly learned programs. Thus, if the system becomes dysfunctional, one would expect to see impaired selection and "sticky" shifting of motor and cognitive behaviors. Moreover, this dysregulation does not necessarily have to occur at just one particular node in the system. It is possible to visualize a variety of different types of OCD. One type might arise as a result of cortical lesions; Ridley (1994) suggests that frontal projections may inhibit stereotypies of this type. Another type (and probably the most common) might result from striatal dysfunction. A third type might be the result of imbalance in hippocampal or amygdalar input. Another possible type might result from dysfunction at the level of the thalamus or thalamocortical projections. Similarly, there may be different genetic forms of OCD. The responses of the immediate early genes in the medium spiny neurons that interact with numerous other neurotransmitter systems serve to perpetuate at a molecular level the disturbed function of these neurons so that repetitive environmental or neurochemical triggers would serve to exacerbate maladaptive motor behaviors and cognitive processes. Graybiel's (2000b) observation that there is a similarity between stereotypies and OCD provides an animal model for OCD which will be as instructive as the experimental PD models and will make it possible to ask more sophisticated questions when setting up research programs relating to OCD in a clinical setting.

REFERENCES

Aizman, O., Brismar, H., Uhlen, P., Zettergren, E., Levey, A.I., Forssberg, H., Greengard, P., and Aperia, A. (2000) Anatomical and physiological evidence for D1 and D2 dopamine receptor colocalization in neostriatal neurons. *Nat Neurosci* 3:226–230.

Alsobrook, I.J., Leckman, J.F., Goodman, W.K., Rasmussen, S.A., and Pauls, D.L. (1999) Segregation analysis of obsessive-compulsive disorder using symptom-based factor scores. *Am J Med Genet* 88:669–675.

Asano, S., Matsuda, T., Nakasu, Y., Maeda, S., Nogi, H., and Baba, A. (1997) Inhibition by nitric oxide of the uptake of [3H]serotonin into rat brain synaptosomes. *Jpn J Pharmacol* 75: 123–128.

Baxter, L.R., Jr. (1992) Neuroimaging studies of obsessive compulsive disorder. *Psychiatr Clin North Am* 15:871–884.

Baxter, L.R., Jr. (1994) Positron emission tomography studies of cerebral glucose metabolism in obsessive compulsive disorder. *J Clin Psychiatry* 55 Suppl:54–59.

Becquet, D., Faudon, M., and Hery, F. (1990) In vivo evidence for an inhibitory glutamatergic control of serotonin release in the cat caudate nucleus: involvement of GABA neurons. *Brain Res* 519: 82–88.

Beers, S.R., Rosenberg, D.R., Dick, E.L., Williams, T., O'Hearn, K.M., Birmaher, B., and Ryan, C.M. (1999) Neuropsychological study of frontal lobe function in psychotropic-naive children with obsessive-compulsive disorder. *Am J Psychiatry* 156:777–779.

Bergqvist, P.B., Bouchard, C., and Blier, P. (1999) Effect of long-term administration of antidepressant treatments on serotonin release in brain regions involved in obsessive-compulsive disorder. *Biol Psychiatry* 45:164–174.

Berke, J.D., Paletzki, R.F., Aronson, G.J., Hyman, S.E., and Gerfen, C.R. (1998) A complex program of striatal gene expression induced by dopaminergic stimulation. *J Neurosci* 18:5301–5310.

Blier, P. and Bouchard, C. (1994). Modulation of 5-HT release in the guinea-pig brain following long-term administration of antidepressant drugs. *Br J Pharmacol* 113:485–495.

Breiter, H.C. and Rauch, S.L. (1996) Functional MRI and the study of OCD: from symptom provocation to cognitive-behavioral probes of cortico-striatal systems and the amygdala. *Neuroimage* 4:S127–S138.

Calabresi, P., Centonze, D, Gubelli, P., Pisani, A., and Bernardi, G. (2000) Acetylcholine-mediated modulation of striatal function. *Trends Neurosci* 23:120–125.

Chacko, R.C., Corbin, M.A., and Harper, R.G. (2000) Acquired obsessive-compulsive disorder associated with basal ganglia lesions. *J Neuropsychiatry Clin Neurosci* 12:269–272.

Chevalier, G. and Deniau, J.M. (1990) Disinhibition as a basic process in the expression of striatal functions. *Trends Neurosci* 13: 277–280.

Cummings, J.L. and Cunningham, K. (1992) Obsessive-compulsive disorder in Huntington's disease. *Biol Psychiatry* 31:263–270.

Denckla, M. (1989) Neurological examination. In: Rapoport, J., ed. *Obsessive-Compulsive Disorder in Children and Adolescents.* Washington, DC: American Psychiatric Press, pp. 107–115.

Eapen, V., Robertson, M.M., Alsobrook, J.P., 2nd, and Pauls, D.L. (1997) Obsessive compulsive symptoms in Gilles de la Tourette syndrome and obsessive compulsive disorder: differences by diagnosis and family history. *Am J Med Genet* 74:432–438.

el Mansari, M. and Blier, P. (1997) In vivo electrophysiological characterization of 5-HT receptors in the guinea pig head of caudate nucleus and orbitofrontal cortex. *Neuropharmacology* 36:577–588.

el Mansari, M., Bouchard, C., and Blier, P. (1995) Alteration of serotonin release in the guinea pig orbito-frontal cortex by selective serotonin reuptake inhibitors. Relevance to treatment of obsessive-compulsive disorder. *Neuropsychopharmacology* 13: 117–127.

Enoch, M., Greenberg, B.D., Murphy, D.L., and Goldman, D. (2001) Sexually dimorphic relationship of a 5-HT(2A) promoter polymorphism with obsessive-compulsive disorder. *Biol Psychiatry*, 49:385–388.

Evans, D.W., Leckman, J.F., Carter, A., Reznick, J.S., Henshaw, D., King, R.A., and Pauls, D. (1997) Ritual, habit, and perfectionism: the prevalence and development of compulsive-like behavior in normal young children. *Child Dev* 68:58–68.

Flament, M.F., Koby, E., Rapaport, J.L., Berg, C.J., Zahn, T., Cox, C., Denckla, M., and Lenane, M. (1990). Childhood obsessive-compulsive disorder: a prospective follow-up study. *J Child Psychol Psychiatry* 31:363–380.

Foote, S.L. and Morrison, J.H. (1987) Development of the noradrenergic, serotonergic, and dopaminergic innervation of neocortex. *Curr Top Dev Biol* 21:391–423.

Frisch, A., Michaelovsky, E., Rockah, R., Amir, I., Hermesh, H., Laor, N., Fuchs, C., Zohar, J., Lerer, B., Buniak, S.F., Landa, S., Poyurovsky, M., Shapira, B., and Weizman, R. (2000) Association between obsessive-compulsive disorder and polymorphisms of genes encoding components of the serotonergic and dopaminergic pathways. *Eur Neuropsychopharmacol* 10:205–209.

Geller, D., Biederman, J., Faraone, S.V., Frazier, J., Coffey, B.J., Kim, G., and Bellordre, C.A. (2000) Clinical correlates of obsessive compulsive disorder in children and adolescents referred to specialized and non-specialized clinical settings [In Process Citation]. *Depress Anxiety* 11:163–168.

Geller, D., Biederman, J., Jones, J., Park, K., Schwartz, S., Shapiro, S., and Coffey, B. (1998a) Is juvenile obsessive-compulsive disorder a developmental subtype of the disorder? A review of the pediatric literature. *J Am Acad Child Adolesc Psychiatry* 37:420–427.

Geller, D.A., Biederman, J., Jones, J., Shapiro, S., Schwartz, S., and Park, K.S. (1998b) Obsessive-compulsive disorder in children and adolescents: a review. *Harv Rev Psychiatry* 5:260–273.

Gerfen, C.R. (1989) The neostriatal mosaic: striatal patch-matrix organization is related to cortical lamination. *Science* 246:385–388.

Graybiel, A.M., Canales, J.J., and Capper-Loup, C. (2000a) Levodopa-induced dyskinesias and dopamine-dependent stereotypies: a new hypothesis. *Trends Neurosci* 23:S71–S77.

Graybiel, A.M., and Rauch, S.L. (2000b) Toward a neurobiology of obsessive-compulsive disorder. *Neuron* 28:343–347.

Greenberg, B.D., Benjamin, J., Martin, J.D., Keuler, D., Huang, S.J., Altemus, M., and Murphy, D.L. (1998) Delayed obsessive-compulsive disorder symptom exacerbation after a single dose of a serotonin antagonist in fluoxetine-treated but not untreated patients. *Psychopharmacology* 140:434–444.

Grofova, I. (1975) The identification of striatal and pallidal neurons projecting to substantia nigra. An experimental study by means of retrograde axonal transport of horseradish peroxidase. *Brain Res* 91:286–291.

Hahm, D.S., Kang, Y., Cheong, S.S., and Na, D.L. (2001) A compulsive collecting behavior following an A-com aneurysmal rupture. *Neurology* 56:398–400.

Hamik, A. and Peroutka, S.J. (1989) 1-(m-chlorophenyl)piperazine (mCPP) interactions with neurotransmitter receptors in the human brain. *Biol Psychiatry* 25:569–575.

Hanna, G.L. (2000) Clinical and family-genetic studies of childhood obsessive-compulsive disorder. In Goodman, W.K., Rudorfer, M.V., and Maser, J.D., eds. *Obsessive-Compulsive Disorder: Contemporary Issues in Treatment.* Mahwah, NJ: Lawrence Erlbaum Associates, pp. 87–103.

Hikosaka, O., Nakahara, H., Rand, M.K., Sakai, K., Lu, X., Nakamura, K., Miyachi, S., and Doya, K. (1999) Parallel neural networks for learning sequential procedures. *Trends Neurosci* 22: 464–471.

Hokfelt, T., Holets, V.R., Staines, W., Meister, B., Melander, T., Schalling, M., Schultzberg, M., Freedman, J., Bjorklund, H., Olson, L., et al. (1986) Coexistence of neuronal messengers—an overview. *Prog Brain Res* 68:33–70.

Hollander, E., Schiffman, E., Cohen, B., Rivera-Stein, M.A., Rosen, W., Gorman, J.M., Fyer, A.J., Papp, L., and Liebowitz, M.R. (1990) Signs of central nervous system dysfunction in obsessive-compulsive disorder. *Arch Gen Psychiatry,* 47:27–32.

Horwitz, B., Swedo, S.E., Grady, C.L., Pietrini, P., Schapiro, M.B., Rapoport, J.L., and Rapoport, S.I. (1991) Cerebral metabolic pattern in obsessive-compulsive disorder: altered intercorrelations between regional rates of glucose utilization. *Psychiatry Res* 40: 221–237.

Jackson, M.E. and Moghaddam, B. (2001) Amygdala regulation of nucleus accumbens dopamine output is governed by the prefrontal cortex. *J Neurosci* 21:676–681.

Jenike, M.A., Breiter, H.C., Baer, L., Kennedy, D.N., Savage, C.R., Olivares, M.J., O'Sullivan, R.L., Shera, D.M., Rauch, S.L., Keuthen, N., Rosen, B.R., Caviness, V.S., and Filipek, P.A. (1996) Cerebral structural abnormalities in obsessive-compulsive disorder. A quantitative morphometric magnetic resonance imaging study. *Arch Gen Psychiatry* 53:625–632.

Jog, M.S., Kubota, Y., Connolly, C.I., Hillegaart, V., and Graybiel, A.M. (1999) Building neural representations of habits. *Science* 286:1745–1749.

Karayiorgou, M., Sobin, C., Blundell, M.L., Galke, B.L., Malinova, L., Goldberg, P., Ott, J., and Gogos, J.A. (1999) Family-based association studies support a sexually dimorphic effect of COMT and MAOA on genetic susceptibility to obsessive-compulsive disorder. *Biol Psychiatry* 45:1178–1189.

Karno, M., Golding, J.M., Sorenson, S.B., and Burnam, M.A. (1988) The epidemiology of obsessive-compulsive disorder in five US communities. *Arch Gen Psychiatry* 45:1094–1099.

Kiss, J.P. and Vizi, E.S. (2001) Nitric oxide: a novel link between synaptic and nonsynaptic transmission. *Trends Neurosci* 24:211–215.

Laplane, D., Levasseur, M., Pillon, B., Dubois, B., Baulac, M., Mazoyer, B., Tran Dinh, S., Sette, G., Danze, F., and Baron, J.C. (1989) Obsessive-compulsive and other behavioural changes with bilateral basal ganglia lesions. A neuropsychological, magnetic resonance imaging and positron tomography study. *Brain* 112: 699–725.

Leckman, J.F., Goodman, W.K., North, W.G., Chappell, P.B., Price, L.H., Pauls, D.L., Anderson, G.M., Riddle, M.A., McSwiggan-Hardin, M., McDougle, C.J., et al. (1994) Elevated cerebrospinal fluid levels of oxytocin in obsessive-compulsive disorder. Comparison with Tourette's syndrome and healthy controls. *Arch Gen Psychiatry* 51:782–792.

Leckman, J.F., Grice, D.E., Boardman, J., Zhang, H., Vitale, A., Bondi, C., Alsobrook, J., Peterson, B.S., Cohen, D.J., Rasmussen, S.A., Goodman, W.K., McDougle, C.J., and Pauls, D.L. (1997)

Symptoms of obsessive-compulsive disorder. *Am J Psychiatry* 154:911–917.

Leckman, J.F. and Mayes, L.C. (1998) Understanding developmental psychopathology: how useful are evolutionary accounts? *J Am Acad Child Adolesc Psychiatry* 37:1011–1021.

Leonard, H.L., Goldberger, E.L., Rapoport, J.L., Cheslow, D.L., and Swedo, S.E. (1990) Childhood rituals: normal development or obsessive-compulsive symptoms? *J Am Acad Child Adolesc Psychiatry* 29:17–23.

Leonard, H.L., Lenane, M.C., Swedo, S.E., Rettew, D.C., Gershon, E.S., and Rapoport, J.L. (1992) Tics and Tourette's disorder: a 2- to 7-year follow-up of 54 obsessive-compulsive children. *Am J Psychiatry* 149:1244–1251.

Leonard, H.L., Swedo, S.E., Lenane, M.C., Rettew, D.C., Hamburger, S.D., Bartko, J.J., and Rapoport, J.L. (1993) A 2- to 7-year follow-up study of 54 obsessive-compulsive children and adolescents. *Arch Gen Psychiatry* 50:429–439.

Lewis, D.A., Foote, S.L., Goldstein, M., and Morrison, J.H. (1988) The dopaminergic innervation of monkey prefrontal cortex: a tyrosine hydroxylase immunohistochemical study. *Brain Res* 449: 225–243.

Lonart, G. and Johnson, K.M. (1994) Inhibitory effects of nitric oxide on the uptake of [3H]dopamine and [3H]glutamate by striatal synaptosomes. *J Neurochem* 63:2108–2117.

Lucey, J.V., Costa, D.C., Busatto, G., Pilowsky, L.S., Marks, I.M., Ell, P.J., and Kerwin, R.W. (1997). Caudate regional cerebral blood flow in obsessive-compulsive disorder, panic disorder and healthy controls on single photon emission computerised tomography. *Psychiatry Res* 74:25–33.

MacMaster, F.P., Keshavan, M.S., Dick, E.L., and Rosenberg, D.R. (1999) Corpus callosal signal intensity in treatment-naive pediatric obsessive compulsive disorders. *Prog Neuropsychopharmacol Biol Psychiatry* 23:601–612.

Mataix-Cols, D., Junque, C., Sanchez-Turet, M., Vallejo, J., Verger, K., and Barrios, M. (1999) Neuropsychological functioning in a subclinical obsessive-compulsive sample. *Biol Psychiatry,* 45: 898–904.

Max, J.E., Smith, W.L., Lindgren, S.D., Robin, D.A., Mattheis, P., Stierwalt, J., and Morrisey, M. (1995). Case study: obsessive-compulsive disorder after severe traumatic brain injury in an adolescent. *J Am Acad Child Adolesc Psychiatry,* 34:45–49.

Modell, J.G., Mountz, J.M., Curtis, G.C., and Greden, J.F. (1989) Neurophysiologic dysfunction in basal ganglia/limbic striatal and thalamocortical circuits as a pathogenetic mechanism of obsessive-compulsive disorder. *J Neuropsychiatry Clin Neurosci* 1:27–36.

Molliver, M.E. (1987) Serotonergic neuronal systems: what their anatomic organization tells us about function. *J Clin Psychopharmacol* 7:3S–23S.

Mordecai, D., Shaw, R.J., Fisher, P.G., Mittelstadt, P.A., Guterman, T., and Donaldson, S.S. (2000) Case study: suprasellar germinoma presenting with psychotic and obsessive-compulsive symptoms. *J Am Acad Child Adolesc Psychiatry* 39:116–119.

Nestadt, G., Samuels, J., Riddle, M., Bienvenu, O.J., Liang, K.Y., LaBuda, M., Walkup, J., Grados, M., and Hoehn-Saric, R. (2000) A family study of obsessive-compulsive disorder. *Arch Gen Psychiatry* 57:358–363.

Obeso, J.A., Rodriguez-Oroz, M.C., Rodriguez, M., Lanciego, J.L., Artieda, J., Gonzalo, N. (2000) Pathophysiology of the basal ganglia in Parkinson's disease. *Trends Neurosci* 23, S8–S19.

O'Donnell, P., Levin, A., Enquist, L.W., Grace, A.A., Card, J.P. (1997) Interconnected parallel circuits between rat nucleus accumbens and thalamus revealed by retrograde transynaptic transport of pseudorabies vaccine. *J. Neurosci* 17, 2143–2167.

Perugi, G., Akiskal, H.S., Gemignani, A., Pfanner, C., Presta, S., Milanfranchi, A., Lensi, P., Ravagli, S., Maremmani, I., and Cassano, G.B. (1998). Episodic course in obsessive-compulsive disorder. *Eur Arch Psychiatry Clin Neurosci* 248:240–244.

Pujol, J., Torres, L., Deus, J., Cardoner, N., Pifarre, J., Capdevila, A., and Vallejo, J. (1999) Functional magnetic resonance imaging study of frontal lobe activation during word generation in obsessive-compulsive disorder. *Biol Psychiatry*, 45:891–897.

Rasmussen, S.A. and Tsuang, M.T. (1984) The epidemiology of obsessive compulsive disorder. *J Clin Psychiatry* 45:450–457.

Rauch, S.L., Jenike, M.A., Alpert, N.M., Baer, L., Breiter, H.C., Savage, C.R., and Fischman, A.J. (1994) Regional cerebral blood flow measured during symptom provocation in obsessive-compulsive disorder using oxygen 15-labeled carbon dioxide and positron emission tomography. *Arch Gen Psychiatry* 51:62–70.

Rauch, S.L., Savage, C.R., Alpert, N.M., Dougherty, D., Kendrick, A., Curran, T., Brown, H.D., Manzo, P., Fischman, A.J., and Jenike, M.A. (1997) Probing striatal function in obsessive-compulsive disorder: a PET study of implicit sequence learning. *J Neuropsychiatry Clin Neurosci* 9:568–573.

Reddy, P.S., Reddy, Y.C., Srinath, S., Khanna, S., Sheshadri, S.P., and Girimaji, S.R. (2001) A family study of juvenile obsessive-compulsive disorder. *Can J Psychiatry* 46:346–351.

Riddle, M.A., Scahill, L., King, R., Hardin, M.T., Towbin, K.E., Ort, S.I., Leckman, J.F., and Cohen, D.J. (1990) Obsessive compulsive disorder in children and adolescents: phenomenology and family history. *J Am Acad Child Adolesc Psychiatry* 29:766–772.

Ridley, R.M. (1994) The psychology of perserverative and stereotyped behaviour. *Prog Neurobiol* 44:221–231.

Robinson, D., Wu, H., Munne, R.A., Ashtari, M., Alvir, J.M., Lerner, G., Koreen, A., Cole, K., and Bogerts, B. (1995) Reduced caudate nucleus volume in obsessive-compulsive disorder. *Arch Gen Psychiatry* 52:393–398.

Rosenberg, D.R., Keshavan, M.S., Dick, E.L., Bagwell, W.W., MacMaster, F.P., and Birmaher, B. (1997a) Corpus callosal morphology in treatment-naive pediatric obsessive compulsive disorder. *Prog Neuropsychopharmacol Biol Psychiatry* 21:1269–1283.

Rosenberg, D.R., Keshavan, M.S., O'Hearn, K.M., Dick, E.L., Bagwell, W.W., Seymour, A.B., Montrose, D.M., Pierri, J.N., and Birmaher, B. (1997b) Frontostriatal measurement in treatment-naive children with obsessive-compulsive disorder. *Arch Gen Psychiatry* 54:824–830.

Rosenberg, D.R., MacMaster, F.P., Keshavan, M.S., Fitzgerald, K.D., Stewart, C.M., and Moore, G.J. (2000) Decrease in caudate glutamatergic concentrations in pediatric obsessive-compulsive disorder patients taking paroxetine. *J Am Acad Child Adolesc Psychiatry* 39:1096–1103.

Saxena, S., Brody, A.L., Schwartz, J.M., and Baxter, L.R. (1998) Neuroimaging and frontal-subcortical circuitry in obsessive-compulsive disorder. *Br J Psychiatry Suppl* 35:26–37.

Schoepp, D.D., Jane, D.E., and Monn, J.A. (1999) Pharmacological agents acting at subtypes of metabotropic glutamate receptors. *Neuropharmacology*, 38:1431–1476.

Sleight, A.J., Cervenka, A., and Peroutka, S.J. (1990). In vivo effects of sumatriptan (GR 43175) on extracellular levels of 5-HT in the guinea pig. *Neuropharmacology* 29:511–513.

Swedo, S.E. (1994) Sydenham's chorea. A model for childhood autoimmune neuropsychiatric disorders. *JAMA* 272:1788–1791.

Swedo, S.E., Pietrini, P., Leonard, H.L., Schapiro, M.B., Rettew, D.C., Goldberger, E.L., Rapoport, S.I., Rapoport, J.L., and Grady, C.L. (1992) Cerebral glucose metabolism in childhood-onset obsessive-compulsive disorder. Revisualization during pharmacotherapy. *Arch Gen Psychiatry* 49:690–694.

Swedo, S.E., Rapoport, J.L., Leonard, H., Lenane, M., and Cheslow, D. (1989a) Obsessive-compulsive disorder in children and adolescents. Clinical phenomenology of 70 consecutive cases. *Arch Gen Psychiatry* 46:335–341.

Swedo, S.E., Schapiro, M.B., Grady, C.L., Cheslow, D.L., Leonard, H.L., Kumar, A., Friedland, R., Rapoport, S.I., and Rapoport, J.L. (1989b) Cerebral glucose metabolism in childhood-onset obsessive-compulsive disorder. *Arch Gen Psychiatry* 46:518–523.

Swoboda, K.J. and Jenike, M.A. (1995) Frontal abnormalities in a patient with obsessive-compulsive disorder: the role of structural lesions in obsessive-compulsive behavior. *Neurology* 45:2130–2134.

Szeszko, P.R., Robinson, D., Alvir, J.M., Bilder, R.M., Lencz, T., Ashtari, M., Wu, H., and Bogerts, B. (1999) Orbital frontal and amygdala volume reductions in obsessive-compulsive disorder. *Arch Gen Psychiatry* 56:913–919.

Tallis, F. (1997) The neuropsychology of obsessive-compulsive disorder: a review and consideration of clinical implications. *Br J Clin Psychol*, 36:3–20.

Thomsen, P.H. (1995a) Obsessive-compulsive disorder in children and adolescents. A 6–22 year follow-up study of social outcome. *Eur Child Adolesc Psychiatry* 4:112–122.

Thomsen, P.H. (1995b) Obsessive-compulsive disorder in children and adolescents: a study of parental psychopathology and precipitating events in 20 consecutive Danish cases. *Psychopathology* 28:161–167.

Weiss, A.P. and Jenike, M.A. (2000) Late-onset obsessive-compulsive disorder: a case series. *J Neuropsychiatry Clin Neurosci* 12:265–268.

Wichmann, T., Bergman, H., and DeLong, M.R. (1994) The primate subthalamic nucleus. III. Changes in motor behavior and neuronal activity in the internal pallidum induced by subthalamic inactivation in the MPTP model of parkinsonism. *J Neurophysiol* 72:521–530.

13 | Neurobiology of tic disorders, including Tourette's syndrome

JAMES F. LECKMAN, CHIN-BIN YEH, AND PAUL J. LOMBROSO

Tic disorders are chronic conditions that are frequently associated with difficulties in self-esteem, family life, social acceptance, or school or job performance that are directly related to the presence of motor and/or phonic tics. Although tic symptoms have been reported since antiquity, systematic study of individuals with tic disorders dates from the nineteenth century.

In addition to tics, individuals with tic disorders may present with a broad array of behavioral difficulties including disinhibited speech or conduct, impulsivity, distractibility, motoric hyperactivity, and obsessive-compulsive symptoms (Leckman and Cohen, 1998). Alternatively, a sizable portion of children and adolescents with tics will be free of coexisting developmental or emotional difficulties. Scientific opinion has been divided on how broadly to conceive the spectrum of maladaptive behaviors associated with Tourette's syndrome (TS) (Comings, 1988; Shapiro et al., 1988).

In this chapter, a presentation of the phenomenology and classification of tic disorders precedes a review of the neurobiological substrates of these conditions. The general perspective presented is that TS and related disorders are model neurobiological disorders in which to study multiple interactive genetic and environmental mechanisms that interact over the course of development.

DEFINITIONS AND CLASSIFICATIONS

A *tic* is a sudden, repetitive movement, gesture, or utterance that typically mimics some fragment of normal behavior. Tics are perhaps best seen as motor primitives that normally are used to construct voluntary movement and vocalizations but that are misplaced in context. Usually of brief duration, individual tics rarely last more than a second. Tics tend to occur in bouts with brief inter-tic intervals (Peterson and Leckman, 1998). Most tics can also be voluntarily suppressed for brief periods of time.

Individual tics can occur singly or together in an orchestrated pattern. They vary in their intensity or forcefulness. Motor tics vary from simple, abrupt movements such as eye blinking, head jerks, or shoulder shrugs to more complex, purposive appearing behaviors such as facial expressions or gestures of the arms or head. In extreme cases, these movements can be obscene or self-injurious. Phonic or vocal tics can range from simple throat-clearing sounds to more complex vocalizations and speech. In severe cases, coprolalia is present.

By the age of 10 years, most individuals with tics are aware of premonitory urges. These urges are typically localized to a particular body region where the tic is about to occur (Leckman et al., 1993). A majority of patients also report a fleeting sense of relief following a tic. These premonitory urges contribute to the understanding that tics are in part an intentional response to unpleasant stimuli. Indeed, most adult subjects describe their tics as either "voluntary" or as having both voluntary and involuntary aspects. In contrast, many younger children are oblivious to their tics and experience them as wholly involuntary movements or sounds.

Clinicians characterize tics by their anatomical location, number, frequency, and duration. The intensity or "forcefulness" of the tic can also be an important characteristic as some tics call attention to themselves simply by virtue of their exaggerated character. Finally, tics vary in terms of their *complexity*, which usually refers to how simple or involved a movement or sound is, ranging from brief, meaningless, abrupt fragments (simple tics) to ones that are longer, more involved, and seemingly more goal directed in character (complex tics). Each of these elements has been incorporated into clinician rating scales that have proven to be useful in monitoring tic severity (Leckman et al., 1989).

Diagnostic Categories

Several widely used diagnostic classifications currently include sections on tic disorders. These include both the classification system published by the American Psychiatric Association (1994) and the criteria by the World Health Organization (1996). A third classification system, the Classification of Tic Disorders (CTD), has been offered by the Tourette Syndrome Classification Study Group (1993). Although clear differences exist comparing these classification schemes, they are broadly congruent.

Prevalence

Transient tic behaviors are commonplace among children. Community surveys indicate that 1% to 13% of boys and 1% to 11% of girls manifest "frequent" "tics, twitches, mannerisms or habit spasms" (see Zohar et al., 1998, for review). Children between the ages of 7 and 11 years appear to have the highest estimated prevalence rates, in the range of 5%. Although boys are more commonly affected with tic behaviors than girls, the malefemale ratio in most community surveys is less than 2 to 1. Similar estimates have been reported from North Carolina (Costello et al., 1996). Although most reports on tics have come from European, American, and Asian sources, race and socioeconomic status have not been shown to influence the point prevalence of tics.

There is less certainty concerning the prevalence of TS. In the largest study to date, Apter and colleagues (1993) have reported a prevalence rate of 4.5 10,000 for full-blown TS among 16- to 17-year-olds in Israel. Using a similar design, Costello et al. (1996) examined 4500 children 9, 11, and 13 years of age in rural North Carolina. The children were directly examined, as was one parent; both were asked about tic symptoms occurring over the preceding 3 months. Altogether, 10/10,000 children met criteria for TS, 13/10,000 for boys and 7/10,000 for girls.

More recently, Mason et al. (1998) completed a study of all pupils, aged 13 to 14 years, in a mainstream secondary school in the United Kingdom. Five subjects were identified as having TS, yielding a prevalence estimate of 299/10,000 pupils in this age group. Similar findings have recently been reported from Sweden (Kadesjo and Gillberg, 2000). The results from these studies suggest that TS in the community is more common and milder than earlier population-based studies would suggest.

Coexisting Conditions

The past decade has seen a renewed emphasis on the range of neurological and psychiatric symptoms seen in TS patients. Symptoms associated with obsessive-compulsive disorder (OCD) and attention-deficit hyperactivity disorder (ADHD) have received the most attention.

Obsessive-compulsive symptoms

Clinical and epidemiological studies indicate that more than 40% of individuals with TS experience recurrent obsessive-compulsive (OC) symptoms (King et al., 1998). Genetic, neurobiological, and treatment response studies suggest that there may be qualitative differences between tic-related forms of OCD and cases of OCD in which there is no personal or family history of tics.

Symptomatically the most common OC symptoms encountered in TS patients are obsessions about aggression, sex, religion, and the body, as well as related checking compulsions; and obsessions concerning a need for symmetry or exactness, repeating rituals, counting compulsions, and ordering/arranging compulsions (Leckman et al., 1997).

Coexisting attention deficit hyperactivity disorder

Clinical and epidemiological studies sharply differ on rates of ADHD seen among individuals with TS (Walkup et al., 1998). Clinical studies vary according to setting and established referral patterns, but it is not uncommon to see reports of 50% or more of referred children with TS diagnosed with comorbid ADHD. In contrast, epidemiological studies typically indicate a much lower rate of comorbidity (Apter et al., 1993).

Although the etiological relationship between TS and ADHD is in dispute, it is clear that those individuals with both TS and ADHD are at a much greater risk for a variety of untoward outcomes (Carter et al., 2000). Uninformed peers frequently tease individuals with TS. They are often regarded as less likeable, more aggressive, and more withdrawn than their classmates (Bawden et al., 1998). These social difficulties are amplified in a child with TS who also has ADHD. In such cases, their level of social skill is often several years behind their peers.

Negative appraisal by peers in childhood is a strong predictor of global indices of psychopathology. This appears to be particularly true for children with TS and ADHD. Longitudinal studies confirm that these individuals are at high risk for anxiety and mood disorders, oppositional defiant disorder, and conduct disorder (Carter et al., 2000). Much of this negative impact appears to be due to the ADHD, as children who just have TS tend to fare better (Spencer et al., 1998); (Carter et al., 2000). Indeed, levels of tic severity are less predictive of peer acceptance than is the presence of ADHD (Bawden et al., 1998).

Other developmental disorders

Children with a range of developmental disorders appear to be at increased risk for tic disorders. Kurlan and colleagues (1994) reported a fourfold increase in the prevalence of tic disorders among children in special educational settings in a single school district in upstate New York. These children were not mentally retarded but did have significant learning disabilities or other physical impairments.

Children with pervasive developmental disorders are also at higher risk for developing TS. In a recent survey of 447 pupils from nine schools for children and adolescents with autism, 19 children were found to have definite TS, yielding a prevalence rate of 4.3% (Baron-Cohen et al., 1999). However, caution is warranted, as complex motor tics can be difficult to distinguish from motor stereotypies, and differentiation among these behaviors may be especially problematic among retarded individuals with limited verbal skills.

NEURAL SUBSTRATES OF HABIT FORMATION AND TICS

Conceptually, tics are best seen as senseless habits that arise in response to a highly selective set of somatic and/or environmental cues. Habits, like tics, are assembled routines that link sensory cues with motor action. The neural substrates of habit formation and tics are neural loops that connect the basal ganglia with the cortex and thalamus (Fig. 13.1; Graybiel, 1998; Leckman and Riddle, 2000).

The motor, sensorimotor, association, and inhibitory neural circuits that course through the basal ganglia are commonly referred to by their successive processing components, and are designated *cortical-striatal-thalamo-cortical* (CSTC) circuits. These circuits are composed of multiple, partially overlapping, but largely "parallel" circuits that direct information from the cerebral cortex to the subcortex, and then back again to specific regions of the cortex, thereby forming multiple cortical–subcortical loops. Although multiple anatomically and functionally related cortical regions provide input, each circuit in turn refocuses its projections back onto only a discrete subset of the cortical regions initially contributing to that circuit's input. Within the basal ganglia and thalamus, each of the circuits appears to be microscopically segregated from others that course through the same macroscopic structure—hence the conceptualization of these overlapping pathways as being parallel.

Advances in neuroimaging and neurophysiological techniques have made it possible to examine these circuits in living subjects. In TS there is preliminary evidence that voluntary tic suppression involves activation of regions of the prefrontal cortex and caudate nucleus and bilateral deactivation of the putamen and globus pallidus (GP) (Peterson et al., 1998a). If confirmed, these findings are consistent with the well-known finding that chemical or electrical stimulation of inputs into the putamen can provoke motor and vocal responses that resemble tics. They also suggest that prefrontal cortex–basal ganglia circuits participate in shaping of the inhibitory influence of the output neurons in the internal segment of the GP and the pars reticulata of the substania nigra. Transcranial magnetic stimulation (TMS) studies have found decreased neuronal inhibition and a reduced cortical silent period in the primary motor area in TS as well as in OCD (Ziemann et al., 1997); (Greenberg et al., 2000). These data suggest abnormal cortical excitability. These findings are consistent with the hypothesis that tics in TS and the obsessions and compulsions in OCD originate either from a primarily subcortical disorder affecting the motor cortex through disinhibited afferent signals or from impaired inhibition directly at the level of the motor cortex or both.

Neuromodulatory and Neurotransmitter Systems

Extensive immunohistochemical studies of the basal ganglia have demonstrated the presence of a wide spectrum of classic neurotransmitters, neuromodulators, and neuropeptides. The functional status of a number of these systems has been evaluated in TS.

Dopaminergic systems

Inputs from ascending dopamine pathways originating in the substania nigra, pars compacta, play a crucial role in coordinating the output from the striatum (Aosaki et al., 1994). Explicit dopamine hypotheses for Tourette's syndrome posit either an excess of dopamine or an increased sensitivity of D_2 dopamine re-

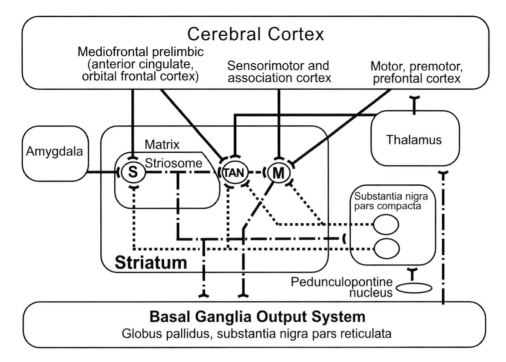

FIGURE 13.1 Cortical–subcortical circuits implicated in tics and stereotypies. Schematic diagram illustrating the organization of the striatum and cortical–subcortical circuits (adapted from Aosaki et al., 1994). Animal models indicate that the medium spiny projection (MSP) neurons of the striatum exist within two intertwined compartments, striosomes (S) and the matrix (M). These two compartments differ with respect to their cortical inputs with the striosomal MSP neurons receiving limbic and prelimbic inputs and the MSP neurons in the matrix receiving inputs from ipsilateral primary motor and sensory motor cortices and contralateral primary motor cortices. An imbalance in the functional activity of the MSP neurons within these two compartments has been implicated in motor stereotypies (Canales and Graybiel, 2000). Similarly, changes in the responsiveness of tonically active neurons located at the boundary between striosomes and matrix could selectively alter behaviors keyed to specific environmental perturbations. Dopaminergic projection neurons from the substania nigra appear to tune this system to respond selectively to certain internal somatosensory or external perceptual cues. Likewise, the antineuronal antibodies found in some TS patients could modulate synaptic transmission and alter the balance between the striosomal and matrisomal compartments of the striatum (see text under Animal models). Key to neurotransmitters: glutamate ▬◀; GABA ▬ · ◀; dopamine ▪▪▪◀; and acetylcholine ▬ ▬◀.

ceptors. These hypotheses are consistent with multiple lines of empirical evidence as well as emerging data from animal models of habit formation. First, data implicating central dopaminergic mechanisms include the results of double-blind clinical trials in which haloperidol, pimozide, tiapride, and other neuroleptics that preferentially block dopaminergic D_2 receptors have been found to be effective in the temporary suppression of tics for a majority of patients (see Chappell et al., 1997, for review). Second, tic suppression has also been reported following administration of agents such as tetrabenazine that reduce dopamine synthesis (see Shapiro and Shapiro, 1988, for review). Third, increased tics have been reported following withdrawal of neuroleptics or following exposure to agents that increase central dopaminergic activity such as lev-

odopa (I-dopa) and central nervous system (CNS) stimulants, including cocaine (see Anderson et al., 1998, for review). Fourth, preliminary positron emission tomography (PET) studies of brain dopamine D_2 receptors provide some evidence that the density and/ or binding of D_2 receptors in the striatum are associated with current levels of tic severity (Wolf et al., 1996). Fourth, postmortem brain and ligand-based neuroimaging studies have reported alterations in the number or affinity of dopamine transporter molecules that act to take released dopamine back into presynaptic terminals in the striatum (Singer et al., 1991; (Malison et al., 1995). Other studies have also implicated the presynaptic processing of dopamine (Ernst et al., 1999). However, a recent assessment of the number of striatal vesicular monoamine transporter type-2 sites found no differences between TS patients and controls (Meyer et al., 1999). In sum, while the evidence that dopaminergic pathways are intimately involved in the formation of habits and the pathobiology of TS is compelling, the exact nature of the abnormality remains to be elucidated.

Excitatory amino acid systems

The excitatory neurotransmitter glutamate is released upon depolarization by the corticostratial, corticosubthalamic, subthalamic, and thalamocortical projection neurons. As such, these excitatory neurons are key players in the functional anatomy of the basal ganglia and the CSTC loops. While the activity of these neurons is likely to be important in TS, only limited data are available to evaluate their role in this disease.

Inhibitory amino acid systems

Neurons containing inhibitory amino acid neurotransmitters, particularly gamma-aminobutyric acid (GABA), also form major portions of CSTC loops. These include GABAergic medium spiny projection (MSP) neurons of the striatum that project to the internal segment of the GP and the pars reticulata of the substantia nigra within the direct pathway. GABAergic neurons are also present in the indirect pathway that relays information from the striatum to the external segment of the GP and from there to the internal segment of the GP. An imbalance between the output from the striosomal compartment and that from the matriosomal striatal compartment has been hypothesized in TS (Fig. 1; Leckman and Riddle, 2000).

Cholinergic systems

The large but rare aspiny interneurons found throughout the striatum are likely to be critically involved in the coordination of striatal response through interactions with central dopaminergic and GABAergic neurons (Aosaki et al., 1994). Specifically, cholinergic tonically active neurons are thought to be present at the striosomal boundaries and likely mediate the functional interface between the striatal compartments. In addition, cholinergic projections from the basal forebrain are found throughout the cortex and within key structures of the basal ganglia and mesencephalon, including the internal segment of the GP, the pars reticulata of the substantia nigra, and the locus coeruleus. Evidence of cholinergic involvement in the pathobiology of TS concerns the reported potentiation of D_2 dopamine receptor blocking agents through the use of transdermal nicotine or nicotine gum (Sanberg et al.,

1997) and more recent reports of the usefulness of a noncompetitive cholinergic agonist, mecamylamine (Silver et al., 2001). Unfortunately, the efficacy of these agents has yet to be evaluated in a double-blind trial.

Endogenous opioid peptides

Endogenous opioid peptides (EOP) are localized in structures of the extrapyramidal system, are known to interact with central dopaminergic and GABAergic neurons, and are likely to be importantly involved in the gating of motor functions. Two of the three families of EOPs, dynorphin and met-enkephalin, are highly concentrated and similarly distributed in the basal ganglia and substantia nigra. In addition, significant levels of opiate receptor binding have been detected in both primate and human neostriatum and substantia nigra.

The EOPs have been directly implicated in the pathophysiology of TS syndrome. Haber and co-workers (1986) reported decreased levels of dynorphin A(1–17) immunoreactivity in striatal fibers projecting to the GP in postmortem material from a small number of Tourette's patients. This observation, coupled with the neuroanatomic distribution of dynorphin, its broad range of motor and behavioral effects, and its modulatory interactions with striatal dopaminergic systems, suggest that dynorphin might have a key role in the pathobiology of TS. However, subsequent studies have failed to confirm these initial observations (van Wattum et al., 1999).

Noradrenergic systems

Noradrenergic projections from the locus coeruleus project widely to the prefrontal and other cortical regions. Noradrenergic pathways are also likely to indirectly influence central dopaminergic pathways via projections to areas near the ventral tegmental area (Grenhoff and Svensson, 1989). Speculation that noradrenergic mechanisms might be relevant to the pathobiology of TS was based initially on the beneficial effects of α_2-adrenergic agonists, including clonidine (Cohen et al., 1979). Although clonidine is one of the most widely prescribed agents for the treatment of tics, its effectiveness remains controversial (Goetz et al., 1987; Leckman et al., 1991). In open and double-blind trials, another related α_2-adrenergic agonist, guanfacine, has been reported to reduce tics and improve ADHD symptoms (Scahill et al., 2001). At the level of receptor function, clonidine has been traditionally viewed as a selective α_2 adrenoceptor agonist active at presynaptic sites, and its primary mode of action may be its ability to reduce the firing rate and the release of norepinephrine from central noradrenergic neurons. However, evidence of heterogeneity among the α_2 class of adrenoceptors and their distinctive distribution within relevant brain regions adds further complexity to treatment of tic disorders. Specifically, differential effects in cortical regions mediated by specific receptor subtypes may account for the differential responsiveness of particular behavioral features of this syndrome to treatment with clonidine versus guanfacine (Arnsten, 2000).

The involvement of the noradrenergic pathways may be one of the mechanisms by which stressors influence tic severity. For example, a series of adult TS patients were found to have elevated levels of cerebrospinal fluid (CSF) norepinephrine (Leckman et al., 1995) and to have excreted high levels of urinary norepinephrine in response to the stress of lumbar puncture (Chappell et al., 1994). These elevated levels of CSF norepinephrine may also contribute to the elevation in CSF corticotopin-releasing factor levels seen in some TS patients (Chappell et al., 1996).

Serotonergic systems

Ascending serotonergic projections from the dorsal raphe have been repeatedly invoked as playing a role in the pathophysiology of both TS and OCD. The most compelling evidence relates to OCD and is based largely on the well-established efficacy of potent serotonin reuptake inhibitors (SRIs) such as clomipramine and fluvoxamine in the treatment of OCD. However, some investigators have reported that the SRIs are less effective in treating tic-related OCD than in treating other forms of OCD (McDougle et al., 1993). Preliminary postmortem brain studies in TS have suggested that serotonin and the related compounds tryptophan and 5-hydroxy-indoleacetic acid may be globally decreased in the basal ganglia and other areas receiving projections from the dorsal raphe (Anderson et al., 1998).

GENETIC SUSCEPTIBILITY

Twin and Family Studies

Tourette's Syndrome is a familial disorder (Pauls et al., 1991; Walkup et al., 1996). Twin and family studies provide evidence that genetic factors are involved in the vertical transmission within families of a vulnerability to TS and related disorders. The concordance rate for TS among monozygotic twin pairs is 50% while the concordance of dizygotic twin pairs is about 10% (Price et al., 1985). If co-twins with chronic motor tic disorder are included, these concordance figures increase to 77% for monozygotic and 30% for dizygotic twin pairs. Differences in the concordance of monozygotic and dizygotic twin pairs indicate that genetic factors play an important role in the etiology of TS syndrome and related conditions. These figures also suggest that nongenetic factors are critical in determining the nature and severity of the clinical syndrome. Other studies indicate that first-degree family members of TS probands are at substantially higher risk for developing TS, chronic motor tic disorder, and OCD than unrelated individuals (Pauls et al., 1991; Walkup et al., 1996). The pattern of vertical transmission among family members has led several groups of investigators to test whether mathematical models of specific genetic hypotheses could be rejected. While not definitive, most segregation analyses could not rule out models of autosomal transmission (Walkup et al., 1996). These studies in turn prompted the identification of large multigenerational families for genetic linkage studies.

Thus far, two areas, one on chromosome 4q and another on chromosome 8p, are suggestive of linkage, based on the results of a genome-wide scan of affected sibling pairs (Tourette Syndrome International Consortium for Genetics, 1999). Through a second genome scan, using data from a large multigenerational Canadian family, a promising region on chromosome 11 (11q23) has been identified (Merrette et al., 2000). Future progress is anticipated. Clarity about the nature and normal expression of even a few of the TS susceptibility genes is likely to provide a major step toward in understanding TS pathogenesis.

ENVIRONMENTAL INFLUENCES

Gender-Specific Endocrine Factors

Males are more frequently affected with TS than females. While this could be due to genetic mechanisms, frequent male-to-male transmissions within families appear to rule out the presence of an X-linked vulnerability gene. This observation has led us to hypothesize that androgenic steroids act at key developmental periods to influence the natural history of TS and related disorders (Peterson et al., 1992). The importance of gender differences in expression of associated phenotypes is also clear, given the observation that women are more likely than men to develop OC symptoms without concomitant tics (Pauls et al., 1991) and that boys are much more likely than girls to display disruptive behaviors (Comings and Comings, 1987).

Surges in testosterone and other androgenic steroids during critical periods in fetal development are known to be involved in the formation of structural CNS dimorphisms (Sikich and Todd, 1988). In recent years, several sexually dimorphic brain regions have been described. These regions contain high levels of androgen and estrogen receptors and are known to influence activity in the basal ganglia both directly and indirectly. Further support for a role for androgens comes from anecdotal reports of tic exacerbation following androgen use and from trials of antiandrogens in patients with severe TS and/or OCD (Peterson and Leckman, 1998). In the most rigorous study to date, Peterson and colleagues (1998b) found that the therapeutic effects of the antiandrogen, flutamide, were modest in magnitude and these effects were short-lived, possibly because of physiologic compensation for androgen receptor blockade.

Perinatal Risk Factors

The search for nongenetic factors that mediate the expression of a genetic vulnerability to TS and related disorders has also focused on the role of adverse perinatal events. This interest dates from the report of Pasamanick and Kawi (1956), who found that mothers of children with tics were 1.5 times more likely to have experienced a complication during pregnancy than the mothers of children without tics. Other investigations have reported that among monozygotic twins discordant for TS syndrome, the index twins with TS had lower birth weights than their unaffected co-twins (Hyde et al., 1992). Severity of maternal life stress during pregnancy and severe nausea and/or vomiting during the first trimester have also emerged as potential risk factors in the development of tic disorders (Leckman et al., 1990). In 1997, Whitaker and co-workers reported that premature and low–birth weight children are at increased risk of developing tic disorders and ADHD. This appears to be especially true of children who had ischemic parenchymal brain lesions. Finally, there is limited evidence that smoking and alcohol use, as well as forceps delivery, can predispose individuals with a vulnerability to TS to develop comorbid OCD (Santangelo et al., 1994). The mechanisms responsible for the impact of these perinatal factors may involve differential ischemic injury to the striatal compartments or the establishment of a heightened degree of stress response that could also lead to the differential activation of striatal compartments.

Psychological Stress and Emotional Arousal

Tic disorders have long been identified as stress-sensitive conditions (Silva et al., 1995). Typically,

symptom exacerbations follow in the wake of stressful life events. These events need not be adverse in character. Clinical experience suggests that, in some unfortunate instances, the family and teachers hope to suppress the symptoms by punishment and humiliation. This can initiate a vicious cycle in which tic symptoms are misunderstood and the stress on the child mounts, which in turn can lead to a further exacerbation of symptoms and further increase in stress in the child's interpersonal environment. Although psychological factors are insufficient to cause TS, the intimate association of the content and timing of tic behaviors and dynamically important events in the lives of children make it difficult to overlook their contribution to the intramorbid course of these disorders (Carter et al., 2000).

In addition to the intramorbid effects of stress and anxiety that have been well characterized, premorbid stress may also play an important role as a sensitizing agent in the pathogenesis of TS among vulnerable individuals (Leckman et al., 1984). It is likely that the immediate family environment, e.g., parental discord, and the coping abilities of family members are factors in TS pathogenesis (Leckman et al., 1990), and these may lead to a sensitization of stress-responsive biological systems such as the hypothalamic–pituitary–adrenal axis and the differential activation of the striosomal striatal compartment (see above, Chappell et al., 1994, 1996; Leckman et al., 1995).

Postinfectious Autoimmune Mechanisms

The past decade has seen the reemergence of an area of research that is examining the hypothesis that postinfectious autoimmune mechanisms contribute to the pathogenesis of some TS cases. Speculation concerning a postinfectious (or at least a post–rheumatic fever) etiology for tic disorder symptoms dates from the late 1800s. It is well established that group A beta hemolytic streptococci (GABHS) can trigger immune-mediated disease in genetically predisposed individuals. Acute rheumatic fever (RF) is a delayed sequela of GABHS, occurring approximately 3 weeks following an inadequately treated upper respiratory tract infection. Rheumatic fever is characterized by inflammatory lesions involving the joints, heart, and/or CNS (Sydenham's chorea [SC]).

Sydenham's chorea and TS share common anatomic areas—the basal ganglia of the brain and the related cortical and thalamic sites. Furthermore, some SC patients display motor and vocal tics, OC, and ADHD symptoms, suggesting the possibility that at least in some instances these disorders share a common etiology. As in SC, antineuronal antibodies have been reported to be elevated in the sera of some patients with TS (Singer et al., 1998). It has been proposed that Pediatric autoimmune neuropsychiatric dissorders associated with streptococcal infections (PANDAS) represent a distinct clinical entity, and includes SC and some cases of TS and OCD. Further suggestive evidence comes from Swedo and colleagues (1998), who reported that in children who met PANDAS criteria, GABHS infection was likely to have preceded neuropsychiatric symptom onset for 44% of the children, whereas pharyngitis (no culture obtained) preceded onset for another 28% of the children.

Although the etiological significance of the antineuronal antibodies and the association with prior GABHS infections remains a topic of considerable debate, it is clear that a minority of TS patients have such antibodies (Singer et al., 1998; Morshed et al., 2001) and that therapeutic interventions based on this mechanism show promise (Perlmutter et al., 1999). Furthermore, if specific immunological alterations are associated with onset or acute clinical exacerbations, then the nature of these alterations should provide insight in to the genetic, neuroanatomic, and immunologic mechanisms involved. This knowledge may provide a basis for the rational design of therapeutic and preventative interventions.

ANIMAL MODELS

Future progress in elucidating the pathogenesis and treatment of TS could be greatly accelerated with the development of animal models. At present, stimulant and stress-induced stereotypies continue to offer the greatest promise (Fig. 13.1; Leckman and Riddle, 2000). If tics, like stereotypies, vary according to the balance of activity of MSP neurons in the striosome and matrix compartments of the striatum (Fig. 13.1; Canales and Graybiel, 2000), then it should be possible to examine the clinical impact of genetic and/or developmental insults that affect the relative number and sensitivity of MSP neurons in the two striatal compartments. For example, perinatal ischemic and hypoxic insults involving parenchymal lesions increase the risk of tic disorders eightfold (Whitaker et al., 1997). Do they also increase an animal's susceptibility to develop stereotypies in response to psychomotor stimulants? If so, is there evidence of a differential injury to MSP neurons in the matrix?

This model may provide a meaningful integration of knowledge about tics that is drawn from a number of perspectives, including the stress responsiveness of tics

(limbic activation), the presence of premonitory sensory urges (as sensory motor and primary motor cortical inputs converge on the fewer MSPs in the matrix), the reduction of tics when an individual is engaged in acts that require selective attention and guided motor action (heightened activity within the matrix compartment), and the need to even up sensory and motor stimuli in a bilaterally symmetrical fashion (convergence of information from both ipsi- and contralateral primary motor neurons on MSP within the matrix). The timing of tics and the course of tic disorders may be reflected in the collective burst firing of dopaminergic neurons.

From a developmental perspective, it is clear that many of the GABAergic interneurons of the cerebral cortex migrate tangentially from the same embryonic regions in the ganglionic eminence that also give rise to the GABAergic MSP neurons of the striatum (Ware et al., 1999). Could adverse events occurring at a specific point in development account for both the striatal imbalance and the intracortical deficits inhibition seen in some patients with TS (Ziemann et al., 1997)?

Finally, it is tempting to speculate that in SC and postinfectious forms of TS the functional activity of the MSP neurons of the matrix is differentially impaired as a result of the autoimmune response. Indeed, preliminary data suggest that either bilateral striatal infusion into rats of antineuronal antibodies from TS patients or the immunization of mice with rat striatal homogenates may produce animal models of TS complete with stereotypical movements and audible vocalizations (Hallett et al., 2000; Hoffman and Lipkin, 2000). One plausible hypothesis is that the antineural antibodies found in a subset of TS patients may modulate synaptic transmission and alter the balance between the striosomal and matrisomal compartments of the striatum (Leckman and Riddle, 2000).

CONCLUSION AND FUTURE PROSPECTS

Current conceptualizations of TS have been shaped by advances in systems neuroscience and the emerging understanding of the role of the basal ganglia in implicit learning and habit formation. Although the evidence that the same mechanisms are involved in both habit formation and tics is circumstantial, recent progress in neuroanatomy, systems neuroscience, and functional in vivo neuroimaging has set the stage for a major advance in our understanding of TS. Continued success in these areas will lead to the targeting of specific brain circuits for more intensive study. Diagnostic, treatment, and prognostic advances can also be anticipated—e.g., which circuits are involved and to what degree? How does that degree of involvement affect the patient's symptomatic course and outcome? Will it be possible to track treatment response using neuroimaging techniques? And will specific circuit-based therapies using deep-brain stimulation emerge to treat refractory cases (Vandewalle et al., 1999)? In addition, a deeper understanding of the factors that alter the functional balance between striatal compartments may lead directly to the testing of novel pharmacological agents.

The identification of susceptibility genes in TS will doubtless point in new therapeutic directions for treatment, as will the characterization of the putative autoimmune mechanisms active in the PANDAS subgroup of patients. Given this potential, TS can be considered a model disorder to study the dynamic interplay of genetic vulnerabilities, epigenetic events, and neurobiological systems active during early brain development. It is likely that the research paradigms used in these studies and many of the empirical findings resulting from them will be relevant to other disorders of childhood onset and to our understanding of normal development.

REFERENCES

American Psychiatric Association (1994) *Diagnostic and Statistical Manual of Mental Disorders, 4th ed.* Washington, DC: American Psychiatric Association Press.

Anderson, G.M., Leckman, J.F., and Cohen, D.J. (1998) Neurochemical and neuropeptide systems. In: Leckman, J.F. and Cohen, D.J. eds. *Tourette's Syndrome Tics, Obsessions, Compulsions—Developmental Psychopathology and Clinical Care.* New York: John Wiley and Sons, pp. 261–281.

Apter, A., Pauls, D., Bleich, A. Zohar, A.H., Kron, S., Ratzoni, G., Dycian, A., Kotler, M., Weizman, A., and Cohen, D.J. (1993) An epidemiological study of Gilles de la Tourette's syndrome in Israel. *Arch Gen Psychiatry* 50:734–738.

Aosaki, T., Graybiel, A.M., and Kimura, M. (1994). Effect of the nigrostriatal dopamine system on acquired neural responses in the striatum of behaving monkeys. *Science* 265:412–415.

Arnsten, A.F. (2000) Through the looking glass: differential noradenergic modulation of prefrontal cortical function. *Neural Plasticity* 7:33–46.

Baron-Cohen, S., Scahill, V.L., Izaguirre, J., Hornsey, H., and Robertson, M.M. (1999) The prevalence of Gilles de la Tourette syndrome in children and adolescents with autism: a large scale study. *Psychol Med* 29:1151–1159.

Bawden, H.N., Stokes, A., Camfield, C.S., Camfield, P.R., and Salisbury, S. (1998) Peer relationship problems in children with Tourette's disorder or diabetes mellitus. *J Child Psychol Psychiatry* 39:663–668.

Canales, J.J. and Graybiel, A.M. (2000) A measure of striatal function predicts motor stereotypy. *Nat Neurosci* 3:377–383.

Carter, A.S., O'Donnell, D.A., Schultz, R.T., Scahill, L., Leckman, J.F., and Pauls, D.L. (2000) Social and emotional adjustment in children affected with Gilles de la Tourette syndrome: associations with ADHD and family functioning. *J Child Psychol Psychiatry* 41:215–223.

Chappell, P., Leckman, J., Goodman, W., Bissette, G., Pauls, D., Anderson, G., Riddle, M., Scahill, L., McDougle, C., and Cohen, D. (1996) Elevated cerebrospinal fluid corticotropin-releasing factor in Tourette's syndrome: comparison to obsessive compulsive disorder and normal controls. *Biol Psychiatry* 39:776–783.

Chappell, P.B., Riddle, M., Anderson, G., Scahill, L., Hardin, M., Walker, D., Cohen, D., and Leckman, J. (1994) Enhanced stress responsivity of Tourette syndrome patients undergoing lumbar puncture. *Biol Psychiatry* 36:35–43.

Chappell, P.B., Scahill, L.D., and Leckman, J.F. (1997) Future therapies of Tourette syndrome. *Neurol Clin* 15:429–450.

Cohen, D.J., Young, J.G., Nathanson, J.A., and Shaywitz, B.A. (1979) Clonidine in Tourette's syndrome. *Lancet* 2:551–553.

Comings, D.E. (1988) *Tourette Syndrome and Human Behavior.* Daurte, CA: Hope Press.

Comings, D.E. and Comings, B.G. (1987) A controlled study of Tourette syndrome. *Am J Hum Genet* 41:701–760.

Costello, E.J., Angold, A., Burns, B.J., Stangl, D.K., Tweed, D.L., Erkanli, A., and Worthman, C.M. (1996) The Great Smoky Mountains Study of Youth. Goals, design, methods, and the prevalence of DSM-III-R disorders. *Arch Gen Psychiatry* 53:1129–1136.

Ernst, M., Zametkin, A.J., Jons, P.H., Matochik, J.A., Pascualvaca, D., and Cohen, R.M. (1999) High presynaptic dopaminergic activity in children with Tourette's disorder. *J Am Acad Child Adolesc Psychiatry* 38:86–94.

Goetz, C.G., Tanner, C.M., Wilson, R.S., Carroll, V.S., Como, P.G., and Shannon, K.M. (1987) Clonidine and Gilles de la Tourette syndrome: double-blind study using objective rating method. *Ann Neurol* 31:307–310.

Graybiel, A.M. (1998). The basal ganglia and chunking of action repertoires. *Neurobiol Learn Memory* 70:119–136.

Greenberg, B.D., Ziemann, U., Cora-Locatelli, G., Harmon, A., Murphy, D.L., Keel, J.C., and Wassermann, E.M. (2000) Altered cortical excitability in obsessive-compulsive disorder. *Neurology* 54:142–147.

Grenhoff, J. and Svensson, T.H. (1989) Clonidine modulates dopamine cell firing in rat ventral tegmental area. *Eur J Pharmacol* 165:11–18.

Haber, S.N., Kowall, N.W., Vonsattel, J.P., Bird, E.D., and Richardson E.P. (1986) Gilles de la Tourette's syndrome: a postmortem neuropathological and immunohistochemical study. *J Neurol Sci* 75:225–241.

Hallett, J.J., Harling-Berg, C.J., Knopf, P.M., Stopa, E.G., and Kiessling, L.S. (2000) Anti-striatal antibodies in Tourette syndrome cause neuronal dysfunction. *J Neuroimmunol* 111:195–202.

Hoffman, K.L. and Lipkin, W.I. (2000) Murine model of autoimmune neuropsychiatric disorders. *Abstr Soci Neurosci* 26: 2310.

Hyde, T.M., Aaronson, B.A., Randolph, C., Rickler, K.C., and Weinberger D.R. (1992) Relationship of birth weight to the phenotypic expression of Gilles de la Tourette's syndrome in monozygotic twins. *Neurology* 42:652–658.

Kadesjo, B. and Gillberg, C. (2000) Tourette's disorder: epidemiology and comorbidity in primary school children. *J Am Acad Child Adolesc Psychiatry* 39:548–555.

King, R.A., Leckman, J.F., Scahill, L.D., and Cohen, D.J. (1998) Obsessive-compulsive disorder, anxiety and depression. In: Leckman, J.F. and Cohen, D.J., eds. *Tourette's Syndrome Tics, Obsessions, Compulsions—Developmental—Psychopathology and Clinical Care.* New York: John Wiley and Sons, pp. 43–62.

Kurlan, R., Whitmore, D., Irvine, C., McDermott, M.P., and Como, P.G. (1994) Tourette's syndrome in a special education population: a pilot study involving a single school district. *Neurology* 44:699–702.

Leckman, J.F. and Cohen, D.J. (1998) *Tourette's Syndrome: Tics, Obsessions, Compulsions—Developmental Psychopathology and Clinical Care.* New York: John Wiley and Sons.

Leckman, J.F., Cohen, D.J., Price, R.A., Minderaa, R.B., Anderson, G.M., and Pauls D.L. (1984) The pathogenesis of Gilles de la Tourette's syndrome: a review of data and hypothesis. In: Shah, A.B., Shah N.S., and Donald, A.G., eds. *Movement Disorders.* New York: Plenum Press, pp. 257–272.

Leckman, J.F., Dolnansky, E.S., Hardin, M.T., Clubb, M., Walkup, J.T., Stevenson, J., and Pauls, D.L. (1990) Perinatal factors in the expression of Tourette's syndrome: an exploratory study. *J Am Acad Child Adolesc Psychiatry* 29:220–226.

Leckman, J.F., Goodman, W.K., Anderson, G.M., Riddle, M.A., Chappell, P.B., McSwiggan-Hardin, M.T., McDougle, C.J., Scahill, L.D., Ort, S.I., Pauls, D.L., and Cohen D.J. (1995) CSF biogenic amines in obsessive compulsive disorder and Tourette's syndrome. *Neuropsychopharmacology* 12:73–86.

Leckman, J.F., Grice, D.E., Boardman, J., Zhang, H., Vitale, A., Bondi, C., Alsobrook, J., Peterson, B.S., Cohen, D.J., Rasmussen, S.A., Goodman, W.K., McDougle, C.J., and Pauls, D.L. (1997) Symptoms of obsessive compulsive disorder. *Am J Psychiatry* 154:911–917.

Leckman, J.F., Hardin, M.T., Riddle, M.A., Stevenson, J., Ort, S.I., and Cohen, D.J. (1991) Clonidine treatment of Gilles de la Tourette's syndrome. *Arch Gen Psychiatry* 48:324–328.

Leckman, J.F. and Riddle, M.A. (2000) Tourette's syndrome: when habit forming systems form habits of their own? *Neuron* 28:349–354.

Leckman, J.F., Riddle, M.A., Hardin, M.T., Ort, S.I., Swartz, K.L., Stevenson, J., and Cohen, D.J. (1989) The Yale Global Tic Severity Scale: initial testing of a clinician-rated scale of tic severity. *J Am Acad Child Adolesc Psychiatry* 28:566–573.

Leckman, J.F., Walker, D.E., and Cohen, D.J. (1993) Premonitory urges in Tourette's syndrome. *Am J Psychiatry* 150:98–102.

Leckman, J.F., Zhang, H., Vitale, A., Lahnin, F., Lynch, K., Bondi, C., Kim, Y.S., and Peterson, B.S. (1998) Course of tic severity in Tourette's syndrome: the first two decades. *Pediatrics* 102:14–19.

Malison, R.T., McDougle, C.J., van Dyck, C.H., Scahill, L., Baldwin, R.M., Seibyl, J.P., Price, L.H., Leckman, J.F., Innis, R.B. (1995) [I^{123}]β-CIT SPECT imaging demonstrates increased striatal dopamine transporter binding in Tourette's syndrome. *Am J Psychiatry* 152:1359–1361.

Mason, A., Banerjee, S., Eapen, V., Zeitlin, H., and Robertson, M.M. (1998) The prevalence of Tourette syndrome in a mainstream school population. *Dev Med Child Neurol* 40:92–296.

McDougle, C.J., Goodman, W.K., Leckman, J.F., Barr, L.C., Heninger, G.R., and Price, L.H. (1993). The efficacy of fluvoxamine in obsessive compulsive disorder: effects of comorbid chronic tic disorder. *J Clin Psychopharmacol* 13:354–358.

Merette, C., Brassard, A., Potvin, A., Bouvier, H., Rousseau, F., Emond, C., Bissonnette, L., Roy, M.A., Maziade, M., Ott, J., and Caron, C. (2000). Significant linkage for Tourette syndrome in a large French Canadian family. *Am J Hum Genet* 67:1008–1013.

Meyer, P., Bohnen, N.I., Minoshima, S., Koeppe, R.A., Wernette, K., Kilbourn, M.R., Kuhl, D.E., Frey, K.A., and Albin, R.L. (1999) Striatal presynaptic monoaminergic vesicles are not increased in Tourette's syndrome. *Neurology* 53:371–374.

Morshed, S.A., Parveen, S., Leckman, J.F., Mercadante, M.T., Bittencourt Kiss, M.H., Miguel, E.C., Yazgan, Y., Fujii, T., Paul, S., Peterson, B.S., Scahill, L., and Lombroso, P.J. (2001) Antibodies against neural, nuclear, cytoskeletal and streptococcal epitopes

in children and adults with Tourette's syndrome, Sydenham's chorea, and autoimmune disorders. *Biol Psychiatry* 50:566–577.

Pasamanick, B. and Kawi, A. (1956) A study of the association of prenatal and paranatal factors in the development of tics in children. *J Pediatr* 48:596–602.

Pauls, D.L., Raymond, C.L., Stevenson, J.F., and Leckman J.F. (1991) A family study of Gilles de la Ttte. *Am J Hum Genet* 48:154–163.

Perlmutter, S.J., Leitman, S.F., Garvey, M.A., Hamburger, S., Feldman, E., Leonard, H.L., and Swedo, S.E. (1999) Therapeutic plasma exchange and intravenous immunoglobulin for obsessive-compulsive disorder and tic disorders in childhood. *Lancet* 354:1153–1158.

Peterson, B.S. and Leckman, J.F. (1998) Temporal characterization of tics in Gilles de la Tourette's syndrome. *Biol Psychiatry* 44:1337–1348.

Peterson, B.S., Leckman, J.F., Scahill, L., Naftolin, F., Keefe, D., Charest, N.J., and Cohen, D.J. (1992) Steroid hormones and sexual dimorphisms modulate symptom expression in Tourette's syndrome. *Psychoneuroendocrinology* 17:553–563.

Peterson, B.S., Skudlarski, P., Anderson, A.W., Zhang, H., Gatenby, J.C., Lacadie, C.M., Leckman, J.F., and Gore, J.C. (1998a) A functional magnetic resonance imaging study of tic suppression in Tourette syndrome. *Arch Gen Psychiatry* 55:326–333.

Peterson, B.S., Zhang, H., Bondi, C., Anderson, G.M., and Leckman, J.F. (1998b) A double-blind, placebo-controlled, crossover trial of an antiandrogen in the treatment of Tourette's syndrome. *J Clin Psychopharmacol* 18:324–331.

Peterson, B.S., Price, A.R., Kidd, K.K., Cohen, D.J., Pauls, D.L., and Leckman, J.F. (1985) A twin study of Tourette's syndrome. *Arch Gen Psychiatry* 42:815–820.

Sanberg, P.R., Silver, A.A., Shytle, R.D., Philipp, M.K., Cahill, D.W., Fogelson, H.M., and McConville, B.J. (1997) Nicotine for the treatment of Tourette's syndrome. *Pharmacol Ther* 74:21–25.

Santangelo, S.L., Pauls, D.L., Goldstein, J.M., Faraone, S.V., Tsuang, M.T., and Leckman, J.F. (1994) Tourette's syndrome: what are the influences of gender and comorbid obsessive-compulsive disorder? *J Am Acad Child Adolesc Psychiatry* 33:795–804.

Scahill, L., Chappell, P.B., Kim, Y-S., Schultz, R.T., Katsovich, L., Shepard, E., Arnsten, A.F.T., Cohen, D.J., and Leckman, J.F. (2001) Guanfacine in the treatment of children with tic disorders and ADHD: a placebo-controlled study. *Am J Psychiatry.* 158:1067–1074.

Shapiro, A.K. and Shapiro, E.S. (1988) Treatment of tic disorders with haloperidol. In: Cohen, D.J., Bruun, R.D., and Leckman, J.F., eds. *Tourette's Syndrome and Tic Disorders.* New York: John Wiley and Sons, pp. 267–280.

Shapiro, A.K., Shapiro, E.S., Young, J.G., and Feinberg, T.E., eds. (1988) *Gilles de la Tourette Syndrome, 2nd ed.* New York: Raven Press.

Sikich, L. and Todd, R.D. (1988) Are neurodevelopmental effects of gonadal hormones related to sex differences in psychiatric illness. *Psychiatr Dev* 6:277–310.

Silva, R.R., Munoz, D.M., Barickman, J., and Friedhoff, A.J. (1995) Environmental factors and related fluctuation of symptoms in children and adolescents with Tourette's disorder. *J Child Psychol Psychiatry* 36:305–312.

Silver, A.A., Shyytle, R.D., and Sanberg, P.R. (2001) Mecamylamine in Tourette's syndrome: a two-year retrospective study. *J Child Adolesc Psychopharmacol.* 40:1103–1110.

Singer, H.S., Giuliano, J.D., Hansen, B.H., Hallett, J.J., Laurino, J.P., Benson, M., and Kiessling, L.S. (1998) Antibodies against human putamen in children with Tourette syndrome. *Neurology* 50: 1618–1624.

Singer, H.S., Hahn, I.-H., and Moran, T.H. (1991) Abnormal dopamine uptake sites in postmortem striatum from patients with Tourette's syndrome. *Ann Neurol* 30:558–562.

Spencer, T., Biederman, J., Harding, M., O'Donnell, D., Wilens, T., Faraone, S., Coffey, B., and Geller, D. (1998) Disentangling the overlap between Tourette disorder and ADHD. *J Child Psychol Psychiatry* 39:1037–1044.

Swedo, S.E., Leonard, H.L., Garvey, M., Mittleman, B., Allen, A.J., Perlmutter, S., Lougee, L., Dow, S., Zamkoff, J., and Dubbert, B.K. (1998) Pediatric autoimmune neuropsychiatric disorders associated with streptococcal infections: clinical description of the first 50 cases. *Am J Psychiatry* 155:264–271.

Tourette Syndrome Classification Study Group (1993) Definitions and classification of tic disorders. *Arch Neurol* 50:1013–1016.

Tourette Syndrome International Consortium for Genetics (1999) A complete genome screen in sib-pairs affected with Gilles de la Tourette syndrome. *Am J Hum Genet* 65:1428–1436.

Vandewalle, V., van der Linden, C., Groenewegen, H.J., and Caemaert, J. (1999) Stereotactic treatment of Gilles de la Tourette syndrome by high frequency stimulation of thalamus. *Lancet* 353: 724.

van Wattum, P.J., Anderson, G.M., Chappell, P.B., Goodman, W.K., Riddle, M.A., and Leckman, J.F. (1999) Cerebrospinal fluid dynorphin A[1–8] and beta-endorphin levels in Tourette's syndrome are unaltered. *Biol Psychiatry* 45:1527–1528.

Walkup, J.T., Khan, S., Schuerholz, L., Paik, Y.-S., Leckman, J.F., and Schultz, R.T. (1998) Phenomenology and natural history of tic-related ADHD and learning disabilities. In: Leckman, J.F. and Cohen, D.J., eds. *Tourette's Syndrome Tics, Obsessions, Com-*

pulsions—Developmental Psychopathology and Clinical Care. New York: John Wiley and Sons, pp. 63–79.

Walkup, J.T., LaBuda, M.C., Singer, H.S., Brown, J., Riddle, M.A., and Hurko, O. (1996) Family study and segregation analysis of Tourette syndrome: evidence for a mixed model of inheritance. *Am J Hum Genet* 59:684–693.

Ware, M.L., Tavazoie, S.F., Reid, C.B., and Walsh, C.A. (1999) Coexistence of widespread clones and large radial clones in early embryonic ferret cortex. *Cereb Cortex* 9:636–645.

Whitaker, A.H., Van Rossem, R., Feldman, J.F, Schonfeld, I.S., Pinto-Martin, J.A., Tore, C., Shaffer, D., and Paneth, N. (1997) Psychiatric outcomes in low-birth-weight children at age 6 years: relation to neonatal cranial ultrasound abnormalities. *Arch Gen Psychiatry* 54:847–856.

Wolf, S.S., Jones, D.W., Knable, M.B., Gorey, J.G., Lee, K.S., Hyde, T.M., Coppola, R., and Weinberger, D.R. (1996) Tourette syndrome: prediction of phenotypic variation in monozygotic twins by caudate nucleus D2 receptor binding. *Science* 273:1225–1227.

World Health Organization (1996) *Multiaxial Classification of Child and Adolescent Disorders: The ICD-10 Classification of Mental and Behavioural Disorders in Children and Adolescents.* Cambridge, UK: Cambridge University Press, pp. 43–45.

Ziemann, U., Paulus, W., and Rothenberger, A. (1997) Decreased motor inhibition in Tourette's disorder: evidence from transcranial magnetic stimulation. *Am J Psychiatry* 154:1277–84.

Zohar, A.H., Apter, A., King, R.A., Pauls, D.L., Leckman, J.F., and Cohen D.J. (1998) Epidemiological studies. In: Leckman, J.F. and Cohen, D.J., eds. *Tourette's Syndrome Tics, Obsessions, Compulsions—Developmental Psychopathology and Clinical Care.* New York: John Wiley and Sons, pp. 177–193.

14 | Neurobiology of immune-mediated neuropsychiatric disorders

MARY LYNN DELL, CHARLOTTE S. HAMILTON, AND
SUSAN E. SWEDO

Obsessive-compulsive, tic, and movement disorders in childhood and adolescence are now recognized as relatively common neuropsychiatric disorders, varying in severity, duration of symptom exacerbations, and degree of disability. In some children, the symptoms of these disorders are distinct and easily defined, whereas others display ever-changing combinations of obsessions, compulsions, abnormal motor movements, and tics that may be a mix of transient, chronic, simple, complex, vocal, or motor tics.

Epidemiological studies from the United States, Germany, New Zealand, and Israel have estimated the prevalence of childhood-onset obsessive-compulsive disorder (OCD) to be from 0.5% to 4.0%, with an average of approximately 2.5% (Anderson et al., 1987; Zohar, 1988; Lewisohn et al., 1993; Reinherz et al 1993, Douglass et al., 1995; Wittchen et al., 1998). Affected males outnumber affected females in the prepubertal years, with an earlier age of onset, greater severity, and higher likelihood of comorbid tics and disruptive behavior disorders (Swedo et al., 1989b; Flament et al., 1990; Geller et al., 1996, 1998). After puberty and into adulthood, the gender ratio equalizes, then eventually demonstrates a higher incidence in females (Leonard et al., 1999).

Generally, childhood-onset OCD symptoms are similar to those in adults, encompassing a wide range of obsessive thoughts and compulsive rituals. Common obsessions involve contamination fears, worries about harm befalling self or others, concerns about morality, and a need for symmetry. Common compulsions include checking, washing, and repeating until "it's just right." Most children experience a combination of obsessions and rituals, and children with rituals only are more common than those with obsessions only. A feature common to this population is the recognition that their symptoms are nonsensical, leading to significant,

often elaborate, attempts to hide the obsessions and compulsions from parents, teachers, and peers (Swedo et al., 1989b).

The clinical course of childhood-onset OCD is usually described as persistent and unremitting. Spontaneous remissions are estimated to occur in fewer than one-third of affected youth (Karno and Goulding, 1990). Although long-term, prospective follow-up studies are rare, studies of adults whose OCD began in childhood show that most patients remain symptomatic throughout their lives, despite improved pharmacotherapies, cognitive, behavioral, and other treatment modalities (Hollingsworth et al., 1980; Honjo et al., 1989; Thomsen and Mikkelsen, 1991; Leonard et al., 1993; Hanna, 1995).

Approximately three-quarters of children with OCD have comorbid diagnoses. These include tic disorders (24%–30%) and mood disorders, especially major depression (26%–29%). Riddle and colleagues (1990) found that 38% of children with OCD have other anxiety disorders, while Swedo (1989) more specifically identified increased rates of simple phobias (17%), overanxious disorder (16%), and separation anxiety disorder (7%). Other reported comorbidities include specific developmental disabilities, adjustment disorder with depressed mood, oppositional defiant disorder, attention-deficit hyperactivity disorder (ADHD), conduct disorder, and enuresis/encopresis (Swedo et al., 1989b; Riddle et al., 1990).

Tics are a heterogeneous group of relatively brief, unvoluntary simple or complex vocalizations or movements that interrupt normal speech or motor activities. Common motor tics include eye blinking and rolling, mouth opening, facial twitching, head nodding, shoulder shrugging, throat clearing, sniffing, and grunting. More complex tics include bending, twisting, touching, echolalia, and coprolalia. Tics may occur intermittently or many times a day. They may be transient, lasting no longer than 12 consecutive months, or chronic, occurring over a time period that exceeds 1 year. When multiple motor tics and one or more vocal tics of varying location, frequency, complexity, and severity have been present for at least 1 year, a diagnosis of Tourette's disorder can be made (American Psychiatric Association, 1994).

Transient tics are thought to be among the most common neuropsychiatric disorders of childhood, although reliable epidemiological data have been difficult to obtain because of methodological constraints. Tics are estimated to occur in 4%–24% of school children (Shapiro and Shapiro, 1982), making the disorder 5–12 times more prevalent among children than adults. Boys are affected twice as often as girls (Burd et al., 1986a,b). Of greatest significance for this discussion is the high rate of comorbidity of OCD and tic disorders. In one study, 23% of 134 individuals with tic disorders had OCD, with an additional 46% having symptoms but not meeting full diagnostic criteria (Leckman et al., 1994). Swedo and colleagues (1989b) found that 20% of patients with OCD have lifetime histories of multiple tics, and 5%–10% meet criteria for Tourette's syndrome at some time during the course of their illness. The group at the National Institute of Mental Health (NIMH) also reported that 56% of children with OCD had developed tics and 14% met criteria for Tourette's disorder during a 2- to 5-year follow-up study (Leonard et al., 1992).

POSTINFECTIOUS SUBTYPE OF OBSESSIVE-COMPULSIVE, TIC, AND MOVEMENT DISORDERS

Supporting evidence for postinfectious OCD and tics comes from studies of patients with Sydenham chorea, a constellation of abnormal movements occurring 1 to 6 months after group A beta hemolytic streptococcal (GABHS) infections (Sydenham, 1848; Taranta and Stollerman, 1956; Ayoub and Wannamaker, 1966). The motor symptoms of Sydenham chorea consist of unilateral or bilateral gait disturbances, ballismus, impairment of fine motor skills, speech abnormalities, tongue fasciculations, and facial grimacing. As early as 1894, Sir William Osler described emotional lability, irritability, and unusual behaviors in patients with Sydenham chorea. Over the ensuing decades, a number of clinicians have continued to observe obsessive-compulsive and other symptoms (Chapman et al., 1958; Grimshaw, 1964; Wilcox and Nasrallah, 1986). Freeman et al. (1965) noted an increased incidence of compulsive personality, phobias, obsessive-compulsive

symptoms, conversion, and anxiety in 40 adults with histories of Sydenham chorea compared to 40 adults hospitalized during the same time period for rheumatic fever without chorea, glomerulonephritis, or osteomyelitis. Most recently, Swedo's group has systematically studied the neuropsychiatric manifestations of Sydenham chorea by comparing two groups of rheumatic fever patients, one group with and the other without chorea. Consistent with historical accounts, the Sydenham group had significantly more obsessive-compulsive symptoms than the group with rheumatic fever alone (Swedo et al., 1989a). Furthermore, at least 70% of Sydenham patients experience obsessive-compulsive symptoms virtually identical to those of individuals with classic, non-postinfectious OCD (Swedo et al., 1993; Asbahr et al., 1998). Among children suffering multiple recrudescences of sydenham chorea, the rate of OCD approaches 100%. (Asbahr et al., 1999)

The complexities and interrelationships of these particular neuropsychiatric disorders have been brought to the forefront once again with the identification of a postinfectious subtype of childhood-onset obsessive-compulsive and tic disorders seemingly separate from classic rheumatic fever and Sydenham chorea. As early as 1929, a case series was published describing three children with tic onset and exacerbations associated with acute sinusitis (Selling, 1929). Brown (1957) also proposed bacterial infection as an etiology for tic disorders nearly 30 years later, based on his observations and experience with 34 patients. Both investigators attributed the tics directly to the sinus infections or to the resultant irritation and discomfort. Since 1978, two separate case reports describing three patients with postinfectious tics have been published (Kondo and Kabasawa, 1978; Matarazzo, 1992). Kiessling and colleagues also noted an abrupt rise in the number of patients presenting with tics following a local outbreak of GABHS infections in Rhode Island (Kiessling, 1989).

Building on the work noted above, Swedo and colleagues at NIMH have described a patient group whose obsessive-compulsive, tic, and movement disorder symptoms are prepubertal in onset and temporally related to GABHS infections. The acronym PANDAS, standing for Pediatric Autoimmune Neuropsychiatric Disorders Associated with Streptococcal infections, has been applied to these postinfectious symptom complexes. Five criteria identify the PANDAS subgroup: (1) presence of OCD and/or tic disorder according to the Diagnostic and Statistical Manual of Mental Disorders, 4th ed. (DSM-IV) criteria; (2) prepubertal onset, or the first appearance of symptoms between the ages of 3 and 12 years of age; (3) an episodic course, character-

TABLE 14.1 *Criteria for Pediatric Autoimmune Neuropsychiatric Disorders Associated with Streptococcal Infections*

1. Presence of OCD and/or a tic disorder (lifetime) according to DSM-IV diagnostic criteria

2. Prepubertal onset: symptoms of the disorder first become evident between age 3 years and the beginning of puberty (approximately age 12 years)

3. Episodic symptom course: characterized by abrupt onset of symptoms and/or dramatic symptom exacerbations

4. Associated neurological abnormalities: adventitious movements, especially choreiform movements, are particularly common

5. Temporal association with GABHS infections

ized by a sudden, dramatic onset of symptoms and abrupt exacerbations occurring during periods when symptoms are in complete or partial remission; (4) adventitious movements, primarily choreiform in nature, which may be accompanied by deterioration in gross and fine motor skills; and (5) temporal association between GABHS infection and the onset or exacerbation of symptoms (Swedo et al., 1997; Table 14.1)

PEDIATRIC AUTOIMMUNE NEUROPSYCHIATRIC DISORDERS ASSOCIATED WITH STREPTOCOCCAL INFECTIONS: COMORBIDITIES AND FAMILY FINDINGS

Studies at the National Institutes of Health (NIH) have detailed the clinical characteristics of patients in the PANDAS subgroup (Swedo et al., 1998). The rate of neuropsychiatric comorbidity in this population is quite striking. Twenty of the 50 children (40%) met DSM-IV criteria for ADHD and/or oppositional defiant disorder (ODD), 18 (36%) for major depressive disorder, 14 (28%) for overanxious disorder, and 10 (20%) for separation anxiety disorder. Six children (12%) were enuretic, often episodically and closely correlated with periods of OCD and tic exacerbations. Depressive symptoms, ADHD, and separation anxiety disorder also waxed and waned in concert with the OCD/tic symptoms. In addition, exacerbations of OCD and tics were accompanied frequently by the acute onset of choreiform movements (clinically distinct from chorea), emotional lability and irritability, tactile/sensory defensiveness, motoric hyperactivity, messy handwriting, and symptoms of separation anxiety (Perlmutter et al., 1998; Becker et al., 2000).

Not surprisingly, the rates of OCD and tic disorders in first-degree relatives of PANDAS patients are higher

than those reported in the general population and are similar to those reported previously for these disorders (Lenane et al., 1990; Riddle et al., 1990; Walkup et al., 1996; (Lougee et al 2000). In the largest family study to date, relatives of 54 probands with PANDAS, 24 with a primary OCD diagnosis and 30 with a primary tic disorder diagnosis, were evaluated for psychiatric morbidity. One hundred fifty-seven first-degree relatives (100 parents [93%] and 57 siblings [100%]) were evaluated for the presence of a tic disorder, and 139 first-degree relatives (100 parents [93%] and 39 of 41 siblings over the age of 6 [95%]) were evaluated with clinical and structured psychiatric interviews to determine the presence of subclinical OCD, OCD, and other DSM-IV axis I disorders. Twenty-one probands (39%) had one or more first-degree relatives with histories of a vocal or motor tic. Fourteen probands (26%) had at least one first-degree relative with OCD, in addition to another 8% of parents ($n = 8$) and 8% of siblings ($n = 3$) who evidenced subclinical forms of OCD. Eleven parents (11%) were diagnosed as having obsessive-compulsive personality disorder (Lougee et al., 2000). These results suggest that genetic vulnerability plays a role in the PANDAS subgroup. However, more research is needed to assess the interactions of genetics, environment, infectious agents, and immunity on symptom expression in children with PANDAS.

BIOLOGICAL BASIS OF POSTINFECTIOUS NEUROPSYCHIATRIC DISORDERS

Before discussing the postulated disease mechanisms in postinfectious OCD and tic disorders, it is necessary to review several related concepts.

Group A Beta-Hemolytic Streptococcal Infections and Host Immune Response

Group A beta hemolytic streptococcus is a gram-positive coccus that differs from other hemolytic streptococci in its unique cell wall carbohydrates. There are over 100 types of GABHS, distinguished by serologically distinct surface proteins. The M protein is largely responsible for GABHS communicability by conveying resistance to phagocytosis. Infections are spread by direct contact with respiratory secretions or large droplets of secretions harboring the bacteria and are most common in the winter and spring in cold and temperate climates. In addition to the high frequency of asymptomatic streptococcal infections, a carrier state may exist in up to 20% of school-age children at any given time (Kaplan, 1971). Prepubertal children are not only quite susceptible to GABHS infections, they also spread the illness quite successfully via asymptomatic carrier states in situations in which they are in close physical proximity with others. Although GABHS can cause impetigo, pyoderma, otitis media, and other infections, the nasopharyngeal and tonsilar infections of school-aged children are most relevant to this discussion (McMillan and Feigen, 1999).

In the normal immune response against GABHS, antibodies against the M proteins in the outer protein layer of the cell wall opsonize the bacteria in the presence of neutrophils. In postinfectious neuropsychiatric diseases, abnormal cell-mediated and humoral immune responses to GABHS cell wall antigens are postulated, analogous to the phenomenon of molecular mimicry thought to occur in rheumatic fever and Sydenham chorea. The antistreptococcal antibodies cross-react with the host tissues implicated in the development of neuropsychiatric symptoms (Lennon, 1998; El-Said, 1999). Husby et al. (1976) first reported the presence of immunoglobulin G (IgG) antibodies in the sera of children with rheumatic fever. These serum antibodies in Sydenham patients were shown to not only recognize components of the streptococcal cell wall but also "cross-react" with the cytoplasm of the subthalamic and caudate nuclei (Husby et al., 1976). Subsequent studies have replicated Husby's findings in Sydenham chorea, and have found elevated rates of antineuronal antibodies in children with post-streptococcal OCD and tic disorders (Kiessling et al., 1994; Swedo, 1994; Swedo et al., 1994).

Clinically, a throat culture, high or rising antistreptolysin O (ASO), antideoxyribonuclease B (anti-DNaseB) titers, or all three may indicate that neuropsychiatric symptoms were precipitated by GABHS infection (American Academy of Child and Adolescent Psychiatry, 1998). However, these laboratory findings are not specific to PANDAS. A finding of a high antistreptococcal antibody titer in a child with tics, obsessions, or compulsions could occur by chance alone, given that the majority of school-age children have evidence of a current or recent streptococcal infection (Kaplan et al., 1998a, b). Antineuronal antibodies have also been found in the sera of 20%–40% of normal controls (Kiessling et al., 1994; Singer et al., 1998). Another complication in the effort to clearly describe and delineate PANDAS is that there may be other infectious triggers for the development of OCD, tics, and movement disorders in addition to streptococcal infections. Lyme borreliosis (Lyme disease) and viral illnesses have been reported to be infectious antecedents to psychiatric and neurologic symptoms, including OCD (Fallon et al., 1993; Fallon and Nields, 1994;

Allen et al., 1995). To increase confidence that an affected child belongs in the PANDAS subgroup, there must be at least two symptom exacerbations occurring subsequently to documented GABHS infections, and one or more periods of partial or complete quiescence of symptoms in the absence of streptococcal pharyngitis.

Brain Systems Implicated

Several lines of evidence support frontal lobe–limbic–basal ganglia dysfunction in obsessive-compulsive and movement disorders. Historically, Constantin von Economo (1931) described the compulsory features of motor tics and ritualistic behaviors in patients with postencephalitic Parkinson's disease. The chief finding on neuropathological examinations of these patients was basal ganglia destruction (von Economo, 1931). Huntington's chorea, another basal ganglia disease, has been associated with an increased rate of obsessive-compulsive symptoms and OCD (Cummings and Cunningham, 1992). Traumatic brain injury, brain tumors, carbon monoxide poisoning, and other neurological injuries leading to basal ganglia insults have been linked to the onset of obsessive-compulsive symptoms and even OCD (Insel, 1992; Max et al., 1995). Additional support for basal ganglia dysfunction includes an increased incidence of choreiform movements and motor tics in children with OCD (Denckla, 1989) and the association of OCD with Tourette's disorder (Frankel et al., 1986; Pauls et al., 1986; Grad et al., 1987).

The most convincing evidence for basal ganglia–frontal lobe dysfunction in OCD is found in neuroimaging studies (Rauch and Baxter, 1998; Fitzgerald et al., 1999). Structural brain imaging studies have revealed volumetric abnormalities of the caudate (Luxenberg et al., 1988), putamen (Rosenberg et al., 1997) and globus pallidus (Giedd et al., 2000). Volumetric changes have also been demonstrated in patients with Sydenham chorea. In a magnetic resonance imaging (MRI) study of 24 Sydenham patients and 48 matched controls, mean volume increases were seen in the SC patient group in the caudate (9%–11%), putamen (6%–8%), and globus pallidus (7%–13%) (Giedd et al., 1995).

Giedd et al. (1996) reported the results of serial head MRI scans of a 12-year-old male who experienced a dramatic exacerbation of OCD and tics following documented GABHS pharyngitis. Imaging was performed before, during, and after immunomodulatory treatment with plasmaphoresis. Initial caudate volume was more than two standard deviations greater than norms for his age, sex, and weight. After treatment, caudate, globus pallidus, and putamen volumes decreased by 24%, 28%, and 12%, respectively. Tics and OC symptoms improved in conjunction with the volumetric decreases. A follow-up study examined basal ganglia volumes in 30 PANDAS children and 56 age- and sex-matched controls (Giedd et al., 2000). No differences in total brain or thalamic volumes were noted between the two groups, but basal ganglia enlargement was demonstrated again in the subjects. Significant increases were noted in the volumes of the caudate nuclei (mean of 13%), putamen (mean of 5%), and globus pallidus (mean of 7%) (Fig. 14.1).

Despite these interesting findings, structural MRI cannot be used as a diagnostic tool or to monitor treatment response because of the large amount of variability of basal ganglia volumes in healthy children and adolescents.

Genetic Vulnerability and Biologic Markers

In 1979, Zabriskie and colleagues discovered a non-HLA DR-positive B-cell surface marker present in over 90% of patients with rheumatic fever, but in only 5%–10% of healthy control populations (Patarroyo et al., 1979; Regelmann et al., 1989; Gibofsky et al., 1991). This surface marker is recognized by a monoclonal antibody labeled D8/17. In view of the large separation between patients and controls and epidemiological studies showing that rheumatic fever affects only 5%–7% of the world's population, the D8/17 marker was anticipated to be a useful trait marker of rheumatic fever susceptibility (Khanna et al., 1989; Feldman et al., 1993; Kemeny et al., 1994). Indeed, over 90% of a NIMH cohort of Sydenham chorea were identified as D8/17 positive, compared to 10% of age- and sex-matched controls (Swedo, 1994). Shortly thereafter, the D8/17 marker was tested in the PANDAS subgroup, with 85% of PANDAS patients being positive compared to 17% of controls (Swedo et al., 1997).

Murphy and colleagues (1997) compared 31 patients with childhood-onset OCD and Tourette's disorder with 21 healthy volunteers. The patient group had 100% positive expression the D8/17 marker, regardless of whether the symptoms were temporally related to

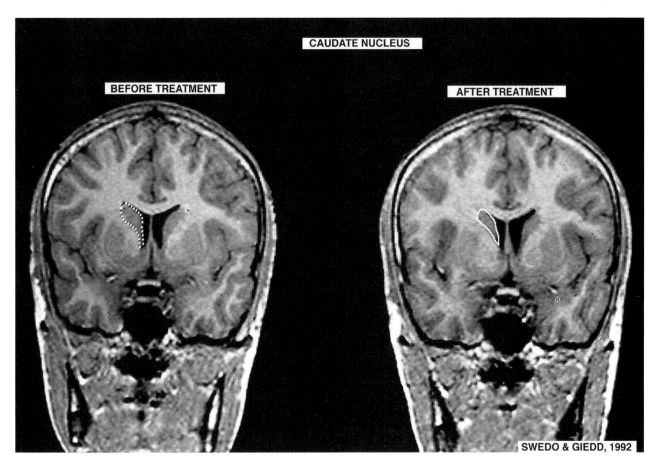

FIGURE 14.1 Caudate size before and after plasma exchange in 14-year-old boy with OCD.

GABHS infections. More recently, high rates of D8/17 expression have been demonstrated in a small sample of autistic patients, with variations in numbers of D8/17 cells linked to severity of compulsions (Hollander et al., 1999). The findings of Murphy and Hollander cast doubt on the specificity of the D8/17 marker for PANDAS susceptibility. Further, recent experience with the D8/17 marker suggests that it's sensitivity may also have declined as fewer than 50% of a cohort of SC patients were found to be D8/17 positive (Swedo, unpublished data, 2001). Additional research is in process to investigate the marker's sensitivity, specificity, and reliability in PANDAS and other disorders.

TREATMENT MODALITIES: INVESTIGATIONAL AND STANDARD

If post-streptococcal autoimmunity is the pathophysiologic mechanism at work in PANDAS, then immunomodulatory therapies may be effective. Results from a controlled trial of plasmapheresis and intravenous immunoglobulin (IVIG) in Sydenham patients demonstrated that both treatments were effective in reducing symptom severity and hastening recovery (Swedo, 1994; Garvey and Swedo, 1997). To determine whether the treatments would also be effective for postinfectious OCD, tic disorder, or Tourette's disorder, 29 children were randomized to receive treatment with plasma exchange, IVIG, or placebo (sham IVIG). Steroid therapy was excluded from consideration for treatment of PANDAS because OCD and tics may be exacerbated by steroids (Jonasson and Wilkinson, 1993). Ten patients received plasmapheresis (five single-volume exchanges over 2 weeks), nine were administered IVIG (1 g/kg on 2 consecutive days), and 10 children received placebo (saline solution given in an identical manner to IVIG). Neuropsychiatric symptom severity was rated at baseline, and then 1 and 12 months after treatment. At the 1-month follow-up, patients in the plasmapheresis and IVIG groups showed striking improvements on ratings of obsessive-compulsive symptoms, anxiety, and overall functioning. Tics improved significantly in the plasma exchange group as well. No change in symptom severity was observed in the placebo group. Twelve months after treatment, symptom improvement continued to be "much" or "very much" improved over baseline by seven of eight patients who had received plasma exchange and seven of nine children who were treated with IVIG, an overall maintenance rate of 82% (Perlmutter et al., 1999). To answer the question of specificity, five children with severe OCD but without streptococcal-related symptom exacerbations underwent a comparable trial of plasma exchange. None of these patients showed significant improvement (Nicolson et al., 2000). Taken together, the studies support the potential utility of immunomodulatory therapies as specific treatments for the PANDAS subgroup of OCD, tics, and movement disorders. However, replicative studies are warranted before therapeutic plasma exchange and IVIG become a standard part of the clinical armamentarium.

Antibiotic prophylaxis has long been used successfully in rheumatic fever patients to protect against streptococcal-induced recrudescences. The similarities in the pathogenesis of Sydenham chorea and PANDAS naturally led to a question regarding the utility of antibiotic prophylaxis for reducing or eliminating neuropsychiatric symptom exacerbations triggered by recurrent streptococcal infections. The NIMH group enrolled 37 children with PANDAS in an 8-month, placebo-controlled, double-blind, balanced crossover study. Patients received 4 months of penicillin V 250 mg twice daily and then 4 months of placebo, or vice versa. Monthly throat cultures and streptococcal antibody titers were obtained. Neuropsychiatric symptoms were also rated at monthly follow-up visits. Although parent ratings of overall behavior and patient ratings of severity of depression and anxiety were improved during the penicillin phase, there were no significant changes in OCD and tic severity. This may have been the result of a failure of penicillin prophylaxis against GABHS infections, as a similar rate of streptococcal infections occurred in both the active and placebo phases of the study. Of concern is the finding that throat cultures were sometimes negative during penicillin administration, despite rising antistreptococcal antibody titers, which suggests that the prophylaxis might obscure clinically significant infections (Garvey et al., 1999). Additional studies of antibiotic prophylaxis are warranted and are currently underway.

At the present time, no PANDAS-specific treatment is indicated for routine clinical care. The patients can benefit from, and should receive anti-obsessional or anti-tic treatment modalities consistent with the guidelines set forth in the American Academy of Child and Adolescent Psychiatry (1998) Practice Parameters for the Assessment and Treatment of Children and Adolescents with OCD and The Expert Concensus Guideline Series on the Treatment of OCD (March et al., 1997). Treatment strategies involving the use of psychopharmacology (selective serotonin reuptake inhibitors, clomipramine, dopamine antagonists, augmentation agents), cognitive-behavioral therapy, and appropriate combination therapies should be used in PANDAS just as they are for other children and adolescents with OCD and tic disorders. Patient and family education about PANDAS and the treatments prescribed for an individual child, as well as active liaison and partnership with the child's school, are also necessary for optimal functioning in all domains of an affected child's life.

REFERENCES

Allen, A.J., Leonard, H.L., and Swedo, S.E. (1995) Case study: a new infection-triggered, autoimmune subtype of pediatric OCD and Tourette's syndrome. *J Am Acad Child Adolesc Psychiatry* 34:307–311.

American Academy of Child and Adolescent Psychiatry (1998) Practice parameters for the assessment and treatment of children and adolescents with obsessive-compulsive disorder. *J Am Acad Child Adolesc Psychiatry* 37:27S–45S.

American Psychiatric Association (1994) *Diagnostic and Statistical Manual of Mental Disorders, 4th ed.* Washington, DC: American Psychiatric Association.

Anderson, J.C., Williams, S., McGee, R., and Silva, P.A. (1987) DSM-III disorders in preadolescent children: prevalence in a large sample from the general population. *Arch Gen Psychiatry* 44:9–76.

Asbahr, F.R., Negrao, A.B., Gentil, V., Zanetta, D.M., da Paz, J.A., Marques-Dias, M.J., and Kiss, M.H. (1998) Obsessive-compulsive and related symptoms in children and adolescents with rheumatic fever with and without chorea: a prospective 6-month study. *Am J Psychiatry* 155:1122–1124.

Asbahr FR, Ramos RT, Negrao AB, and Gentil V. (1999) Case Series: increased vulnerability to obsessive-compulsive symptoms with repeated episodes of Sydenham chorea. *J Am Acad Child Adolesc Psychiatry* 38:1522–1525.

Ayoub, E.M. and Wannamaker, L.W. (1966) Streptococcal antibody titers in Sydenham's chorea. *Pediatrics* 38:946–956.

Becker, D., Swedo, S.E., and Garvey, M.A. (2000) Abnormal motor performance during streptococcal-triggered exacerbations of neuropsychiatric symptoms [abstract]. *Neurology* 54:A318.

Brown, E.E. (1957) Tics (habit spasms) secondary to sinusitis. *Arch Pediatr* 74:39–46.

Burd, L., Kerbeshian, L., Wikenheiser, M., and Fisher, W. (1986a) Prevalence of Gilles de la Tourette's syndrome in North Dakota adults. *Am J Psychiatry* 143:787–788.

Burd, L., Kerbeshian, L., Wikenheiser, M., and Fisher, W. (1986b) A prevalence study of Gilles de la Tourette's syndrome in North Dakota school-age children. *J Am Acad Child Adolesc Psychiatry* 25:552–553.

Chapman, A.H., Pilkey, L., and Gibbons, M.J. (1958) A psychosomatic study of eight children with Sydenham chorea. *Pediatrics* 30:582–595.

Cummings, J.L. and Cunningham, K. (1992) Obsessive-compulsive disorder in Huntington's disease. *Biol Psychiatry* 31:263–270.

Denckla, M.B. (1989) Neurological examination. In: Rapoport, J.L., ed. *Obsessive-Compulsive Disorder in Children and Adolescents.* Washington, DC: American Psychiatric Press, pp. 107–118.

Douglass, H.M., Moffit, T.E., Dar, R., McGee, R., and Silva, P. (1995) Obsessive-compulsive disorder in a birth cohort of 18 year olds: prevalence and predictors. *J Am Acad Child Adoles Psychiatry* 34:1424–1431.

El-Said, G.M. (1999) Rheumatic fever. In: McMillan, J.A., De-Angelis, C.D., Feigen, R.D., and Warshaw, J.B., eds. *Oski's Pediatrics: Principles and Practice, 3rd ed.* Philadelphia: Lippincott, Williams, and Wilkins, pp. 1417–1428.

Fallon, B.A. and Nields, J.A. (1994) Lyme disease: a neuropsychiatric illness. *Am J Psychiatry* 151:1571–1583.

Fallon, B.A., Nields, J.A., Parsons, B., Liebowitz, M.R., and Klein, D.F. (1993) Psychiatric manifestations of Lyme borreliosis. *J Clin Psychiatry* 54:263–268.

Feldman, B.M., Zabriskie, J.B., Silverman, E.D., and Laxer, R.M. (1993) Diagnostic use of B-cell alloantigen D8/17 in rheumatic chorea. *J Pediatr* 123:84–86.

Fitzgerald, K.D., MacMaster, F.P., Paulson, L.D., and Rosenberg, D.R. (1999) Neurobiology of childhood obsessive-compulsive disorder. *Child Adolesc Psychiatr Clin North Am* 8:533–575.

Flament, M.F., Koby, E., Rapoport, J.L., Berg, C.J., Zahn, T., Cox, C., Denckla, M., and Lenane, M. (1990) Childhood obsessive compulsive disorder: a prospective follow-up study. *J Child Psychol Psychiatry* 31:363–380.

Frankel, M., Cummings, J.L., Robertson, M.M., Trimble, M.R., Hill, M.A., and Benson, D.F. (1986) Obsessions and compulsions in Gilles de la Tourette's syndrome. *Neurology* 36:378–382.

Freeman, J.H., Aron, A.M., Collard, J.E., and MacKay MC (1965) The emotional correlates of Sydenham's chorea. *Pediatrics* 35:42–49.

Garvey, M.A., Perlmutter, S.J., Allen, A.J., Hamburger, S., Lougee, L., Leonard, H.L., Witowski, M.E., Dubbert, B., and Swedo, S.E. (1999) A pilot study of penicillin prophylaxis for neuropsychiatric symptom exacerbations triggered by streptococcal infections. *Biol Psychiatry* 45:1564–1571.

Garvey, M.A. and Swedo, S.E. (1997) Sydenham's chorea: clinical and therapeutic update. *Adv Exp Med Biol* 418:115–120.

Geller, D.A., Biederman, J., Griffin, S., Jones, J., and Lefkowitz, T.R. (1996) Comorbidity of juvenile obsessive-compulsive disorder with disruptive behavior disorders. *J Am Acad Child Adoles Psychiatry* 35:1637–1646.

Geller, D., Biederman, J., Jones, J., Park, K., Schwartz, S., Shapiro, S., and Coffey, B. (1998) Is juvenile obsessive-compulsive disorder a developmental subtype of the disorder? A review of the pediatric literature. *J Am Acad Child Adoles Psychiatry* 37:420–427.

Gibofsky, A., Khanna, A., Suh, E., and Zabriskie, J.B. (1991) The genetics of rheumatic fever: relationship to streptococcal infection and autoimmune disease. *J Rheumatol* (Suppl 30) 18:1–5.

Giedd, J.N., Rapoport, J.L., Garvey, M.A., Perlmutter S., and Swedo, S.E. (2000) MRI assessment of children with obsessive compulsive disorder or tics associated with streptococcal infection. *Am J Psychiatry* 157:281–283.

Giedd, J.N., Rapoport, J.L., Kruesi, M.J.P., Parker, C., Schapiro, M.B., Allen, A.J., Leonard, H.L., Kaysen, D., Dickstein, D.P., Marsh, W.L., Kozuch, P.L., Vaituzis, A.C., Hamburger, S.D., and Swedo, S.E. (1995) Sydenham's chorea: magnetic resonance imaging of the basal ganglia. *Neurology* 45:2199–2202.

Giedd, J.N., Rapoport, J.L., Leonard, H.L., Richter D., and Swedo, S.E. (1996) Case study: acute basal ganglia enlargement and obsessive-compulsive symptoms in an adolescent boy. *J Am Acad Child Adolesc Psychiatry* 35:913–915.

Grad, L.R., Pelcovitz, D., Olson, M., Mathews, M., and Grad, G.J. (1987) Obsessive-compulsive symptomatology in children with Tourette's syndrome. *J Am Acad Child Adolesc Psychiatry* 26:69–73.

Grimshaw, L. (1964) Obsessional disorder and neurological illness. *J Neurol Neurosurg Psychiatry* 27:229–231.

Hanna, G.L. (1995) Demographic and clinical features of obsessive-compulsive disorder in children and adolescents. *J Am Acad Child Adolesc Psychiatry* 34:19–27.

Hollander E., DelGiudice-Asch, G., Simon, L., Schmeidler J., Cartwright, C., DeCaria, C.M., Kwon, J., Cunningham-Rundles, C., Chapman, F., and Zabriskie, J.B. (1999) B lymphocyte antigen D8/17 and repetitive behaviors in autism. *Am J Psychiatry* 156: 317–320.

Hollingsworth, C.E., Tanguay, P.E., Grossman, L., and Pabst, P. (1980) Long-term outcome of obsessive-compulsive disorder in childhood. *J Am Acad Child Adolesc Psychiatry* 19:134–144.

Honjo, S., Hirano, C.C., Murase, S., Kaneko, T., Sugiyama, T., Ohtaka, K., Aoyama, T., Takei, Y., Inoko, K., and Wakabayashi, S. (1989) Obsessive compulsive symptoms in childhood and adolescence. *Acta Psychiatr Scand* 80:83–91.

Husby, G., van de Rijn, I., Zabriskie, J.B., Abdin, Z.H., and Williams, R.C., Jr. (1976) Antibodies reacting with cytoplasm of subthalamic and caudate nuclei neurons in chorea and acute rheumatic fever. *J Exp Med* 144:1094–1110.

Insel, T.R. (1992) Toward a neuroanatomy of obsessive-compulsive disorder. *Arch Gen Psychiatry* 49:739–744.

Jonasson, G. and Wilkinson, S.R. (1993) Prednisolone-induced obsessive-compulsive behaviour in a child. *Tidsskr Nor Laegeforen* 113:3162–3166.

Kaplan, E.L. (1971) Diagnosis of streptococcal pharyngitis: differentiation of active infection from carrier state in the symptomatic child. *J Infect Dis* 123:490–501.

Kaplan, E.L. and Gerber, M.A. (1998a) Group A, group C and group G beta hemolytic streptococcal infections. In: Feigen, R.D. and Cherry, J.D., eds. *Textbook of Pediatric Infectious Diseases*. Philadelphia: W.B. Saunders, pp. 1076–1088.

Kaplan, E.L., Rothermel, C.D., and Johnson, D.R. (1998b) Antistreptolysin O and anti-deoxyribonuclease B titers: normal values for children ages 2 to 12 in the United States. *Pediatrics* 101:86–88.

Karno, M. and Golding, J. (1991) Obsessive compulsive disorder. In: Robins L. and Regrer, D.A., eds. *Psychiatric Disorders in America: The Epidemiological Catchment Area Study*. New York: The Free Press, pp. 204–219.

Kemeny, E., Husby, G., Williams, R.C., Jr., and Zabriskie, J.B. (1994) Tissue distribution of antigen(s) defined by monoclonal antibody D8/17 reacting with B lymphocytes of patients with rheumatic heart disease. *Clin Immunol Immunopathol* 72:35–43.

Khanna, A.K., Buskirk, D.R., Williams, R.C., Jr., Gibofsky, A., Crow, M.K., Menon, A., Fotino, M., Reid, H.M., Poon-King, T., Rubinstein, P., and Zabriskie, J.B. (1989) Presence of a non-HLA B cell antigen in rheumatic fever patients and their families as defined by a monoclonal antibody. *J Clin Invest* 83:1710–1716.

Kiessling, L.S. (1989) Tic disorders associated with evidence of invasive group A beta hemolytic streptococcal disease. *Dev Med Child Neurol* 31 (Suppl 59):48.

Kiessling, L.S., Marcotte, A.C., and Culpepper, L. (1994) Antineuronal antibodies: tics and obsessive-compulsive symptoms. *J Dev Behav Pediatr* 15:421–425.

Kondo, K. and Kabasawa, T. (1978) Improvement in Gilles de la Tourette syndrome after corticosteroid therapy. *Ann Neurol* 4: 387.

Leckman, J.F., Walker, D.E., Goodman, W.K., Pauls, D.L., and Cohen, D.J. (1994) "Just right" perceptions associated with compulsive behavior in Tourette's syndrome. *Am J Psychiatry* 151: 675–680.

Lenane, M.C., Swedo, S.E., Leonard, H.L., Pauls, D.L., Sceery, W., and Rapoport, J.L. (1990) Psychiatric disorders in first-degree relatives of children and adolescents with obsessive compulsive disorder. *J Am Acad Child Adolesc Psychiatry* 29:407–412.

Lennon, D. (1998) Acute rheumatic fever. In: Feigen, R.D. and Cherry, J.D., eds. *Textbook of Pediatric Infectious Diseases, 4th ed.* Philadelphia: W.B. Saunders, pp. 371–384.

Leonard, H.L., Lenane, M.C., Swedo, S.E., Rettew, D.C., Gershon, E.S., and Rapoport, J.L. (1992) Tics and Tourette's syndrome: a 2- to 7-year follow-up of 54 obsessive compulsive children. *Am J Psychiatry* 149:1244–1251.

Leonard, H.L., Swedo, S.E., Garvey, M.A., Beer, D., Perlmutter, S., Lougee, L., Karitani, M., and Dubbert, B. (1999) Postinfectious and other forms of obsessive-compulsive disorder. *Child Adolesc Psychiatr Clin North Am* 8:497–511.

Leonard, H.L., Swedo, S.E., Lenane, M.C., Rettew, D.C., Hamburger, S.D., Bartko, J.J., and Rapoport, J.L. (1993) A 2- to 7-year follow-up study of 54 obsessive compulsive children and adolescents. *Arch Gen Psychiatry* 50:429–439.

Lewinsohn, P.M., Hops, H., Roberts, R.E., Seeley, J.R., and Andrews, J.A. (1993) Adolescent psychopathology: I. Prevalence and incidence of depression and other DSM-III-R disorders in high school students. *J Abnorm Psychol* 102:133–144.

Lougee, L., Perlmutter, S.J., Nicolson, R., Garvey, M.A., and Swedo, S.E. (2000) Psychiatric disorders in first-degree relatives of children with pediatric autoimmune neuropsychiatric disorders associated with streptococcal infections (PANDAS). *J Am Acad Child Adolesc Psychiatry* 39:1120–1126.

Luxenberg, J.S., Swedo, S.E., Flament, M.F., Friedland, R.P., Rapoport, J., and Rapoport, S.I. (1988) Neuroanatomic abnormalities in obsessive-compulsive disorder detected with quantitative x-ray computed tomography. *Am J Psychiatry* 145:1089–1094.

March, J., Frances, A., Kahn, D., and Carpenter, D. (1997) Expert consensus guidelines: treatment of obsessive-compulsive disorder. *J Clin Psychiatry* 58 (Suppl 4):1–72.

Matarazzo, E.B. (1992) Tourette's syndrome treated with ACTH and prednisone: report of two cases. *J Child Adolesc Psychopharmacol* 2:215–226.

Max, J.E., Smith, W.L., Lindgen, S.D., Robin, D.A., Mattheis, P., Stierwalt, J., and Morrisey, M. (1995) Case study: obsessive-compulsive disorder after severe traumatic brain injury in an adolescent. *J Am Acad Child Adolesc Psychiatry* 34:45–49.

McMillan, J.A. and Feigen, R.D. (1999) Group A streptococcal infections. In: McMillan, J.A., DeAngelis, C.D., Feigen, R.D., and Warshaw, J.B., eds. *Oski's Pediatrics: Principles and Practice, 3rd ed.* Philadelphia: Lippincott, Williams, and Wilkins, pp. 1012–1017.

Murphy, T.K., Goodman, W.K., Fudge, M.W., Williams, R.C., Jr., Ayoub, E.M., Dalal, M., Lewis, M.H., and Zabriskie, J.B. (1997) B lymphocyte antigen D8/17: a peripheral marker for childhood-onset obsessive-compulsive disorder and Tourette's syndrome? *Am J Psychiatry* 154:402–407.

Nicolson, R., Swedo, S.E., Lenane, M., Bedwell, J., Wudarsky, M., Gochman, P., Hamburger, S.D., and Rapoport, J.L. (2000) An open trial of plasma exchange in childhood-onset obsessive-compulsive disorder without poststreptococcal exacerbations. *J Am Acad Child Adolesc Psychiatry* 39:1313–1315.

Osler, W. (1894) *On Chorea and Choreiform Affections*. Philadelphia: H.K. Lewis, pp. 33–35.

Patarroyo, M.E., Winchester, R.J., Vejerano, A., Gibofsky, A., Chalem, F., Zabriskie, J.B., and Kunkel, H.G. (1979) Association of a B-cell alloantigen with susceptibility to rheumatic fever. *Nature* 278:173–174.

Pauls, D.L., Towbin, K.K., Leckman, J.F., Zahner, G.E.P., and Cohen, D. (1986) Gilles de la Tourette's syndrome and obsessive-compulsive disorder: evidence supporting a genetic relationship. *Arch Gen Psychiatry* 43:1180–1182.

Perlmutter, S.J., Garvey, M.A., Castellanos, X., Mittleman, B.B., Giedd, J., Rapoport, J.L., and Swedo, S.E. (1998) A case of pediatric autoimmune neuropsychiatric disorders associated with streptococcal infections. *Am J Psychiatry* 155:1592–1598.

Perlmutter, S.J., Leitman, S.F., Garvey, M.A., Hamburger S., Feldman, E., Leonard, H.L., and Swedo, S.E. (1999) Therapeutic plasma exchange and intravenous immunoglobulin for obsessive-compulsive disorder and tic disorders in childhood. *Lancet* 354: 1153–1158.

Rauch, S.L. and Baxter, L.R. (1998) Neuroimaging of OCD and related disorders. In: Jenike, M.A., Baer, L., and Minichiello, W.E., eds. *Obsessive-Compulsive Disorders: Practical Management.* Boston: Mosby, pp. 222–253.

Regelmann, W.E., Talbot, R., Cairns, L., Martin, D., Miller, L.C., Zabriskie, J.B., Braun, D., and Gray, E.D. (1989) Distribution of cells bearing rheumatic antigens in peripheral blood of patients with rheumatic fever/rheumatic heart disease. *J Rheumatol* 16: 931–935.

Reinherz, H.Z., Giaconia, R.M., Lefkowitz, E.S., Pakiz, B., and Frost, A.K. (1993) Prevalence of psychiatric disorders in a community population of older adolescents. *J Am Acad Child Adolesc Psychiatry* 32:369–377.

Riddle, M., Scahill, L., King, R., Hardin, M.T., Towbin, K.E., Ort, S.I., Leckman, J.F., and Cohen, D.J. (1990) Obsessive compulsive disorder in children and adolescents: phenomenology and family history. *J Am Acad Child Adolesc Psychiatry* 29:766–772.

Rosenberg, D.R., Keshavan, M.S., O'Hearn, K.M., Dick, E.L., Bagwell, W.W., Seymour, A.B., Montrose, D.M., Pierri, J.N., and Birmaher, B. (1997) Fronto-striatal morphology of treatment-naïve pediatric obsessive compulsive disorder. *Arch Gen Psychiatry* 54: 831–838.

Selling, L. (1929) The role of infection in the etiology of tics. *Arch Neurol Psychiatry* 22:1163–1171.

Shapiro, A.K. and Shapiro, E. (1982). Clinical efficacy of haloperidol, pimozide, penfluridol, and clonidine in the treatment of Tourette syndrome. *Adv Neurol* 35:383–386.

Singer, H.S., Giuliano, J.D., Hansen, B.H., Hallett, J.J., Laurino, J.P., Benson, M., and Kiessling, L.S. (1998) Antibodies against human putamen in children with Tourette syndrome. *Neurology* 50: 1618–1624.

Swedo, S.E. (1989) Rituals and releasers: an ethological model of OCD. In: Rapoport, J.L., ed. *Obsessive Compulsive Disorder in Children and Adolescents.* Washington, DC: American Psychiatric Press, pp. 269–288.

Swedo, S.E. (1994) Sydenham's chorea: a model for childhood autoimmune neuropsychiatric disorders. *JAMA* 272:1788–1791.

Swedo, S.L., Leonard, H.L., Garvey, M., Mittleman, B., Allen, A.J., Perlmutter, S., Lougee, L., Dow, S., Zamkoff, J., and Dubbert, B.K. (1998) Pediatric autoimmune neuropsychiatric disorders associated with streptococcal infections: clinical description of the first 50 cases. *Am J Psychiatry* 155:264–271.

Swedo, S.E., Leonard, H.L., and Kiessling, L.S. (1994) Speculations on antineuronal antibody-mediated neuropsychiatric disorders of childhood. *Pediatrics* 93:323–326.

Swedo, S.E., Leonard, H.L., Mittleman, B.B., Allen, A.J., Rapoport, J.L., Dow, S.P., Kanter, M.E., Chapman, F., and Zabriskie, J. (1997) Identification of children with pediatric autoimmune neuropsychiatric disorders associated with streptococcal infections by a marker associated with rheumatic fever. *Am J Psychiatry* 154: 110–112.

Swedo, S.E., Leonard, H.L., Schapiro, M.B., Casey, B.J., Mannheim, G.B., Lenane, M.C., and Rettew, D.C. (1993) Sydenham's chorea: physical and psychological symptoms of St. Vitus dance. *Pediatrics* 91:706–713.

Swedo, S.E., Rapoport, J.L., Cheslow, D.L., Leonard, H.L., Ayoub, E.M., Hosier, D.M., and Wald, E.R. (1989a) High prevalence of obsessive-compulsive symptoms in patients with Sydenham's chorea. *Am J Psychiatry* 146:246–249.

Swedo, S.E., Rapoport, J.L., Leonard, H.L., Lenane, M., and Cheslow, D. (1989b) Obsessive-compulsive disorder in children and adolescents: clinical phenomenology of 70 consecutive cases. *Arch Gen Psychiatry* 46:335–341.

Sydenham, T. (1848) *The Entire Works of Thomas Sydenham*, Vols. 1–2. London: Sydenham Society.

Taranta, A. and Stollerman, G.H. (1956) The relationship of Sydenham's chorea to infection with group A streptococci. *Am J Med* 20:170.

Thomsen, P.H. and Mikkelsen, H.U. (1991) Children and adolescents with obsessive-compulsive disorder: the demographic and diagnostic characteristics of 61 Danish patients. *Acta Psychiatr Scand* 83:262–266.

von Economo, C. (1931) The sequelae of encephalitis lethargica. In: *Encephalitis Lethargica: Its Sequelae and Treatment.* London: Oxford University Press, pp. 111–134.

Walkup, J.T., LaBuda, M.C., Singer, H.S., Brown, J., Riddle, M.A., and Hurko, O. (1996) Family study and segregation analysis of Tourette syndrome: evidence for a mixed model inheritance. *Am J Hum Genet* 59:684–693.

Wilcox, J.A. and Nasrallah, H.A. (1986) Sydenham's chorea and psychosis. *Neuropsychobiology* 15:13–14.

Wittchen, H.U., Nelson, C.B., and Lachner, G. (1998) Prevalence of mental disorders and psychosocial impairments in adolescents and young adults. *Psychol Med* 28:109–126.

Zohar, A.H., Ratzoni, G., Pauls, D.L., Apter, A., Bleich, A., Kron, S., Rappaport, M., Weizman, A., and Cohen, D.G. (1988) An epidemiological study of obsessive-compulsive disorder and related disorders in Israeli adolescents. *J Am Acad Child Adolesc Psychiatry* 31:1057–1061.

15 | Neurobiology of childhood schizophrenia and related disorders

ROB NICOLSON AND JUDITH L. RAPOPORT

Schizophrenia has been described as one of the worst diseases affecting humankind. It is found in about 1 in 100 people worldwide, generally becoming manifest in late adolescence or early adulthood. Because it begins so early and usually interferes with education, employment, and interpersonal functioning, schizophrenia burdens not only those who suffer from it but also their families and society. Most affected individuals have substantial lifelong impairment, and more than one-half require continuous support, whether living in the community or in institutions. The chronic suffering of people with schizophrenia is highlighted by the fact that 10%–15% ultimately commit suicide and that many are homeless.

Although childhood cases are rare (McKenna et al., 1994), schizophrenia has been identified in children since its earliest descriptions. Despite this, the nosological status of schizophrenia in children was controversial for many years, and the *Diagnostic and Statistical Manual of Mental Disorders, 2nd ed.* (DSM-II) category "childhood schizophrenia" included other psychotic disorders in children as well as autistic disorder, limiting the usefulness of early studies. The landmark studies by Kolvin (1971), however, clearly differentiated schizophrenia with onset in childhood from pervasive developmental disorders.

CLINICAL PHENOTYPE OF SCHIZOPHRENIA IN CHILDREN AND ADOLESCENTS

The schizophrenia syndrome is characterized by a variety of cognitive and emotional impairments that may be conceptualized as falling into three broad categories: positive symptoms, negative symptoms, and disorganization. Positive symptoms (hallucinations and delusions) appear to reflect an excess or distortion of normal functions and are often the most obvious symptoms. Disorganized speech and behavior are sometimes conceived of as positive symptoms, although factor analyses suggest that it might be a separate symptom domain (Arndt et al., 1991). Negative symptoms, including affective flattening, alogia, and avolition, probably reflect low levels of emotional arousal, mental activity, and social drive, and can be the most debilitating symptoms for many patients. The DSM-IV requires that two of the above symptoms be present in association with impaired social or occupational functioning. However, if the delusions are bizarre or if hallucinations involve two or more voices conversing with each other or a voice maintaining a running commentary on the patient's thoughts or behavior, that symptom alone can satisfy the criteria for schizophrenia.

While early studies of children with schizophrenia were plagued by problems of diagnostic heterogeneity, recent studies have demonstrated that schizophrenia can be diagnosed reliably in children, using unmodified adult criteria (McKenna et al., 1994; Spencer and Campbell, 1994). Although developmental differences need to be considered in the evaluation of schizophrenic symptoms in very young patients, careful assessment permits the reliable identification of the characteristic symptoms of the illness (McKenna et al., 1994; Spencer and Campbell, 1994). However, childhood-onset schizophrenia (COS) is rare, with a rate of probably less than 1 in 10,000 (McKenna et al., 1994), and a detailed history is required to make the diagnoses accurately. Of the first 217 children referred for an ongoing study of COS at the National Institute of Mental Health (NIMH), only 69 received this diagnosis following extensive screening. A significant proportion (n = 45) of the patients excluded from the study of COS had transient, rather than pervasive, psychotic symptoms and severely disruptive behaviour. These patients with atypical psychotic disorders have been labeled provisionally by our group as "multidimensionally impaired" (Kumra et al., 1998b).

There was no excess of undifferentiated and disorganized subtypes among the NIMH sample of childhood-onset schizophrenics, and, surprisingly, the paranoid subtype was as frequent as in adult-onset patients. As patients in the NIMH study were all treatment-refractory, it is not surprising that they resemble adult patients with poor outcome in various ways. Others, however, using unselected series of patients, have also found COS to be a severe disorder with a generally poor outcome (Hollis, 2000). A preliminary analysis of 4-year outcome data on the NIMH cohort has similarly found that a systematic diagnosis of COS is stable over time, with a chronic illness being the rule (M. Lenane, unpublished data).

Comorbidity among patients with COS is exceptionally common (50% of patients), probably reflecting the severity of the underlying abnormalities of neurodevelopment. The comorbid diagnoses of the NIMH sample included approximately 20% with an anxiety disorder and a further 10% with a premorbid diagnosis of attention-deficit hyperactivity disorder (ADHD). Of particular interest are the nine patients (nearly 20%) who met criteria for a pervasive developmental disorder years before the onset of psychotic symptoms. In addition, a number of other COS patients had subthreshold symptoms of pervasive developmental disorders premorbidly. This high rate of pervasive developmental disorders among patients with COS has been reported by other groups (Watkins et al., 1988), and is inconsistent with findings among autistic adolescents and adults, among whom a diagnosis of schizophrenia is very rare (Volkmar and Cohen, 1991). This discrepancy may reflect the extreme rarity of COS.

NEUROANATOMICAL STUDIES OF CHILDHOOD-ONSET SCHIZOPHRENIA

Structural brain abnormalities are seen consistently in schizophrenia (Wright et al., 2000). Common findings include enlargement of the lateral and third ventricles and reduced volume of the total brain volume, cortical gray matter, medial temporal lobe structures, and thalamus. Most of these abnormalities have been found in first-episode, never-medicated adults with schizophrenia, suggesting that they are not a consequence of the disorder or of its treatment. The finding of similar abnormalities in relatives of patients with schizophrenia (Lawrie et al., 1999) further suggests that the brain anatomic abnormalities in schizophrenia represent a true biological marker of the illness.

Although animal models of psychiatric disorders have inherent limitations (Lipska and Weinberger, 2000), newer models of schizophrenia have implicated brain regions found to be abnormal in adult patients. Lipska and Weinberger (2000), for example, have reported that neonatal lesions to the ventral hippocampus in rats produce a range of dopamine-related behavioral and physiological abnormalities during adolescence in these animals that are similar to those seen in animals exposed to high doses of stimulants. The conclusion drawn by this group is that neonatal lesions of the hippocampus can produce a host of neurodevelopmental abnormalities, particularly a dysconnection between the hippocampus and prefrontal cortex. This model and others mimic some of the neurobiological phenomena associated with schizophrenia (Lipska and Weinberger, 2000), suggesting that they merit consideration in the development of new therapies, in identifying candidate genes, and in providing new insights about the pathophysiology and etiology of the disorder. However, studies of COS suggest that temporal lobe changes may be later developmental abnormalities (see next section), a finding not supportive of current models, and which will need to be considered in future animal models.

Brain Morphology in Childhood-Onset Schizophrenia

Patients with COS have morphometric abnormalities similar to those seen in adult patients with the disorder (Kumra et al., 2000; Sowell et al., 2000). Initial scans of 46 COS patients and 82 matched healthy control subjects showed, as expected, reduced total cerebral volume (secondary to gray matter loss) and midsagittal thalamic area, and increased lateral ventricular volume (Kumra et al., 2000; see Table 15.1). While volumetric reductions in medial temporal lobe structures are found consistently in studies of adults with schizophrenia (Wright et al., 2000), differences between patients with COS and controls in these structures were not significant at the time of the initial scan (Jacobsen et al., 1996a; Kumra et al., 2000).

As part of the NIMH study of COS, patients and controls have been asked to return for follow-up magnetic resonance imaging (MRI) scans on every 2 years. Given the prevailing neurodevelopmental hypothesis of schizophrenia (Murray and Lewis, 1987; Weinberger, 1987) and other theories about the role of synaptic pruning during adolescence in the onset of schizophrenia (Feinberg, 1982–1983), longitudinal studies of these patients during adolescence would seem to be particularly important in understanding the pathogenesis of the disorder. During adolescence, COS patients showed an exaggerated loss of hippocampal and amyg-

TABLE 15.1 *Brain Magnetic Resonance Imaging Volumes for Patients with Childhood-Onset Schizophrenia (n = 46) and Controls (n = 82)*

Brain Region	COS Patients (Mean ± SD)	Controls (Mean ± SD)	F_a	df	p
Total cerebral volume	1073.0 ± 123.3	1102.2 ± 113.0	6.3	1134	0.05
Total white matter	389.3 ± 51.8	383.8 ± 50.5	13.3	1133	0.001
Total gray matter	683.7 ± 81.4	718.0 ± 76.3	13.3	1133	0.001
Frontal gray matter	210.5 ± 23.9	223.1 ± 21.7	16.9	1133	0.001
Temporal gray matter	177.2 ± 22.0	182.8 ± 18.1	0.6	1133	0.4
Parietal gray matter	111.9 ± 14.7	120.3 ± 12.6	16.9	1133	0.001
Occipital gray matter	61.6 ± 9.5	64.4 ± 10.8	0.4	1133	0.5
Lateral ventricles	15.7 ± 7.8	11.1 ± 6.2	19.0	1133	0.001
Hippocampus	8.8 ± 1.2	9.1 ± 0.9	0.9	1121	0.4
Amygdala	4.9 ± 1.3	4.8 ± 1.0	1.8	1121	0.2

COS, childhood-onset schizophrenia.

[a]All *F* values, except total cerebral volume, are for analysis of covariance (ANCOVA) using total cerebral volume as a covariate. Adapted from Kumra et al. (2000)

dala volumes so that by late adolescence their scans resembled those of adult patients with respect to these structures (Jacobsen et al., 1998a; Giedd et al., 1999). Repeat scans of these childhood-onset patients have also revealed a more general progressive loss of gray matter volume, particularly in the frontal and temporal regions (Rapoport et al., 1999), and progressive increases in ventricular volume (Rapoport et al., 1997). These results are more striking than those seen in the few prospective brain MRI studies of adult patients that have found progressive changes (Gogate et al., in press) and demonstrate that the study of very early–onset patients provides a unique and important opportunity to further our understanding of the neurodevelopmental abnormalities hypothesized to underlie schizophrenia.

While brain changes, particulary in the basal ganglia, have been noted after treatment with atypical antipsychotics (Chakos et al., 1995; Frazier et al., 1996), the differential progression for the NIMH patients does not appear to be accounted for by such confounds, as it is time limited (chiefly between ages 13 and 18) and occurs independent of the dose and type of antipsychotic, or of clinical condition. Most intriguing is the significant correlation found between the reduction in hippocampal volume and a reduced ability to learn new information, as demonstrated by a smaller increase in raw scores on the information subtest of the Wechsler Intelligence Scale for Children (Bedwell et al., 1999).

While the role of medication in these changes appears to be insignificant, the COS studies could not exclude this completely. However, another group of patients treated with antipsychotics for behavioral dyscontrol and transient psychotic symptoms have also been followed clinically and with longitudinal MRI scans at the NIMH (Kumra et al., 1998b). An analysis of the longitudinal brain changes of these patients did not find any progressive reductions in gray matter volume or increases in ventricular volume, indicating that antipsychotic medications are unlikely to cause the progressive brain changes seen in COS (Nicolson et al., 2000a)

Functional and Metabolic Brain Imaging

Although studies of resting brain metabolism in adults with schizophrenia have produced conflicting results, studies during activation tasks have more consistently revealed frontal hypometabolism. Patients with COS were noted to have somewhat similar (but not more severe) abnormalities in a positron emission tomography (PET) study, although interpretation was limited as these severely ill patients could not adequately perform the activation task (Jacobsen et al., 1997b).

Magnetic resonance spectroscopy studies of COS patients revealed decreases in the ratio of *N*-acetyl aspartate to creatine (a putative marker of neuronal density) in the frontal cortex (Thomas et al., 1998) and hippocampus (Bertolino et al., 1998). These results were similar in direction and extent to those seen in adult patients.

NEUROPHYSIOLOGICAL STUDIES OF CHILDHOOD-ONSET SCHIZOPHRENIA

Autonomic Functioning

High levels of resting peripheral indicators of autonomic activity and reduced responsiveness of these indicators (including skin conductance and heart rate) have been found in adult-onset schizophrenia. Similar patterns were seen for COS patterns in the NIMH sample.

Smooth Pursuit Eye Movements

From 40% to 80% of patients with adult-onset schizophrenia have abnormalities in smooth pursuit eye movements (Holzman, 2000). Here, too, studies of COS find abnormalities similar to those reported in adult patients: decreased gain (ratio of eye speed to target speed), increased root mean square error (a global level of aberrant tracking reflecting the average distance from the target), and increased anticipatory saccades (Jacobsen et al., 1996b; Kumra et al., 2001). Sixty-seven percent of childhood-onset schizophrenics had qualitatively poor eye tracking. While these results are similar to those of adult patients, Ross et al. (1999) reported an increased rate of anticipatory saccades in a small group of childhood-onset probands (n = 10) when compared with adult-onset patients.

Neurotransmitters

Several neurotransmitters, most prominently dopamine and glutamate, have been implicated in schizophrenia. Dopaminergic hyperactivity in the mesencephalic projections to the limbic striatum has long been suspected. Indirect evidence for this includes the positive correlation between the clinical potency and D_2 binding affinity of antipsychotic drugs and the ability of dopamine agonists to induce psychotic symptoms. Although both postmortem and PET studies of schizophrenia patients found increased D_2 receptor density, the possible etiological role of antipsychotic drug treatment could not be ruled out (Davis and Lieberman, 2000).

Recently, however, direct evidence of dopamine hyperactivity has emerged from both preclinical and clinical studies. Several functional imaging studies have found elevated synaptic concentrations of dopamine and exaggerated stimulation of dopaminergic transmission in response to administration of amphtamines.

The results of these studies implicate dysfunctions in presynaptic storage, release, reuptake, and metabolic mechanisms in dopamine mesolimbic systems (Davis and Lieberman, 2000).

Glutamate was initially implicated in schizophrenia by studies of the behavioral effects of N-methyl-D-aspartate (NMDA) receptor antagonists (e.g., PCP, ketamine), which produce psychotic symptoms and cognitive dysfunction in healthy subjects and exacerbate psychotic, negative, and cognitive symptoms in patients with schizophrenia. Studies show that acute administration of NMDA antagonists causes NMDA receptor dysfunction, resulting in decreased inhibition of subcortical dopamine neurons and consequent increased mesolimbic dopamine release. Chronic administration produces decreased release, or hypoactivity, of dopamine in the prefrontal cortex (Davis and Lieberman, 2000).

Although the role of neurotransmitter dysfunction in schizophrenia remains an exciting and important avenue of exploration, we are only aware of one study of neurotransmitters in COS. Jacobsen and colleagues (1997a) measured cerebrospinal fluid (CSF) levels of HVA and 5-HIAA, metabolites of dopamine and serotonin, respectively. While the concentrations of these monoamine metabolites were similar to that seen in adults with schizophrenia, they did not change significantly with treatment.

Genetic Factors in Childhood-Onset Schizophrenia

Genetic factors are important in the pathogenesis of schizophrenia (Karayiorgou and Gogos, 1997), and the notion that such factors may be more salient in very early onset–cases fueled two classic family studies of childhood-onset cases (Kallmann and Roth, 1956; Kolvin et al., 1971).

In studies of adult patients, age of onset in schizophrenia has a lower correlation for affected siblings (approximately 0.26) and concordant dizygotic twins (approximately 0.30) than between concordant monozygotic twins (r = 0.68) (Kendler et al., 1987), suggesting a genetic influence on age of onset. Although some studies find a relationship between pedigree density and age of onset (Pulver and Liang, 1991; Suvisaari et al., 1998; Asarnow, 1999), others have not (Kendler et al., 1987, 1996). This inconsistency, in combination with the higher correlation between age of onset in concordant monozygotic twins than in concordant dizygotic twins, suggests that age of onset might be influenced by genetic factor(s) independent of disease liability. However, there are no published studies of the relationship between age of onset and family loading in childhood-onset samples, and the possibility remains that very early–onset cases may reveal more unique or potent genetic factors.

Schizophrenia and spectrum disorders (schizoaffective disorder and schizotypal and paranoid personality disorders) are increased in the relatives of patients with schizophrenia, and adoption studies document the genetic basis of these disorders (Karayiorgou and Gogos, 1997). To assess the rate of familial schizophrenia spectrum disorders in COS, available parents (n = 92) of the NIMH cohort were administered the Schedule for Affective Disorders and Schizophrenia and the Structured Interview for DSM-IV Personality Disorders. Using a hierarchical method to assign diagnoses, 26 (28%) parents met criteria for schizophrenia or a spectrum disorder: 1 one for schizophrenia, 9 for schizotypal personality disorder, and 16 for paranoid personality disorder. Twenty (48%) of the probands had at least one relative with a spectrum disorder (Nicolson et al., 2000b). When compared with parents of patients with adult-onset schizophrenia (n = 87) and parents of community controls (n = 129), parents of COS patients had a significantly higher rate of schizophrenia spectrum disorders, who in turn had a higher rate of these disorders than parents of community controls (Nicolson et al., 2000b) (see Table 15.2).

The rates of the more disabling disorders (schizophrenia and schizoaffective disorder) in relatives of the childhood-onset patients were similar to those seen in relatives of adult-onset patients, perhaps because of a sampling bias inherent in a national study of a rare disorder, which involves long distance travel and parental participation. As such, severely ill parents and their children would be unlikely to participate. However, there appears to be a striking excess of schizotypal and paranoid personality disorders in the relatives of these patients. Although these data are preliminary and based on unblinded interviews, they are in accordance with results from the ongoing University of California at Los Angeles study of COS (Asarnow, 1999). Together, these studies indicate more salient genetic factors for the very early–onset disorder.

Neurophysiological Measures

Another measure of familial risk for schizophrenia is abnormalities of smooth pursuit eye movements, which are increased in unaffected relatives of adult probands (Holzman, 2000). To date, 56 relatives (age

TABLE 15.2 *Schizophrenia Spectrum Disorders in Parents of Childhood-Onset Schizophrenia Patients, Parents of Adult-Onset Schizophrenia Patients, and Parents of Community Controls*

Diagnosis[a]	COS Parents n (%)	AOS Parents n (%)	Control Parents n (%)
Schizophrenia	1/92 (1.1)	1/89 (1.1)	0
Schizoaffective disorder	0	0	0
Schizotypal personality disorder	9/91 (9.9)	4/88 (4.5)	1/129 (0.8)
Paranoid personality disorder	16/82 (19.5)	8/82 (9.8)	2/128 (1.6)
Any schizophrenia spectrum disorder[b]	26/92 (28.3)	13/89 (14.6)	3/129 (2.3)

AOS, adult-onset schizophrenia; COS, childhood-onset schizophrenia. [a]Rates of all diagnoses were determined hierarchically, whereby a person could only receive one of the four schizophrenia spectrum diagnoses. [b]COS parents > AOS parents > control parents (χ^2 = 30.3, df = 2, p < 0.001). Adapted from Nicolson et al. (2000b)

14 and over) of our COS probands have been examined and, with the use of qualitative ratings, 8 (14.3%) were determined to have abnormal eye tracking, whereas only 1 of 42 control subjects (2.4%) had similar results (p = 0.04). The COS relatives also had greater root mean square errors (p = 0.02) (Nicolson et al., 1999b). However, these abnormalities in the parents of the NIMH COS probands do not appear to be increased in comparison with the relatives of adult-onset patients, although Ross et al. (1999) reported that anticipatory saccades were greater in a small sample (n = 24) of parents of childhood-onset patients than in parents of adult-onset patients, and that childhood-onset patients also had a greater likelihood of having both parents exhibit this abnormality (bilineality).

Other Genetic Studies

An increased rate of chromosomal abnormalities has been reported for adult-onset schizophrenia (Karayiorgou and Gogos, 1997; Bassett et al., 2000). Cytogenetic abnormalities have been examined in the NIMH COS cohort. Five of our initial 54 patients had cytogenetic abnormalities (a girl with Turner's syndrome, a boy with a balanced translocation of chromosomes 1 and 7, and two girls and a boy with velocardiofacial syndrome [deletion 22q11]) (Nicolson et al., 1999a), a rate that appears to be higher than that seen in adult-onset schizophrenia. In particular, the rate of deletions of 22q11 may be increased over that seen among adult-onset patients, a finding that is of great interest, given that genetic studies in adult patients have reported linkage to this region (Owen, 2000).

Trinucleotide repeats, human leukocyte antigen (HLA), and apolipoprotein (APO) E4 have been investigated as possible etiologic factors in adult-onset schizophrenia, with conflicting results (Karayiorgou and Gogos, 1997). For the NIMH cohort, no association was seen for APOE4 (Fernandez et al., 1999), HLA (Jacobsen et al., 1998b), or trinucleotide repeats (Sidransky et al., 1998). These findings are consistent with observations in studies of adults, which generally do not support a role of APOE4, HLA, or trinucleotide repeats in schizophrenia.

Recent Linkage and Molecular Studies of Schizophrenia

A number of linkage studies have been undertaken in an attempt to identify candidate regions in which susceptibility genes may reside. Although most of these studies await replication, potentially important regions include 5q21–q31, 6p24–22, 8p22–21, 10p15–p11, 13q14.1–q32, 18p 22–21, and 22q11–12 (Owen, 2000).

Association studies, which can be used to identify genes of small effect, have also been used in studies of adult-onset schizophrenics to identify polymorphisms in the *5HTA* receptor gene and the *DRD3* receptor gene, which may be involved in schizophrenia (Owen, 2000).

Because of the rarity of COS, there have been no large-scale molecular genetic studies of COS. However, at least two collaborative studies are planned for the coming years.

ENVIRONMENTAL FACTORS

Environmental factors, such as prenatal maternal infections and perinatal complications, have been implicated in the pathogenesis of schizophrenia. Also, the correlation of only 0.6 for age of onset in monozygotic twins concordant for schizophrenia suggests that nongenetic factors play a role in determining the age of onset (Kendler et al., 1987). A greater frequency or severity of these factors could conceivably result in an earlier onset of schizophrenia.

Patients with adult-onset schizophrenia have been reported to have an increased rate of obstetric complications in both case–control and epidemiological studies (when compared with siblings or community controls) (Jones et al., 1998; Geddes et al., 1999; Dalman et al., 1999), although not all studies have found this (Done et al., 1991). A recent reanalysis of the original data from a number of studies found those schizophrenia patients with birth complications to have an earlier age of onset of illness (Verdoux et al., 1997).

Blinded scoring of the birth records of 36 patients with COS and 35 sibling controls found no significant differences between the groups (Nicolson et al., 1999c). Moreover, the rate of complications in the early-onset patients of the NIMH study was similar to that seen in adult-onset patients. These preliminary results, as well as the work of others (Frangou, 1999), suggest that, while obstetric complications may play a role in the development of schizophrenia in some patients, they are not more salient in childhood-onset cases.

Other environmental factors have been examined in the NIMH cohort, with similarly negative results. Patients with COS do not have an exaggerated rate of psychosocial stressors (M. Lenane, unpublished data), and the timing of the onset of puberty in COS patients did not differ from that of their siblings or national norms (Frazier et al., 1997).

The role of other factors in the pathogenesis of schizophrenia, such as prenatal nutritional deprivation or prenatal maternal infections, have, to our knowledge, not been investigated in patients with childhood-onset schizophrenia. Given the rarity of this condition, such studies are unlikely.

PREMORBID DEVELOPMENT

Premorbid Course

Patients with adult-onset schizophrenia have been shown to have subtle but demonstrable impairments in premorbid language as well as in motor and social development (Davies et al., 1998), and a poor outcome in schizophrenia is correlated with more pronounced early developmental abnormalities. Several independent studies have found that very early–onset schizophrenia is associated with similar but more pronounced abnormalities (Watkins et al., 1988; Alaghband-Rad et al., 1995; Hollis, 1995).

The prepsychotic developmental course of the first 49 patients in the NIMH COS study confirms and extends these findings. Of these patients, 55% had language abnormalities, 57% had motor abnormalities, and 55% had social abnormalities years before the onset of psychotic symptoms. There was also an exceedingly high rate of educational underachievement among these patients: 31 (63.3%) had either failed a grade or required placement in a special education setting before the onset of their illness (Nicolson et al., 2000c).

In the NIMH study, a family history of schizophrenia spectrum disorders was related to premorbid impairment in the proband. Seventeen of the 22 patients (77.3%) with relatives with schizophrenia spectrum disorders had premorbid language abnormalities, whereas only 10 of the 26 subjects (38.5%) without a similar family history had early speech and language difficulties (p = 0.007) (Nicolson et al., 2000c). This relationship is intriguing, as British and American birth cohort studies (Done et al., 1994; Jones et al., 1994; Bearden et al., 2000) have found aberrant speech and language development in infancy and childhood to be significantly increased in those who later developed schizophrenia. In the National Collaborative Perinatal Project, children with abnormalities of language had a 14-fold greater risk of later developing schizophrenia than children without such abnormalities (Bearden et al., 2000). Early language impairments also appear to be predictive of schizophrenia as well as other disorders: Howlin and colleagues (2000) reported that 2 of 25 children with severe receptive language disorders developed schizophrenia during adolescence. Our finding of an association between premorbid language impairments and schizophrenia spectrum disorders in relatives suggests that either specific disease-related factors interact with a more general liability or, more interestingly, that genes involved in the etiology of schizophrenia interfere with the development of language-related brain regions.

CONCEPTUAL MODELS

The neurodevelopmental hypothesis of schizophrenia posits that the disorder is due to a subtle defect in prenatal brain development but is not clinically manifest until many years later (Murray and Lewis, 1987; Weinberger, 1987). This theory has two essential components: a presumption of developmental neuropathology and an expectation that this developmental neuropathology results in a pattern of brain malfunction which ultimately produces the symptoms of schizophrenia.

Some features of patients with COS are consistent with this prenatal hypothesis. However, other data from patients with a very early onset of the disorder suggest that they may have both more severe early as well as more striking late neurodevelopmental abnormalities. Consistent with the "prenatal lesion" model, patients with COS have a range of early cognitive, motor, and language deficits, strongly suggestive of anomalous brain development (Nicolson et al., 2000c). On initial scan, these patients also have a variety of morphometric brain abnormalities, detected by MRI, which are best interpreted as indicative of abnormal brain development rather than neurodegeneration. However, at initial scan, these abnormalities were not more striking than those seen in adults with schizophrenia and were less striking than those seen later in adolescence in COS patients. Clearly, there is a continuing abnormal developmental process, which may be a later effect of a single neurotrophin or peptide. Models supporting this possibility are already described. For example, a mutant mouse strain with reduced postnatal levels of transforming growth factor alpha (a nervous system growth factor) is found at a young age to have relatively normal brain morphology. However, as the mouse develops (and levels of transforming growth factor fall), the total cerebral volume decreases relative to normal mice and they also demonstrate an increase in ventricular volume (Burrows et al., 2000).

One weakness of the neurodevelopmental hypothesis is the lack of a convincing explanation for abnormal neuronal networks present since fetal life not causing psychosis until much later in life in most patients. One model for the onset of the disorder in late adolescence in most patients has been aberrant synaptic pruning (Feinberg, 1982–1983; McGlashan and Hoffman, 2000), which is normally increased during later adolescence. The findings of progressive volumetric changes in patients with COS (Rapoport et al., 1997, 1999; Giedd et al., 1999) are consistent with the aberrant pruning hypothesis and suggest that childhood and adolescence are a particularly important period when this may be observed. Only later in adolescence, for example, do temporal lobe deficits become significant (Jacobsen et al., 1998a; Gogate et al., in press). On a molecular level, these findings are consistent with the postmortem findings of Lewis and his group (Mirnics et al., 2000), in which decreased expression of synapsin (a transcript encoding a protein involved in the regulation of presynaptic function) was prominent in a wide microarray analysis of gene expression in the prefrontal cortex.

RELEVANCE TO PHARMACOTHERAPY

Patients with COS may be more resistant to treatment than adults with the disorder (Meltzer et al., 1997), possibly because their neurodevelopmental abnormalities render them less amenable to drug treatment.

In addition, early-onset patients seem to have a higher rate of adverse drug effects (Kumra et al., 1996; 1998a), with a greater risk of dyskinesias (Kumra et al., 1998a) and of prolactin-related adverse effects (Wudarsky et al., 1999). Although the mechanisms for this are not clear, developmental aspects may play a role: dopamine receptors are more dense early in life (Seeman et al., 1987) and thus effects of blockade of these receptors by antipsychotic medications may be augmented.

CONCLUSIONS

Childhood-onset schizophrenia is a rare and severe form of the disorder. Study of these patients may provide us with information that is integral to understanding the pathogenesis of the disorder (see Table 15.3). For example, greater understanding of their progressive brain changes will be enabled by continuing to follow up these patients with serial MRI scans and more sophisticated localization and timing of progressive brain changes (e.g., Thompson et al., 2000, 2001).

Emerging evidence suggests that patients with a very early onset of schizophrenia have greater levels of both early and later neurodevelopmental abnormalities. Environmental factors are not increased, while genetic risk seems heightened (Asarnow, 1999; Frangou, 1999; Nicolson et al., 2000b). Multicenter genetic linkage studies of these patients are expected to be particularly informative in uncovering genes involved in the etiology of schizophrenia. Furthermore, because of the elevated rate of deletions of chromosome 22q11 in these patients, this region is a prime area of interest for association studies. From results of our imaging studies, it is anticipated that relevant genes will have roles in both prenatal and postnatal brain development.

TABLE 15.3 *Risk Factors for Schizophrenia in Patients with Childhood Onset of the Disorder*

Risk Factor	Abnormality Relative to controls	More Striking Than in Adult-Onset Patients
Cytogenetic abnormalities	Increased	Yes
Familial schizophrenia spectrum disorders	Increased	Yes
Smooth pursuit eye movement abnormalities	Increased	No
Obstetrical complications	Not different	No
Premorbid developmental abnormalities	Increased	Yes
Onset of puberty	Not different	No

Adapted from Nicolson and Rapoport (1999).

REFERENCES

Alaghband-Rad, J., McKenna, K., Gordon, C.T., Albus, K.E., Hamburger, S.D., Rumsey, J.M., Frazier, J.A., Lenane, M.C., and Rapoport, J.L. (1995) Childhood-onset schizophrenia: the severity of premorbid course. *J Am Acad Child Adolesc Psychiatry* 34: 1273–1283.

Arndt, S., Alliger, R.J., and Andreasen, N.C. (1991) The distinction of positive and negative symptoms: the failure of a two-dimensional model. *Br J Psychiatry* 158:317–322.

Asarnow, R.F. (1999) What are the boundaries of the schizophrenia phenotype? *Biol Psychiatry* 45:12S.

Bassett, A.S., Chow, E.W.C., and Weksburg R (2000). Chromosomal abnormalities and schizophrenia. *Am J Med Genet* 97:45–51.

Bearden, C.E., Rosso, I.M., Hollister, J.M., Sanchez, L.E., Hadley, T., and Cannon, T.D. (2000) A prospective cohort study of childhood behavioral deviance and language abnormalities as predictors of adult schizophrenia. *Schizophr Bull* 26:395–410.

Bedwell, J.S., Keller, B., Smith, A.K., Hamburger, S., Kumra, S., and Rapoport, J.L. (1999) Childhood-onset schizophrenia: why does post-psychotic full-scale IQ decline? *Am J Psychiatry* 156:1996–1997.

Bertolino, A., Kumra, S., Callicott, J.H., Mattay, V.S., Lestz, R.M., Jacobsen, L., Barnett, I.S., Duyn, J.H., Frank, J.A., Rapoport, J.L., and Weinberger, D.R. (1998) Common pattern of cortical pathology in childhood-onset and adult-onset schizophrenia as identified by proton magnetic resonance spectroscopic imaging. *Am J Psychiatry* 155:1376–1383.

Burrows, R.C., Levitt, P., and Shors, T.J. (2000) Postnatal decrease in transforming growth factor alpha is associated with enlarged ventricles, deficient amygdaloid vasculature and performance deficits. *Neuroscience* 96:825–836.

Chakos, M.H., Lieberman, J.A., Alvir, J., Bilder, R., and Ashtari, M. (1995) Caudate nuclei volumes in schizophrenic patients treated with typical antipsychotics or clozapine. *Lancet* 345:456–457.

Dalman, C., Allebeck, P., Cullberg, J., Grunewald, C., and Koster, M. (1999) Obstetric complications and the risk of schizophrenia: a longitudinal study of a national birth cohort. *Arch Gen Psychiatry* 56:234–240.

Davies, N., Russell, A., Jones, P., and Murray, R.M. (1998) Which characteristics of schizophrenia predate psychosis? *J Psychiatr Res* 32:121–131.

Davis, D.A. and Lieberman, J.A. (2000) Catching up on schizophrenia: natural history and neurobiology. *Neuron* 28:325–334.

Done, D.J., Crowe, T.J., Johnstone, E.C., and Sacker, A. (1994) Childhood antecedents of schizophrenia and affective illness: social adjustment at ages 7 and 11. *BMJ* 309:699–703.

Done, D.J., Johnstone, E.C., Frith, C.D., Golding, J., Shepherd, P.M., and Crow, T.J. (1991) Complications of pregnancy and delivery in relation to psychosis in adult life: data from the British perinatal mortality survey sample. *BMJ* 302:1576–1580.

Feinberg, I. (1982–1983) Schizophrenia: caused by a fault in programmed synaptic elimination during adolescence? *J Psychiatr Res* 17:319–334.

Fernandez, T., Yan, W.L., Hamburger, S., Rapoport, J.L., Saunders, A.M., Schapiro, M., Ginns, E.I., and Sidransky, E. (1999) Apolipoprotein E alleles in childhood-onset schizophrenia. *Am J Med Genet* 88:211–213.

Frangou, S. (1999) The Maudsley early onset schizophrenia study: abnormal genes, abnormal brains, abnormal families. *Biol Psychiatry* 45:12S.

Frazier, J.A., Alaghband-Rad, J., Jacobsen, L., Lenane, M.C., Hamburger, S., Albus, K., Smith, A., McKenna, K., and Rapoport, J.L. (1997) Pubertal development and onset of psychosis in childhood onset schizophrenia. *Psychiatry Res* 70:1–7.

Frazier, J.A., Giedd, J.N., Kaysen, D., Albus, K., Hamburger, S., Alaghband-Rad, J., Lenane, M.C., McKenna, K., Breier, A., and Rapoport, J.L. (1996) Childhood-onset schizophrenia: brain MRI rescan after 2 years of clozapine maintenance treatment. *Am J Psychiatry* 153:564–566.

Geddes, J.R., Verdoux, H., Takei, N., Lawrie, S.M., Bovet, P., Eagles, J.M., Heun, R., McCreadie, R.G., McNeil, T.F., O'Callaghan, E., Stober, G., Willinger, U., and Murray, R.M. (1999) Schizophrenia and complications of pregnancy and labor: an individual patient data meta-analysis. *Schizophr Bull* 25:413–423.

Giedd, J.N., Jeffries, N.O., Blumenthal, J., Castellanos, F.X., Vaituzis, A.C., Fernandez, T., Hamburger, S.D., Liu, H., Nelson, J., Bedwell, J., Tran, L., Lenane, M.C., Nicolson, R., and Rapoport, J.L. (1999) Childhood-onset schizophrenia: progressive brain changes during adolescence. *Biol Psychiatry* 46:892–898.

Gogate, N., Giedd, J.N., Janson, K., Rapoport, J.L. (in press) Normal and abnormal brian development: new perspectives for child psychiatry. *Clin Neurosci Res*.

Hollis, C. (1995) Child and adolescent (juvenile onset) schizophrenia: a case–control study of premorbid developmental impairments. *Br J Psychiatry* 166:489–495.

Hollis, C. (2000) Adult outcomes of child- and adolescent-onset schizophrenia: diagnostic stability and predictive validity. *Am J Psychiatry* 157:1652–1659.

Holzman, P.S. (2000) Eye movements and the search for the essence of schizophrenia. *Brain Res Brain Res Rev* 31:350–356.

Howlin, P., Mawhood, L., and Rutter, M. (2000) Autism and developmental receptive language disorder—a follow-up comparison in early adult life. II: Social, behavioural, and psychiatric outcomes. *J Child Psychol Psychiatry* 41:561–578.

Jacobsen, L.K., Frazier, J.A., Malhotra, A.K., Karoum, F., McKenna, K., Gordon, C.T., Hamburger, S.D., Lenane, M.C., Pickar, D., Potter, W.Z., and Rapoport, J.L. (1997a) Cerebrospinal fluid monoamine metabolites in childhood-onset schizophrenia. *Am J Psychiatry* 154:69–74.

Jacobsen, L.K., Giedd, J.N., Castellanos, F.S., Vaituzis, A.C., Hamburger, S.D., Kumra, S., Lenane, M.C., and Rapoport, J.L. (1998a) Progressive reduction of temporal lobe structures in childhood-onset schizophrenia. *Am J Psychiatry* 155:678–685.

Jacobsen, L.K., Giedd, J.N., Vaituzis, A.C., Hamburger, S.D., Rajapakse, J.C., Frazier, J.A., Kaysen, D., Lenane, M.C., McKenna, K., Gordon, C.T., and Rapoport, J.L. (1996a) Temporal lobe morphology in childhood-onset schizophrenia. *Am J Psychiatry* 153:355–361.

Jacobsen, L.K., Hamburger, S.D., Van Horn, J.D., Vaituzis, A.C.,

McKenna, K., Frazier, J.A., Gordon, C.T., Lenane, M.C., Rapoport, J.L., and Zametkin, A.J. (1997b) Cerebral glucose metabolism in childhood-onset schizophrenia. *Psychiatry Res* 75:131–144.

Jacobsen, L.K., Hong, W.L., Hommer, D.W., Hamburger, S.D., Castellanos, F.X., Frazier, J.A., Giedd, J.N., Gordon, C.T., Karp, B.I., McKenna, K., and Rapoport, J.L. (1996b) Smooth pursuit eye movements in childhood-onset schizophrenia: comparison with attention-deficit hyperactivity disorder and normal controls. *Biol Psychiatry* 40:1144–1154.

Jacobsen, L.K., Mittleman, B.B., Kumra, S., Lenane, M.C., Barracchini, K.C., Adams, S., Simonis, T., Lee, P.R., Long, R.T., Sharp, W., Sidransky, E., Ginns, E.I., and Rapoport, J.L. (1998b) HLA antigens in childhood-onset schizophrenia. *Psychiatry Res* 78:123–132.

Jones, P., Rodgers, B., Murray, R., and Marmot, M. (1994) Child development risk factors for schizophrenia in the British 1946 birth cohort. *Lancet* 344:1398–1402.

Jones, P.B., Rantakallio, P., Hartikainen, A.L., Isohanni, M., and Sipila, P. (1998) Schizophrenia as a long-term outcome of pregnancy, delivery, and perinatal cmplications: a 28-year follow-up of the 1966 north Finland general population birth cohort. *Am J Psychiatry* 155:355–364.

Kallmann, F.J. and Roth, B. (1956) Genetic aspects of preadolescent schizophrenia. *Am J Psychiatry* 112:599–606.

Karayiorgou, M. and Gogos, J.A. (1997) A turning point in schizophrenia genetics. *Neuron* 19:967–979.

Kendler, K.S., Karkowski-Shuman, L., and Walsh, D. (1996) Age at onset in schizophrenia and risk of illness in relatives. Results from the Roscommon Family Study. *Br J Psychiatry* 169:213–218.

Kendler, K.S., Tsuang, M.T., and Hays, P. (1987) Age at onset in schizophrenia. A familial perspective. *Arch Gen Psychiatry* 44:881–890.

Kolvin, I. (1971) Studies in the childhood psychoses. I. Diagnostic criteria and classification. *Br J Psychiatry* 118:381–384.

Kolvin, I., Garside, R.F., and Kidd, J.S. (1971) Studies in the childhood psychoses. IV. Parental personality and attitude and childhood psychoses. *Br J Psychiatry* 118:403–406.

Kumra, S., Frazier, J.A., Jacobsen, L.K., McKenna, K., Gordon, C.T., Lenane, M.C., Hamburger, S.D., Smith, A.K., Albus, K.E., Alaghband-Rad, J., and Rapoport, J.L. (1996) Childhood-onset schizophrenia. A double-blind clozapine-haloperidol comparison. *Arch Gen Psychiatry* 53:1090–1097.

Kumra, S., Giedd, J.N., Vaituzis, A.C., Jacobsen, L.K., McKenna, K., Bedwell, J., Hamburger, S., Nelson, J.E., Lenane, M., and Rapoport, J.L. (2000) Childhood-onset psychotic disorders: magnetic resonance imaging of volumetric differences in brain structure. *Am J Psychiatry* 157:1467–1474.

Kumra, S, Hommer, D.W., Nicolson, R., Thaker, G., Israel, E., Lenane, M., Bedwell J., Jacobsen, L.K., McKenna, K., Hamburger, S., and Rapoport, J.L. (2001). Childhood-onset psychotic disorders: smooth pursuit eye tracking impairment. *Am J Psychiatry* 158:1291–1298.

Kumra, S., Jacobsen, L.K., Lenane, M., Smith, A., Lee, P., Malanga, C.J., Karp, B.I., Hamburger, S., and Rapoport, J.L. (1998a) Case series: spectrum of neuroleptic-induced movement disorders and extrapyramidal side effects in childhood-onset schizophrenia. *J Am Acad Child Adolesc Psychiatry* 37:221–227.

Kumra, S., Jacobsen, L.K., Lenane, M., Zahn, T.P., Wiggs, E., Alaghband-Rad, J., Castellanos, F.X., Frazier, J.A., McKenna, K., Gordon, C.T., Smith, A., Hamburger, S., and Rapoport, J.L. (1998b) "Multidimensionally impaired disorder": is it a variant of very early-onset schizophrenia? *J Am Acad Child Adolesc Psychiatry* 37:91–99.

Lawrie, S.M., Whalley, H., Kestelman, J.N., Abukmeil, S.S., Byrne, M., Hodges, A., Rimmington, J.E., Best, J.J., Owens, D.G., and Johnstone, E.C. (1999) Magnetic resonance imaging of brain in people at high risk of developing schizophrenia. *Lancet* 353:30–33.

Lipska, B.K. and Weinberger, D.R. (2000) To model a psychiatric disorder in animals: schizophrenia as a reality test. *Neuropsychopharmacology* 23:223–239.

McGlashan, T.H. and Hoffman, R.E. (2000) Schizophrenia as a disorder of developmentally reduced synaptic connectivity. *Arch Gen Psychiatry* 57:637–648.

McKenna, K., Gordon, C.T., Lenane, M., Kaysen, D., Fahey, K., and Rapoport, J.L. (1994) Looking for childhood-onset schizophrenia: the first 71 cases screened. *J Am Acad Child Adolesc Psychiatry* 33:636–644.

Meltzer, H.Y., Rabinowitz, J., Lee, M.A., Cola, P.A., Ranjan, R., Findling, R.L., and Thompson, P.A. (1997) Age at onset and gender of schizophrenic patients in relation to neuroleptic resistance. *Am J Psychiatry* 154:475–482.

Mirnics, K., Middleton, F.A., Marquez, A., Lewis, D.A., and Levitt P. (2000) Molecular characterization of schizophrenia viewed by microarray analysis of gene expression in prefrontal cortex. *Neuron* 28:53–67.

Murray, R.M. and Lewis, S.W. (1987) Is schizophrenia a neurodevelopmental disorder? *BMJ* 295:681–682.

Nicolson, R., Giedd, J.N., Blumenthal, J., Hamburger, S., Vaituzis, A.C., Nelson, J., Lenane, M., Wudarsky, M., Gochman, P., and Rapoport, J.L. (2000a) A longitudinal MRI study of children and adolescents with atypical psychotic disorders. *Biol Psychiatry* 47:494S.

Nicolson, R., Giedd, J.N., Lenane M., Hamburger, S., Singaracharlu, S., Bedwell, J., Fernandez, T., Thaker, G.K., Malaspina, D., and Rapoport, J.L. (1999a) Clinical and neurobiological correlates of cytogenetic abnormalities in childhood-onset schizophrenia. *Am J Psychiatry* 156:1575–1579.

Nicolson, R., Gochman, P., Lenane, M., Brookner, F., Egan, M.F., Pickar, D., Weinberger, D.R., and Rapoport, J.L. (2000b) Familial schizophrenia spectrum disorders in childhood- and adult-onset schizophrenia. *Biol Psychiatry* 47:12S–13S.

Nicolson, R., Hommer, D., Thaker, G., Brown, M., Bedwell, M., Lenane, M., Fernandez, T., and Rapoport, J.L. (1999b) Smooth pursuit eye movements in the relatives of patients with childhood-onset schizophrenia. Schizophr Res 36:93.

Nicolson, R., Lenane, M., Singaracharlu, S., Malaspina, D., Giedd, J.N., Hamburger, S.D., Gochman, P., Bedwell, J., Thaker, G.K., Fernandez, T., Wudarsky, M., Hommer, D.W., and Rapoport, J.L. (2000c) Premorbid speech and language impairments in childhood-onset schizophrenia: association with risk factors. *Am J Psychiatry* 157:794–800.

Nicolson, R., Malaspina, D., Giedd, J.N., Hamburger, S., Lenane, M., Bedwell, J., Berman, A., Susser, E., and Rapoport, J.L. (1999c) Obstetrical complications in childhood-onset schizophrenia. *Am J Psychiatry* 156:1650–1652

Nicolson, R. and Rapoport, J.L. (1999) Childhood-onset schizophrenia: rare but worth studying. *Biol Psychiatry* 46:1418–1428.

Owen, M.J. (2000) Molecular genetic studies of schizophrenia. *Brain Res Brain Res Rev* 31:179–186.

Pulver, A.E. and Liang, K.Y. (1991) Estimating effects of proband characteristics on familial risk: II. The association between age at onset and familial risk in the Maryland schizophrenia sample. *Genet Epidemiol* 8:339–350.

Rapoport, J.L., Giedd, J., Blumenthal, J., Hamburger, S., Jeffries, N., Fernandez, T., Nicolson, R., Bedwell, J., Lenane, M., Zijdenbo, A., Paus, T., and Evans, A. (1999) Progressive cortical change during adolescence in childhood-onset schizophrenic subjects: a longitudinal study. *Arch Gen Psychiatry* 56:649–654.

Rapoport, J.L., Giedd, J., Kumra, S., Jacobsen, L., Smith, A., Lee, P., Nelson, J., and Hamburger, S.D. (1997) Childhood-onset schizophrenia: progressive ventricular change during adolescence. *Arch Gen Psychiatry* 54:897–903.

Ross, R.G., Olincy, A., Harris, J.G., Radant, A., Hawkins, M., Adler, L.E., and Freedman, R. (1999) Evidence for bilineal inheritance of physiological indicators of risk in childhood-onset schizophrenia. *Am J Med Genet* 88:188–199.

Seeman, P., Bzowej, N.H., Guan, H.C., Bergeron, C., Becker, L.E., Reynolds, G.P., Bird, E.D., Riederer, P., Jellinger, K., Watanabe, S., et al. (1987) Human brain dopamine receptors in children and aging adults. *Synapse* 1:399–404.

Sidransky, E., Burgess, C., Ikeuchi, T., Lindblad, K., Long, R.T., Philibert, R.A., Rapoport, J., Schalling, M., Tsuji, S., and Ginns, E.I. (1998) A triplet repeat on 17q accounts for most expansions detected by the repeat-expansion-detection technique. *Am J Hum Genet* 62:1548–1551.

Sowell, E.R., Levitt, J., Thompson, P.M., Holmes, C.J., Blanton, R.E., Kornsand, D.S., Caplan, R., McCracken, J., Asarnow, R., and Toga, A.W. (2000). Brain abnormalities observed in early onset schizophrenia spectrum disorder observed with statistical parametric mapping of structural magnetic resonance images. *Am J Psychiatry* 157:1475–1484.

Spencer, E.K. and Campbell, M. (1994) Children with schizophrenia: diagnosis, phenomenology, and pharmacotherapy. *Schizophr Bull* 20:713–725.

Suvisaari, J.M., Haukka, J., Tanskanen, A., and Lonnqvist, J.K. (1998) Age at onset and outcome in schizophrenia are related to the degree of familial loading. *Br J Psychiatry* 173:494–500.

Thomas, M.A., Ke, Y., Levitt, J., Caplan, R., Curran, J., Asarnow, R., and McCracken, J. (1998) Preliminary study of frontal lobe H-1 MR spectroscopy in childhood-onset schizophrenia. *J Magn Reson Imaging* 8:841–846.

Thompson, P.M., Giedd, J.N., Woods, R.P., MacDonald, D., Evans, A.C., and Toga, A.W. (2000) Growth patterns in the developing brain detected by using continuum mechanical tensor maps. *Nature* 404:190–193.

Thompson, P.M., Mega, M.S., Vidal, C., Rapoport, J.L., and Toga, A.W. (in 2001) Detecting disease-specific patterns of brain structure using cortical pattern matching and a population-based probabilistic brain atlas. In: *Proceedings of the 17th International Conference on Information Processing in Medical Imaging* (IPMI 2001). Eds. Insana MF, Leahy, R.M. Springer-Verlag, Berlin, pp. 488–501.

Verdoux, H., Geddes, J.R., Takei, N., Lawrie, S.M., Bovet, P., Eagles, J.M., Heun, R., McCreadie, R.G., McNeil, T.F., O'Callaghan, E., Stober, G., Willinger, M.U., Wright, P., and Murray, R.M. (1997) Obstetric complications and age at onset in schizophrenia: an international collaborative meta-analysis of individual patient data. *Am J Psychiatry* 154:1220–1227.

Volkmar, F.R. and Cohen, D.J. (1991) Comorbid association of autism and schizophrenia. *Am J Psychiatry* 148:1705–1707.

Watkins, J.M., Asarnow, R.F., and Tanguay, P.E. (1988) Symptom development in childhood-onset schizophrenia. *J Child Psychol Psychiatry* 29:865–878.

Weinberger, D.R. (1987) Implications of normal brain development for the pathogenesis of schizophrenia. *Arch Gen Psychiatry* 44: 660–669.

Wright, I.C., Rabe-Hesketh, S., Woodruff, P.W., David, A.S., Murray, R.M., and Bullmore, E.T. (2000) Meta-analysis of regional brain volumes in schizophrenia. *Am J Psychiatry* 157:16–25.

Wudarsky, M., Nicolson, R., Hamburger, S.D., Spechler, L., Gochman, P., Bedwell, J., Lenane, M.C., and Rapoport, J.L. (1999) Elevated prolactin in pediatric patients on typical and atypical antipsychotics. *J Child Adolesc Psychopharmacol* 9:239–245.

16 | Neurobiology of affiliation: implications for autism spectrum disorders

SHERIE NOVOTNY, MARTIN EVERS, KATHERINE BARBOZA, RON RAWITT, AND ERIC HOLLANDER

In human beings and most mammals, affiliation is an essential part of the life process, as it is necessary for both reproduction and survival. There are nonetheless instances in nature of profound lack of affiliative behavior. For example, children with autism spectrum disorders have significant difficulties in social skills, including lack of positive reinforcement from social interaction, poor eye gaze, impairment in social interactions, difficulties in attachment, and difficulties in nonverbal and, often, verbal communication. Deficits of this kind have led us to the study of the neurobiology underlying attachment and affiliation.

Attachment takes many forms, including affiliative (mates) and maternal and infant bonding. Much of what follows in this chapter concerns maternal–infant bonding, as this is most relevant to the subject of child psychiatry. Information on the neurobiology, neurocircuitry, and genetics of affiliative processes is integrated in this chapter, and the clinical relevance of these areas is highlighted.

NEUROCIRCUITS AND PATHOLOGY

Hypothalamic Circuitry

Medial preoptic areas

What is known about the neural circuitry for mammalian maternal behavior has been delineated using animal models, predominantly the rat. The medial preoptic area (MPOA) of the hypothalamus is important in reproductive function—i.e., in sexual behavior, gonadotrophin secretion, and the expression of normal maternal behavior (Numan, 1974). Maternal behaviors

include nursing, retrieving pups, and nest building. Lesion studies show that damage to either neuronal cell bodies or axons in the MPOA will disrupt maternal behavior, indicating that MPOA neurons and their efferent connections are important for maternal behavior (Numan, 1988, Numan et al., 1988). Lesions of the medial preoptic area severely disrupt maternal behaviors of postpartum lactating female rats (Numan, 1974). Cuts severing mediolateral connections of the preoptic anterior hypothalamic continuum result in disruption of normal maternal behavior (Numan, 1974). Cuts posterior to the MPOA–anterior hypothalamic continuum disrupt female sexual behavior (Numan, 1974). Severance of the lateral connections of the MPOA cause profound disruption of maternal behavior (Numan and Callahan, 1980), most notably pup retrieval behavior (Numan, 1990). This disruption is not due to a general oral motor deficit (Numan and Corodimas, 1985). While preoptic damage interferes with all aspects of maternal behavior, retrieval behavior seems to be the most permanently and severely affected (Numan, 1990).

Lateral efferents of the MPOA innervate septum, amygdala, other hypothalamic regions, ventral tegmental area (VTA) of the midbrain, and midbrain central gray matter (Numan, 1986). Studies have shown that the MPOA–VTA–basal ganglia (BG) circuit is believed to be of importance in maternal behavior because the BG is a major component of the extrapyramidal system (EPS) (Numan, 1986). Perhaps MPOA neurons relevant to maternal behavior via the BG to EPS promote the somatic-motor processes underlying maternal responsiveness (Numan, 1986).

The MPOA is acted on by estrogen to facilitate the

195

onset of maternal behavior (Numan et al., 1977). The ovarian steroid changes of pregnancy may increase oxytocin (OT) synthesis, transport, and release, hastening the onset of maternal behavior (Pedersen, 1997). Injections of estradiol or prolactin into the MPOA activate maternal behavior (Bridges et al., 1990; Numan, 1994). The onset of maternal behavior in virgin female rats presented with pup stimulation is a function of the MPOA; this can be disrupted by MPOA lesioning (Numan et al., 1977). The MPOA is the site of the onset and maintenance of maternal behavior and this induction of maternal behavior may have long-lasting effects on the subsequent responsiveness of maternal behavior to the facilitatory effects of pup stimulation (Numan et al., 1977). The OT receptor levels are enhanced in the rat and sheep MPOA and increase following parturition (Fleming et al., 1989). Infusion of OT into the MPOA increases maternal behavior (Pedersen and Prange 1991).

Fos-like immunoreactivity in the MPOA and lateral preoptic area (LPOA) is associated with maternal behavior in both virgin female rats exposed to pups and lactating postpartum females (Numan and Numan, 1992). The observed induction of fos activity in the POA is likely partially due to the receipt of olfactory and ventral tactile and suckling-related sensory stimulation from pups. The POA also receives suckling-related sensory data related to lactation. However, because maternal behavior occurs in females who have been thelectomized (nipple removal) or olfactory bulbectomized, a population of POA output cells exists that is essential for the performance of maternal duties in the absence of the usual sensory inputs (Numan, 1994).

Androgenic stimulation of the MPOA often stimulates the display of male-typical behaviors. The MPOA is consistently androgen-responsive and has been implicated in different species in the motor performance of copulatory behavior (Christensen and Clemens, 1974), scent marking (Thiessen and Yahr, 1970), and aggressive behaviors. The MPOA may be involved in appetitive sexual motivation, although several studies point to the amygdala's performance in this role.

Paraventricular nucleus

The paraventricular nucleus (PVN) is the major source of OT input to other brain regions, and oxytocinergic neurons projecting to the VTA are located in the PVN (Numan 1994). Lesioning the PVN disrupts the postpartum initiation of maternal behavior (Insel and Harbaugh, 1989), but does not result in any defect in ma-

ternal behavior in lactating rats with 5 days at least of postpartum experience (Numan and Corodimas, 1985). This suggests that oxytocinergic neural pathways are crucial for initiation of maternal behavior, but are not critical in the maintenance of postpartum maternal behaviors (Numan and Corodimas, 1985).

Limbic areas

Amygdala

The medial amygdala (MA) has an inhibitory role in maternal behavior (Numan, 1994). This inhibition is thought to be mediated by the olfactory system (Numan, 1994). Ablation of olfactory neurons will allow for the development of maternal behavior in nulliparous rats exposed to rat pups, whereas nulliparus rats with intact olfaction will avoid pups altogether. N-methyl-D,L-aspartic acid (NMA)-induced lesions of the MA influenced maternal behavior by removing neural inhibition and inducing a hormonal state arousing maternal behavior through neural excitation that facilitates prolactin release (Numan et al., 1993).

Odor cues eliciting withdrawal and avoidance of rat pups by virgin females are transmitted through both the vomeronasal (arising in the amygdala) and accessory olfactory bulb projections to the MPOA. The MA receives a significant source of its neural input from the olfactory bulbs; it has therefore been suggested that the MA plays a role in this olfactory inhibition of maternal behavior by relaying olfactory input to the MPOA (Fleming et al., 1980). Anosmic female rats have a reduced latency to maternal behavior, and lesions of the amygdala enhance maternal behavior in virgin females (Fleming et al., 1980). The amygdala-to-hypothalamus circuit most likely dampens maternal behavior by triggering a central aversion system that is down-regulated by the endocrine events of late pregnancy (Numan and Sheehan, 1997).

The OT receptor levels are enhanced in the rat central amygdala and increase following parturition (Fleming et al., 1989). Reduced OT receptor levels in the central amygdala are observed in rat mothers who spend less time licking and grooming offspring (Francis et al., 1999b). Infusion of OT into the central amygdala has an anxiolytic effect in female rats; it has been suggested that OT might promote maternal behavior by inhibiting fear-related neural activity.

An enhanced level of corticotropin-releasing hormone (CRH) receptors is found in the central amygdala of rat mothers who spend relatively less time licking and grooming offspring (Francis et al., 1999a), this suggests a possible role for the amygdala in the fearfulness-response mechanisms that may affect maternal behaviors in rats.

It has been suggested that the basolateral amygdala is involved in appetitive behaviors reflective of sexual motivation (Everitt, 1990). The amygdala may be involved in hormonal activation of certain male-typical behaviors. The amygdala has significant levels of androgen and estrogen receptors and aromatase enzyme (Matochik et al., 1994). In addition, pheremonal information, necessary to inducing male-typical behaviors in mice, is processed by olfactory pathways through the amygdala.

Hippocampus

The dorsal and ventral hippocampus is involved in the formation of social memory (van Wimersma Greidanus and Maigret, 1996). Neonatal ablations of hippocampal regions can lead to decreased and abnormal social behavior in rhesus monkeys that is reminiscent of severe neuropsychiatric disorders in humans such as autism and schizophrenia (Bachevalier et al., 1999). These monkeys are often withdrawn socially and will develop locomotoric stereotypies a pattern similar to that found in autistic children.

Ventral bed nucleus of the stria terminalis

The junction between the MPOA and lateral preoptic areas is the ventral part of the bed nucleus of the stria terminalis (ventral BST), and excitotoxic lesions disrupt retrieval behaviors and other aspects of maternal behavior in postpartum rats (Numan and Numan, 1996). Strong ventral BST projections to the lateral septum, substantia innominata, PVN, VTA, periaquedutal gray matter, retrorubral field, and the region surrounding the locus coeruleus (Numan and Numan, 1996).

The MA projects to the MPOA indirectly through a synapse in the BST (Numan, 1994). Thus, the BST may be part of the neural circuitry involved in olfactory inhibition of maternal behavior in rats. Fos-like immunoreactivity in the VBST, MPOA, and LPOA is associated with maternal behavior in both virgin female rats exposed to pups and lactating postpartum females (Numan and Numan, 1992). Oxytocinergic neurons projecting to the VTA are located in the BST (Numan, 1994). Concentrations of OT in sheep BST are elevated at parturition and with vaginocervical stimulation (Kendrick et al., 1992). Arginine Vasopressin (AVP)-containing fibers of the lateral septum, involved in social recognition, originate in the BST and MA (De Vries et al., 1985). Prolactin and μ-opioid receptors (discussed in Opioids and μ-Opioid Receptors, below) are distributed across the ventral BST.

Other brain regions

Other brain regions are undoubtedly involved in affiliative behaviors. For example, the ventral temporal area of the cortex appears to be involved in facial discrimination in humans, and abnormalities in the activation of this area during facial discrimination tasks are present in individuals with autism (Schultz et al., 2000). In rats and other mammals, the olfactory bulb and entorhinal cortex also appear to be involved in affiliative behaviors, including maternal behaviors (Numan, 1994).

NEUROCHEMISTRY AND GENETICS OF AFFILIATION

Oxytocin

Peptide

Oxytocin, a nine amino acid peptide, is synthesized primarily in the paraventricular and supraoptic (SON) nuclei of the hypothalamus, from which it is released to the general circulation through the posterior pituitary (Insel et al., 1997). However, oxytocinergic fibers have also been found to project from the PVN to the limbic system and several autonomic centers in the brain stem. This "central" OT pool appears to be independent of pituitary OT release; cerebrospinal fluid (CSF) and plasma OT responses to numerous stimuli are not correlated (Insel, 1997). Oxytocin and its analog (or partner) peptide vasopressin are found only in mammals. A related peptide, vasotocin, thought to be the evolutionary precedent of these peptides, is found in reptiles and birds. The first known actions of OT were its peripheral effects on the physiology of new mothers. In mammals, OT stimulates milk ejection and uterine contraction, essential aspects of maternal physiology (Insel et al., 1997).

In different species, the OT has been found to influence a wide range of social behaviors, including maternal and paternal behavior, sexual, aggressive and affiliative behaviors, olfactory investigation, and social recognition memory. These relationships are complex, with OT effects, dose–response relationships, and directionality differing across species. In a number of studies, OT infusion has had contrasting effects on the social behaviors of various species (Winslow et al.,

2000). Oxytocin typically has a facilitative effect on affiliative behaviors (Witt et al., 1992), including parental and reproductive behaviors and infant–mother attachment. Oxytocin facilitates social memory, with knockout mice displaying social memory deficits; it facilitates conditioning to maternal-related olfactory cues (Nelson and Panksepp, 1996).

The effects of OT appear to be species-specific (Wang et al., 2000). Thus, while OT appears not to be essential for the onset of maternal behavior in mice (Barnes and Pompeiano, 1991), it may be essential for the onset of maternal behavior in species that become maternal at parturition, such as rats and sheep (Wang et al., 2000). In sheep, the central release of OT, prompted by parturition and/or stimulation of the vagina and cervix, has been implicated in the induction of maternal behavior; OT release increases with maternal experience (Levy et al., 1995). This enhanced OT release at parturition is associated with elevated acetylcholine, noradrenaline, and GABA release, which are in turn associated with olfactory memory; this may explain the shorter period of time needed by multiparous ewes to selectively bond with lambs.

Central infusion of OT will stimulate the rapid induction of maternal behavior in estrogen-primed virgin rats (Bridges, 1998); central infusion into the hypothalamus also facilitates sexual behavior in female rats primed with estrogen. Oxytocin has also been linked to maternal aggression and reduced separation anxiety in rats (Winslow et al., 2000). Rat pups have a significantly decreased amount of distress calls after injection with OT (Insel and Winslow, 1991). Central OT infusion induced paw sucking (an affiliative behavior) in infant rats while an OT antagonist reduced these behaviors (Nelson and Alberts, 1997). Oxytocin is an anxiolytic agent in infant rats and adult female rodents (Winslow et al., 2000), and facilitates sexual and affiliative behaviors in rats (Witt et al., 1992).

The exact role of the peptide in human social bonding is unclear, secondary to multiple difficulties in studying OT in humans (McCarthy and Altemus, 1997). Oxytocin peaks have been observed in women in the first hour postpartum (Nissen et al., 1995), a time essential for facilitating mother–offspring bonding. It has been suggested that OT promotes attachment by making affiliation or friendly social contact pleasant and rewarding (Insel, 1997). In normally cycling women, elevated plasma OT levels have been associated with relaxation massage, while decreased OT levels have been associated with sad emotion (Turner et al., 1999). Oxytocin responses to emotional stimuli in this study were highly individualized. In men, an

increase in mean plasma OT is seen at ejaculation (Winslow et al., 1993). Autistic children have roughly half the plasma OT levels of normal controls, and don't show a normal developmental increase of plasma OT with age or interpersonal skills (Insel and Winslow, 1991). As OT and AVP are critical in pathways of social behavior, learning, and memory, and deficits in these abilities are seen in autism, some speculation centers on a role for OT and/or AVP, or their receptors, in autism. Because there is little relationship between plasma and CSF OT, the meaning of associations between plasma OT and human behavior is uncertain, particularly associations between plasma OT and human psychological traits.

In addition, the neuroanatomy of OT receptor distribution patterns is species-specific. Wide variability in patterns of receptor distribution exists across even closely related species (Insel and Shapiro, 1991 Insel et al., 1999). These cross-species disparities necessitate caution when one makes general statements about the relationships between OT and specific behaviors. For example, primates and humans have a circadian rhythm of CSF OT, while rodents do not (McCarthy and Altemus, 1997). There are important limits to the extent to which the results of specific gene knockout models may be extrapolated to other species. Ultimately, primate models may be necessary to assess the functions of OT in the primates and humans.

Characterization of OT knockout models in animals is being used to develop an understanding of the specific function of OT in maternal, social bonding and other behaviors. An OT knockout mouse has been created that completely lacks the nucleotide sequences encoding the OT peptide. No OT mRNA is detectable in the brain of these homozygous (−/−) knockout mice, while some OT mRNA can be picked up by infrared stain in heterozygotes (+/−). This graded genotype-dependent expression of OT mRNA allows for the study of the effects on behavior of partial as well as complete OT deficits. The OT knockout mice show no difference from wild-type mice in OT receptor distribution; this finding suggests that differences in presynaptic OT do not influence OT receptor distribution. This similarly infers that differences in the distribution of oxytocinergic neurons do not account for interspecies differences in OT receptor patterns (Young et al, 1997). Of note, OT knockout mice do not display deficiencies in any of the commonly quantified measures of maternal behavior, except lactation (Bridges, 1998).

Compared to wild-type mice, knockout homozygotes and heterozygotes show decreased olfactory social investigation, less fearfulness, and increased aggression toward intruders (Winslow et al., 2000). There are quantitative differences in the social behavior displayed by homozygous (−/−) and heterozygous (+/−) knockout mice. Observed levels of social investigation positively correlate with OT expression, while aggressiveness is negatively correlated with OT expression. In addition, knockout mice derived from obligate (homozygous × homozygous) litters displayed significantly less fear and more aggression than knockout mice derived from nonobligate litters (heterozygous × heterozygous). This suggests that some behavioral differences may be influenced by differing postnatal environments (mothering styles litter composition) associated with the obligate and nonobligate litters (Winslow et al., 2000).

Male OT knockout mice fail to develop social memory, defined as a reliable decrease in olfactory investigation as a result of repeated or prolonged encounters with a conspecific (Ferguson et al., 2000). Olfactory investigation of nonsocial stimuli, as assessed by olfactory foraging and habituation studies, was intact in the knockout animals. In addition, spatial memory was not impaired. This indicates that social memory has a different neural basis than nonsocial memory. Treatment with OT rescued social memory in these animals, while administration of an OT antagonist produced some characteristics of social amnesia and impaired social memory in normal mice. This suggests that OT is necessary for the development of normal social memory (Ferguson et al., 2000).

Separation distress, as measured by the frequency of isolation distress calls emitted by pups separated from their mothers, was decreased in knockout pups, relative to wild-type youngsters. The level of decrease in OT expression paralleled the decrease in distress call frequency (Winslow et al., 2000). This suggests that youngsters with OT deficits do not form proper social attachments early in life; consequently, they are not as distressed as wild-type pups by separation from their mothers. Alternatively, reduced vocalization in OT knockout pups may relate to reduced fearfulness in general, as well as to reduced sensitivity to maternal separation (Winslow et al., 2000). Administration of OT to infant rats had a quieting effect on pups separated from their mothers.

There are some genotype-independent differences in behavior between mice reared by heterozygous (+/−) mothers and those reared by wild-type mothers. Both heterozygous and knockout males raised by wild-type mothers tended to have higher anxiety indices than those raised by heterozygous mothers, indicating some role for environment in the shaping of emotional phe-

notype. However, evidence from other studies suggests that behavioral phenotype is for the most part dependent on genotype rather than litter environment (Winslow et al., 2000).

Receptors

Oxytocin receptors are widely distributed in the brain (Insel et al., 1997). Brain receptors are biochemically identical to receptors found in uterine myometrium and mammary myoepithelium. There is a remarkable diversity across species in the neuroanatomical distribution and regulation of OT receptors. These receptors are heavily controlled by gonadal steroids, and the pattern of steroid regulation of OT receptor expression varies across species as well. This diversity of receptors may be the mechanism through which OT function, and thus the social behaviors influenced by that function vary across species.

It has been observed that interspecies differences in social organization and behavior are associated with differences in OT receptor distribution. The most compelling example of this phenomenon is seen in the contrasting social behaviors of two different species of vole. Prairie voles, which are monogamous (pairbond), parental, and highly affiliative, show markedly different patterns of OT receptor expression in the brain from those of montane voles, which are promiscuous, minimally parental, and asocial (Insel et al., 1997). Significant differences lie in the distribution, rather than the total number, of OT receptors. Examination of receptor patterns in other vole species has confirmed a correlation between specific receptor distributions and levels of social organization. By contrast, few differences in OT-producing cells or fibers have been found among the different species (Insel et al., 1997), suggesting strongly that the differences in receptor expression are critical. This has lead to the suggestion that the OT receptor gene is a candidate gene for monogamy.

Prairie vole young show high levels of stress in response to social isolation, while montane vole offspring show minimal behavioral or physical response to separation (Insel et al., 1997). Prairie voles are much more vocal than montane voles during social separation (Winslow et al., 2000). It is suggested that this difference is related to diversity in OT receptor distribution across vole species. This phenomenon is an interesting parallel to the differences in pup vocalization (and therefore socialization) seen between OT knockout pups and their wild-type counterparts.

In sheep, oxytocinergic terminals and OT receptors

have been localized to a number of parts of the olfactory processing system, including the olfactory bulb and secondary and tertiary olfactory processing sites such as the piriform cortex, frontal cortex, and hippocampus. Release of OT modulates the formation of olfactory memory by regulating the release of norepinephrine, acetylcholine, and GABA (which are essential in memory formation) and works in the olfactory bulb to reduce rejection behavior toward lambs (Broad et al., 1999).

Previous maternal experience affects the expression of OT receptors in the sheep PVN (Broad et al., 1999). Oxytocin receptor expression is enhanced in several areas of the olfactory processing, limbic, and diencephalic regions of the brain on parturition in primiparous sheep, while parturition leads to even more enhanced expression of OT receptors including receptors in the PVN, in maternally experienced sheep. This may partially explain why inexperienced sheep do not exhibit maternal behavior as readily as experienced sheep. Specifically, it is suggested that the enhancement of OT receptor expression in the PVN of experienced mothers leads to a more efficient release of OT or the potentiation of OT release at lower thresholds (Broad et al., 1999). Ewe–lamb bonding (dependent on olfactory recognition) is slower to occur in inexperienced mothers; as an increase in the ability of the olfactory bulbs to process incoming information is seen with maternal experience. Maternal inexperience has been associated with severe deficits in maternal behavior in sheep, rats, pigs, and humans, while an experience-dependent facilitation of maternal behavior has been reported in sheep, rats, mice, fur seals, pigs, and humans (Broad et al., 1999).

Differences in receptor distribution are due to species differences in region-specific gene expression. Across vole species, OT receptor coding sequences and promoter sequences are virtually identical; species diversity in receptor expression appears to relate to quantitative and regional differences rather than qualitative aspects of the receptor when expressed (Insel et al., 1997).

Because fundamental differences in social behaviors across species are based on differences in the distribution of OT receptors, it may be possible in animal studies to manipulate brain OT receptor expression to examine the effects of this manipulation on behavior.

Vasopressin

Arginine-vasopressin, a nine amino acid peptide, facilitates the formation of social recognition and social memory in rats, and AVP antagonists block such facilitation (Winslow et al., 1993). It has been suggested that the neurohypophyseal peptides (OT as well as AVP) have a prepotent role in the modulation of mnemonic processing of chemosensory information associated with social interactions (Winslow et al., 1993). Vasopressin weakly stimulates the onset of maternal behavior (Pedersen et al., 1982), and may influence paternal behavior. In the rat, AVP release is enhanced at parturition, and intracerebrovascular infusions shorten latency to maternal behavior (Levy et al., 1995).

Research suggests a sexual dimorphism: that AVP is important for pair bonding in male prairie voles, while OT is important for pair bonding in female prairie voles (Insel and Hulihan, 1995). Arginine-vasopressin is secreted during sexual arousal in humans. However, the exact role of the peptide in social bonding among humans remains unclear.

Prolactin

Prolactin is a polypeptide hormone secreted by the pituitary gland and (to a lesser extent) peripheral tissues. It is involved in over 300 separate functions in vertebrates (Goffin et al., 1999), with the most important functions relating to lactation and reproduction. Studies in rats indicate that prolactin facilitates, but is not essential for, the induction of parental behavior in pup-stimulated animals and is important in priming pregnant females for the induction of postpartum parental behavior (Stack and Numan, 2000). Prolactin appears to act centrally in the stimulation of maternal behavior in female rats (Bridges et al., 1990). Infusion of prolactin into the MPOA at doses lacking effect when injected elsewhere stimulates maternal behavior toward foster young. Numerous studies show that prolactin can enter CSF from the blood; in addition, elevated CSF prolactin levels are associated with suckling and higher blood prolactin levels (Login and Macleod 1977).

In the brain, the V-shaped distribution of prolactin receptors and prolactin-like immunoreactive fibers extends from the medial preoptic nucleus (MPN) of the MPOA of the rodent brain to the ventral bed of the stria terminalis (vBST). This distribution parallels that of mu-opioid and progesterone receptors. It has therefore been speculated that activation of mu-receptors may inhibit prolactin priming and the induction of parental behavior (see discussion of μ-receptors, below). Similarly, the distribution of prolactin receptor mRNA in the MPOA and VBST match the distribution of cells displaying enhanced c-fos and FosB expression during maternal behavior, which has led to the suggestion that expression of c-fos and FosB play a regulatory role in prolactin activities (Numan et al., 1998).

Knockout of the prolactin receptor, rather than knockout of prolactin, is necessary to explore the role of the hormone and its receptor in maternal behavior because several molecules other than prolactin, including growth hormone (GH) and placental lactogens, may stimulate the prolactin receptor. Disruption of the prolactin receptor gene in a mouse model has allowed for assessment of phenotypes associated with partial and complete prolactin receptor deficits (Goffin et al., 1999). Prolactin receptor knockout mice have severe reproductive deficits. Heterozygous mothers (receptor −/+) were also unable to lactate (Bridges, 1998).

Maternal behavior is also severely deficient in both heterozygous and homozygous prolactin receptor knockouts (Goffin et al., 1999). Primiparous heterozygous females displayed deficits in the retrieval of foster pups (Goffin et al., 1999; Lucas et al., 1998). Significant differences have been seen in pup contact–induced maternal behavior in virgin females. One study found that maternal behavior was displayed by wild-type virgin females within 1–2 days of pup exposure. Heterozygotes exhibited a latency of 4 days, while the homozygote knockouts did not exhibit this maternal behavior at all (Goffin et al., 1999). Lack of prolactin receptor activation may lead to reduced release of GABA, which functions in the reduction of fearfulness and anxiety (Lucas et al., 1998). It has been suggested that the resultant increased level of fear and anxiety in mutants may explain the enhanced latency to approach and accept foster pups.

Opioids and μ-Opioid Receptors

Opioids are important in fostering social attachment. Opioid agonists have decreased separation calling in most young animals studied (Nelson and Panksepp, 1996). Additionally, opiate levels are increased during social contact in many species. The reward aspects of opioids can create odor and place preference, and low levels of endogenous opioids can increase social motivation (Nelson and Panksepp, 1996). Species differences in separation calling may reflect species differences in patterns of receptor expression in the developing brain (Insel and Winslow et al., 1998). In stable pairs of talapoin monkeys, naloxone (an opioid antagonist) increases grooming invitations, while morphine decreases grooming invitations and increases refusals to be groomed (Keverne et al., 1989).

μ-Opioid receptors are present in abundance in the MPOA of the rodent brain, which has been widely implicated in control of maternal behavior. The density of receptors in the MPOA is responsive to gonadal steroid hormones. Activation of μ-receptors by morphine and other μ-receptor agonists inhibits parental behavior in juvenile and adult rats. Opiate inhibition of maternal behavior is associated with a reduced ability of pup stimulation to induce c-fos expression in the MPOA of postpartum rats (Stack and Numan, 2000). In addition, suckling promotes the release of opioids in the medial preoptic area of the sheep. Plasma levels of endorphins double in lactating women when their infants are nursing. Researchers have suggested that activation of the endogenous opioid system in late pregnancy and suckling promote the positive affect arising from maternal behavior. In Keverne et al.'s study (1997), naloxone-treated rhesus monkey mothers were significantly less caregiving and protective toward their infants. In the infants' first few weeks, when infant retrieval is normally very high, naloxone-treated mothers neglected their infants and showed less retrieval when their infants went away. These mothers also permitted other females to groom their infants, while saline-treated control mothers were very possessive and protective of their infants. Therefore, it seems that the mother–infant bond does not develop normally when the opioid receptors are blocked. These studies demonstrate the significance of the brain's opioid system for the affective component of relationships in social development.

Steroids and Gonadal Hormones

Progesterone has a dual effect on maternal behavior. A decline in progesterone from high levels (progesterone withdrawal) is facilitatory, potentiating the facilitatory effects of estradiol and prolactin exposure on maternal behavior (Numan et al., 1999). Conversely, high levels of progesterone may inhibit maternal behavior (Numan et al., 1999). Progesterone also binds to the intracellular glucocorticoid receptor (GR), albeit with less affinity than for the progesterone receptor (PR). It is possible that progesterone moderates maternal behavior by binding to GRs rather than PRs (Numan et al., 1999).

Estrogen is involved in both the stimulation (Moltz et al., 1970) and inhibition (Leon et al., 1973) of maternal behavior in female rats. Increasing estrogen titers before birth, in the presence of declining serum progesterone, facilitates the onset of maternal behavior in female rats (Numan, 1978). Response to estrogen is dependent on endogenous physiologic and hormonal conditions and the pattern of estrogen secretion in the animal. Additionally, estrogen induces OT receptor gene expression.

Cortisol and CRH mediate behavioral, emotional, autonomic, and endocrine responses to environmental and emotional stresses. The cortisol system also plays a role in both maternal and afiliative behavior. Much of this information is covered in Chapter 9 in this volume.

Serotonin

Serotonin (5-hydroxytryptamine [5-HT]) influences a number of social behaviors including separation calls, allogrooming, and social dominance. Mammalian infants give calls when they are initially separated from their families, which are a powerful stimulus for maternal retrieval (Newman, 1988). Studies have shown that highly affiliative species of voles call more in response to social isolation (Shapiro and Insel, 1990). Thus isolation calls have been used to measure affiliation in rat pups. Insel and Winslow (1998) found that drugs that blocked 5-HT uptake decreased the number of calls after a single administration, whereas norepinephrine (NE) or dopamine (DA)-uptake blockers increased them. Insel and Winslow also discovered that rat pup separation calls were decreased by serotogenic lesions, 5-HT agonists, and 5-HT_2 antagonists, and were increased by 5-HT_{1b} agonists. Studies by Smythe and colleagues (1994) showed that daily separation from the mother and handling of pups increased 5-HT_{1b} turnover in the hippocampus (but not in the amygdala or hypothalamus). Handling seemed to induce an increase in hippocampal glucocorticoid and 5-HT_2 receptors, which altered stress responses in adulthood. Furthermore, neonatal treatment with a serotonin neurotoxin decreased hippocampal glucocorticoid receptors in young rats, while in cultured hippocampal neurons serotonin treatment doubled the number of receptors. Thus, it appears that 5-HT release as a consequence of handling, or from later effect of maternal care, may have long-term consequences for hippocampal function, stress responsiveness, and adult behavior (Insel and Winslow, 1998).

Serotonin in non-human primates has been studied from CSF levels of the metabolite 5-HIAA, a marker of CNS serotonin activity. In both humans and non-human primates, CSF 5-HIAA has been negatively correlated with aggression or impaired impulse control. In free-ranging adolescent male rhesus monkeys, it has been reported that 5-HIAA in CSF is positively correlated with time spent in close proximity with other members of the social group and time spent grooming (Higley et al, 1993). 5-HIAA levels in vervets have been associated with social dominance (Raleigh et al., 1983). Among males of uncertain social status, those treated with serotonergic enhancers achieved social dominance through increased affiliative interactions (including

grooming) with females (Raleigh et al., 1991). Among humans, paroxetine treatment has been associated with increased social interaction on problem-solving tasks (Knutson et al., 1997). Serotonin abnormalities have also been associated with autism (Hollander et al., 1998), a disorder with severe abnormalities of social behavior.

The neurotransmitter 5-HT acts through seven distinct receptor families (5-HT_1, 5-HT_2, etc.). There is a high degree of homology between mouse and human 5-HT receptors, as they differ by a single amino acid. This homology suggests that rodent studies have relevance for human function; accordingly, the 5-HT_1 family, specifically the 5-HT_{1B} receptor, has been the subject of investigation using knockout mice.

In a variety of knockout mouse studies, reduced serotonergic activity in knockout mice has been associated with increased aggression and impulsiveness, reduced anxiety, and increased addictive behavior. The relationship between between anxiety and aggression is complex, however; analyses of 5-HT receptor function generally support the view that serotonergic activity is positively associated with anxiety. The 5-HT_{1B} receptor is anxiogenic, and murine anxiety has been associated with 5-HT_{1B} receptor density. Stimulation of serotonergic receptors in certain brain regions has been associated with anxiogenesis. Pharmacologic agents stimulating the 5-HT_{1A} autoreceptor have an anxiolytic effect, probably because of the resultant reduction of 5-HT transmission. Allelic variation in human 5-HT transporter genes, which affect 5-HT transmission, has been associated with increased anxiety (Brunner et al., 1999; Zuang et al., 1999).

5-HT_{1B} knockout mouse studies have been used in research on murine maternal–infant interactions. Knockout pups exhibit reduced anxiety and increased motor activity. They vocalize less and probably emit fewer ultrasonic signals to their mothers. Knockout mothers are hyperactive and spend up to 20% less time with their litters. In wild-type mice, prolonged separation of the pup from its mother can have numerous deleterious effects on the pup, including temperature and weight loss, delayed development, motor difficulties, decreased sensitivity to reward, and overreaction to stress. However, 5-HT_{1B} knockout mice display none of these difficulties, and even thrive, compared to wild-type mice; they have increased weight gain, less reaction to stress, and enhanced sensitivity to reward. The hyperactivity of the knockout mother and developmental adaptation to the absence of 5-HT_{1B} receptor may play roles in this scenario. Knockout adults exhibit reduced emotionality and increased motor activity. As was noted above, the effects of 5-HT and 5-HT receptors on behavior are complex and not fully understood. Similarly, the 5-HT$_{1B}$ knockout mice exhibit physiologic and behavioral adaptations to their mutant status that confound the quest for simple relationships drawn from knockout studies (Brunner et al., 1999; Zuang et al., 1999).

Norepinephrine and Dopamine

The dopamine beta-hydroxylase (*Dbh*) gene is necessary for the production of NE and epinephrine. Disruption of this gene results in the absence of NE and epinephrine production and is therefore used in studies determining the roles of these neurotransmitters. This approach is favored over the knockout of adrenergic receptors because of the multiplicity of receptor types for NE and epinephrine.

Norepinephrine appears to trigger numerous maternal behaviors in mice (Gammie and Nelson, 1999). *Dbh−/−* knockout mice (which lack NE and epinephrine) show clear deficits in maternal behavior (Thomas and Palmiter, 1997a). Knockout females show very low rates of retrieval of pups into nests, and may fail to give pups proper instructional cues for nursing; in addition, often pups are not cleaned or their placenta is still attached. A high rate of pup mortality is seen in young fostered by *Dbh−/−* mice. This mortality appears to be secondary to the poor maternal behavior of *Dbh* knockout females, as the children of *Dbh−/−* females thrive when fostered by *Dbh+/−* females. Mortality does not appear to be secondary to deficiencies in lactation or other physiologic function.

Restoration of NE via the injection of dihydroxyphenylsevine (DOPS), a precursor of NE, into *Dbh* knockout mice shortly before birth results in the rescue of maternal behavior (Thomas and Palmiter, 1997b). Additionally, this rescue carries over to subsequent pregnancies, even when NE is no longer present. Use of DOPS at any point subsequent to birth does not achieve the rescue of maternal behavior. Thus, it appears that the presence of NE at birth promotes long-lasting facilitation of the expression of maternal behavior. It further appears that NE contributes to the development of pathways mediating maternal behavior.

It has been postulated that NE is important for olfactory recognition of newborns in mice (as well as in other species), which may be essential for postpartum maternal behavior. For instance, depletion of NE in the mouse olfactory bulb via infusion of 6-hydroxydopamine (6-OHDA) has deleterious effects on maternal behavior that are similar to, though not as severe as, those brought on by *Dbh* disruption.

However, *Dbh* knockout mice retain normal olfactory response to novel odors (Bridges, 1998).

Norepinephrine may also play a role in the induction of immediate early genes in response to pup exposure (Thomas and Palmiter, 1997). Norepinephrine has been linked to maternal behavior in certain other animal models, such as sheep and rats. It may also play a role in olfactory recognition and memory in rats. Intraventricular administration of 6-OHDA prior to birth has been noted to impair postpartum maternal behavior; administration after birth had no such effect.

Dopamine also appears to be important in affiliative behaviors. Dopamine is well known for its role in the reward systems of the brain, and this role most likely extends to social behaviors as well. In prairie voles, the D$_2$ receptors appear to play an important role in partner preference formation after mating (Insel and Young, 2001). The specific role has yet to be elucidated, however, agonists can facilitate this behavior and antagonists of the D$_2$ receptor can inhibit it.

Neuronal Nitric Oxide Synthase and Maternal Aggression

Maternal aggression is defined as aggression toward intruders displayed by mothers who are lactating and/or raising pups. This aggression, which is highly conserved among mammals and has survival benefit for offspring, appears to be controlled by a different neural mechanism than that for territorial aggression (Gammie and Nelson, 1999). Although it is well known that female mice and rats exhibit maternal aggression, the proximal neurochemical causes of this aggression are not totally clear. Nor is much known about the initiation of this behavior in mice; as discussed above, it is suspected that NE plays a role in the onset of a variety of maternal behaviors in mice. Steroid hormones facilitate maternal aggression and other maternal behaviors in rats; however, it is not clear whether hormonal input is necessary once lactation has begun (Gammie and Nelson, 1999). The suckling of rat pups is involved in the initiation and maintenance of maternal aggression. Changes in central 5-HT and OT levels have been implicated in rat maternal aggression; 5-HT and AVP have been implicated in the regulation of male aggression among rodents (Gammie and Nelson, 1999).

Nitric oxide (NO) has also been implicated in certain maternal behaviors, including the timing of parturition in rats and olfactory memory formation in lactating sheep (Gammie and Nelson, 1999), as well as aggression and maternal aggression. Nitric oxide is produced from L-arginine by three different tissue-localized nitric oxide synthase (NOS) enzymes: neuronal (nNOS), en-dothelial (eNOS), and inducible (iNOS), NOS enzymes. The specific actions of NO depend ultimately on its enzymatic source. Deletion of the nNOS gene and inhibition of nNOS with pharmacologic agents both yield increased aggression in male mice (Gammie and Nelson, 1999). However, female nNOS knockout mice exhibit deficits in maternal aggression. Other aspects of maternal behavior, such as pup retrieval, are unaffected in the knockout strains. This suggests, indirectly, that NO release is associated with maternal aggression. However, without direct evidence or deduction of a mechanism, the relationship between NO and maternal aggression is a (statistically significant) association rather than a proof of causation.

GENETIC DETERMINANTS OF AFFILIATION

Immediate early genes (IEGs) code for proteins that serve as transcription factors, controlling the expression of downstream genes and coupling extracellular signals to long-term genomic responses within the cell. The IEGs are widely used as markers of neuroactivation secondary to hormonal challenges, aggressive and sexual behaviors, and long-term potentiation and/or learning and memory. Immediate early gene expression is seen in association with sensory stimulation, motor output, and behavioral performance (Numan and Numan, 1994).

Immediate early gene expression in certain brain regions is necessary for, and indicative of, aspects of maternal behavior. The IEGs that have been studied include c-fos, fosB, zif/268 (egr-1), c-jun, mest, and peg3. Of these, c-fos is the most studied, and appears to be particularly important in inducing maternal behavior in both rats and sheep (Da Costa et al., 1997). Although this IEG and others have been extensively studied with regard to maternal behavior and social attachment, a detailed review of this research is beyond the scope of this chapter.

ENVIRONMENTAL FACTORS

Variations in maternal care may serve as the basis for a nongenomic behavioral transmission of individual differences in stress reactivity across multiple generations. Researchers have found evidence of such transmission in mother–pup contact of rats. Variations in maternal licking/grooming and arched back nursing (LG-ABN) given by the mother to her pups have been associated with the development of individual differ-

ences in hypothalamic-pituitary-adrenal (HPA) and behavioral responses to stress in offspring (Caldji, et al., 1998). It has also been found that repeated periods of prolonged maternal separation resulted in decreased GABAergic (GABA$_A$) receptor binding and diminished central type I benzodiazepine receptor levels (Caldji, et al., 2000). This system is a potent source of inhibitory regulation of emotional, behavioral, and endocrine responses to stress. These relationships are covered in Chapters 9 and 10 in this volum and thus will not be covered here.

Studies with rhesus monkeys have shown similar evidence of transmission of individual differences through parenting styles. Berman (1990) found that the rate of mothers rejecting their infants was correlated with the rejection rate of the mothers' mothers. Individual differences in fearfulness or maternal behavior have been mapped onto those of the rearing mother, rather than the biological mother.

INTERFACE WITH HUMAN PATHOLOGY

Although social attachment and impairment of social behaviors are evident in a wide range of psychopathology, including childhood trauma, personality disorders, and anxiety disorders, an extensive review of this subject is beyond the scope of this chapter. The focus of this section will thus be primarily limited to the neurobiology of affiliation as it relates to autism spectrum disorders.

Autism

Symptoms and criteria

Autism is a developmental disorder of early childhood, characterized by social impairment, communication deficits, and compulsive behavior. The diagnostic criteria, epidemiology, and treatment of this disorder are covered elsewhere in this book (see chapter 42). This section focuses primarily on the dimension of social impairment and the neurobiology relevant to this aspect of autism.

Neurobiology relevant to social abnormalities

Oxytocin involvement. The function of central OT in the human brain is not known. However, it has been suggested that OT released during sexual activity may influence selective pair bonds between partners, and when the hormone is released during childbirth and lactation, it may play a role in the selective bond between mother and child (Turner et al., 1999). Insel (1992) has suggested that OT may release social behavior sequences or may promote and reinforce social contact. Elevated OT in the CSF of a subset of obsessive-compulsive disorder patients has also been found (Leckman et al., 1994). Modahl et al. (1998) hypothesized that abnormal OT system function might be found in autistic individuals. They also suggest that localized dysfunction of OT receptor sites in the limbic tissue could disrupt the perception of the significance of others and disrupt normal affiliative behaviors. In their study, they found that autistic children as a group showed lower OT levels than normal children. Greater deficits in social awareness were correlated with higher OT in autism. Greater language deficits, however, were significantly correlated with lower OT. Researchers suggest that this finding may reflect the fact that only higher-functioning autistic children had enough spoken language for specific language abnormalities to appear. In addition, Hollander et al. (submitted) have found that intravenous OT infusion in adults with autistic spectrum disorders leads to a decrease in repetitive and compulsive behaviors over the course of the infusion. In one clinical population, a higher level of induction (of labor) with Pitocin (synthetic oxytocin) has been found in people with autism (60 %) than in the general population (20 %), although this information has yet to be replicated. For example, another survey done by Fein et al. (1997) does not show a significant increase in the rate of induction in autistic children. In each of these studies, various factors, such as other medication and birth difficulties were not assessed and may be confounding factors in understanding the relationship between Pitocin induction and the development of autism. In addition, it is not clear whether Pitocin induction is a factor causing the disorder; or if the need for induction with Pitocin results from abnormalities already present in a baby who will go on to develop autism. Therefore, more research is needed to understand the relationship of Pitocin induction and autism. Taken together, however, these findings may be viewed as preliminary indications that OT may play a role in autism.

Serotonin involvement. There is substantial evidence supporting abnormal 5-HT function in autism, particularly with regard to both the social deficit and repetitive behavior dimensions of this disorder. Many studies of the neurobiology of autism have focused on 5-HT, which is implicated in the regulation of many functions relevant to autism, such as learning, memory, repetitive behaviors, sensory, social and motor processes (Ciaranello et al., 1982). Serotonin function also plays an important role in modulating anxiety, depression, and obsessive compulsive behavior.

Studies of 5-HT in whole-blood and plasma suggest an elevation of whole-blood 5-HT in some autistic individuals (Ritvo et al., 1970; Hoshino et al., 1984; Anderson et al., 1987), and in some studies, an association between hyperserotonemia and greater cognitive impairment, increased stereotypies, and more severe behavioral disturbance (Campbell and Plij, 1985; Ritvo et al., 1986). However, other studies have not shown 5-HT levels to correlate with specific clinical features (Schain and Freedman, 1961; Young et al., 1987). In autistic individuals with affected relatives, 5-HT blood levels were significantly higher than those without affected relatives (Kuperman et al., 1985; Piven et al., 1991). In addition, relatives of autistic probands with normal 5-HT levels were found to have normal 5-HT levels (Abrahamson et al., 1989; Cook et al., 1990). Thus, 5-HT blood levels may be familial and possibly associated with a genetic liability to specific subtypes of autism.

Preliminary studies on pharmacological manipulation of the serotonergic system in autism suggest that acute depletion of the 5-HT precursor tryptophan can exacerbate many behavioral symptoms of autistic disorder (McDougle et al., 1996). McBride et al. (1989) showed decreased central 5-HT responsiveness in autistic adults via blunted prolactin response to fenfluramine, a 5-HT-releasing agent.

A recent positron emission tomography (PET) study in which the radiolabeled serotonin precursor alpha C^{11} methyl tryptophan was used provides empirical evidence of decreased 5-HT synthesis in frontal and thalamic regions and increased 5-HT synthesis in contralateral cerebellar dentate regions (Chugani et al., 1997). These findings are consistent with findings of increased 5-HT$_{1d}$ inhibitory autoreceptor sensitivity in adult autistic patients (Hollander et al., 2000; Novotny et al., 2000), since these receptors are prevalent in frontal and thalamic, but not cerebellar, regions.

Studies with the 5-HT$_{1d}$ agonist sumatriptan demonstrated that altered neuroendocrine response reflecting 5-HT$_{1d}$ sensisitivy significantly correlates with severity of the repetitive behavior domain (Hollander et al., 2000). In addition, there is evidence for improvement in global severity as well as improvements in both social deficits and decreased repetitive behavior in autistic individuals with serotonin reuptake inhibitor (SRI) treatment (Gordon et al., 1993, McDougle et al., 1996, Hollander et al, 1998). There is substantial evidence to support the involvement of 5-HT dysfunction in the social deficit domain of autism.

Opioid involvement. Although the definitive role of opioid hormones in reinforcing social and maternal behavior has not been delineated, researchers have suggested a role for the opioid system in autistic disorders. Abnormalities of the opioid system have been documented in some subgroups of the autistic population and include predominantly reduced beta endorphin plasma levels in autistic individuals in most studies (although more recent studies have found elevated levels of plasma beta endorphin), and increased beta endorphin levels in the CSF of autistic individuals in some studies (Gillberg, 1995; Brambilla et al, 1997). There is some suggestion that levels of endgenous endorphins correlate with self-injurious behavior. Abnormalities in the opioid system could be correlated with abnormalities in the 5-HT system, although the complex nature of this interaction has yet to be fully understood.

Additionally, an opioid antagonist, naltrexone, has been used to treat children with autism. The results from these studies have been mixed, with some studies showing a mild decrease in hyperactivity and self-injurious behavior, and improved attention (Gillberg, 1995). The children who respond best to this medication appear to have more severe abnormalities in their beta endorphin levels (Bouvard et al., 1995). Overall, the research suggests that the endogenous opioid system, which is important in the reward aspects of affiliation, may also play a role in the neurobiology of autism.

CONCLUSIONS

The neurobiology of affiliation and attachment is a vast and complicated topic. Despite the significant amount of work that has already been completed in this field, there is still much to learn about the various complex behaviors that comprise affiliation, as well as the neurobiology that underlies these behaviors. The importance of studying these behaviors is apparent when one views the damage that occurs when these systems do not function normally, particularly in disorders such as autism and childhood trauma. Although not enough is understood about either of these disorders, the potential for understanding some of the pathology of these disorders through further research on the neurobiology of affiliation is in the least intriguing and at best may help to elucidate specific domains of select neuropsychiatric disorders, potentially leading to new and better treatments.

REFERENCES

Abrahamson, R.K., Wright, H.H., Carpenter, R., Brennan, W., Lumpuy, O., Cole, E., and Young, S.R. (1989) Elevated blood serotonin in autistic probands and their first-degree relatives. *J Autism Dev Disorder* 19:397–407.

Anderson, G.M., Freedman, D.X., Cohen, D.J., Volkmar, F.R., Hoder, E.L., McPhedran, P., Minderaa, R.B., Hansen, C.R., and Young, J.G. (1987) Whole blood serotonin in autistic and normal subjects. *J Child Pscyhol Psychiatry* 28:885–900.

Bachevalier, J., Alvarado, M.C., and Malkova, L. (1999) Memory and socioemotional behavior in monkeys after hippocampal damage incurred in infancy or in adulthood. *Biol Psychiatry* 46:329–339.

Barnes, C.D., and Pompeiano, O., eds. (1991) *Progress in Brain Research 99, Neurobiology of the Locus Coeruleus* London: Elsevier Science Publishing.

Berman, C.M. (1990) Intergenerational transmission of maternal rejection rates among free-ranging rhesus monkeys on Cayo Santiago. *Anim Behav*, 44:247–258.

Bouvard, M.P., Leboyer, M., Launay, J.M., Recasens, C., Plumet, M.H., Waller-Perotte, D., Tabuteau, F., Bondoux, D., Dugas, M., Lensing, P., et al. (1995) Low-dose naltrexone effects on plasma chemistries and clinical symptoms in autism: a double-blind, placebo-controlled study. *Psychiatry Res* 58:191–201.

Brambilla, F., Guareschi-Cazzullo, A., Tacchini, C., Musetti, C., Panerai, A.E., and Sacerdote, P. (1997) Beta-endorphin and cholecystokinin 8 concentrations in peripheral blood mononuclear cells of autistic children. *Neuropsychobiology* 35:1–4.

Bridges, R.S. (1998) The genetics of motherhood. *Nat Genet* 20:108–109.

Bridges, R.S., Numan, M., Ronsheim, P.M., Mann, P.E., and Lupini, C.E. (1990) Central prolactin infusions stimulate maternal behavior in steroid-treated, nulliparous female rats. *Proc Natl Acad Sci USA* 87:8003–8007.

Broad, K.D., Levy, F., Evans, G., Kimura, T., Keverne, E.B., and Kendrick, K.M. (1999). Previous maternal experience potentiates the effect of parturition on oxytocin receptor mRNA expression in the paraventricular nucleus. *Eur J Neurosci* 11:3725–3737.

Brunner, D., Buhot, M.C., Hen, R., and Hofer, M. (1999). Anxiety, motor activation, and maternal-infant interactions in 5HT1B knockout mice. *Behav Neurosci* 113:587–601.

Caldji, C., Diorio, J., and Meaney, M.J. (2000) Variations in maternal care in infancy regulate the development of stress reactivity. *Soc Biol Psychiatry* 49:1164–1174.

Caldji, C., Tannenbaum, B., Sharma, S., Francis, D., Plotsky, P.M., and Meaney M.J. (1998) Maternal care during infancy regulates the development of neural systems mediating the expression of behavioral fearfulness in adulthood in the rat. *Proc Natl Acad Sci* 95:5335–5340.

Campbell, M., and Plij, M. (1985) Behavioral and cognitive measures used in psychopharmacological studies of infantile autism. *Psychopharmacol Bull* 21:1047–1053.

Christensen, L.W., and Clemens, L.G. (1974) Intrahypothalamic implants of testosterone or estradiol and resumption of masculine sexual behavior in long-term castrated male rats. *Endocrinology* 95:984–990.

Chugani, D.C., Muzik, O., Rothermel, R., Behen, M., Chakraborty, P., Mangner, T., da Silva, E.A., and Chugani, H.T. (1997) Altered serotonin synthesis in the dentathalamocortical pathway in autistic boys. *Ann Neurol* 42:666–669.

Ciarenello, R.D., Vanderberg, S.R., and Anders T.F. (1982) Intrinsic and extrinsic determinants of neuronal development: relevance to infantile autism. *J Autism Dev Disorders* 12:115–145.

Cook, E.H., Leventhal, B.L., Hellar, W., Metz, J., Wainwright, M., and Freedman, D.X. (1990) Relationships between serotonin and norepinephrine levels and intelligence. *J Neuropsychiatry Clin Neurosci* 2:268–274.

Da Costa, A.P., Broad, K.D., and Kendrick, K.M. (1997). Olfactory memory and maternal behaviour-induced changes in c-fos and zif/268 mRNA expression in the sheep brain. *Brain Res Mol Brain Res*, 46:63–76.

Da Costa, A.P., De La Riva, C., Guevara-Guzman, R., and Kendrick, K.M. (1999) C-fos and c-jun in the paraventricular nucleus play a role in regulating peptide gene expression, oxytocin and glutamate release, and maternal behaviour. *Eur J Neurosci* 11:2199–2210.

DeVries, G.J., Buijs, R.M., Van Leeuwen, F.W., Caffe, A.R., and Swaab, D.F. (1985) The vasopressinergic innervation of the brain in normal and castrated rats. *J Comp Neurol* 233:236–254.

Everitt, B.J. (1990) Sexual motivation: a neural and behavioural analysis of the mechanisms underlying appetitive and copulatory responses of male rats. *Neurosci Biobehav Rev* 14:217–232.

Fein, D., Allen, D., Dunn, M., Feinstein, C., Green, L., Morris, R., Rapin, I., and Waterhouse, L. (1997) Pitocin induction and autism. *Am J Psychiatry* 154:438–9.

Ferguson, J.N., Young, L.J., Hearn, E.F., Matzuk, M.M., Insel, T.R., and Winslow, J.T. (2000) Social amnesia in mice lacking the oxytocin gene. *Nat Genet* 25:284–288.

Fleming, A.S., Cheung, U., Myhal, N., and Kessler, Z. (1989) Effects of maternal hormones on 'timidity' and attraction to pup-related odors in female rats. *Physiol Behav* 46:449–453.

Fleming, A.S., Vaccarino, F., and Luebke, C. (1980) Amygdaloid inhibition of maternal behavior in the nulliparous female rat. *Physiol Behav* 25:731–743.

Francis, D.D., Caldji, C., Champagne, F., Plotsky, P.M., and Meaney, M.J. (1999a) The role of corticotropin-releasing factor–norepinephrine systems in mediating the effects of early experience on the development of behavioral and endocrine responses to stress. *Biol Psychiatry* 46:1153–1166.

Francis, D.D., Champagne, F.A., Liu, D., and Meaney, M.J. (1999b) Maternal care, gene expression, and the development of individual differences in stress reactivity. *Ann NY Acad Sci* 896:66–84.

Gammie, S.C., and Nelson R.J. (1999) Maternal aggression is reduced in neuronal nitric oxide synthase-deficient mice. *J Neurosci* 19:8027–8035.

Gillberg, C. (1995) Endogenous opioids and opiate antagonists in autism: brief review of empirical findings and implications for clinicians. *Dev Med Child Neurol* 37:239–245.

Goffin, V., Binart, N., Clement-Lacroix, P., Bouchard, B., Bole-Feysot, C., Edery, M., Lucas, B.K., Touraine, P., Pezet, A., Maaskant, R., Pichard, C., Helloco, C., Baran, N., Favre, H., Bernichtein, S., Allamando, A., Ormandy, C., and Kelly P.A. (1999) From the molecular biology of prolactin and its receptor to the lessons learned from knockout mice models. *Genet Anal* 15:189–201.

Gordon, C.T., State, R.C., Nelson, J.E., Hamburger, S.D., and Rapoport J.L. (1993) A double-blind comparison of clomipramine, desipramine, and placebo in the treatment of autistic disorder. *Arch Gen Psychiatry* 50:441–447.

Higley, J.D., Thompson, W.W., Champoux, M., Goldman, D., Hasert, M.F., Kraemer, G.W., et al. (1993). Paternal and maternal genetic and environmental contributions to cerebrospinal fluid monoamine metabolites in rhesus monkeys (macaca mulatta). *Arch Gen Psychiatry* 50:615–623.

Hollander, E., Cartwright, C., Wong, C.M., DeCarla, C.M.,

DelGiudice-Asch, G., Buchsbaum, M.S., and Aronowitz, B. (1998) A dimensional approach to the autism spectrum. *CNS Spectrums* 3:22–39.

Hollander, E., Novotny, S., Allen, A., Aronowitz, B., and DeCaria, C. (2000) The relationship between repetitive behaviors and growth hormone response to sumatriptan challenge in adult autistic disorders. *Neuropsychopharmacology* 22:163–167.

Hollander, E., Novotny, S., Hanratty, M., Allen, A., Yafte, R., De Caria, e., Aronowitz, B., Moscovish, S. Oxytocin infusion reduces repetitive behaviors in adults with autism spectrum disorders. *Neuropsychopharmacology* (submitted).

Hoshino, Y., Yamamoto, T., Kaneko, M., Tachibana, R., Wantabe, M., Ono, Y., and Kumashiro, H. (1984) Blood serotonin and free tryptophan concentration in autistic children. *Neuropsychobiology* 11:22–27.

Insel, T.R. (1992) OT—a neuropeptide for affiliation. *Psychoneuroendocrinology* 17:3–35.

Insel, T.R. (1997) A neurobiological basis of social attachment. *Am J Psychiatry* 154:726–735.

Insel, T.R., and Harbaugh C.R. (1989) Lesions of the hypothalamic paraventricular nucleus disrupt the initiation of maternal behavior. *Physiol Behav* 45:1033–1041.

Insel, T.R., and Hulihan T.J. (1995) A gender-specific mechanism for pair bonding: Oxytocin and partner preference formation in monogamous voles. *Behav Neurosci* 109:782–789.

Insel, T.R., O'Brien, D.J., and Leckman, J.F. (1999) Oxytocin, vasopressin, and autism: is there a connection? *Biol Psychiatry* 45:145–157.

Insel, T.R., and Shapiro, L.E. (1991) Oxytocin receptor distribution reflects social organization in monogamous and polygamous voles. *Proc Natl Acad Sci USA* 89:5981–5985.

Insel, T.R., and Winslow, J.T. (1991) Central administration of oxytocin modulates the infant rat's response to social isolation. *Eur J Pharmacol* 203:149–152.

Insel, T.R., and Winslow J.T. (1998) Serotonin and neuropeptides in affiliative behaviors. *Biol Psychiatry* 443:207–219.

Insel, T.R., and Young, L.J. (2001) The neurobiology of attachment. *Nat Rev Neurosci* 2:129–136.

Insel, T.R., Young, L., and Wang, Z. (1997) Molecular aspects of monogamy. *Ann NY Acad Sci* 807:302–316.

Kendrick, K.M., Keverne, E.B., Hinton, M.R., and Goode J.A. (1992) Oxytocin, amino acid and monoamine release in the region of the medial preoptic area and bed nucleus of the stria terminalis of the sheep during parturition and suckling. *Brain Res* 569:199–209.

Keverne, E.B., Martensz, N.D., and Tuite, B. (1989) Beta-endorphin concentrations in Cerebrospinal fluid of monkeys are influenced by grooming relationships. *Psychoneuroendocrinology* 14:155–161.

Keverne, E.B., Nevison, C.M., and Martel, F.L. (1997) Early learning and the social bond. *Ann NY Acad Sci* 807:329–339.

Knutson, B., Cole, S., Wolkowitz, O., Reus, V., Chan, T., and Moore, E. (1997) Serotonergic intervention increases affiliative behavior in humans. *Ann NY Acad Sci* 807:492–493.

Kuperman, S., Beeghly, J.H., Burns, T.L., and Tsai, L.Y. (1985) Serotonin relationships of autistic probands and their first-degree relatives. *J Am Acad Child Adolesc Psychiatry* 24:186–190.

Leckman, J.F., Goodman, W.K., North, W.G., Chappell, P.B., Price, L.H., Pauls, D.L., et al. (1994) Elevated cerebrospinal fluid levels of oxytocin in obsessive-compulsive disorder. *Arch Gen Psychiatry* 51:782–792.

Leon, M., Numan, M., and Moltz, H. (1973) Maternal behavior in the rat: facilitation through gonadectomy. *Science* 179:1018–1019.

Levy, F., Kendrick, K.M., Goode, J.A., Guevara-Guzman, R., and Keverne, E.B. (1995) Oxytocin and vasopressin release in the olfactory bulb of parturient ewes: changes with maternal experience and effects on acetylcholine, gamma-aminobutyric acid, glutamate and noradrenaline release. *Brain Res* 669:197–206.

Login, I.S. and MacLeod, R.M. (1977) Prolactin in human and rat serum and cerebrospinal fluid. *Brain Res* 132:477–483.

Lucas, B.K., Ormandy, C.J., Binart, N., Bridges, R.S., and Kelly, P.A. (1998) Null mutation of the prolactin receptor gene produces a defect in maternal behavior. *Endocrinology* 139:4102–4107.

Matochik, J.A., Sipos, M.L., Nyby, J.G., and Barfield, R.J. (1994) Intracranial androgenic activation of male-typical behaviors in house mice: motivation versus performance. *Behav Brain Res* 60:141–149.

McBride, P.A., Anderson, G.M., Hertzig, M.E., Sweeney, J.A., Kleam J., Cohen, D.J., and Mann, J.J. (1989) Serotonergic response in male young adults with autistic disorder. *Arch Gen Psychiatry* 46:205–212.

McCarthy, M.M. and Altemus M. (1997) Central nervous system actions of oxytocin and modulation of behavior in humans. *Mol Med Today* 3:269–275.

McDougle, C.J., Naylor, S.T., Cohen, D.J., Volkmar, F.R., Heninger, G.R., and Price, L.H. (1996) A double-blind placebo-controlled study of fluvoxamine in adults with autistic disorder. *Arch Gen Psychiatry* 53:1001–1008.

Modahl, C., Green, L., Fein, D., Morris, M., Waterhouse, L., Feinstein, C., and Levin, H. (1998) Plasma oxytocin levels in autistic children. *Biol Psychiatry* 43:270–277.

Nelson, E. and Alberts, J.R. (1997) Oxytocin-induced paw sucking in infant rats. *Ann NY Acad Sci* 807:543–545.

Nelson, E. and Panksepp, J. (1996) Oxytocin mediates acquisition of maternally associated odor preferences in preweaning rat pups. *Behav Neurosci* 110:583–592.

Newman, J.D. (1988) *The Physiologic Control of Mammalian Vocalization.* New York: Plenum Press.

Nissen, E., Lilja, G., Widstrom, A.M., and Uvnas-Moberg, K. (1995) Elevation of oxytocin levels early post partum in women. *Acta Obstet Gynecol Scand* 74:530–533.

Novotny, S., Hollander, E., Allen, A., Mosovich, S., Aronowitz, B., Cartwright, C., DeCaria, C., and Dolgoff-Kaspar, R. (2000) Increased growth hormone response to sumatriptan challenge in adult autistic disorders. *Psychol Res* 44:173–177.

Numan, M. (1974) Medial preoptic area and maternal behavior in the female rat. *J Comp Physiol Psychol* 87:746–759.

Numan, M. (1978) Progesterone inhibition of maternal behavior in the rat. *Horm Behav* 11:209–231.

Numan, M. (1986) The role of the medial preoptic area in the regulation of maternal behavior in the rat. *Ann NY Acad Sci* 474:226–233.

Numan, M. (1988) Maternal behavior. In: Knobil, E. and Neill, J., eds. *The Physiology of Reproduction, Vol. 2.* New York: Raven Press, pp. 1569–1645.

Numan, M. (1990) Long-term effects of preoptic area knife cuts on the maternal behavior of postpartum rats. *Behav Neural Biol* 53:284–290.

Numan, M. (1994) A neural circuitry analysis of maternal behavior in the rat. *Acta Pediatr Suppl* 397:19–28.

Numan, M. and Callahan, E.C. (1980) The connections of the medial preoptic region and maternal behavior in the rat. *Physiol Behav* 25:653–665.

Numan M. and Corodimas K.P. (1985) The effects of paraventricular hypothalamic lesions on maternal behavior in rats. *Physiol Behav* 35:417–425.

Numan, M., Corodimas, K.P., Numan, M.J., Factor, E.M., and Piers, W.D. (1988) Axon-sparing lesions of the preoptic region and substantia innominata disrupt maternal behavior in rats. *Behav Neurosci* 102:381–396.

Numan, M. and Numan, M.J. (1992) Maternal behavior in female rats is associated with increased numbers of Fos containing neurons in the medial preoptic area. *Soc Neurosci Abstr* 18:892.

Numan, M. and Numan, M.J. (1994) Expression of Fos-like immunoreactivity in the preoptic area of maternally behaving virgin and postpartum rats. *Behav Neurosci* 108:379–394.

Numan, M. and Numan, M.J. (1996) A lesion and neuroanatomical tract-tracing analysis of the role of the bed nucleus of the stria terminalis in retrieval behavior and other aspects of maternal responsiveness in rats. *Dev Psychobiol* 29:23–51.

Numan, M., Numan, M.J., and English, J.B. (1993) Excitotoxic amino acid injections into the medial amygdala facilitate maternal behavior in virgin female rats. *Horm Behav* 27:56–81.

Numan, M., Numan, M.J., Marzella, S.R., and Palumbo, A. (1998) Expression of c-*fos*, *fos* B, and *egr-1* in the medial preoptic area and bed nucleus of the stria terminalis during maternal behavior in rats. *Brain Res* 792:348–352.

Numan, M., Roach, J.K., del Cerro, M.C., Guillamon, A., Segovia, S, Sheehan, T.P., and Numan, M.J. (1999) Expression of intracellular progesterone receptors in rat brain during different reproductive states, and involvement in maternal behavior. *Brain Res* 830:358–371.

Numan, M., Rosenblatt, J.S., and Komisaruk, B.R. (1977) Medial preoptic area and onset of maternal behavior in the rat. *J Comp Physiol Psychol* 91:146–164.

Numan, M. and Sheehan, T.P. (1997) Neuroanatomical circuitry for mammalian maternal behavior. *Ann NY Acad Sci* 807:101–125.

Pedersen, C.A. (1997) Oxytocin control of maternal behavior. Regulation by sex steroids and offspring stimuli. *Ann NY Acad Sci* 807:126–145.

Pedersen, C.A., Ascher, J.A., Monroe, Y.L., and Prange, A.J., Jr. (1982) Oxytocin induces maternal behavior in virgin female rats. *Science* 216:648–650.

Pedersen, C.A., and Prange, A.J., Jr. (1991) Induction of maternal behavior in virgin rats after intracerebroventricular administration of oxytocin. *Proc Natl Acad Sci USA* 76:6661–6665.

Piven, J., Chase, G.A., Landa, R., Wzorek, M., Gayle, J., Cloud, D., and Folstein, S. (1991) Psychiatric disorders in the parents of autistic individuals. *J Am Acad Child Adolesc Psychiatry* 30:471–478.

Raleigh, M.J., Brammer, G.L., and McGuire, M.T. (1983) Male dominance, serotonergic systems, and the behavioral and physiological effects of drugs in vervet monkeys (*Cercopithecus aethiops sabaeus*). *Prog Clin Biol Res* 131:185–197.

Raleigh, M.J., McGuire, MT., Brammer, G.L., Pollack, D.B., and Yuwiler, A. (1991) Serotonergic mechanisms promote dominance acquisition in adult male vervet monkeys. *Brain Res* 559:181–190.

Ritvo, E.R., Freeman, B.J., Yuwiler, A., Geller, E., Schroth, P., Yokota, A., Mason-Biothers, A., August, G.J., Klykylo, W., Leventhal, B. Lewis, K., Piggott, L., Realmutto G., Stubbs E.G., and Umansky, R. (1986) Fenfluramine treatment of autism: UCLA Collaborative study of 81 patients at nine medical centers. *Psychopharmacol Bull* 22:133–140.

Ritvo, E.R., Yuwiler, A., Geller, E., Ornitz, E.M., Saeyer, K., and Plotkin, S. (1970) Increased blood serotonin and platelets in early infantile autism. *Arch Gen Psychiatry* 23:566–572.

Schain, R.J., and Freedman, D.X. (1961) Studies on 5-hydroxyindoleamine metabolism in autistic and other mentally retarded children. *J Pediatr* 58:315–320.

Schultz, R.T., Gauther, I., Klin, A., Fulbright, R.K., Anderson, A.W., Volkmar, F., Skudlarski, P., Lacadie, C., Cohen, D.J., and Gore, J.C. (2000) Abnormal ventral temporal cortical activity during face discrimination among individuals with autism and Asperger syndrome. *Arch Gen Psychiatry* 57:331–340.

Shapiro, L.E., and Insel, T.R. (1990) Infant's response to social separation reflects adult differences in affiliative behavior: a comparative developmental study in prairie and montane voles. *Dev Psychobiol* 23:374–394.

Smythe, J.W., Rowe, W.B., and Meaney, M.J. (1994) Neonatal handling alters serotonin (5-HT) turnover and 5-HT₂ receptor binding in selected brain regions: relationship to the handling effect of glucocorticoid receptor expression. *Brain Res* 80:183–189.

Stack, E.C. and Numan, M. (2000) The temporal course of expression of c-Fos and Fos B within the medial preoptic area and other brain regions of postpartum female rats during prolonged mother–young interactions. *Behav Neurosci* 14:609–622.

Thiessen, D.D. and Yahr, P. (1970) Central control of territorial marking in the mongolian gerbil. *Physiol Behav* 5:275–278.

Thomas, S.A. and Palmiter, R.D. (1997a) Impaired maternal behavior in mice lacking norepinephrine and epinephrine. *Cell* 91:583–592.

Thomas, S.A., Palmiter, R.D. (1997) Disruption of the dopamine beta-hydroxylase gene in mice suggests roles for neuropinephrine in motor function, learning & memory. *Behav Neurosci* 1110:579–89.

Turner, R.A., Altemus, M., Enos, T., Cooper, B., and McGuinness, T. (1999) Preliminary research on plasma oxytocin in normal cycling women: investigating emotion and interpersonal distress. *Psychiatry* 62:97–113.

van Wimersma Greidanus, T.B. and Maigret, C. (1996) The role of limbic vasopressin and oxytocin in social recognition. *Brain Res* 713:153–159.

Wang, Z.X., Liu, Y., Young, L.J., and Insel, T.R. (2000) Hypothalamic vasopressin gene expression increases in both males and females postpartum in a biparental rodent. *J Neuroendocrinol* 12:111–120.

Winslow, J.T., Hastings, N., Carter, C.S., Harbaugh, C.R., and Insel, T.R. (1993) A role for central vasopressin in pair bonding in monogamous prairie voles. *Nature* 365:545–548.

Winslow, J.T., Hearn, E.F., Ferguson, J., Young, LJ., Matzuk, M.M., Insel, T.R. (2000) Infant vocalization, adult aggression, and fear behavior of an oxytocin null mutant mouse. *Horm Behav* 37:145–155.

Witt, D.M., Winslow, J.T., and Insel, T.R. (1992) Enhanced social interactions in rats following chronic, centrally infused oxytocin. *Pharmacol Biochem Behav* 43:855–861.

Young, J.G., Level, L.I., Newcorn, J.H., and Knott, P.J. (1987) Genetic and neurobiological approaches to the pathophysiology of autism and the pervasive developmental disorders. In: Meltzer, H.Y., ed. *Psychopharmacology: The Third Generation of Progress.* New York: Raven Press, pp. 825–836.

Young, L.J., Winslow, J.T., Wang, Z., Gingrich, B., Guo, Q., Matzuk, M.M., and Insel, T.R. (1997) Gene targeting approaches to neuroendocrinology: oxytocin, maternal behavior, and affiliation. *Horm Behav* 31:221–231.

Zhuang, X., Gross, C., Santarelli, L., Compan, V., Trillat, A.C., and Hen, R. (1999) Altered emotional states in knockout mice lacking 5-HT1A or 5-HT1B receptors. *Neuropsychopharmacology* 21(2 Suppl):52S–60S.

17 | Neurobiology of aggression

MARKUS J.P. KRUESI, SONDRA KELLER, AND MARK W. WAGNER

L.F. socked him in the mouth, chipping tooth.
—*Narrative account from a randomly selected
school accident report, Johnson et al. (1974)*

Fundamentally, all behaviors rely on a neurobiologic substrate for expression. In this chapter, we will focus on information about the neurobiology of aggression. Here, *aggression* is defined as physical violence that is an associated feature or symptom of a psychiatric disorder. This definition is intended to include aggression often described as impulsive or affective, in contrast to that described as predatory. A clinical belief exists that medication is more likely to impact affective aggression (Vitiello et al., 1990). In this chapter, we will review the neurobiology of both impulsive and predatory types of aggression. We will also touch on pharmacologic treatment used attempting to alter pathophysiologic relationships. Human psychopharmacology treatment studies are covered in greater detail in Chapter 50 in this volume.

PREVALENCE OF AGGRESSION AND COMORBIDITY OF AGGRESSION AND PSYCHIATRIC ILLNESS

Aggression often prompts requests for intervention. Depending on the setting and the youth involved, the probability of observing aggression will vary; in some sites, it is virtually a daily occurrence. For example, a state-wide prevalence survey of institutionalized mentally retarded individuals found that 13.6% engaged in self-injurious behavior (Griffin et al., 1986), with over half engaging in such behavior daily. Even in mainstream school settings, aggression that causes injury is common. Three decades before shootings at school were a national focus, a study in Seattle public schools found that aggressive behavior (mainly fights, pushing, and throwing objects) caused 13% of all reported school injuries (Johnson et al., 1974).

Aggression can occur as either an essential or associated feature of a psychiatric disorder. The diagnoses in each of these categories, according to the *Diagnostic and Statistical Manual of Mental Disorders*, 4th ed. (American Psychiatric Association 1994), are listed in

Table 17.1. In this context, mental retardation deserves special comment. Although most persons with mental retardation are not violent, there is an increased risk of inappropriate aggression among individuals with psychiatric diagnoses in general, including mental retardation. Most research on associations between violence and mental illness has focused on adults. To assess the relationship between aggressive behaviors and psychiatric disorders, it is useful to look at the prevalence of psychiatric disorders in those who have committed violent acts, and to examine the prevalence of violence in psychiatric patients in different settings.

Adult Jail Detainees

In a 1994 study Teplin evaluated 728 male jail detainees, and found that nearly two-thirds of this population had a psychiatric disorder with antisocial personality disorder (ASP), the most common diagnosis at 50%. However, 35% of the population had a current diagnosis other than ASP, and two-thirds had previously been given a lifetime diagnosis other than ASP. Substance abuse was common, with a 62% lifetime prevalence. More than one out of three detainees had a severe mental disorder (schizophrenia, bipolar affective disorder, or major depression). In another study, 693 homicide offenders were evaluated and elevated rates of schizophrenia and ASP were found (Eronen et al., 1996). Earlier studies found schizophrenia in 29%–75% and affective disorders in 4%–35% of prisoners.

Most of such studies have excluded women. In one study of 1272 female pretrial detainees, over 80% met criteria for at least one psychiatric disorder, with substance abuse and post-traumatic stress disorder (PTSD) being the most common (Teplin et al., 1996). Similar results were found in 805 women felons, with high rates of substance abuse, borderline personality disorders, and ASP, compared to respective rates in the community (Jordan et al., 1996).

Inpatient Adults

Most studies of violent behavior in adults focus on inpatient or recently discharged patients. As a group,

TABLE 17.1 *DSM-IV Disorders with Aggression*

As a Diagnostic Feature	As an Associated Feature
Antisocial personality disorder	Attention-deficit hyperactivity disorder
Borderline personality disorder	Bipolar affective disorder
Conduct disorder	Mental retardation
Intermittent explosive disorder	Psychoactive substance abuse disorder
	Psychotic disorder

schizophrenics, consistently tend to be more violent than other patients. In a review of 13 studies involving over 20,000 inpatient hospitalizations (Krakowski et al., 1986), schizophrenia was the diagnosis associated with aggression in inpatient settings; however, no subtype predominated. Two recent studies using large Danish birth cohorts ($n > 324,000$) found that (*1*) persons with a history of psychiatric hospitalization were more likely to have been confined for a criminal offense than those without a psychiatric hospitalization (Hodgins et al., 1996); and (*2*) individuals hospitalized with schizophrenia and men with organic psychosis had the highest rate of arrest for violence (Brennan et al., 2000).

Children and Adolescents

Aggressive behavior and conduct problems are a common presentation for pediatric psychiatric referrals, as one-third to one-half of such patients present with these symptoms (Kazdin, 1987). Conduct disorder is the only childhood disorder with aggression as a criterion symptom. However, conduct disorder has significant comorbidity with other disorders, including attention-deficit hyperactivity disorder (ADHD), and affective and psychotic disorders. Aggression is a common complaint in children presenting with ADHD (Conner and Steingard, 1996). In mood and psychotic disorders in children and adolescents, irritability and aggression may be common symptoms (Conner and Steingard, 1996). In contrast to adults, data on aggression in childhood schizophrenia are limited, probably because of the rarity of the disorder. Up to 29% of children suffering from schizophrenia have a history of conduct disorder (Russell, 1994; Spenser and Campbell, 1994).

In examining different disorders, it is important to consider the clinical setting in which they are studied and the informant involved. Report of aggression is a

major determinant of placement (e.g. home, hospital, residential treatment). According to teacher reports, children in outpatient settings exhibited more aggressive behavior. This observation is most likely a reflection of the difference in the amount of time the teachers spent with the children in the different settings (Zimet et al., 1994a, b).

In most studies of childhood aggression, the children are in inpatient settings, where the most aggressive individuals would be placed. The aggressive inpatient is most likely to be diagnosed with conduct disorder. In a study of 163 hospitalized adolescents (Apter et al., 1995), violent behaviors were significantly higher in conduct disorders, compared to other diagnostic groups, including schizophrenia, anxiety, and mood disorder; however, ADHD was not included. Gabel and Shindledecker (1991) found similar results in a study of 348 youth in inpatient and day treatment. A significant number of the aggressive patients had conduct disorder, compared to ADHD and depressive disorders. Vivona et al. (1995) found that in 89 hospitalized youth, histories of antisocial behaviors, foster home placement, and abuse were more often found in the aggressive population, compared to the nonaggressive group.

DEFINITIONS OF AGGRESSION

Definitions of aggression are critical to the interpretation of studies of the neurobiology of aggression and for identifying targets for psychopharmacologic intervention. Items on aggression rating scales often include emotions, thoughts, and activity associated with anger; however, their relevance to physical aggression per se has been viewed as speculative (Edmunds and Kendrick, 1980; Kay et al., 1988). More recently, however, individual differences in emotion regulation skills, particularly as they apply to suppression of negative affect, are thought to be particularly important in determining vulnerability to aggression and violence (Davidson et al., 2000). The measurement of aggression is often described as problematic (Kruesi et al., 1994). Sources of difficulty include (*1*) the definition of aggression; (*2*) choices between frequency- and severity-based ratings; (*3*) low frequencies of certain types of aggressive acts, particularly severe physical aggression; (*4*) different weighting of specific behaviors; (*5*) information source; (*6*) lack of empirical validation for many of the measures of aggression; (*7*) failure to differentiate between predatory and affective violence; and (*8*) ethical concerns.

Another conceptual advance in understanding aggression and its neurobiology is the distinction between predatory and affective/impulsive aggression. Studies of youth and adults indicate that impulsive and premeditated aggression are independent constructs (Dodge and Coie, 1987; Vitiello et al., 1990; Barratt et al., 1999). Contrasts between predatory and impulsive aggression are discussed below.

Differentiating between types of aggression can be pertinent to medication trials. Chronic inhibition of monoamine oxidase or serotonin (5-hydroxtryptamine [5-HT]) uptake, with antidepressant treatment, reliably facilitates defensive aggression but not attack behavior in rodents (Miczek et al., 1994). Thus, at least in animal studies, affective and predatory types of aggression differ in their psychopharmacologic response.

ANIMAL MODELS

Many behavioral concepts in ethological and psychiatric inquiries into aggression are derived from early observations on brain stimulation–evoked behaviors in cats (Hess and Brugger, 1943). One influential distinction regarding types of aggression concerns that between predatory and affective subtypes (Moyer, 1968). Synonyms for *predatory aggression* include instrumental, goal-directed, offensive, and premeditated. *Affective aggression* is often described as impulsive, reactive, or defensive. Predatory aggression is linked to parasympathetic activity and affective aggression to sympathetic activity, as evidenced by the need for lowered heart rate during some hunting activities, in contrast to the rage and sympathetic discharge that accompanies affective aggression. As described later, stimulation studies have also demonstrated anatomic differences between the two types.

Animals fight or threaten another animal for diverse reasons. Brain (1984) identified five categories: (1) *predation*, which generally involves efficient killing and is often followed by feeding; (2) *infanticide*, which for males may be a method of increasing reproductive fitness, whereas for females it is more likely a response to stress; (3) *self-defense*, behaviors that protect from predators or attacking conspecifics; (4) *parental defense*, which serves to protect the young or the nest from potential intruders; and (5) *social conflict*, or intraspecific competition for something (mate, territory, food, etc.), the possession of which increases the organism's fitness. Social conflict often involves generalized ritualized behaviors that do not lead to severe damage. Four major categories of experimental manipulations for aggression in animals are described in Table 17.2.

Cross-species comparisons are complicated by differences between species, their context, and conventions regarding description, as well as problems in using response patterns to categorize aggression. In reviewing three decades of research using brain stimulation in cats and rats, Siegel et al. (1999) point to a number of germane differences: (1) the responses to stimulation of the periaqueductal gray of the midbrain and the hypothalmus differ between cats and rats; (2) cats and rats occupy different ecological niches—solitary carnivore versus colony-dwelling, opportunistic omnivore; and (3) threat in defense of a territory is termed "defensive" in the cat but "offensive" in the rat. The motivational state of animals is inferred on the basis of releasing and directing stimuli in the specific space–time sequence in the animal's natural state. Critics have argued that because motivational states are constructs derived from behavioral observations, they may not relate neatly to a specific brain mechanism (Kruk 1991). Hence, classifying behaviors produced by electrical stimulation of discrete areas into motivational categories may be risky.

Development of psychopharmacologic agents using animal models of aggression has encountered a lack of enthusiasm from major research funding sources, including both the National Institutes of Health (NIH) and industry. Obstacles in the U.S. Food and Drug Administration (FDA) approval process have led to the scuttling of the only industry program aimed at developing a class of aggression-reducing drugs (Enserink, 2000).

BRAIN SYSTEMS IMPLICATED IN AGGRESSION

Anatomic Evidence

Historically, lesions (often due to accident or tumor), trauma history, and findings on neurological exam or neuropsychological testing have furnished evidence regarding localization. Two regions have most consistently been implicated: the prefrontal cortex and temporal lobe.

Evidence is strongest and most consistent for involvement of prefrontal regions. Prefrontal cortex lesions generally increase aggression (Mirsky and Siegel, 1994). The Phineas Gage case is well known as evidence of traumatic frontal lesion leading to impulsivity and rage (Damasio et al., 1994). Subsequent cases have offered confirmation that frontal lesions are associated with hostile, impulsive, aggressive behavior (Grafman et al., 1996; Anderson et al., 1999). Violent psychopaths display clear evidence of orbitofrontal dysfunction

TABLE 17.2 *Experimental Models of Aggression in Laboratory Animals*

Model	Procedure	Biologic Function	Behavior
Killing			
Muricide in rats or cats	Food deprivation, presence of prey	Food source	Stalk, seize, kill, sometimes consume prey
Ethological situations			
Aggression by resident toward intruder (most species)	Unfamiliar conspecific adult	Territorial or group defense, rivalry between same gender animals	Attack and threat vs. defense, submission, flight
Female aggression, maternal rodents	Lactating female with litter present confronts intruding male	Defense of young, competition for resources	Attack and/or threaten intruder
Dominance-related, in mice, rats, monkeys	Maintenance or formation of social group	Social cohesion and dispersion	Signals (display, sounds, odor) between group members of different social rank, low-level/intensity of aggression
Aversive environmental manipulation			
Isolation-induced aggression, mostly in mice	Isolation housing prior to confrontation with another isolate or group-housed animal	Territorial defense or pathologic behavior	Full agonistic pattern: the isolate attacks, threatens, pursues opponent
Shock–or pain-induced, mostly in rats, also monkeys	Electric shock via grid floor or to tail to pairs of animals	Somewhat similar to reaction to predator or large opponent	Defensive reactions, including upright posture, bites toward opponent's face and inanimate objects, audible vocalization
Aggression due to omission of reward, mostly in pigeons, also monkeys	Conditioned history, schedule-controlled operant behavior, omit or infrequent reinforcement	Competition for resources: food, sex, protected niches	Attack pecks or bites, threat display toward conspecific or suitable object
Brain manipulations			
Lesion-induced aggression, mostly in rats, also cats	Destruction of neural tissue, plus subsequent environmental or social changes	Neurologic disease	Defensive reactions, biting
Stimulation-induced aggression, mostly in cats, also rats	Direct electrical stimulation of diencephalon and mesencephalon, also other limbic or cerebellar areas	Defense against attacker; Predatory attack	Defensive reactions accompanied by autonomic arousal Predatory attack and killing

Adapted from Miczek et al. (1994)

on neuropsychological tests (LaPierre et al., 1995). However, clinical observation suggests that the social inappropriateness of patients with adult-onset prefrontal damage tends not to include violent and criminal behavior (Damasio, 2000). In contrast, early-onset prefrontal cortex lesions (before 16 months) are associated with defective social and moral reasoning, in addition to insensitivity to future consequences, defective autonomic responses to punishment, and failure to respond to behavioral interventions despite normal basic cognitive abilities (Anderson et al., 1999).

Involvement of the temporal lobe is less clear, but warrants additional attention. Medial temporal damage may reduce aggression (Geschwind, 1973), but abnormal neuronal activity in the temporal lobe as seen in temporal lobe epilepsy can result in increased aggression (Bear and Fedio, 1977). A study of 372 male maximum-security patients found that high violence scores correlated with computed tomography (CT) scan and electroencephalogram (EEG) abnormalities in the temporal lobes (Wong et al., 1994). More recently, neuroimaging techniques have provided more convincing support for the role of frontal and temporal regions in aggression (see next section).

Frontal and/or temporal locations associated with aggression need to be thought of as interconnected or interdependent, rather than isolated independent structures. This point is illustrated by a study of temporal lobe epilepsy (TLE) patients. Analysis of magnetic resonance imaging (MRI) from 35 controls, 24 TLE patients with a history of repeated, interictal episodes of aggression, and 24 TLE patients without aggression found that patients with TLE with aggressive episodes had less gray matter, particularly in the left frontal lobe, than each of the other groups (Woermann et al., 2000). Although the temporal lobe is a site of obvious pathology, the epileptic focus, findings suggest that structures elsewhere (frontal lobe) underlie the pathophysiology of aggression in TLE.

Human Neuroimaging Studies

There have been recent advances in the understanding in brain structure and function of some childhood psychiatric disorders; however, no controlled neuroimaging studies involving aggressive childhood disorders and conduct disorders have been published (Peterson, 1995). Despite the fact that ADHD and conduct disorders are commonly comorbid, existent imaging studies of ADHD are not informative, because typically these studies have excluded youths with conduct disorder.

Most neuroimaging data regarding aggression involve adult-only samples. One exception is a study of single photon emission compute tomograph (SPECT) findings in 40 aggressive adolescents and adults with various diagnoses (Amen et al., 1996). The authors found significantly decreased activity in the prefrontal cortex and increased activity in the anteriomedial portion of the frontal lobe and left side basalganglia in the aggressive patients. Focal abnormalities were also seen in the left temporal lobe. The prefrontal cortex is involved in impulse control, critical thinking, and concentration. Another SPECT study (Soderstrom et al., 2000) included a mixed adolescent and adult sample of 21 nonpsychotic violent offenders. In 16 of these subjects, some hypoperfusion was noted in the frontal or temporal lobes. Importantly, the abnormalities were as severe in the subgroup ($n = 7$) without major mental disorders or substance abuse as they were in those with those diagnoses.

Adult-only neuroimaging

One of the earliest neuroimaging studies of adults was that of four psychiatric patients with histories of repetitive purposeless violence; EEG, CT scan, and positron emission tomography (PET) were the means of imaging used (Volkow and Tancredi 1987). Three patients showed spiking activity in left temporal regions, and two showed CT abnormalities. The PET scans showed blood flow and metabolic abnormalities in the left temporal lobe. Two patients also had derangement in the frontal cortex. Patients showing the largest defects on PET scans were those whose CT scans were reported to be normal. A subsequent PET study found lower metabolic rates in medial temporal and frontal regions of violent patients than those in controls, although the location of abnormalities were not consistent from patient to patient (Volkow et al., 1995).

More recent PET studies have also identified functional abnormalities associated with violence. Murderers ($n = 41$) had reduced glucose metabolism compared to controls in the prefrontal cortex, superior parietal gyrus, left angular gyrus, and the corpus callosum, while abnormal asymmetries of activity (left hemisphere lower than right) were also found in the amygdala, thalamus, and medial temporal lobe (Raine et al., 1997). In a subsequent analysis, some subjects were classified as predatory murderers ($n = 15$) and others as affective murderers ($n = 9$) (Raine et al., 1998). Paralleling studies of predatory versus affective aggression in cats, functional differences were seen: affective murderers, relative to comparisons, had lower left and right prefrontal functioning, higher right hemisphere subcortical functioning, and lower right hemisphere prefrontal/subcortical ratios. In contrast, predatory murderers had prefrontal functioning more equivalent to that of comparisons, while also having high right subcortical activity. These results support the hypothesis that emotional, unplanned impulsive murderers are less able to regulate and control aggressive impulses generated from subcortical structures because of deficient prefrontal regulation. The excessive subcortical activity associated with violence is consistent with other suggestions that neural overactivity can increase violence risk.

Recent functional studies examined emotional states salient to affective aggression. A PET study measured regional cerebral blood flow (rCBF) in eight men during anger simulation and found activation of the left orbitofrontal cortex, right anterior cingulate, and bilateral temporal poles (Dougherty et al., 1999). In another PET study, self-induced anxiety and anger in 16 adults were contrasted. Both emotions were associated with increased rCBF in the left inferior frontal and left temporal regions, and decreased rCBF in right posterior temporal/parietal and right superior frontal cortex, compared to PET findings during an emotionally neutral condition (Kimbrell et al., 1999). Anger was uniquely associated with increased rCBF in the right temporal pole and thalamus. A third study found rCBF reductions in the ventromedial prefrontal cortex of 15 volunteers during imagined aggressive behavior (Pietrini et al., 2000). This suggests a possible role for functional deactivation of the area during aggression.

Additional studies suggest relationships between diminished frontal lobe function and poorly modulated aggression. Using MRI, Raine et al., (2000) found an 11% reduction in the prefrontal gray matter volume in 21 subjects with ASP, compared to 34 healthy controls, 26 substance abusers, and 21 psychiatric controls. Thus, it appears that ASP with violent behavior is associated with reduced frontal lobe volume.

A magnetic resonance spectroscopy (MRS) study examined correlates of repetitive violence in 13 mildly mentally retarded individuals and 14 controls (Critchley et al., 2000). Concentrations and ratios of N-acetyl aspartate (NAA) and creatine phosphocreatine (Cr+PCr) were assayed. The NAA and CR+CR concentrations reflect neuronal density and high-energy phosphate metabolism, respectively. Violent patients had lower prefrontal concentrations of NAA and Cr+PCr and a lower NAA/Cr+PCr ratio in the amygdalohippocampal complex than that in controls. Within the violent group, prefrontal NAA concentration correlated with aggression frequency.

ELECTROPHYSIOLOGY

Animal Models

Both predatory and defensive types of aggression can be produced in the cat by stimulation of discrete brain areas (Siegel et al., 1999). "Quiet biting" attack behavior can be induced by electrical stimulation of the perifornical lateral hypothalmus. The behavior consists of "stalking" a prey object such as an anesthetized rat, followed by biting the back of the prey's neck, and looks remarkably like the predatory actions seen under natural conditions. In contrast, defensive rage (sham rage) has an affective appearance in cats that includes piloerection, arching of the back, retraction of the ears, pupil dilatation, vocalization, and unsheathing of the claws. Defensive rage or affective defense consists of threat postures, which may be followed by strikes upon provocation. The natural counterpart is seen when a mother cat perceives that another animal endangers her kittens. Two distinct neural circuits involving the hypothalmus and periaqueductal gray and which have been identified subserve the two different types of aggression. At the hypothalamic level, predatory attack sites are lateral to stimulation sites associated with defensive rage. At the level of the periaqueductal gray, defensive rage sites are dorsal to predatory attack sites.

Human Psychophysiology

The most common psychophysiologic measures recorded from antisocial populations have been EEG and event-related potentials (ERPs), heart rate (HR), and skin conductance (SC) (Scarpa and Raine, 1997).

Frequencies of EEG activity are beta (13–30 Hz), alpha (8–12 Hz), theta (4–8 Hz), and delta (0–4 Hz). Greater predominance of higher frequencies is thought to represent greater levels of cortical arousal. Adult psychopathy studies find three relatively consistent abnormalities: (1) generalized excess theta activity; (2) foci of 6–8/second, 14–16/second bilateral or right temporal activity; and (3) localized slow-wave activity in the temporal lobe (Dolan, 1994). The comparatively slower EEGs are consistent with underarousal theories of psychopathy. However, often the EEG studies include psychopaths or criminals, but may not represent aggression or violence. For example, two prospective studies by Volavka (1987), which tracked Scandinavian boys and followed up their criminal records, found relatively slower childhood EEG frequencies in those with repetitive theft, but did not mention a specific link to violence. However, a study of 372 male maximum-security mental hospital patients found more EEG abnormalities (slowing and/or sharp waves) in the temporal lobes of the most violent patients than in those of the least violent: 20% versus 2.4% (Wong et al., 1994). Overall rates of EEG abnormalities (meaning without regard to location) were higher (43%) in the most violent patients than in the least violent patients (24%–26%).

Event-related potentials are averaged changes of the brain's electrical activity in response to specific stimuli. Late, middle, and early components are believed to be associated with attention, cortical augmenting, and environmental filtering. Studies (of psychopathic subjects (Raine and Lencz, 1993), support three findings: (1) enhanced late-latency ERP P300 amplitudes to stimuli of interest, suggesting enhanced attention for stimulating events; (2) heightened middle-latency ERP amplitudes to stimuli of increasing intensity, consistent with sensation seeking; and (3) long early-latency brain stem average evoked responses, consistent with decreased arousal and excessive environmental filtering.

Heart rate reflects sympathetic and parasympathetic activity. The common view is that high HR is associated with anxiety, whereas low HR reflects underarousal. Fourteen studies of resting HR in young noninstitutionalized individuals reported consistently and significantly lower HR in antisocial groups (Raine and Lencz, 1993). Only three studies addressed violence. All reported that lower HRs were associated with aggression (Farrington 1987, Wadsworth 1976, Pitts 1993). A lone doctoral dissertation has examined aggression typology (reactive, proactive, and nonaggressive control boys) in relation to HR (Pitts, 1993) Only those with reactive aggression had increased HR in response to provocation, but both aggressive groups had a lower HR than controls. A caveat regarding the childhood results is that adult studies have not found criminals or psychopaths to have a lower HR.

Skin conductance represents changes in the electrical activity of skin. Resting skin conductance level (SCL) and the number of nonspecific fluctuations (spontaneous skin conductance responses [SCRs] seen in a resting state) are thought to reflect arousal. Skin conductance responses are also seen 1 to 3 seconds after stimulus onset, when they index the *orienting reflex*, which measures allocation of attention to the stimulus. Although SC arousal studies show some consistency, 4 out of 10 showed underarousal in antisocial-spectrum subjects; no specific links to violence are reported (Scarpa and Raine, 1997).

NEUROTRANSMITTERS AND NEUROMODULATORS

Because body fluids are remote from many relevant sites of neurotransmitter action and confounded by multiple events, it is all the more impressive when substantial consistency in results is seen.

Dopamine

All three major brain dopamine (DA) systems (nigrostriatal, mesocortical, and mesolimbic) have been implicated in aggression in animal studies (Miczek et al., 1994). Brain DA systems appear to be involved in (1) the rewarding or reinforcing aspects of aggression, possibly via mesolimbic and mesocortical DA systems; and (2) the initiation, execution, and termination of aggressive behavior patterns, possibly via the nigrostriatal and mesolimbic DA systems.

Low cerebrospinal fluid (CSF) concentrations of homovanillic acid, a dopamine metabolite, were associated with suicide attempts in two pediatric studies (Kruesi et al., 1992; L. Greenhill, personal communication).

Serotonin

In essentially all species of animals, including humans, serotonin is important in aggression (Kravitz, 2000). Relationships between CSF concentrations of a serotonin metabolite, 5-hydroxyindoleacetic acid (5-HIAA), and human aggression were described in Asberg et al.'s landmark study (1976), which showed a bimodal distribution among depressed patients. A meta-analysis of 27 studies, involving 1202 psychiatric patients, showed an association between attempted suicide and low levels of CSF 5-HIAA (Lester, 1995).

Consensus exists that low CSF 5-HIAA is associated with poorly modulated, socially unproductive, impulsive, and/or affect-laden types of aggression (Kruesi and Jacobsen, 1997). A significant inverse correlation between CSF 5-HIAA and a lifetime history of aggression was initially established in adults (Brown et al., 1979) and later in children and adolescents (Kruesi et al., 1990, 1992). Other investigations showed that it is impulsive/affective aggression, rather than more predatory aggression, that is linked with low CSF 5-HIAA (Linnoila et al., 1983; Virkkunen et al., 1994, 1995; Mehlman et al., 1994).

Following the initial CSF findings, other serotonergic methods have added to our knowledge of its role in aggression. Tryptophan, the essential amino acid precursor to serotonin, has been studied via depletion and augmentation and naturalistically. Depletion increased competitive and spontaneous aggression in non-human primates (Chamberlin et al., 1987) and laboratory aggression in human males (Bjork et al., 1999). In a within-subjects design in which seasonal variation in plasma L-tryptophan availability and relationships to violent suicide occurrence were investigated (Maes et al., 1995), 26 adults had monthly blood samplings drawn. Results showed that L-tryptophan and the L-tryptophan/competing amino acid ratio were significantly lower in the spring. The bimodal pattern of plasma L-tryptophan concentrations mirrored seasonal patterns for violent suicide.

Pharmacologic challenge studies provide additional evidence associating serotonin with aggression. In these studies, the prolactin response to the indirect serotonin agonist dl-fenfluramine has been used. Adult personality disorders have shown decreased prolactin responses, which correlate with impulsive aggression (Coccaro et al., 1989). Lower prolactin response is also associated with violence in ASP (O'Keane et al., 1992), as well as with suicide (Coccaro et al., 1989). A PET study of five borderline patients and eight controls, with and without fenfluramine, found diminished metabolism in the right orbital and medial prefrontal region of borderline subjects when challenged with fenfluramine (Soloff et al., 2000). This suggests a diminished response to serotonergic stimulation in a brain area implicated in impulsive aggression.

In contrast, pediatric challenge studies present a less consistent picture. One study of 25 boys with ADHD found that the aggressive subgroup had a significantly greater prolactin response (Halperin et al., 1994). However, another study found fenfluramine-induced prolactin release was not correlated with aggression in disruptive behavior disorder (DBD) and did not differ significantly between individuals with DBD and controls (Stoff et al., 1992). A study of 18 adolescent/early adult individuals with early-onset alcoholism found no significant difference in prolactin response to fenfluramine, compared to matched controls (Soloff et al., 2000). A study of 34 younger brothers of convicted delinquents found that increasing degrees of aggressive behavior were positively correlated with the prolactin response to fenfluramine challenge (Pine et al., 1997).

Testosterone and Sex Steroids

In most species, androgens appear to exert a significant influence on the form and degree of aggressive behavior (Rubinow and Schmidt, 1996). Steroid hormones are thought to play two distinct roles in modulating be-

havior: an organizational as well as an activational role. Gonadal steroids act around the time of birth in organizing which tissues will be steroid-responsive. Later in life, the hormone will activate behavioral patterns, such as mating behavior.

Body fluid findings have linked testosterone concentrations with aggression in humans. For example, higher CSF testosterone was associated with increased aggression among alcoholic offenders (Virkkunnen et al., 1994). Yet, aggression–testosterone relationships are not simply linear. Increasingly there is evidence that androgens modify or interact with neurotransmitters in modifying or modulating aggression. For example, the increased aggression evident in genetically altered neuronal nitrous oxide–negative male mice appears to be modulated by testosterone (Kriegsfeld et al., 1997). Castration reduced aggression in neuronal nitrous oxide–negative mice and wild-type mice to equally low levels. Testosterone replacement restored aggression to pre-castration levels, suggesting testosterone dependence.

GENETICS

Both genetic and environmental factors contribute to aggressive behavior. Genetic determinism has been replaced by more current research suggesting that the expression of a specific gene on the spectrum of aggressive behavior is dependent upon the interaction between genetic predisposition and environmental factors. Twin and adoption studies are useful to parse the proportions of variance attributable to environment and to genetics. The measure most frequently used to evaluate childhood and adolescent aggression in genetic studies is the Child Behavior Checklist (CBCL) (Achenbach and Edelbrock, 1983). Caveats about use and interpretation of the CBCL aggressive subscale for measurement of aggression include (1) only two items on the scale directly refer to physical aggressiveness, and (2) in a study of disruptive children, CBCL aggressive scale scores did not correlate significantly with severity of physical aggressiveness (Kruesi et al., 1994). This suggests caution when using the CBCL to discriminate among pathological forms of aggression. In contrast, the CBCL is well suited to epidemiological designs because of documented psychometric properties and population-based norms.

Most pediatric twin studies argue for significant genetic contributions to CBCL aggression. Ghodesian-Carpy and Baker (1987) studied aggression in 21 monozygotic and 17 dizygotic twin pairs. Twin correlations of 0.78 for monozygotic and 0.31 for dizygotic pairs were found on CBCL aggression. In the Oregon Twin Project's 151 pairs (Leve et al., 1998), correlations of 0.83 for monozygotic twins and 0.62 for dizygotic twins were found, using CBCL aggression. A study of 111 biologic and 221 nonbiologic sibling pairs found that genetics accounted for 90% of the variance in CBCL aggression (van den Oord et al., 1994).

In contrast, a study by Plomin et al. (1981) used hitting Bobo the clown as a measure of aggression in 54 monozygotic and 33 dizygotic pairs, and found that genetic variability does not play a great role in behavior. Data from adult twin studies support the heritability of aggressive behavior. In the largest twin sample ($n = 4997$ pairs) to measure violent behavior (Cloninger and Gottsman, 1987), court records of crimes were used. For monozygotic pairs who committed offenses against persons a correlation of 0.77, and for dizygotic pairs, 0.52. Monozygotic twins committing property offenses had a correlation of 0.67 and dizygotic twins, 0.29. Both the person and property crime data suggest genetic effects, accounting for 60% to 70% of the variance. These results have been consistent in later adult twin studies. McGue et al. (1993) examined 79 monozygotic and 48 dizygotic twin pairs, using the Multiple Personality Dimension Questionnaire aggression scale, and found that in 20-year-olds genetic variability accounted for 61% of the variance. When reassessed at age 30, genetic variability accounted for 38% of the variance. Thus, genetic influence on aggression decreased with age. This finding is in contrast to the general maxim that genetic expression increases with age. If replicated, the findings suggest that contributions of genetic and environmental variance may change over a person's life span.

Huesmann et al. (1984) suggest that the nature of aggressive behavior may change as a person ages. Measuring individual aggression both across generations and within individuals over time, they found that the highest stability coefficients were between the proband's level of aggression at age 8 and the proband's child's aggression when that child was 8 years old; this finding also suggests genetic mechanisms. To more fully explicate the genetic and environmental contribution and interaction, Cadoret et al. (1995) followed up an adoption sample ($n = 197$) whose biologic parents had been diagnosed as ASP or alcoholic according to prison or hospital records. Adverse adoptive home environments were assessed. Adoptees raised in an adverse adoptive environment and who had antisocial or alcoholic biologic parents were more likely to demonstrate aggressive behavior. These data suggest that interaction between environmental and genetic factors accounts for variation in childhood and adolescent aggression. Moreover, these findings are highly consistent with earlier findings by the same investigator (Cadoret et al., 1983).

Molecular genetics provides much evidence to support the hypothesis that aggression and violent behavior are heritable. In animal models, behaviors can be altered significantly by modifying specific neurotransmitter systems (Hen, 1996). The focus in such studies has been primarily on serotonin. Pucilowski and Kostowsk reported initial relevant studies in mice in 1983. Subsequent studies verified the role of serotonin and its relation to aggression (Vergnes et al., 1986; Molina et al., 1987). Data supported the suggestion that decreases in serotonin correlate strongly with increased aggression, and increased serotonin correlate with decrease aggression. Advances in molecular genetics have furthered these ideas with the development of the transgenic mouse line, in which specific genes can be induced, and the knockout model, in which specific genes can be turned off. Gene coding for 5-HT$_{1B}$ mediates aggressive behavior in mouse models (Saundou et al., 1994; Lucas and Hern, 1995). Another model uses the transgenetic mouse line lacking the gene for monamine oxidase A (MAOA) and MAOB enzyme. The MAOA knockout mouse line indicated a ninefold increase in brain serotonin and a twofold increase in norepinephrine. The MAOA knockout mouse also demonstrated a high degree of abnormal aggression in male mice, particularly high levels of aggression with high levels of brain serotonin. These findings were consistent with earlier reports on a large Dutch family with a specific mutation in the *MAOA* gene that appeared to correlate with the behavioral phenotype indicating inability to control impulsive aggression (Brunner et al., 1993). A subsequent study of 52 Danish men and women indicated a significant positive correlation in aggression with both CSF serotonin levels and the serotonin precursor tryptophan (Moller et al, 1996).

Although serotonin remains a central figure, other systems have also been recently implicated using gene knockout models. Chen et al. (1994) produced transgenetic mice deficient for the gene encoding for α-calcium-calmodulin-dependent kinase II (CaMK II). This mouse line had an abnormally low fear response and increased aggression. CaMK II facilitates presynaptic neurotransmitter release and CAMK II–mediated phosphorylation is required for activation of tryptophan hydroxylase, the rate-limiting enzyme in serotonin biosynthesis.

Evidence of a behavioral role for central neuronal nitric oxide synthetase has been reported. A knockout mouse deficient in the gene encoding for this enzyme had a significant increase in aggression, as well as excessive inappropriate sexual behavior (Nelson et al., 1995).

ENVIRONMENTAL INFLUENCES

Environmental events or stimuli are often necessary ingredients for aggression or violence, as seen in the animal models described in Table 17.2. The introduction of an intruder near a mother cat's litter will provoke certain aggressive responses. This environmental influence on aggression has a relatively short time frame and is readily apparent. However, other environmental influences may be less obvious. Weather conditions have long been thought to be linked to violence and evidence suggests possible mechanisms. A within-subjects design found 12% to 14% of the variance in L-tryptophan availability could be explained by the composite effects of present and past atmospheric factors; higher ambient temperature and relative humidity with lower air pressure are the most important predictors of low L-tryptophan availability (Maes et al., 1995). This suggests that weather conditions influence serotonergic status. Firearm availability, an environmental variable, increases the likelihood of adolescent homicide or suicide and is the rationale for restricting access to lethal means as a prevention strategy (Kruesi et al., 1999).

Evidence that social experience modifies aggression risk is growing. A seminal study by Widom (1989) found that exposure to violence, as in abuse or neglect, increases a child's subsequent risk for violence. Based upon epidemiological data, some have argued that television exposure early in life, particularly during infancy, may increase violence risk later in life (Centerwall, 1992). Biologic factors and environmental circumstances, such as rearing, interact in altering risk of violence. A study of 4269 males in Denmark found that birth complications interacted with early maternal rejection in predisposing individuals to violence as young adults (Raine et al., 1997).

Animal models make a case that previous social experience alters the propensity for subsequent aggression and the biology that underlies that aggression. A clever study by Raleigh et al. (1983, 1991) on the effects of pharmacologic manipulation of serotonin upon dominance in non-human primates suggests that relationships between serotonin and behavior are modifiable with a combination of social and pharmacologic maneuvers. A monkey's stature in a dominance hierarchy may determine whether the monkey is the exhibitor or recipient of aggression. In the Raleigh study, 36 adult male monkeys were housed in 12 social groups, containing 3 adult males, at least 3 adult females, and immature offspring. After the dominant males were removed from each social group, for the next 4 weeks, one of the remaining subordinate males in each group received tryptophan and fluoxetine to increase serotonin, or they received fenfluramine or cyproheptadine to decrease serotonin. Increasing serotonergic activity facilitated the acquisition of dominance in males. Once the treated subjects became dominant, they *also remained so* during the entire experiment. Treatment with fenfluramine or cyproheptadine, however, decreased the likelihood of becoming dominant. Behavioral changes exhibited by tryptophan/fluoxetine-treated subjects paralleled those shown by animals that acquired dominance in drug-free conditions. However, the pharmacologic effects were apparently mediated by the males' relationship to females in the group. Raleigh et al. (1991) concluded that serotonergic systems may promote the acquisition of male dominance in unstable social conditions.

Recent study of crayfish indicates that the modulatory effect of serotonin on dominance aggression behavior depends on social experience (Yeh et al., 1996). Serotonin injected into the circulatory system causes crayfish to assume a dominant posture. When a pair of previously isolated crayfish are placed together, the pair will agonistically interact to determine which crayfish is dominant. After the agonistic interaction, the subordinate moves by retreating or tail-flipping to avoid contact with the dominant animal. The effect of serotonin on the neural circuit for tail-flip behavior was found to depend on the animal's social experience. Serotonin persistently enhanced the response to sensory stimuli of the lateral giant tail-flip command neuron in socially isolated crayfish, reversibly inhibited it in subordinate animals, and reversibly enhanced it in socially dominant crayfish. Serotonin receptor agonists had opposing effects: m-CPP, a 5-HT-1 agonist, had no effect on the lateral giant neuron's responses in social isolates but it reduced excitatory postsynaptic evoked potentials in both dominant and subordinate crayfish. In contrast, a 5-HT-2 agonist produced similar electrophysiologic changes in isolates, dominants, and subordinates. Yeh et al. (1996) demonstrated that the modulatory effect of serotonin can depend on not only the crayfish's current social status but also its *prior* status. Provocative as these findings are in arguing for social experience as a modulator of serotonergic neural plasticity relevant to aggressive behavior, they must be viewed with some caution. The serotonergic receptors in the stomatogastric nervous system of crustaceans differ from vertebrate types (Zhang and Harris-

Warrick, 1994). And, perhaps more importantly, the aggression involved in sorting "pecking-order" conflicts among conspecifics is not equivalent to violence.

CONCLUSIONS AND IMPLICATIONS

Persons with psychiatric disorders, particularly ASP/conduct disorder or schizophrenia, are at increased risk for aggression. The aggression found in psychiatric or forensic samples often includes a spectrum ranging from affective to predatory, with many individuals showing both types (Vitiello et al., 1990; Barrat et al., 1999). Recent critics of predatory–affective dichotomies suggest that knowledge structure models of aggression can better handle the complex multiple motives seen in much human aggression (Bushman and Anderson, 2001). Relationships between knowledge structure models of aggression and neurobiology are, as yet, unexplored.

In terms of anatomy, orbital frontal regions are most consistently implicated in aggression modulation. Less attention has been directed to temporal regions, but there are intimations of involvement. Thus far, serotonin is more consistently implicated in aggression modulation than any other neurotransmitter. Electrophysiologic studies suggest that excess activity, whether seizure-like focus or increased HR following provocation, may relate to poorly modulated reactive/affective aggression rather than more predatory violence, whereas underarousal is linked more to criminal behavior that may be viewed as predatory. Evidence hints at a relatively early postnatal developmental influence upon aggression and that neurobiologic relationships with aggression may change across a person's life span.

Current pediatric psychopharmacologic practice does not integrate well with most current foci in neurobiologic research. Neuroleptics are often thought of in terms of dopamine and serotonin receptors. Yet, our scientific understanding of the relevance of dopamine receptors to human violence is meager. The relevance of physiologic overactivity to aggression raises intriguing (and unanswered) questions about the clinical use of α-agonists.

Environmental stimuli and context are relevant to the occurrence of aggression. The interaction between environment and genetic risk factors may offer new opportunities for intervention. For example, individuals with family histories of suicide are at increased risk for suicide. However, even individuals with low levels of 5-HIAA generally do not make daily or even monthly attempts—so what is it that relates to an attempt happening on one day and not another? Maes et al. (1995)

would argue that environmentally mediated tryptophan availability plays a role in this timing. Are there atmospheric conditions in which those at risk should have a brief pharmacologic boost? Will there be a place for medication delivery systems with barometric tryptophan availability feedback loops? We still have much to learn in this area.

REFERENCES

Achenbach, T.M. and Edelbrock, C.S. (1983) *Manual for the Child Behavior Checklist and Revised Child Behavior Profile.* Burlington, VT: Department of Psychiatry, University of Vermont.

Amen, D., Stubblefield, M., Carmichael, B., and Thisted, R. (1996) Brain SPECT findings and aggression. *Ann Clin Psychiatry* 8:129–137.

American Psychiatric Association (1994) *Diagnostic Statistical Manual of Mental Disorders, 4th ed.* Washington, DC:American Psychiatric Association Press.

Anderson, S.W., Bechara, A., Damasio, H., Tranel, D., and Damasio, A.R. (1999) Impairment of social and moral behavior related to early damage in human prefrontal cortex. *Nat Neurosci* 2:1032–1037.

Apter, A., Gothelf, D., Orbach, I., Weizman, R., Ratzoni, G., Har-Even, D., and Tgano, S. (1995) Correlation of suicidal and violent behavior in different diagnosis categories in hospitalized adolescent patients. *J Am Acad Child Adolesc Psychiatry* 34:912–918.

Asberg, M., Traskman, L., and Thoren, P. (1976) 5-HIAA in the cerebrospinal fluid. A biochemical suicide predictor? *Arch Gen Psychiatry* 33:1193–1197.

Barratt, E.S., Stanford, M.S., Dowdy, L., Liebman, M.J., and Kent, T.A. (1999) Impulsive and premeditated aggression: a factor analysis of self-reported acts. *Psychiatry Res* 86:163–173.

Bear, D.M. and Fedio, P. (1977) Quantitative analysis of interictal behavior in temporal lobe epilepsy. *Arch Neurol* 34:454–467.

Bjork, J.M., Dougherty, D.M., Moeller, F.G., Cherek, D.R., and Swann, A.C. (1999) The effects of tryptophan depletion and loading on laboratory aggression in men: time course and a food-restricted control. *Psychopharmacology* 142:24–30.

Brain, P.F. (1984) Comments on laboratory-based "aggression" tests. *Anim Behav* 32:1256–1257.

Brennan. P., Mednick, S., and Hodgins, S. (2000) Major mental disorders and criminal violence in a danish birth cohort. *Arch Gen Psychiatry* 57:494–500.

Brown, G.L., Goodwin, F.K., Ballenger, J.C., Goyer, P.F., and Major, L.F. (1979) Aggression in humans correlates with cerebrospinal fluid amine metabolites. *Psychiatry Res* 1:131–139.

Brunner, H.G., Nelen, M., Breakefield, X.O., Roper, H.H., and van Oost, H.A. (1993) Abnormal behavior associated with a point mutation in the structural gene for monoamine oxidase A. *Science* 262(5133):578–580.

Bushman, B.J., and Anderson, C.A. (2001) Is it time to pull the plug on the hostile versus instrumental aggression dichotomy? *Psychol Rev* 108:273–279.

Cadoret, R.J., Cain, C.A., and Crowe, R.R. (1983) Evidence for gene–environment interaction in development of adolescent antisocial behavior. *Behav Genet* 13:301–310.

Cadoret, R.J., Yates, W.R., Troughton, E., Woodworth, G., and Stewart, M.A.(1995) Genetic–environmental interaction in the genesis of aggressivity and conduct disorders. *Arch Gen Psychiatry* 52:916–924.

Centerwall, B.S. (1992) Television and violence. The scale of the problem and where to go from here. *JAMA* 267:3059–3063.

Chamberlain, B., Ervin, F.R., Pihl, R.L., and Young, S.N. (1987) The effect of raising or lowering tryptophan levels on aggression in vervet monkeys. *Pharmacol Biochem Behav* 18:503–510.

Chen, C., Rainvie, D.G., Greene, R.W., and Tonegawa, S. (1994) Abnormal fear response and aggressive behavior in mutant mice deficient for calcium-calmodulin kinase: II. *Science* 266:291.

Cloninger, C.R. and Gottesman, I.I. (1987) Genetic and environmental factors in antisocial behavior disorders. In: Mednick, S.A., Moffitt, T.E., and Stark, S.A., eds. *The Causes of Crime: New Biological Approaches.* New York: Cambridge University Press, pp. 92–109.

Coccaro, E.F., Siever, L.J., Klar, H.M. Maurer, G., Cochrane, K. Cooper, T.H., Mohs, R.C., and Davis, K.L. (1989) Serotonergic studies in affective and personality disorder patients: correlations with behavioral aggression and impulsivity. *Arch Gen Psychiatry* 46:587–599.

Conner, D. and Steingard, R.J. (1996) A clinical approach to the pharmacotherapy of aggression in children and adolescents. *Ann NY Acad Sci* 794:290–307.

Critchley, H.D., Simmons, A., Daly, E.M., Russell, A., van Amelsvoort, T., Robertson, D.M., Glover, A., and Murphy, D.G.M. (2000) Prefrontal and medial temporal correlates of repetitive violence to self and others. *Biol Psychiatry* 47:928–934.

Damasio, A.R. (2000) A neural basis for sociopathy. *Arch Gen Psychiatry* 57:118–135.

Damasio, H, Grabowski, T., Frank, R., Galaburda, A.M., and Damasio, A.R. (1994) The return of Phineas Gage: clues about the brain from a skull of a patient. *Science* 264:1102–1105.

Davidson, R.J., Putnam, K.M., and Larson, C.L. (2000) Dysfunction in the neural circuitry of emotion regulation—a possible prelude to violence. *Science* 289(5479):591–594.

Dodge, K.A. and Coie, J.D. (1987) Social information processing factors in reactive and proactive aggression in children's peer groups. *J Pers Soc Psychol* 53:1146–1158.

Dolan, M.(1994) Psychopathy—a neurobiological perspective. *Br J Psychiatry* 165:151–159.

Dougherty, D.D., Shin, L.M., Alpert, N.M., Pitman, R.K., Orr, S.P., Lasko, M., Macklin, M.L., Fischman, A.J., and Rauch, S.L. (1999) Anger in health men: a PET study using script-driven imagery. *Biol Psychiatry* 46:466–472.

Edmunds, G. and Kendrick, D.C. (1980) *The Measurement of Human Aggressiveness.* Chichester, UK: Ellis Horwood.

Enserink, M. (2000) Searching for the mark of Cain. *Science* 289:575–579.

Eronen, M., Hakola, P., and Tiihonen, H.J. (1996) Mental disorders and homicidal behavior in Finland. *Arch Gen Psychiatry* 53:497–501.

Farrington, D.P. (1987) Implications of biological findings for criminological research. In: Mednisk, S.A., Moffitt, T.E., Stack, S.A., eds. *The Causes of Crime: New Biological Approaches.* New York, Cambridge University Press, pp. 42–64.

Gabel, S. and Shindledecker, R. (1991) Aggressive behavior in youth: characteristics, outcomes and psychiatric diagnosis. *J Am Acad Child Adolesc Psychiatry* 30:982–988.

Geschwind, N. (1973) Effects of temporal-lobe surgery on behavior. *N Engl J Med* 289:480–481.

Ghodesian-Carpey, J. and Baker, L.A. (1987) Genetic and environmental influences on aggression in 4- to 7-year-old twins. *Aggressive Behav* 13:173.

Graffman, J., Schwab, K. Warden, D., Pridgen, A., Brown, H.R., and Salazar, A.M. (1996) Frontal lob injuries, violence and aggression: a report of the Vietnam Head Injury Study. *Neurology* 46:1231–1238.

Griffin, J.C., Williams, D.E., Stark, M.T., Altmeyer, H.K., and Mason, M. (1986) Self-injurious behavior: a state-wide prevalence survey of the extent and circumstances. *Appl Res Ment Retard* 7:105–16.

Halperin, J.M., Sharma, V., Siever, L.J., Schwartz, S.T., Matier, K., Wornell, G., and Newcorn, J.H. (1994) Serotonergic function in aggressive and nonaggressive boys with attention deficity hyperactivity disorder. *Am J Psychiatry* 151:243–248.

Hen, R. (1996) Mean genes. *Neuron* 16:17–21.

Hess, W.R. and Brugger, M. (1943) Das subkortikale Zentrum der affektiven Abwehrreaktion. *Hel Physiol Pharmcol Acta* 1:33–52.

Hodgins, S., Mednick, S., Brennan, P., Schulsinger, F., and Engberg, M. (1996) Mental disorder and crime. *Arch Gen Psychiatry* 53:489–496.

Huesmann, L.R., Eron, L.D., Lefkowitz, M.M., and Walder, L.ú(1984) Stability of aggression over time and generations. *Dev Psychol* 20:1120–1134.

Johnson, C.J., Carter, A.P., Harlin, V.K., and Zoller, G. (1974) Student injuries due to aggressive behavior in the Seattle Public School during the school year 1969–1970. *Am J Public Health* 64:904–906.

Jordan, K., Schlengerm, W., Fairbank, J., and Caddell, J. (1996) Prevalence of psychiatric disorders among incarcerated women. *Arch Gen Psychiatry* 53:513–519.

Kay, S.R., Wolkenfeld, F., and Murril, L.M. (1988) Profiles of aggression among psychiatric patients II. Nature and prevalence. *J Nerv Ment Dis* 176:539–546.

Kazdin, A. (1987) Treatment of antisocial behaviors in children: current status and future directions. *Psychol Bull* 102:187–203.

Kimbrell, T.A., George, M.S., Parekh, P.I., Ketter, T.A., Podell, D.M., Danielson, A.L., Repella, J.D., Benson, B.E., Willis, M.W., Herscovitch, P., and Post, R.M. (1999) Regional brain activity during transient self-induced anxiety and anger in healthy adults. *Biol Psychiatry* 46:454–465.

Krakowski, M., Volavka, J., and Brizer, D. (1986) Psychopathology and violence: a review of the literature. *Compr Psychiatry* 27:131–146.

Kravitz, E.A. (2000) Serotonin and aggression: insights gained from a lobster model system and speculations on the role of amine neurons in a complex behavior. *J Comp Physiol* A 186:221–238.

Kriegsfeld, L.J., Dawson, T.M., Dawson, V.L., Nelson, R.J. and Snyder, S.H. (1997) Aggressive behavior in male mice lacking the gene for neuronalnitric oxide synthase requires testosterone. *Brain Research* 769:66–70.

Kruesi, M.J., Grossman, J., Pennington, J.M., Woodward, P.J., Duda, D., and Hirsch, J.G. (1999) Suicide and violence prevention: parent education in the emergency department. *J Am Acad Child Adolesc Psychiatry* 38:250–255.

Kruesi, M.J.P., Hibbs, E.D., Hamburger, S.D., Rapoport, J.L., Keysor, C.S., and Elia, J. (1994) Measurement of aggression in children with disruptive behavior disorders. *J Offender Rehab* 21:159–172.

Kruesi, M.J.P., Hibbs, E.D., Zahn, T.P., Keysor, C.S., Hamburger, S.D., Bartko, J.J., and Rapoport, J.L. (1992) A 2-year prospective follow-up study of children and adolescents with disruptive behavior disorders: prediction by cerebrospinal fluid 5-hydroxyindoleacetic acid, homovanillic acid, and autonomic measures. *Arch Gen Psychiatry* 49:429–435.

Kruesi, M.J.P. and Jacobsen, T. (1997) Serotonin and human violence: do environmental mediators exist? In: Raine, A., Farrington, D., Brennan, P., and Mednick, S.A., eds. *Biosocial Bases of Violence.* New York: Plenum Publishing, pp. 189–205.

Kruesi, M.J.P., Rapoport, J.L., Hamburger, S., Hibbs, E., Potter, W.Z., Lenane, M., and Brown, G.L. (1990). Cerebrospinal fluid monoamine metabolites, aggression, and impulsivity in disruptive behavior disorders of children and adolescents. *Arch Gen Psychiatry* 47:419–426.

Kruk, M.R. (1991) Ethology and pharmacology of hypothalamic aggression in the rat. *Neurosci Biobehav Rev* 15:527–538.

LaPierre, D., Braun, C.M.J., and Hodgins, S. (1995) Ventral front deficits in psychopathy: neuropsychological test findings. *Neuropsychologia* 131:39–151

Lester, D. (1995) The concentration of neurotransmitter metabolites in the cerebrospinal fluid of suicidal individuals: a meta-analysis. *Pharmacopsychiatry* 28(2):45–50.

Leve, L.D., Winebarger, A.A., Fagot, B.I., Reid, J.B., and Goldsmith, H.H. (1998) Environmental and genetic variance in children's observed and reported maladaptive behavior. *Child Dev* 69(5): 1286–98.

Linnoila, M., Virkkunen, M., Scheinin, M., Nuutila, A., Riman, R., and Goodwin, F.K. (1983) Low cerebrospinal fluid 5-hydroxyindoleacetic acid concentration differentiates impulsive from nonimpulsive violent behavior. *Life Sci* 33:2609–2614.

Lucas, J.J. and Hern, R. (1995) New players in the 5-HT receptor field: genes and knockouts. *Trends Pharmacol Sci* 16:246–252.

Maes, M., Scharpe, S., Verkerk, R., D'Hondt, P., Peeters, D., Cosyns, P., Thompson, P., De Meyer, F., Wauters, A., and Neels, H. (1995) Seasonal variation in plasma L-tryptophan availability in healthy volunteers. *Arch Gen Psychiatry* 52:937–946.

McGue, M., Bacon, S., and Lykken, D.T. (1993) Personality stability and change in early adulthood: a behavioral genetic analysis. *Dev Psychol* 29:96.

Mehlman, P.T., Higley, J.K., Faucher, I., Lilly, A.A., Taub, D.M., Vickers, J., Suomi, S.J., and Linnoila, M. (1994) Low CSF 5-HIAA concentrations and severe aggression and impaired impulse control in nonhuman primates. *Am J Psychiatry* 151:1485–1491.

Miczek, K., Haney, M., Tidey, J., Vivian, J., and Weerts, E. (1994) Neurochemistry and pharmacotherapeutic management of Aggression and violence. In: Reiss, A.J., Miczek, K.A. and Roth and J.A., eds. *Understanding and Preventing Violence, Vol. 2.* Washington, DC: National Academy Press, pp. 245–514.

Mirsky, A.F. and Siegel, A. (1994) The neurobiology of violence and aggression. In: Reiss, A.J., Miczek, K.A., and Roth, J.A., eds. *Understanding and Preventing Violence, Vol. 2.* Washington, DC: National Academy Press, pp. 59–111.

Molina, V., Ciesielski, L., Gobaiile, S., Isel, F., and Mandel, P. (1987) Inhibition of mouse killing behavior by serotonin-mimetic drugs: effects of partial alterations of serotonin neurotransmission. *Pharmcol Biochem Behav* 27:123–131.

Moller, S.E., Mortensen, E.L., Breum, L., Alling, C., Larsen, O.G., Boge-Rasmussen, T., Jensen, C., and Bennicke, K. (1996) Aggression and personality: association with amino acids and monoamine metabolites. *Psychol Med* 26:323–331.

Moyer, K.E. (1968) Kinds of aggression and their physiological basis. *Communication Behav Bio* 2:65–87.

Nelson, R.J., Demas, G.E., Huang, P.L., Fishman, M.C., Dawson, V.L., Dawson, T.M., and Snyder, S.H. (1995) Behavioral abnormalities in male mice lacking neuronal nitric oxide synthase. *Nature* 378(6555):383–386.

O'Keane, V., Moloney, E., O'Neill, H., O'Connor, A., Smith, C., and Dinan, T.G. (1992) Blunched prolactin responses to d-fenfluramine in sociopathy: evidence for subsensitivity of central serotonergic function. *Br J Psychiatry* 160:643–646.

Peterson, B.F. (1995) Neuroimaging in child and adolescent neuropsychiatric disorders. *J Am Acad Child Adolesc Psychiatry* 34: 1650–1676.

Pietrini, P., Guazzelli, M. Basso, G., Jaffe, K., and Grafman, J. (2000) Neural correlates of imaginal aggressive behavior assessed by positron emission tomography in health subjects. *Am J of Psychiatry* 157:1772–1781

Pine, D.S., Coplan, J.D., Wasserman, G.A., Miller, L.S., Fried, J.E., Davies, M., Cooper, T.B., Greenhill, L., Shaffer, D., and Parsons, B. (1997) Neuroendocrine response to fenfluramine challenge in boys. Associations with aggressive behavior and adverse rearing. *Arch Gen Psychiatry* 54:839–846.

Pitts, T.B. (1993) Cognitive and psychophysiological differences in proactive and reactive aggressive boys [doctoral dissertation]. Department of Psychology, University of Southern California, Los Angeles.

Plomin, R., Foch, T.T., and Rowe, D.C. (1981) Bobo clown aggression in childhood: environment not genes. *J Res Pers* 15:331.

Pucilowski, O. and Kostowski, W. (1983) Aggressive behavior and the central serotonergic system. *Brain Res* 9:33–48.

Raine, A., Buchsbaum, M., and LaCasse, L. (1997) Brain abnormalities in murderers indicated by positron emission tomography. *Biol Psychiatry* 42:495–508.

Raine, A. and Lencz, T. (1993) Brain imaging research on electrodermal activity in humans. In: Roy, J.C. and Boucsein, W., ed., et al. *Progress in Electrodermal Research. NATO ASI Series: Series A: Life Sciences, Vol. 249.* New York: Plenum Press, pp. 115–135.

Raine, A., Lencz, T., Bihrle, S., LaCasse, L., and Colletti, P. (2000) Reduced prefrontal gray matter volume and reduced autonomic activity in antisocial personality disorder. *Arch. Gen Psychiatry* 57:119–127.

Raine, A., Meloy, J.R., Bihrle, S., Stoddard, J., LaCasse, L., and Buchsbaum, M.S. (1998) Reduced prefrontal and increased subcortical brain functioning assessed using positron emission tomography in predatory and affective murderers. *Behav Sci Law* 16:319–332.

Raleigh, M.J., Brammer, G.L., and McGuire, M.T. (1983) Male dominance, serotonergic systems, and the behavioral and physiological effects of drugs in vervet monkeys (*cercopithecus aethiops sabaeus*). In: Miczek, K., ed. *Ethopharmacology: Primate Models of Neuropsychiatric Disorders.* New York: Alan R. Liss, pp. – .

Raleigh, M.J., McGuire, M.T., Brammer, G.L., Pollack, D.B., and Yuwiler, A. (1991) Serotonergic mechanisms promote dominance acquisition in adult male vervet monkey. *Brain Res* 559:181–190.

Rubinow, D.R. and Schmidt, P.J. (1996) Androgens, brain and behavior. *Am J Psychiatry* 153:974–984.

Russell, A. (1994) The clinical presentation of childhood onset schizophrenia. *Schizophr Bull* 20:631–646.

Saudou, F., Amara, D., Dierick, A., LeMeur, M., Ramboz, S., Segu, L., Buhot, M.C., and Hen, R. (1994) Enhanced aggressive behavior in mice lacking 5-HT1B receptor. *Science* 265(5180): 1875–1878.

Scarpa, A. and Raine, A. (1997) Psychophysiology of anger and violent behavior. *Psychiatr Clin North Am* 20:375–394.

Siegel, A., Roeling, T.A.P., Gregg, T.R., and Kruk, M.R. (1999) Neuropharmacology of brain-stimulation-evoked aggression. *Neurosci Biobehav Rev* 23:359–389.

Soderstrom, H., Tullberg, M., Wikkelso, C., Ekholm, S., and Forsman, A. (2000) Reduced regional cerebral blood flow in nonpsychotic violent offenders. *Psychiatry Res Neuroimaging* 98:29–41.

Soloff, P.H., Meltzer, C.C., Greer, P.J., Constantine, D., and Kelly, T.M. (2000) A fenfluramine-activated FDG-PET study of borderline personality disorder. *Biol Psychiatry* 47:540–547.

Spenser E. and Campbell, M. (1994) Children with schizophrenia: diagnosis, phenomenology, and pharmocotherapy. *Schizophr Bull* 20:713–725.

Stoff, D.M., Pasatiempo, A.P., Yeung, J., Cooper, T.B., Bridger, W.H., and Rabinovich, H. (1992) Neuroendocrine responses to challenge with dl-fenfluramine and aggression in disruptive behavior disorders of children and adolescents. *Psychiatry Res* 43:263–276.

Teplin, L. (1994) Psychiatric and substance abuse disorders among male urban jail detainees. *Am J Public Health* 84:290–293.

Teplin, L., Abram, K., and McClelland, G. (1996) Prevalence of psychiatric disorders among incarcerated women pretrail jail detainees. *Arch Gen Psychiatry* 53:505–512.

van den Oord, E.J.C.G., Boomsma, D.I., and Verhulst, F.C. (1994) A study of problem behaviors in 10- to 15-year-old biologically related and unrelated international adoptees. *Behav Genet* 24: 193–205.

Vergnes, M., Depaulis, A., and Boehrer, A. (1986) Parachlorophenyl-alanine-induced serotonin depletion increases offensive but not defensive aggression in male rats. *Physiol Behav* 36:653.

Virkkunen, M., Goldman, D., Nielsen, D.A., and Linnoila, M. (1995) Low brain serotonin turnover rate (low CSF 5-HIAA) and impulsive violence. *J Psychiatry Neurosci* 20:271–275.

Virkkunen, M., Rawlings, R., Tokola, R., Poland, R.E., Guidotti, A., Nemeroff, C., Bissette, G. Kalogeras, K., Karonen, S.L., and Linnoila, M. (1994) CSF biochemistries, glucose metabolism and diurnal activity rhythms in alcoholic, violent offenders, fire setters, and health volunteers. *Arch Gen Psychiatry* 51:20–27.

Vitiello, B., Behar, D., Hunt, J., Stoff, D., and Ricciuti, A. (1990) Subtyping aggression in children and adolescents. *J Neuropsychiatry Clin Neurosci* 2:189–192.

Vivona, J., Ecker, B., Haligin, R., Cates, D., Garrison, W., and Friedman, M. (1995) Self and other directed aggression in child and adolescent psychiatric inpatients. *J Am Acad Child Adolesc Psychiatry* 34:434–444.

Volavka, J. (1987) Electroencephalogram among criminals. In: Mednick, S.A., Moffitt, E.E., Stack, S.A., eds. *Causes of Crime.* Cambridge, UK: Cambridge University Press, pp. 137–145.

Volkow, N.D. and Trancredi, L. (1987) Neural substrates of violent behavior: a preliminary study with positron emission tomography. *Br J Psychiatry* 151:668–673.

Volkow, N.D., Trancredi, L., Grant, C., Gillespie, H., Valentine, A., Mullani, N., Wange, G.J., and Hollister L. (1995) Brain glucose metabolism in violent psychiatric patients: a preliminary study. 61:243–253.

Wadsworth, M.E.J. (1976) Delinquency,pulse rate and early emotional deprivation. *Br J Criminology* 16:245–256.

Widom, C.S. (1989) The cycle of violence. *Science* 244(4901):160–166.

Woermann, F.G., van Elst, L.T., Koepp, M.J., Free, S.L., Thompson, P.J., Trimble, M.R., and Duncan, J.S. (2000) Reduction of frontal neocortical grey matter associated with affective aggression in patients with temporal lobe epilepsy: an objective voxel by voxel analysis of automatically segmented MRI. *J Neurol Neurosurg Psychiatry* 68:162–169.

Wong, M.T.H., Lumsden, J., Fenton, G.W., and Fenwick, P.B.C. (1994) Electroencephalography, computer tomography and violence rating of male patients in a maximum-security mental hospital. *Acta Psychiatr Scand* 90:97–101.

Yeh, S., Fricke, R.A., and Edwards, D.H. (1996) The effect of social experience on serotonergic modulation of the escape circuit of crayfish. *Science* 271:366–369.

Zhang, B. and Harris-Warrick, R.M. (1994) Multiple receptors mediate the modulatory effects of serotonergic neurons in a small neural network. *J Exp Biol* 190:55–77.

Zimet, S., Farley, G., and Zimet, G. (1994a) Home behaviors of children in three settings: an outpatient clinic, a day hospital and an inpatient hospital. *J Am Acad Child Adolesc Psychiatry* 33: 56–59.

Zimet, S., Fraley, G., and Zimet, G. (1994b) The school behaviors of children in three psychiatric settings: an outpatient clinic, a day hospital, and an inpatient hospital. *Child Psychiatry Hum Dev* 24:265–274.

18 | Neurobiology of eating disorders

WALTER KAYE, MICHAEL STROBER, AND KELLY L. KLUMP

Anorexia nervosa (AN) and bulimia nervosa (BN) are disorders characterized by aberrant patterns of feeding behavior and weight regulation, and disturbances in attitudes and perceptions toward body weight and shape. In AN, there is an inexplicable fear of weight gain and unrelenting obsession with fatness even in the face of increasing cachexia. Bulimia nervosa usually emerges after a period of dieting, which may or may not have been associated with weight loss. Binge eating is followed by either self-induced vomiting or some other means of compensation for the excess of food ingested. Most people with BN have irregular feeding patterns and satiety may be impaired. Although abnormally low body weight is an exclusion for the diagnosis of BN, some 25% to 30% of bulimics presenting to treatment centers have a prior history of AN; however, all bulimics have pathological concern with weight and shape. Common to individuals with AN or BN are low self-esteem, depression, and anxiety.

In certain respects, both diagnostic labels are misleading. Individuals affected with AN rarely have complete suppression of appetite, but rather exhibit a volitional, and more often than not, ego syntonic resistance to feeding drives while eventually becoming preoccupied with food and eating rituals to the point of obsession. Similarly, BN may not be associated with a primary, pathological drive to overeat; rather, like individuals with AN, bulimics have a seemingly relentless drive to restrain their food intake, an extreme fear of weight gain, and often have a distorted view of their actual body shape. Loss of control with overeating usually occurs intermittently and typically only some time after the onset of dieting behavior. Episodes of binge eating ultimately develop in a significant proportion of people with AN (Halmi et al., 1991), and some 5% of those with BN will eventually develop AN. Because restrained eating behavior and dysfunctional cognitions relating weight and shape to self-concept are shared by patients with both of these syndromes, and transitions between syndromes occur in many, it has been argued that AN and BN share at least some risk and liability factors in common.

The etiology of AN and BN is presumed to be complex and multiply influenced by developmental, social, and biological processes (Treasure and Campbell, 1994). However, the exact nature of these interactive processes remains incompletely understood. Certainly, cultural attitudes toward standards of physical attractiveness have relevance to the psychopathology of eating disorders, but it is unlikely that cultural influences in pathogenesis are very prominent. First, dieting behavior and the drive toward thinness are quite commonplace in industrialized countries throughout the world, yet AN and BN affect only an estimated 0.3% to 0.7% and 1.7% to 2.5%, respectively, of females in the general population. Moreover, numerous clear descriptions of AN date from the middle of the nineteenth century (Treasure and Campbell, 1994), suggesting that factors other than our current culture play an etiologic role. Secondly, these syndromes, particularly AN, have a relatively stereotypic clinical presentation, sex distribution (90 to 95% female), and age of onset, supporting the possibility of some biologic vulnerability.

This chapter begins with a brief overview of the phenomenology of AN and BN and then summarizes current knowledge of genetic and neurobiological risk and vulnerability factors in the development of AN and BN.

CLINICAL PHENOMENOLOGY

Variations in feeding behavior have been used to subdivide individuals with AN into two meaningful diagnostic subgroups that have been shown to differ in other psychopathological characteristics (Garner et al., 1985). In the *restrictor subtype*, subnormal body weight and an ongoing malnourished state are maintained by unremitting food avoidance; in the *bulimic* subtype of AN, there is comparable weight loss and malnutrition, yet the course of illness is marked by supervening episodes of binge eating, usually followed by some type of compensatory action such as self-induced vomiting or laxative abuse. Individuals with the bulimic subtype of AN are also more likely to exhibit histories of behavioral dyscontrol, substance abuse, and overt family conflict than those with the restricting subtype. Particularly common in individuals with AN are personality traits of marked perfectionism, conformity, obsessionality, constriction of affect and emotional expressiveness, and reduced social spontaneity; these traits typically appear in advance of the onset of illness and persist even after long-term weight recovery, indicating that they are not merely epiphenomena of acute malnutrition and disordered eating behavior (Strober, 1980; Casper, 1990; Srinivasagam et al., 1995).

Individuals with BN remain at normal body weight, although many aspire to ideal weights far below the range of normalcy for their age and height. The core features of BN include repeated episodes of binge eating followed by compensatory self-induced vomiting, laxative abuse, or pathologically extreme exercise, as well as abnormal concern with weight and shape. The *Diagnostic and Statistical Manual on Mental Disorders, 4th ed.* (DSM-IV) has specified a distinction within this group between those bulimics who engage in self-induced vomiting or laxative, diuretic, or enema abuse (purging type), and those who exhibit other forms of compensatory action such as fasting or exercise (nonpurging type). Beyond these differences, it has been speculated (Vitousek and Manke, 1994) that there are two clinically divergent subgroups of individuals with BN differing significantly in psychopathological characteristics: a so-called multi-impulsive type, in whom bulimia occurs in conjunction with more pervasive difficulties in behavioral self-regulation and affective instability, and a second type, whose distinguishing features include self-effacing behaviors, dependence on external rewards, and extreme compliance. Bulimics of the multi-impulsive type are far more likely to have histories of substance abuse and display other impulse control problems such as shoplifting and self-injurious behaviors. Considering these differences, it has been postulated that multi-impulsive bulimics rely on binge eating and purging as a means of regulating intolerable states of tension, anger, and fragmentation; in contrast, bulimics of the latter type may have binge episodes precipitated through dietary restraint with compensatory behaviors maintained through reduction of guilty feelings associated with fears of weight gain.

COURSE OF ILLNESS

Most cases of AN emerge during the period of adolescence, although the condition can be observed in chil-

dren; there is no clear consensus yet on whether prepubertal onset of the illness confers a more or less ominous prognosis. Recovery from the illness tends to be protracted, but studies of long-term outcome show the illness course to be highly variable: roughly 50% of individuals will eventually have reasonably complete resolution of the illness, whereas another 30% will have lingering residual features that wax and wane in severity long into adulthood. Once developed, AN will pursue a chronic, unremitting course in some 10% of individuals and the remaining 10% of those affected will eventually die from the disease.

Bulimia nervosa is usually precipitated by dieting and weight loss, yet it can occur in the absence of apparent dietary restraint. The frequency of binge episodes, their duration, and amount of food consumed during any one episode all vary considerably among patients. Age of onset is somewhat more variable in BN than in AN, with most cases developing during the period from mid- to late adolescence through the mid-20s. Follow-up studies of clinic samples 5 to 10 years after presentation showed a 50% rate of recovery while nearly 20% continued to meet full criteria for BN (Keel and Mitchell, 1997). Following onset, disturbed eating behavior tends to wax and wane over the course of several years in a high percentage of clinic cases. In the above follow-up studies, approximately 30% of women who had been in remission experienced relapse into bulimic symptoms.

EVIDENCE FOR HERITABILITY: FAMILY AND TWIN STUDIES

Family studies provide a necessary first step in determining whether a disorder is genetic by establishing whether it clusters among biologically related individuals. These studies have generally found an increased rate of eating disorders in AN and BN relatives compared to control relatives. Findings from the largest and most systematic studies (Lilenfeld et al., 1998; Strober et al., 2000) suggest a 7 to 12-fold increase in the prevalence of AN and BN in relatives of eating disordered probands compared to controls. This significantly increased clustering of eating disorders in families of AN and BN individuals provides strong support for familial transmission of both disorders. However, given that first-degree relatives share both genes and environments, these studies are unable to differentiate genetic from environmental causes for familial clusters. Researchers have turned to twin studies to disentangle genetic and environmental effects.

Unlike family studies, twin studies are able to differentiate genetic from environmental effects by comparing similarity for a trait or disorder between identical (monozygotic [MZ]) and fraternal (dizygotic [DZ]) twins. This comparison is based on the fact that MZ twins share roughly double the amount of genetic material as that in DZ twins; consequently, MZ twin correlations that are ≥2 times DZ twin correlations suggest genetic effects. Several twin studies of eating disorders have now been published, and greater MZ than DZ twin similarity for AN and BN has generally been found. Indeed, studies have shown that 58%–76% of the variance in AN (Wade et al., 2000; Klump et al., 2001) and 54%–83% of the variance in BN (Kendler et al., 1991; Bulik et al., 1998) can be accounted for by genetic factors. These heritability estimates are similar to those found in studies of schizophrenia and bipolar disorder, suggesting that AN and BN may be as genetically influenced as disorders traditionally viewed as biological in nature.

Cumulating evidence suggests that AN and BN likely share some etiologic features. Family and twin studies indicate an increased risk of both AN and BN in relatives of AN and BN probands (Walters and Kendler, 1995; Lilenfeld et al., 1998; Strober et al., 2000), suggesting a shared familial component between the two disorders. In addition, subthreshold forms of eating disorders appear to lie on a continuum of liability with full eating disorders. These findings suggest the existence of a broad eating disorder phenotype with possible shared genetic predispositions.

Recent studies have provided further support for the heritability of eating disorders by showing that eating disorder symptoms themselves have a heritable component. Twin studies of eating disorder attitudes, such as body dissatisfaction, eating and weight concerns, and weight preoccupation, suggest that 32%–72% of the variance in these attitudes can be accounted for by genetic factors (Wade et al., 1998; 1999; Klump et al., 2000b). Likewise, binge eating, self-induced vomiting, and dietary restraint have all been found to have heritabilities between 46% and 72% (Sullivan et al., 1998; Klump et al., 2000b). Taken together, findings suggest a significant genetic component to AN and BN as well as to the attitudes and behaviors that contribute to, and correlate with, clinical eating pathology.

Recent studies (Klump et al., 2000b) from the Minnesota Twin Family Study (MTFS) have raised the question of whether there are developmental changes in genetic and environmental influences on eating pathology. In the first of these studies, the relative influence of genetic factors on eating attitudes and behaviors was compared between 680 11-year-old twins and 602 17-year-old twins. Essentially no genetic influence was found for weight preoccupation scores and overall eating pathology in the 11-year-old twins, whereas 52%–57% of the variance in these attitudes and behaviors could be accounted for by genetic factors in the 17-year-old twin cohort (Klump et al., 2000b). The authors hypothesized that genetic relationships may exist between eating pathology and the ovarian hormones activated during puberty that could account for the observed age differences.

TRANSMISSION OF OTHER TRAITS AND DISORDERS

A range of psychiatric symptoms and psychological traits are commonly found in patients with AN or BN. In many cases, they develop secondarily to malnutrition and other effects of aberrant eating; yet, in some, they clearly antedate disordered eating, or arise following recovery from low body weight or binge eating. Determining whether particular psychiatric disorders or traits are expressions of a shared genetic diathesis is one strategy for identifying the nature of genetic influence on eating pathology.

Several family and twin studies have examined the covariation between eating disorders and various other psychiatric conditions that co-occur with AN and BN. These studies have been reviewed in detail (Lilenfeld et al., 1998; Strober, 2000). With regard to major affective illness, studies of AN probands have yielded familial risk estimates in the range of 7% to 25%, with relative risk estimates in studies employing normal controls in the range of 2.1 to 3.4. Likewise, studies of BN probands have shown, with rare exception, that their first-degree relatives are several times more likely to develop affective disorders than relatives of control subjects. At the same time, most studies considering the effects of proband comorbidity on familial risk have shown that affective illness is more likely to occur in probands with this same diagnostic comorbidity. Two recent twin studies support this conclusion, as both found evidence for shared as well as unique genetic influences on major depression and both AN and BN (Kendler et al., 1995; Wade et al., 2000). In short, although AN and BN often co-occur with major mood disorders, unipolar depression in particular, the two conditions do not seem to express a single, shared transmitted liability.

Family studies investigating rates of substance use disorders suggest relatively low rates among relatives of restricting AN probands. In contrast, rates are elevated in relatives of probands with BN. However, several studies (Kaye et al., 1996; Schuckit et al., 1996) indicate that there is no evidence of a cross-transmission of BN and substance use disorder in families, and twin data (Kendler et al., 1995) have shown that the genes influencing susceptibility to alcoholism were independent of those underlying risk to BN.

Independent familial transmission of obsessive-compulsive disorder (OCD) and both AN and BN was recently found in a controlled family study of eating disorders (Lilenfeld et al., 1998). By contrast, shared transmission was found between broadly defined AN and BN and the childhood anxiety disorders separation anxiety and overanxious disorder (Miller et al., 1998), and shared genetic transmission was found between BN and both phobia and panic disorder (Kendler et al., 1995). Preliminary data suggest common familial transmission of AN and obsessive-compulsive personality disorder (OCPD; Lilenfeld et al., 1998). Findings indicated an increased risk of OCPD in relatives of AN probands compared to controls, even after accounting for the effects of proband comorbidity for these disorders. These results suggest the possible existence of a broad, genetically influenced phenotype with core features of rigid perfectionism and propensity for extreme behavioral constraint.

BEHAVIORAL CHARACTERISTICS

People who have eating disorders often have a variety of symptoms aside from pathological eating behaviors. Physiological symptoms include an abundance of neuroendocrine, autonomic, and metabolic disturbances. Psychological symptoms include depression, anxiety, substance abuse, and personality disorders. Determining whether such symptoms are a consequence or a potential cause of pathological feeding behavior or malnutrition is a major methodological issue in the study of eating disorders. It is impractical to study eating disorders prospectively because of the young age of onset and difficulty in premorbid identification of people who will develop eating disorders. However, subjects can be studied after long-term recovery from an eating disorder. The assumed absence of confounding nutritional influences in women who have recovered from an eating disorder raises a possibility that persistent psychobiological abnormalities might be trait related and contribute to the pathogenesis of this disorder. A limited number of studies have investigated people who have recovered from AN and BN. While the definition of recovery from an eating disorder has not been formalized, investigators tend to include people formerly ill with AN after they were at a stable and healthy body weight for months or years and had not been malnourished or engaged in pathological eating

behavior during that period of recovery. For BN, investigators tend to include subjects who have been abstinent from bingeing and purging for months or years. Some investigators include a criterion of normal menstrual cycles and a minimal duration of recovery, such as 1 year.

Individuals with both AN and BN exhibit characteristic personality traits that include high levels of harm avoidance, stress reactivity, and negative emotionality (Bulik et al., 1995; Klump et al., 2000a). These characteristics persist after recovery from the disorder and are independent of body weight (Klump et al., 2000a), thus they may be trait disturbances contributing to the disorders' pathogenesis. The moderately heritable nature of these characteristics (Tellegen et al., 1988) suggests that etiologic relationships may be genetic in nature.

Investigators (Strober, 1980; Casper, 1990; Srinivasagam et al., 1995; Kaye et al., 1998) have found that women who have recovered long term from AN and BN persist in obsessional behaviors as well as inflexible thinking, restraint in emotional expression, and a high degree of self and impulse control. In addition, they exhibit social introversion, overly compliant behavior, and limited social spontaneity as well as greater risk avoidance and harm avoidance. Moreover women who are long-term recovered from AN or BN had continued core eating disorder symptoms, such as ineffectiveness, a drive for thinness, and significant psychopathology related to eating habits. Recovered AN and BN patients showed increased perfectionism and their most common obsessional symptom was the need for symmetry, accompanied by the compulsion to order and arrange. Considered together, these residual behaviors can be characterized as overconcerns with body image and thinness, obsession with symmetry exactness, perfectionism, and dysphoric/negative affect. In general, pathological eating behavior and malnutrition appear to exaggerate the magnitude of these concerns. Thus, the intensity of these symptoms is less after recovery but the content of these concerns remains unchanged. The persistence of these symptoms after recovery raises a question of whether a disturbance of such behaviors may in fact occur premorbidly and contribute to the pathogenesis of AN and BN.

STUDIES OF NEUROTRANSMITTERS

The role of biology in the etiology of AN has been proposed for the past 60 years (Treasure and Campbell, 1994). Earlier theories questioned whether people with AN had a pituitary or hypothalamic disturbance.

More recently, a growing understanding of neurotransmitter modulation of appetitive behaviors has pointed to some disturbance of neurotransmitter function as the cause of AN and/or BN (Morley and Blundell, 1988; Fava et al., 1989). It is possible that disturbances of brain neuropeptides and/or monoamines could contribute to other symptoms and behaviors, such as neuroendocrine or autonomic abnormalities, or alterations of mood and behavior in people with AN or BN. It is important to emphasize that monoamine or neuropeptide disturbances could be a consequence of dietary abnormalities, or premorbid traits that contribute to a vulnerability to develop AN or BN. One way to tease apart cause and effect is to study people with AN or BN at various stages in their illness—that is, while symptomatic and after recovery.

Neuropeptides

Multiple neuroendocrine abnormalities have been documented in AN and BN (Rubin and Kaye, 2001), including alteration of the hypothalamic–pituitary–gonadal axis, the hypothalamic-pituitary-adrenal (HPA) axis, thyroid system, growth hormone (GH) secretion and fluid conservation, as well as autonomic instability and reduced metabolic function. For the most part, these neuroendocrine disturbances are state related and tend to normalize after clinical recovery. In the past decade, studies have questioned whether alterations in brain neuropeptides contributed to disturbed neuroendocrine function in AN and BN. Neuropeptides also play a role in feeding behavior. The mechanisms for controlling food intake involve a complicated interplay between peripheral (taste, gastrointestinal peptides, vagal afferent nerves) and central nervous system (CNS) neuropeptides and/or monoamines. In fact, neuropeptides have specific roles in regulating the structure of feeding—that is, studies in animals show that neuropeptides, such as opioids, neuropeptide Y (NPY), and peptide YY (PYY), regulate the rate, duration, and size of meals, as well as macronutrient selection (Morley and Blundell, 1988). Thus it is theoretically possible that alterations in neuropeptide function could contribute to disturbances in the form or structure of feeding behavior in AN and BN.

Corticotropin-releasing hormone

When underweight people with AN have increased plasma cortisol secretion (Walsh et al., 1978) that is thought to be a consequence of hypersecretion of endogenous corticotropin-releasing hormone (CRH) (Gold et al., 1986; Kaye et al., 1987b Fig. 18.1) Both measures normalize after weight restoration, thus activation of the HPA axis may be precipitated by weight loss. Still, increased CRH activity is of great theoretical interest in anorexia since intracerebroventricular CRH administration in experimental animals produces many of the physiologic and behavioral changes associated with AN, including hypothalamic hypogonadism, decreased sexual activity, decreased feeding behavior, and hyperactivity.

Opioid peptides

Studies in animals (Morley et al., 1983) raise the possibility that altered endogenous opioid activity might contribute to pathological feeding behavior in eating disorders, since opioid agonists generally increase food intake and opioid antagonists decrease it. Reduced concentrations of cerebrospinal fluid (CSF) β-endorphin concentrations have been found in both underweight AN and ill BN subjects (Kaye et al., 1987a; (Brewerton et al., 1992); these concentrations normalize after recovery. If β-endorphin activity is a facilitator of feeding behavior, then reduced CSF (Fig. 18.1) concentrations could reflect decreased central activity of this system, which then maintains or facilitates inhibition of feeding behavior in the eating disorders. Less is known about other opioid systems in AN or BN.

Neuropeptide Y and peptide YY

These peptides are of considerable theoretical interest as they are among the most potent endogenous stimulants of feeding behavior within the CNS (Morley et al., 1985; Stanley et al., 1986). They have neuroanatomically separate systems and presumably have different roles. Peptide YY is three times as potent as NPY in stimulating food intake; both are selective for carbohydrate-rich foods. Animal studies also suggest that increased NPY activity may represent a homeostatic mechanism to stimulate feeding, as it has been observed that intracerebroventricular injection of PYY in rats precipitated massive increases in food ingestion to which tolerance did not develop, prompting speculation that this peptide may have relevance to the pathophysiology of binge eating (Morley et al., 1985; Stanley et al., 1986).

Underweight anorexics have been shown to have elevations of CSF NPY, but normal PYY (Kaye et al., 1990b; Fig. 18.1). Clearly, elevated NPY does not stimulate feeding in underweight anorexics; however, the possibility that increased NPY activity underlies the ob-

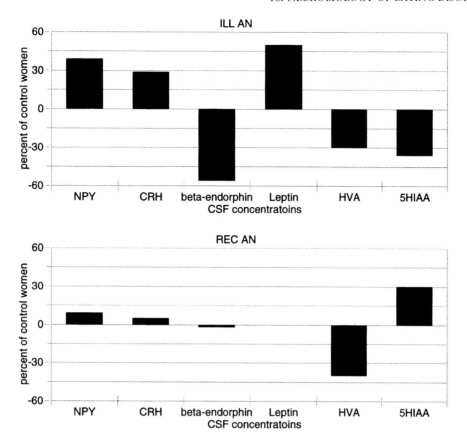

FIGURE 18.1 Comparison of cerebrospinal fluid (CSF) concentrations of neuropeptide and monoamine metabolites in people who were ill (underweight) and in those with long-term recovery from anorexia nervosa (AN). The CSF values in AN compared to healthy control women, where control mean values are set to 0. CRH, corticotropin-releasing hormone; HVA, homovanillic acid; NPY, neuropeptide Y; REC, recovered; SHIAA, 5-hydroxyindolacetic acid.

sessive and paradoxical interest in dietary intake and food preparation is a hypothesis worth exploring. In this regard, intracerebroventricular NPY administration to experimental animals produces many of the physiological and behavioral changes associated with AN, including gonadal steroid–dependent effects on luteinizing hormone secretion, suppression of sexual activity, increased release of CRH in the hypothalamus, and hypotension. By contrast, CSF levels of NPY and PYY have been reported to be normal in women with BN who are acutely ill. Levels of PYY only increased above normal when subjects were reassessed after 1 month of abstinence from bingeing and vomiting, but normalized in the long term (Gendall et al., 1999). Whether the transient elevation of PYY arises merely as an epiphenomenon of pathological eating or emesis, whether it is a compensatory response to normalization of feeding patterns and the arrest of binge eating and purging, or whether it expresses an underlying patho-

physiological susceptibility are questions that remain unanswered.

Cholecystokinin

Cholecystokinin (CCK) is a peptide secreted by the gastrointestinal system in response to food intake. Release of CCK is thought to be one means of transmitting satiety signals to the brain by way of vagal afferents. Its role in satiety is supported by findings that exogenously administered CCK reduces food intake in animals and humans (Baile et al., 1986). In addition, CNS CCK has been implicated in the modulation of anxiety (Bradwejn and de Montigny, 1984).

Some (Geracioti and Liddle, 1988; Pirke et al., 1994), but not all (Philipp et al., 1991) studies have shown that bulimics have reduced plasma CCK after a test meal. Lower-than-average basal levels of CSF CCK have also been found in women with BN (Lydiard et al., 1993). In comparison, some (Philipp et al., 1991; Tamai et al., 1993), but not all (Pirke et al., 1991; Geracioti et al., 1992) studies have found elevations of basal and post-prandial plasma CCK in underweight anorexics. Levels of CCK and blunting of CCK response to an oral glucose load have been shown to normalize in anorexics after partial restoration of body weight (Tamai et al., 1993). These data raise the question of whether CCK plays a role in the perpetuation of pathologic eating in AN and BN. The inconsistent findings may, be related in part, to the fact that there are several different molecular forms of CCK, which studies to date have not been able to measure.

Leptin

Leptin is secreted predominantly by adipose tissue cells; it is thought to act as an afferent signal and regulator of body fat stores (Zhang et al., 1994). In rodent models, defects in the leptin coding sequence resulting in leptin deficiency or defects in leptin receptor (Chen et al., 1996) are associated with obesity. In humans, leptin is positively correlated with fat mass in individuals in all weight ranges and women tend to have higher concentrations than men of the same weight, presumably because of the higher proportion of body fat in females (Considine et al., 1996). Obesity in humans is not thought to be a result of leptin deficiency per se, but it is postulated that obesity may be associated with leptin resistance (Hamann and Matthaei 1996).

Malnourished and underweight patients with AN have consistently been found to have significantly reduced plasma and CSF leptin concentrations (Hebebrand et al., 1995; Grinspoon et al., 1996; Ferron et al., 1997; Mantzoros et al., 1997) compared to normal-weight controls. This binding strongly implies a normal physiological response to starvation. Mantzoros et al. (1997) also reported an elevated CSF-to-plasma leptin ratio in AN patients compared to controls, suggesting that the proportional decrease in leptin levels with weight loss is greater in plasma than in CSF. As in normal control women, leptin levels in AN patients are correlated with body weight and fat mass (Grinspoon et al., 1996); (Mantzoros et al., 1997). A longitudinal investigation during refeeding in AN patients has shown that CSF leptin concentrations reach normal values before full weight restoration, possibly as a consequence of the relatively rapid and disproportionate accumulation of fat during refeeding (Mantzoros et al., 1997). This finding led the authors to suggest that premature normalization of leptin concentration might contribute to difficulty in achieving and sustaining a normal weight in AN.

The leptin status of individuals with BN has been less examined. To date, one study has found that serum leptin concentrations in ill bulimics are similar to those of normal control women and are correlated with body mass (Ferron et al., 1997). Recent studies from our group (Gendell et al., 1999) show that plasma and CSF leptin levels are normal in long-term recovered AN and BN subjects. Taken together, these data on AN and BN suggest that, as in normal individuals, leptin is correlated with body weight and is not involved in the etiology of these disorders. However, leptin may still play a role in the development of symptoms when patients are ill with these disorders.

Leptin appears to play an important role in triggering an adaptive response to starvation (Ahima et al., 1996; Boden et al., 1996). Under conditions of intense food deprivation, leptin may act as an initial warning signal, instigating metabolic responses to "famine," even before a significant weight or fat loss has occurred. Indeed, reduced leptin concentrations have been found to be a critical signal that initiates the neuroendocrine response to starvation, including limiting procreation, decreasing thyroid thermogenesis, and increasing secretion of stress steroids. In summary, these changes in leptin may play an important role in the well known hormonal and metabolic response to starvation found in AN.

Relationship of neuropeptide alterations to symptoms in eating disorders

Multiple neuroendocrine and neuropeptide disturbances occur when people with AN and BN are engaged in pathological eating behaviors and/or are malnourished. While there are relatively few relevant studies to date, data tend to suggest that such disturbances normalize after recovery (Fig. 18.1). The correction of these disturbances after recovery suggests that such disturbances are secondary to malnutrition and/or weight loss and are not their cause. Still, an understanding of these neuropeptide disturbances may shed light on the difficulty many people with AN or BN have in "reversing" their illness. In AN, malnutrition may contribute to entering a downward spiraling circle, with malnutrition sustaining and perpetuating the desire for more weight loss and dieting. Symptoms such as increased satiety, as well as obsessions and dysphoric mood, may be exaggerated by these neuropeptide alterations and thus contribute to this downward spiral. Even after improved nutrition and weight gain, many people with AN have much difficulty normalizing their behavior. For example, menstrual dysfunction may persist for some months after weight restoration.

While these disturbances do not appear to be a permanent feature or cause of AN, they are strongly entrenched and are not easily corrected by improved nutrition or short-term weight normalization.

Monoamine Systems

The most compelling evidence for a disturbance of serotonin and/or norepinephrine in eating disorders is that people with BN (Walsh, 1991; (Mitchell et al., 1993) and AN (Kaye et al., 2001) respond to antidepressants in placebo-controlled trials. Numerous studies have also shown alterations in these monoamines in the ill state. While less well studied, monoamine disturbances appear to persist after recovery.

Dopamine

Altered dopamine activity has been found among ill AN and BN individuals. Homovanillic acid (HVA), the major metabolite of dopamine (DA) in humans, was decreased in CSF of underweight AN subjects (Kaye et al., 1984). While ill BN subjects, as a group, have normal CSF HVA, several studies have shown a significant reduction of CSF HVA in BN patients with high binge frequency (Kaye et al., 1990a; Jimerson et al., 1992). Dopamine metabolism in the CNS may explain differences in symptoms between AN, BN-AN, and BN subjects. Our group found that recovered AN subjects had significantly reduced concentrations of CSF HVA, compared to recovered BN-AN or BN women (Kaye et al., 1999; Fig 18.1). Dopamine neuronal function has been associated with motor activity (Kaye et al., 1999a), reward (Blum et al., 1995; Salamone, 1996), and novelty seeking. Individuals with AN have stereotyped and hyperactive motor behavior, anhedonic, restrictive personalities, and reduced novelty seeking. Whether individuals with AN have an intrinsic disturbance of dopamine remains uncertain.

Serotonin

Serotonin (5-hydroxytryptamine [5-HT]) pathways play an important role in postprandial satiety. Treatments that increase intrasynaptic serotonin or directly activate serotonin receptors tend to reduce food consumption, whereas interventions that dampen serotonergic neurotransmission or block receptor activation reportedly increase food consumption and promote weight gain (Blundell, 1984; Leibowitz, 1986). Moreover, CNS serotonin pathways have been implicated in the modulation of mood, impulse regulation and behavioral constraint, and obsessionality, and they affect a variety of neuroendocrine systems.

There has been considerable interest in the role that serotonin may play in AN and BN (Jimerson et al., 1990; Kaye et al., 1991, 1998; Treasure and Campbell, 1994; Brewerton, 1995). This is related in part to the fact that studies have found that AN and BN have alterations in serotonin metabolism. When underweight, anorexics have a significant reduction in basal concentrations of the serotonin metabolite 5-hydroxyindolacetic acid (5-HIAA) in the CSF compared to healthy controls, as well as blunted plasma prolactin response to drugs with serotonin activity, and reduced ^{3}H-imipramine binding. Together, these findings suggest reduced serotonergic activity, although this may arise secondarily from reductions in dietary supplies of the serotonin-synthesizing amino acid tryptophan. By contrast, CSF concentrations of 5-HIAA are reported to be elevated in long-term weight-recovered anorexics. These contrasting findings of reduced and heightened serotonergic activity in acutely ill and long-term recovered anorexics, respectively, may seem counterintuitive; however, since dieting lowers plasma tryptophan levels in otherwise healthy women (Anderson et al., 1990), resumption of normal eating in anorexics may unmask intrinsic abnormalities in serotonergic systems that mediate certain core behavioral or temperamental underpinnings of risk and vulnerability.

Considerable evidence also exists of dysregulation of serotonergic processes in BN. Examples includes blunted prolactin response to the serotonin receptor agonists m-chlorophenylpiperazine (m-CPP) 5-hydroxytrytophan, and dl-fenfluramine, and enhanced migraine-like headache response to m-CPP challenge. Acute perturbation of serotonergic tone by dietary depletion of tryptophan has also been linked to increased food intake and mood irritability in bulimics compared to healthy controls. And, like women who have recovered from AN, women with long-term recovery from BN have been shown to have elevated concentrations of 5-HIAA in the CSF. Recently, our group (Kaye et al., 2001) found that recovered BN patients had a reduction of medial orbital frontal cortex 5-HT$_{2A}$ binding, which, theoretically, could be related to vulnerabilities for impulse dyscontrol and mood. In addition, control women, but not recovered BN women, had an age-related decline in 5-HT$_{2A}$ binding. Taken together, these data provide further evidence of persistent serotonin alterations after recovery from BN.

It has been found that *low* levels of CSF 5-HIAA are associated with impulsive and non-premeditated aggressive behaviors (Stein et al., 1993), which cut across traditional diagnostic boundaries. Thus, it is of interest that recovered AN and BN women had elevated CSF 5-HIAA concentrations. Behaviors found after recovery from AN and BN, such as obsession with symmetry and exactness, and perfectionism, tend to be opposite in character to behaviors displayed by people with low 5-HIAA levels. These studies contribute to a growing literature suggesting that CSF 5-HIAA concentrations may correlate with a spectrum of behavior. Reduced CSF 5-HIAA levels appear to be related to behavioral undercontrol, whereas increased CSF 5-HIAA concentrations may be related to behavioral overcontrol.

The possibility of a common vulnerability for BN and AN may seem puzzling, given well-recognized differences in behavior in these disorders. However, recent studies suggest that AN and BN have a shared etiologic vulnerability. That is, there is a familial aggregation of a range of eating disorders in relatives of probands with either BN or AN and these two disorders are highly comorbid in twin studies. Both disorders respond to serotonin-specific medications and both disorders have high levels of harm avoidance (see Klump et al., 2000b), a personality trait hypothesized to be related to increased serotonin activity. These data raise the possibility that a disturbance of serotonin activity may create a vulnerability for the expression of a cluster of symptoms common to both AN and BN. Other factors that are *independent* of a vulnerability for the development of an eating disorder may contribute to the development of eating disorder subgroups. For example, people with restrictor-type AN have extraordinary self-restraint and self-control. The risk for OCPD is elevated only in this subgroup and in their families and shows a shared transmission with restrictor-type AN (Lilenfeld et al., 1998). In other words, an additional vulnerability for behavioral overcontrol and

rigid and inflexible mood states, combined with a vulnerability for an eating disorder, may result in restrictor-type AN.

The contribution of serotonin to specific human behaviors remains uncertain. Serotonin has been postulated to contribute to temperament or personalty traits such as harm avoidance (Cloninger, 1987) or behavioral inhibition (Soubrie, 1986), or to categorical dimensions such as OCD (Barr et al., 1992), anxiety and fear (Charney et al., 1990), or depression (Grahame-Smith, 1992), as well as to satiety for food consumption. It is possible that separate components of serotonin neuronal systems (i.e., different pathways or receptors) are coded for such specific behaviors. However, that may not be consistent with the neurophysiology of serotonin neuronal function.

IMAGING STUDIES

Brain Imaging Studies of Eating Disorders

It is well known that ill AN subjects have enlarged ventricles and sulci widening (see review by Ellison and Fong, 1998). ^{1}H magnetic resonance spectroscopy (^{1}H-MRS) revealed reduced lipid signals in the frontal white matter and occipital gray matter, and was associated with decreased body mass index (Roser et al., 1999). These alterations have been thought to be reversible after recovery but recent data suggest persistent changes after recovery (Katzman et al., 1997; (Lambe et al., 1997). A number of studies (see Table 18.1) using single photon emission computed tomography (SPECT) or photon emission tomography (PET) with 2-deoxy-glucose have shown temporal alterations and less frequently frontal or cingulate changes. Of particular interest are several recent relevant studies.

TABLE 18.1 *Brain Imaging Studies in Anorexia Nervosa*

Year	Author	Method	Subjects	Frontal	Temporal	Cingulate
1995	Nozoe S	SPECT	ill AN	X	X	
1995	Delvenne	PET	ill AN	X		
1996	Herholtz	PET	ill AN			
1997	Gordon	SPECT	ill AN, rec AN		X	
1998	Ellison	f MRI	ill AN		X	X
1998	Kuruoglu	SPECT	ill AN, rec AN	X	X	
1999	Delvenne	PET	ill AN	X		
1999	Hirano	SPECT	ill BN-AN		X	
2000	Rauch	PET	ill AN		X	

AN, anorexia nervosa; BN-AN, bulimia nervosa-anorexia nervosa; fMRI, functional magnetic resonance imaging; PET, positron emission tomography; rec, recovered; SPECT, single photon emission computed tomography.

Using SPECT, Gordon et al., (1997) found ill anorectics to have unilateral temporal lobe hypoperfusion that persisted in subjects studied after weight restoration. Ellison et al. (1998), using functional magnetic resonance imaging (fMRI) found that when ill AN subjects viewed pictures of high-caloric drinks, they had increased signal changes in the left insular, cingulate gyrus, and left amygdala–hippocampus region and increased anxiety. Using PET O-15 and pictures of high-calorie food, Gordon et al. (2001) found that ill AN subjects had elevated cerebral blood flow (rCBF) in bilateral medial temporal lobes and increased anxiety. Naruo et al., (2000), who used SPECT to investigate the effects of imagining food, found that ill BN-AN subjects had a significantly higher percent change in the inferior, superior, prefrontal, and parietal regions of the right brain than AN subjects or controls, as well as the highest level of apprehension about food intake. In our laboratory (unpublished data), we used PET to investigate 5-HT_{1A} and 5-HT_{2A} binding, and found alterations in temporal and other regions in recovered AN subjects. Taken together, these studies support involvement of the temporal cortex in AN. Few studies to date have used brain imaging to investigate BN.

MOLECULAR GENETIC STUDIES

Researchers have recently begun to examine genetic influences through association and linkage studies. Association studies, focus on the relative influence of a specific gene or genetic marker (candidate gene) on the development of eating disorders. This is accomplished by either comparing the frequency of the gene's alleles in individuals with and without the disorder or examining the frequency of transmission of alleles from parents to children with either AN or BN. By contrast, linkage analyses identify contributing genetic loci by examining allele sharing among family members at a number of genetic markers across the genome. Instead of focusing on one particular gene, traditionally researchers use this approach to examine all identified genetic markers in the genome. A number of association studies of both AN and BN have now been conducted, some with promising results. Linkage studies have been much less common, although recent studies funded by the Price Foundation of Switzerland are likely to provide novel and interesting results.

Association Studies

Evidence linking AN and BN to monoamine functioning (see Monoamine Systems,) have led researchers to target serotonin- and dopamine-related genes in association analyses. Several studies have now shown an increase in the $-1438/A$ allele of the 5-HT_{2A} receptor gene in AN women compared to controls (Collier et al., 1997; Enoch et al., 1998; Sorbi et al., 1998; Nacmias et al., 1999). However, additional studies of this and other serotonin-related genes ($5\text{-HT}_{1D\beta}$, 5-HTT, 5-HT7, tryptophan hydroxylase [TPH] receptor have failed to find significant associations in AN (Hinney et al., 1997a; 1997b; 1999a; Campbell et al., 1998; (Han et al., 1999; Ziegler et al., 1999) or BN (Burnet et al., 1999; Nacmias et al., 1999) subjects. Studies have also failed to find increased allele frequencies of the dopamine D_3 (Bruins-Slot et al., 1998) and D_4 (Hinney et al., 1999b) receptor genes in AN subjects compared to control subjects. These genes have not yet been examined in subjects with BN.

The primary role of weight control, feeding, and energy expenditure in the pathology of AN and BN has lead researchers to examine genes related to these processes. Findings suggest possible associations between the UCP-2/UCP-3 gene (Campbell et al., 1999) and the estrogen receptor β gene (Rosenkrantz et al., 1998) in AN. Additional research is necessary to clarify conflicting findings and replicate initial results. Moreover, association studies of BN are needed, as this disorder has been much less studied than AN and findings thus far have been generally negative.

Linkage Analysis

The authors of this chapter are part of a multicenter international collaboration that has collected 192 families composed of at least one affected relative pair with anorexia nervosa and related eating disorders (Kaye et al, 2000). For the entire sample, there was only modest evidence for linkage, with the highest non-parametric linkage (NPL) score of 1.80 on chromosome 4 at marker D4S2367 (Grice et al. 2002). However, a linkage analysis in a subset (n=37) of families where at least two affected relatives had diagnoses of anorexia nervosa, showed a multipoint NPL score of 3.03 on chromosome 1p at marker D1S3721. Genotyping additional markers in this region led to a peak multipoint NPL score of 3.45, providing suggestive evidence for the presence of a susceptibility locus for anorexia nervosa on chromosome 1p. Other analysis have focused on psychiatric, personality and temperament phenotypes. A multipoint Affected Sibling Pair (ASP) linkage analysis was done using a novel method that incorporates covariates (Devlin, 2002). By exploring seven attributes thought to typify individuals with eating disorders, we identified two variables, drive-for-thinness and obsessionality, which delimit populations among the ASP. When we incorporated these covariates into the ASP linkage analysis, we found several regions of suggestive linkage: one close to genome-wide significance on Chromosome 1 (at 202 cM, D1S1660; LOD = 3.46, p= 0.00003); another on Chromosome 2 (at 102 cM, D2S1779; LOD = 2.22; p = 0.00070); and a third region on Chromosome 13 (at 102 cM, GATA121A08; LOD = 2.50; p = 0.00035). By comparing our results to those implemented using more standard linkage methods, we find the covariates convey substantial information for the linkage analysis.

We have recently completed a larger, genome-wide linkage study of approximately 400 families with two or more family members with AN, BN, or EDNOS (W. Kaye et al., unpublished results). This larger study will enable us to detect linkage and may prove to be the first study to identify susceptibility loci for these disorders. In addition, we are currently in the process of collecting genetic data on approximately 700 AN individuals and their parents. This homogeneous sample will be used to conduct association analyses such as those described above and will be a stronger aid in detecting genes of modest to large effect.

SUMMARY

Daunting challenges remain in the investigation of neurobiological mediators of risk and clinical pathology in AN and BN. The extent to which these abnormalities are consequences of pathological eating behavior, malnutrition, or long-term sequelae of either condition remains speculative. Data on the functional status of these neurobiological systems are too sparse to allow for definitive conclusions regarding the possible etiological significance of differences reported between individuals with eating disorders and normal controls.

Clearly, many of the alterations in neuropeptide and monoaminergic function in eating disorders are state-dependent; however, given the effects of these systems on mood, anxiety, memory organization, and body physiology, they may well have significant pathogenic influence, both sustaining and exacerbating certain psychological and cognitive elements of these syndromes. Thus, neurobiologically mediated effects may be contributing factors to the frequently long-term, pernicious, and self-sustaining course of illness, at least in many patients. These associations, while remaining speculative, nevertheless underscore the importance of aggressive and sustained treatment of both the nutritional and behavioral–psychological elements

of the syndromes to allow for a truly sustained normalization of neuropeptidergic and monoaminergic functions.

REFERENCES

Ahima, R.S, Prabakaran, D., Mantzoros, C., Qu D., Lowell, B, Maratos-Flier, E. and Flier, J.S. (1996) Role of leptin in the neuroendocrine response to fasting. *Nature* 382:250–252.

Anderson, I.M., Parry-Billings, M., Newsholme, E.A., et al. (1990) Dieting reduces plasma tryptophan and alters brain 5-HT function in women. *Psychol Med* 20:785–791.

Baile, C.A., McLaughlin, C.L., and Della-Fera, M.A. (1986) Role of cholecystokinin and opioid peptides in control of food intake. *Physiol Rev* 66:172–234.

Barr, L.C., Goodman, W.K., Price, L. H., McDougle, C.J. and Charney, D.S. (1992) The serotonin hypothesis of obsessive compulsive disorder: implications of pharmacologic challenge studies. *J Clin Psychiatry* 53(4, Suppl):17–28.

Blum, K., Sheridan, P.J., Wood, R.C., Braverman, E.R., Chen, T.J., and Comings, D.E. (1995) Dopamine D2 receptor gene variants: association and linkage studies in impulsive addictive-compulsive behavior. *Pharmacogenetics* 5:121–141.

Blundell, J.E. (1984) Serotonin and appetite. *Neuropharmacology* 23:1537–1551.

Boden, G., Chen, X., Mozzoli, M., and Ryan, I. (1996) Effect of fasting on serum leptin in normal subjects. *J Clin Endocrinol* 81: 3419–3423.

Bradwejn, J. and de Montigny, C. (1984) Benzodiazepines antagonize cholecystokinin-induced activation of rat hippocampal neurones. *Nature* 312(5992):363–364.

Brewerton, T.D. (1995) Toward a unified theory of serotonin dysregulation in eating and related disorders. *Psychoneuroendocrinology* 20:561–590.

Brewerton, T.D., Lydiard, R.B., Laraia, M.T., Shook J.E. and Ballenger, J.C. (1992) CSF beta-endorphin and dynorphin in bulimia nervosa. *Am J Psychiatry* 149:1086–1090.

Bruins-Slot, L., Gorwood, P., Bouvard, M., Blot, P., Ades, J., Feingold, J., Schwartz, J.C., Mouren, S., and Marie, C. (1998) Lack of association between anorexia nervosa and D3 dopamine receptor gene. *Biol Psychiatry* 43:76–78.

Bulik, C.M., Sullivan, P.F., and Kendler, K.S. (1998) Heritability and reliability of binge-eating and bulimia nervosa. *Biol Psychiatry* 44:1210–1218.

Bulik, C.M., Sullivan, S.A. Weltzin, T.E., and Kaye, W.H. (1995) Temperament in eating disorders. *Int. J. Eating Disord.* 17:251–261.

Burnet, P.W., Smith, K.A., Cowen, P.J., Fairburn, C.G., and Harrison, P.J. (1999) Allelic variation of the 5-HT2C receptor (HTR2C) in bulimia nervosa and binge eating disorder. *Psychiatr Genet*, 9: 101–104.

Campbell, D.A., Sundaramurthy, D., Gordon, D., Markham, A.F., and Pieri, L.F. (1999) Association between a marker in the UCP-2/UCP-3 gene cluster and genetic susceptibility to anorexia nervosa. *Mol Psychiatry* 4:68–70.

Campbell, D.A., Sundaramurthy, D., Gordon, D., Markham, A.F., and Pieri, L.F. (1998) Lack of association between 5-HT2A gene promoter polymorphism and susceptibility to anorexia nervosa. *Lancet* 351:499.

Casper, R.C. (1990) Personality features of women with good outcome from restricting anorexia nervosa. *Psychosom Med*, 52(2): 156–170.

Charney, D.S., Woods, S.W., Krystal, J.H., and Heninger, G.R. (1990) Serotonin function and human anxiety disorders. *Ann NY Acad Sci* 600:558–573.

Chen, H., Charlat, O., Tartaglia, L.A., Woolf, E.A., Weng, X., Ellis, S.J., Lakey, N.D., Culpepper, J., Moore, K.J., Breitbart, R.E., Duyk, G.M., Tepper, R.I., and Morgensten, J.P. (1996) Evidence that the diabetes gene encodes the leptin receptor: identification of a mutation in the leptin receptor gene in *db/db* mice. *Cell* 84:491–495.

Cloninger, C.R. (1987) A systematic method for clinical description and classification of personality variants. *Arch Gen Psychiatry* 44:573–588.

Collier, D.A., Arranz, M.J., Li, T., Mupita, D., Brown, N., and Treasure, J. (1997) Association between 5-HT2A gene promoter polymorphism and anorexia nervosa. *Lancet* 350:412.

Considine, R.V., Sinha, M., Heiman, M.L., Kriauciunas, A., Stephens, T.W., Nyce, M.R. Ohannesian, J.P., Marco C.C., McKee, L.J., and Bauer, T.L. (1996) Serum immunoreactive-leptin concentrations in normal-weight and obese humans. *N Engl J Med* 334:292–295.

Devlin, B., Bacanu, S., Klump, K.L., Bulik, C.M., Fichter, M., Halmi, K.A., Kaplan, A.S., Strober, M., Treasure, J., Woodside, D.B., Berrettini, W.H., and Kaye, W.H. (2002). Linkage analysis of anorexia nervosa incorporating behavioral covariates. *Hum Mol Genet* (in press).

Ellison, A.R., and Fong, J., Neuroimaging in eating disorders. In: Hoek, H.W., Treasure, J.L., and Katzman, M.A. eds. *Neurobiology in the Treatment of Eating Disorders*. Chichester: John Wiley and Sons, pp. 255–261.

Ellison, Z., Fong, J., Howard, R., Bullmore, E., Williams, S., and Treasure, J. (1998) Functional anatomy of calorie fear in anorexia nervosa. *Lancet* 352:1192.

Enoch, M., Kaye, W., Ozaki, N., Mazzanti, C., Rotondo, A., Greenberg, B., Altemus, M., Murphy, D., and Goldman, D. (1998) Replication of an association between 5-HT2A promoter polymorphism −1438G/A and anorexia nervosa, and association with obsessive-compulsive disorder. *Lancet* 351:1785–1786.

Fava, M., Copeland, P.M., Schweiger, U., and Herzog, D.B. (1989) Neurochemical abnormalities of anorexia nervosa and bulimia nervosa. *Am J Psychiatry* 146:963–971.

Ferron, F., Considine, R.V., Peino, R., Lado, I.E., Dieguez, C., and Casanueva, F.F. (1997). Serum leptin concentrations in patients with anorexia nervosa, bulimia nervosa and non-specific eating disorders correlate with body mass index but are independent of the respective disease. *Clin Endocrinol* 46:289–293.

Garner, D.M., Garfinkel, P.E., and O'Shaughnessy, M. (1985) The validity of the distinction between bulimia with and without anorexia nervosa. *Am J Psychiatry* 142:581–587.

Gendall, K.A., Kaye, W.H., Altemus, M., McConaha, C.W., and La Via, M.C. (1999) Leptin, NPY and PYY in long term recovered eating disorders patients. *Biol Psychiatry* 46:292–299.

Geracioti, T.D. and Liddle, R.A. (1988) Impaired cholecystokinin secretion in bulimia nervosa. *N Engl J Med* 319:683–688.

Geracioti, T.D., Liddle, R.A., Altemus, M., et al. (1992) Regulation of appetite and cholecystokinin secretion in anorexia nervosa. *Am J Psychiatry*, 149:958–961.

Gold, P.W., Gwirtsman, H., Avgerinos, P.C., Nieman, L.K., Gallucci, W.T., Kaye, W., Jimerson. D. Ebert, M., Rittmaster, R., and Loriaux, D.L. (1986) Abnormal hypothalamic-pituitary-adrenal function in anorexia nervosa. Pathophysiologic mechanisms in underweight and weight-corrected patients. *N Engl J Med*, 314:1335–42.

Gordon, J., Lask, B., Bryant-Waugh, R., Christie, D., and Timimi, S.

(1997) Childhood-onset anorexia nervosa: towards identifying a biological substrate. *Int J Eat Disord* 22:159–165.

Gordon, C.M., Dougherty, D.D., Fischmann, A.J., Emans, S.J., Grace, E., Lamm, R., Alpert, N.M., Majzoub, J.A., and Rausch, S.L. (2001) Neural substrates of anorexia nervosa: a behavioral challenge study with positron emission tomography. *J. Pediatr* 139:51–57.

Grahame-Smith, D.G. (1992) Serotonin in affective disorders. *Int J Clin Psychopharmacol*, 6(4):S5-S13.

Grice, D.E., Halmi, K.A., Fichter, M., Strober, M., Woodside, D.B., Treasure, J., Kaplan, A.S., Magistretti, P.J., Goldman, D., Kaye, W.H. Bulik, C.M., and Berrettini, W.H. (2002). Evidence for a susceptibility gene for anorexia nervosa on Chromosome 1. *Am J Human Genet* (in press).

Grice, D.E., Berrettini, W.H., Halmi, K.A., Fichter, M., Strober, M., Woodside, D.B., Treasure, J., Kaplan, A.S., Magistretti, P.J., and Goldman, D., and Kaye, W.H. (in press). Genome-wide affected relative pair analysis of anorexia nervosa and related eating disorders. *Am J Hum Genet*

Grinspoon, S., Gulick, T., Askari, H., Landt, M., Lee, K., Anderson, E., Ma, Z., Vignati, L., Bowsher, R., and Herzog, D. (1996) Serum leptin levels in women with anorexia nervosa. *J Clin Endocrinol Metab* 81:3861–3864.

Halmi, K.A., Eckert, E., Marchi, P., et al. (1991) Comorbidity of psychiatric diagnoses in anorexia nervosa [see comments]. *Arch Gen Psychiatry*, 48:712–718.

Hamann, A., and Matthaei, S. (1996) Regulation of energy balance by leptin. *Exp Clin Endocrinol Diabetes* 104:293–300.

Han, L., Nielson, D.A., Rosenthal, N.E., Jefferson, K., Kaye, W., Murphy, D., Altemus, M., Humphries, J., Casssano, G., Rotondo, A., Virkkhunen, M., Linnoila, M., and Goldman, D. (1999) No coding variant of the tryptophan hydroxylase gene detected in seasonal affective disorder, obsessive-compulsive disorder, anorexia nervosa, and alcoholism. *Biol Psychiatry* 45:615–619.

Hebebrand, J., Van der heyden, J, Devos, R., Kopp, W., Herpertz S., Remschmidt, H., and Herzog, D. (1995) Plasma concentrations of obese protein in anorexia nervosa. *Lancet* 346:1624–1625.

Hinney, A., Barth, N., Ziegler, A., von-Prittwitz, S., Hamann, A., Hennighausen, K., Pirke, K.M., Heils, A., Rosenkranz, K., Roth, H., Coners, H., Mayer, H., Herzog, W., Siegfried, A., Lehmkuhl, G., Poustka, F., Schmidt, M.H., Schafer, H., Grzeschik, K.H., Lesch, K.P., Lentes, K.U., Remschmidt, H., and Hebebrand, J. (1997a) Serotonin transporter gene-linked polymorphic region: allele distributions in relationship to body weight and in anorexia nervosa. *Life Sci* 61(21):295–303.

Hinney, A., Herrmann, H., Lohr, T., Rosenkranz, K., Ziegler, A., Lehmkuhl, G., Poustka, R., Schmidt, M.H., Mayer, H., Siegfried, W., Remschmidt, H., and Hebebrand, J. (1999a). No evidence for involvement of alleles of polymorphisms in the serotonin 1Dbeta and 7 receptor genes in obesity, underweight or anorexia nervosa. *Int J Obes Rel Metab Disord* 23:760–763.

Hinney, A., Schneider, J., Ziegler, A., Lehmkuhl, G., Poustka, F., Schmidt, M.H., Mayer, H., Siegfried, W., Remschmidt, H., and Hebebrand, J. (1999b) No evidence for involvement of polymorphisms of the dopamine D4 receptor gene in anorexia nervosa, underweight, and obesity. *Am J Med Genet*, 88:594–597.

Hinney, A., Ziegler, A., Nothen, M.M., Remschmidt, H., and Hebebrand, J. (1997b) 5-HT2A receptor gene polymorphisms, anorexia nervosa, and obesity. *Lancet* 350:1324–1325.

Jimerson, D.C., Lesem, M.D., Kaye, W.H., Hegg, A.P., and Brewerton, T.D (1990) Eating disorders and depression: is there a serotonin connection? *Biol Psychiatry* 28:443–454

Jimerson, D.C., Lesem, M.D., Kaye, W.H., and Brewerton, T.D.

(1992) Low serotonin and dopamine metabolite concentrations in cerebrospinal fluid from bulimic patients with frequent binge episodes. *Arch Gen Psychiatry* 49:132–138.

Katzman, D.K., Zipursky, R.B., Lambe, E.K., Mikulis, D.J. (1997) A longitudinal magnetic resonance imaging study of brain changes in adolescents with anorexia nervosa. *Arch Pediatr Adolesc Med* 151:793–797.

Kaye, W.H., Ballenger, J.C., Lydiard, R.B., Stuart, G.W., Laraia, M.T., O'Neil, P., Fossey, M.D., Stevens, V., Lesser, S., and Hsu, L.K.G. (1990a) CSF monoamine levels in normal-weight bulimia: evidence for abnormal noradrenergic activity. *Am J Psychiatry* 147:225–229.

Kaye, W.H., Berrettini, W.H., Gwirtsman, H.E., Chretien, M., Gold, P.W., George, D.T., Jimerson, D.C., and Ebert, M.H. (1987a) Reduced cerebrospinal fluid levels of immunoreactive pro-opiomelanocortin related peptides (including beta-endorphin) in anorexia nervosa. *Life Sci* 41:2147–2155.

Kaye, W.H., Berrettini, W., Gwirtsman, H., and George, D.T. (1990b) Altered cerebrospinal fluid neuropeptide Y and peptide YY immunoreactivity in anorexia and bulimia nervosa. *Arch Gen Psychiatry* 47:548–556.

Kaye, W.H., Ebert, M.H., Raleigh, M., and Lake, R. (1984) Abnormalities in CNS monoamine metabolism in anorexia nervosa. *Arch Gen Psychiatry* 41:350–355.

Kaye, W.H., Frank, G.K.W., and McConaha, C. (1999) Altered dopamine activity after recovery from restricting-type anorexia nervosa. *Neuropsychopharmacology* 21:503–506.

Kaye, W.H., Frank, G.K., Meltzer, C.C., Price, J.C., McConaha, C.W., Crossan, P.J., Klump, K.L. (in press) Altered medial orbital frontal serotonin receptor activity after recovery from bulimia nervosa. *Am J Psychiatry*.

Kaye, W.H., Greeno, C.G., Moss, H., Fernstrom, J., Fernstrom, M., Lilenfeld, L.R., Weltzin, T.E., and Mann, J. (1998) Alterations in serotonin activity and psychiatric symptomatology after recovery from bulimia nervosa. *Arch Gen Psychiatry* 55:927–935.

Kaye, W.H., Gwirtsman, H.E., George, D.T., and Ebert, M.H. (1991) Altered serotonin activity in anorexia nervosa after long-term weight restoration: does elevated cerebrospinal fluid 5-hydroxyindoleacetic acid level correlate with rigid and obsessive behavior? *Arch Gen Psychiatry* 48:556–562.

Kaye, W.H., Gwirtsman, H.E., George, D.T., Ebert, M.H., Jimerson, D.C., Tonnai, T.P., Chrousos, G.P., and Gold, P.W. (1987b) Elevated cerebrospinal fluid levels of immunoreactive corticotropin-releasing hormone in anorexia nervosa: relation to state of nutrition, adrenal function, and intensity of depression. *J Clini Endocrinol Metab* 64:203–208.

Kaye, W.H., Lilenfeld, L.R.R., Berrettini, W.H., Strober, M., Devlin, B., Klump, K.L., Goldman, D., Bulik, C.M., Halmi, K.A., Fichter, M.M., Kaplan, A., Woodside, D.B., Treasure, J., Plotnicov, K.H., Pollice, C, Rao, R., and McConaha, C. (2000) A search for susceptibility loci for anorexia nervosa: methods and sample description. *Biol Psychiatry* 47:794–803.

Kaye, W.H., Lilenfeld, L.R., Plotnicov, K., Merikangas, K.R., Nagy, L., Strober, M. Bulik, C.M., Moss, H. and Greeno, C.G. (1996) Bulimia nervosa and substance dependence: association and family transmission. *Alcohol Clin Exp Res* 20:878–881.

Kaye, W.H., Weltzin, T.E., Nagata, T., Hsu, L.K.G., Sokol, M.S., McConaha, C., Plotnicov, K.H., Weise J., and Deep, D. (2001) Double-blind placebo-controlled administration of fluoxetine in restricting and restricting-purging-type anorexia nervosa. *Biol Psychiatry* 49:644–652.

Keel, P.K. and Mitchell, J.E. (1997) Outcome in bulimia nervosa. *Am J Psychiatry* 154:313–321.

Kendler, S.K., MacLean, C., Neale, M., Kessler, R.C., Heath, A.C., and Eaves, L.J. (1991) The genetic epidemiology of bulimia nervosa. *Am J Psychiatry* 148:1627–1637.

Kendler, K.S., Walters, E.E., Neale, M.C., Kessler, R.C., Heath, A.C., and Eaves, L.J. (1995) The structure of the genetic and environmental risk factors for six major psychiatric disorders in women. *Arch Gene Psychiatry* 52:374–383.

Klump, K.L., Bulik, C.M., Pollice, C., Halmi, K.A., Fichter, M.M., Berrettini, W., Devlin, B., Goldman, D., Strober, M., Kaplan, A., Woodside, D.B., Treasure, J., Shabbout, M., Lilenfeld, L.R.R., Plotnicov, K.H., Kaye, W.H. (2000a). Temperament and character in women with anorexia nervosa. *J Nerv Ment Dis* 188:559–567.

Klump, K.L., McGue, M., and Iacono, W.G. (2000b) Age differences in genetic and environmental influences on eating attitudes and behaviors in preadolescent and adolescent twins. *J Abnorm Psychol* 109:239–251.

Klump, K.L., McGue, M., and Iacono, W.G. (2001) Genetic and environmental influences on anorexia nervosa syndromes in a population-based sample of twins. *Psychol Med.* 31:737–740.

Lambe, E.K., Katzman, D.K., Mikulis, D.J., Kennedy, S.H., and Zipursky, R.B. (1997) Cerebral gray matter volume deficits after weight recovery from anorexia nervosa. *Arch Gen Psychiatry* 54:537–542.

Leibowitz, S.F. (1986) Brain monoamines and peptides: role in the control of eating behavior. *Fed Proc* 45:1396–1403.

Lilenfeld, L.R., Kaye, W.H., Greeno, C.G., Merikangas, K.R., Plotnicov, K., Pollice, C., Rao, R., Strober, M., Bulik, C.M., and Nagy, L. (1998) A controlled family study of anorexia nervosa and bulimia nervosa: psychiatric disorders in first-degree relatives and effects of proband comorbidity. *Arch Gen Psychiatry* 1998; 55:603–610.

Lydiard, R.B., Brewerton, T.D., Fossey, M.D., Laraia, M.T., Stuart, G., Beinfeld, M.C., and Ballenger, J.C. et al. (1993) CSF cholecystokinin octapeptide in patients with bulimia nervosa and in normal comparison subjects [see comments]. *Am J Psychiatry* 150:1099–1101.

Mantzoros, C., Flier, J.S., Lesem, M.D., Brewerton, T.D., and Jimerson, D.C. (1997) Cerebrospinal fluid leptin in anorexia nervosa: correlation with nutritional status and potential role in resistance to weight gain. *J Clin Endocrinol Metab* 82:1845–1851.

Miller, K.B., Klump, K.L., Keel, P.K., McGue, M., and Iacono, W.G. (1998) A population-based twin study of anorexia and bulimia nervosa: heritability and shared transmission with anxiety disorders. Presented at the Eating Disorder Research Society Meeting, Boston, MA.

Mitchell, J.E., Raymond, N., and Specker, S. (1993). A review of the controlled trials of pharmacotherapy and psychotherapy in the treatment of bulimia nervosa. *Int J Eat Disord* 14:229–247.

Morley, J.E. and Blundell, J.E. (1988) The neurobiological basis of eating disorders: some formulations. *Biol Psychiatry* 23:53–78.

Morley, J.E., Levine, A.S., Grace, M., and Kreip, J. (1985) Peptide YY (PYY), a potent orexigenic agent. *Brain Res* 341:200–203.

Morley, J.E., Levine, A.S., Yim, G.K., et al. (1983) Opiod modulation of appetite. *Neurosci Biobehav Revi* 7:281–305.

Nacmias, B., Ricca, V., Tedde, A., Mezzani, B., Rotella, C.M., and Sorbi, S. (1999) 5HT$_{2A}$ receptor gene polymorphisms in anorexia nervosa and bulimia nervosa. *Neurosci Lett* 277:134–136.

Naruo, T., Nakabeppu, Y., Sagiyama, K., Munemoto, T., Homan, N., Deguchi, D., Nakajo, M., and Nosoe, S. (2000) Characteristics regional cerebral blood flow patterns in anorexia nervosa patients with binge/purge behavior. *Am J Psychiatry* 157:1520–1522.

Philipp, E., Pirke, K.-M., Kellner, M.B., and Krieg, J.C. (1991) Disturbed cholecystokinin secretion in patients with eating disorders. *Life Sci* 48:2443–2450.

Pirke, K.M., Kellner, M.B., Friess, E., Krieg, J.C., and Fichter, M.M. (1994) Satiety and cholecystokinin. *Int J Eat Disord* 15: 63–69.

Pirke, K.M., Trimborn, P., Platte, P., et al. (1991) Average total energy expenditure in anorexia nervosa, bulimia nervosa, and healthy young women. *Biol Psychiatry* 30:711–718.

Rosenkranz, K., Hinney, A., Ziegler, A., Hermann, H., Fichter, M., Mayer, H., Siegfried, W., Young, J.K., Remschmidt, H., and Hebebrand, J. (1998) Systematic mutation screening of the estrogen receptor beta gene in probands of different weight extremes: identification of several genetic variants. *J Clin Endocrinol Metab* 83: 4524–4527.

Roser, W., Bubl, R., Buergin, D., Seelig, J., Radue, E.W., and Rost, B. (1999) Metabolic changes in the brain of patients with anorexia and bulimia nervosa as detected by proton magnetic resonance spectroscopy. *Int J Eat Disord* 26:119–136.

Rubin, R.T. and Kaye, W.H. (2001) Anorexia nervosa and other eating disorders. In: DeGroot, L.J., and Jameson, J.L. eds. *Endocrinology, 4th ed.* Philadelphia: W.B. Saunders, pp. 215–225.

Salamone, J.D. (1996) The behavioral neurochemistry of motivation: methodological and conceptual issues in studies of the dynamic activity of nucleus accumbens dopamine. *J Neurosci Methods* 64: 137–149.

Schuckit, M.A., Tipp, J.E., Anthenelli, R.M., Bucholz, K.K., Hesselbrock, V.M., and Nurnberger, J.I. Jr., Anthenelli, R.M., et al. (1996) Anorexia nervosa and bulimia nervosa in alcohol-dependent men and women and their relatives. *Am J Psychiatry* 153:74–82.

Schweiger, U. and Fichter, M. (1997) Clinical presentation, classification and etiologic models. In: Kaye, W.H. and Jimerson, D.C., eds. *Eating Disorders.* Balliere's Clinical Psychiatry, Balliere's Tindall, pp. 199–216.

Sorbi, S., Nacmias, B., Tedde, A., Ricca, V., Mezzani, B., and Rotella, C.M. (1998) 5-HT2A promoter polymorphism in anorexia nervosa. *Lancet* 351:1785.

Soubrie, P. (1986) Reconciling the role of central serotonin neurosis in human and animal behavior. *Behav Brain Sci* 9:319–363.

Srinivasagam, N.M., Kaye, W.H., Plotnicov, K.H., Greeno, C, Weltzin, TE, and Rao, R. (1995) Persistent perfectionism, symmetry, and exactness after long-term recovery from anorexia nervosa. *Am J Psychiatry* 152:1630–1634.

Stanley, B.G., Kyrkouli, S.E., Lampert, S., et al. (1986) Neuropeptide Y chronically injected into the hypothalamus: a powerful neurochemical inducer of hyperphagia and obesity. *Peptides* 7:1189–1192.

Stein, D.J., Hollander, E., and Liebowitz, M.R. (1993) Neurobiology of impulsivity and impulse control disorders. *J Neuropsychiatry Clin Neurosci* 5:9–17.

Strober, M. (1980) Personality and symptomatological features in young, nonchronic anorexia nervosa patients. *J Psychosom Res* 24:353–359.

Strober, M., Freeman, R., Lampert, C., Diamond, J., and Kaye, W. (2000) A controlled family study of anorexia nervosa and bulimia nervosa: evidence of shared liability and transmission of partial syndromes. *Am J Psychiatry* 157:393–401.

Sullivan, P.F., Bulik, C.M., and Kendler, K.S. (1998) The epidemiology and classification of bulimia nervosa. *Psychol Med* 28:599–610.

Tamai, H., Takemura, J., Kobayashi, N., Matasubayashi, S., Matasukura, S., and Nakagawa, T. (1993) Changes in plasma cholecystokinin concentrations after oral glucose tolerance test in anorexia nervosa before and after therapy. Metab Clini Exp 42: 581–584.

Tellegen, A., Lykken, D.T., Bouchard, T.J., Wilcox, K.J., Segal, N.L., and Rich, S. (1988) Personality similarity in twins reared apart and together. *J Soc Pers Psychol* 54:1031–1039.

Treasure, J. and Campbell, I. (1994) The case for biology in the aetiology of anorexia nervosa. Psychol Med 24:3–8.

Treasure, J., Schmidt, U., Troop, N., Tiller J., Todd, G., and Turnbull, S. (1996) Sequential treatment for bulimia nervosa incorporating a self-care manual. *Br J Psychiatry* 168:94–98.

Vitousek, K. and Manke, F. (1994) Personality variables and disorders in anorexia nervosa and bulimia nervosa. *J Abnorm Psychol* 103:137–47.

Wade, T., Martin, N.G., and Tiggeman, M. (1998) Genetic and environmental risk factors for the weight and shape concerns characteristic of bulimia nervosa. *Psychol Med* 28:761–771.

Wade, T., Martin, N.G., Neale, M.C., Tiggemann, M., Treloar, S.A., Bucholz, K.K., Madden, P.A., and Heath, A.C. (1999) The structure of genetic and environmental risk factors for three measures of disordered eating. *Psychol Med* 29:925–934.

Wade, T.D., Bulik, C.M., Neale, M., and Kendler, K.S. (2000) Anorexia nervosa and major depression: an examination of shared genetic and environmental risk factors. *Am J Psychiatry* 157:469–471.

Walsh, B.T. (1991) Psychopharmacologic treatment of bulimia nervosa. *J Clin Psychiatry* 52(Suppl):34–38.

Walsh, B.T., Katz, J.L., Levin, J., Kream, J., Fukushima, D.K., Hellman, L.D., Weiner, H., and Zumoff, B. (1978) Adrenal activity in anorexia nervosa. *Psychosom Med* 40:499–506.

Walters, E.E. and Kendler, K.S. (1995) Anorexia nervosa and anorexic-like syndromes in a population-based twin sample. *Am J Psychiatry* 152:64–71.

Zhang, Y., Proenca, R., Maffei, M., Barone, M., Leopold, L., and Friedman, J.M. (1994) Positional cloning of the mouse obese gene and its human homologue. *Nature* 372:425–432.

Ziegler, A., Hebebrand, J., Gorg, T., Rosenkranz, K., Fichter, M.M., Herpertz-Dahlmann, B., Remschmidt, H., and Hinney, A. (1999) Further lack of association between the 5-HT2A gene promoter polymorphism and susceptibility to eating disorders and a meta-analysis pertaining to anorexia nervosa. *Mol Psychiatry* 4:410–412.

19 | Neurobiology of substance abuse and dependence disorders

LESLIE K. JACOBSEN

Substance abuse and dependence disorders occurring during childhood or adolescence, just as other psychiatric disorders that develop during this period, are associated with significant functional impairment and, in some cases, mortality. However, a critical difference between these and other psychiatric disorders is that the existence of substance abuse and dependence disorders requires an external agent that is available and potent, and a host who is willing to self-administer the agent. This key difference shapes both the neurobiologic and the psychosocial underpinning of this class of disorders.

DEFINITIONS

The fourth edition of the *Diagnostic and Statistical Manual of Mental Disorders* (DSM-IV) (American Psychiatric Association, 1994) defines *substance dependence* as a pattern of substance use leading to clinically significant impairment or distress, which can be manifested by tolerance (need for increased amounts of the substance to achieve intoxication), withdrawal, taking of larger amounts of the substance than intended, unsuccessful efforts to control substance use, expenditure of a great deal of time procuring, using, and recovering from the substance, and resulting abandonment of social, occupational, and recreational activities, or continued use of the substance despite awareness of problems that it is creating in the user's life. The DSM-IV definition of *substance abuse* is similar to that of substance dependence but does not include tolerance, withdrawal, or a pattern of compulsive use. However, these criteria may not be completely appropriate for teenagers. In particular, children and adolescents are less likely than adults to be able to link specific sequelae to substance use and thus may never be aware of the contribution of substance use to their problems.

Furthermore, these definitions do not capture differences between ramifications of the use of widely available substances, such as tobacco and ethanol, and ramifications of the use of less widely available substances, such as heroin.

PREVALENCE AND PATTERNS OF SUBSTANCE USE

Most epidemiologic studies of substance use among United States youth have focused upon adolescents (ages 12 to 18). Ethanol and tobacco are the most frequently used substances by adolescents, with 51% of 12th graders, 40% of 10th graders, and 24% of 8th graders reporting that they consumed at least one alcoholic beverage in the preceding 30 days in the 1999 Monitoring the Future Survey (Johnston et al., 2000). *Binge drinking,* defined as consuming five or more drinks in a row during the prior 2-week interval, was reported by 30.8% of 12th graders, 25.6% of 10th graders, and 15.2% of 8th graders in 1999. The prevalence of tobacco use among adolescents has been increasing steadily since 1992. In 1999, the National Youth Tobacco Survey indicated that 34.8% of 11th graders reported current tobacco use (MMWR, 2000). In contrast, the rate of current tobacco use among United States adults is 23% (http://www2.cdc.gov).

Marijuana has been the most widely used illicit substance by adolescents for the past 25 years, with annual prevalence rates in grades 12, 10, and 8 in 1999 of 37.8%, 32.1%, and 16.5%, respectively (Johnston et al., 2000). Current daily prevalence rates (defined as the proportion using it on 20 or more occasions in the prior 30 days) were 6% among 12th graders, 3.8% among 10th graders, and 1.4% among 8th graders in 1999. The annual prevalence rate of use of all other substances was less than 10% among all grades surveyed in 1999, with the exception of inhalants (annual prevalence rate of 5.6%, 7.2%, and 10.3% among 12th, 10th, and 8th graders, respectively) and non-prescribed use of amphetamines (annual prevalence rate of 10.2%, 10.4%, and 6.9% among 12th, 10th and 8th graders, respectively) (Johnston et al., 2000).

Although surveys such as the Monitoring the Future Survey and the National Youth Tobacco Survey provide the most accurate prevalence estimates available for substance use among adolescents, these surveys are restricted to adolescents attending school and so exclude truants and school dropouts. Because these excluded groups are also at increased risk for substance use, the prevalence rates provided by these surveys very likely underestimate the true prevalence rates.

Longitudinal studies of substance use have supported the existence of sequential stages of substance use, beginning with the use of licit substances, such as tobacco and ethanol, and progressing to illicit substances, particularly marijuana (Kandel et al., 1992).

NEUROANATOMICAL SUBSTRATES OF REWARD

The neuropharmacologic profiles of the different classes of abused substances, including sedative-hypnotics, opiates, psychostimulants, and cannabinoids, are vastly different. Not surprisingly, each class is associated with a distinct syndrome of intoxication and of withdrawal. Yet, despite their distinct pharmacologic profiles, the rewarding properties of these drugs appear to involve activation of common brain reward circuits. These circuits are also activated by conventional reinforcers, such as food, water, and sex. Adaptation of this reward circuitry to chronic drug use leads to the development of tolerance to the euphorigenic effects of the drug and the consequent need to consume increasing amounts of the drug to experience a "high." In addition, neuroadaptation of this circuitry to chronic substance use mediates the emergence of intense negative affective motivational states, including dysphoria, depression, irritability, and anxiety, when drug use is terminated (Koob, 1999b).

Preclinical Studies

Animal studies have provided compelling evidence supporting a central role for the mesocortical dopamine system in drug reward. The chief components of this circuit are the ventral tegmental area, the basal forebrain (including the nucleus accumbens, frontal cortex, and amygdala), and the dopaminergic connections between the ventral tegmental area and the basal fore-

brain (Koob, 1999b). Recent work has supported the importance of a second system, termed the *extended amygdala*, in drug reward. The extended amygdala is a network of basal forebrain structures including the bed nucleus of the stria terminalis, the central medial amygdala, the shell of the nucleus accumbens, and the sublenticular substantia innominata (Koob, 1999b).

Enhancement of dopamine neurotransmission in the mesocorticolimbic dopamine system is critical for the acute reinforcing action of psychostimulants. The reinforcing properties of opiates, ethanol, and tetrahydrocannabinol (the chief psychoactive component of cannabis and hashish) also involve facilitated mesocorticolimbic dopaminergic neurotransmission, as well as facilitation of other neurotransmitter systems within the mesocorticolimbic dopamine system, including gamma-aminobutyric acid (GABA), glutamate, serotonin, and opioid peptide systems. Most major drugs of abuse also activate dopaminergic neurotransmission in the shell of the nucleus accumbens (Koob and LeMoal, 1997).

Clinical Studies

Functional imaging studies that have examined brain response to drug administration in humans have corroborated the importance of the mesocorticolimbic system in response to drug administration and in drug craving. The effects of nicotine and cocaine administration have both been examined using functional magnetic resonance imaging (fMRI), a method of imaging with high temporal (on the order of seconds) and spatial (on the order of millimeters) resolution. Both agents were found to activate nucleus accumbens. In addition, both activated cingulate and frontal lobe cortical regions (Breiter et al., 1997; Stein et al., 1998). The effects of tetrahydrocannabinol (THC) administration in marijuana abusers has been examined using ^{18}F-fluorodeoxyglucose and positron emission tomography (PET), a lower-resolution imaging modality. During THC intoxication, activation of basal ganglia (spatial resolution is too low to distinguish nucleus accumbens from basal ganglia), prefrontal, and orbitofrontal cortices was observed (Volkow et al., 1996a). Imaging studies examining cerebral response to ethanol intoxication have shown that ethanol decreases global and regional brain glucose metabolism with sparing of basal ganglia and corpus callosum (de Wit et al., 1990; Volkow et al., 1990). The pattern of decreases in regional brain glucose metabolism with ethanol administration parallels the distribution of benzodiazepine receptors (Volkow et al., 1990). In contrast, regional cerebral blood flow is increased by acute administration of ethanol, particularly in the prefrontal cortex (Netrakom et al., 1999).

NEUROBIOLOGY OF SUBSTANCE ABUSE AND DEPENDENCE: ANIMAL MODELS

Although there is no animal model that incorporates all elements of substance dependence, animal models have been developed and validated for specific key dimensions of substance dependence. The development and maintenance of substance dependence has been conceptualized to result from both positive and negative reinforcing effects of substance use (Koob, 2000b). The existence of positive reinforcing effects is required for the initiation of substance self-administration and for vulnerability to relapse to substance self-administration. Because of the potent positive reinforcing effects of substances with abuse potential, both animals and humans will self-administer these agents in the nondependent state. Indeed, the degree to which animals will self-administer a substance is predictive of abuse potential in humans (Collins et al., 1984). Three of the most widely used animal models to study the neurobiology of the positive reinforcing effects of substances are oral or intravenous (IV) drug self-administration, conditioned place preference, and intracranial self-stimulation (ICSS).

In drug self-administration paradigms, animals are trained to emit a certain behavior, such as pressing a lever, in order to receive an oral or injected dose of the drug under study. The frequency and duration of the behavior while it is paired with drug administration, as well as the persistence of the behavior after it is no longer paired with drug administration, are both strongly correlated with abuse liability (Collins et al., 1984). In conditioned place preference paradigms, drug administration is paired with an environment with distinct sensory cues while saline administration is paired with a second environment with different sensory cues. After repeated exposure to the drug–environment pairing, the duration of time that animals spend in each environment is measured in the absence of drug or saline administration. The degree to which animals prefer the environment paired with drug exposure is strongly correlated with the abuse liability of the drug (Tzschentke, 1998). The ICSS, or brain stimulation reward, paradigm involves unilateral implantation of an electrode into the medial forebrain bundle. Animals experience pulses of current delivered through the electrode as highly rewarding and will work (e.g., press a

lever or rotate a wheel) to receive current pulses. Drugs of abuse reliably lower the current intensity level prompting animals to work for more stimulation (Kornetsky et al., 1979), which is generally considered an index of the rewarding properties of the drug.

Animal models of the negative reinforcing properties of drugs of abuse include self-administration of drug during withdrawal in dependent animals, self-administration of increasingly larger amounts of drug in dependent animals (tolerance), and ICSS. Self-administration during drug deprivation has shown, for example, that ethanol-dependent animals will significantly increase their intake of ethanol after a period of forced abstinence from regular drinking. This has been termed the *ethanol deprivation effect* and is considered a useful model for testing anti craving/antirelapse compounds (Koob, 2000a). The ICSS paradigms have shown that withdrawal from chronic administration of drugs with abuse liability reliably increases the current intensity level prompting animals to work for more stimulation. This is considered to be an index of the negative affective and motivational state induced by drug withdrawal (Schulteis et al., 1995).

ACUTE ACTIONS OF DRUGS OF ABUSE

Psychostimulants

Psychostimulant reinforcement is mediated by the central monoamines, particularly dopamine. Cocaine binds to presynaptic dopamine, serotonin, and norepinephrine transporters, thereby inhibiting reuptake of all three monoamines from the synaptic cleft and potentiating monaminergic neurotransmission. Amphetamine and its derivatives (e.g., methamphetamine, methylenedioxy-methamphetamine, or ecstasy) potentiate monoaminergic neurotransmission by increasing monoamine release. Amphetamine is transported into nerve terminals by monoamine transporters where it interacts with vesicles storing monoamine transmitters, leading to release of these transmitters and their reverse transport into the synaptic cleft (Koob, 1999b).

Self-administration of psychostimulants by humans produces a syndrome of intoxication, the symptoms of which can include elevated pulse and blood pressure, pupillary dilation, euphoria, and psychomotor agitation. Ingestion of excessive amounts can result in compulsive behavior, psychotic symptoms that include auditory and visual hallucinations and paranoid delusions, chest pain, arrhythmias, dyskinesias, and seizures.

Nicotine

Nicotine is a psychostimulant that binds stereoselectively to nicotinic acetylcholine receptors (nAChRs) in the brain, autonomic ganglia, adrenals, and at the neuromuscular junction. Nicotine exerts an excitatory effect on dopamine neurons of the ventral tegmentum. Neuronal nAChRs consist of combinations of α (2–9) and β (2–4) subunits arranged to form a pentameric receptor. Evidence suggests that excitation of dopaminergic neurons in the ventral tegmental area by nicotine is mediated directly by the action of nicotine at high-affinity nAChRs on these neurons and by the action of nicotine at nAChRs at presynaptic sites, which may modulate glutamatergic inputs to these dopaminergic neurons (Mansvelder and McGehee, 2000).

Nicotine is typically self-administered via smoking tobacco, however, it is readily absorbed through the oral (chew) and nasal (snuff) mucosa. Among adolescents, nicotine is the most widely abused substance. Acute administration produces both stimulating and rewarding effects. Animal and some human studies have shown that nicotine improves both memory and attention.

Ingestion of excessive amounts of nicotine can result in nicotine poisoning, the signs and symptoms of which include pallor, diaphoresis, nausea, vomiting, salivation, abdominal pain, diarrhea, headache, dizziness, auditory and visual disturbance, tremor, confusion, and weakness. Hypotension and respiratory failure develop with large overdoses. The minimum oral acute lethal dose for nicotine in adult humans is estimated to be only 40 to 60 mg.

Opioids

Three principle types of opioid receptors have been identified; μ, δ, and κ. All three types are coupled to G proteins that have seven transmembrane segments. Stimulation of these receptors by opioid agonists inhibits adenylyl cylclase, leading to reduced intracellular levels of cyclic adenosine monophosphate (AMP), altered protein phosphorylation, and changes in gene transcription. These changes in gene expression appear to mediate long-term effects of chronic opioid use. Acutely, activation of opioid receptors increases K^+ conductance, leading to hyperpolarization and inhibition of firing. This action is critical to the reinforcing properties of opioids, which are mediated by activation of dopaminergic neurons of the ventral tegmental area. For example, local GABA-releasing interneurons in the ventral tegmental area have μ-opioid receptors. When

these receptors are stimulated by morphine, for example, inhibitory GABA release onto ventral tegmental dopaminergic cells diminishes and their firing rate consequently increases (Di Chiara and North, 1992).

Acute administration of opioids, particularly in non-tolerant individuals, produces a syndrome of intoxication characterized by pupillary dilation and initial euphoria, followed by apathy, psychomotor retardation, slurred speech, and impaired attention and memory. Opioid overdose can produce fatal respiratory depression and thus is a medical emergency.

Ethanol and Sedative Hypnotics

The acute effects of ethanol and other sedative-hypnotics are mediated by actions at a number of receptor systems. For example, ethanol inhibits several excitatory receptor systems, including N-methyl-D-aspartate (NMDA) receptors, kainate receptors, and Ca^{2+} channels. In addition, ethanol enhances the action of GABA at $GABA_A$ receptors and appears to modulate serotonergic neurotransmission. Although a component of ethanol reinforcement is mediated by the activation of mesocorticolimbic dopamine neurons, activation of these neurons may not be necessary for ethanol reinforcement, as ethanol remains reinforcing in the absence of these neurons (Samson and Harris, 1992; Koob, 2000b).

Ethanol and sedative hypnotic intoxication are both characterized by behavioral disinhibition, which can be manifested as inappropriate aggressive or sexual behavior, mood lability, and impaired judgement. Associated signs include slurred speech, incoordination, unsteady gait, nystagmus, and impaired attention and memory. Ingestion of excessive amounts can result in stupor, coma, and death from respiratory depression.

Cannabis

Cannabis sativa plants contain at least 400 different compounds, of which as many as 60 are structurally related to δ⁹-tetrahydrocannabinol (δ⁹-THC), the primary psychoactive constituent of cannabis. When cannabis is smoked, hundreds of additional compounds are produced by pyrolysis, which may contribute to both acute and chronic effects (Abood and Martin, 1992). The central nervous system actions of cannabinoids are mediated primarily through the CB_1 receptor. A second type of cannabinoid receptor, termed the CB_2 receptor, is distributed primarily in the periphery (Gifford et al., 1999). Activation of central cannabinoid receptors modulates neurotransmitter release at the presynaptic level, inhibiting glutamate and acetylcholine release in hippocampus and GABA release in substantia nigra (Gifford et al., 1999), and activating dopaminergic neurons in the ventral tegmentum and substantia nigra (Wu and French, 2000). Activation of midbrain dopaminergic neurons likely mediates the euphorigenic properties of exogenous cannabinoids and, in the case of the ventral tegmentum, does not appear to attenuate with chronic exposure to the drug (Wu and French, 2000).

δ^9-THC is usually consumed via smoking cannabis, but it can also be ingested orally. Cannabis intoxication is typically characterized by an initial period of euphoria, followed by a period of drowsiness or sedation. Impaired motor coordination, anxiety, a sensation of slowed time, impaired judgement, social withdrawal, conjunctival injection, increased appetite, dry mouth, and tachycardia are frequently observed during cannabis intoxication. Use of excessive amounts has been associated with development of panic attacks and paranoia.

NEUROBIOLOGY OF CHRONIC EFFECTS OF DRUG USE

The neurobiology of drug use initiation rests upon the acute reinforcing effects of drugs of abuse. In contrast, the core features of drug addiction, which include development of a withdrawal syndrome upon cessation of drug use and heightened vulnerability to relapse, reflect the effects of neuroadaptation to chronic drug use. The molecular actions of the different classes of abused drugs differ widely, so that chronic use of each drug is associated with a distinct pattern of brain changes, including distinctive changes in receptor density and function. However, recent work has highlighted the importance of neuroadaptive changes that appear to be a common result of chronic use of all abused substances. Specifically, chronic use of drugs of abuse results in adaptive changes within the same reward circuits mediating reinforcing effects of drugs—the mesocortical dopamine system and the extended amygdala. In animals, these chronic changes increase the level of stimulation required to prompt an animal to work for more stimulation in ICSS paradigms. In humans, neuroadaptation of reward circuitry resulting from chronic drug use is believed to mediate the negative affective states, including dysphoria, depression, irritability, and anxiety, associated with acute drug withdrawal (Koob, 2000b). These negative affective states play a prominent role in drug withdrawal syndromes, craving, and

vulnerability to relapse and, as a result, are a focus of treatment.

A second common adaptive response to chronic drug use involves chronic changes in brain and pituitary stress systems. Pituitary adrenal function is altered in response to chronic drug use. Extrapituitary brain corticotropin-releasing factor (CRF) systems are activated during acute withdrawal from psychostimulants, opiates, ethanol, and cannabis and this activation may mediate the anxiogenic and stress-like symptoms of acute withdrawal (Koob, 2000b). Microinjection of CRF antagonist into the central nucleus of the amygdala can reverse these aversive symptoms of acute withdrawal in animals (Koob, 2000b).

Psychostimulants

Receptor studies

Both postmortem and in vivo studies have demonstrated significantly increased dopamine transporter and serotonin transporter binding sites in cocaine-dependent patients (Jacobsen et al., 2000; Mash et al., in press). The bulk of evidence suggests that dopamine D_1 receptor density is decreased, but dopamine D_2 receptor density is unchanged after chronic cocaine exposure (Staley, 1998). Postmortem studies have also found evidence for elevation of κ-opioid receptor binding sites in anterior and ventral striatum and nucleus accumbens in human cocaine overdose victims (Staley, 1998). Finally, preclinical studies have provided evidence for increased cortical and ventral tegmental NMDA receptor binding following chronic cocaine exposure.

Human postmortem studies of tobacco smokers have shown significant increases in nAChR binding in hippocampus, caudate, and cortex, with the amount of up-regulation being positively correlated with the amount of tobacco used (Breese et al., 2000). Although nicotine is an nAChR agonist, this up-regulation likely reflects adaptation to the rapid desensitization of nAChR receptors following stimulation with nicotine.

Brain morphology

Brain morphometric studies of cocaine abusers have revealed evidence for enlargement of caudate and putamen during initial abstinence, but no evidence for changes in total brain volume or volume of medial temporal lobe structures (Jacobsen et al., 2001 a,b). Enlargement of basal ganglia structures likely reflects dopamine depletion that appears to develop following cessation of chronic cocaine use.

Cerebral blood flow, metabolism, and function

The effects of chronic cocaine use on brain function have been studied during both acute and extended abstinence from cocaine. Early in abstinence, regional cerebral glucose metabolism is increased in orbitofrontal cortex and basal ganglia (Volkow et al., 1991). These differences appear to normalize after 2 to 4 weeks of abstinence (Volkow et al., 1991). Chronic cocaine use is associated with decreased cerebral blood flow in frontal, temporal, parietal, and striatal regions (Holman et al., 1991). Abstinence coupled with treatment with buprenorphine, a mixed opioid agonist-antagonist, has been shown to improve regional cerebral blood flow in these patients, although it is not clear whether this improvement would occur with abstinence from cocaine alone (Holman et al., 1993).

Ethanol

Receptor studies

In vivo studies of alcoholics have shown marked reductions in striatal dopamine transporter binding upon admission for detoxification, with recovery of dopamine transporter binding to normal levels after a 4-week period of abstinence (Laine et al., 1999). Brain stem serotonin transporter binding has been found to be reduced in alcoholics during withdrawal, with the reduction being correlated with withdrawal-associated depression and anxiety (Heinz et al., 1998). Benzodiazepine receptor binding has been found to be reduced in frontal, anterior cingulate, and cerebellar cortices in alcoholics (Abi-Dargham et al., 1998). Although two studies have found decreased dopamine D_2 receptor binding availability in alcoholics, others have observed increased or unchanged D_2 receptor binding availability in this population (Volkow et al., 1996b).

Brain morphology

Interest in changes in brain morphology associated with alcoholism was initially stimulated by the increased incidence of frank encephalopathy among these patients. In patients with chronic alcoholism, including those without cognitive deficits, brain volume and brain weight are decreased. Postmortem studies have shown that both white matter and neuronal density of gray matter are decreased. Cortical volume loss appears to be most pronounced in the frontal lobes. Heavy drinking accelerates age-related myelin loss and cerebellar atrophy is common. Reduction in the volume of subcortical structures, such as the hippocampus, appears to be proportional, and not disproportionately greater than, reduction in cortical volume (Agartz et al., 1999). Women may be more vulnerable to ethanol-induced central nervous system (CNS) damage, as studies have demonstrated evidence of decreased brain volume and decreased midsagittal corpus callosum area in female alcoholics of a magnitude similar to that seen in male alcoholics, despite shorter durations and lower levels of drinking in women. This gender difference in vulnerability may be mediated by several factors, including lower body weight and lower total body water volume in women than in men. In addition, women have less gastric alcohol dehydrogenase than men (Ragan et al., 1999). Longitudinal studies have documented partial recovery of brain volume loss with extended abstinence from ethanol (Muuronen et al., 1989).

Cerebral blood flow, metabolism, and function

The spectrum of cognitive deficits associated with chronic alcohol use extends to the extreme of Wernicke's encephalopathy and Korsakoff's psychosis. *Wernicke's encephalopathy* is an acute neurologic syndrome caused by thiamine deficiency. Symptoms include mental confusion, ophthalmoplegia, and ataxia. Many of these symptoms reverse with administration of thiamine; however; about 50% of patients are left with some degree of ataxia. Left untreated, Wernicke's encephalopathy can progress to stupor, coma, and death. Approximately 80% to 90% of alcoholics treated for Wernicke's encephalopathy are left with *Korsakoff's psychosis*, a syndrome of impaired learning and recent memory produced by lesions of the medial dorsal nuclei of the thalamus.

Ethanol-related cognitive deficits in the absence of Wernicke's encephalopathy also improve with extended abstinence. Most functional neuroimaging studies of abstinent alcoholics have shown decreases in both cerebral glucose metabolism and blood flow, with the decreases being greatest in the frontal lobes (Netrakom et al., 1999).

Opiates

Receptor studies

Postmortem studies of humans with opiate dependence have shown that μ-opiate receptor density is unchanged in frontal cortex, thalamus, and caudate. In contrast, α_{-2} adrenoceptor density is decreased in these regions, while Gα-protein density in frontal cortex may be increased (Gabilondo et al., 1994; Garcia-Sevilla et al., 1997).

Brain morphology

Few brain morphometric studies of opiate abusers have been conducted and these have been poorly controlled and have utilized lower-resolution technologies, such as computed tomography. These preliminary studies have suggested that brain volume may be decreased in chronic opiate abusers.

Cannabis

Receptor studies

To date, little postmortem work has been done in human cannabis abusers. Preclinical studies indicate that chronic treatment with δ^9-THC markedly reduces CB_1 receptor binding in all brain areas containing this receptor (cerebellum, hippocampus, cortex, globus pallidus, striatum), and enhances the cAMP pathway (Rubino et al., 2000). Other preclinical work has shown that the cannabinoid receptor reserve is larger than that for most other G protein–coupled receptor systems (Gifford et al., 1999). This means that at occupancies as low as 0.13%, 50% of maximal inhibition of Ach release is achieved.

Brain morphology

As in the case of chronic opiate abuse, few brain morphometric studies of human cannabis abusers have been conducted. However, recent preclinical work has demonstrated that δ^9-THC concentrations as low as 0.5 to 1 μM, which are compatible with plasma δ^9-THC levels achieved by humans ingesting marijuana, are toxic to hippocampal neurons (Chan et al., 1998). This hippocampal toxicity may underlie the cognitive deficits observed in chronic marijuana users, which have been shown to persist after abstinence (Pope and Yurgelun-Todd, 1996).

RISK FACTORS FOR DEVELOPMENT OF SUBSTANCE ABUSE AND DEPENDENCE

Genetic Vulnerabilities

Twin, family, and adoption studies

Twin, family, and adoption studies have suggested that heritable factors are important in the development of

substance abuse and dependence. Grove and colleagues (1990) studied 32 sets of monozygotic (MZ) twins reared apart, using blind structured interviews. Significantly less variance in scores for drug-related problems was observed between members of the same MZ twin pairs than between members of different MZ twin pairs. Heath and colleagues (1991b) examined self-report data on alcohol consumption from 3810 adult MZ and dizygotic (DZ) twin pairs. Results of their analysis suggested that the frequency of alcohol consumption and quantity that subjects tended to consume are inherited as independent factors (Heath et al., 1991a), with heritability estimates of 0.66 in females and 0.42–0.75 in males for frequency; and 0.57 in females and 0.24–0.61 in males for quantity, depending on the model used. Pickens and colleagues (1991) found modest estimates of heritability of alcohol abuse or dependence (0.35 for males, 0.24 for females) in a study involving structured interviews of 81 MZ and 88 DZ twin pairs. However, later reanalysis of their data suggested that heritability of risk for alcohol abuse or dependence was much greater (0.73) in males with early age of onset, relative to males with later onset or to females (McGue et al., 1992).

Kendler and colleagues (1992), conducting structured blind interviews of 1030 female–female MZ and DZ twin pairs, found estimates of heritability of risk for alcoholism in women of 0.50 to 0.60. Recently, Kendler and colleagues (1997) examined 8935 male–male twin pairs of known zygosity, and estimated from these data that heritability of risk for alcohol abuse was 0.54. Tsuang and colleagues (1996) examined 3372 twin pairs and found evidence that 34% of the observed variance in drug abuse was due to genetic factors. Thus, estimates of heritability of alcoholism and drug abuse from twin studies range from modest to strong, with stronger estimates of heritability emerging when phenotypic subgroups are considered.

A recent series of twin studies has examined genetic contributions to tobacco smoking. Data from these studies suggest that as much as 50% of the variance in smoking initiation may be due to variance in genetic factors (True et al., 1997; Han et al., 1999). Evidence from these studies further suggests that separate genetic factors may contribute to the persistence of smoking behavior, explaining as much as 70% of the variance in nicotine dependence (Han et al., 1999; Kendler et al., 1999).

Cross-fostering adoption studies have similarly demonstrated support for a genetic contribution to risk for developing alcohol or drug abuse problems. In an examination of 913 women adopted by nonrelatives at an early age Bohman and colleagues (1981) found a threefold excess of alcohol abusers among adopted daughters of alcoholic biological mothers relative to other daughters. This group (Cloninger et al., 1981) also examined 862 men adopted by nonrelatives at an early age and identified a highly heritable form of alcoholism related to severe alcohol abuse, severe criminality, and extensive treatment in the biological father (type 2 alcoholism). In two large studies of children adopted at birth, Cadoret and colleagues (1986; 1995) found that alcoholism and antisocial personality disorder in biological parents significantly increased the risk of substance abuse among adoptees. Finally, a controlled family study (Rounsaville et al., 1991) found significantly increased relative risk for substance abuse, alcoholism, antisocial personality, and major depression among first-degree relatives of opiate-addicted probands compared to relatives of controls.

Candidate gene studies have focused on genes coding for proteins involved in reward neurocircuitry. These studies have provided evidence that carriers of the 9-repeat allele of the dopamine transporter gene (*SLC6A3*) and the A2 allele of the D_2 receptor gene may be less likely to use tobacco (Lerman et al., 1999). Other studies have provided evidence for an association between the A1 allele of the D_2 receptor gene and alcoholism (Comings and Blum, 2000).

Quantitative trait loci

Quantitative trait loci (QTL) mapping is a method in which inbred strains of mice with differing preferences for drugs or alcohol are bred and the drug or alcohol preference of the resulting progeny is measured. The QTL mapping of those animals exhibiting extreme levels of drug or alcohol consumption is then used to identify chromosomal locations of genes contributing to drug or alcohol preference. Using this method, genes have been identified that influence morphine preference (Berrettini et al., 1994), sensitivity to ethanol (Browman and Crabbe, 2000), and sensitivity to cocaine (Jones et al., 1999).

Environmental Factors

While genetic studies provide clear evidence that a substantial proportion of the variation in risk for developing a substance abuse or dependence disorder is accounted for by genetic variation, these studies also point to a significant environmental contribution. Although environmental determinants of risk for substance abuse or dependence are undoubtedly complex, recent work has indicated that environmental stress can

play a pivotal role at multiple stages in the development of substance dependence.

Role of Stress in Initiation of Drug Use

Both clinical and epidemiological studies have provided evidence for a link between trauma and later substance abuse and dependence. Adolescents with alcohol and/or substance dependence disorders are 6 to 21 times more likely to have a physical and/or sexual abuse history than adolescents without a substance dependence disorder (Clark et al., 1997; Anda et al., 1999). In addition, rates of lifetime post-traumatic stress disorder have been estimated to be as high as 29% in this population (Deykin and Buka, 1997). High rates of other anxiety disorders, such as social phobia, have also been observed among adults with substance dependence and a history of childhood trauma (de Wit et al., 2000). These observations have led to the proposal that persons with stress-related anxiety disorders may both use drugs to control their symptoms of anxiety (self medication) and/or experience greater reward associated with drug use (modulation of reward circuitry by prior exposure to trauma) (Jacobsen et al., in 2001c).

Preclinical work has provided further support for the notion that stress may modulate the response of reward neurocircuitry to drugs of abuse. Both prenatal stress, such as maternal restraint during the third and fourth week of gestation, and neonatal isolation stress have been found to increase proclivity toward psychostimulant self-administration in rats (Deminiere et al., 1992; Kosten et al., 2000). Similarly, in adult animals naive to illicit substances, a large range of stressors increase proclivity toward psychostimulant self administration (Schenk et al., 1987; Piazza et al., 1990; Maccari et al., 1991; Deroche et al., 1994; Goeders and Guerin, 1994).

Role of stress in progression from substance use to dependence

The neurobiology mediating the transition from experimentation to compulsive drug use and dependence remains incompletely understood. Preclinical studies suggest that stress can play an important role in this transition. In addition to the abovementioned studies showing that stress can enhance proclivity toward drug self-administration, other work has shown that animals demonstrating a more sustained corticosterone secretion following stress are more likely to spontaneously self-administer psychostimulants (Piazza et al., 1989).

While much preclinical work has focused on corticosterone as mediating proclivity toward drug self-administration, other work has highlighted the importance of corticotropin-releasing hormone (CRH), which is the primary physiological regulator of adrenocorticotropic hormone (ACTH) and β-endorphin release from the anterior pituitary during stress. However, the distribution of CRH in the CNS far exceeds that required for its role in ACTH and β-endorphin release. The CRH-containing cells and fibers exist in the paraventricular nucleus of the hypothalamus, central nucleus of the amygdala, prefrontal cortex, cingulate cortex, bed nucleus of the stria terminalis, substantia innominata, locus coeruleus, and the parabrachialis nucleus (Koob, 1999a). Central, but not peripheral, administration of CRH induces a long lasting enhancement (sensitization) of the locomotor response to D-amphetamine (Cador et al., 1993), while pretreatment with a CRH antagonist blocks the development of stress induced sensitization to D-amphetamine (Cole et al., 1990).

Stress, craving, and relapse to drug use

Clinical studies have demonstrated that humans with alcohol or drug dependence most frequently identify stress and negative mood states as reasons for relapse and ongoing drug and alcohol abuse (Ludwig and Wikler, 1974; Litman et al., 1977; Bradley et al., 1989; Wallace, 1989; Brewer et al., 1998). In fact, stressful events and negative mood states, such as anger, fear, and sadness, often coincide when craving is precipitated. Recently, a personalized stress imagery task was shown to reliably increase ratings of cocaine craving and subjective anxiety in cocaine addicts (Sinha et al., 1999). Stress imagery induction of craving was also associated with significant increases in salivary cortisol in this study.

Animal studies have shown that stress reliably precipitates relapse to heroin and to cocaine self-administration in rats trained to self-administer these drugs and then subjected to extinction and to prolonged drug-free periods (Shaham and Stewart, 1995; Erb et al., 1996).

IMPACT OF DRUGS OF ABUSE ON DEVELOPING BRAIN: STUDIES OF PRENATAL EXPOSURE

Brain development occurs in a complex series of events regulated by cellular and environmental interactions (Levitt, 1998). Most abused substances readily cross the placenta. Many are concentrated in the amniotic fluid and metabolized less efficiently by the fetus, exacerbating the teratogenic consequences of exposure. The effects of prenatal exposure to drugs of abuse

upon brain development have been shown to be highly variable. This variability is due to a number of factors—most importantly, timing of exposure, magnitude of exposure (amount and duration), and genetic vulnerability of the mother and fetus. Human studies of prenatal exposure to drugs of abuse are often complicated by confounding effects of poor prenatal care, poor maternal nutrition, and greater maternal psychosocial stress.

Ethanol

Prenatal exposure to ethanol results in a spectrum of abnormalities including, at one extreme, fetal alcohol syndrome, which includes growth retardation, facial anomalies, mental retardation, and microencephaly. Children with less severe prenatal exposures often lack the characteristic facial features of fetal alcohol syndrome, but suffer from a similar pattern of cognitive deficits (Berman and Hannigan, 2000). Mild exposures are associated with variable deficits in motor development and functional delays (Levitt, 1998).

Data from preclinical studies suggests that CNS abnormalities resulting from prenatal ethanol exposure stems from abnormal development of neurons and glia as well as ethanol-induced cell death. Ethanol has differential effects on progenitor cells surrounding the neural tube, reducing proliferation of cells in the ventricular zone, which give rise to neurons, and increasing proliferation of cells in the subventricular zone, which give rise to glia (Levitt, 1998). Ethanol-induced reduction in brain size appears to be a result of altered cell cycle kinetics, leading to a larger than normal loss of ventricular zone cells (Levitt, 1998). This line of work has shown that restricting ethanol exposure to the proliferative phase (roughly corresponding to the first trimester in humans) can produce the same brain abnormalities as those from longer-term prenatal exposure. Preclinical studies examining the impact of late gestational exposure (roughly corresponding to the third trimester in humans) have provided evidence that ethanol exposure during this time may be particularly toxic to hippocampal neurons. The resulting abnormal number, morphology, and function of hippocampal neurons appear to mediate deficits in spatial learning and memory that may correspond to the more subtle cognitive deficits seen in children with late-gestational ethanol exposure (Berman and Hannigan, 2000).

Tobacco Smoke

Tobacco smoke contains more than 2000 compounds, of which, nicotine and carbon monoxide have received the greatest attention in the literature on effects of prenatal exposure. Nicotine and cotinine, the major metabolite of nicotine, concentrate in the amniotic fluid. Nicotine is also secreted in breast milk. Smoking during pregnancy decreases fetal breathing movements and increases fetal heart rate. Smokers have a 1.2- to 1.7-fold increased risk of spontaneous abortion relative to nonsmokers. Tobacco smoking is also associated with decreased fetal growth and preterm delivery. The increased risk of low birth weight is not present in women who stop smoking by the third trimester. Pre- and postnatal exposure to tobacco smoke has been linked to an increased risk of sudden infant death syndrome (SIDS; Lee, 1998). Smoking during pregnancy has also been linked to a four-fold increased risk of prepubertal onset of conduct disorder in boys and a five-fold increased risk of adolescent-onset drug dependence in girls (Weissman et al., 1999).

Preclinical studies have shown that prenatal exposure to nicotine reduces brain weight, decreases cortical thickness, and produces abnormalities of pyramidal neuron maturation (Lee, 1998). Reduction in CNS markers of catecholamine activity, such as tyrosine hydroxylase activity, have been observed; however, these appear to normalize by adolescence (Levitt, 1998).

Cocaine

Abuse of cocaine during pregnancy is associated with increased rates of prematurity, low birth weight, respiratory distress, bowel and cerebral infarctions, reduced head circumference, and increased risk of seizures (Keller and Snyder-Keller, 2000). Infants prenatally exposed to cocaine show abnormal habituation and impaired attention.

Preclinical work has shown that prenatal exposure to cocaine produces anatomical and neuropharmacological changes that are specific to anterior cingulate and medial prefrontal cortices (Levitt, 1998). Alterations include abnormal morphology of pyramidal neuron dendrites in anterior cingulate cortex and a large reduction in dopamine D_1 receptor–G protein coupling in mesocortical and striatal regions. Behaviorally, prenatally exposed animals show a disruption in discrimination learning that may serve as a model for the attentional deficits of children following prenatal exposure to cocaine (Levitt, 1998).

Cannabis

Findings from human studies of the impact of prenatal exposure to cannabis have been inconsistent. Cannabis users tend to have lower–birth weight infants, but the relationship between prenatal cannabis use and prematurity has not been consistent (Lee, 1998).

Preclinical studies have shown that fetal tetrahydrocannabinoid levels remain lower than maternal plasma levels, indicating that the placenta may act as a partial barrier to this class of compounds. Decreased birth weight and postnatal growth have been observed in rats prenatally exposed to cannabis. Some studies have observed learning deficits in prenatally exposed animals, while others have not (Lee, 1998).

Opiates

Prenatal exposure to opiates has been linked to mild psychomotor developmental delays. Administration of methadone to pregnant opiate-dependent women significantly improves pregnancy outcome by providing more controlled exposure to an opiate with a longer elimination half-life, and by providing a context for delivery of prenatal care. However, as with neonates prenatally exposed to illicit opiates, a neonatal abstinence syndrome typically develops following birth, which usually requires pharmacological management. Methadone maintenance does not appear to completely eliminate the risk for developmental delay (Bunikowski et al., 1998).

Preclinical studies have found reductions in brain acetylcholine content and disruption of the activity of cholinergic neurons following prenatal exposure to opiates (Robinson, 2000). Other work has documented increased hypothalamic norepinephrine content and tyrosine hydroxylase immunoreactivity following prenatal exposure to opiates (Vathy et al., 2000).

CONCLUSIONS

Both preclinical and clinical studies have demonstrated the importance of mesocortical brain reward circuitry in mediating the acute reinforcing properties of abused substances, thereby mediating initiation of drug use. Adaptation of this circuitry to chronic drug use, in turn, appears to mediate the emergence of negative affective and motivational states following cessation of drug use that constitute core symptoms of withdrawal and place patients at heightened vulnerability for relapse.

Both twin studies and quantitative trait loci mapping methods have provided evidence for a significant genetic contribution to the risk of developing a substance dependence disorder. However, both of these lines of research have underscored the importance of environmental factors. A rich body of preclinical work has demonstrated that stress delivered at a wide range of time points in development can modulate proclivity towards drug self-administration. Evidence has suggested the importance of both corticosterone and CRH in mediating these effects of stress.

Clinical studies have also provided evidence for a role of stress in the development of substance dependence disorders and in relapse in those individuals who manage to become abstinent. However, much work remains to be done toward achieving an adequate understanding of what brain changes are induced by stress that result in substance use, dependence, and relapse. More specifically, research is needed that will clarify the differential impact of stress on brain function and the neuroendocrine axes in individuals at high and low genetic risk for substance dependence. In addition, tracer imaging studies need to be done in humans to clarify how stress modulates response of brain dopamine systems to dopaminergic agents. Such studies will need to characterize type, duration and timing of stress to be meaningful.

ACKNOWLEDGMENTS
This work was supported in part by grant DA00167 from the National Institute on Drug Abuse.

REFERENCES

Abi-Dargham, A., Krystal, J.H., Anjilvel, S., Scanley, B.E., Zoghbi, S., Baldwin, R.M., Rajeevan, N., Ellis, S., Petrakis, I.L., Seibyl, J.P., Charney, D.S., Laruelle, M., and Innis, R.B. (1998) Alterations of benzodiazepine receptors in type II alcoholic subjects measured with SPECT and [^{123}I]iomazenil. *Am J Psychiatry* 155: 1550–1555.

Abood, M.E. and Martin, B.R. (1992) Neurobiology of marijuana abuse. *Trends Pharmacol Sci* 13:201–206.

Agartz, I., Momenan, R., Rawlings, R.R., Kerich, M.J., and Hommer, D.W. (1999) Hippocampal volume in patients with alcohol dependence. *Arch Gen Psychiatry* 56:356–363.

American Psychiatric Association (1994) *Diagnostic and Statistical Manual of Mental Disorders, 4th ed.* (DSM-IV). Washington, DC: American Psychiatric Association.

Anda, R.F., Croft, J.B., Felitti, V.J., Nordenberg, D., Giles, W.H., Williamson, D.F., and Giovino, G.A. (1999) Adverse childhood experiences and smoking duing adolescence and adulthood. *JAMA* 282:1652–1658.

Berman, R.F. and Hannigan, J.H. (2000) Effectsof prenatla alchol expsure on the hippocampus: spatial behavior, electrophysiology, and neuroanatomy. *Hippocampus* 10:94–110.

Berrettini, W.H., Ferraro, T.N., Alexander, R.C., Buchberg, A.M., and Vogel, W.H. (1994) Quantitative trait loci mapping of three loci controlling morphine preference using inbred mouse strains. *Nat Geneti* 7:54–58.

Bohman, M., Sigvardsson, S., and Cloninger, C.R. (1981) Maternal inheritance of alcohol abuse: cross-fostering analysis of adopted women. *Arch Gen Psychiatry* 38:965–969.

Bradley, B.P., Phillips, G., Green, L., and Gossop, M. (1989) Circumstances surrounding the initial lapse to opiate use following detoxification. *Br J Psychiatry* 154:354–359.

Breese, C.R., Lee, M.J., Adams, C.E., Sullivan, B., Logel, J., Gillen, K.M., Marks, M.J., Collins, A.C., and Leonard, S. (2000) Abnormal regulation of high-affinity nicotinic receptors in subjects with schizophrenia. *Neuropsychopharmacology* 23:351–364.

Breiter, H.C., Gollub, R.L., Weisskoff, R.M., Kennedy, D.N., Makris, N., Berke, J.D., Goodman, J.M., Kantor, H.L., Gastfriend, D.R., Riorden, J.P., Mathew, R.T., Rosen, B.R., and Hyman, S.E. (1997) Acute effects of cocaine on human brain activity and emotion. *Neuron* 19:591–611.

Brewer, D.D., Catalano, R.F., Haggerty, K., Gainey, R.R., and Fleming, C.B. (1998) A meta-analysis of predictors of continued drug use during and after treatment for opiate addiction. *Addiction* 93:73–92.

Browman, K.E. and Crabbe, J.C. (2000) Quantitative trait loci affecting ethanol sensitivity in BXD recombinant inbred mice. *Alcohol Clin Exp Res* 24:17–23.

Bunikowski, R., Grimmer, I., Heiser, A., Metze, B., Schafer, A., and Obladen, M. (1998) Neurodevelopmental outcome after prenatal exposure to opiates. *Euro J Pediatr* 157:724–730.

Cador, M., Cole, B.J., Koob, G.F., Stinus, L., and Le Moal, M. (1993) Central administration of corticotropin releasing factor induces long-term sensitization to D-amphetamine. *Brain Res* 606:181–186.

Cadoret, R.J., Troughton, E., O'Gorman, T.W., and Heywood, E. (1986) An adoption study of genetic and environmental factors in drug abuse. *Arch Gen Psychiatry* 43:1131–1136.

Cadoret, R.J., Yates, W.R., Troughton, E., Woodworth, G., and Stewart, M.A. (1995) Adoption study demonstrating two genetic pathways to drug abuse. *Arch Gen Psychiatry* 52:42–52.

Chan, G.C., Hinds, T.R., Impey, S., and Storm, D.R. (1998) Hippocampal neurotoxicity of δ9-tetrahydrocannabinol. *J Neurosci* 18:5322–5332.

Clark, D.B., Lesnick, L., and Hegedus, A.M. (1997) Traumas and other adverse life events in adolescents with alcohol abuse and dependence. *J Am Acad Child Adolesc Psychiatry* 36:1744–1751.

Cloninger, C.R., Bohman, M., and Sigvardsson, S. (1981) Inheritance of alcohol abuse: cross-fostering analysis of adopted men. *Arch Gen Psychiatry* 38:861–868.

Cole, B.J., Cador, M., Stinus, L., Rivier, J., Vale, W., Koob, G.F., and Le Moal, M. (1990) Central administration of a CRF antagonist blocks the development of stress-induced behavioral sensitization. *Brain Res* 512:343–346.

Collins, R.J., Weeks, J.R., Cooper, M.M., Good, P.I., and Russell, R.R. (1984) Prediction of abuse liability of drugs using IV self-administration by rats. *Psychopharmacology* 82:6–13.

Comings, D.E. and Blum, K. (2000) Reward deficiency syndrome: genetic aspects of behavioral disorders. *Prog Brain Res* 126:325–341.

Deminiere, J.M., Piazza, P.V., Guegan, G., Abrous, N., Maccari, S., Le Moal, M., and Simon, H. (1992) Increased locomotor response to novelty and propensity to intravenous amphetamine self-administration in adult offspring of stressed mothers. *Brain Res* 586:135–139.

Deroche, V., Piazza, P.V., Le Moal, M., and Simon, H. (1994) Social isolation-induced enhancement of the psychomotor effects of morphine depends on corticosterone secretion. *Brain Res* 640: 136–139.

de Wit, D.J., MacDonald, K., and Offord, D.R. (2000) Childhood stress and symptoms of drug dependence in adolscence and early adulthood: social phobia as a mediator. *Am J Orthopsychiatry* 69:61–72.

de Wit, H., Metz, J., Wagner, N., and Cooper, M. (1990) Behavioral and subjective effects of ethanol: relationship to cerebral metabolism using PET. *Alcohol Clin Exp Res* 14:482–489.

Deykin, E.Y. and Buka, S.L. (1997) Prevalence and risk factors for posttraumatic stress disorder among chemically dependent adolescents. *Am J Psychiatry* 154:752–757.

Di Chiara, G. and North, R.A. (1992) Neurobiology of opiate abuse. *Trends Pharmacol Sci* 13:185–193.

Erb, S., Shaham, Y., and Stewart, J. (1996) Stress reinstates cocaine-seeking behavior after prolonged extinction and a drug-free period. *Psychopharmacology* 128:408–412.

Gabilondo, A.M., Meana, J.J., Barturen, F., Sastre, M., and Garcia-Sevilla, J.A. (1994) mu-opioid receptor and alpha 2-adrenoceptor agonist binding sites in the postmortem brain of heroin addicts. *Psychopharmacology* 115:135–140.

Garcia-Sevilla, J.A., Ventayol, P., Busquets, X., La Harpe, R., Walzer, C., and Guimon, J. (1997) Regulation of immunolabelled mu-opioid receptors and protein kinase C-alpha and zeta isoforms in the frontal cortex of human opiate addicts. *Neurosci Lett* 226: 29–32.

Gifford, A.N., Bruneus, M., Gatley, S.J., Lan, R., Makriyannis, A., and Volkow, N.D. (1999) Large receptor reserve for cannabinoid actions in the central nervous system. *J Pharmacol Exp Ther* 288: 478–483.

Goeders, N.E. and Guerin, G.F. (1994) Non-contingent electric footshock facilitates the acquisition of intravenous cocaine self-administration in rats. *Psychopharmacology* 114:63–70.

Grove, W.M., Eckert, E.D., Heston, L., Bouchard, T.J., Segal, N., and Lykken, D.T. (1990) Heritability of substance abuse and antisocial behavior: a study of monozygotic twins reared apart. *Biol Psychiatry* 27:1293–1304.

Han, C., McGue, M.K., and Iacono, W.G. (1999) Lifetime tobacco, alcohol and other substance use in adolescent Minnesota twins: univariate and multivariate behavioral genetic analyses. *Addiction* 94:981–993.

Heath, A.C., Meyer, J., Eaves, L.J., and Martin, N.G. (1991a) The inheritance of alcohol consumption patterns in a general population twin sample: I. Multidimensional scaling of quantity/frequency data. *J Stud Alcohol* 52:345–352.

Heath, A.C., Meyer, J., Jardine, R., and Martine, N.G. (1991b) The inheritance of alcohol consumption patterns in a general population twin sample: II. Determinants of consumption frequency and quantity consumed. *J Stud Alcohol* 52:425–433.

Heinz, A., Ragan, P., Jones, D.W., Hommer, D., Williams, W., Knable, M.B., Gorey, J.G., Doty, L., Geyer, C., Lee, K.S., Coppola, R., Weinberger, D.R., and Linnoila, M. (1998) Reduced central serotonin transporters in alcoholism. *Am J Psychiatry* 155:1544–1549.

Holman, B.L., Carvalho, P.A., Mendelson, J., Teoh, S.K., Nardin, R., Hallgring, E., Hebben, N., and Johnson, K.A. (1991) Brain perfusion is abnormal in cocaine-dependent polydrug users: a study using technetium-99m-HMPAO and ASPECT. *J Nucl Med* 32: 1206–1210.

Holman, B.L., Mendelson, J., Garada, B., Teoh, S.K., Hallgring, E., Johnson, K.A., and Mello, N.K. (1993) Regional cerebral blood flow improves with treatment in chronic cocaine polydrug users. *J Nucl Med* 34:723–727.

Jacobsen, L.K., Giedd, J.N., Gottschalk, C., Kosten, T.R., and Krystal, J.H. (2001 a) Quantitative morphology of the caudate and putamen in cocaine dependence. *Am J Psychiatry*: 158:486–489.

Jacobsen, L.K., Giedd, J.N., Kreek, M.J., Gottschalk, C., and Kosten, T.R (2001 b) Quantitative medial temporal lobe brain morphology and hypothalamic-pituitary-adrenal axis function in cocaine dependence: a preliminary report. *Drug Alcohol Depend*: 62:49–56.

Jacobsen, L.K., Southwick, S.M., and Kosten, T.R. (2001 c) Sub-stance use in patients with posttraumatic stress disorder: a review of the literature. *Am J Psychiatry*: 158:1184–1190.

Jacobsen, L.K., Staley, J.K., Malison, R.T., Zoghbi, S.S., Seibyl, J.P., Kosten, T.R., and Innis, R.B. (2000) Elevated central serotonin transporter binding availability in acutely abstinent cocaine-dependent patients. *Am J Psychiatry* 157:1134–1140.

Johnston, L.D., O'Malley, P.M., and Bachman J.G. (2000) *Monitoring the Future: National Results on Adolescent Drug Use.* Bethesda, MD: U.S. Department of Health and Human Services.

Jones, B.C., Tarantino, L.M., Rodriguez, L.A., Reed, C.L., McClearn, G.E., Plomin, R., and Erwin, V.G. (1999) Quantitative-trait loci analysis of cocaine-related behaviours and neurochemistry. *Pharmacogenetics* 9:607–617.

Kandel, D.B., Yamaguchi, K., and Chen, K. (1992) Steps in the progression in drug involvement from adolescence to adulthood: further evidence for the gateway theory. *J Stud Alcohol* 53:447–457.

Keller, R.W. and Snyder-Keller, A. (2000) Prenatal cocaine exposure. *Ann NY Acad Sci* 909:217–232.

Kendler, K.S., Heath, A.C., Neale, M.C., Kessler, R.C., and Eaves, L.J. (1992) A population-based twin study of alcoholism in women. *JAMA* 268:1877–1882.

Kendler, K.S., Neale, M.C., Sullivan, P., Corey, L.A., Gardner, C.O., and Prescott, C.A. (1999) A population-based twin study in women of smoking initiation and nicotine dependence. *Psychol Med* 29:299–308.

Kendler, K.S., Prescott, C.A., Neale, M.C., and Pedersen, N.L. (1997) Temperance board registration for alcohol abuse in a national sample of Swedish male twins, born 1902 to 1949. *Arch Gen Psychiatry* 54:178–184.

Koob, G.F. (1999a) Corticotropin-releasing factor, norepinephrine and stress. *Biol Psychiatry* 46:1167–1180.

Koob, G.F. (1999b) The role of the striatopallidal and extended amygdala systems in drug addiction. *Ann NY Acad Sci* 877:445–460.

Koob, G.F. (2000a) Animal models of craving for ethanol. *Addiction* 95:S73-S81.

Koob, G.F. (2000b) Neurobiology of addiction: toward the development of new therapies. *Ann NY Acad Sci* 909:170–185.

Koob, G.F. and LeMoal, M. (1997) Drug abuse: hedonic, hoeostatic dysregulation. *Science* 278:52–58.

Kornetsky, C., Esposito, R.U., McLean, S., and Jacobson, J.O. (1979) Inracranial self-stimulation thresholds: a model for the hedonic effects of drugs of abuse. *Arch Gen Psychiatry* 36:289–292.

Kosten, T.A., Miserendino, M.J., and Kehoe, P. (2000) Enhanced acquisition of cocaine self-administration in adult rats with neonatal isolation stress experience. *Brain Res* 875:44–50.

Laine, T.P.J., Ahonen, A., Torniainen, P., Heikkila, J., Pyhtinen, J., Rasanen, P., Niemela, O., and Hillbom, M. (1999) Dopamine transporters increase in human brain after alcohol withdrawal. *Mol Psychiatry* 4:189–191.

Lee, M.J. (1998) Marihuana and tobacco use in pregnancy. *Obstet Gynecol Clini North Am* 25:65–83.

Lerman, C., Caporaso, N.E., Audrain, J., Main, D., Bowman, E.D., Lockshin, B., Boyd, N.R., and Shields, P.G. (1999) Evidence suggesting the role of specific genetic factors in cigarette smoking. *Health Psychol* 18:14–20.

Levitt, P. (1998) Prenatal effects of drugs of abuse on brain development. *Drug Alcohol Depend* 51:109–125.

Litman, G.K., Eiser, J.R., Rawson, N.S., and Oppenheim, A.N. (1977) Towards a typology of relapse: a preliminary report. *Drug Alcohol Depend* 2:157–162.

Ludwig, A.M. and Wikler, A. (1974) "Craving" and relapse to drink. *Q J Stud Alcohol* 35:108–130.

Maccari, S., Piazza, P.V., Deminiere, J.M., Lemaire, V., Mormede, P., Simon, H., Angelucci, L., and Le Moal, M. (1991) Life events–induced decrease of type I corticosteroid receptors is associated with reduced corticosterone feedback and enhanced vulnerability to amphetamine self-administration. *Brain Res* 547:7–12.

Mansvelder, H.D. and McGehee, D.S. (2000) Long-term potentiation of excitatory inputs to brain reward areas by nicotine. *Neuron* 27:349–357.

Mash, D.C., Staley, J.K., Izenwasser, S., Basile, M., and Ruttenber, A.J. (2000) Serotonin transporters upregulate with chronic cocaine abuse. *J Chemi Neuroanat*. 20:271–280.

McGue, M., Pickens, R.W., and Svikis, D.S. (1992) Sex and age effects on the inheritance of alcohol problems: a twin study. *J Abnorm Psychol* 101:3–17.

MMWR (2000) Tobacco use among middle and high school students—United States, 1999. *JAMA* 283:1134–1136.

Muuronen, A., Bergman, H., Hindmarsh, T., and Telakivi, T. (1989) Influence of improved drinking habits on brain atrophy and cognitive performance in alcoholic patients: a 5-year follow-up study. *Alcohol Clin Exp Res* 13:137–141.

Netrakom, P., Krasuski, J.S., Miller, N.S., and O'Tuama, L.A. (1999) Structural and functional neuroimaging findings in substance-related disorders. *Psychiatr Clin North Am* 22:313–329.

Piazza, P.V., Deminiere, J.M., Le Moal, M., and Simon, H. (1989) Factors that predict individual vulnerability to amphetamine self-administration. *Science* 245:1511–1513.

Piazza, P.V., Deminiere, J.M., Le Moal, M., and Simon, H. (1990) Stress- and pharmacologically induced behavioral sensitization increases vulnerability to acquisition of amphetamine self-administration. *Brain Res* 514:22–26.

Pickens, R.W., Svikis, D.S., McGue, M., Lykken, D.T., Heston, L.L., and Clayton, P.J. (1991) Heterogeneity in the inheritance of alcoholism. *Arch Gen Psychiatry* 48:19–28.

Pope, H.G. and Yurgelun-Todd, D. (1996) The residual cognitive effects of heavy marijuana use in college students. *JAMA* 275: 521–527.

Ragan, P.W., Singleton, C.K., and Martin, P.R. (1999) Brain injury associated with chronic alcoholism. *CNS Spectrums* 4:66–87.

Robinson, S.E. (2000) Effect of prenatal opioid exposure on cholinergic development. *J Biomed Sci* 7:253–257.

Rounsaville, B.J., Kosten, T.R., Weissman, M.M., Prusoff, B., Pauls, D., Anton, S.F., and Merikangas, K. (1991) Psychiatric disorders in relatives of probands with opiate addiction. *Arch Gen Psychiatry* 48:33–42.

Rubino, T., Vigano, D., Massi, P., Spinello, M., Zagato, E., Giagnoni, G., and Parolaro, D. (2000) Chronic delta-9-tetrahydrocannabinol treatment increases cAMP levels and cAMP-dependent protein kinase activity in some rat brain regions. *Neuropharmacology* 39:1331–1336.

Samson, H.H. and Harris, R.A. (1992) Neurobiology of alcohol abuse. *Trends Pharmacol Sci* 13:206–211.

Schenk, S., Lacelle, G., Gorman, K., and Amit, Z. (1987) Cocaine self-administration in rats influenced by environmental conditions: implications for the etiology of drug abuse. *Neurosci Lett* 81:227–231.

Schulteis, G., Markou, A., Cole, M., and Koob, G.F. (1995) Decreased brain reward produced by ethanol withdrawal. *Proc Natl Acad Sci USA* 92:5880–5884.

Shaham, Y. and Stewart, J. (1995) Stress reinstates heroin-seeking in drug-free animals: an effect mimicking heroin, not withdrawal. *Psychopharmacology* 119:334–341.

Sinha, R., Catapano, D., and O'Malley, S. (1999) Stress-induced craving and stress response in cocaine dependent individuals. *Psychopharmacology* 142:343–351.

Staley, J.K. (1998) Neurochemical adaptations and cocaine dependence. In: Karch S.B., ed. *Drug Abuse Handbook*. New York: CRC Press, pp. 420–441.

Stein, E.A., Pankiewicz, J., Harsch, H.H., Cho, J.K., Fuller, S.A., Hoffmann, R.G., Hawkins, M., Rao, S.M., Bandettini, P.A., and Bloom, A.S. (1998) Nicotine-induced limbic cortical activation in the human brain: a functional MRI study. *Am J Psychiatry* 155: 1009–1015.

True, W.R., Heath, A.C., Scherrer, J.F., Waterman, B., Goldberg, J., Lin, N., and Eisen, S.A. (1997) Genetic and environmental contributions to smoking. *Addiction* 92:1277–1287.

Tsuang, M.T., Lyons, M.J., Eisen, S.A., Goldberg, R., True, W., Lin, N., Meyer, J.M., Toomey, R., Faraone, S.V., and Eaves, L. (1996) Genetic influences on DSM-III-R drug abuse and dependence: a study of 3,372 twin pairs. *Am J Med Genet* 67:473–477.

Tzschentke, T.M. (1998) Measuring reward with the conditioned place preference paradigm: a comprehensive review of drug effects, recent progress and new issues. *Prog Neurobiol* 56:613–672.

Vathy, I., He, H.J., Iodice, M., Hnatczuk, O.C., and Rimanoczy, A. (2000) Prenatal morphine exposure differentially alters TH-immunoreactivity in the stress-sensitive brain circuitry of adult male and female rats. *Brain Res Bull* 51:267–273.

Volkow, N.D., Fowler, J.S., Wolf, A.P., Hitzemann, R., Dewey, S., Bendriem, B., Alpert, R., and Hoff, A. (1991) Changes in brain glucose metabolism in cocaine dependence and withdrawal. *Am J Psychiatry* 148:621–626.

Volkow, N.D., Gillespie, H., Mullani, N., Tancredi, L., Grant, C., Valentine, A., and Hollister, L. (1996a) Brain glucose metabolism in chronic marijuana users at baseline and during marijuana intoxication. *Psychiatry Res* 67:29–38.

Volkow, N.D., Hitzemann, R., Wolf, A.P., Logan, J., Fowler, J.S., Christman, D., Dewey, S.L., Schlyer, D., Burr, G., and Vitkun, S. (1990) Acute effects of ethanol on regional brain glucose metabolism and transport. *Psychiatry Res* 35:39–48.

Volkow, N.D., Wang, G.J., Fowler, J.S., Logan, J., Hitzemann, R., Ding, Y.S., Pappas, N., Shea, C., and Piscani, K. (1996b) Decreases in dopamine receptors but not in dopamine transporters in alcoholics. *Alcohol Clin Exp Res* 20:1594–1598.

Wallace, B.C. (1989) Psychological and environmental determinants of relapse in crack cocaine smokers. *J Subst Abuse Treat* 6:95–106.

Weissman, M.M., Warner, V., Wickramaratne, P.J., and Kandel, D.B. (1999) Maternal smoking during pregnancy and psychopathology in offspring followed to adulthood. *J Am Acad Child Adolesc Psychiatry* 38:892–899.

Wu, X. and French, E.D. (2000) Effects of chronic delta9-tetrahydrocannabinol on rat midbrain dopamine neurons: an electrophysiological assessment. *Neuropharmacology* 39:391–398.

II | SOMATIC INTERVENTIONS

Our cerebrospinal fluid (CSF) observations and . . . studies of the locus ceruleus (LC) and clonidine call for the assessment of noradrenergic metabolism and clonidine in Tourette's syndrome.

D.J. Cohen, J.G. Young, J.A. Nathanson, and B.A. Shaywitz (1979) Clonidine in Tourette's syndrome.
Lancet, *September 15, p. 551*

IN addition to covering traditional areas such as mechanism of action, structure–function relationships, and drug disposition and toxicity, this part of the volume reviews drug-specific data that are specifically pertinent to children and adolescents. Age and developmental phase as critical variables relevant to dosing schemes and side effect liabilities are two recurring themes. Clinical "mechanics" for using these drugs in children, such as initiation, laboratory monitoring, and discontinuation, are spelled out in detail. The nine chapters that comprise this section's first part cover all currently employed psychotropic drugs; readers are also referred to the volume's *Appendix* for a quick "bird's eye view" and cross-reference source for these agents and their specific characteristics.

A second part consists of two chapters covering other somatic interventions, including complementary, alternative, and naturopathic medicine approaches (such as St. John's wort), as well as more "aggressive" treatments less commonly used in children and adolescents, such as electroconvulsive therapy (ECT) and transcranial magnetic stimulation (TMS).

PART

II-A | PSYCHOTROPIC AGENTS

20 | **Stimulants**

REBECCA E. FORD, LAURENCE L. GREENHILL, AND KELLY POSNER

The increasing use of stimulants in the United States to treat attention deficit hyperactivity disorder (ADHD) has aroused parental concern and compelled both medical professionals and the media to question the safety and efficacy of this type of treatment. Because ADHD is among the most common reasons for seeking mental health services for children, these questions are more pertinent than ever. This chapter will examine the history of stimulant use, the mechanism of action, pharmacokinetics, side effects, and issues related to their clinical use in children and adolescents. More detailed information on clinical applications is provided in Section III.

HISTORY AND OVERVIEW

Stimulants are considered to be among the safest and most effective psychotropic medications prescribed. This view is based on a history of over 60 years of research and clinical use for a variety of physiological and psychiatric conditions. In a ground-breaking article, Bradley (1937) reported that D, L-amphetamine diminished motor activity, increased compliance, and improved academic performance in hyperactive children. Continuing his research throughout the next two decades, Bradley published more case reports of successful amphetamine treatments in children (Bradley and Bowen, 1941).

Stimulant treatment of ADHD has generated the largest body of treatment literature of any childhood psychiatric disorder. Between 1962 and 1993, over 250 reviews and over 3000 articles were published on stimulant effects (Swanson, 1993). By 1996, 161 randomized controlled trials (RCTs) had been published, encompassing 5 preschool, 150 school-age, 7 adolescent, and 9 adult studies. Improvement occurred in 65%–75% of the children randomized to stimulants (methylphenidate) [MPH]: *n* = 133 trials; dextroamphetamine [DEX]: *n* = 22 trials; pemoline [PEM]: *n* = 6 trials) compared to 5%–30% of those assigned to placebo (Spencer et al., 1996b). Other reviews have previously summarized this trial literature (Barkley, 1977; Schmidt et al., 1984; Gittelman-Klein, 1987; American Academy of Child and Adolescent Psychiatry, 1997; DuPaul and Barkley, 1998; Greenhill et al., 1999; Jadad et al., 1999.

The benefits of stimulant use in children with ADHD are evident both in school and at home. In the classroom, stimulants decrease interrupting and motor restlessness, increase on-task behavior, and consistently reduce symptoms of ADHD on standardized rating scales completed by parents and teachers (Conners et al., 1967). In addition, stimulants decrease response variability and impulsivity on laboratory cognitive tasks, increase performance precision, and improve short-term memory, reaction time, math computation, problem solving, and sustained attention. At home, stimulants improve parent–child interactions, on-task behavior, homework completion, and compliance. Socially, children with ADHD taking stimulants receive better peer nominations and show increased attention during sports activities. Moreover, in the presence of other comorbid axis I disorders, stimulants prove to be effective in ameliorating the symptoms of ADHD and possibly of the comorbid conduct disorder (Klein et al., 1997) or comorbid anxiety disorder (MTA Cooperative Group, 1999).

Despite the overwhelming evidence for short-term effectiveness, only recently have studies begun to address long-term benefits of stimulant treatments. Prospective randomized controlled trials with durations of 12 to 24 months and doses up to 60 mg/day of MPH have been conducted to address this issue. The largest of these studies, the National Institute of Mental Health (NIMH)-sponsored Multimodal Treatment Study of Attention-Deficit Hyperactivity Disorder (MTA Study), showed that stimulants (either by themselves or in combination with behavioral treatments) lead to stable, long-term improvements in ADHD symptoms as long as the medication is taken (MTA Cooperative Group, 1999).

In the United States, clinicians have steadily increased their stimulant prescribing over the past decade. Outpatient visits to primary practitioners for ADHD-related problems have increased from 1.6 to 4.2 million per year between 1990 and 1993 (Swanson et al., 1995). During these visits, 90% of the children were given prescriptions, 71% of which were for the stimulant MPH. Further evidence of increased stimulant use is that MPH production in the United States increased from 1784 kg/year to 5110 kg/year during the same 3-year period. Over 10 million prescriptions for MPH were written in 1996 (Vitiello and Jensen 1997).

The exact causes of the increased stimulant production and use remain elusive. A 1998 Consensus Development Conference (CDC) on ADHD, sponsored by the National Institutes of Health (NIH) (NIH Consensus Statement, 1998), found "wide variations in the use of psychostimulants across communities and physicians." Such variability suggests that either physicians are becoming better educated about ADHD or they are over prescribing. One epidemiological survey in four different communities found that only one-eighth of the children who met criteria for ADHD were receiving adequate stimulant treatment (Jensen et al., 1999). Alternatively, and also of concern, a survey in rural North Carolina found 72% of school-aged children receiving stimulants did not even meet criteria for ADHD (Angold et al., 2000). This discrepancy only serves to underline the need for further research on the correlates of prescribing practices in pediatric populations.

MECHANISM OF ACTION

Despite the documented efficacy and safety of the psychostimulants, their mechanism of action is not fully understood. Stimulants affect central nervous system (CNS) dopamine (DA) and norepinephrine (NE) pathways crucial in frontal lobe function. The stimulants act by causing release of catecholamines from the DA axons and blocking their reuptake. Methylphenidate releases catecholamines from long-term stores, so its effects can be blocked by pretreatment with reserpine. Amphetamines, on the other hand, release catecholamines from recently formed storage granules near the surface of the presynaptic neuron, so their action is not blocked by reserpine. In addition, the stimulants bind to the DA transporter in striatum (see Figures 2.6 and 2.7) and block the reuptake of both DA and NE. This action reduces the rate that catecholamines are removed from the synapse back into the axon and leads to an increase in synaptic DA concentration in the striatum (Volkow et al., 1998).

The increased availability of DA in striatum is presumed to enhance prefrontal cortical function through striatal–frontal pathways. Prefrontal dysfunction, including deficits in inhibitory control and working memory, has been linked to NE and DA dysfunction, leading to ADHD-associated impairments (Douglas et al., 1988; Barkley, 1997).

PHARMACOKINETICS AND DRUG DISPOSITION

The pharmacokinetics of stimulants are characterized by rapid absorption, low plasma protein binding, and quick extracellular metabolism (Patrick et al., 1987). Although some investigators claim that the dose–response relationship is affected by the child's weight, others have shown that individual dose–response stimulant effects are independent of the child's weight (Rapport et al., 1989).

Rapidly absorbed from the gut, immediate-release (IR) stimulants begin to act about 30 minutes after ingestion. Both the absorption and bioavailability of MPH may increase after a meal Chan et al., 1983). This rapid increase in IR stimulant plasma concentrations was thought necessary for the most enhanced therapeutic effect. However, IR stimulants are short-acting, so that multiple doses at 4-hour intervals are required to sustain the behavioral improvements across the day throughout school, recreational activities, and homework. The necessity of this bolus, or "ramp effect" (Birmaher et al., 1989), was thrown into question by a newer study. A gradual increase in stimulant concentration over the day (without a sharp ramp-up in absorption) produced the best control of attention and deportment compared to alternative plasma level curves, such as a "flat" plasma level or a "decreasing" concentration (Swanson et al., 1999a).

Generic MPH and the brand name drug products show similar, although not identical, pharmacokinetic profiles. Generic MPH is generally absorbed more quickly and peaks sooner (Vitiello and Burke, 1998).

Methylphenidate and DEX elevate glucose metabolism in the brains of rats, although subjects with schizophrenia given DEX show decreased glucose metabolism. Studies using positron emission tomography (PET) scanning have demonstrated that untreated adults with a past history of ADHD show 8.1% lower levels of cerebral glucose metabolism than controls (Zametkin et al., 1991), with the greatest differences in the superior prefrontal cortex and premotor areas. No changes in cerebral glucose metabolism were found in PET scans when 19 MPH-treated and 18 DEX-treated adults with ADHD were compared, even though the adults showed significant changes in behavior (Matochik et al., 1993).

Although the IR preparations of the major stimulants last between 3 hours (MPH) and 11 hours (DEX), behavioral improvements last only 3 to 5 hours. Plasma levels of MPH do not correlate with clinical response (Gualtieri et al., 1982) and provide less predictive power for clinical improvement than do teacher and parent global rating forms (Sebrechts et al., 1986). Several pathways, including p-hydoxylation, N-demthylation, deamination, and conjugation, are involved in the metabolism of stimulants. Up to 80% may be excreted unchanged in the urine in the case of amphetamine (Weiner, 1991). Methylphenidate undergoes de-esterification in plasma (Patrick et al., 1987). The concentration-enhancing and activity-reducing effects of MPH disappear well before the medication leaves the plasma. This is known as *clockwise hyperesis* (Cox, 1990).

Similar to MPH, the effects of PEM on cognitive processing begin within the first 2 hours after ingestion (Sallee et al., 1992). In contrast to MPH, however, the behavioral effects of PEM last up to 6 hours. Although the therapeutic effects of MPH and DEX are concentrated during absorption, PEM has significant effects lasting into the post-distribution phase. Previously believed to require 3–6 weeks to work (Page et al., 1974), PEM has been shown to be effective after the first dose (Sallee et al., 1985); (Pelham et al., 1995). Despite these potential advantages, PEM usage has decreased markedly because of reports of hepatic failure.

LONG-ACTING STIMULANTS

Pragmatic issues associated with IR preparations, such as the need for frequent doses and resulting problems in compliance, have led to the development of long-duration stimulants. Ritalin-SR (MPH-SR20) uses a wax-matrix vehicle for slow release (SR). The DEX "spansule" accomplishes longer duration coverage by using small medication particles in a capsule. The DEX spansule vehicle has been studied in pharmacokinetic–pharmacodynamic single-site trials, and found to exert most of the ADHD symptoms reduction during the period that the amphetamine is increasing in concentration (Brown et al., 1980). Slow-release, "branded" generics, such as Metadate-ER and Methylin, use the same wax-matrix vehicle as Ritalin-SR.

Although these long-duration versions of stimulant medications have been available for more than a decade, their clinical use has been limited. Expert raters reviewing behavioral and continuous performance test (CPT) data first reported that MPH-SR20 was less effective than the standard MPH at 10 mg two times a day, when both were used to treat 13 children with ADHD in a summer program (Pelham et al., 1989). This reduced effect may be related to delayed onset of action and its lower plasma level peak (Birmaher et al., 1989).

The recently introduced product Concerta is a once-a-day administration MPH delivery system called *OROS* (osmotically released). This delivery system creates an ascending plasma level pattern instead of the peak-and-valley pharmacokinetic profile seen in the IR preparations. Similar extended-delivery bead-technology, double-pulse preparations have been introduced for Metadate-CD at 10, 20, and 30 mg (Greenhill et al., 2002, in press) for the spheroidal technology of Ritalin-LA, and for Adderall-XR preparations (McGough et al., 2002, in press). Beaded stimulant preparations mix IR and delayed-release beads in a capsule. The patient can swallow the capsule whole or sprinkle the contents in food if pill taking is difficult for the child.

The IR version of Adderall, which has been on the market under that name since 1994, has a duration of action of 5 hours only (Swanson et al., 1998), so it required a double-pulse, bead-technology delivery system to enable one dosing administration to cover the entire day (Greenhill et al., 2001b).

Drug Interactions

The prevalence of concurrent prescriptions raises concern regarding drug interactions with stimulants. Stimulants, especially MPH, have been used to augment the effects of tricyclic antidepressants in the treatment of refractory depression. Although one early report claimed that circulating levels of imipramine can rise seven fold when taken concurrently with MPH (Wharton et al., 1971), a more recent study found that combining stimulants with desipramine (DMI) did not increase the plasma level of DMI relative to children treated with DMI alone (Cohen et al., 1999).

In two double-blind, placebo-controlled crossover studies (Pataki et al., 1993; Rapport et al., 1993), DMI and MPH were used alone and in combination in an inpatient population to discover potential side effects. The 16 subjects, ages 7–12, had comorbid mood disorders and ADHD and received careful electocardiographic (EKG) and tricyclic antidepressant (TCA) blood level monitoring. The mean daily dosage of DMI was 4.04 mg/kg/day, with a range of 2.4 to 6.1 mg/kg/day. The DMI plasma levels ranged from 121 to 291 ng/mL. The dose range of MPH was 10–40 mg/day. Although clinical response was not measured, computerized assessments of attention and impulsivity indicated that the combination was superior on some measures and inferior on others when compared to either medication alone. Side effects such as nausea, dry mouth, and tremor were twice as common when the medications were combined than either alone, but remained relatively mild. The authors concluded that "there was no clinical evidence of unique or serious side effects in combining desipramine and MPH beyond those attributable to desipramine alone" (Rapport et al., 1993).

Can antidepressants such as tricyclics or buproprion augment the effect of stimulants on nondepressed children with ADHD? Randomized controlled trials have yet to address this question. Nonetheless, such combinations are common in clinical practice. One case report showed leukopenia in a child treated with a combination of MPH and tricyclics for 4 months, although the doses were not specified (Burke et al., 1995). Another case report indicated that obsessive-compulsive symptoms developed secondary to the combination of MPH and tricyclics (Pataki et al., 1993). On a cautionary note, MPH has been found to interact with guanethidine to produce paradoxical hypotension. Patients on monoamine oxidose (MAO) inhibitors are likely to develop hypertensive crises if given a stimulant.

Although tricyclics continue to be used today to treat childhood depression (Zito et al., 2000), the use in children with ADHD has decreased, most likely because of its association with the sudden deaths of five children (Biederman, 1991). Furthermore, the Physician's Desk Reference (PDR) warns that MPH may inhibit the metabolism of tricyclics, but no such warning exists for DEX or (AMP). Due to the concern that children on this combination of medications are prone to develop more side effects, it is not a recommended form of treatment. Instead, MPH combined with a selective serotonin reuptake inhibitor is preferable for treating a child with ADHD and comorbid depression.

Methylphenidate also has been combined with clonidine, the α_2 agonist, to reduce aggression, to provide better control of ADHD symptoms after the stimulant wears off, and to counteract insomnia associated with stimulant treatment (Wilens et al., 1994). The report of four deaths on the Federal Drug Administration (FDA)'s MEDWATCH surveillance network, however,

has prompted concern among clinicians. Although subsequent review of these cases did not conclude that either medication or the combination was responsible for any of these deaths, some experts warn against the combination of these two medications (Swanson et al., 1999b). Electrocardiographic monitoring will not directly address this concern, as the rate of adverse events such as bradycardia, hypotension, and hypertension reported during treatment with this combination of drugs is infrequent, with less than 50 cases reported in the literature.

A recent study of 136 children with ADHD and Tourette's syndrome evaluated the safety and efficacy of MPH ($n = 37$), clonidine ($n = 34$), and the combination ($n = 33$) against placebo ($n = 32$) (TACT, 2002). Each of the active medications alone and the combination were superior to placebo. The average dose of clonidine was 0.26 mg/day when given alone or when given in combination with methylphenidate. When given in combination, clonidine appeared to confer additive benefit for disruptive behavior. There were no serious side effects in any of the treatments and EKG monitoring did not reveal any evidence of cardiac toxicity. Sedation was common in the clonidine-treated group, affecting 64% of subjects. This reportedly had a dose-limiting effect in half of the subjects in the clonidine group. Although only 19% of the MPH-treated subjects reported an increase in tics, the tics limited dosage increases in just over a third of the MPH-only group. By contrast, tics limited dosage increase in 18% in the clonidine-only group and 15% in the clonidine + MPH group. The authors concluded that MPH and clonidine, alone or in combination, are safe and effective for the short-term treatment of children with ADHD and tics.

SIDE EFFECTS AND TOXICITY

With an estimated 3 million children and adolescents in the United States taking stimulants daily, the management of side effects is a significant clinical issue. Psychostimulant use is associated with several minor negative side effects in 10% to 15% of children treated that respond to adjustments in dose or in time of administration. Delay of sleep onset, reduced appetite, headache, and jitteriness are the most frequently cited stimulant-related side effects that have been identified in placebo-controlled trials Barkley et al., 1990. No additional delay in sleep onset was seen after adding a third, mid-afternoon dose of MPH to standard bid dosing regimens (Kent et al., 1995). Some children experience motor tics while on stimulants, but the mechanism for this is unclear. Out of 23 controlled studies, no differences in side effects were reported among various stimulants. Only abdominal discomfort, delay of sleep onset, and headache occurred more often for stimulant than placebo treatments (McMaster University Evidence-Based Practice Center, 1998).

Animal toxicity studies reveal other abnormal findings. These results have not been reported in humans because of differences of species, dosage, route of administration, and end point selected. For example, Sprague-Dawley rats given a high subcutaneous dose of 25 mg/kg of DEX, MPH, and 3,4-methylene-dioxymethamphetamine (MDMA) (as opposed to 0.3 mg/kg given orally in children) later showed a loss of serotonin reuptake sites (Battaglia et al., 1987). Hepatic tumor rates increased in mice (a strain known to have genetic diathesis for liver tumors), while tumor rates decreased in rats (reflected also in human data) when treated with high oral MPH doses of 4–47 mg/kg (Dunnick and Hailey, 1995). In very high doses (e.g., 20–100 mg/kg), stimulants can induce stereotypies in animals (e.g., licking, grooming). These repetitive behaviors may be analogous to the involuntary, repetitive movements seen in children who develop tics during treatment with stimulants.

The 1998 NIH Consensus Development Conference on ADHD cautioned that extremely high doses of stimulants may cause central nervous system damage, cardiovascular damage, and hypertension (NIH Consensus Statement, 1998). As a curious historical example, Japanese factory workers developed brain lesions leading to death when chronically self-administering toxic doses of amphetamines in order to work long hours in post-war Japan. Likewise, paranoid hallucinations have been produced in normal adult volunteers after taking single doses of 300 mg of amphetamine (Angrist and Gershon, 1972). These observations suggest that toxic responses to stimulants are dose related and occur most often during overdose, not in standard practice.

Although side effects of other stimulants respond to dose reduction or change in time of administration, PEM use can be associated with serious, irreversible liver damage. Postmarketing surveillance revealed abnormalities in liver function tests in 44 children receiving PEM acutely or chronically (Berkovitch et al., 1995). Even more disturbing, 13 children on PEM experienced total liver failure—11 resulting in death or transplant within 4 weeks of failure. This exceeds the rate in the normal population by 4 to 17 times. Pemoline, therefore, is reserved for alternative treatment only if the patient fails to tolerate all three stimulants (MPH, DEX, and AMP) and subsequent trials of an-

tidepressants (bupropion or tricyclics) or other agents (such as the α agonists).

CLINICAL USE IN CHILDREN AND ADOLESCENTS

Uses in Young Children

Although the bulk of the research available on psychostimulant treatment of ADHD focuses on prepubescent school-age children, new attention has been turned to the preschool population. To date, there are no data on pharmacokinetics, phamacodynamics, peak and duration of behavioral effects, interaction between drug and the developing brain, guidelines for dose response, and side effects of short- and long-term exposure for preschool-age children on MPH. Despite this lack of safety and efficacy information, the amount of off-label MPH prescriptions for preschool-age children increased three-fold between 1991 and 1995, and experts currently estimate that 1.2% of this population is on MPH (Zito et al., 2000). Three principal challenges confront the treatment of such young children with stimulants: (1) the actual diagnosis according to DSM-IV criteria is difficult to discern from developmentally appropriate behavior in this population; (2) determining an appropriate dosage is challenging because of the absence of data; and (3) preschoolers may encounter difficulty swallowing pills as compared to older children.

Before Starting the Drug

There is not an empirically proven threshold of ADHD symptoms that can guide the decision about whether a particular child should be started on a stimulant, or what the initial dosage should be. Only those patients with moderate to severe impairment should be considered. Even though children diagnosed with ADD, predominantly inattentive type, might not experience impairment socially or at home, they may benefit academically from stimulant treatment. To qualify for stimulant treatment, the child must be living with a responsible adult who can administer the medication. In the case of multiple daily dosing schedules, it is necessary for school personnel to administer the mid-day dose.

The literature is of little assistance in determining the best stimulant for an individual patient, starting dosage, or the dosing regimen. Also, the clinician must determine the best timing of doses during the day. Because only a small proportion of children with ADHD show a sufficiently positive response to daily dosing with IR MPH (Pliszka, 2000), most clinicians use a bid or tid schedule. A recent pharmacodynamic study in a laboratory classroom setting revealed that if children receive increasing doses of IR MPH over the day, their ADHD symptoms remain low. Most clinicians in the United States adjust the dosage in escalating steps involving whole or half MPH pills (10–60 mg range) until the child shows improvement or side effects (Greenhill, 1998; Barkley et al., 1999). Maximum daily doses for most pediatric patients are 60 mg of MPH or 40 mg of DEX/AMP. Once a child responds, there is no universally accepted criterion for the amount of symptom reduction that must occur before the clinician ceases to increase the dosage. According to the mean change in placebo-controlled studies, positive response is in the range of 40% reduction on a teacher rating and slightly less on parent ratings (Barkley et al., 1990).

Sustained-release stimulants

Children naive to stimulant treatment may be started directly on a sustained-release formulation. Starting doses could be any of the following: 5 mg of Dexedrine spansules once in the morning, or 5 mg of Adderall bid, or 18 mg of Concerta, which is equivalent to MPH 5 mg tid. Before the availability of Concerta, it had become common practice to combine short-acting MPH with MPH-SR20 to increase efficacy and duration of effect and to allow for more flexible dosing.

Monitoring

Once the child has been stabilized on a stimulant medication, the child should come in for regular medication management. This may be as frequent as once a month for children with adverse events or unstable symptoms, or once every other month for those who are stable.

Blood levels are not informative. Assessment of stimulant blood levels is not helpful in clinical practice. The short half-life makes it difficult to select the best time to draw a blood sample to monitor levels of medication in the patient. A half-hour variation can make a significant difference, especially if only one blood sample is drawn.

Special laboratory tests are not necessary for monitoring. With over 30 years of use in millions of children, no hematologic abnormalities have been associated with stimulant use. Despite stimulant effects on blood pressure and pulse when first used, no long-lasting changes have been noted. Therefore, no routine blood or ECG tests are recommended during long-term monitoring.

Long-Term Use Considerations

Does stimulant treatment retard normal physical growth? Statistically significant but clinically small weight decrements are reported during short-term trials (Gittelman-Klein et al., 1988), but prospective follow-up into adult life shows no significant, long-term impairment in terms of height achieved (Manuzza et al., 1991). In the NIMH MTA Study, ADHD children treated with stimulants for 14 months had significant decrements in rates of weight gain compared to those receiving a nonmedication treatment, but differences between groups in rates of height acquisition were not significant (Greenhill and MTA Cooperative Group, 1999). Growth rate delays attributed to medication may be a developmental artifact associated with the disorder (Spencer et al., 1996a).

Mounting concern for abuse potential of MPH has paralleled the increasing production and use of the medication. Stimulant medications are classified as drugs of abuse by the U.S. Drug Enforcement Administration. In laboratory experiments, animals often self-administered and chose DEX, MPH, and Adderall over food—a behavior associated with addiction. Some have worried that long-term treatment with MPH might predispose children with ADHD to abuse cocaine or other illicit drugs (Goldman et al., 1998; Lambert and Hartsough, 1998).

Several considerations assuage these concerns. First, stimulants used for treatment are limited in their ability to induce euphoria when administered orally. As shown in PET scans, compared to intravenous cocaine, oral MPH is absorbed more slowly, binds to the DA transporter for longer periods, and does not produce euphoria (Volkow et al., 1995). Moreover, although MPH does appear in emergency room mentions in the Drug Abuse Warning Network (DAWN), its mention rate is only 1/40th the rate for cocaine (Goldman et al., 1998). There have been reports that adolescents with ADHD treated with stimulants show lower rates of substance use disorder (SUD) than adolescents with ADHD not in treatment (Molina and Pelham, 1999). Furthermore, there is little evidence of the development of long-term tolerance to stimulants as shown by the need to increase the dosage to get the same response (Safer and Allen, 1989). Despite concerns about the risk of psychostimulant abuse and recreational use, analyses of annual school surveys of drug use and the DAWN data on emergency room visit monitoring have not suggested an increase in either.

The Drug Enforcement Administration has been supportive of a public education program about the diversion and sale of stimulants as drugs of abuse. At present, there has been no evidence from follow-up studies, surveys of high school students, or mentions in emergency room visits that stimulant medications have been primary drugs of abuse. Of course, the absence of evidence does not constitute *proof*, and all stimulants have some abuse potential. Thus, pill usage should be followed, and the practitioner should be wary of patients who request multiple prescriptions during a month. Schools are encouraged to keep the medication in locked cabinets, to maintain careful dispensing records, and never to use one child's medication to treat another. To avoid drug diversion and peer ridicule of the child, the practitioner can avoid administering stimulant medications in school by using longer-duration drugs such as Concerta, Metadate-CD, Adderall-XR, or Dexedrine spansules.

Discontinuation

The effects of stimulant medication generally cease upon discontinuation of the treatment. One double-blind study, however, did not find this to be necessarily true for DEX (Gillberg et al., 1997). Many patients favor a period off the medication, a "drug holiday," to deal with the partial suppression of weight gain, worries about long-term effects, or to assess the need for staying on medication. This type of trial is best done when the child is not scheduled for important school tests or social activities (e.g., summer camp).

FUTURE RESEARCH

An improved understanding of the neurobiological substrates underlying attentional mechanisms, as well as the mechanisms of stimulant action, could aid in the development of future medication formulations. The lack of data on stimulant use in particular populations, especially among preschoolers and children with developmental disabilities, and questions regarding the safety and efficacy of long-term stimulant treatment underscore the need for further research.

REFERENCES

American Academy of Child and Adolescent Psychiatry (1997). Practice parameters for the assessment and treatment of attention-deficit/hyperactivity disorder. *Acad Child Adolesc Psychiatry* 36: 85s–121s.

Angold, A., Erkanli, A., Egger, H., and Costello, J. (2000) Stimulant treatment for children: a community perspective. *Acad Child Adolesc Psychiatry* 39:975–983.

Angrist, B.M., and Gershon, S. (1972) Psychiatric sequalae of am-

phetamine use. In: Shader, R.I., ed. *Psychiatric Complications of Medical Drugs, 1st. ed.* New York: Raven Press, pp. 175–199

Barkley, R., DuPaul, G., and Connor, D.F. (1999) Stimulants. In: Werry, J. and Aman, M., eds. *Practitioner's Guide to Psychoactive Drugs for Children and Adolescents. 2nd ed.* New York: Plenum, Press, pp. 205–237.

Barkley, R., McMurray, M., Edelbroch, C., and Robbins, K. (1990) Side effects of MPH in children with attention deficit hyperactivity disorder: a systematic placebo-controlled evaluation. *Pediatrics* 86:184–192.

Barkley, R.A. (1977) A review of stimulant drug research with hyperactive children. *Child Psychol Psychiatry* 18:137–165.

Barkley, R.A. (1997) *ADHD and the Nature of Self-Control,* New York: Guilford.

Barkley, R.A., Edwards, G., Laneri, M., Fletcher, K., and Metevia, I. (2001) Executive functioning, temporal discounting, and sense of time in adolescents with attention-deficit/ hyperactivity disorder (ADHD) and Oppositional-Defiant Disorder (ODD), *Abnorm Child Psychol* 29:541–556.

Battaglia, G., Yeh, S., O'Hearn, E., Molliver, M., Kuhar, M., and De Souza, E. (1987) 3,4-methyoxydioxymethamphetamine and 3,4-methylenedioxyamphetamine destroy serotonin terminals in rat brain: quantification of neurodegeneration by measurement of [3H] paroxetine-labeled serotonin uptake sites. *Pharmacol Exp Ther*, 242:911–916.

Berkovitch, M., Pope, E., Phillips, J., and Koren, G. (1995) Pemoline-associated fulminant liver failure: testing the evidence for causation. *Clini Pharmacol Ther* 57:696–698.

Biederman, J. (1991) Sudden death in children treated with a tricyclic antidepressant: a commentary. *Biol Ther Psychiatry Newsletter* 14:1–4.

Birmaher, B.B., Greenhill, L., Cooper, T., Fried, J., and Maminski, B. (1989) Sustained release methylphenidate: pharmacokinetic studies in ADDH males. *J Am Acad Child Adolesc Psychiatry* 28: 768–772.

Bradley, C. (1937). The behavior of children receiving Benzedrine. Am J Psychiatry 94:577–585.

Bradley, C., and Bowen, M. (1941) Amphetamine (benzedrine) therapy of children's behavior disorders. *Am Orthopsychiatry* 11:92–103.

Brown, G.L., Ebert, M.H., Mikkelsen, E.I., and Hunt R.D. (1980) Behavior and motor acitivity response in hyperactive children and plasma amphetamine levels following a sustained release preparation. *J Am Acad Child Adolesc Psychiatry* 19:225–239.

Burke, M.S., Josephson, A., and LIghtsey, A. (1995) Combined methylphenidate and imipramine complication [letter]. *Am Acad Child Adolesc Psychiatry* 34:403–404.

Chan, Y.P., Swanson, J.M., Soldin, S.S., Thiessen, J.J., and Macleod, S.M. (1983) Methylphenidate hydrochloride given with or before breakfast: II. Effects on plasma concentration of methylphenidate and ritalinic acid. *Pediatrics* 72:56–59.

Cohen, L.G., Prince, J., Wilens, T., Faraone, S., Whitt, S., Mick, E., Spencer, T., and Meyer, M.C. (1999) Absence of effect of stimulants on the pharmacokinetics of desipramine in children. *Pharmacotherapy* 19:746–752.

Conners, C.K., Eisenberg, L., and Barcai, A. (1967) Effect of dextroamphetamine on children: studies on subjects with learning disabilities and school behavior problems. *Arch Gen Psychiatry* 17: 478–485.

Cox, B.M. (1990) Drug tolerance and physical dependence. In: Pratt, W.B. and Taylor, P., eds. *Principles of Drug Action: The Basis of Pharmacology, 1st ed.* New York: Churchill Livingstone, pp. 639–690.

Douglas, V.I., Barr, R.G., Amin, K., O'Neill, M.E., and Britton, B.G. (1988) Dose effects and individual responsivity to methylphenidate in attention deficit disorder. *J Child Psychol Psychiatry* 29: 453–475.

Dunnick, J., and Hailey, J. (1995) Experimental studies on the long-term effects of methylphenidate hydrochloride. *Toxicology* 103: 77–84.

DuPaul, G.J., and Barkley, R.A. (1998) Medication therapy. In: Barkley, R.A., ed. *Attention Deficit Hyperactivity Disorder: A Handbook for Diagnosis and Treatment, 2nd ed.* New York: Guilford Press, pp. 573–612.

Gillberg, C., Melander, H., von Knorring, A., Janols, L., Thernlund, G., Heggel, B., Edievall-Walin, L., Gustafsson, P., and Kopp, S. (1997) Long-term central stimulant treatment of children with attention-deficit hyperactivity disorder. A randomized double-blind placebo-controlled trial. *Arch Gen Psychiatry* 54:857–864.

Gittelman-Klein, R. (1987) Pharmacotherapy of childhood hyperactivity: an update. In: Meltzer, H.Y., ed. *Psychopharmacology: The Third Generation of Progress.* New York: Raven Press, pp. 000–000.

Gittelman-Klein, R., Landa, B., Mattes, J.A., and Klein, D.F. (1988) Methylphenidate and growth in hyperactive children. *Arch Gen Psychiatry* 45:1127–1130.

Goldman, L., Genel, M., Bazman, R., and Stanetz, P. (1998) Diagnosis and treatment of attention-deficit/hyperactivity disorder. *JAMA* 279:1100–1107.

Grace, T. (2000) Cellular and molecular neurochemistry of psychostimulant effects on dopamine. In: Solanto, M. and Castellanos, X., eds. *The Neuropharmacology of Psychostimulant Drugs: Implications for ADHD, 1st ed.* New York: Oxford University Press, pp. 85–100.

Greenhill, L. (1998) Childhood attention deficit hyperactivity disorder: pharmacological treatments. In: Nathan, P.E. and Gorman, J., eds. *Treatments That Work, 1st ed.* Philadephia: W.B. Saunders, pp. 42–64.

Greenhill, L., Findling, R., Swanson, J., and Metadate Study Group. A double-blind, placebo-controlled, study of modified-release MPH MR in children with attention-deficit/hyperactivity disorder. *Pediatrics, in Press.*

Greenhill, L.L. and MTA Cooperative Group. (1999) Chronic stimulant treatment effects of weight acquisition rates of ADHD children. 39:26–27.

Greenhill, L., Swanson, J., Steinhoff K, Tullock S, Clausen S, Zhang Y (2002 b), A pharmacokinetic/pharmacodynamic study comparing a single morning dose of Adderall to twice daily dosing in children with attention-deficit/hyperactivity disorder. *J Am Acad Child Adolesc (in press). Psychiatry.*

Gualtieri, C.T., Wargin, W., Kanoy, R., Patrick, K., Shen, C.D., Youngblood, W., Mueller, R.A., and Breese, G.R. (1982) Clinical studies of methylphenidate serum levels in children and adults. *Child Psychiatry* 21:19–26.

Jadad, A.R., Boyle, M, Cunningham, C. et al. (1999) Treatment of Attention-Deficit/Hyperactivity Disorder: Evidence Report/Technology Assessment No. 11 (Prepared by McMaster University under Contract No. 290-97-0017). AHRQ Publication No. 00-E005. Rockville, Maryland: Agency for Healthcare Research and Quality. November.

Jensen, P., Kettle, L., Roper, M., Sloan, M., Dulcan, M., Hoven, C., Bird, H., Bauermeister, J., and Payne, J. (1999) Are stimulants overprescribed? Treatment of ADHD in 4 US communities. *J Am Acad Child Adolesc Psychiatry* 38:797–804.

Kent, J., Blader, J., Koplewicz, H., Abikoff, H., and Foley, C. (1995) Effects of late-afternoon methylphenidate administration on be-

havior and sleep in attention-deficit hyperactivity disorder. *Pediatrics* 96:320–325.

Klein, R., Abikoff, H., Klass, E., Ganales, D., Seese, L., and Pollack, S. (1997) Clinical efficacy of methylphenidate in conduct disorder with and without attention deficit hyperactivity disorder. *Arch Gen Psychiatry* 54:1073–1080.

Lambert, N.M., and Hartsough, C.S. (1998) Prospective study of tobacco smoking and substance dependence among samples of ADHD and non-ADHD subjects. *J Learn Disord* 31:533–544.

Manuzza, S., Klein, R., Bonagura, N., Malloy, P., Giampino, T., and Addlii, K. (1991) Hyperactive boys almost grown up: V. Replication of psychiatric status. *Arch Gen Psychiatry* 48:77–83.

Matochik, J., Nordahl, T., Gross, M., Semple, M., King, A., and Cohen, R., Zametkin, A. (1993) Effects of acute stimulant medication on cerebral metabolism in adults with hyperactivity. *Neuropsychopharmacology* 8:377–386.

McGough, J.J., Biederman, J., Greenhill, L.L., McCracken, J., Spencer, T.J., Posner, K., Wigal, S., Gornben, J., Tullock, S., and Swanson, J. (2002) Pharmacokinetics of Adderall and Adderall XR. *J Am Acad Child Adolesc Psychiatry*, in press.

McMaster University Evidence-Based Practice Center (1998). The treatment of attention-deficit/hyperactivity disorder: an evidence report (contract 290-97-0017).

Molina, B. and Pelham, W. (1999) ADHD, alcoholism, and drug abuse: a review of the literature. Unpublished report.

MTA Cooperative Group (1999) Moderators and mediators of treatment response for children with ADHD: the MTA study. *Arch Gen Psychiatry* 56:1088–1096.

National Institutes of Health (2000). The National Institutes of Health Consensus Development Conference Statement: Diagnosis and treatment of Attention-Deficit / Hyperactivity Disorder (ADHD). *J Am Acad Child Adolesc Psychiatry* 39:182–193.

Page, J.G., Bernstein, J.E., Janicki, R.S., and Michelli, F.A. (1974) A multicenter trial of pemoline (cylert) in childhood hyperkinesis. In: Conners, C.K., ed. *Clinical Use of Stimulant Drugs in Children.* The Hague, Netherlands: Excerpta Medica, pp. 98–124.

Pataki, C., Carlson, G., Kelly, K., and Rapport, M. (1993) Side effects of methylphenidate and desipramine alone and in combination in children. *J Am Acad Child Adolesc Psychiatry* 32:1065–1072.

Patrick, K.S., Mueller, R.A., Gualtieri, C.T., and Breese, G.R. (1987) Pharmacokinetics and actions of methyphenidate. In: Meltzer, H.Y., ed. *Psychopharmacology: A Third Generation of Progress, 3rd ed.* New York: Raven Press, pp. 1387–1395.

Pelham, W.E., Sturges, J., and Hoza, J. (1989) The effects of sustained release 20 and 10 mg Ritalin bid on cognitive and social behavior in children with attention deficit disorder. *Pediatrics* 80: 491–501.

Pelham, W.E., Swanson, J., Furman, M., and Schwindt, H. (1995) Pemoline effects of children with ADHD: a time-reponse by dose–response analysis on classroom measures. *J Am Acad Child Adolesc Psychiatry* 34:1504–1513.

Pliszka, S.R. (2000) Comparing the effects of stimulant and nonstimulant agents on catecholamine function: implications for theories of attention deficit hyperactivity disorder (ADHD). In: Solanto, M. and Castellanos, X., eds. *The Neuropharmacology of Psychostimulant Drugs: Implications for AD/HD, 1st ed.* New York: Oxford University Press, pp. 141–160.

Rapport, M.D., DuPaul, G.J., and Kelly, K.I. (1989) Attention deficit hyperactivity disorder and methylphenidate: the relationship between gross body weight and drug response in children. *Psychopharm Bull,* 25:285–290.

Rapport, M., Carlson, G., Kelly, K., and Pataki, C. (1993) Methylphenidate and desipramine in hospitalized children. I. Separate and combined effects on cognitive function. *J Am Acad Child Adolesc Psychiatry* 32:333–342.

Safer, D.J., and Allen, R.P. (1989). Absence of tolerance to the beharioral effects of methylphenidate and inattentive children. *J Pediatr* 115:1003–1008.

Sallee, F., Stiller, R., and Perel, J. (1992) Pharmacodynamics of pemoline in attention deficit disorder with hyperactivity. *J Am Acad Child Adolesc Psychiatry* 31:244–251.

Sallee, F.R., Stiller, R., Perel, J., and Bates, T. (1985) Oral pemoline kinetics in hyperactive children. *Clini Pharmacol Ther* 37:606–609.

Schmidt, K., Solanto, M.V., and Sanchez, M. (1984) The effect of stimulant medication of academic performance, in the context of multimodal treatment, in attention deficit disorders with hyperactivity. *J Clin Psychopharm* 4:100–103.

Sebrechts, M.M., Shaywitz, S.E., Shaywitz, B.A., Jatlow, P., Anderson, G.M., and Cohen, D.J. (1986) Components of attention, methylphenidate dosage, and blood levels in children with attention deficit disorder. *Pediatr* 77:222–228.

Spencer, T., Biederman, J., Harding, M., Faraone, S., and Wilens, T. (1996a) Growth deficits in ADHD children revisited: evidence for disorder related growth delays. *J Am Acad Child Adolesc Psychiatry* 35:1460–1467.

Spencer T., Biederman, J., Wilens, T., Harding, M., O'Donnell, D., and Griffin, S. (1996b) Pharmacotherapy of attention-deficit hyperactivity disorder across the life cycle. *J Am Acad Child Adolesc Psychiatry* 35:409–432.

Swanson, J. (1993) Effect of stimulant medication on hyperactive children: a review of reviews. *Exceptional Child* 60:154–162.

Swanson, J., Gupta, S., Guinta, D., Flynn, D., Agler, D., Lerner, M., Williams, L., Shoulson, I., Wigal, S. (1999a) Acute tolerance to methylphenidate in the treatment of attention deficit hyperactivity disorder in children. *Clin Pharmacol Ther* 66:295–305.

Swanson, J., Lerner, M., and Williams, L. (1995) More frequent diagnosis of attention deficit-hyperactivity disorder. *New Engl J Med* 333:944–944.

Swanson, J.M., Connor, D.F., and Cantwell, D. (1999b) Combining methylphenidate and clonidine: ill-advised. *J Am Acad Child Adolesc Psychiatry* 38:617–619.

TACT Study Group, (2002) Treatment of ADHD in children with Tourette's syndrome (TACT Trial). (2002), in press.

Vitiello, B., and Burke, L. (1998) Generic methylphenidate versus brand Ritalin: which should be used. In: Greenhill, L. and Osman, B., eds. *Ritalin: Theory and Practice, 2nd ed.* Larchmont, NY: Mary Ann Liebert, Inc., pp. 221–226.

Vitiello, B. and Jensen, P. (1997) Medication development and testing in children and adolescents. *Arch Gen Psychiatry* 54:871–876.

Volkow, N., Ding, J., Fowler, G., Wang, J., Logan, J., Gatley, J., Dewey, S., Ashby, C., Lieberman, J., Hitzemann, R., and Wolf, A. (1995) Is methylphenidate like cocaine? *Arch Gen Psychiatry* 52:456–464.

Volkow, N., Wang, G., Fowler, J., Gatley, S., Logan, J., Ding, Y., Hitzemann, R., and Pappas, N. (1998) Dopamine transporter occupancies in the human brain induced by therapeutic doses of oral methylphenidate. *Am J Psychiatry* 155:1325–1331.

Weiner, N. (1991) Drugs that inhibit adrenergic nerves and block adrenergic receptors. In: Gilman, A. and Goodman, L., eds. *Norepinephrine, Epinephrine and the Sympathomimetic Amines, 7th ed.* New York: The Pharmacological Basis of Therapeutics, pp. 145–180.

Wharton, R.W., Perel, J.M., Dayton, P.G., and Malitz, S.A. (1971) Potential clinical use for methylphenidate with tricyclic antidepressants. *Am J Psychiatry* 127:55–61.

Wilens, T., Biederman, J., and Spencer, T. (1994) Clonidine for sleep disturbances associated with attention deficit hyperactivity disorder. *J Am Acad Child Adolesc Psychiatry* 33:424–427.

Zametkin, A.J., Nordahl, T.E., Gross, M., King, A.C., Semple, W.E., Rumsey, J., Hamburger, S., and Cohen, R.M. (1991) Cerebral glucose metabolism in adults with hyperactivity of childhood onset. *New Engl J Med* 323:1361–1366.

Zito, J., Safer, D., dosReis, S., Gardiner, J., Boles, M., and Lynch, F. (2000) Trends in the prescribing of psychotropic medications to preschoolers. *JAMA* 283:1025–1030.

21 | Adrenergic agonists: clonidine and guanfacine

JEFFREY H. NEWCORN, KURT P. SCHULZ, AND JEFFREY M. HALPERIN

The alpha-2 (α_2) adrenergic agonists clonidine and guanfacine were first developed as anti-hypertensive agents. However, these have agents secondary uses in psychiatry because of their effects on norepinephrine (NE) and other neurotransmitter systems. Efficacy of the α_2 agonists in child and adolescent psychiatric disorders is principally derived from open studies, retrospective reviews, and case reports. There have been several controlled studies as well, but most are plagued by small sample size. Conditions in children that have been found to respond to the α_2 agonists include Tourette's disorder (TS), attention-deficit/hyperactivity disorder (ADHD), aggression, and post-traumatic stress disorder (PTSD) (Newcorn et al., 1998). Nevertheless, the α_2-adrenergic agonists are not approved by the Food and Drug Administration (FDA) for any of these indications and, because the number of studies examining efficacy and safety remains quite limited, there are not yet clear-cut guidelines to inform clinical usage.

Initial use of the α_2 agonists in child psychiatry can be traced as far back as the 1970s. Cohen and colleagues (1979) first noted beneficial effects of clonidine in the amelioration of tics, (Cohen et al., 1979), and began to use it as an alternative to neuroleptic treatment in TS. Several smaller studies and a larger controlled trial by Leckman and colleagues (1991) further supported the role of clonidine in TS. Benefits were also observed in reducing motor activity and impulsive behavior in ADHD in several studies by Hunt and colleagues (1985; 1987), although results were better for treatment of hyperactivity, impulsivity, and aggression than they were for inattention, and samples were small. Several subsequent studies examined the utility of clonidine in the treatment of ADHD + TS, with most reporting at least moderate improvement (Connor et al., 1999). More recently, several studies have demonstrated similar and possibly superior effects using the newer $\alpha_2$adrenergic agonist guanfacine in the treatment of ADHD (Horrigan and Barnhill, 1995; Hunt et al., 1995; Taylor and Russo, 2001) or ADHD + TS (Chappell et al., 1995; Scahill et al., 2001). Because guanfacine is a more specific α_{2A} agonist and has a longer half-life, it holds the prospect of more specific and sustained duration of action, with fewer adverse effects.

Clonidine has also been used in the treatment of aggression, generally with positive results. In addition to the fact that most studies with ADHD samples report lower ratings of aggression, pilot studies of children with oppositional defiant disorder or conduct disorder have consistently shown a reduction in aggression (Kemph et al., 1993; Schvela et al., 1994; Connor et al., 2000). Clonidine has also been used successfully to treat aggression in children with developmental disorders (Jaselskis et al., 1992). Finally, initial reports indicate that α_2 agonists can ameliorate anxiety and overarousal linked to the occurrence of severe stress or traumatic events (Pynoos and Nader, 1993; Perry, 1994; Horrigan, 1996). However, there have not been adequate data to address this question.

Interest in the psychiatric applications of α_2-adrenergic agonists is driven not only by initial reports of efficacy but also by the recognition of problems associated with more established treatments. In the case of ADHD, there is considerable interest in developing nonstimulant treatments, particularly in the wake of reports of overprescription and/or abuse of stimulants (LeFever, et al., 1999). Further, because the α_2 agonists do not cause insomnia, and may even be sedating, they can be used in the evening, and are sometimes given to minimize stimulant induced insomnia (Wilens et al., 1994; Prince et al., 1996). In the case of TS and other conditions linked to behavioral dysregulation, the α_2 agonists have commanded interest because of the desire to identify alternatives

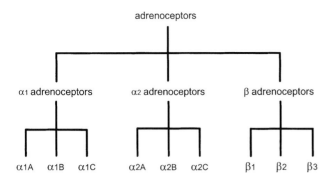

FIGURE 21.1 β-adrenergic receptors and subtypes.

to neuroleptic use in children. Finally, because NE innervation affects diverse brain regions and is likely involved in numerous psychiatric disorders, noradrenergic medications such as the α_2 agonists hold the prospect of being particularly useful when symptoms of multiple disorders are present.

Pharmacoepidemiologic data indicate that use of the α_2-adrenergic agonists has increased dramatically in the past decade. Swanson et al. (1995) estimated that in 1994, approximately 89,000 prescriptions were written for clonidine monotherapy for the treatment of ADHD, and another 61,000 prescriptions were written for the combination of methylphenidate and clonidine. Another review reported that over 100,000 children in the United States were medicated with the combination of methylphenidate and clonidine (Cantwell et al., 1997). In contrast, approximately 20,000 prescriptions were written for clonidine in 1990, suggesting a seven-fold increase from 1990 to 1995. More recently, Zito et al. (2000) reported that the use of clonidine increased 6 to 28 fold among preschool children from 1991 to 1995, depending on the database sampled. However, the number of preschool children actually being treated with this medication was still quite low, with 1–2 children treated per 1000 population.

Some authors have questioned whether there is sufficient efficacy and safety data to support widespread use of the α_2-adrenergic agonists (Cantwell et al., 1997), a position which intensified following the report of several sudden deaths of children who were medicated with clonidine and methylphenidate in combination (Popper, 1995). Although the FDA could not establish a causal link between the medications and these catastrophic outcomes, clearly more research is needed. At the same time, interest at the national level in establishing a more extensive scientific database to support the use of previously off-label prescription patterns, and interest on the part of industry to obtain FDA approval for new indications, suggests that larger

and more systematic trials of the α_2-adrenergic agonists are likely to be undertaken.

This chapter will review the characteristics and regulatory properties of α_2 receptors, neuropharmacology of the α_2-adrenergic agonists, hypothesized mechanisms by which these medications alter central nervous system (CNS) activity, as well as a variety of issues related to their clinical use, including safety and adverse effects, dosing, and medication interactions.

BASIC PROPERTIES OF α_2 ADRENOCEPTORS

Receptor Subtypes

The α_2-adrenergic agonists modulate central noradrenergic activity primarily through their effects on α_2 receptors, which are broadly distributed throughout the brain. The α_2 receptor is one of five adrenergic receptors (α_1, α_2, β_1, β_2, β_3), and is itself differentiated into three distinct subtypes: α_{2A}, α_{2B}, and α_{2C} (Fig. 21.1) (MacDonald et al., 1997). All three receptor subtypes transduce their signals via the $G_{i/o}$ protein signaling system, suppressing adenyl cyclase activity, inhibiting the opening of voltage-gated Ca^{2+} channels, and activating K^+ channels (MacDonald et al., 1997). The three receptor subtypes are encoded by distinct intronless genes, located in humans on chromosomes 10, 2, and 4, respectively.

Regulatory Properties

Biochemical properties of G proteins enable the α_2 adrenoceptors to adapt to fluctuations in synaptic activity and integrate the myriad of received signals (Böhm et al., 1997). The triggered intracellular responses of α_{2A} and α_{2B} receptors are diminished within seconds to minutes of exposure to agonists, a phenomenon known as *desensitization* (Eason and Liggett, 1992). Agonist-occupied receptors are reversibly phosphorylated by G protein–coupled receptor kinases (GRK), which uncouple the receptors from their G proteins and effectively terminate signaling. However, the extent of phosphorylation varies among agonists of different chemical structures (Jewell-Motz et al., 2000). Continued exposure to agonists results in a net reduction in all three α_2 adrenoceptor subtypes (Heck and Bylund, 1997). Down-regulation to 50% of pretreatment values occurs in approximately 2.5 hours. Interestingly, down-regulation of the α_{2A} receptor requires 100-fold more agonist than down-regulation of the α_{2B} and α_{2C} subtypes (Pleus et al., 1993).

Prolonged exposure to agonists is rare under normal physiological conditions, but may occur during stress (Nisenbaum and Abercrombie, 1993) or in response to pharmacological treatment. Receptor down-regulation is believed to be responsible for the development of drug tolerance or tachyphylaxis. Recovery from down-regulation necessitates the synthesis of new receptors and proceeds over hours to days. Differences in signaling and regulatory properties among the three α_2 adrenoceptor subtypes account for their distinct physiological profiles, and may help to explain pharmacodynamic differences between different α_2 agonists. These differences also raise the possibility that new α_2-adrenergic agonists with custom-designed characteristics can be developed in the future.

Anatomical Distribution

The α_{2A} adrenoceptor resides in the plasma membrane and is the predominant α_2 subtype in the brain, with large numbers found in the locus ceruleus (LC) and other noradrenergic brain stem nuclei, cerebellum, striatum, hypothalamus, thalamus, amygdala, hippocampus, septum, and cerebral cortex (Aoki et al., 1994). The α_{2B} adrenoceptor subtype also resides in the plasma membrane, but the expression of this receptor is limited mainly to the thalamus (Scheinin et al., 1994). In contrast, the α_{2C} adrenoceptor is localized primarily intracellularly and has little cell surface localization (Olli-Lähdesmäki et al., 1999), but is widely distributed in the striatum, the hippocampus, the cerebral cortex, and the LC (Scheinin et al., 1994). Given that agonist–receptor interactions occur at the cell surface, the distribution of the three α_2 adrenoceptors suggests that the α_{2A} subtype may mediate most of the central effects of α_2-adrenergic agonists.

NEUROPHARMACOLOGY OF α_2 AGENTS: CLONIDINE AND GUANFACINE

Chemical Structure

The α_2-adrenergic agonists clonidine and guanfacine are structurally different compounds. As denoted by their chemical names, clonidine, or 2-(2,6-dichlorophenylamino)-2-imidazoline, is an imidazoline derivative, while guanfacine, or N-amidino-2-(2,6-dichlorophenyl) acetamide, is not. However, clonidine and guanfacine have structurally similar elements. Both compounds contain a guanidine structure, but in the case of clonidine the guanidine is part of a ring structure in the form of imidazoline (see Fig. 21.2).

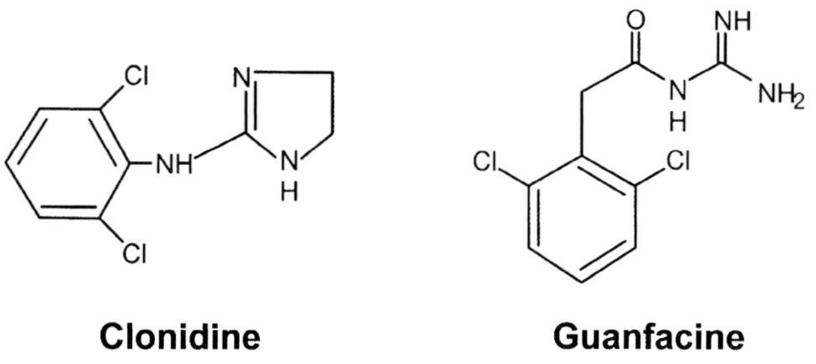

Clonidine   **Guanfacine**

FIGURE 21.2 Chemical structure of clonidine and guanfacine.

Binding Properties

Guanfacine is relatively specific in its effects on α_2 receptors, while clonidine is less selective. Guanfacine has nanomolar affinity for the α_{2A} receptor, with 100-fold lower affinity for the α_{2B} receptor and 40-fold lower affinity for the α_{2C} receptor (Uhlén et al., 1995). Moreover, guanfacine demonstrates little nonspecific binding to other receptors. In comparison, the affinity of clonidine for the α_{2A} receptor is only 4-fold and 10-fold greater than its affinity for the α_{2B} and α_{2C} receptors, respectively (MacDonald et al., 1997). Furthermore, clonidine also binds with moderate to high affinity to α_1 adrenoceptors and nonadrenergic imidazoline sites (Uhlén et al., 1995).

Pharmacokinetic and Pharmacodynamic Properties

Clonidine is highly lipid soluble and is completely absorbed after oral administration, with peak plasma levels occurring within 3 to 5 hours. In contrast, the absolute oral bioavailability of guanfacine is approximately 80% of an equivalent intravenous dose, with peak plasma concentrations occurring within 1 to 4 hours (mean = 2.6 hours) (Physician's Desk Reference, 2001). In addition to being more rapidly absorbed into circulation, guanfacine has a longer elimination half-life than clonidine. The plasma half-life of guanfacine is approximately 17 hours (range = 10 to 30 hours) in healthy adults, but tends to be shorter in younger individuals (range = 13 to 14 hours). In comparison, clonidine has a half-life of 12 to 16 hours in adults and 8 to 12 hours in children.

Elimination of clonidine is 65% by renal excretion and 35% by liver metabolism, while guanfacine and its metabolites are excreted primarily in the urine, with approximately 50% as unchanged drug. These differences in elimination may account for differences in the pharmacodynamic properties of the two drugs. The behavioral effects of clonidine last only 3 to 6 hours and oral medication is usually given on a tid or qid schedule (Hunt et al., 1985; 1990), while guanfacine tends to have a slightly longer behavioral effect that may permit a bid or tid dosing schedule (Chappell et al., 1995; Scahill et al., 2001). Differences in the regulatory properties of the various α_2 adrenoceptors may also account for the observed differences in behavioral half-life between clonidine and guanfacine. Since greater amounts of agonist are required for down-regulation of the α_{2A} receptor than other α_2 receptor subtypes, the more α_{2A}-selective guanfacine may take longer to down-regulate than the relatively nonselective clonidine.

Pharmacologic Activity

The α_{2A} adrenoceptor functions as an autoreceptor and mediates the potent inhibitory effects of α_2 agonists on noradrenergic metabolism through actions at the LC (Lakhlani et al., 1997; Feuerstein et al., 2000). Somatodendritic α_{2A} autoreceptors suppress the excitability of LC neurons (Arima et al., 1998), while presynaptic α_{2A} autoreceptors mediate the autoinhibition of NE release (Boehm and Huck, 1996). These inhibitory effects on LC activity are believed to produce the calming and sedative effects of α_2-adrenergic agonists (De Sarro et al., 1987; Nacif-Coelho et al., 1994), and may explain the role for these medications in treating states of overarousal, excitability, and aggression.

Prejunctional α_{2A} adrenoceptors are also widely expressed on nonnoradrenergic terminals throughout the brain (Aoki et al., 1994), and inhibit the release of several neurotransmitters, including dopamine (Hertel et al., 1999) and glutamate (Boehm, 1999). α_{2A} heteroreceptor–mediated inhibition of glutamate release is thought to be associated with inhibition of kindling in the amygdalohippocampal area (Boehm, 1999), gating of corticothalamic synapses (Castro-Alamancos and Calcagnotto, 2001), and reduction of sympathetic outflow in the rostral ventrolateral medulla (Milner et al., 1999), all of which are consistent with the general calming affects of α_2 agonists. Inhibition of kindling in the amygdalohippocampal area might further suggest a possible role for α_2 agonists in the treatment of PTSD, while the modulation of dopaminergic neurotransmission might partially explain the beneficial effects of α_2 agonists on inattention (Coull et al., 1995).

The clinical effects of α_2-adrenergic receptor agonists may also derive from the action of postsynaptic α_{2A} adrenoceptors, which modulate the excitability of target neurons in select noradrenergic terminal fields in the neocortex (Pralong and Magistretti, 1995; Carette, 1999). α_2 adrenoceptor–mediated inhibition of neuronal excitability in the amygdala is responsible for the antiepileptogenic effect of α_2-adrenergic agonists (Gellman et al., 1987). The stimulatory effect of α_2-adrenergic agonists on growth hormone (GH) secretion is also mediated by the postsynaptic α_{2A} adrenoceptor, which regulates the release of growth hormone releasing factor (GHRF) in the ventromedial and arcuate nuclei of the hypothalamus (Cella et al., 1987). Measuring GH release following acute administration of clonidine or guanfacine can therefore be used as an indirect probe of central α_{2A} activity (Balldin et al., 1993).

The cognitive-enhancing effects of the α_2-adrenergic agonists may also be mediated by postsynaptic α_{2A} adrenoceptors (Arnsten et al., 1996). Stimulation of postsynaptic α_{2A} adrenoceptors in the prefrontal cortex enhances task-related firing relative to background activity, thereby improving mnemonic and inhibitory functions (Sawaguchi, 1998). This cognitive-enhancing effect of α_2-adrenergic agonists has been noted on several tasks involving delayed responding and inhibitory control (Arnsten and Goldman-Rakic, 1985; Sawaguchi 1998), and may partially explain the beneficial effects of α_2 agonists in the treatment of ADHD (Arnsten et al., 1996).

Consistent with the limited expression of the α_{2B} adrenoceptor, the role of this subtype seems to be restricted to cardiovascular function (Kable et al., 2000). The α_{2B} adrenoceptor mediates the initial, transient hypertensive response to α_2-adrenergic agonists through actions in the vascular smooth muscle cells in the arterial wall (Link et al., 1996). Consistent with this, guanfacine, which is relatively selective for the α_{2A} subtype, seems less often to be associated with cardiovascular adverse effects such as hypotension and bradycardia in clinical studies (Scahill et al., 2001; Taylor and Russo, 2001), while clonidine, which has mixed $\alpha_{2A/2B/2C}$ binding properties, has been more highly associated with cardiovascular changes (Cantwell et al., 1997; Connor, et al., 1999). In contrast to the α_{2A} and α_{2B} adrenoceptors, the α_{2C} receptor does not seem to be involved in cardiovascular regulation or other classical actions of α_2-adrenergic agonists. However, this receptor may play a minor role in the modulation of dopamine metabolism (Sallinen et al., 1997; Hein et al., 1999); which may partially explain the slight cognitive-enhancing effect of α_{2C} adrenoceptor stimulation (Bjorklund et al., 1999, 2000). Yet, the physiological function of the α_{2C} adrenoceptor, and the role that this receptor plays in various behavioral paradigms, has yet to be adequately determined.

CLINICAL USE OF α₂ AGONISTS

α₂ Agonist Medications: Description and Administration

Clonidine is manufactured in 0.1, 0.2, and 0.3 mg tablets. There is also a transdermal therapeutic (TTS) system (clonidine patch), which provides more sustained coverage and eliminates the need for frequent daily oral doses. Transdermal therapeutic system dosing is determined from the equivalent daily oral clonidine dose. As with the tablets, patches come in doses of 0.1, 0.2, and 0.3 mg daily (i.e., TTS-1, TTS-2, and TTS-3). Each patch lasts about 5 days, although the product labeling indicates 1 week activity (Hunt, 1987). Guanfacine can only be taken orally, and tablets are 1 mg and 2 mg. Guanfacine is 10 times less potent than clonidine, and a 1 mg guanfacine tablet is comparable in potency and physiologic effect to a 0.1 mg clonidine tablet. It is important to be mindful of the awkward 0.1 mg clonidine dose, and the potential for confusion with the more user-friendly 1 mg guanfacine dose, particularly when switching from clonidine to guanfacine, or vice versa.

Application of the clonidine patch requires a certain degree of knowledge and vigilance (Hunt et al., 1990). The patch is placed on a clean, dry, and hairless section of skin, usually on the back. If the patch comes off repeatedly—as a result of either bathing, sweating, swimming, or other physical activity—it may limit utility. Often, multiple patches are used to achieve the optimal therapeutic dose, which offers protection against dose reduction if a patch does fall off. Patches are optimally applied at different times of the week, since relatively newer patches may take 2–3 days to reach their full activity. Patches may be cut and sealed to give doses as low as 0.05 mg. However, the control membrane in the TTS system must remain sealed for the patch to perform optimally. Damage to the membrane has been associated with accidental overdose (Broderick-Cantwell, 1999). It is generally recommended to titrate with oral clonidine and switch to the TTS system once the optimal dose is determined. Combination of TTS and oral forms may be used.

Dosing

Recommended dosing schedules for clonidine and gunafacine have varied considerably across studies. A standard clonidine dose for ADHD is approximately 3–5 µg/kg/day, with a range of 0.1–0.3 mg/day (Hunt et al., 1990). Some studies have employed doses as high as 0.4 to 0.5 mg (Wilens et al., 1994; Prince et al., 1996), often to induce sleep. However, the risk of adverse effects may increase at higher doses. It is usually recommended to begin with low doses and titrate slowly because of sedation and possible cardiovascular effects. A general rule is to not increase the dose by more than 0.05 mg every 3 days. There is some evidence that severity of dose-dependent adverse effects decreases over time (Physicians Desk Reference, 2001).

Dosing of guanfacine reflects its lower potency and longer duration of action. Doses range from 0.5 to 4 mg/day (Chappell et al., 1995; Hunt et al., 1995; Scahill et al., 2001), generally administered on a bid or tid schedule. Like clonidine, the dose can be increased by 0.5 mg every 3 to 4 days. The modal total daily dose used by Scahill and colleagues (2001) in a controlled study of ADHD + TS was 2.5 mg/day, given tid.

Adverse Effects

Commonly reported adverse effects of clonidine include dry mouth (40%), drowsiness (33%), dizziness (16%), sedation (10%), weakness (10%), and fatigue (4%). Nervousness, agitation, headache, nightmares and frequent waking, weight gain, nausea, and vomiting are reported but less frequently so (Physician's Desk Reference, 2001). Hypotension and bradycardia are also commonly observed (Connor, et al., 1999), but are less consistently present. An asymptomatic 10% decrease in systolic blood pressure (BP) has been reported by Hunt et al. (1990), with orthostatic hypotension present in less than 5% of cases. Electrocardiographic (EKG) abnormalities can be secondary to rhythm changes, or may be idiosyncratic. Prolongation of PR and QTc intervals have been reported in some individuals treated with clonidine, but systematic investigation has not supported consistent medication effects (Connor et al., 1999, 2000; Kofoed et al., 1999). Depression has also been reported (McCracken and Martin, 1997); and the related symptom of irritability may be more common in children (Connor et al., 1999). Dermatitis may develop when the adhesive agents are used, although this can often be managed by premedicating with hydrocortisone cream (Hunt et al., 1990). A variety of other adverse effects have been reported infrequently, including changes in blood counts and in hepatic and urinary function.

The adverse effect profile of guanfacine is similar, with the exception that dry mouth and sedation are less common (Wilson et al., 1986). Blood pressure was not different from placebo in initial controlled studies of children with ADHD ± TS (Scahill et al., 2001; Taylor and Russo, 2001), but this may reflect the low number of subjects or the short duration of treatment. Orthostatic hypotension has also not been reported thus far, although bradycardia apparently occurs rarely. One case series reported the occurrence of mania and hypomania in several children following treatment with guanfacine (Horrigan and Barnhill, 1999); however, on closer inspection these children had various risk factors for bipolar disorder. It should be remembered that the adverse effects listed in the PDR for the α_2-adrenergic agonists generally refer to their use in the treatment of hypertension in adults, often at higher doses than are used in children.

Premedication Work-up, Ongoing Monitoring, and Contraindications to Treatment

Careful review of medical and cardiac history, and a screening physical exam, are reommended before initiating clonidine or guanfacine treatment. Cardiac murmurs should be evaluated to determine their hemodynamic significance. Sinus node and atrioventricular (AV) node disease are relative contraindications, as they can present with syncope and bradycardia, which may be exacerbated by α_2 agonist treatment. Renal disease is also a relative contraindication due to the association with hypertension and cardiovascular disease, although guanfacine has been used safely to treat hypertension in adults with renal disease (Sorkin and Heel, 1986).

Baseline resting pulse and BP should be monitored both prior to and during treatment (Hunt et al., 1990; Oesterheld and Tervo, 1996). If the baseline pulse is less than 60, or if BP is greater or less than 2 standard deviations from age- and gender-adjusted means on two repeated evaluations, more detailed evaluation should be obtained. Orthostatic pulse or BP changes of greater than 10% should raise concern as to whether the dose should be decreased.

It is generally recommended that an EKG be obtained at baseline and when on a stable dosage (Dulcan et al., 1997), although a recent review by the American Heart Association did not recommend EKG monitoring (Gutgessell et al., 1999), and most studies of clonidine efficacy did not monitor EKG (Connor et al., 1999). If the EKG shows bradycardia, impaired AV conduction (first-degree, second-degree, or complete heart block), or QRS interval >120 msec, it is advisable to obtain further consultation. Other laboratory studies recommended as part of the initial medical work-up (Hunt et al., 1990) include complete blood cell count (CBC) with differential, electrolytes, fasting blood glucose, thyroid function tests, liver function tests (serum glutamic-oxaloacetic transaminase [SGOT], serum glutamic-pyruvic transaminase [SGPT], bilirubin), and renal function tests (blood urea nitrogen [BUN]/creatinine).

Once on medication, it is important to evaluate any new onset of treatment-emergent symptoms, especially if they are exercise related. Acute onset of dizziness, fatigue, light-headedness, sedation, syncope, and near-syncope (especially if exercise related) require close clinical monitoring and possible evaluation using Holter monitor and/or echocardiogram (Oesterheld and Tervo, 1996).

Two different patterns of clonidine-induced cardiovascular complications have been described (Swanson et al., 1995). One is characterized by decreased pulse and BP, often with associated EKG changes, fatigue, and sedation, and responds to a decrease in dosage. The other presents with tachycardia, tachypnea, with or without fever, anxiety, panic, and acute mental status changes, and is often associated with a missed dose or an abrupt taper. This pattern often responds to reinstituting the dosage and slowly tapering as necessary.

Discontinuation

It is necessary to taper clonidine rather than abruptly discontinuing it to decrease the risk of rebound hypertension (Leckman et al., 1986). Hunt et al. (1990) recommend that if the medication has been used for only 1 week, it can be discontinued immediately. If it has been prescribed for 1–4 weeks, it can be tapered by 0.05 mg daily; and if it has been prescribed for over 4 weeks, it should be tapered by 0.05 mg every third day. The possibility of rebound hypertension should also be evaluated in patients on clonidine who are not consistent in their medication-taking behavior. Less is known about the likelihood of rebound hypertension following discontinuation of guanfacine. Although the PDR lists this as possible, one study found this not to be the case (Wilson et al., 1986), possibly because of its longer duration of action.

Drug interactions

There are few absolute contraindications, but several points should be considered. Medications that produce changes in sinus node or AV nodal conduction may potentiate the cardiovascular adverse effects of the α_2 agonists. This may be particularly relevant for concomitant administration of beta-blockers, which, similar to the α_2 agonists, have been used to treat aggression.

Coadministration of beta-blockers can potentiate rebound hypertension upon discontinuation of α_2 medications, and it is therefore recommended that the beta-blocker be withdrawn before the α_2 agonist (Physicians Desk Reference, 2001). Tricyclic antidepressants may also produce changes in sinus node and AV conduction, and it is recommended that they be used cautiously in combination with α_2 agonists (Physicians Desk Reference, 2001). However, in child psychiatric practice, there has been debate about whether there are adverse interactions related to concomitant use of tricyclics and α_2 agonists. Finally, the α_2 agonists may potentiate the effects of CNS depressants (e.g., barbiturates) or other medications that produce sedation, so lower doses of each may be warranted.

Reports of Sudden Death with Combined Clonidine–Methylphenidate Treatment

A flurry of clinical and media reports surfaced in 1995 publicizing the death of four children receiving combination treatment with methylphenidate and clonidine. The circumstances surrounding the deaths are difficult to fully ascertain, but were briefly described in a review conducted by the FDA (Fenichel, 1995). Of note, all of the deaths had multiple confounding variables that precluded attributing their cause to the drug combination. Although hypotension was present in virtually all the cases, this does not necessarily suggest an adverse drug interaction. Consistent with this conclusion, Swanson et al. (1995) reported on 19 cases of adverse events associated with clonidine, generally involving cardiovascular function, and most often following a change in use (either prescribed, accidental or a cessation of medication). Further, Chandran (1994) reported on EKG changes following clonidine administration in 3/60 children treated, all of which responded to dose reduction or discontinuation.

One hypothesized mechanism of methylphenidate-clonidine toxicity involves the concomitant use of methylphenidate during the day, for control of ADHD symptoms, and clonidine at night, to minimize stimulant use late in the day and to promote sleep. Swanson et al. (1995) reasoned that if methylphenidate is administered in the morning after an evening dose of clonidine is wearing off, each of the medications could independently contribute to increased BP—clonidine through rebound, and methylphenidate through its usual effect of slightly raising BP.

Since the mid-1990's, there have been no further reports of serious methylphenidate–clonidine toxicity, possibly owing to less frequent use of this medication combination. However, more recent studies have questioned whether the α_2 agonists are indeed associated with substantial cardiovascular toxicity. Kofoed et al. (1999) examined pre- and post-treatment EKGs of children and adolescents treated with clonidine, alone or in combination with stimulants. No consistent abnormalities in PR or QTc intervals were identified in either the clonidine monotherapy or combination therapy groups. Of note, there was considerable variability in EKG findings across multiple time points, and minor abnormalities normalized following treatment approximately as often as new problems developed. Additionally, Connor and colleagues (2000) followed EKG parameters in children treated with clonidine alone ($n = 8$) or clonidine and methylphenidate ($n = 8$), and found no consistent abnormalities associated with treatment. However, there was lengthening of the PR interval, more prominent with the combination, but not reaching criteria for first-degree AV block. Finally, open (Chappel et al., 1995; Horrigan and Barnhill, 1995; Hunt et al., 1995) and controlled (Scahill et al., 2001) treatment trials with guanfacine have identified little or no hypotension and no EKG changes following treatment.

In summary, the α_2 agonists do not seem to be associated with an adverse profile of cardiovascular effects for the majority of individuals, whether given alone or in combination with short-acting stimulants. However, there may be a small number of individuals who are sensitive to these medications, particularly clonidine, and who may be at increased risk. Although serious adverse interactions with methylphenidate have not been substantiated, additional caution may be warranted. For those children in whom combined stimulant/α_2 treatment is being considered, it may be prudent to use longer-acting medications, such as dextroamphetamine, newer sustained-release stimulant preparations, and guanfacine. This should, at least theoretically, reduce the concern that hypertension may develop as a function of on–off effects of medication.

SUMMARY AND CONCLUSIONS

The α_2-adrenergic agonists are promising agents for the treatment of many frequently occurring child psychiatric syndromes, including hyperactivity, aggression, tics and other conditions characterized by overarousal and traumatic stress, consistent with hypothesized noradrenergic mechanisms in these conditions. However, their profiles of clinical and adverse effects have been inadequately researched. Although they cannot be considered a first-line treatment for any disorder, they may be particularly useful as second-line treatments, adjunctive therapy in partial responders, and treatment of cases in which comorbidity is present. The safety profiles of the α_2 agonists, and their potential for coadministration with other psychotropics, suggest that they may be well suited for this purpose, although careful assessment and monitoring of cardiovascular status is required. Guanfacine is a particularly promising treatment, in terms of its more specific α_{2A} activity and preliminary reports of efficacy, safety, and tolerability. However, more extensive study is required.

REFERENCES

Aoki, C., Go, C.G., Venkatesan, C., and Kurose, H. (1994) Perikaryal and synaptic localization of α_{2A}-adrenergic receptor–like immunoreactivity. Brain Res 650:181–204.

Arima, J., Kubo, C., Ishibashi, H., and Akaike, N. (1998) α-2 Adrenoceptor-mediated potassium currents in acutely dissociated rat LC neurones. J Physiol 508:57–66.

Arnsten, A.F.T. and Goldman-Rakic, P.S. (1985) α-2 Adrenergic mechanisms in prefrontal cortex associated with cognitive decline in aged nonhuman primates. Science 230:1273–1276.

Arnsten, A.F.T., Steere, J.C., and Hunt, R.D. (1996) The contribution of α_2 noradrenergic mechanisms to prefrontal cortical cognitive functions: potential significance to attention-deficit hyperactivity disorder. Arch Gen Psychiatry 53:448–455.

Balldin, J., Berggren, U., Eriksson, E., Lindstedt, G., and Sundkler, A. (1993) Guanfacine as an alpha-2-agonist inducer of growth hormone secretion: a comparison with clonidine. Psychoneuroendocrinology 18:45–55.

Bjorklund, M., Sirvio, J., Riekkinen, M., Sallinen, J., Scheinin, M., and Riekkinen, P., Jr. (2000) Overexpression of α_{2C}-adrenoceptors impairs water maze navigation. Neuroscience 95:481–487.

Bjorklund, M., Sirvio, J., Sallinen, J., Scheinin, M., Kobilka, B.K., and Riekkinen, P., Jr. (1999) α_{2C}-Adrenoceptor overexpression disrupts execution of spatial and non-spatial search patterns. Neuroscience 88:1187–1198.

Boehm, S. (1999) Presynaptic α_2-adrenoceptors control excitatory, but not inhibitory, transmission, at rat hippocampal synapses. J Phsyiol 519:439–449.

Boehm, S., and Huck, S. (1996) Inhibition of N-type calcium channels:the only mechanism by which presynaptic α_2-autoreceptors control sympathetic transmitter release. Eur J Neurosci 8:1924–1931.

Böhm, S.K., Grady, E.F., and Bunnett, N.W. (1997) Regulatory mechanisms that modulate signalling by G-protein–coupled receptors. Biochem J 322:1–18.

Broderick-Cantwell, J.J. (1999) Case study: accidental clonidine patch overdose in attention-deficit/hyperactivity disorder patients. J Am Acad Child Adolesc Psychiatry 38:95–98.

Cantwell, D.P., Swanson, J., and Connor, D.F. (1997) Case study: adverse response to clonidine. J Am Acad Child Adolesc Psychiatry 36:539–544.

Carette, B. (1999) Noradrenergic responses of neurones in the mediolateral part of the lateral septum: α_1-adrenergic depolarization and rhythmic bursting activities, and α_2-adrenergic hyperpolarization from guinea pig brain slices. Brain Res Bull 48:263–276.

Castro-Alamancos, M.A. and Calcagnotto, M.E. (2001) High-pass filtering of corticothalamic activity by neuromodulators released in the thalamus during arousal: in vitro and in vivo. J Neurophysiol 85:1489–1497.

Cella, S.G., Locatelli, V., De Gennaro, V., Wehrenberg, W.B., and Muller, E.E. (1987) Pharmacological manipulations of α-adrenoceptors in the infant rat and effects on growth hormone secretion. Study of the underlying mechanisms of action. Endocrinology 120:1639–1643.

Chandran, K.S. (1994) ECG and clonidine. J Am Acad Child Adolesc Psychiatry 33:1351–1352.

Chappell, P.B., Riddle, M.A., Scahill, L., Lynch, K.A., Schultz, R., Arnsten, A., Leckman, J.F., and Cohen, D.J. (1995) Guanfacine treatment of comorbid attention-deficit hyperactivity disorder and Tourette's syndrome:preliminary clinical experience. J Am Acad Child Adolesc Psychiatry 34:1140–1146.

Cohen, D.J., Young, J.G., Nathanson, J.A., and Shaywitz, B.A. (1979) Clonidine in Tourette's syndrome. Lancet, 2:551–553.

Connor, D.F., Barkley, R.A., and Davis, H.T. (2000) A pilot study of methylphenidate, clonidine, or the combination in ADHD comorbid with aggressive oppositional defiant or conduct disorder. Clin Pediatr 39:15–25.

Connor, D.F., Fletcher, K.E., and Swanson, J.M. (1999) A meta-analysis of clonidine for symptoms of attention-deficit hyperactivity disorder. J Am Acad Child Adolesc Psychiatry 38:1551–1559.

Coull, J.T., Sahakian, B.J., Middleton, H.C., Young, A.H., Park, S.B., McShane, R.H., Cowen, P.J., and Robbins, T.W. (1995) Differential effects of clonidine, haloperidol, diazepam and tryptophan depletion on focused attention and attentional search. Psychopharmacology 121:222–230.

De Sarro, G.B., Ascioti, C., Froio, F., Libri, V., and Nistico, G. (1987) Evidence that LC is the site where clonidine and drugs acting at alpha 1- and alpha 2-adrenoceptors affect sleep and arousal mechanisms. Br J Pharmacol 90:675–685.

Dulcan, M. (American Academy of Child and Adolescent Psychiatry) (1997) Practice parameters for the assessment and treatment of children, adolescents and adults with attention-deficit/hyperactivity disorder. J Am Acad Child Adolesc Psychiatry 36(Suppl):85S–121S.

Eason, M.G., and Liggett, S.B. (1992) Subtype-selective desensitization of α_2-adrenergic receptors. Different mechanisms control short and long term agonist promoted desensitization of α_{2C10}, α_{2C4} and α_{2C2}. J Biol Chem 267:25473–25479.

Fenichel, R.R. (1995) Combining methylphenidate and clonidine: the role of post-marketing surveillance. J Child Adolesc Psychopharmacol, 5:155–156.

Feuerstein, T.J., Huber, B., Vetter, J., Aranda, H., van Velthoven, V., and Limberger, N. (2000) Characterization of the α_2-adrenoceptor subtype, which functions as α_2-autoreceptor in human neocortex. J Pharmacol Exp Ther 294:356–362.

Gellman, R.L., Kallianos, J.A., and McNamara, J.O. (1987) Alpha-2 receptors mediate and endogenous noradrenergic suppression of kindling development. J Pharmacol Exp Ther 241:891–898.

Gutgesell, H., Atkins, D., Barst, R., Buck, M., Franklin, W., Humes, R., Ringel, R., Shaddy, R., and Taubert, K. (1999) Cardiovascular monitoring of children and adolescents receiving psychotropic drugs. Circulation 99:979–982.

Heck, D.A., and Bylund, D.B. (1997) Mechanism of down-regulation of alpha-2 adrenergic receptor subtypes. J Pharmacol Exp Ther 282:1219–1227.

Hein, L., Altman, J.B., and Kobilka, B.K. (1999) Two functionally distinct α_2-adrenergic receptors regulate sympathetic neurotransmission. Nature 402:181–184.

Hertel, P., Nomikos, G.G., and Svensson, T.H. (1999) Idazoxan preferentially increases dopamine output in the rat medial prefrontal cortex at the nerve terminal level. Eur J Pharmacol 371:153–158.

Horrigan, J.P. (1996) Guanfacine for PTSD nightmares. *J Am Acad Child Adolesc Psychiatry* 35:975–976.

Horrigan, J.P. and Barnhill, L.J. (1995) Guanfacine for treatment of attention-deficit hyperactivity disorder in boys. *J Child Adolesc Psychopharmacol* 5:215–223.

Horrigan, J.P. and Barnhill, L.J. (1999) Guanfacine and secondary mania in children. *J Affect Disord* 54:309–314.

Hunt, R.D. (1987) Treatment effects of oral and transdermal clonidine in relation to methylphenidate—an open pilot study in ADDH. *Psychopharmacol Bull* 27:111–114.

Hunt, R.D., Arnsten, A.F.T., and Asbell, M. (1995) An open trial of guanfacine in the treatment of attention-deficit hyperactivity disorder. *J Am Acad Child Adolesc Psychiatry* 34:50–54.

Hunt, R.D., Capper, L., and O'Connell, P. (1990) Clonidine in child and adolescent psychiatry. *J Child Adolesc Psychopharmacol* 1: 87–102.

Hunt, R.D., Minderaa, R.B., and Cohen, D.J. (1985) Clonidine benefits children with attention deficit disorder and hyperactivity:report of a double-blind placebo-crossover therapeutic trial. *J Am Acad Child Adolesc Psychiatry* 24:617–629.

Jaselskis, C.A., Cook, E.H., Fletcher, K.E., and Leventhal, B.L. (1992) Clonidine treatment of hyperactive and impulsive children with autistic disorder. *J Clin Psychopharmacol* 12:322–327.

Jewell-Motz, E.A., Small, K.M., Theiss, C.T., and Liggett, S.B. (2000) $\alpha_{2A/2C}$-Adrenergic receptor third loop chimera show that agonist interaction with receptor backbone establishes G protein–coupled receptor kinase phosphorylation. *J Biol Chem* 275: 28989–28993.

Kable, J.W., Murrin, L.C., and Bylund, D.B. (2000) In vivo gene modification elucidates subtype-specific functions of α_2-adrenergic receptors. *J Pharmacol Exp Ther* 293:1–7.

Kemph, J.P., DeVane, C.L., Levin, G.M., Jarecke, R., and Miller, R.L. (1993) Treatment of aggressive children with clonidine: results of an open pilot study. *J Am Acad Child Adolesc Psychiatry* 32:577–581.

Kofoed, L., Tadepalli, G., Oesterheld, J.R., Awadallah, S., and Shapiro, R. (1999) Case series: clonidine has no systematic effects on PR or QTc intervals in children. *J Am Acad Child Adolesc Psychiatry* 38:1193–1196.

Lakhlani, P.P., MacMillan, L.B., Guo, T.Z., McCool, B.A., Lovinger, D.M., Maze, M., and Limbird, L.E. (1997) Substitution of a mutant α_{2A}-adrenergic receptor via "hit and run" gene targeting reveals the role of this subtype in sedative, analgesic, and anesthetic-sparing responses in vivo. *Proc Natl Acad Sci USA* 94: 9950–9955.

Leckman, J.F., Hardin, M.T., Riddle, M.A., Stevenson, J., Ort, S.I., and Cohen, D.J. (1991) Clonidine treatment of Gilles de la Tourette's syndrome. *Arch Gen Psychiatry* 48:324–328.

Leckman, J.F., Ort, S., Caruso, K.A., Anderson, G.M., Riddle, M.A., and Cohen, D.J. (1986) Rebound phenomena in Tourette's syndrome after abrupt withdrawal of clonidine. *Arch Gen Psychiatry* 43:1168–1176.

LeFever, G.B., Dawson, K.V., and Morrow, A.L. (1999) The extent of drug treatment for attention deficit–hyperactivity disorder among children in public schools. *Am J Public Health* 89:1359–1364.

Link, R.E., Desai, K., Hein, L., Stevens, M.E., Chruscinski, A., Bernstein, D., Barsh, G.S., and Kobilka, B.K. (1996) Cardiovascular regulation in mice lacking α_2-adrenergic receptor subtypes b and c. *Science* 273:803–805.

MacDonald, E., Kobilka, B.K., and Scheinin, M. (1997) Gene targeting-homing in on α_2-adrenoceptor-subtype function. *Trends Pharmacol Sci* 18:211–219.

McCracken, J.T. and Martin, W. (1997) Clonidine side effect. *J Am Acad Child Adolesc Psychiatry* 36:160–161.

Milner, T.A., Rosin, D.L., Lee, A., and Aicher, S.A. (1999) α_{2A}-Adrenergic receptors are primarily presynaptic heteroreceptors in the C1 area of the rat rostral ventrolateral medulla. *Brain Res* 821:200–211.

Nacif-Coelho, C., Correa-Sales, C., Chang, L.L., and Maze, M. (1994) Perturbation of ion channel conductance alters the hypnotic response to the α_2-adrenergic agonist dexmedetomidine in the LC of the rat. *Anesthesiology* 81:1527–1534.

Newcorn, J.H., Schulz, K., Harrison, M., De Bellis, M.D., Udarbe, J.K., and Halperin, J.M. (1998) α_2-adrenergic agonists: neurochemistry, efficacy and clinical guidelines for use in children. *Pediatr Clin North Am* 45:1099–1122.

Nissenbaum, L.K., and Abercrombie, E.D. (1993) Presynaptic alterations with enhancement of evoked release and synthesis and release of norepinephrine in hippocampus of chronically cold-stressed rats. *Brain Res* 608:280–287.

Oesterheld, J. and Tervo, R. (1996) Clonidine: a practical guide for usage in children. *S D J Med* 49:234–237.

Olli-Lähdesmäki, T., Kallio, J., and Scheinin, M. (1999) Receptor subtype-induced targeting and subtype-specific internalization of human α_2-adrenoceptor in PC12 cells. *J Neurosci* 19:9281–9289.

Perry, B.D. (1994) Neurobiological sequelae of childhood trauma: PTSD in children. In: Murburg, M.M., ed., *Catecholamine Function in Posttraumatic Stress Disorder: Emerging Concepts*. Washington DC: American Psychiatric Press, pp. 235–255.

Physician's Desk Reference 55th ed.. (2001), Montvale, NJ: Medical Economics Data.

Pleus, R.C., Schreve, P.E., Toews, M.L., and Bylund, D.B. (1993) Down-regulation of α_2-adrenoceptor subtypes. *Eur J Pharmacol* 244:181–185.

Popper, C.W. (1995) Combining methylphenidate and clonidine: pharmacologic questions and news reports about sudden death. *J Child Adolesc Psychopharmacol* 5:157–166.

Pralong, E. and Magistretti, P.J. (1995) Norepinephrine increases K-conductance and reduces glutamatergic transmission in the mouse entorhinal cortex by activation of α_2-adrenoreceptors. *Eur J Neurosci* 7:2370–2378.

Prince, J.B., Wilens, T.E., Biederman, J., Spencer, T.J., and Wozniak, J.R. (1996) Clonidine for sleep disturbances associated with attention-deficit hyperactivity disorder: a systematic chart review of 62 cases. *J Am Acad Child Adolesc Psychiatry* 35:599–605.

Pynoos, R.S. and Nader, K. (1993) Issues in the treatment of posttraumatic stress disorder in children and adolescents. In: Wilson, J. and Raphael, B., eds. *The International Handbook of Traumatic Stress Syndromes* Washington, DC: American Psychiatric Press, pp. 535–549.

Sallinen, J., Link, R.E., Haapalinna, A., Viitamaa, T., Kulatunga, M., Sjöholm, B., MacDonald, E., Pelto-Huikko, M., Leino, T., Barsch, G.S., Kobilka, B.K., and Scheinin, M. (1997) Genetic alteration of α_{2C}-adrenoceptor expression in mice: influence on locomotor, hypothermic, and neurochemical effects of dexemedetomidine, a subtype-nonselective α_2-adrenoceptor agonist. *Mol Pharmacol* 36:36–46.

Sawaguchi, T. (1998) Attenuation of delay-period activity of monkey prefrontal neurons by an α_2-adrenergic antagonist during an oculomotor delayed response task. *J Neurophysiol* 80:2200–2205.

Scahill, L., Chappell, P.B., Kim, Y.S., Schultz, R.T., Katsovich, L., Shepherd, E., Arnsten, A.F.T., Cohen, D.J., and Leckman, J.F. (2001) A placebo-controlled study of guanfacine in the treatment of children with tic disorders and attention deficit hyperactivity disorder. *Am J Psychiatry* 158:1067–1074.

Scheinin, M., Lomasney, J.W., Hayden-Hixson, D.M., Schambra, U.B., Caron, M.G., Lefkowitz, R.J., and Fremeau, R.T., Jr. (1994) Distribution of α_2-adrenergic receptor subtype gene expression in rat brain. *Brain Res Mol Brain Res* 21:133–149.

Schvehla, T.J., Mandoki, M.W., and Sumner, G.S. (1994) Clonidine therapy for comorbid attention deficit hyperactivity disorder and conduct disorder: preliminary findings in a children's inpatient unit. *South Med J* 87:692–695.

Sorkin, E.M. and Heel, R.C. (1986) Guanfacine: a review of the pharmacodynamic and pharmacikinetic properties, and therapeutic efficacy in the treatment of hypertension. *Drugs* 31:301–336.

Swanson, J.M., Flockhart, D., Udrea, D., Cantwell, D.P., Connor, D., and Williams, L. (1995) Clonidine in the treatment of ADHD: questions about safety and efficacy. *J Child Adolesc Psychopharmacol* 5:301–304.

Taylor, F.B. and Russo, J. (2001) Comparing guanfacine and dextroamphetamine for the treatment of adult attention-deficit/hyperactivity disorder. *J Clin Psychopharmacol* 21:1–6.

Uhlén, S., Muceniecce, R., Rangel, N., Tiger, G., and Wikberg, J.E.S. (1995) Comparison of the binding activities of some drugs on α_{2A}, α_{2B} and α_{2C}-adrenoceptors and non-adrenergic imidazoline sites in the guinea pig. *Pharmacol Toxicol* 76:353–364.

Wilens, T.E., Biederman, J., and Spencer, T. (1994) Clonidine for sleep disturbances associated with attention-deficit hyperactivity disorder. *J Am Acad Child Adolesc Psychiatry* 33:424–426.

Wilson, M.F., Haring, O., Lewin, A., Bedsole, G., Stepansky, W., Fillingim, J., Hall, D., Roginsky, M., McMahon, F.G., Jagger, P., and Strauss, M. (1986) Comparison of guanfacine versus clonidine for efficacy, safety and occurrence of withdrawal syndrom in step-2 treatment of mild to moderate essential hypertension. *Am J Cardiol* 57:43E–49E.

Zito, J.M., Safer, D.J., dos Rios, S., Gardner, J.F., Boles, M., and Lynch, F. (2000) Trends in the prescribing of psychotropic medications to preschoolers. *JAMA* 283:1025–1030.

22 | Antidepressants I: selective serotonin reuptake inhibitors

SUFEN CHIU AND HENRIETTA L. LEONARD

The selective serotonin reuptake inhibitors (SSRI) have been used in adults for a wide variety of disorders, including major depression, social anxiety (social phobia), generalized anxiety disorder (GAD), eating disorders, premenstrual dysphoric disorder (PMDD), post-traumatic stress disorder (PTSD), panic, obsessive-compulsive disorder (OCD), trichotillomania, and migraine headaches. Some of the specific SSRI agents have an approved indication in adults for some of these disorders, as reviewed later in this chapter. The SSRIs have also been tried in children and in adults for symptomatic treatment of pain syndromes, aggressive or irritable ("short fuse") behavior, and for self-injurious and repetitive behaviors. This chapter will review general aspects of the SSRIs and discuss their approved indications in children and adolescents.

OVERVIEW OF SELECTIVE SEROTONIN REUPTAKE INHIBITOR MEDICATIONS IN CHILD PSYCHIATRY

The prototypical serotonin reuptake inhibitor (SRI) medication is the non-selective agent clomipramine, a tricyclic antidepressant (TCA). The Selective SRIs (SSRIs) include fluoxetine (Prozac), sertraline (Zoloft), paroxetine (Paxil), fluvoxamine (Luvox), and citalopram (Celexa). The Food and Drug Administration (FDA) approved clinical indications for these medications are described in Table 22.1.

GENERAL PROPERTIES OF SELECTIVE SEROTONIN REUPTAKE INHIBITOR MEDICATIONS

SSRI medications differ greatly in their chemical structures and composition. For example, citalopram is a tertiary amine with 2 N-metabolites. All three compounds are racemic, which means that there are S- and R-enantiomer forms for each compound. Only the S-citalopram is thought to be clinically active. The ratio of $S/(S+R)$ citalopram varies from 0.35 to 1 (Rochat et al., 1995a,b).

Fluoxetine is a secondary amine, which is demethylated to norfluoxetine. Norfluoxetine is clinically active. Both compounds have S- and R- enantiomers (Wong et al., 1990, 1993). Unlike citalopram, S- and R-fluoxetine and S-norfluoxetine are active forms. R-fluoxetine is much less potent than the other two compounds. In addition, it appears that R-fluoxetine and R-norfluoxetine are metabolized more rapidly than the S-enantiomers (Torok-Both et al., 1992).

Paroxetine and sertraline are chiral drugs as well, but only one enantiomer form of each has been marketed. Fluvoxamine is notably different in that it is achiral (Baumann, 1996). Table 22.2 summarizes active metabolites and elimination half-lives of each SSRI. Much of this information does not distinguish between the different enantiomer forms of each drug.

The presence of an active metabolite and the duration of parent compound and metabolite half-life all impact the clinical interpretation of dosing, side effects, and potential for withdrawal. Fluoxetine and its active metabolite, both of which have a relatively long half-life, remain in the system for a long time after discontinuation. Industry prescribing instructions for fluvoxamine recommend a bid dosing regimen, in part because of the absence of an active metabolite. Paroxetine, without an active metabolite and with a relatively short half-life, has been anecdotally associated with late-day withdrawal effects.

Relative Selectivity of Serotonin Reuptake Inhibition

Paroxetine and sertraline are the most potent inhibitors of serotonin reuptake among the five approved SSRI

TABLE 22.1 *Food and Drug Administration–Approved Indications for Serotonin Reuptake Inhibitor and Selective Serotonin Reuptake Inhibitor Agents*

| SRI or SSRI | Adult FDA Indications | | | | Pediatric FDA Indications |
	Depression	OCD	Panic	Other	
Citalopram	X				None
Clomipramine		X			OCD in patients ≥10 years old
Fluoxetine	X	X		Bulimia nervosa PMDD	None
Fluvoxamine		X			OCD in patients ≥8 years old
Paroxetine	X	X	X	Social anxiety GAD	None
Sertraline	X	X	X	PTSD	OCD ≥6 years old

FDA, Food and Drug Administration; GAD, general anxiety disorder; OCD, obsessive-compulsive disorder; PMDD, Premenstrual dysphoric disorder; PTSD, post-traumatic stress disorder; SRI, serotonin reuptake inhibitor; SSRI, selective serotonin reuptake inhibitor.

TABLE 22.2 *Selective Seratonin Reuptake Inhibitor Active Metabolites*

Antidepressant Drugs	Main Active Metabolites	Elimination Half-life[a]	Reference
Fluoxetine	Norfluoxetine	2 to 7 days	Schenker et al., 1988
Fluvoxamine	None	17 to 22 hours	Hrdina, 1991; Spigset et al., 1998
Paroxetine	None	24 hours	Lund et al., 1982
Sertraline	Desmethylsertraline	26 hours	Ronfeld et al., 1997
Citalopram	Desmethylcitalopram	1 to 2.5 days	Overo, 1978

[a] The elimination half-life includes the metabolite if it is a significant one by prolonging the parent compound's clinical effect.

medications, whereas citalopram is the most selective (Sanchez and Hyttel, 1999). The selectivity differences among SSRIs are not clinically significant, but may have an impact on side effect profile and drug interaction patterns (Leonard et al., 1997). Among the SSRI medications, sertraline has the greatest potency at the dopamine uptake pump. Clinically, this effect is not apparent because the concentration of sertraline needed to bind to the dopamine uptake pump is twofold higher than that needed to saturate the serotonin reuptake pump (Preskorn, 2000).

ADVERSE EFFECTS

Specific Considerations for Pediatric Use

As early as 1987, Teicher and Baldessarini predicted on the basis of animal studies that SSRI agents may be more agitating in healthy, younger children (Teicher and Baldessarini, 1987), and this concern has been discussed in the pediatric literature (Riddle et al., 1991). The standard study of sertraline for pediatric OCD reported that 13% of the patients treated experienced agitation, as compared to 2% of those on placebo (March et al., 1998). The study of fluvoxamine for OCD reported that 12.3% of patients on active medication (versus 3.2% on placebo) experienced agitation or hyperkinesia (Riddle et al., 2001). Those numbers raise the question of whether the pediatric ages may be more vulnerable to activation or agitation on the SSRIs, but until populations are compared side by side, it is not possible to draw conclusions.

Fluoxetine's most notable side effect is nervousness (>10% in adults) (Preskorn, 2000), which may be more common in the pediatric population (Teicher and Baldessarini, 1987). Fluvoxamine is less stimulating than fluoxetine but is a significant inhibitor of CYP3A4, which metabolizes common pediatric medications (Michalets and Williams, 2000). Fluvoxamine is most likely to cause constipation in adults (>10%) (Preskorn, 2000). This is an important consideration in children, given the often comorbid symptoms of encopresis from overflow constipation.

General Adverse Effects

The most common adverse side effects of SSRI medications, in decreasing order, include sexual dysfunction (30%), nausea, drowsiness, constipation, nervousness, and fatigue (>10%) (Preskorn, 2000). Nervousness includes anxiety, agitation, hostility, akathisia, and central nervous system (CNS) stimulation. Other adverse effects reported include headache, dizziness, dry mouth, insomnia, restlessness, tremor, and abdominal discomfort. Studies in children have generally reported similar same side effect profiles (e.g., Emslie et al., 1997; March et al., 1998; Keller et al., 2001; Walkup et al., 2001). Nausea most frequently occurred with fluvoxamine (>25%), likely mediated by excessive serotonin activity at the 5-HT$_3$ receptor.

In general, one of the advantages of the SSRIs is that electrocardiographic (EKG) monitoring is not required. Few, if any, cardiac adverse events are reported on SSRI monotherapy. Recently, Wilens and colleagues (1999) reported that there were no changes in EKG indices or vital signs in children and adolescents on sertraline at doses up to 200 mg/day.

In general, the SSRIs have a more tolerable side effect profile than the tricyclic antidepressants with their anticholinergic effects. Review of the rate that subjects in the controlled studies discontinued a SSRI because of adverse effects provides some perspective on how well tolerated the medications are, although the specifics may vary according to dosage and design (e.g., forced titration) and are not directly comparable. The rate of discontinuation was reported to be 12% (4/48) for fluoxetine (Emslie et al., 1997), 9.7% for paroxetine (Keller et al., 2001), 13% (12/92) for sertraline (March et al., 1998), and 33% (19/57) (Riddle et al., 2001) and 7.9% (5/63) for fluvoxamine (Walkup et al., 2001).

Neurological Side Effects

Movement disorders and extrapyramidal signs and symptoms

Extrapyramidal side effects (EPS) associated with SSRI medications used as single agents were reported as early as 1979 (Meltzer et al., 1979). Since then, several case reports have been published on use of fluoxetine (Hamilton and Opler, 1992), paroxetine (Nicholson, 1992), and sertraline (Opler 1994). The SSRI medications in combination with neuroleptics can cause severe EPS (Tate, 1989; Ketai, 1993) above and beyond what may be associated with increased levels of antipsychotic medications (Goff et al., 1991), and are perhaps related to pharmacokinetic drug interactions.

Neuropsychiatric and behavioral effects

Initial worsening of symptoms. Any of the SSRIs may initially worsen symptoms of anxiety, particularly in patients with OCD or panic disorder (Pohl et al., 1988). This phenomenon is different from the behavioral activation sometimes seen in subsequent treatment. Starting with lower doses of medications may alleviate these phenomena.

Behavioral activation. Adverse effects while on the SSRIs may include anxiety, restlessness, agitation, akathisia, jitteriness, disinhibition, and/or activation. The development of anxiety, restlessness, and agitation while on an antidepressant has been described as "part of the complex and poorly self-described syndrome of akathisia" (Kalda, 1993). "Behavioral activation" is variously reported as akathisia, jitteriness, disinhibition, activation, or agitation, and may represent overlapping or different phenomena. It is important for clinicians to discuss these potential symptoms with children and their parents, as the symptoms certainly can occur in the pediatric age group, and it is not known if there is an additional age-related risk.

Mania. Mania and hypomania can also occur in children and adolescents on SSRIs, and, again, it is not known if there is an added developmental risk (Venkataraman et al., 1992). In a fluoxetine treatment study for depression, 3 (of 48) patients developed manic symptoms, even after excluding patients with psychotic depression, bipolar symptoms, or a family history of bipolar disorder (Emslie et al., 1997). In a paroxetine treatment study for depression, 5 adolescents (of 93) were removed for emotional lability and 1 for euphoria/expansive mood (Keller et al., 2001).

Apathy and frontal lobe-like syndromes. A reversible, dose-related frontal lobe–like syndrome characterized by apathy, indifference, loss of initiative, and/or disinhibition has been reported in adults on SSRI therapy (Hoehn-Saric et al.1990, 1991). Recently, five cases of "amotivational syndrome" in youths, 10 to 17 years of age, were reported (Garland Baerg, 2001). Symptoms had a delayed onset, were dose related, and were reversible. The authors caution that such presentation may go underrecognized or may be mistakenly attributed to residual depression or to avoidance rather than to a medication side effect.

Sleep. All of the SSRIs can potentially alter sleep architecture and decrease sleep efficiency, which may manifest itself as daytime sedation or trouble concentrating. The SSRIs may have differing effects on sleep. Fluoxetine has been reported to increase rapid eye movement (REM) latency, increase the number of awakenings, decrease sleep efficiency, and suppress

REM sleep (Rush et al., 1998). In one of the few sleep studies of children and adolescents treated with fluoxetine, similar findings were noted, with increased light stage 1 sleep, increased number of arousals and REM density, and a largely unaffected REM latency (Armitage et al., 1997). One must keep in mind that studies of depressed children and adolescents suggest that subjects may have sleep polysomnographic abnormalities associated with depression itself (Emslie et al., 2001).

Bleeding complications. Lake and colleagues (2000) reported five children (ages 8–15 years of age) who developed bruising (1) or epistaxis (4) 1 week to 3 months after starting SSRI treatment. In all cases, bleeding ceased fairly abruptly when the medication was discontinued or the dose was reduced. All of the five children were taking sertraline, although there is no evidence to suggest that it may have a greater propensity to cause bleeding than the other SSRIs. For patients using SSRIs, physicians should be attentive to signs of possible abnormal bleeding, including easy bruisability, menorrhagia, and epistaxis. Additionally, SSRIs should be used cautiously in patients with thrombocytopenia or platelet disorders. The fact that Lake et al.'s study is the only case report to date suggests that it is a rare adverse reaction, although it may be underreported. Vascular complications include vasodilation, which could lead to hypotension, especially in cases of overdose (Fraser and South, 1999).

Discontinuation Syndrome

In a randomized, double-blind, placebo-controlled study of paroxetine treatment of panic disorder in adults, 12 weeks of treatment was followed by 2 weeks of placebo (Oehrberg et al., 1995). In this placebo period, 19 patients out of 55 (34.5%) who had received paroxetine reported an adverse event on discontinuation, compared to 7 out of 52 (13.5%) patients who had received placebo. The most common discontinuation complaint was dizziness.

In a retrospective chart review of 352 adult patients treated in an outpatient clinic with SSRI medications, 171 patients who had supervised discontinuation of their medication were compared to those who stayed on medication (Coupland et al., 1996). The most common withdrawal symptom was, again, dizziness, but paresthesias, asthenia, nausea, visual disturbances, and headache were also common. Movement-induced exacerbation of symptoms were associated with discontinuation of paroxetine (16.0%) and fluvoxamine (7.0%). It seems prudent to recommend gradual titration of SSRIs. Fluoxetine, with its long metabolite half-life, may be the exception to this general rule.

Selective Serotonin Reuptake Inhibitor Overdose

Lethal overdosages are extremely rare (Barbey and Roose, 1998), but have been reported for fluoxetine (260 to 6000 mg), sertraline (1100 mg), paroxetine (530 to 600 mg), and fluvoxamine (unknown dose). Many of these lethal doses occurred in adults; reports of lethal overdose in children occur even less frequently. One report of a 4-year-old boy who ingested 400 mg of fluvoxamine described life-threatening complications requiring respiratory and inotropic support (Fraser and South, 1999). The boy presented in a coma with hypotension and bradycardia. After 24 hours, he recovered.

In general, SSRI doses of 50 to 75 times the common daily doses result in minor symptoms. Higher doses cause serious symptoms of seizure, arrhythmias, and decreased consciousness; only doses greater than 150 times the common daily therapeutic dose can result in death (Barbey and Roose, 1998). Overdose in combination with alcohol or other drugs increases toxicity and accounts for most fatalities involving the SSRIs. Nevertheless, compared to TCA medications, which annually results in 100 to 150 fatal overdoses reported to the American Association of Poison Control Centers (AAPCC), the SSRI agents accounted for only 16 fatal overdoses reported to that organization between 1987 and 1996 (Barbey and Roose, 1998).

Drug–Drug Interactions

The SSRIs bind tightly to plasma proteins and may interfere with other protein-bound drugs (e.g., warfarin, digitoxin), causing a shift in plasma concentrations that can potentially result in adverse effects (Schrefer, 2001). As mentioned above, the SSRI medications can

TABLE 22.3 *Cytochrome P450 Enzyme Inhibition by Selective Serotonin Reuptake Inhibitor Agents*

	Enzyme System Inhibited				
SSRI	CYP1A2	CYP2C9	CYP2C19	CYP2D6	CYP3A4
Citalopram	X		X	X	
Fluoxetine		X		X	X
Fluvoxamine	X	X			X
Paroxetine				X	
Sertraline		X		X	X

Adapted from Nemeroff et al. (1996) and Schrefer (2001)

increase levels of antipsychotic medications. Addition of SSRI agents to TCAs increases serum TCA levels (40%–300%) and therefore may increase cardiac conduction abnormalities (Preskorn et al., 1994; Burke et al., 1996; Alderman et al., 1997).

As summarized in Table 22.3, All SSRIs interact with cytochrome P450 function to various degrees. These interactions and their clinical implications are extensively covered in Chapter 5 in this volume.

The interaction of SSRI agents with other drugs administered breast-feeding women warrants clinical attention. The degree to which SSRI medications are present in breast milk or in infant plasma remains poorly understood (Yoshida et al., 1999; Burt et al., 2001). For example, sertraline does not appear at high enough levels in breast-fed infants ($n = 11$) to alter their platelet serotonin levels (Epperson et al., 2001).

Serotonin Syndrome

Sternbach (1991) originally defined the clinical symptoms of the serotonin syndrome (Table 22.4). Table 22.5 lists medications that have been implicated in causing serotonin syndrome.

Other etiologies need to be ruled out because many of the symptoms of serotonin syndrome overlap with those of early sepsis or neuroleptic malignant syndrome, conditions associated with significant mortality. It is critical to evaluate for sepsis and to determine that a neuroleptic has not been started or increased prior to the onset of

TABLE 22.4 *Symptoms of Serotonin Syndrome*

Coincident with the addition (or increase) of a known serotonergic agent to an established medication regimen, at least 3 of the following:

Mental status changes	Shivering
Agitation	Tremor
Myoclonus	Diarrhea
Hyperreflexia	Incoordination
Diaphoresis	Fever

Adapted from Sternbach (1991)

signs and symptoms. Serotonin syndrome and neuroleptic malignant syndrome share common symptoms of altered consciousness, diaphoresis, autonomic disturbances, hyperthermia, extrapyramidal symptoms, and elevated creatine kinase (Lane 1997; Keck and Arnold, 2000). For more information on this syndrome and differential diagnosis, the reader is directed to the Neuroleptic Malignant Syndrome Information Service (1–888-NMS-TEMP or www.nmsis.org).

In general, herbal remedies, including St. John's wort, echinacea, kava kava, and ginkgo, should be avoided. St John's wort is considered an herbal remedy with some serotonergic reuptake inhibition properties and is purported to be helpful with depression. It is sometimes used concurrently with SSRI medications by patients who assume it is relatively free of adverse side effects.

TABLE 22.5. *Drugs that Potentiate Serotonin in the Central Nervous System and Could Be Associated with Serotonin Syndrome*

Enhances Serotonin Synthesis	Increases Serotonin Release	Serotonin agonist	Inhibits Serotonin Catabolism	Inhibits Serotonin Reuptake
L-tryptophan	Cocaine	Buspirone	Tranylcypromine	Bromocriptine
	Amphetamines	Lithium	Phenelzine	Dextromethorphan
	Stimulants	Sumatriptan	Moclobemide	Flenfluramine
	Sibutramine	Dihydroergotamine (DHE)	Isocarboxazid	Meperidine
	Fenfluramine	Meta-chlorophenylpiperazine (mCPP)	Selegiline	Nefazodone
	Dextromethorphan			Trazodone
	Meperidine	Trazodone (mCPP)		Pethidine
	Methylene dioxymethamphetamine			Tramadol
				Mirtazapine
				TCA medications
				Venlafaxine
				SSRI agents

Adapted from Keck and Arnold (2000) and Sternbach (1991)

No cases of serotonin syndrome associated with St. John's wort have been reported to date. St. John's wort does not produce clinically evident inhibition of CYP2D6 or CYP3A4 (Markowitz et al., 2000). However, recent reports highlight that St. John's wort has clinically significant effects via induction of CYP3A4 by binding activation of steroid X receptors known to bind pregnanes (Moore et al., 2000; Wentworth et al., 2000).

PEDIATRIC PHARMACOKINETIC SELECTIVE SEROTONIN REUPTAKE INHIBITOR STUDIES

Paroxetine pharmacokinetics in 30 depressed children and adolescents of ages 6 to 17 demonstrated substantial interindividual variability and more rapid clearance in youths than in adults (Findling et al., 1999). Nevertheless, paroxetine may be given once daily in the pediatric population.

Sertraline pharmacokinetics were described in 61 children and adolescents (ages 6 to 17) with depression or OCD (Alderman et al., 1998). Mean area under the plasma concentration–time curve, peak plasma concentration, and elimination half-life for sertraline and desmethylsertraline were similar to previously reported adult values. No differences between children and adolescents were apparent when values were normalized for body weight.

Wilens and colleagues (Wilens, 2001) studied the pharmacokinetics of fluoxetine pharmacokinetics in 21 children and adolescents (ages 6 to 18). Mean steady-state fluoxetine and norfluoxetine were achieved in children and adolescents with major depressive disorder after 4 weeks of treatment, with high variability among patients. Fluoxetine serum levels were two-fold higher and nor-fluoxetine serum levels were 1.7-fold higher in children relative to adolescents. As with sertraline, when normalized to body weight, serum levels of fluoxetine and nor-fluoxetine were similar for both age groups. Estimates of fluoxetine clearance and apparent volume of distribution exhibited high between-patient variability, similar to that reported in adults.

RISK/BENEFIT AND FUTURE DIRECTIONS OF SELECTIVE SEROTONIN REUPTAKE INHIBITOR MEDICATIONS IN PEDIATRIC POPULATIONS

The long-term effects of SSRI medications on the developing brain remain to be explored. A preliminary study on developing rodent brains reported a persistent increase in serotonin transporter density in the frontal cortex of rat pups treated with fluoxetine for 2 weeks, during the early time of developing central serotonergic and nonadrenergic systems (Wegerer et al., 1999). In contrast, rats given fluoxetine at a later point in development (during their prepubertal period) showed only a temporary increase in serotonin density. This was the first demonstration of long-lasting effects of a SSRI administration during juvenile life on the maturation of the central serotonergic system.

A neuroanatomical magnetic resonance imaging (MRI) brain study compared treatment naive pediatric patients with OCD ($n = 21$) and healthy volunteers ($n = 21$) (Gilbert et al., 2000). Treatment naive pediatric patients with OCD had statistically larger thalamic volumes than healthy controls. A subgroup of the pediatric patients with OCD ($n = 10$) were treated with paroxetine for 12 weeks. After 12 weeks, thalamic volumes were significantly decreased to levels comparable to those of controls. These studies mark the advent of new technologies to better assess treatment effects. It is premature to generalize these findings to the general pediatric population.

In Emslie's (1999) thoughtful commentary on these studies, he raised several issues. Is the neurobiology of childhood-onset disorders different from that in adults, and does this affect presentation and treatment response? What are the consequences of developmental differences related to side effects and are they irreversible? What might the positive impact of early treatment of disorders be, before the disorders themselves cause changes in brain functioning? To date, there is no evidence that early treatment with SSRIs has any negative long-term impact on patients. Importantly, one must consider that we may even identify positive effects of treatment during an important period of brain development.

COMMENTARY

Consideration of the use of medications in children requires a careful discussion with the child and the child's family of the risks and benefits potentially associated with the treatment. The AACAP Practice Parameters address the issue of informed consent, and how children, parents, and clinicians might reach a consensus on the use of medications (King, 1997). Children should have the opportunity to assent to the use of medications at a developmentally appropriate level. In general, pharmacotherapy should not be used as the sole intervention for a child's disorder but should be integrated into a comprehensive treatment plan.

REFERENCES

Alderman, J., Preskorn, S.H., Greenblatt, D.J., Harrison, W., Penenberg, D, Allison, J., Chung, M. (1997). Desipramine pharmacokinetics when coadministered with paroxetine or sertraline in extensive metabolizers. *J Clin Psychopharmacol* 17:284–291.

Alderman, J., Wolkow, R., Chung, M., and Johnston, H.F. (1998) Sertraline treatment of children and adolescents with obsessive-compulsive disorder or depression: pharmacokinetics, tolerability, and efficacy. *J Am Acad Child Adolesc Psychiatry* 37:386–394.

Armitage, R., Emslie, G., and Rintelmann, J. (1997) The effect of fluoxetine on sleep EEG in childhood depression: a preliminary report. *Neuropsychopharmacology* 17:241–245.

Barbey, J.T. and Roose, S.P. (1998) SSRI safety in overdose. *J Clin Psychiatry* 59 (Suppl 15):42–48.

Baumann, P. (1996) Pharmacokinetic–pharmacodynamic relationship of the selective serotonin reuptake inhibitors. *Clin Pharmacokinet* 31:444–469.

Bell, C.J. and Nutt, D.J. (1998) Serotonin and panic. *Br J Psychiatry* 172:465–471.

Bernstein, G.A., Borchardt, C.M., and Perwien, A.R. (1996) Anxiety disorders in children and adolescents: a review of the past 10 years. *J Am Acad Child Adolesc Psychiatry* 1996; 35:1110–1119.

Birmaher B., Waterman GS, Ryan N, Cully M, Balach L, Ingram J, Brodsky M. Fluoxetine for childhood anxiety disorders. *J Am Acad Child Adolesc Psychiatry* 33:993–999.

Black, B. and Robbins D.R. (1990) Panic disorder in children and adolescents. *J Am Acad Child Adolesc Psychiatry* 29:36–44.

Black, B. and Uhde, T.W. (1994) Treatment of elective mutism with fluoxetine: a double-blind, placebo controlled study. *J Am Acad Child Adolesc Psychiatry* 33:1000–1006.

Bryant, R.A. and Friedman, MBc. (2001) Medication and non-medication treatments of post-traumatic stress disorder. *Current Opinion in Psychiatry* 14:119–123.

Burke, M.J.M.D.P. and Harvey, A.T.P., (1996) Pharmacokinetics of the Newer antidepressants. *Am J Med* 100:119–121.

Chappell, P.B., Scahill, L.D., and Leckman, J.F. (1997) Future therapies of Tourette syndrome. *Neurol Clin* 15:429–450.

Cohen, J.A., Mannarino, A.P., and Rogal, S. (2001) Treatment practices for childhood posttraumatic stress disorder. *Child Abuse Negl*; 25:123–135.

Cook, E.H., Jr., Rowlett, R., Jaselskis, C., and Leventhal, B.L. (1992) Fluoxetine treatment of children and adults with autistic disorder and mental retardation. *J Am Acad Child Adolesc Psychiatry* 31:739–745.

Coupland, N.J., Bell, C.J., and Potokar, J.P. (1996) Serotonin reuptake inhibitor withdrawal. *J Clin Psychopharmacol* 16:356–362.

Cunningham, M., Cunningham, K., Lydiard, R.B. (1990) Eye tics and subjective hearing impairment during fluoxetine therapy. *Am J Psychiatry* 147:947–948.

Davies, T.S. and Kluwe W.M. (1998) Preclinical toxicological evaluation of sertraline hydrochloride. *Drug Chem Toxicol* 21:521–537.

DeVeaugh-Geiss, J., Moroz, G., Biederman, J., Cantwell, D., Fontaine, R., Greist, J.H., Reichler, R., Katz, R., and Landau, P. (1992) Clomipramine hydrochloride in childhood and adolescent obsessive-compulsive disorder—a multicenter trial. *J Am Acad Child Adolesc Psychiatry* 31:45–49.

Dulcan, M.K., Bregman, J., Weller, E.B., and Weller, R. (1998) *Treatment of childhood and adolescent disorders*. 2nd ed. Washington, D.C.: American Psychiatric Press.

Dummit, E.S., 3rd, Klein, R.G., Tancer, N.K., Asche, B., and Martin, J. (1996) Fluoxetine treatment of children with selective mutism: an open trial. *J Am Acad Child Adolesc Psychiatry* 35:615–621.

Elko, C.J., Burgess, J.L., and Robertson, W.O. (1998) Zolpidem-associated hallucinations and serotonin reuptake inhibition: a possible interaction. *J Toxicol Clin Toxicol* 36:195–203.

Emslie, G.J., Rush, A.J., Weinberg, W.A., Kowatch, R.A., Hughes, C.W., Carmody, T., and Rintelmann, J.A. (1997) double-blind, randomized, placebo-controlled trial of fluoxetine in children and adolescents with depression. *Arch Gen Psychiatry* 54:1031–1037.

Emslie, G.J., Armitage, R., Weinberg, W.A., Rush, A.J., Mayes, T.L., and Hoffmann, R.F. (2001) Sleep polysomnography as a predictor of recurrence in children and adolescents with major depressive disorder. *Int J Neuropsychopharmacol* 4:159–168.

Emslie, G.J., Rush, A.J., et al. (1997) A double-blind, randomized, placebo-controlled trial of fluoxetine in children and adolescents with depression. *Arch Gen Psychiatry* 54:1031–1037.

Findling, R.L., Reed, M.D., Myers, C., O'Riordan, M.A., Fiala, S., Branicky, L, Waldorf, B., and Blumer, J.L. (1999) Paroxetine pharmacokinetics in depressed children and adolescents. *J Am Acad Child Adolesc Psychiatry* 38:952–959.

Fraser, J. and South, M. (1999) Life-threatening fluvoxamine overdose in a 4-year-old child. *Intensive Care Med* 25:548.

Garland, E.J. and Weiss, M. (1996) Case study: obsessive difficult temperament and its response to serotonergic medication. *J Am Acad Child Adolesc Psychiatry* 35:916–920.

Garland, E.J. and Baerg, E.A. (2001) Amotivational syndrome associated with selective serotonin reuptake inhibitors in children and adolescents. *J Child Adolesc Psychopharmacol* 11:181–186.

Gilbert, A.R., Moore, G.J., Keshavan, M.S., Paulson, L.A., Narula, V., Mac Master, F.P., Stewart, C.M., and Rosenberg, D.R. (2000) Decrease in thalamic volumes of pediatric patients with obsessive-compulsive disorder who are taking paroxetine. *Arch Gen Psychiatry* 57:449–456.

Goff, D.C., Midha, K.K., Brotman, A.W., Waites, M., and Baldessarini, R.J. (1991) Elevation of plasma concentrations of haloperidol after the addition of fluoxetine. *Am J Psychiatry* 148:790–792.

Greenspan, S.I. and Weider, S. (1991) Regulatory Disorders. In: C.H. Z, ed. *Handbook of Infant Mental Health*. New York: Guildford Press, pp. 280–290.

Guyatt, G.H. and Rennie, D. (1993) Users' guides to the medical literature. *Jama* 270:2096–2097.

Hamilton, M.S. and Opler, L.A. (1992) Akathisia, suicidality, and fluoxetine. *J Clin Psychiatry* 53:401–406.

Hoehn-Saric, R., Harris, G.J., Pearlson, G.D., Cox, C.S., Machlin, S.R., and Camargo, E.E. (1991) A fluoxetine-induced frontal lobe syndrome in an obsessive compulsive patient. *J Clin Psychiatry* 52:131–133.

Hoehn-Saric, R., Lipsey, J.R., and McLeod, D.R. (1990) Apathy and indifference in patients on fluvoxamine and fluoxetine. *J Clin Psychopharmacol* 10:343–345.

Hostetter, A., Stowe, Z.N., Strader, J.R., Jr., McLaughlin, E., Llewellyn, A. (2001) Dose of selective serotonin uptake inhibitors across pregnancy: clinical implications. *Depress Anxiety*; 11:51–57.

Hrdina, P.D. (1991) Pharmacology of serotonin uptake inhibitors: focus on fluvoxamine. *J Psychiatry Neurosci* 16(Suppl 1):10–18.

Iancu, I., Ratzoni, G., Weitzman, A., and Apter, A. More fluoxetine experience. *J Am Acad Child Adolesc Psychiatry* 31:755–756.

Kalda, R. (1993) Media-or fluoxetine-induced akathisia? *Am J Psychiatry* 150:531–532.

Keck, P.E., Jr. and Arnold, L.M. (2000) The serotonin syndrome. *Psychiatr Ann* 30:333–343.

Keller, M.B., Ryan, N.D., Strober, M., Klein, R.G., Kutcher, S.P., Birmaher, B., Hagino, O.R., Koplewicz, H., Carlson, G.A., Clarke, G.N., Emslie, G.J., Feinberg, D., Geller, B., Kusumakar, V., Papatheodorou, G., Sack, W.H., Sweeney, M., Wagner, K.D., Weller, F.B., Winters, N.C., Oakes, R., McCafferty, and J.P. (2001) Efficacy of paroxetine in the treatment of adolescent major depression: a randomized, controlled trial. *J Am Acad Child Adolesc Psychiatry* 40:762–772.

Kent, J.M., Coplan, J.D., and Gorman, J.M. (1998) Clinical utility of the selective serotonin reuptake inhibitors in the spectrum of anxiety. *Biol Psychiatry* 44:812–824.

Ketai, R. (1993) Interaction between fluoxetine and neuroleptics. *Am J Psychiatry* 150:836–837.

King, R.A. (1997) Practice parameters for the psychiatric assessment of children and adolescents. American Academy of Child and Adolescent Psychiatry. *J Am Acad Child Adolesc Psychiatry* 36(10 Suppl):4S–20S.

Kurlan, R., Como, P.G., Deeley, C., McDermott, M., McDermott, M.P. (1993) A pilot controlled study of fluoxetine for obsessive-compulsive symptoms in children with Tourette's syndrome. *Clin Neuropharmacol* 16:167–172.

Labellarte, M.J., Ginsburg, G.S., Walkup, J.T., and Riddle, M.A. (1999) The treatment of anxiety disorders in children and adolescents. *Biol Psychiatry* 46:1567–1578.

Lake, M.B., Birmaher, B., Wassick, S., Mathos, K., and Yelovich, A.K. (2000) Bleeding and selective serotonin reuptake inhibitors in childhood and adolescence. *J Child Adolesc Psychopharmacol* 10:35–38.

Lane, R. and Baldwin, D. (1997) Selective serotonin reuptake inhibitor-induced serotonin syndrome: review. *J Clin Psychopharmacol* 17:208–221.

Leonard, H.L., March, J., Rickler, K.C., and Allen, A.J. (1997) Pharmacology of the selective serotonin reuptake inhibitors in children and adolescents. *J Am Acad Child Adolesc Psychiatry* 36:725–736.

Liu, B.A., Mittmann, N., Knowles, S.R., and Shear, N.H. (1996) Hyponatremia and the syndrome of inappropriate secretion of antidiuretic hormone associated with the use of selective serotonin reuptake inhibitors: a review of spontaneous reports. *CMAJ*; 155: 519–527.

Lund, J., Thayssen, P., Mengel, H., Pedersen, O.L., Kristensen, C.B., and Gram L.F. (1982) Paroxetine: pharmacokinetics and cardiovascular effects after oral and intravenous single doses in man. *Acta Pharmacol Toxicol (Copenh)* 51:351–357.

March, J., Frances, A., Docherty, J.P., and Kahn, D.A. (1997) Expert Consensus Guidelines: Treatment of obsessive-compulsive disorder. *J Clin Psychiatry*, 58(Suppl 4):1–72.

March, J.S., Biederman, J., Wolkow, R., Safferman, A., Mardekian, J., Cook, E.H., Cutler, N.R., Dominguez, R., Ferguson, J., Muller, B., Riesenberg, R., Rosenthal, M., Sallee, F.R., Wagner, K.D., and Steiner, H. (1998) Sertraline in children and adolescents with obsessive-compulsive disorder: a multicenter randomized controlled trial. *JAMA* 280:1752–1756.

Markowitz, J.S., DeVane, C.L., Boulton, D.W., Carson, S.W., Nahas, Z., and Risch, S.C. (2000) Effect of St. John's wort (*Hypericum perforatum*) on cytochrome P-450 2D6 and 3A4 activity in healthy volunteers. *Life Sci* 66:PL133–PL139.

McDougle, C.J., Goodman, W.K., Price, L.H., Delgado, P.L., Krystal, J.H., Charney, D.S. and Heninger, G.R. (1990) Neuroleptic addition in fluvoxamine-refractory obsessive-compulsive disorder. *Am J Psychiatry* 147:652–654.

McDougle, C.J., Goodman, W.K., Leckman, J.F., Lee, N.C., Heninger, G.R., and Price, L.H. (1994) Haloperidol addition in fluvoxamine-refractory obsessive-compulsive disorder. A double-blind, placebo-controlled study in patients with and without tics. *Arch Gen Psychiatry* 51:302–308.

McDougle, C.J., Kresch, I.E., Goodman, W.K., Naylor, S.T., Volkmar, F.R., Cohen, D.J., and Price L.H. (1995) A case-controlled study of repetitive thoughts and behavior in adults with autistic disorder and obsessive-compulsive disorder. *Am J Psychiatry* 152: 772–777.

McDougle, C.J., Brodkin, E.S., Naylor, S.T., Carlson, D.C., Cohen, D.J., and Price, L.H. (1998) Sertraline in adults with pervasive developmental disorders: a prospective open-label investigation. *J Clin Psychopharmacol* 18:62–66.

McDougle, C.J., Epperson, C.N., Pelton, G.H., Wasylink, S., and Price, I.H. (2000) A double-blind, placebo-controlled study of risperidone addition in serotonin reuptake inhibitor-refractory obsessive-compulsive disorder. *Arch Gen Psychiatry*; 57:794–801.

McDougle, C.J., Kresch, L.E., and Posey, D.J. (2000) Repetitive thoughts and behavior in pervasive developmental disorders: treatment with serotonin reuptake inhibitors. *J Autism Dev Disord* 30:427–435.

Meltzer, H.Y., Young, M., Metz, J., Fang, V.S., Schyve, P.M., and Arora, R.C. (1979) Extrapyramidal side effects and increased serum prolactin following fluoxetine, a new antidepressant. *J Neural Transm* 45:165–175.

Michalets, E.L. and Williams, C.R. (2000) Drug interactions with cisapride: clinical implications. *Clin Pharmacokinet* 39:49–75.

Moore, L.B., Goodwin, B., Jones, S.A., Wisely, G.B., Serabjit-Singh, C.J., Willson, T.M., Collins, J.L., and Kliewer, S.A. (2000) St. John's wort induces hepatic drug metabolism through activation of the pregnane X receptor. *Proc Natl Acad Sci USA* 97:7500–7502.

Moreau, D., Weissman, M.M. (1992) Panic disorder in children and adolescents: a review. *Am J Psychiatry* 149:1306–1314.

Nemeroff, C.B., DeVane, C.L., and Pollock, B.G. (1996) Newer antidepressants and the cytochrome P450 system. *Am J Psychiatry* 153:311–320.

Nicholson, S.D. (1992) Extrapyramidal side effects associated with paroxetine. *N Engl Med J* 107:90–91.

Oehrberg, S., Christiansen, P.E., and Behnke, K., Borup, A.L., Severin, B., Soegaard, J., Calberg, H., Judge, R., Ohrstrom, J.K., and Manniche, P.M. (1995) Paroxetine in the treatment of panic disorder. A randomised, double-blind, placebo-controlled study. *Br J Psychiatry* 167:374–379.

Ollendick, T.H., Mattis, S.G., and King, N.J. (1994) Panic in children and adolescents: a review. *J Child Psychol Psychiatry* 35:113–134.

Opler, L.A. (1994) Sertraline and akathisia. *Am J Psychiatry* 151: 620–621.

Overo, K.F. (1978) Preliminary studies of the kinetics of citalopram in man. *Eur J Clin Pharmacol* 14:69–73.

Perrin, S., Smith, P., and Yule, W. (2000) The assessment and treatment of Post-traumatic Stress Disorder in children and adolescents. *J Child Psychol Psychiatry* 41:277–289.

Pfefferbaum, B., (1997) Posttraumatic stress disorder in children: a review of the past 10 years. *J Am Acad Child Adolesc Psychiatry* 36:1503–1511.

Piscitelli, S.C., Burstein, A.H., Chaitt, D., Alfaro, R.M., and Falloon, J. (2000) Indinavir concentrations and St John's wort. *The Lancet.* 355:547–548.

Pohl, R., Yeragani, V.K., Balon, R., and Lycaki, H. (1988) The jitteriness syndrome in panic disorder patients treated with antidepressants. *J Clin Psychiatry* 49:100–104.

Preskorn, S.H. (2000) The adverse effect profiles of the selective serotonin reuptake inhbitors: relationship to in vitro pharmacology. *J Psychiatri Practi* 6:153–157.

Preskorn, S.H., Alderman, J., et al. (1994) Pharmacokinetics of desipramine coadministered with sertraline or fluoxetine. *J Clin Psychopharmacol* 14:90–98.

Riddle, M.A., King, R.A., Hardin, M.T., and Scahill, L. (1991) Behavioral side effects of fluoxetine in children and adolescents. *J Child Adolesc Psychopharmacol* 1:

Riddle, M.A., Reeve, E.A., Yaryura-Tobias, J.A., Yang, H.M., Claghorn, J.L., Gaffney, G., Greist, J.H., Holland, D., McConville, B.J., Pigott, T., and Walkup, J.T. (2001) Fluvoxamine for children and adolescents with obsessive-compulsive disorder: a randomized, controlled, multicenter trial. *J Am Acad Child Adolesc Psychiatry* 40:222–229.

Rochat, B., Amey, M., and Baumann, P. (1995a) Analysis of enantiomers of citalopram and its demethylated metabolites in plasma of depressive patients using chiral reverse-phase liquid chromatography. *Ther Drug Monit* 17:273–279.

Rochat, B., Amey, M., Van Gelderen, H., Testa, B., and Baumann, P. (1995b) Determination of the enantiomers of citalopram, its demethylated and propionic acid metabolites in human plasma by chiral HPLC. *Chirality* 7:389–395.

Ronfeld, R.A., Tremaine, L.M., and Wilner, K.D. (1997) Pharmacokinetics of sertraline and its *N*-demethyl metabolite in elderly and young male and female volunteers. *Clin Pharmacokinet* 32(Suppl 1): 22–30.

Rosenberg, D.R., Benazon, N.R., Gilbert, A., Sullivan, A., and Moore, G.J. (2000) Thalamic volume in pediatric obsessive-compulsive disorder patients before and after cognitive behavioral therapy. *Biol Psychiatry*; 48:294–300.

Ruschitzka, F., Meier, P.J., Turina, M., Luscher, T.F., and Noll, G. (2000) Acute heart transplant rejection due to Saint John's wort. *Lancet* 355:548–549.

Rush, A.J., Armitage, R., Gillin, J.C., Yonkers, K.A., Winokur, A., Moldofsky, H., Vogel, G.W., Kaplita, S.B., Fleming, J.B., Montplaisir, J., Erman, M.K., Albala, B.J., and McQuade, R.D. (1998) Comparative effects of nefazodone and fluoxetine on sleep in outpatients with major depressive disorder. *Biol Psychiatry* 44:3–14.

Ryan, N.D. and Varma, D. (1998) Child and adolescent mood disorders—experience with serotonin-based therapies. *Biol Psychiatry* 44:336–340.

Sackett, D.W.R. (1997) *Evidence-Based Medicine*. London: Churchill Livingston.

Sallee FR, DeVane CL, Ferrell RE. Fluoxetine-related death in a child with cytochrome P-450 2D6 genetic deficiency. *J Child Adolesc Psychopharmacol*. 2000; 10(1): 27–34.

Sanchez, C. and Hyttel, J. (1999) Comparison of the effects of antidepressants and their metabolites on reuptake of biogenic amines and on receptor binding. *Cell Mol Neurobiol* 19:467–489.

Sands, M.A. (1994) *Diagnostic Classification: Zero to Three: Diagnostic Classification of Mental Health in Developmental Disorders in Infancy and Early Childhood*. Arlington, VA: Zero to Three/National Center for Clinical Infant Programs.

Scahill, L., Riddle, M.A., King, R.A., Hardin, M.T., Rasmusson, A., Makuch, R.W., and Leckman, J.F. Fluoxetine has no marked effect on tic symptoms in patients with Tourette's syndrome: a double-blind placebo-controlled study. *J Child Adolesc Psychopharmacol* 7:75–85.

Schenker, S., Bergstrom, R.F., Wolen, R.L., and Lemberger, L. (1988) Fluoxetine disposition and elimination in cirrhosis. *Clin Pharmacol Ther* 44:353–359.

Simeon, J.G., Dinicola, V.F., Ferguson, H.B., and Copping, W. (1990)

Adolescent depression: a placebo-controlled fluoxetine treatment study and follow-up. *Prog Neuropsychopharmacol Biol Psychiatry* 4:791–795.

Skop, B.P. and Brown, T.M. (1996) Potential vascular and bleeding complications of treatment with selective serotonin reuptake inhibitors. *Psychosomatics* 37:12–16.

Spearing, M.K., Post, R.M., Leverich, G.S., Brandt, D., and Nolen, W., (1997) Modification of the Clinical Global Impressions (CGI) Scale for use in bipolar illness (BP): the CGI-BP. *Psychiatry Res* 73:159–171.

Spigset, O. and Mjorndal, T. (1997) The effect of fluvoxamine on serum prolactin and serum sodium concentrations: relation to platelet 5-HT2A receptor status. *J Clin Psychopharmacol* 17: 292–297.

Spigset, O., Granberg, K., et al. (1998) Non-linear fluvoxamine disposition. *Br J Clin Pharmacol* 45:257–263.

Spigset, O., Granberg, K., Hagg, S., Soderstrom, E., and Dahlqvist, R. (1998) Non-linear fluvoxamine disposition. *Br J Clin Pharmacol* 45:257–263.

Steele, M. and Couturier, J. (1999) A possible tetracycline-risperidone-sertraline interaction in an adolescent. *Can J Clin Pharmacol* 6:15–17.

Sternbach, H. (1991) The serotonin syndrome. *Am J Psychiatry* 148: 705–713.

Tanguay, P.E. (2000) Pervasive development disorders: a 10-year review. *J Am Acad Child Adolesc Psychiatry* 39:1079–1095.

Tate, J.L. (1989) Extrapyramidal symptoms in a patient taking haloperidol and fluoxetine. *Am J Psychiatry* 146:399–400.

Teicher, M.H. and Baldessarini, R.J. (1987) Developmental pharmacodynamics. In: Popper, C., ed. *Psychiatric Pharmacosciences of Children and Adolescents*. Washinton, DC: American Psychiatric Association Press, pp. 47–80.

Ten Eick, A.P., Nakamura, H., and Reed, M.D. (1998) Drug-drug interactions in pediatric psychopharmacology. *Pediatr Clin North Am* 45:1233–1264, x–xi.

Torok-Both, G.A., Baker, G.B., Coutts, R.T., McKenna, K.F., and Aspeslet, I.J. (1992) Simultaneous determination of fluoxetine and norfluoxetine enantiomers in biological samples by gas chromatography with electron-capture detection. *J Chromatogr* 579: 99–106.

Turner, S. (1999) Place of pharmacotherapy in post-traumatic stress disorder. [Editorial]. *Lancet* 354:1404–1405.

Venkataraman, S., Naylor, M.W., and King, C.A. (1992) Mania associated with fluoxetine treatment in adolescents. *J Am Acad Child Adolesc Psychiatry* 31:276–281.

Walkup, J.T., Labellarte, M.J., Riddle, M.A., Pine, D.S., Greenhill, L., Klein, R., Davies, M., Sweeney, M., Abikoff, H., Hack, S., Klee, B., McCracken, J., Bergman, L., Piacentini, J., March, J., Compton, S., Robinson, J., O'Hara, T., Baker, S., Vitiello, B., Ritz, L.A., and Roper, M. (2001) Fluvoxamine for the treatment of anxiety disorders in children and adolescents. *N Engl J Med* 344:1279–1285.

Wegerer, V., Moll, G.H., Bagli, M., Rothenberger, A., Ruther, E., and Huether, G. (1999) Persistently increased density of serotonin transporters in the frontal cortex of rats treated with fluoxetine during early juvenile life. *J Child Adolesc Psychopharmacol* 9: 13–24.

Wentworth, J.M., Agostini, M., Love, J., Schwabe, J.W., and Chatterjee, V.K. (2000) St John's wort, a herbal antidepressant, activates the steroid X receptor. *J Endocrinol* 166:R11–R16.

Wilens, TE. (2001) Pharmacokinetics of fluoxetine pediatric patients (personal communication).

Wong, D.T., Bymaster, F.P., Reid, L.R., Mayle, D.A., Krushinski,

J.H., and Robertson, D.W. (1993) Norfluoxetine enantiomers as inhibitors of serotonin uptake in rat brain. *Neuropsychopharmacology* 8:337–344.

Wong, D.T., Fuller, R.W., and Robertson DW. (1990) Fluoxetine and its two enantiomers as selective serotonin uptake inhibitors. *Acta Pharm Nord* 2:171–180.

Wudarsky, M., Nicolson, R., (1999) Hamburger, S.D., Spechler, L., Gochman, P., Bedwell, J., Lenane, M.C., and Rapoport, J.L. (1999) Elevated prolactin in pediatric patients on typical and atypical antipsychotics. *J Child Adolesc Psychopharmacol*, 9: 239–245.

Yoshida, K., Smith, B., et al. (1999) Psychotropic drugs in mothers' milk: a comprehensive review of assay methods, pharmacokinetics and of safety of breast-feeding. *J Psychopharmacol* 13: 64–80.

23 | Antidepressants II: tricyclic agents

KARL GUNDERSEN AND BARBARA GELLER

Tricyclic antidepressants (TCA) were first synthesized in the 1940s by chemists looking for drugs to act as sedatives, antihistamines, and anti-parkinsonian drugs (Baldessarini, 1996). Use in depression was first reported in the late 1950s, and hundreds of studies have confirmed their effectiveness in adult populations. In the mid-1960s, TCAs were first studied as an alternative to stimulant medication in the treatment of childhood attention-deficit hyperactivity disorder, (ADHD). To date, TCAs have been used in multiple psychiatric disorders in children, including obsessive-compulsive disorder (OCD), major depressive disorder (MDD), anxiety, and enuresis. The Food and Drug Administration (FDA) has approved TCAs only for use in the treatment of OCD (clomipramine) and enuresis (imipramine).

This chapter describes the structure and neurochemical function of TCAs, metabolism and significant interactions with other medications, side effects, and specific recommendations for monitoring of side effects in children and adolescents. Because of the recent concern regarding the sudden deaths of children stabilized on TCAs, particular attention will be paid to the potential cardiovascular effects of these medications. The chapter will focus on the five TCA medications that have been most widely used in children: amitriptyline (AMI), nortriptyline (NT), imipramine (IMI), desipramine (DMI), and clomipramine (CMI).

STRUCTURE

Tricyclic antidepressants have a basic three-ring structure with attached amine groups. Differences between each drug are in the attached amine and whether it is tertiary (three methyl groups attached to a nitrogen) or secondary (two methyl groups attached to a nitrogen). Tertiary amines include IMI, AMI, and CMI, and secondary amines, DMI and NT. The two secondary amines are demethylated metabolites of tertiary amines and are themselves active chemical compounds. Thus, DMI is the metabolite of IMI, and NT is the metabolite of AMI. For details of the chemical structure of TCAs, see Figure 23.1.

MECHANISM OF ACTION

Tricyclic antidepressants act both presynaptically and postsynaptically on two major systems, the noradernergic and the serotonergic. The actions of TCAs in each system will be discussed separately. Figure 23.2 shows an overall schematic of the receptor blockade of TCAs.

Noradrenergic System

Tricyclic antidepressants exert their primary effect by blocking the reuptake transporter protein for norepinephrine, which is the normal degradation pathway. The TCAs also bind to presynaptic α_2 receptors, increasing release of norepinephrine into the synapse. Postsynaptically, TCAs bind to α_1 receptors, leading to activation and increased postsynaptic activity (Sugrue, 1983). Tricyclic antidepressants have been reported to bind to postsynaptic α_2 receptors, but the significance of this event is unclear (Svensson, 1984). There is also binding to postsynaptic β-adrenergic receptors. Chronic TCA treatment leads to decreased numbers of β-receptors and further alteration in postsynaptic transmission (Sugrue, 1983).

Serotonergic System

Tricyclic antidepressants bind presynaptically to the 5-HT_1 autoreceptor site, leading to decreased serotonin reuptake and degradation. Postsynaptically TCAs bind to 5-HT_2 receptors, leading to increased activity.

The tertiary amine tricyclics have similar effects on norepinephrine and serotonin transmission, while the two secondary amines have more specific effects on norepinephrine, with much smaller effects on serotonin. This can be seen in the K_i (inhibitory constant) values for the TCAs, as listed in Table 23.1. K_i is the concentration of drug required to block transport of the neurotransmitter (in this case, norepinephrine or serotonin). Lower K_i equals greater relative ability to block transport. Desipramine and NT have the greatest inhibitory effects at the α_1 receptor site, while CMI has

Tertiary Amines

Imipramine

Amitriptyline

Clompiramine

Secondary Amines

Desipramine

Nortriptyline

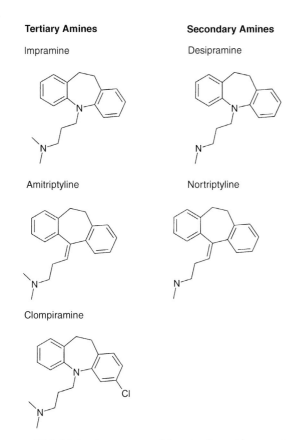

FIGURE 23.1 Molecular structure of the tricyclic antidepressants.

the greatest inhibition of the 5-HT$_1$ autoreceptor (Richelson and Pfenning, 1984).

None of the TCAs seem to have an effect on dopaminergic neurotransmission in the central nervous system (CNS). This has been supported by the lack of alterations in dopamine receptor sensitivity in chronically treated patients who have shown response to treatment (Sugrue, 1983). More recent investigations have also shown that administration of DMI to depressed subjects had no effect on levels of homovanillic acid, the principal metabolite of dopamine, in a measure of brain neurotransmitter production. In this investigation, DMI administration did increase norepinephrine production and overall cerebral metabolism (Lambert, 2000).

The binding sites of TCAs in the brain appear to be localized to hypothalamus, frontal cortex, hippocampus, and caudate nucleus. Least binding is observed in the white matter and cerebellum (Langer et al., 1981).

In addition to their effects on norepinephrine and serotonin, TCAs have significant antagonistic effects at muscarinic and histaminic receptors. While TCAs appear to bind equally to all subtypes of the muscarinic receptor, they show preferential affinity for the histaminic H$_1$ receptor over the H$_2$ receptor subtype. The

tertiary amines are significantly more active at muscarinic receptors than the secondary amines, and typically show much more anticholinergic side effects, including dry mouth, tachycardia, and delirium (Sugrue, 1983).

Postsynaptic Effects

The significance of the effects of the TCAs on receptor sensitivity and subsequent antidepressant effects remains unclear. Other agents that possess similar receptor interactions to TCAs (such as cocaine and the α_2 receptor) are devoid of antidepressant activity. In addition, receptor blockade is seen with initial doses of medication, while changes in mood symptoms have considerable lag time. The lag phase of clinical effectiveness appears to be due to changes in receptor density and postsynaptic activity associated with chronic administration of TCAs (Sugrue, 1983).

Recent investigations into intracellular events have begun to define the postsynaptic events through which TCAs appear to exert their effects (Morinobu et al., 1995). One of the observations made was downregulation of transcription factors for early gene products such as c-Fos. C-Fos is normally produced in response to periods of stress. In research with rats, TCAs as well as other antidepressants have been shown to decrease the expression of c-Fos in areas of frontal cortex after chronic but not acute treatment. Other psychotropic medications (e.g., cocaine and haloperidol) with similar acute effects on norepinephrine/serotonin neurotransmission have not shown this same chronic effect. It has been speculated that the decreased production of c-Fos is the end product of a cascade of events stimulated by increased norepinephrine levels (Morinobu et al., 1995).

More recent studies have begun to more precisely define this pathway, which results in altered gene expression at its final point. For example, research has recently shown that TCA treatment and subsequent activation of the cyclic adenosine monophosphate (cAMP) cascade results in up-regulation of the production of cAMP response element–binding protein (CREB) and brain-derived neurotrophic factor (BDNF). In rats, chronic, but not acute, treatment with TCA leads to increased expression of CREB, which then acts on various gene targets, including BDNF. The increased activity of BDNF is thought to lead to neurogenesis of cells affected by depression in the hippocampus and prefrontal cortex and possibly helps protect cells that would otherwise undergo death in the presence of stress or depression (Duman et al., 1999; see also Chapter 3 in this volume). In addition, the time course for activation of CREB activity is consistent with the lag time seen for full treatment with antidepressants (Thome et al., 2000). Fur-

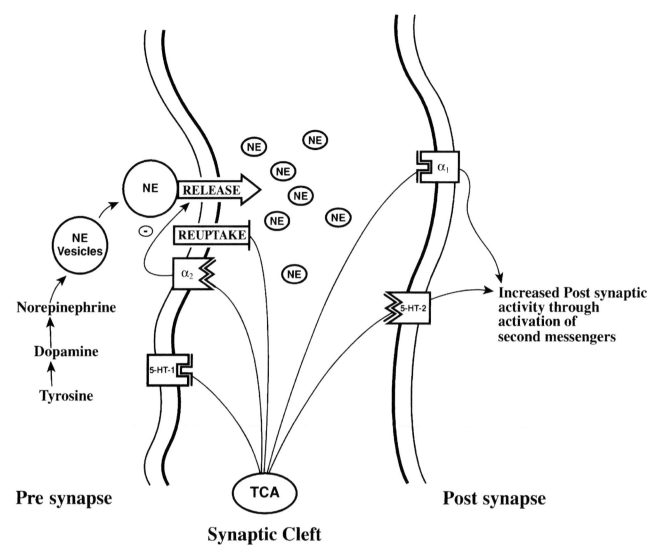

FIGURE 23.2 Sites of action of tricyclic antidepressants at the synaptic junction. (Modified from Baldessarini (1996).

thermore, the brain areas where CREB and BDNF show greatest activity are similar to those where TCAs have the highest receptor binding affinity. Chronic treatment with TCAs may also show protective effects on hippocampus cells. In this regard, chronic TCA treatment in rats blocked the down-regulation of BDNF seen in response to an acute stressor (Nibuya et al., 1995).

PHARMACOKINETICS

Absorption

In adults, all TCAs are rapidly and completely absorbed from the gastrointestinal tract, and reach peak levels in the blood relatively quickly (2–4 hours) following administration of a single dose of medication. They then pass through the liver via the portal circulation and undergo extensive initial metabolism (40%–70%) by the cytochrome P450 (CYP) enzyme system before being distributed to the rest of the body (Janicak et al., 1997).

Distribution

In adults, TCAs are highly protein-bound medications. At any one time 75%–95% of the drug in the body will be bound to circulating α_1 glycoprotein. Competition for binding sites on α_1 glycoprotein by drugs such as aspirin, phenytoin, and some phenothiazines

TABLE 23.1 *Receptor Blockade Profile of Tricyclics*

Drug	Class of Amine	Major Mechanism of Action	Reuptake Receptor Blockade Profile [$K_i \pm SEM$ (nM)]		FDA-Approved Uses in Children
			NE	5-HT	
Imipramine	Tertiary	Blockade of norepinephrine reuptake at α_2 autoreceptor and blockade of serotonin reuptake at 5-HT$_1$ autoreceptor	13 ± 2	42 ± 2	Enuresis, age 6+ years
Desipramine	Secondary	Same as imipramine (above)	0.9 ± 0.2	340 ± 60	None
Amitriptyline	Tertiary	Same as imipramine (above)	24 ± 6	66 ± 3	None
Nortriptyline	Secondary	Same as imipramine (above)	4 ± 1	260 ± 40	None
Clomipramine	Tertiary	Same as imipramine (above)	28 ± 7	5.4 ± 0.2	Obsessive-compulsive disorder, age 12+ years

$K_i \pm SEM$ = inhibitory constant for blockade of receptor; NE = α-2 autoreceptor blockade value; 5-HT = 5-HT$_1$ autoreceptor blockade value; From Richelson and Pfenning (1984).

can increase the amount of free TCA that is present in the body. Febrile illnesses also have been noted to increase total levels of TCA. This may be due to increased circulating protein and subsequent increase in binding sites (Geller et al., 1985a).

The TCAs are highly lipophilic medications, causing a wide distribution in the body and allowing medications to cross the blood–brain barrier into the central nervous system.

Metabolism

Tricyclic antidepressants undergo metabolism primarily by microsomal enzymes in the liver. The primary isoenzyme for metabolism is CYP2D6, although other enzymes are involved in the biotransformation of individual compounds. Specifically, IMI uses the CYP1A2 and CYP2C19 isoenzymes, and AMI uses the CYP1A2 isoenzyme. The tertiary amines (AMI and IMI) undergo demethylation to their secondary amine equivalents. Imipramine undergoes demethylation to DMI, while AMI is metabolized to NT. Another major metabolic pathway involves hydroxylation, and all TCAs are then glucoronidated to final deactivation.

Children are much more efficient metabolizers of TCAs than adults because of their larger hepatic capacity relative to body size. It has been noted that there is a relatively large percentage (5%–10%) of children, similar to adults, who can be characterized as being "slow metabolizers." In these populations, genetic variances in the CYP enzyme activity can be extremely low and administration of a single dose of medication can result in blood plasma levels that differ as much as 10- to 15-fold (de Gatta et al., 1984; Geller et al., 1987b).

Excretion

Most (up to 95%) of a dose of a single TCA is eliminated through the urine as an inactive metabolite. A smaller amount of excretion occurs in the feces. Half-life for NT has been established through careful investigation in children, and ranges from 10 to 30 hours (Geller et al., 1987b). In general, half-lives of tricyclics in children are shorter than in adults. This is due to more efficient hepatic metabolism as well as to more rapid renal clearance (Geller, 1991). The therapeutic range in children for TCAs has not been established, in part because no systematic efficacy study has shown superiority of TCA to placebo in major depression. Elimination of TCA in children shows linear pharmacokinetics within the adult therapeutic range of plasma level, meaning that the amount of drug excreted is proportional to the amount present in the bloodstream. It also means that at steady state, as long as the total dose stays within the therapeutic range, the amount of drug ingested is proportional to the amount found in the bloodstream (Fetner and Geller, 1992).

Drug Interactions during Metabolism

Tricyclics interact with other drugs and substances at a variety of points during distribution and metabolism. Most interactions occur at the CYP isoenzyme complex in the liver. Other interactions occur at peripheral sites and involve interaction at the noradernergic receptors (α and β). A summary of major TCA drug interactions is given in Table 23.2.

SIDE EFFECTS

General Effects

Because of the multiple receptor sites that TCAs bind to, there are a variety of possible side effects that can be seen in treatment. The blockade of muscarinic receptors leads to increased anticholinergic tone and subsequent anti-cholinergic side effects, especially in the gastrointestinal system. These include delirium, dry mouth, tachycardia, constipation, and urinary retention in adults. In children, anticholinergic side effects are often not seen with treatment (Geller et al., 1992). Tricyclic antidepressant blockade of the presynaptic α_2 receptors leads to increased autonomic tone throughout the body, causing elevations in heart rate and blood pressure.

Sedation is often seen in adults as a side effect of treatment. It is presumably related to a combination of anticholinergic, antihistaminic, and serotonergic effects of this medication. Sedation is seen more often with the tertiary amines than with the secondary amines (Baldessarini, 1996).

Tricyclic antidepressants also have a documented syndrome associated with withdrawal from medications (Petti and Law, 1981). This syndrome can mimic appendicitis or the flu, and can include such symptoms as nausea and vomiting, headache, lethargy, and abdominal pain. If a child on TCAs presents with withdrawal symptoms, questions of compliance must be addressed.

Other frequently occurring side effects that have been reported in the adult literature include changes in weight, jaundice, changes in hematological parameters, and alteration in seizure threshold (Blackwell, 1981). Specific side effects seen with TCA treatment and their management are summarized in Table 23.3.

Cardiac Effects

Cardiovascular effects of TCAs have been of concern since recent reports of sudden death in children undergoing treatment. This effect may be due to pharmacological similarities between the tricyclics and the type 1A antiarrhythmics, which cause prolongation of conduction indices and possible arrhythmias with use. The question of a possible relationship between TCA treatment and sudden unexplained death was first reported in the early 1990s (Abramowicz, 1990; Biederman, 1991; Riddle et al., 1993; Varley and McClellan, 1997). The cases in question, about which little information was available, noted that the children were on stable regimens of DMI.

Tricyclic antidepressants have effects on heart rate (HR), blood pressure (BP), and three distinct measures of the electrocardiogram (EKG). The EKG parameters affected are (1) the PR interval, which represents depolarization of the atria; (2) the QRS duration, which represents intraventricular conduction time; and (3) the QTc, which represents the depolarization and subsequent repolarization of the ventricles, corrected for cardiac rate.

A survey of the literature by Wilens et al. (1996) noted statistically significant increases in some cardiac measures, including BP, HR, and EKG conduction parameters in children undergoing TCA treatment. The changes appeared to be related to plasma level. There appeared to be few differences between effects seen in children and those seen in adolescents. Long-term monitoring (24-hour) and monitoring with exercise tests revealed similar asymptomatic changes in EKG parameters. The long-term clinical significance of these cardiac changes is not fully understood.

The American Heart Association has also done a review of potential cardiac effects of TCAs (Gutgessel et al., 1999). This review notes similar effects of TCA administration on EKG parameters, including an increase in the QTc interval, and recommends stricter guidelines for EKG monitoring than those in the Wilens et al. article, as summarized in Table 23.4.

Toxicity and Overdose

Overdose with TCAs causes tachycardia, hypotension, prolonged EKG intervals, and fatal arrhythmias, including ventricular tachycardias and bundle branch blocks (lack of conduction of the cardiac impulse). Conduction deficits alone and in combination with hypotension account for most of the morbidity and mortality associated with TCA overdose (Baldessarini, 1996).

Other symptoms of toxicity that can be seen include sedation or paradoxical excitability, signs of anticholinergic blockade including delirium and tachycardia, dry skin, blurred vision, hyperpyrexia, and flushing of the skin, and seizures.

It is difficult to estimate the risk of seizures in children with toxic levels of TCAs. In adults, studies have been done that show a correlation between a QRS complex length 100 msec and an increased risk of seizures. Increased risk of seizures was not related to other monitored parameters, including plasma blood level, and patients with QRS duration within normal limits (<100 msec) had no incidence of seizures or arrhythmias (Boehnert and Lovejoy, 1985). It is unclear

TABLE 23.2 *Drug Interactions of Tricyclics with Other Compounds*

Interacting Agent	Mechanism of Interaction	Clinical Presentation	Management	Reference
Acetylsalicylic acid, phenytoin, phenothiazines	Competition for binding to α_1 glycoprotein	TCA toxicity (cardiac effects, delirium, sedation) due to increased amount of free TCA	Lower TCA dose	Baldessarini, 1996
Neuroleptics	Competition for metabolism at CYP2D6 isoenzyme	TCA toxicity due to possible 30% increase in TCA levels with coadministration	Lower TCA dose or neuroleptic dose	Geller, 1991
Low-potency neuroleptics (e.g., chlorpromazine)	Additive effects of blockade of muscarinic cholinergic receptors	Anticholinergic effects (dry mouth, tachycardia, possible hyperpyrexia, and delirium)	Lower doses of both agents	Geller, 1991
SSRIs—fluvoxamine, fluoxetine, and paroxetine, more than sertraline and citalopram	Inhibition of metabolism at CYP2D6 isoenzyme	TCA toxicity due to up to 10-fold increase in TCA levels with coadministration	Lower TCA dose	Baumann, 1996
Oral contraceptives	Inhibition of metabolism at CYP2D6 isoenzyme	Possible TCA toxicity increased amount of active TCA varies can be up to 30%	Lower TCA dose	D'Arcy, 1986
Alcohol	Inhibition of metabolism at CYP2D6 isoenzyme	TCA toxicity due to possible 30% increase in TCA levels with coadministration	Caution patients against use Obtain history of use prior to drug trial	Dorian et al., 1983
Alcohol	Theories include combination of effects at H_1 receptor and β_1 adernergic agonism leading to GABA receptor sensitization to ethanol	Sedation and hypotension with coadministration	Caution patients to avoid coadministration	Lin et al., 1994
Carbamazepine	Induction of CYP isoenzymes	Decreased clinical effect due to decreased levels of TCA	Increase TCA dose	Spina et al., 1996
Cimetidine	Inhibition of metabolism at CYP2D6 isoenzyme	Sudden TCA toxicity	No coadministration	Henauer and Hollister, 1984
Dexedrine, methylphenidate	Inhibition of metabolism at 2D6 enzyme seen in vitro	Potential TCA toxicity, none reported in literature	Currently theoretical interaction only	Fawcett, 2000
Clonidine	TCA postsynaptic α_1-adrenergic receptor antagonism blocks the α_1 agonist effect of clonidine	Decrease in hypotensive effect of clonidine can be seen within days	Increased doses of clonidine to continue	van Zwieten, 1975
Bupropion	Potential additive effect on lowering of seizure threshold	Increased risk of seizure with coadministration	Avoid in history of seizure disorder	Rosenstein et al., 1993
MAOI	Increased levels of norepinephrine due to combined reuptake blockade (TCA) and degradation pathway blockade (MAOIs)	Increased rates of hypertensive crisis; also convulsions and hyperpyrexia; in severe states can lead to coma	Recommend avoiding administration of drugs within 2 weeks of each other	Baldessarini, 1996
Quinidine	Similar class 1A antiarrhythmic effect, leading to EKG parameter changes (e.g., longer QRS)	Palpitations, bradycardia	Need frequent monitoring of EKG parameters when drugs are used in combination	Glassman and Preud'homme, 1993

CYP, cytochrome P450; EKG, electrocardiogram; MAOI, monoamine oxydase inhibitor; SSRI, selective serotonin reuptake inhibitor; TCA, tricyclic antidepressant.

TABLE 23.3 *Major Side Effects Seen in Tricyclic Treatment of Children and Adolescents*

Side Effects	Mechanism of Action	Clinical Presentation	Management/Comments	Reference
Cardiac changes, including tachycardia and arrhythmias	Blockade of presynaptic α_2 autoreceptors	Palpitations, fainting	Lower dose of TCA	Wilens et al., 1996
Hypertension		Headaches due to increased blood pressure	Switch to TCA with less NE receptor potency	
Heart rate changes	Blockade of muscarinic receptors, possibly M_2 and M_3	Tachycardia Nausea and vomiting Diarrhea Sedation	Lower dose or switch to alternate antidepressant May respond to HS dosing	Richelson, 1990
Dental caries, dry mouth		Dry mouth	Use candies, gum potential for tooth decay in long-term use	
Constipation		Constipation	Use suppositories May lead to paralytic ileus in toxicity	
Urinary symptoms Complaints of fatigue		Urinary retention		

EKG changes
    PR prolongation
    QT prolongation
    QRS prolongation
	Increased anticholinergic and noradrenergic tone at the His bundle, leading to blockade of electrical impulses	Bradycardia
		Palpitations
		Fainting
		Sudden death
			Monitor EKG parameters frequently	Wilens et al., 1996

Postural hypotension	Post-synaptic alpha-1 blockade	Fainting	Lower TCA dose Behavioral modification (slow rising from a lying position)	Glassman and Preud'homme, 1993
Seizures	Unknown, occurs in 0.1% to 4% of patients on TCA	Seizures	Use with care in patients with known seizure disorder Increase anticonvulsant levels for continued control	Rosenstein et al., 1993
Flu-like symptoms with abrupt withdrawal	Cholinergic sensitization and rebound hyperactivity	Nausea/vomiting Headache Lethargy Diarrhea	Taper TCA over a period of time Avoid abrupt discontinuation	Petti and Law, 1981
Neutropenia Agranulocytosis Thrombocytopenia	Unknown, rare	Bleeding, bruising Unexplained infections	Monitor CBC frequently	Blackwell, 1981
Jaundice	Unknown, rare	Jaundice	Monitor liver function periodically	Blackwell, 1981

CBC, complete blood cell count; EKG, electrocardiogram; HS, *hora somnis*, bedtime administration; NE, norepinephrine; TCA, tricyclic antidepressant.

whether this particular report's findings are applicable to the treatment of children.

A detailed discussion of the treatment of TCA overdose is beyond the scope of this chapter. Important principles of TCA overdose include removal of drug if possible, intensive cardiac monitoring, and support of respiratory, cardiac, and CNS functions. For a detailed discussion of the treatment of overdose, readers are referred to Rogers and Nichols' *Textbook of Pediatric Intensive Care* (1996).

USES IN CHILDREN AND ADOLESCENTS

Since their introduction, TCAs have been studied for use in a variety of clinical situations, some of which have been related to the use of these medications in adults (e.g., major depression and OCD). They have also been studied in areas where first-line agents have been not tolerated (e.g., ADHD). Because of their side effect profile and possibly serious cardiac effects, however, these agents should probably not be considered first-line med-

TABLE 23.4 *Suggested Guidelines for Cardiovascular Parameters in Children and Adolescents Treated with Tricyclics*

	Parameter	Children	Adolescents
Wilens et al., 1996			
Vital signs	Heart rate	≤110–130 beats/min	≤110–120 beats/min
	Blood Pressure	<120/80 mmHg	<140/90 mmHg
Electrocardiogram	PR interval	<200 msec	<200 msec
	QRS interval	≤120 msec	≤120 msec
	QTc interval	≤460–480 msec	≤460–480 msec
American Heart Association, 1999			
Vital signs	Heart rate	<130 beats/min	—
Electrocardiogram	PR interval	<200 msec	—
	QRS interval	<120 msec	—
	QTc interval	<460 msec	—

Data from Wilens et al. (1996) and Gutgessel et al. (1999)

ications for most disorders of child psychiatry. Studies that used a double-blind, placebo-controlled design will be reviewed briefly.

School Phobia and Separation Anxiety

Because of the hesitancy to use normal anxiolytic substances (benzodiazepines) in children, TCAs were first studied in the use of school refusal and separation anxiety disorder in the 1970s. There have been both positive (Gittleman-Klein and Klein, 1973, Bernstein et al., 2000, 2001) and negative studies for this indication (Berney et al., 1981; Klein et al., 1992).

Attention-Deficit Hyperactivity Disorder

Attention-deficit hyperactivity disorder has been treated with TCAs since the 1960s. The initial rationale for studies in this area rose from two separate medication needs: (1) medications with longer effective half-lives (before the introduction of extended-release stim-

ulants); and (2) the need for medications in children who were unresponsive to or intolerant of the side effects of stimulant medications.

Studies have compared IMI, DMI, or AMI and stimulant to placebo, and found efficacy on standard measures (Winsberg et al., 1972; Yepes et al, 1977; Donnelly et al., 1986).

Major Depressive Disorder

Most of the TCAs have been studied in children with major depression. These studies followed from the noted efficacy of these medications in adult populations, and it was surmised that they would show similar efficacy in children. This has not proved to be the case. In seven double-blind placebo-controlled studies using oral medication, no TCA has shown efficacy over placebo (Geller et al., 1999).

One study did find efficacy of intravenous pulse-dose CMI over placebo in depressed adolescents (Sallee et al., 1997). It was initially unclear why an intermittent dosing regimen was effective where "normal" dosing regimens were not. It has recently been speculated that the positive results may be due to a phenomenon known as *time-dependent sensitization* (TDS). In other studies, pulse-type dosing of medication has been as efficacious as regular dosing schedules. This appears to be due to a long-term response of the body to stressors (e.g., drugs) that results in induction of neuronal and behavioral effects even in the absence of continued drug exposure (Antelman et al., 2000).

Obsessive-Compulsive Disorder

The study of TCAs in children with OCD led directly from the use of these medications in adults with similar symptoms. Findings have shown significant advantage with both CMI and DMI over placebo in the treatment of this illness (Flament et al., 1985; deVaugh-Geiss et al., 1992). Clomipramine is the only TCA with a distinct indication from the FDA for the treatment of OCD. Use of TCAs has recently been supplanted by selective serotonin reuptake inhibitor (SSRI) medications that may have a more favorable side effect profile.

Autism and Pervasive Developmental Disorders

The ritualistic, repetitive behaviors in autism are often seen as parallel to some of the behaviors seen in OCD spectrum disorders. Because of this, CMI was initially compared with both DMI and placebo in the treatment of children with autism. Clomipramine showed superior efficacy to both DMI and to placebo (Gordon et al., 1993). The SSRIs have also been used in this population, and may be better tolerated by children and adolescents.

Nocturnal Enuresis

Multiple studies have been done of TCAs in the treatment of nocturnal enuresis, and all consistently show effect over placebo. Most notably, Rapoport et al. (1978) found a significant relationship between IMI plasma level and response to medication. Imipramine is the only medication with FDA approval for treatment of this condition.

It should be noted that TCA dosages for the treatment of enuresis are often lower than those seen with the treatment of other disorders. It has been presumed that this level of dosing is efficacious because the TCAs are acting directly in the CNS, and the benefits seen not due to a peripheral anticholinergic side effect seen only at higher doses.

CLINICAL USE IN CHILDREN AND ADOLESCENTS

Before Starting the Drug

Prior to starting TCAs, all children should undergo a thorough history and medical examination. Particular emphasis should be placed on any history of cardiac disease, either in the patient or the family. In all cases of TCA use, the potential risks and benefits of using this class of medications should be carefully thought out and discussed with the parents as well as the patient; they should also be informed of the potential lethal consequences of using this medication. Documentation of the risks of using TCAs is imperative for both quality clinical care and for medicolegal reasons.

Because of the risk of compromise of cardiac status, it is currently recommended that baseline HR, BP readings, and EKGs be obtained from all potential TCA patients. Both Wilens et al. (1996) and the American Heart Association (Gutgessel et al., 1999) have proposed guidelines for EKGs based on age-normal values and clinical experience. These are summarized in table 23.4.

In the case of abnormal EKGs at baseline, the use of a TCA, as well as potential risks and benefits, needs to be carefully reevaluated. In addition, a family history of premature cardiac problems or a personal history of cardiac disease, especially structural and conduction abnormalities, should warrant consultation with a pediatric cardiologist before starting medications. Parents and patients should be aware of the potential risk for

sudden death with TCAs, and should be apprised of clinical signs suggestive of cardiac abnormalities, including palpitations, lightheadedness, and headaches.

Baseline laboratory assessment should also include a complete blood count with differential, and a hepatic function panel. These are recommended because of the side effects of the medications, as well as the importance of the liver as the sole source of metabolism.

Dosages

Two methods of deriving an initial dosage have been used clinically: (1) plasma level, and (2) fixed dose. The plasma level method takes into account the linear pharmacokinetics in children who take TCAs. In this method, children are given an initial dose of medication and a blood level of medication is drawn 24 hours later. For IMI and NT, tables have been created which allow determination of final dosage based on this plasma level and the initial dosage (de Gatta et al., 1984; Geller et al., 1985b.) Subsequent blood levels should then be within the normal therapeutic range.

Other clinicians use the fixed dosage method, in which patients are begun on a dose of 1.5 mg/kg/day of medication after baseline laboratory assessment is completed and results are within normal limits. Increases in total daily dose are then done gradually. Electrocardiogram should be done after each change in dosage. Blood levels should also be monitored so that putative therapeutic ranges are not exceeded. The patient is continued on to a maximum of 5 mg/kg/day (3 mg/kg/day for NT or CMI) and adjustments are made following a check of blood levels. For children who are on NT and CMI, these initial increments should likely be halved, given the approximately twofold increase in potency of these medications. The clinician should be aware that this method could quickly lead to toxic levels in slow metabolizers.

Monitoring for plasma levels should be done when the TCA has reached steady state in the body, an average of approximately 5 days in most children.

Monitoring

Electrocardiograms, HR, and BP measurements should be performed at baseline and after every change in dosage. In addition, EKGs should be monitored when medications or agents that are thought to interact with TCA levels are added to the medical regimen of the patient.

In addition to monitoring for EKG changes, it is also recommended that monitoring of plasma levels of the TCA medications be done after every change in dosage, or when medications that have the potential to interact with TCAs are introduced to the regimen. Levels should also be obtained when there is clinical suspicion of toxicity. Routine plasma levels for monitoring of TCAs should be done 9–11 hours after a dose.

Discontinuation

Given the presence of a known withdrawal syndrome in abrupt discontinuation of the TCAs, it is advised that the medications be slowly discontinued over a period of time, giving the body an opportunity to adjust to the increased cholinergic activity. A gradual taper of the medication, where the dose is dropped by 10–25 mg not sooner than every 2–3 days until discontinuation, will decrease these effects. If symptoms do occur, the addition of one dose of medication or a lengthening of the taper will likely relieve symptoms. In one open study of NT discontinuation using this schedule, there was minimal distress and alterations in the planned taper were not needed (Geller et al., 1987a).

REFERENCES

Abramowicz, M. (1990) Sudden death in children treated with a tricyclic antidepressant. *Med Lett Drug Ther* 32:53.

Antelman, S.M., Levine, J., and Gershon, S. (2000) Time-dependent sensitization: the odyssey of a scientific heresy from the laboratory to the door of the clinic. *Mol Psychiatry* 5:350–356.

Baldessarini, R.J. (1996) Drugs and the treatment of psychiatric disorders: depression and mania. In: Hardman, J.G. and Limbird, L.E., eds. *Goodman and Gilman's The Pharmacological Basis of Therapeutics, 9th ed.* New York: McGraw Hill pp. 431–459.

Baumann, P. (1996) Pharmacokinetic–pharmacodynamic relationship of the selective serotonin reuptake inhibitors. *Clin Pharmacokinet* 31:444–469.

Berney, T., Kolvin, I., Bhate, S.R., Garside R.F., Jeans, J., Kay, B., and Scarth, L. (1981) School phobia: a therapeutic trial with clomipramine and short-term outcome. *Br J Psychiatry* 138:110–118.

Bernstein, G.A., Borchardt, C.M., Perwien, A.R., Crosby, R.D., Kushner, M.G., Thuras, P.D., and Last, C.G. (2000) Imipramine plus cognitive-behavioral therapy in the treatment of school refusal. *J Am Acad Child Adolesc Psychiatry* 39:276–283

Bernstein, G.A., Hektner, J.M., Borchardt, C.M., and McMillan, M.H. (2001) Treatment of school refusal: one-year follow-up. *J Am Acad Child Adolesc Psychiatry* 40:206–213.

Biederman, J. (1991) Sudden death in children treated with a tricyclic antidepressant. *J Am Acad Child Adolesc Psychiatry* 30:495–497.

Blackwell, B. (1981) Adverse effects of antidepressant drugs. Part 1: monoamine oxidase inhibitors and tricyclics. *Drugs* 21:201–219.

Boehnert, M.T. and Lovejoy, F.H. (1985) Value of the QRS duration versus the serum drug level in predicting seizures and ventricular arrhythmias after and acute overdose of tricyclic antidepressants. *N Engl J Med* 313:474–479.

Cowen, P.J. (1990) A role for 5-HT in the action of antidepressant drugs. *Pharmacol Ther* 46:43–51.

Daly, J.M. and Wilens, T. (1998) The use of tricyclic antidepressants in children and adolescents. *Pediatr Clin North Am.* 45:1123–1135.

D'Arcy, P.F. (1986) Drug interactions with oral contraceptives. *Drug Intell Clin Pharm* 20:353–362.

de Gatta, M.F., Garcia, M.J., Acosta, A., Rey, F., Gutierrez, J.R., and Dominguez-Gill, A. (1984) Monitoring of serum levels of imipramine and desipramine and individualization of dose in enuretic children. *Ther Drug Monit* 6:438–443.

deVaugh-Geiss, J., Moroz, G., Biederman, J., Cantwell, D., Fontaine, R., Greist, J.H., Reichler, R., Katz, R. and Landau, P. (1992) Clomipramine hydrochloride in childhood and adolescent obsessive-compulsive disorder—a multicenter trial. *J Am Acad Child Adolesc Psychiatry* 31:45–49.

Donnelly, M., Zametkin, A.J., Rapoport, J.L., Ismond, D.R., Weingartner, H., Lane, E., Oliver, J., Linnoila, M., and Potter, W.Z. (1986) Treatment of childhood hyperactivity with desipramine: plasma drug concentration, cardiovascular effects, plasma and urinary catecholamine levels, and clinical response. *Clin Pharmacol Ther* 39:72–81.

Dorian, P., Sellers, E.M., Reed, K.L., Warsh, J.J., Hamilton, C., Kaplan, H.L., and Fan, T. (1983) Amitriptyline and ethanol: pharmacokinetic and pharmacodynamic interaction. *Eur J Clin Pharmacol* 25:325–331.

Duman, R.S., Malberg, J., and Thome, J. (1999) Neural plasticity to stress and antidepressant treatment. *Biol Psychiatry* 46:1181–1191.

Fawcett, J. (2000) Sympathomimetics. In: Sadock, B.J. and Sadock, V.A., eds. *Kaplan and Sadock's Comprehensive Textbook of Psychiatry, 7th ed.* Philadelphia: Lippincott Williams and Wilkins; pp. 2474–2478.

Fetner, H.F. and Geller, B. (1992) Lithium and tricyclic antidepressants. *Psychiatr Clin North Am* 15:223–241.

Flament, M.F., Rapoport, J.L., Berg, C.J., Sceery, W., Kilts, C., Mellstrom, B., and Linnoila, M. (1985) Clomipramine treatment of childhood obsessive-compulsive disorder. A double-blind controlled study. *Arch Gen Psychiatry* 42:977–983.

Geller, B. (1991) Psychopharmacology of children and adolescents: pharmacokinetics and relationships of plasma/serum to response. *Psychopharmacol Bull* 27:401–409.

Geller, B., Cooper, T.B., Carr, L.G., Warham, J.E., and Rodriguez, A. (1987a) Prospective study of scheduled withdrawal from nortriptyline in children and adolescents. *J Clin Psychopharmacol* 7:252–254.

Geller, B., Cooper, T.B., and Chestnut, E.C. (1985a) Serial monitoring and achievement of steady state nortriptyline plasma levels in depressed children and adolescents: preliminary data. *J Clin Psychopharmacol* 5:213–216.

Geller, B. Cooper, T.B., Chestnut, E.C., Anker, J.A., Price D.T., and Yates, E. (1985b) Child and adolescent nortriptyline single dose kinetics predict steady state plasma levels and suggested dose: preliminary data. *J Clin Psychopharmacol* 5:154–158.

Geller, B., Cooper, T.B., Graham, D.L., Fetner, H.H., Marsteller, F.A., and Wells, J.M. (1992) Pharmacokinetically designed double-blind placebo-controlled study of nortriptyline in 6- to 12-year-olds with major depressive disorder. *J Am Acad Child Adolesc Psychiatry* 31:34–44.

Geller, B. Cooper, T.B., Schluchter, M.D., Warham, J.E., and Carr, L.G. (1987b) Child and adolescent nortriptyline single dose pharmacokinetic parameters: final report. *J Clin Psychopharmacol* 7:321–323.

Geller, B., Reising, D. Leonard, H.L., Riddle, M.A,. and Walsh, B.T. (1999) Critical review of tricyclic antidepressant use in children and adolescents. *J Am Acad Child Adolesc Psychiatry* 38:513–516.

Gittleman-Klein, R. and Klein, D.F. (1973) School phobia: diagnostic considerations in the light of imipramine effects. *J Nerv Ment Dis* 156:199–215.

Glassman, A.H. and Preud'homme, X.A. (1993) Review of the cardiovascular effects of heterocyclic antidepressants. *J Clin Psychiatry* 54(suppl):16–22.

Gordon, C.T., State, R.C., Nelson, J.E., Hamburger, S.D. and Rapoport, J.L. (1993) A double-blind comparison of clomipramine, desipramine, and placebo in the treatment of autistic disorder. *Arch Gen Psychiatry* 50:441–447.

Gutgessel, H., Atkins, D., Barst, R., Buck, M., Franklin, W., Humes, R., Ringel, R., Shaddy, R., and Taubert, K.A. (1999) AHA Scientific Statement: cardiovascular monitoring of children and adolescents receiving psychiatric drugs. *J Am Acad Child Adolesc Psychiatry* 38:1047–1050.

Henauer, S.A. and Hollister, L.E. (1984) Cimetidine interaction with imipramine and nortriptyline. *Clin Pharmacol Ther* 35:183–187.

Janicak, P.G., Davis, J.M., Preskorn, S.H., and Ayd, F.J., Jr. (1997) *Principles and Practice of Psychopharmacotherapy, 2nd ed.* Baltimore: Williams and Wilkins.

Klein, R.G., Koplewicz, H.S., and Kanner, A. (1992) Imipramine treatment of children with separation anxiety disorder. *J Am Acad Child Adolesc Psychiatry* 31:21–28.

Lambert, G., Johansson, M., Agren, H., and Friberg, P. (2000) Reduced brain norepinephrine and dopamine release in treatment-refractory depressive illness. *Arch Gen Psychiatry* 57:787–793.

Langer, S.Z., Javoy-Agid, F., Raisman, R., Briley, M., and Agid, Y. (1981) Distribution of specific high-affinity binding sites for [3H]imipramine in human brain. *J Neurochem* 37:267–271.

Lin, A.M., Freund, R.K., Hoffer, B.J., and Palmer, M.R. (1994) Ethanol-induced depressions of cerebellar purkinje neurons are potentiated by beta-adrenergic mechanisms in rat brain. *J Pharmacol Exp Ther* 271:1175–1180.

Morinobu, S., Nibuya, M., and Duman, R.S. (1995) Chronic antidepressant treatment down-regulates the induction of c-Fos mRNA in response to acute stress in rat frontal cortex. *Neuropsychopharmacology* 12:221–228.

Nibuya, M., Morinobu, S., and Duman, R.S. (1995) Regulation of BDNF and trkB mRNA in rat brain by chronic electroconvulsive seizure and antidepressant drug treatments. *J Neurosci* 15:7539–7547.

Petti, T.A. and Law, W., 3rd. (1981) Abrupt cessation of high-dose imipramine treatment in children. *JAMA.* 246:768–769.

Rapoport, J.L., Mikkelsen, E.J., and Zavadil, A.P. (1978) Plasma imipramine and desmethylimipramine concentration and clinical response in childhood enuresis. *Psychopharmacol Bull* 14:60–61.

Richelson, E. (1990) Antidepressants and brain neurochemistry. *Mayo Clin Proc* 65:1227–1236.

Richelson, E. and Pfenning, M. (1984) Blockade by antidepressants and related compounds of biogenic amine uptake into rat brain synaptosomes: most antidepressants selectively block norepinephrine uptake. *Eur J Pharmacol* 104:277–286.

Riddle, M.A., Geller, B., and Ryan, N. (1993) Case study: another sudden death in a child treated with desipramine. *J Am Acad Child Adolesc Psychiatry* 32:792–797.

Rogers, M.C. and Nichols, D.G., eds. (1996) *Textbook of Pediatric Intensive Care, 3rd ed.* Baltimore: Williams and Wilkins.

Rosenstein, D.L., Nelson, J.C., and Jacobs, S.C. (1993) Seizures associated with antidepressants: a review. *J Clin Psychiatry* 54:289–299.

Sallee, F.R., Vrindavanam, N.S., Deas-Nesmith, D. Carson, S.W., and Sethuraman, G. (1997) Pulse intravenous clomipramine for depressed adolescents: double-blind, controlled trial. *Am J Psychiatry* 154:668–673.

Spina, E., Pisani, F., and Perucca, E. (1996) Clinically significant pharmacokinetic drug interactions with carbamazepine. An update. *Clin Pharmacokinet* 31:198–214.

Sugrue, M.F. (1983) Chronic antidepressant therapy and associated changes in central monoaminergic receptor functioning. *Pharmacol Ther* 21:1–33.

Svensson, T.H. (1984) Central alpha-adrenoceptors and the mechanisms of action of antidepressant drugs. *Adv Biochem Psychopharmacol* 39:241–248.

Thome, J., Sakai, N., Shin, K., Steffen, C., Zhang, Y.J., Impey, S., Storm, D., and Duman, R.S. (2000) cAMP response element–mediated gene transcription is upregulated by chronic antidepressant treatment. *J Neurosci* 20:4030–4036.

Tollefson, G.D. and Senogles, S.E. (1983) A comparison of first and second generation antidepressants at the human muscarinic cholinergic receptor. *J Clin Psychopharmacol* 3:231–234.

van Zwieten, P.A. (1975) Interaction between centrally acting hypotensive drugs and tricyclic antidepressants. *Arch Int Pharmacodyn Ther* 214:12–30.

Varley, C.K. and McClellan, J. (1997) Case study: two additional sudden deaths with tricyclic antidepressants. *J Am Acad Child Adolesc Psychiatry* 36:390–394.

Wilens, T.E., Biederman, J., Baldessarini, R.J., Geller, B., Schleifer, D., Spencer, T.J., Birmaher, B., and Goldblatt, A. (1996) Cardiovascular effects of therapeutic doses of tricyclic antidepressants in children and adolescents. *J Am Acad Child Adolesc Psychiatry* 35:1491–1501.

Winsberg, B.G., Bialer, I., Kupietz, S., and Tobias, J. (1972) Effects of imipramine and dextroamphetamine on behavior of neuropsychiatrically impaired children. *Am J Psychiatry* 128:1425–1431.

Yepes, L.E., Balka, E.B., Winsberg, B.G., and Bialer, I. (1977) Amitriptyline and methylphenidate treatment of behaviorally disordered children. *J Child Psychol Psychiatry* 18:39–52.

24 | Antidepressants III: other agents

JOHN T. WALKUP, JULIA RITTER-WELZANT, ELIZABETH KASTELIC, NANDITA JOSHI, AND EMILY FROSCH

The low side effect profile, ease of use, and powerful clinical effect of the selective serotonin reuptake inhibitors (SSRIs) revolutionized the treatment of depression and anxiety in the 1990s. The success of the SSRIs shifted the focus from noradrenergic to serotonergic mechanisms in these common disorders.

As we move into the new millennium, the focus is shifting to antidepressants considered more atypical. These antidepressants have either mixed receptor functioning (noradrenergic, serotonergic, and dopaminergic), selective impact on noradrenergic or dopaminergic function, or impact on neural systems via less conventional mechanisms. The combined noradrenergic and serotonergic reuptake inhibitors (NSRIs) offer advantages over more selective antidepressants. Although not necessarily considered first-line treatments, the NSRIs may be used as first line and may be particularly helpful for more severe depressions (e.g., venlafaxine) or offer a profile of effects that aid in the treatment of specific patients (e.g., the sedative effects of mirtazapine). The NSRIs also offer an improved side effect profile with fewer anticholinergic and antihistaminic effects than tricyclic antidepressants.

Currently there are no available antidepressants that are selective noradrenergic reuptake inhibitors (SNRIs), but a few are involved in clinical testing, such as reboxetine, atomoxetine, and duloxetine. Reboxetine is available in Europe and Federal Drug Administration (FDA) approval of the drug is being sought in the United States for treatment of adult depression. Atomoxetine is also being tested in clinical trials in the United States for treatment of attention-deficit hyperactivity disorder (ADHD) symptoms. Duloxetine is currently under investigation for treatment of depression in adults.

Despite the success of bupropion for depression, there has been little progress or apparent interest in antidepressants focused on dopaminergic activity or potentiation. The impact of more dopaminergic medications can be inferred from the unique clinical uses of bupropion for depression, nicotine addiction, ADHD symptoms, and possibly dopaminergic augmentation of more traditional antidepressants.

Other available antidepressants have unique mechanisms of action that may have an impact on norepinephrine, serotonin, or dopamine indirectly through other mechanisms. For example, mirtazapine's direct antagonism of presynaptic α_2-adrenergic receptors results in an indirect increase in central noradrenergic and serotonergic activity.

The future of antidepressant development will likely lead to the further refinement of selective reuptake inhibitors and agonists, development of agents with mixed receptor activity, and agents with a novel impact on central nervous system (CNS) functioning. In addition, drug development will include drug delivery strategies that may be more convenient for specific patient groups, such as the weekly form of fluoxetine, or the mirtazapine dissolvable tablets for the elderly and perhaps pediatric populations.

This chapter will review available atypical antidepressants and will specifically discuss their uses in children and adolescents. At this time, it is important to note that none of the agents discussed in the chapter have an FDA indication for use in children and adolescents; however, the use of these agents in children and adolescents is increasing, and knowledge of these agents is critical for both research and clinical practice.

MONOAMINE OXIDASE INHIBITORS

History

Similar to the discovery of other psychiatric medications, the mood-enhancing effects of monoamine oxidase inhibitors (MAOIs) were identified serendipitously: mood improvements were observed in patients with tuberculosis treated with iproniazid (Bloch et al., 1954) The early enthusiasm for the MAOIs was based on significant and unprecedented antidepressant effects and the link between antidepressant efficacy and their role in metabolism of serotonin and norepinephrine in presynaptic neurons. This link was a critical step in developing the monoamine hypothesis for mood disorders.

The enthusiasm for MAOIs was tempered by the observation of serious side effects. MAOIs, when combined with tyramine containing food, such as aged meats, cheeses, wine, and some legumes (Blackwell, 1963), or medications with monoamine agonist activity, can cause large, even life-threatening, increases in blood pressure. Concerns regarding dietary noncompliance and the inaccurate perception that all interactions are catastrophic have limited their use. Although there is a range of severity associated with MAOI–food and MAOI–drug interactions, clinicians tend to polarize around this issue, with some never using the MAOIs and others using them in patients with a history of adherence to treatment and partially responsive or refractory mood and anxiety disorders. The response to combination MAOIs–monoamine agonist medication may be beneficial. Some clinicians intentionally use MAOIs in combination with other neurotransmitter agonists because of the potent interactional effects of these medications on mood and anxiety disorders.

In the United States, the three MAOIS available for the treatment of psychiatric conditions are phenelzine (Nardil), tranylcypromine (Parnate), and isocarboxazid (Marplan). All three agents have indications for adult major depression (>16 years old) and, more specifically, atypical depression (anergia, hypersomnia, hyperphagia, somatization, and anxiety symptoms). Although not indicated for anxiety, the MAOIs can also be particularly helpful in treatment of these disorders. Selegiline or L-deprenyl (Eldepryl) is also available in the United States and indicated for symptoms of Parkinson's disease and depression.

Mechanism of Action

Monoamine oxidase (MAO) is an enzyme that is found on the outer membrane of mitochondria and widely distributed in the CNS and other organs. Its function is to inactivate endogenous and exogenous biogenic amines. In the liver and gastrointestinal tract, MAO degrades exogenous amines from food, beverages, medicines, and toxins. In the CNS, MAO functions to catabolize neurotransmitters. Monoamine oxidase enzyme activity varies across the life span and increases with age.

There are two types of MAO: MAO-A and MAO-B. Monoamine oxidase A preferentially deaminates norepinephrine and serotonin, while MAO-B prefer-

entially deaminates phenylethylamine and benzylamine. Both MAO-A and MAO-B deaminate certain amines, such as dopamine and tyramine. Monamine oxidase A is found predominantly in the gut and sympathetic nerve terminals, and accounts for ~20% of CNS MAO. Monoamine oxidase B is primarily located in the CNS and accounts for ~80% of CNS MAO.

As a class, MAOIs inhibit one or both MAO-A and MAO-B, resulting in elevated levels of neurotransmitters and other biogenic amines. Specific MAOIs can be subdivided on the basis of selectivity for inhibition of MAO-A or MAO-B and the reversibility of the enzyme–drug bond. Given concerns about adverse events associated with irreversible bonding and a desire to specifically target CNS neurotransmitter function, pharmaceutical development of MAOIs has focused on selectivity for MAO-A and reversibility.

Nonselective and Irreversible Inhibitors of Monoamine Oxidase A and Monoamine Oxidase B

The earliest and most studied MAOIs in the United States, phenelzine, tranlycypromine, and isocarboxazid, are thought to irreversibly inhibit both MAO-A and MAO-B. This inhibition results in significant food–drug and drug–drug interactions, as described above. It has been postulated that these MAOIs exert their antidepressant and anxiolytic effects by increasing intracellular levels of neurotransmitters, leading to increased intercellular release. Acute intercellular increases of neurotransmitters may account for early side effects associated with these medications, but prolonged increases are probably necessary to obtain the delayed (up to 8 weeks) antidepressant effect.

Selective and Irreversible Inhibitors of Monoamine Oxidase B

Recently, selegiline has been made available in the United States for the treatment of Parkinson's disease. At the low doses used in Parkinson's (10 mg/day), selegiline selectively inhibits MAO-B, which results in elevated levels of neurotransmitters in the CNS, especially dopamine. Ironically, selegiline does not appear to have antidepressant effects at low doses. To achieve antidepressant effects, higher doses of selegiline are necessary (> 10 mg/day). At the higher dosage, however, like phenelzine and tranylcypromine, selegiline becomes nonselective, with no clear side effect advantage (Mann et al., 1989).

Optimism regarding the impact of selective inhibition of MAO-B on dopamine led to trials of selegiline (and pargyline, which is not available in the U.S.) for treatment of adult and pediatric ADHD (Wender et al., 1983; Wood et al., 1983; Feigin et al., 1996; Ernst et al., 1997). Results of these studies were mixed, with some investigators finding selegiline to have no effect (Ernst et al., 1997), and others finding both selegiline (Feigin et al., 1996) and pargyline to be a promising treatment for ADHD (Feigin et al., 1996).

Selective and Irreversible Inhibitors of Monoamine Oxidase A

Inhibition of the MAO-A enzyme for the treatment of depression is appealing because MAO-A is specifically responsible for the degradation of serotonin and norepinephrine. There was initial interest in clorgyline for treatment of adult depression and childhood ADHD (Potter et al., 1982; Zametkin et al., 1985). Clorgyline was found to be beneficial in a small, double-blind, crossover study for the treatment of ADHD in children, but adverse events associated with irreversibility resulted in the lack of an industry sponsor for further trials (Zametkin et al., 1985).

Selective and Reversible Inhibitor of Monoamine Oxidase A

Increasing interest has been placed on the third generation of MAOIs, the reversible inhibitors of MAO-A (RIMAs). The potential advantage of the RIMAs is their impact on important neurotransmitters without the side effects associated with irreversibility. Meclobemide, the prototypical RIMA, has been efficacious in international controlled trials of depressed adults (Angst and Stabl, 1992; Versiani et al., 1997; Sogaard et al., 1999), but results for adult anxiety disorders (social phobia and agoraphobia) are mixed (Versiani et al., 1992; Schneier et al., 1998; Loerch et al., 1999). Moclobemide, the most promising selective and reversible inhibitor of MAO-A, for the treatment of depression, is not available in the United States.

Structure

Structurally, all MAOIs are either hydralazines or non-hydralazines. Iproniazid, the first MAOI used for depression, is a hydralazine. There are currently two hydralazines available, phenelzine and isocarboxazid. Tranylcypromine is a nonhydralazine with a unique structure. Although tranylcypromine is considered to be a reversible inhibitor of MAO, clinically, the return of normal enzymatic activity is delayed, similar to phe-

nelzine—non-reversible inhibitor. Tranylcypromine structurally resembles amphetamine, which may account for its stimulant-like effects in the treatment of depression.

Pharmacokinetics and Drug Distribution

In adults, phenelzine, tranylcypromine, and isocarboxazid are rapidly absorbed and have short half-lives, requiring more than once-a-day dosing. For example, the half-life of phenelzine ranges from 1.5 to 4 hours and the half-life for tranylcypromine ranges from 1.54 to 3.15 hours (Mallinger and Smith, 1991).

MAOI half-lives are, however, less important then their enzyme inhibition. MAOIs have enduring effects beyond their half-life because of the irreversible nature of their enzyme inhibition. With discontinuation, MAOIs are usually cleared within 24 hours, but the regeneration of MAO may take as long 1–2 weeks. Similarly, the maximal inhibition of the MAO enzyme typically requires several days to weeks of treatment (Tollefson, 1983).

Efforts to determine optimal dosing have not focused on serum drug levels, as drug levels do not reflect enzyme inhibition. Rather, to establish dosing for effective treatment, levels of platelet MAO enzyme inhibition associated with dosage and treatment outcome have been used. The MAOIs appear to be most effective when at least 80% of platelet MAO is inhibited.

The liver appears to be the primary site of metabolism for MAOIs. However, metabolism of MAOIs is poorly understood.

Food and Drug Interactions

The most common reason for the underutilization of MAOIs is the potential for serious consequences of MAOI drug–food and drug–drug interactions. Combined MAOI treatment with (1) foods or medications involved in monoamine synthesis; (2) monoamines themselves; or (3) other sympathomimetics routinely found in over-the-counter medications can result in hyperadrenergic crises or serotonin toxicity (Blackwell, 1991).

Hypertensive–adrenergic crisis

The ingestion of dietary amines is associated with increased production and release of central monoamines such as norepinephrine, but is usually not clinically significant. The first generation of MAOIs irreversibly inhibited the degradation of dietary amines in the gut, liver, and CNS. When patients ingest food containing dietary amines while taking MAOIs, they experience increases in central monoamine release through two mechanisms. *(1)* the dietary amines directly promote production and release of monoamines, and *(2)* the MAOI inhibits the metabolism of monoamines leading to additional release. The amount of dietary amines ingested accounts for the monoamine excess and drug–food interactions.

Hypertensive crises are characterized initially by headache, but can evolve to include neck stiffness, chest discomfort, palpitations, confusion, and, ultimately, hemorrhage or stroke. Treatment of MAOI-associated hypertension may include a watch-and-wait stance by the patient if the symptoms are mild. Some patients have the ability to check and monitor their own blood pressure. Others may consult with a physician for blood pressure checks and observation, but if symptoms are severe, the patient may need to go to an emergency room or self-medicate. Standard emergency room treatment is intravenous phentolamine, an α-adrenergic blocker, continuous monitoring and management until blood pressure is normalized without medication. Some doctors will provide patients with small doses of chlorpromazine or nifedipine to treat hypertension if a problem arises.

Self-medication of a MAOI-induced hypertensive crisis is controversial. In a hypertensive crisis the lack of access to medical services may lead to even greater complications. A small dose of medication taken as part of a larger plan to blunt the rise in blood pressure may prevent serious complications. However, headache is common, has multiple causes, and patients may not accurately identify a headache due to hypertension without a blood pressure check. In addition, self-administration of nifedipine, especially sublingually, may result in needless and perhaps dangerous drops in blood pressure.

To prevent and manage hypertensive crises, patients need to consult with their doctors about avoiding tyramine-containing food and drink, and medications with monoamine agonist activity. The list of tyramine containing foods has become less restrictive, but the list of prescription and over-the-counter medications is expanding as more agents with CNS activity come on the market. Self medicating strategies need to be discussed in detail to assure the patient is fully aware of risks and benefits involved.

Serotonin syndrome

The second major drug interaction involves combining MAOIs with serotonergic drugs, resulting in excessive central release of serotonin. Excess CNS serotonin is characterized by delirium, hyperthermia, autonomic instability, fever, and neuromuscular excitability, and may be associated with coma and death. Combinations of MAOIs with sertononergic agonists, including the SRIs, NSRIs, and other serotonergic medications such as trazadone, nefazadone, buspirone, and mirtazapine, to be avoided.

Medications with serotonergic activity may also have other monaminergic or sympathomimetic activity. Combining MAOIs with these medications may result in a complex side effect profile. For example, combining meperidine or dextromethorphan with MAOIs may result in respiratory depression, in addition to symptoms of serotonin excess. Furthermore, interactions between MAOIs and tricyclic antidepressants (TCAs) more commonly result in potentiating shared adverse events such as othostatic hypotension, as opposed to hyperadrenergic crises or the serotonin syndrome.

Unlike the hypertensive crisis, all the available MAOIs, reversible and irreversible, can induce serotonin excess when used in combination with serotonergic drugs. To avoid such problems, when switching from a MAOI to another antidepressant (including a second MAOI), a 2-week interval is recommended. Similarly, when switching from a SSRI to a MAOI, a 2-week interval is also required, with the exception of patients on a long-acting SSRI, fluoxetine, who need to wait 5 weeks prior to initiating a MAOI. A long washout period can cause other complications. Patients off the medication may suffer a recurence of symptoms, yet not be able to start a new medication. The difficulty with transitioning patients to and from MAOIs may also limit the MAOIs' usefulness.

Side effects and toxicity

Although the MAOIs can have serious and potentially life-threatening adverse effects, it is the more common and less dramatic side effects that often lead to the discontinuation of MAOIs. These side effects include orthostatic hypotension, drowsiness, insomnia, edema, weight gain, sexual dysfunction, and precipitation of mania. Rare side effects include hepatitis and leukopenia. Parasthesias may develop secondary to a MAOI-induced pyridoxine deficiency, which responds to oral pyridoxine supplementation. Overall, phenelzine appears to be more sedating, whereas trancylpromine is more activating because of its stimulant-like properties. Meclobomide has more excitatory side effects, such as restlessness and insomnia.

The MAOIs are dangerous in overdose either alone and in combination with other medications. Overdosage can result in severe autonomic and CNS insta-bility. Symptoms of CNS toxicity includes confusion, coma, involuntary movements, and seizures. In the context of an overdose, patients should be taken to the emergency room and treated for cardiovascular insta-bility and CNS excitation. The signs and symptoms may not be present until 12 hours after ingestion and require ongoing observation and medical management until the patient is stable.

USE IN CHILDREN AND ADOLESCENTS

Understandably, there are only a limited number of studies investigating the benefit of MAOIs in children and adolescents. Studies have focused on depression and ADHD. In a chart review of 23 depressed teen-agers with partial or nonresponse to TCAs, phenelzine and tranylcypromine were prescribed alone or in com-bination with TCAs. The majority of teenagers had clear improvement (17/23) on the MAOIs. However, 7/23 exhibited dietary noncompliance resulting in side effects. Despite the demonstrated benefit of MAOIs in this chart review, the authors cautioned that there may be the potential for adverse events in impulsive or non-compliant adolescents (Ryan et al., 1988). The use of MAOIs in depressed adolescents should be limited to severe depression refractory to other antidepressant treatments. Furthermore, adherence to diet, abstinence from amphetamine-like drugs (including stimulants), and monitoring by parents are important variables to consider in the prescribing of MAOIs to adolescents with depression.

More studies have investigated the role of MAOIs in the treatment of chidren with ADHD than in childhood depression Rapoport, et al., 1985; Zametkin et al., 1985; Ryan et al., 1988; Trott, et al., 1992; Jankovic, 1993; Feigin et al., 1996). Both clorgyline (MAO-A in-hibitor) and phenelzine (nonselective inhibitor) were as effective and well tolerated in a controlled comparison with dextroamphetamine (n = 14)(Zametkin et al., 1985). In contrast, preliminary analysis of a crossover study comparing low-dose selegiline (MAO-B inhibi-tor) to dextroamphetamine suggests that selegiline was less efficacious (Rapoport et al., 1985). Some investi-gators posit that the lack of an ADHD response to a MAO-B suggests that targeting the noradrenergic sys-tem is more important.

Physicians have searched for alternatives to stimu-lants in the treatment of ADHD in Tourette's syn-drome. Two studies have examined the benefit of MAOIs in the treatment of ADHD in children with Tourette's syndrome (Jankovic, 1993; Feigin et al.,

1996). Children with Tourette's syndrome and ADHD refractory to other ADHD medication (n = 29) were treated openly with an average deprenyl dose of 8 mg/day (Jankovic, 1993). The vast majority of patients (26/29) reported clinical improvement with no serious adverse outcomes. Mild side effects that did not require discontinuation of the drug were noted in six patients. Two patients had exacerbations of their tics. A later controlled trial of low-dose selegiline (10 mg/day) did not demonstrate statistically significant improvement of ADHD symptoms in children with Tourette's syn-drome (Feigin et al., 1996).

Clinical Use in Children and Adolescents

Starting monoamine oxydase inhibitors

The patient's psychiatric history should be comprehen-sively reviewed to determine whether a MAOI is the next best step in treatment. The patient should have failed a number of medications and sophisticated psy-chotherapy and family treatment trials (i.e., manual-based type psychotherapies for depression or anxiety). The child and family should be assessed for their com-prehensive understanding of the risks, potential bene-fits, and procedures for a safe trial, including their ca-pacity to maintain compliance with the medication and special MAOI diet; and their capacity to manage hy-pertensive crises should they occur. Patient and family functioning should be stable enough to adequately al-low for assessment of baseline symptomatology and, ultimately, outcome. Instability in psychosocial func-tioning that interferes with the assessment of baseline status and treatment outcome should be addressed prior to initiating treatment. If the patient and family are too unstable, consideration should be given to treating in a structured treatment setting. Many seri-ously ill children who are candidates for MAOIs will be on other medications. The treating clinician needs to evaluate and inform the patient and family regarding problems associated with discontinuing the current medications in the trasition to an MAOI and potenten-tial for the return of depressive symptoms (e.g., suicide) during discontinuation.

Monitoring during treatment

There are no specific requirements for safe follow-up of patients on a MAOI. However, at each follow-up visit it could be considered prudent to evaluate com-pliance, adverse events, clinical response, and concom-itant medications and repeated blood pressures (high and low values are both a concern). Electrocardiographic (EKG) assessment for changes in cardiac conduction times and liver function tests should occur during the period of follow-up. Blood levels and platelet-binding studies are not routinely helpful in administering a MAOI.

Discontinuation

Although abrupt discontinuation is never an optimal treatment strategy, it can occur when patients do not take their medication as a result of a hypertensive crisis. Abrupt discontinuation, especially at higher doses, may be associated with medication withdrawal symptoms. For those who have had a good response to a MAOI and continue on the medication for an extended period of time, tapering of medication would likely be slow, to both avoid any withdrawal symptoms and assess for return of symptoms at lower doses. Follow-up after discontinuation of any medication is prudent, to assess for the subtle or subclinical return of symptoms when the patient is off the medication.

NEFAZODONE (SERZONE)

Nefazodone was introduced for clinical use in the United States in 1995.

Mechanism of Action

Nefazodone is a phenylpiperazine with a chemical structure related to that of trazadone. Nefazodone achieves its antidepressant efficacy through inhibiting reuptake at both the norepinephrine and serotonin receptors, as well as preferential blockade of the 5-HT$_2$ receptor (Ayd, 1995). Furthermore, m-chlorophenylpeperazine (m-CPP), one of nefazodone's active metabolites, serves as a powerful 5-HT$_{2c}$ agonist. Nefazadone's receptor binding profile suggests a lack of affinity for muscarinic, D$_2$, and histamine receptors and less α$_1$-adrenergic antagonist activity than trazodone (Taylor et al., 1995). Although the α$_1$-adrenergic affinity for nefazadone is less than that for trazodone, it may be sufficient to account for the orthostatic hypotension associated with nefazodone.

Pharmacokinetics and Drug Disposition

Nefazodone is rapidly absorbed after oral administration. It undergoes extensive first-pass metabolism in the liver, causing bioavailability to be limited to approximately 20%. Peak plasma levels are achieved between 1 and 3 hours. The pharmacokinetics of nefazodone are nonlinear in nature, resulting in greater than expected plasma concentrations in relation to incremental increases in dosage. The elimination half-life of nefazodone is approximately 4 hours. The parent drug is metabolized by CYP-3A3/4, to form three metabolites. The first, m-CPP, acts as a 5-HT$_{2c}$ agonist and is anxiogenic. m-CPP is metabolized by CYP2D6, and has a half-life of 4–9 hours. The remaining metabolites are hydroxynefazodone and triazolodione. Hydroxynefazodone exerts its action in a manner similar to that of nefazodone, and its half-life is 3–4 hours. Triazolodione is a 5-HT$_{2A}$-antagonist. It is particularly significant because of its longer half-life of 18–30 hours, which may allow for once-daily dosing.

Drug Interactions

Presently available data indicate that nefazodone and hydroxynefazodone are metabolized by, and inhibitors of, the CYP3A4 system. Nefazodone and m-CPP are also weak inhibitors of the CYP2D6 system. Therefore, a significant potential exists for interactions with substrates metabolized through the CYP3A4 system. Specifically, when nefazodone is administered in conjunction with triazolam or alprazolam, significantly elevated levels of these benzodiazepine agents result. Use of nefazodone in combination with cisapride is contraindicated, as elevated levels may result in abnormal cardiac conduction, or torsades de pointes. The interaction of digoxin and nefazodone results in modest increases in the level of digoxin; however, even modest increases could be a concern, given the narrow therapeutic index of digoxin.

Side Effects and Toxicity

Nefazodone is generally well tolerated. It has been shown to improve sleep architecture (Armitage et al., 1994), and has minimal associated sexual dysfunction. The adverse effects associated with nefazodone, in descending order of frequency, are dry mouth, somnolence, dizziness, nausea, constipation, blurred vision, and postural hypotension (Preskorn, 1993). Nefazodone does not slow cardiac conduction; therefore, it has been tolerated in intentional overdoses of up to 11,200 mg.

More recently, the FDA required a "black box" warning be added to the product information regarding nefazadone therapy, which has been associated with liver abnormalities ranging from asymptomatic reversible serum transaminase increases to cases of liver failure resulting in transplant and/or death. As per the black box warning, the reported rate in the United States is about one case of liver failure resulting in death or transplant per 250,000–300,000 patient-years of nefazodone. Treatment with nefazodone should not be initiated in patients with active liver disease or elevated baseline serum transaminase levels. Patients should be advised to be alert for signs of liver dysfunction such as anorexia, jaundice, gastrointestinal complaints, or malaise, and to report them to their doctor immediately if they occur. Nefazodone should be discontinued if clinical signs or symptoms indicate liver failure. Patients who while on nefazodone develop signs of hepatocellular injury such as serum transaminase levels more than three times the upper limit of normal should be withdrawn from the medication. These patients should be presumed to be at risk for liver damage if nefazodone is reintroduced. As such, these patients should not be considered for retreatment with nefazodone (http://www.serzone-side-effects-law.com 2002).

It may be prudent to consider liver function testing of patients being treated with nefazodone. Periodic serum transaminase testing has not been proven to prevent serious injury, but it is generally believed that early detection of drug-induced hepatic injury, along with immediate discontinuation of the medication enhances the likelihood for recovery.

Uses in Children and Adolescents

Nefazodone is not approved by the FDA for use in children, and the literature on its efficacy in the pediatric population is limited. A small case study of children and adolescents who suffered from treatment-refractory depressive disorders ($n = 7$; mean age of 12.4) were treated with a mean daily dose of 357 ± 151 mg (3.4 mg/kg) for 13 ± 8 weeks. Over half of the subjects (4/7) were judged to be much to very much improved as rated by the Clinical Global Impression (CGI) (Wilens et al., 1997). More recently, an open-label study of nefazodone in children and adolescents ($n = 28$) with depression yielded significant improvement in depressive symptoms as measured by the Children's Depression Rating Scale, Revised (Findling et al., 2000).

A recent report on a large, multisite, industry-sponsored, randomized, controlled trial suggests that nefazadone is more effective than placebo in the treatment of depression in adolescents. Nefazadone was well tolerated. No subject experienced a significant el-

evation of liver function enzymes during the trial (Emslie et al., personal communications 2002).

Future Clinical Use in Children and Adolescents

Given its therapeutic profile, nefazadone might be useful in children with depression or anxiety who have prominent sleep problems, or who were activated or energized on SSRIs.

TRAZODONE

Trazodone represents the first antidepressant that structurally differs from the existing heterocyclics. Although it was synthesized in Italy in the mid-1960s, it did not receive FDA approval until 1991.

Mechanism of Action

Trazodone is a triazolopyridine derivative, with relatively weak serotonin reuptake inhibition. Trazodone also has antagonist activity at 5-HT_{1A} and 5-HT_{1C} sites (Haria et al., 1994). Trazodone's active metabolite, m-CPP, serves as a direct serotonin agonist.

Trazodone shows significant blockade of peripheral α-adrenergic receptors and moderate antihistamine properties that may account for priapism and somnolence, respectively. Trazodone is almost entirely devoid of anticholinergic activity (Cusack et al., 1994).

Pharmacokinetics and Drug Disposition

Trazodone is well absorbed after oral administration. It achieves peak plasma levels 1–2 hours following ingestion. The bioavailability of trazodone is 60%–80% with doses between 100 and 200 mg. Trazodone exhibits nonlinear pharmacokinetics because of saturable first-pass metabolism in the liver. Trazodone is metabolized by CYP450-3A4, and its active metabolite, m-CPP, is metabolized through CYP450-2D6. The half-life of the parent compound is 5 to 9 hours, and the half-life of m-CPP is 4 to 9 hours. It is excreted primarily in the urine (Preskorn, 1993).

Drug Interactions

Trazodone has relatively few drug interactions. Medications that induce or inhibit first-pass metabolism may affect trazodone's plasma concentration. Even though trazodone is commonly used for SSRI-induced insomnia, it may be counter productive. Compounds such as fluoxetine or paroxetine, inhibitors of CYP450-2D6, may result in elevated levels of trazadone metabolite, m-CPP (Preskorn, 1993), and result in increased anxiety. Because orthostatic hypotension is associated with trazodone, caution is warranted when combining this medication with antihypertensive agents.

Side Effects and Toxicity

Histamine blockade is responsible for the sedation associated with trazodone. Furthermore, priapism and orthostatic hypotension are mediated by α-adrenergic antagonism. There have been over 200 case reports of priapism (Thompson et al., 1990). Prevalence estimates of priapism suggest that 1/6000 men treated with trazodone will be affected. Other side effects include dry mouth, nausea, and vomiting. Because of trazodone's wide therapeutic window, it is relatively safe in overdosage. There are case reports of patients surviving intentional overdoses of up to 9 (Gamble and Peterson, 1986).

Uses in Children and Adolescents

Although trazodone has not received an FDA indication for use in children and adolescents, it has enjoyed some success in the treatment of disruptive behavior disorders in this population. An aggressive 15-year-old male inpatient was treated with trazodone at a dosage of 200 mg/day, which resulted in decreased disruptive behavior. Following discharge from the hospital, trazodone was discontinued and the patient's violent behavior resumed. Upon return to his previous dose of 200 mg, the aggressive behavior again remitted (Fras, 1987). In 1992, an open study of 22 psychiatric inpatients, ages 5 to 12 years, with disruptive behavioral and mood disorders were treated with trazodone. The results revealed a significant decrease in aggressive and impulsive behaviors in 13 of the patients following therapy with trazodone (Zubieta and Alessi, 1992).

Trazodone has been used therapeutically, but because of low potency and marked sedative effects, its use has been mostly restricted to a sleeping aid in doses of 50–100 mg at bedtime. It has been routinely used in adults on SSRIs, who develop sleep problems. The concern about priapism even at low doses may reduce enthusiasm for its use in male children and adolescents.

Clinical Use in Children and Adolescents

Starting trazodone

Similar starting strategies are required for nefazodone and trazodone. However, the dose adjustment of tra-

zodone is more difficult, as the clinician must generally pursue higher doses of medication and likely will need to adjust for sedative effects. The interplay of low potency and sedative profile may leave children at higher risk for undertreatment.

BUPROPION

History

Bupropion was developed over 30 years ago in an attempt to synthesize a novel antidepressant. Researchers wanted the agent to be efficacious for the existing screening models, but be different structurally and biochemically from the tricyclics and MAOIs. The compound was to be devoid of sympathomimetic, anticholinergic, and cardiac depressant effects (Soroko and Maxwell, 1983).

In 1986, just prior to its release, seizures were reported in a small number of nondepressed, bulimic patients taking bupropion. Bupropion was removed from the market by the manufacturer until it was determined that seizures in this vulnerable population appeared to be related to high doses (>450 mg) of bupropion used in the context of metabolic instability. The drug was finally released in the United States in 1989.

Mechanism of Action

Bupropion is an aminoketone that exerts its therapeutic effect through the inhibition of norepinephrine and dopamine reuptake. Bupropion's receptor occupancy profile shows an absence of anticholinergic and antihistaminic effects (Cusack et al., 1994). Bupropion is absorbed rapidly from the gastrointestinal tract, and peak blood levels are achieved within 2 hours for regular release and 3 hours for sustained-release preparations ($t_{1/2}$ = 10 hours). Bupropion undergoes extensive first-pass metabolism in the liver, yielding three active metabolites: hydrobupropion, threohydroxybupropion, and erythrohydrobupropion. The half-lives of the active metabolites are approximately 20 + hours (Preskorn, 1993).

Because bupropion is metabolized in the liver, medications that alter hepatic enzyme metabolism, such as carbamazepine or cimetidine, may effect blood concentrations. Bupropion should not be administered in combination with the MAOIs because of risk of hypertensive crisis. Levo-dopa use in conjunction with bupropion has been associated with confusion, hallucinations, and dyskinesia. Although generally well tolerated, there are case reports documenting that the coadministration of lithium and bupropion resulted in altered lithium levels and three cases of seizures. The addition of fluoxetine to bupropion has led to delirium and seizures (Goodnick, 1991).

Side Effects and Toxicity

The most common associated adverse effects include appetite suppression, restlessness, activation, tremor, insomnia, and nausea (Preskorn and Othmer, 1984). Delusions and hallucinations (Golden et al., 1985) as well as tic exacerbations have been observed in children with ADHD and Tourette's syndrome (Spencer et al., 1993).

One of the more worrisome adverse effects of bupropion is seizures. At dosages of 450 mg/day or less, the rate of seizures is 0.4% for individuals without risk factors (Davidson, 1989). Because of this risk, a single dose of bupropion should not exceed 150 mg and a second dose should be separated in time by a minimum of 8 hours. Also, patients who are metabolically unstable (i.e., have bulimia) should be carefully assessed for the risk of seizures before initiating medication. Finally, bupropion is not associated with sexual side effects.

Bupropion overdose ($n = 58$) and combined overdoses of bupropion and benzodiazepines ($n = 9$) have been associated with symptoms of neurological toxicity, including lethargy, tremors, and seizures, and an absence of cardiovascular toxicity (Spiller et al., 1994).

Uses in Children and Adolescents

Bupropion is not approved by the FDA for use in children below the age of 18 years; however, it has been used to treat depression and ADHD in this population. A double-blind, placebo-controlled study of the efficacy of bupropion in children with ADHD showed . . . bupropion doses of up to 6 mg/kg to be clearly superior to placebo in decreasing hyperactivity and improving behavior (Casat et al., 1987). A double-blind, crossover design was used to compare the efficacy of bupropion with that of methylphenidate in the treatment of ADHD. Following a 14-day medication washout, 15 subjects with ADHD (ages 7 to 17 years) were randomized to bupropion or methylphenidate for a 6-week period, followed by another 2-week washout, and then crossed over to the other medication. Dosage of methylphenidate ranged from 0.4 to 1.3 mg/kg (mean dosage, 0.7 mg/kg/day) and bupropion was adjusted to doses ranging from 1.4 to 5.7 mg/kg (mean dosage 3.3 mg/kg/day). Both bupropion and methylphenidate were found to produce significantly greater ($p < 0.001$) and equivalent improvement on the Iowa–

Conners Teacher's Rating Scale according to subject, parent, and teacher ratings (Barrickman et al., 1995). A larger, double-blind, placebo-controlled study comparing bupropion and placebo in ADHD subjects (ages 6 through 12 years) found bupropion to be clearly superior to placebo (Conners et al., 1996). More recently, an open trial of bupropion was conducted on adolescents with ADHD and comorbid diagnoses of substance use and conduct disorders. The dosage of bupropion was adjusted to a maximum of 300 mg/day. Subjects showed less hyperactivity and improved attention and overall CGI score (Riggs et al., 1998).

Clinical Use in Children and Adolescents

Particular attention should be paid to the risk of seizure. Education of the patient and family regarding dosing too closely in time (< 8 hours) and not doubling up on doses after a missed dose are critical to the safe use of bupropion.

MIRTAZAPINE

Mirtazapine was first marketed in the United States in 1996.

Mechanism of Action

Mirtazapine is a member of the chemical class of compounds known as *piperazinoazepines* and exerts its therapeutic effect through the blockade of serotonin and adrenergic receptors. However, the manner in which mirtazapine achieves this effect is unique. Mirtazapine is a presynaptic α_2 antagonist that causes an increase in norepinephrine and indirectly increases serotonin through adrenergic stimulation of raphe neurons (Janicak et al., 1997). In addition, mirtazapine blocks 5-HT_{2A} and 5-HT_{2c} receptors. Mirtazapine's receptor occupancy profile shows a strong affinity for H_1 blockade, but only moderate affinity for muscarinic receptors.

Pharmacokinetics and Drug Disposition

Mirtazapine is rapidly absorbed from the gastrointestinal tract and achieves peak plasma concentrations within 2 hours of oral administration. It exhibits linear pharmacokinetics and is metabolized through the CYP450-2D6, CYP450-3A4, and, possibly, CYP450-1A2 systems (Owen and Nemeroff, 1998). Mirtazapine does not induce or inhibit any of the cytochrome systems. Only one of mirtazapine's metabolites, desmethyl-mirtazapine shows significant pharmacological activity ($t_{1/2}$ = 20 hours) (Sitsen and Zikov, 1995).

Mirtazapine has been found to have synergistic depressant effects on motor and cognitive performance when used in conjunction with benzodiazepines or alcohol (Kuitunen, 1994). Somnolence and increased appetite accompanied by weight gain are common adverse effects. Lower doses are clearly associated with more sedative effects than those with higher doses. It is unclear if a similar pattern is noted for appetite and weight gain.

There are reports of transient increases in liver enzymes occurring in 2% of patients receiving mirtazapine. Because of mirtazapine's wide therapeutic window, it is considered generally safe in overdose (Nelson, 1997).

Clinical Use in Children and Adolescents

Genetic and environmental risk factors for obesity should be considered before starting mirtazapine. If the clinical impression is correct that somnolence and appetite increases are greatest at lower doses, the clinician should consider not starting mirtazapine at too low a dosage or maintain a low dose for too long. For adults, some clinicians skip the 15 mg/day dose and start at 30 mg/day. Mirtazapine comes in a fruit-flavored, dissolvable tablet. Initially, this dissolvable tablet was intended for use in the elderly, but it may also be a form of medication useful in children and adolescents who have difficulty swallowing pills. For children on the fruit-flavored dissolvable form of medication, more intensive monitoring of the medication at home may be required to prevent misuse (as candy) by the patient or other children in the family.

REBOXETINE

History

Reboxetine was first introduced to the European market in 1997 for the treatment of depression; it is not yet available in the United States. Reboxetine represents a novel antidepressant class, the selective noradrenaline reuptake inhibitors (NRIs).

Mechanism of Action

Reboxetine achieves its antidepressant effect through selective inhibition of norepinephrine reuptake. Reboxetine's receptor occupancy profile shows little or no af-

finity for muscarinic, histaminergic, α_1-adrenergic, and dopaminergic (D_2) receptors (Wong et al., 2000).

Pharmacokinetics

Reboxetine is well absorbed after oral administration and peak plasma levels are achieved within 2.5 hours. The half-life of the agent ranges from 12 to 16 hours, and steady-state levels are achieved within 5 days (DeVane, 1998). Reboxetine is metabolized by the CYP450-3A4 system to O-desmethylreboxetine and three lesser metabolites. Reboxetine is a weak competitive inhibitor of CYP450-2D6 and CYP450-3A4 (Wienkers, et al. 1999). Significant drug interactions appear to be uncommon.

Side Effects and Toxicity

Reboxetine is generally well tolerated. Compared to placebo, most frequently reported adverse effects in the reboxetine group are dry mouth and insomnia (Versiani et al., 2000). There are also reports of tremor, hypertension, and somnolence in association with reboxetine use. Reboxetine has a wide therapeutic index and does not appear to increase the QTc or alter cardiac conduction.

Future Clinical Use in Children and Adolescents

There are no current data supporting the use of reboxetine in the child and adolescent population. However, given its noradrenergic profile, it may be useful for ADHD and perhaps for depression, and anxiety.

VENLAFAXINE

History

Venlafaxine is one of the first selective serotonin and norepinephrine reuptake inhibitors developed for the treatment of depression. It was originally released in the United States in 1994.

Mechanism of Action

Venlafaxine, a bicyclic phenylethlamine, exerts its therapeutic effect through the reuptake inhibition of serotonin and norepinephrine and, to a lesser degree, dopamine (Thase, 1996). Serotonergic reuptake appears most prominent at lower doses, and noradrenergic activity is more prominent at higher doses. It has no significant affinity for muscarinic, cholinergic, histaminic, or α-₁ receptors (Cusack et al., 1994).

Pharmacokinetics and Drug Disposition

Venlafaxine is rapidly absorbed following oral administration. Venlafaxine ($t^{1/2}$ = 5 hours) is metabolized through the CYP450-2D6 and CYP450-3A4 systems to its active metabolite, O-desmethylvenlafaxine ($t^{1/2}$ = 11 hours), and is excreted through the kidney (Klamerus et al., 1992).

The coadministration of venlafaxine and MAOIs is contraindicated because of the risk of serotonin syndrome. Venlafaxine is a relatively weak inhibitor of the CYP450-2D6 system, therefore it has few drug interactions (Ball et al. 1997).

Side Effects and Toxicity

Venlafaxine is generally well tolerated. The most common adverse effects include nausea, drowsiness, insomnia, dizziness, headache, and dry mouth. At higher doses, elevations in blood pressure have been observed.

Uses in Children and Adolescents

Venlafaxine is not FDA approved for use in children below the age of 18; however, it has been used in this population as an antidepressant as well as treatment for ADHD. In 1997, a placebo-controlled trial for children and adolescents (n = 32) diagnosed with major depression failed to show a difference between the control and venlafaxine groups (Mandoki, et al., 1997), possibly because of subtherapeutic doses of venlafaxine. A 5-week open trial of venlafaxine (n = 14) in children and adolescents (ages 8–14) with ADHD yielded significant improvements in parent ratings of hyperactivity and impulsivity on the Conners Parent rating scales (Olvera et al., 1996).

Future Clinical Use in Children and Adolescents

Given the use of venlafaxine for treatment-refractory depression in adults, it is likely that it will be used for similar purposes in children. In addition, it is likely that venlafaxine will be used for childhood anxiety disorders. It is unclear whether venlafaxine is serotonergically powerful enough to be useful in OCD. The lack of significant drug–drug interactions may facilitate its use in patients for whom antidepressant medication combinations are anticipated.

Monitoring during treatment

With its prominent noradrenergic activity at higher doses, and with reports of associated hypertension, blood pressure monitoring and EKGs should be considered for some patients.

ATOMOXETINE

History

Atomoxetine was originally developed as an antidepressant agent (tomoxetine), but failed to realize this potential. It was abandoned until its use for ADHD was conceived and clinical trials were initiated. During clinical trials its name was changed to atomoxetine to avoid confusion with other medications with similar names (e.g., tamoxifen). It is not currently FDA approved for any indication and is not commercially available anywhere. Materials to support an FDA indication for ADHD were submitted in October, 2001.

Mechanism of Action

Atomoxetine exerts its therapeutic efficacy through the selective reuptake inhibition of norepinephrine. Its receptor occupancy profile shows minimal affinity for cholinergic, histaminic, serotonergic, or α-adrenergic receptors (Spencer et al., 1998).

Pharmacokinetics and Drug Disposition

Atomoxetine is well absorbed ($t^{1/2}$ = 4.3 hours) following oral administration (Farid, et al., 1985). It is metabolized through the CYP450-2D6 system and excreted in the urine.

Side Effects and Toxicity

Atomoxetine is generally well tolerated. Its side effect profile includes anorexia, nausea, headache, insomnia, and rhinitis. In terms of toxicity, there is no evidence of cardiac conduction delay or repolarization abnormalities associated with atomoxetine treatment (Spencer et al., 1998). Atomoxetine is metabololized by CYP450-2D6. Hypothetically, hypometabolizers of CYP450-2D6 might be at risk for increased side effects at routine doses and may require dosage adjustment. In addition, increased adverse events might occur if atomoxetine is coadministered with medications that inhibit CYP450-2D6. Final treatment recommendation will be provided if and when atomoxetine is approved for use.

Uses in Children and Adolescents

Atomoxetine is not commercially available but is currently undergoing investigational use as treatment for ADHD in children and adults. A recent randomized placebo-controlled trial was conducted in a pediatric outpatient population with ADHD (N = 297), and results suggest that atomoxetine is superior to placebo in reducing ADHD symptoms and in improving social and family functioning (Michelson et al., 2001).

Clinical use in Children and Adolescents

Although purely speculative, atomoxetine may have uses in the treatment of depression and/or anxiety, either alone or in combination with other medications.

SUMMARY

In this chapter the basics of the available atypical antidepressants and those that may soon to come on the market have been reviewed. The atypical antidepressants are less readily used, and their benefits for treating depression and anxiety are not fully appreciated. The atypical antidepressants may provide benefit for conditions such as ADHD or offer an alternative to other antidepressants with problematic side effects (i.e., activation on SSRIs). They may also provide specific relief for troublesome symptoms (i.e., nefazodone's normalization of sleep architecture).

The future of atypical antidepressants in the treatment of psychiatric disorders is bright. Advances in neuroscience are being followed closely by those involved in drug development. It is likely that in the future more unique, novel agents will be developed. Such collaborative efforts will make safer and more effective medications for childhood psychiatric disorders possible.

REFERENCES

Angst, J. and Stabl, M. (1992) Efficacy of moclobemide in different patient groups: a meta-analysis of studies. *Psychopharmacology (Berl)* 106 (*Suppl*), S109–S113.

Armitage, R., Rush, A.J., Trivedi, M., Cain, J., and Roffwarg, H.P. (1994) The effects of nefazodone on sleep architecture in depression. *Neuropsychopharmacology* 10:123–127.

Ayd, F.J. (1995) Nefrazodone: the latest FDA approved antidepressant. *Int Drug Ther* Newsletter 30:17–20.

Ball, S.E., Ahern, D., Scatina, J., and Kao, J. (1997) Venlafaxine: in vitro inhibition of CYP2D6 dependent imipramine and desipramine metabolism; comparative studies with selected SSRIs, and effects on human hepatic CYP3A4, CYP2C9 and CYP1A2. *Br J Clin Pharmacol* 43:619–626.

Barrickman, L.L., Perry, P.J., Allen, A.J., Kuperman, S., Arndt, S.V., Herrmann, K.J., and Schumacher, E. (1995) Bupropion versus methylphenidate in the treatment of attention-deficit hyperactivity disorder. *J Am Acad Child Adolesc Psychiatry* 34:649–657.

Blackwell, B. (1963) Hypertensive crisis due to monoamine-oxidase inhibition. *Lancet* 2:849–851.

Blackwell, B. (1991) Monoamine oxidase inhibitor interactions with other drugs. *J Clin Psychopharmacol* 11:55–59.

Bloch, R.G., Dooneief, A.S., Buchberg, A.S., and Spellman, S. (1954) The clinical effect of isoniazid and iproniazid in the treatment of pulmonary tuberculosis. *Ann Intern Med* 40:881–900.

Casat, C.D., Pleasants, D.Z., and Van Wyck Fleet, J. (1987) A double-blind trial of bupropion in children with attention deficit disorder. *Psychopharmacol Bull* 23:120–122.

Conners, C.K., Casat, C.D., Gualtieri, C.T., Weller, E., Reader, M., Reiss, A., Weller, R.A., Khayrallah, M., and Ascher, J. (1996). Bupropion hydrochloride in attention deficit disorder with hyperactivity. *J Am Acad Child Adolesc Psychiatry* 35:1314–1321.

Cusack, B., Nelson, A., and Richelson, E. (1994) Binding of antidepressants to human brain receptors: focus on newer generation compounds. *Psychopharmacology (Berl)* 114:559–565.

Davidson, J. (1989) Seizures and bupropion: a review. *J Clin Psychiatry* 50:256–261.

DeVane, C.L. (1998) Differential pharmacology of newer antidepressants. *J Clin Psychiatry* 59 (*Suppl 20*):85–93.

Ernst, M., Liebenauer, L.L., Tebeka, D., Jons, P.H., Eisenhofer, G., Murphy, D.L., and Zametkin, A.J. (1997) Selegiline in ADHD adults: plasma monoamines and monoamine metabolites. *Neuropsychopharmacology* 16:276–284.

Farid, N.A., Bergstrom, R.F., Ziege, E.A., Parli, C.J., and Lemberger, L. (1985) Single-dose and steady-state pharmacokinetics of tomoxetine in normal subjects. *J Clin Pharmacol* 25:296–301.

Feigin, A., Kurlan, R., McDermott, M.P., Beach, J., Dimitsopulos, T., Brower, C.A., Chapieski, L., Trinidad, K., Como, P., and Jankovic, J. (1996) A controlled trial of deprenyl in children with Tourette's syndrome and attention deficit hyperactivity disorder. *Neurology* 46:965–968.

Findling, R.L., Preskorn, S.H., Marcus, R.N., Magnus, R.D., D'Amico, F., Marathe, P., and Reed, M.D. (2000) Nefazodone pharmacokinetics in depressed children and adolescents. *J Am Acad Child Adolesc Psychiatry* 39:1008–1016.

Food Drug Administration. (2002) Black Box Warning For Serzon http://www.gene-sideeffects-law.com,

Fras, I. (1987) Trazodone and violence. *J Am Acad Child Adolesc Psychiatry* 26:453.

Gamble, D.E., and Peterson, L.G. (1986) Trazodone overdose: four years of experience from voluntary reports. *J Clin Psychiatry* 47:544–546.

Golden, R.N., James, S.P., Sherer, M.A., Rudorfer, M.V., Sack, D.A., and Potter, W.Z. (1985) Psychoses associated with bupropion treatment. *Am J Psychiatry* 142:1459–1462.

Goodnick, P.J. (1991) Pharmacokinetics of second generation antidepressants: bupropion. *Psychopharmacol Bull* 27:513–519.

Haria, M., Fitton, A., and McTavish, D. (1994) Trazodone. A review of its pharmacology, therapeutic use in depression and therapeutic potential in other disorders. *Drugs Aging* 4:331–355.

Jankovic, J. (1993). Deprenyl in attention deficit associated with Tourette's syndrome. *Arch Neurol* 50:286–288.

Klamerus, K.J., Maloney, K., Rudolph, R.L., Sisenwine, S.F., Jusko,

W.J., and Chiang, S.T. (1992) Introduction of a composite parameter to the pharmacokinetics of venlafaxine and its active O-desmethyl metabolite. *J Clin Pharmacol* 32: 716–724.

Kuitunen, T. (1994) Drug and ethanol effects on the clinical test for drunkeness: single doses of ethanol, hypnotic drugs, and antidepressant drugs. *Pharmacol Toxicol* 75:91.

Loerch, B., Graf-Morgenstern, M., Hautzinger, M., Schlegel, S., Hain, C., Sandmann, J., and Benkert, O. (1999) Randomised placebo-controlled trial of moclobemide, cognitive-behavioural therapy and their combination in panic disorder with agoraphobia. *Br J Psychiatry* 174:205–212.

Mallinger, A.G., and Smith, E. (1991). Pharmacokinetics of monoamine oxidase inhibitors. *Psychopharmacol Bull* 27:493–502.

Mandoki, M.W., Tapia, M.R., Tapia, M.A., Sumner, G.S., and Parker, J.L. (1997) Venlafaxine in the treatment of children and adolescents with major depression. *Psychopharmacol Bull* 33:149–154.

Mann, J.J., Aarons, S.F., Wilner, P.J., Keilp, J.G., Sweeney, J.A., Pearlstein, T., Frances, A.J., Kocsis, J.H., and Brown, R.P. (1989) A controlled study of the antidepressant efficacy and side effects of (−)-deprenyl. A selective monoamine oxidase inhibitor. *Arch Gen Psychiatry* 46:45–50.

Michelson, D., Faries, D., Wernicke, J., Kelsey, D., Kendrick, K., Sallee, F.R., Spencer, T. (2001) Atomoxetine in the treatment of children and adolescents with attention deficit / hyperactivity disorder: a randomized place to controlled, dose response study. *Pediatrics* 108:E83.

Nelson, J.C. (1997) Safety and tolerability of the new antidepressants. *J Clin Psychiatry* 58 (Suppl 6):26–31.

Olvera, R.L., Pliszka, S.R., Luh, J., and Tatum, R. (1996) An open trial of venlafaxine in the treatment of attention-deficit/hyperactivity disorder in children and adolescents. *J Child Adolesc Psychopharmacol* 6:241–250.

Owen, J.R. and Nemeroff, C.B. (1998) New antidepressants and the cytochrome P450 system: focus on venlafaxine, nefazodone, and mirtazapine. *Depress Anxiety* 7 (Suppl 1):24–32.

Potter, W.Z., Murphy, D.L., Wehr, T.A., Linnoila, M., and Goodwin, F.K. (1982) Clorgyline. A new treatment for patients with refractory rapid-cycling disorder. *Arch Gen Psychiatry* 39:505–510.

Preskorn, S.H. (1993) Pharmacokinetics of antidepressants: why and how they are relevant to treatment. *J Clin Psychiatry* 54 (Suppl): 14–34; discussion 55–16.

Preskorn, S.H., and Othmer, S.C. (1984) Evaluation of bupropion hydrochloride: the first of a new class of atypical antidepressants. *Pharmacotherapy* 4:20–34.

Rapoport, J.L., Zametkin, A., Donnelly, M., and Ismond, D. (1985) New drug trials in attention deficit disorder. *Psychopharmacol Bull* 21:232–236.

Riggs, P.D., Leon, S.L., Mikulich, S.K., and Pottle, L.C. (1998) An open trial of bupropion for ADHD in adolescents with substance use disorders and conduct disorder. *J Am Acad Child Adolesc Psychiatry* 37:1271–1278.

Ryan, N.D., Puig-Antich, J., Rabinovich, H., Fried, J., Ambrosini, P., Meyer, V., Torres, D., Dachille, S., and Mazzie, D. (1988). MAOIs in adolescent major depression unresponsive to tricyclic antidepressants. *J Am Acad Child Adolesc Psychiatry* 27:755–758.

Schneier, F.R., Goetz, D., Campeas, R., Fallon, B., Marshall, R., and Liebowitz, M.R. (1998) Placebo-controlled trial of moclobemide in social phobia. *Br J Psychiatry* 172:70–77.

Sitsen, J.M.A., and Zikov, M. (1995) Mirazapine: clinical profile. *CNS Drugs* 4(Suppl 1):39–48.

Sogaard, J., Lane, R., Latimer, P., Behnke, K., Christiansen, P.E., Nielsen, B., Ravindran, A.V., Reesal, R.T., and Goodwin, D.P. (1999) A 12-week study comparing moclobemide and sertraline in the treatment of outpatients with atypical depression. *J Psychopharmacol* 13:406–414.

Soroko, F.E., and Maxwell, R.A. (1983) The pharmacologic basis for therapeutic interest in bupropion. *J Clin Psychiatry* 44(5 Pt 2): 67–73.

Spencer, T., Biederman, J., Steingard, R., and Wilens, T. (1993) Bupropion exacerbates tics in children with attention-deficit hyperactivity disorder and Tourette's syndrome. *J Am Acad Child Adolesc Psychiatry* 32:211–214.

Spencer, T., Biederman, J., Wilens, T., Prince, J., Hatch, M., Jones, J., Harding, M., Faraone, S.V., and Seidman, L. (1998) Effectiveness and tolerability of tomoxetine in adults with attention deficit hyperactivity disorder. *Am J Psychiatry* 155:693–695.

Spiller, H.A., Ramoska, E.A., Krenzelok, E.P., Sheen, S.R., Borys, D.J., Villalobos, D., Muir, S., and Jones-Easom, L. (1994) Bupropion overdose: a 3-year multi-center retrospective analysis. *Am J Emerg Med* 12:43–45.

Taylor, D.P., Carter, R.B., Eison, A.S., Mullins, U.L., Smith, H.L., Torrente, J.R., Wright, R.N., and Yocca, F.D. (1995) Pharmacology and neurochemistry of nefazodone, a novel antidepressant drug. *J Clin Psychiatry* 56 (Suppl 6):3–11.

Thase, M.E. (1996) Antidepressant options: venlafaxine in perspective. *J Clin Psychopharmacol* 16(3 Suppl 2): 10S–18S; discussion 18S–20S.

Thompson, J.W., Jr., Ware, M.R., and Blashfield, R.K. (1990) Psychotropic medication and priapism: a comprehensive review. *J Clin Psychiatry* 51:430–433.

Tollefson, G.D. (1983) Monoamine oxidase inhibitors: a review. *J Clin Psychiatry* 44(8):280–288.

Trott, G.E., Friese, H.J., Menzel, M., and Nissen, G. (1992) Use of moclobemide in children with attention deficit hyperactivity disorder. *Psychopharmacology (Berl)* 106 (Suppl):S134–136.

Versiani, M., Amin, M., and Chouinard, G. (2000) Double-blind, placebo-controlled study with reboxetine in inpatients with severe major depressive disorder. *J Clin Psychopharmacol* 20:28–34.

Versiani, M., Amrein, R., and Stabl, M. (1997) Moclobemide and imipramine in chronic depression (dysthymia): an international double-blind, placebo-controlled trial. International Collaborative Study Group. *Int Clin Psychopharmacol* 12:183–193.

Versiani, M., Nardi, A.E., Mundim, F.D., Alves, A.B., Liebowitz, M.R., and Amrein, R. (1992) Pharmacotherapy of social phobia. A controlled study with moclobemide and phenelzine. *Br J Psychiatry* 161:353–360.

Wender, P.H., Wood, D.R., Reimherr, F.W., and Ward, M. (1983) An open trial of pargyline in the treatment of attention deficit disorder, residual type. *Psychiatry Res* 9:329–336.

Wienkers, L.C., Allievi, C., Hauer, M.J., and Wynalda, M.A. (1999) Cytochrome P-450-mediated metabolism of the individual enantiomers of the antidepressant agent reboxetine in human liver microsomes. *Drug Metab Dispos* 27:1334–1340.

Wilens, T.E., Spencer, T.J., Biederman, J., and Schleifer, D. (1997) Case study: nefazodone for juvenile mood disorders. *J Am Acad Child Adolesc Psychiatry* 36:481–485.

Wong, E.H., Sonders, M.S., Amara, S.G., Tinholt, P.M., Piercey, M.F., Hoffmann, W.P., Hyslop, D.K., Franklin, S., Porsolt, R.D., Bonsignori, A., Carfagna, N., and McArthur, R.A. (2000) Reboxetine: a pharmacologically potent, selective, and specific norepinephrine reuptake inhibitor. *Biol Psychiatry* 47:818–829.

Wood, D.R., Reimherr, F.W., and Wender, P.H. (1983) The use of
L-deprenyl in the treatment of attention deficit disorder, residual
type. *Psychopharmacol Bull* 19:627–629.

Zametkin, A., Rapoport, J.L., Murphy, D.L., Linnoila, M., and Ismond, D. (1985) Treatment of hyperactive children with monoamine oxidase inhibitors. I. Clinical efficacy. *Arch Gen Psychiatry*
42:962–966.

Zubieta, J.K., and Alessi, N.E. (1992) Acute and chronic administration of trazodone in the treatment of disruptive behavior disorders in children. *J Clin Psychopharmacol* 12:346–351.

25 | Mood stabilizers: lithium and anticonvulsants

PABLO DAVANZO AND JAMES McCRACKEN

In this chapter we review the mechanisms of action, pharmacokinetics, side effects, and uses of lithium and the anticonvulsants as they apply to child psychiatric clinical practice.

LITHIUM

In the process of studying the toxicity of uric acid from patients with manic–depressive illness in guinea pigs, the Australian physician John Cade noted in 1949 that animals became lethargic after injection with lithium carbonate, a monovalent cation (Cade, 1978). This led to the administration of lithium citrate to a manic adult patient who had a marked clinical improvement (Cade, 1978). Twenty years later, lithium was approved by the Federal Drug Administration (FDA) for the treatment of mania in adults. Since then, it has traditionally been used as the preferred treatment of mania in adults (Post et al., 1997) and adolescents (Strober et al., 1990) with bipolar disorder (BD). One double-blind, placebo-controlled study of adolescent mania showing a 43% response efficacy (Geller et al., 1998a) suggests that adolescents with BD may have a similar or even lower response efficacy to lithium compared with adults.

Lithium has numerous pharmacologic effects. It is able to cross through sodium channels, competing with monovalent and divalent cations in cell membranes (AHFS, 2000). Animal studies have shown that lithium at a serum level of 0.66 +/− 0.08 mEq/L can increase the amphetamine-induced release of serotonin (5-hydroxytryptamine [5-HT]) and the concentrations of a serotonin metabolite (e.g., 5-hydroxyindoleacetic acid [5-HIAA]) in the perifornical hypothalamus (PFH) of rats before and after chronic lithium chloride administration (Baptista et al., 1990), a mechanism possibly involved in lithium's antidepressant effect. The precise neurobiological mechanisms through which lithium reduces acute mania and protects against recurrence of illness remain uncertain (Lenox and Hahn,

2000). It is apparent that lithium exerts an effect on intracellular second messenger systems in which activated receptor–ligand complexes stimulate the turnover of inositol-containing phospholipids (Soares et al., 2000). Lithium's inhibitory action on receptor-mediated signal–transduction pathways has been demonstrated in vitro (Atack et al., 1995), showing that it reduces *myo*-inositol levels by noncompetitively inhibiting the enzyme inositol monophosphate, a catalyst for converting inositol monophosphate hydroxyls to *myo*-inositol (Manji et al., 1996). Since the phosphoinositide (PI) cycle regulates a wide variety of neuronal functions, including intracellular calcium mobilization and protein kinase C (PKC) activity (Lenox and Hahn, 2000), lithium-induced modification of the PI cycle has been proposed as one of the main potential therapeutic mechanism underlying its mood-stabilizing effect (Berridge et al., 1982). Although brain tissue can synthesize *myo*-inositol de novo, the ability of neurons to maintain a steady-state supply of cytosolic *myo*-inositol appears to be crucial to the resynthesis of PI. Dampening of PI-mediated signal transduction in excitatory neurons would therefore result in an antimanic effect (Lenox and Hahn, 2000). Lithium also interacts with cyclic adenosine monophosphate (cAMP) second messengers (Mork, 1993). By inhibiting adenylate cyclase, lithium reduces intracellular concentrations of cAMP. One of the most important targets for cAMP is cAMP-dependent protein kinases (PKA) (Mork, 1993). A decrease in levels of cAMP results in changes in PKA-mediated phosphorylation (Jensen and Mork, 1997). These interactions may be involved in lithium's overall stabilizing effect in neurotransmitter function.

Pharmacokinetics

Absorption

Lithium is readily absorbed from the gastrointestinal (GI) tract. Food or antacids (Goode et al., 1984) do not appear to affect the bioavailability of lithium. Absorption of lithium carbonate from extended-release tablets (60%–90% absorbed) is delayed, with peak serum lithium concentrations occurring within 4 to 12 hours (AHFS, 2000). The velocity of absorption depends on the route of administration. The more rapid the absorption, the shorter will be the time (t_{max}) required to reach the peak plasma level (C_{max}) (Feldman et al., 1997). A comparison of 300 mg immediate-release lithium carbonate tablets (Lithotab), 450 mg extended-release lithium carbonate tablets (Eskalith CR), and 300 mg extended-release lithium carbonate tablets (Lithobid) has shown that C_{max} differed significantly among all three lithium carbonate products (Kirkwood, et al., 1994). Eskalith CR produced a 40% lower C_{max} and Lithobid a 25% lower C_{max} than that of Lithotab (Kirkwood et al., 1994). Similarly, significantly lower serum lithium levels achieved with lithium citrate than with lithium carbonate preparation have been described (Tyrer et al., 1982).

Distribution

Lithium is initially distributed into extracellular fluid and the cation is rapidly distributed into thyroid, bone, and brain tissue at concentrations 50% greater than serum concentrations (AHFS, 2000). Lithium initially distributes into an apparent volume that is about 25%–40% of body weight, and later into a volume that is equal to that of total body water. Steady-state distribution volumes of about 0.7–1 L/kg have been reported in adults (Jermain et al., 1991). Children of ages 9 to 12 years may have a shorter elimination half-life and higher total clearance (Vitiello et al., 1988), with a fast-phase half-life of 6.0 +/− 1.8 hour, and a slow-phase half-life of 17.9 +/− 7.4 hour in the serum (Vitiello et al., 1988). Pediatric patients may also have larger volumes of distribution (AHFS, 2000), unlike geriatric patients, in whom the apparent volume of distribution (0.64 +/− 0.16 L/kg) is significantly reduced compared to that in younger adults (Hardy et al., 1987). Lithium is not bound to plasma proteins. Lithium freely crosses the placenta, following a concentration gradient instead of an active transport mechanism (Krachler et al., 1999). The milk of nursing women contains lithium concentrations that are approximately 33%–50% of those in serum (AHFS, 2000).

Elimination

Serum concentrations of lithium decline in a biphasic manner. An initial half-life ($t_{1/2}\alpha$) of 0.8–1.2 hours and a mean terminal elimination half-life ($t_{1/2}\beta$) of 20–27 hours have been observed following single-dose administration of lithium syrup, as well as after tablet dosing (Goode et al., 1984). Lithium is not metabolized; it is excreted almost entirely in the urine. About 80% of the lithium that is filtered by the renal glomeruli is reabsorbed in the proximal renal tubules. The renal plasma clearance of lithium is 20–40 mL/min (AHFS, 2000), and is not enhanced by polyuria or diuretics (Stone, 1999). In patients with normal renal function, about 30%–70% of a single dose is excreted in urine within 6–12 hours (AHFS, 2000); the remainder is excreted slowly over 10–14 days. Pediatric patients (and pregnant women) may have higher lithium renal clearances (AHFS, 2000).

Side Effects

Hagino et al. (1995) gave a test dose of 600 mg of lithium to 20 children ages 4–6, with an initial dose of 30 mg/kg/day (achieving levels of 0.6–1.2 mEq/L in 2 weeks), and found that the average dose preceding side effects was 39 ± 9.5 mg/kg/day. The most commonly reported side effects were neuronal, GI, ocular, and urinary (Hagino et al., 1995). We briefly review here lithium's side effects by system.

Neurologic effects

Hand tremor occurs in about 45%–50% of patients during initiation of lithium therapy and is usually benign (AHFS, 2000). The tremor is a fine, rapid-intention tremor, which generally resolves during continued therapy with the drug. After 1 year of lithium therapy, less than 10% of patients exhibit tremor (Gelenberg et al., 1989). A reduction in lithium dosage or low doses of a β-adrenergic blocking agent (e.g., propranolol) may be beneficial. The tremor is not responsive to antimuscarinic or other antiparkinsonian drugs (Hagino et al., 1995).

Gastrointestinal effects

Lithium reduces intestinal absorption of glucose and water (AHFS, 2000). These actions may be responsible for the osmotic diarrhea and other mild and reversible adverse GI effects that frequently occur during initiation of lithium therapy. Nausea, anorexia, epigastric bloating, diarrhea, vomiting, or abdominal pain occur in about 10%–30% of patients (AHFS, 2000). Taking the drug with meals, dividing dosage, or using an extended-release preparation often alleviates these effects.

Renal effects

A decrease in renal-concentrating ability occurs in 30%–50% of patients shortly after starting lithium therapy and persists in about 25% of treated patients after 1–2 years of lithium therapy (AHFS, 2000). Lithium in children often produces a mild nephrogenic diabetes insipidus manifested as polyuria (Hagino et al., 1995). Polyuria is usually treated with lithium dosage reduction (AHFS, 2000). Anecdotally, this potential side effect may be difficult to treat in children. However, high serum concentrations of lithium have been associated with increased renin release and resultant inhibition of sodium reabsorption in the proximal and distal renal tubules (AHFS, 2000). Sclerosis of 10%–20% of glomeruli has been noted in some patients (AHFS, 2000). These nonspecific changes have not been associated with a decrease in renal function. Studies of pediatric patients on chronic lithium therapy have not been conducted.

Endocrine effects

Lithium blocks the release of thyroxine (T_4) and triiodothyronine (T_3) mediated by thyrotropin (Kleiner et al., 1999). This results in a decrease in circulating T_4 and T_3 concentrations and a feedback increase in serum thyrotropin concentration. It also inhibits thyrotropin-stimulated adenylate cyclase activity (Kleiner et al., 1999). Lithium has varying effects on carbohydrate metabolism. Increased and decreased glucose tolerance and decreased sensitivity to insulin have been observed (Van derVelde & Gordon, 1969). In animals, lithium decreases hepatic cholesterol and fatty acid synthesis.

Cardiac effects

Reversible electrocardiographic (EKG) T-wave depression occurs frequently with therapeutic serum lithium concentrations. Arrhythmias have occurred rarely. The cardiac effects of lithium may result partly from displacement of potassium from intracellular myocardial sites by lithium, resulting in a slow, partial depletion of intracellular potassium (Kawata, 1979).

Hematologic effects

Lithium produces neutrophilia and may also increase platelet counts, perhaps because of lithium's stimulation of the pluripotent stem cell (AHFS, 2000). Neutrophilia is seen generally within 3–7 days after lithium therapy is initiated and rapidly reverses when the drug is discontinued (AHFS, 2000).

Acute lithium intoxication

The acute lethal dose of lithium is generally associated with a dose that produces serum lithium concentrations greater than 3.5 mEq/L 12 hours after ingestion (AHFS, 2000). Acute ingestion of a single massive dose of lithium may produce only vomiting and diarrhea usually within 1 hour of ingestion. Death has occurred in adults who ingested single 10 to 60 g doses of lithium (AHFS, 2000). The treatment is acute and should be conducted on an emergency basis. The stomach should be emptied immediately by inducing emesis or by gastric lavage, and followed by the treatment described for chronic intoxication.

Pediatric Uses

Disorders of impulse control

Some (Campbell et al., 1995; Malone, et al., 2000) but not all (Rifkin et al., 1997), controlled studies of lithium among children with conduct disorder (CD) appear to support lithium's efficacy in the treatment of aggression in this population. Both aggression and irritability are symptoms that cut across diverse disorders and are important confounders in studies of impulse dyscontrol. Double-blind controlled studies are needed to further validate the choice of lithium for patients with BD presenting with excessive irritability and anger outbursts (Fava, 1997).

Mood disorders

Lithium has been used to treat children with mixed BD symptomatology. One prospective controlled study of lithium in adolescents with BD (and substance dependence) has been reported at the time of this writing (Geller et al., 1998a). Forty-six percent of the subjects (in the intent-to-treat group) were responders to lithium, compared to 8.3% who responded to placebo, a significant finding. Kowatch and colleagues (2000) recently completed an open randomized trial of mood stabilizers in children with type I and type II BD. The investigators found no significant differences between the groups at the completion of the study. Indeed, the reported effect size of 1.63 for divalproex sodium (DVP), 1.06 for lithium, and 1.00 for carbamazepine (CBZ), suggested better efficacy for DVP than for lithium in this population, which had a mean age of 11.4 years (Kowatch et al., 2000).

The treatment of children with bipolar II disorder, depressed phase, has been studied by Geller and colleagues (1998b) who hypothesized that lithium would be efficacious for the treatment of prepubertal major depressive disorder (PMDD) in children who had a family history of bipolarity. This lack of statistically significant difference between active and placebo groups on either categorical or continuous measures was concordant with previous controlled studies of MDD in children (Puig-Antich, 1986).

Dosage and Administration

Lithium is approved by the FDA for the treatment of manic episodes in individuals 12 years of age and older with a diagnosis of BD, and for the maintenance of patients with a history of mania. It is supplied as lithium carbonate in 300 mg capsules and tablets, lithium carbonate in slow-release 300 and 450 mg tablets, and as lithium citrate syrup, 8 mEq/5 mL (equal to one 300 mg tablet) (AHFS, 2000). The larger fluid intake, total body water, and increased glomerular filtration rate may account for children's higher lithium excretion rate and shorter half-life (10–12 hours) than those of adults (Vitiello and Jenson, 1995). A lithium titration schedule based on data from Weller and colleagues (1986), or the Cooper nomogram method (Cooper and Simpson, 1976) has shown good predictive values for serum lithium in adults (Cooper and Simpson, 1976) and children (Geller and Fetner, 1989a). The usual starting dosage for preadolescent and adolescents is 30/mg/kg/day (see Table 25.1).

ANTICONVULSANTS

Carbamazepine (CBZ) and divalproex sodium (DVP) are the most common anticonvulsant agents prescribed for adult BD (Bowden et al., 1994); Post et al., 1998b) and pediatric epileptic disorders (Trimble, 1990; Dunn et al., 1998). As a consequence of their documented efficacy in these populations, their use has been extended to pediatric behavioral and mood disorders (Biederman et al., 1998). We review here their mechanisms of action, pharmacokinetics, side effects, and pediatric uses. The multiple cytochrome P450 (CYB)-mediated potential drug interactions of CBZ and DVP are not covered in detail in this chapter. For a comprehensive review of this subjects the reader is referred to a recent publication by Flockhart and Oesterheld (2000).

CARBAMAZEPINE

Carbamazepine is an iminostilbene derivative used as an anticonvulsant and for the relief of pain associated with trigeminal neuralgia (AHFS, 2000). It is structurally related to the tricyclic antidepressants. The anticonvulsant properties of CBZ are most probably dependent on its inhibitory effects on voltage-dependent sodium (Na) channels (Van Calker et al., 1991). Some of the first clinical observations about CBZ in nonepileptic children were noted by Groh (1976), who reported significant improvement in "a multitude of behavior problems" in 20 children and adolescents with CD treated with CBZ. Years later, Trimble and Cull (1988) reported that higher serum levels of CBZ, i.e., 8–12 µg/mL, were associated with decreased behavior problems in children. Results from these uncontrolled studies were not replicated by Cueva and colleagues (1996) in a parallel-group double-blind, placebo-controlled study of 22 hospitalized children diagnosed with CD and treated with CBZ for 6 weeks. Carbamazepine at an optimal mean daily dose of 683 mg, with serum levels of 4.98 to 9.1 µg/mL, was not superior to placebo.

Mechanism of Action

Despite the widespread use of CBZ, the molecular mechanisms underlying its mood-stabilizing effects have not been identified (Post et al., 1998a). Carbamazepine has been described to have antikindling activity, probably via potentiation of γ-aminobutyric acid (GABA)B receptor agonists (Granger, et al., 1995). There is also evidence to suggest that CBZ may act as an antagonist of A1 adenosine receptors (Van Calker et al., 1991), a somewhat paradoxical property, as the clinicals characteristics of CBZ are similar to the sedative and anxiolytic effects of adenosine agonists (Van Calker et al., 1991). However, CBZ has been shown to attenuate the effects of adenosine on the formation of inositol-phosphates (IP) in the brain, via its A1-antagonistic activity, a possible mechanism that would explain its sedative effect (i.e., via dampening of the IP–Ca second messenger system) only selectively for overactive neuronal circuits (Van Calker et al., 1991). Carbamazepine may also inhibit α_2 adrenergic receptors, therefore increasing the release of norepinephrine into the synaptic cleft. It can also reduce calcium influx into glial cells and neurons through the N-methyl-D-aspartate (NMDA) receptor and block sodium channels in many brain regions (Hough et al., 1996).

Pharmacokinetics

The pharmacokinetic parameters of CBZ are similar in children and in adults; however, there is a poor correla-

TABLE 25.1 *Treatment Guidelines for Mood Stabilizers in Children and Adolescents*

Medication	Initial Daily Dose (given bid or tid)		Titration	Half-life (hours)	Target Dose (daily)	Desired Serum Level	Laboratory Testing	Side Effects
Lithium	<25 kg	300 mg	Every 3–5 days	10–12	600 mg 30 mg/kg/day	0.6–1.2 mEq/L Lower levels have fewer side effects but more relapse	CBC, BUN, creatinine (i.e., renal function), urinalysis, thyroid function tests; EKG Serum lithium level (drawn 12 hours after dose) every 1–2 weeks until stable; every 1–2 months during continuation phase Repeat thyroid function testast and urinalysis every 3–6 months	Nausea, vomiting, diarrhea, tremor, weight gain, polydipsia, polyuria, enuresis; fatigue, ataxia; acne, hair loss; elevated TSH; rarely cardiac conduction; impact on skeletal maturation
	25–40 kg	600 mg			750–900 mg			
	>40 kg	900 mg		20–24	1200 mg			
DVP	<25 kg	250 mg	Every 3 days	8–20	500 mg	50–125 µg/mL 10–20 mg/kg/day = therapeutic levels (>50 µg/mL)	CBC, baseline liver function tests, coagulation tests; serum levels (5 days to reach steady state) 8–12 hours after administration	Nausea/vomiting, weight gain, drowsiness skin rash, muscle weakness, hair loss
	25–40 kg	375 mg			750 mg			Rarely, decreased platelets, hepatic toxicity in infants, polycystic ovaries?
	>40 kg	500 mg			>1000 mg			Avoid during first trimester; associated with neural tube defects
CBZ	<25 kg	100 mg	Every 5 days	12–60	400 mg	4–14 µg/mL 10–20 mg/kg/day (200–1200 mg)	CBC, liver function tests; blood levels weekly to adjust dosage, then every 3–6 months	Transient but marked leukopenia, skin rash, dizziness, diplopia, headache; SIADH neutropenia (d/c <1500) agranulocytosis rarely, usually within first 3 months but not predictable
	25–40 kg	200 mg			800 mg			Periodic monitoring does not catch agranulocytosis, so advise family to watch for easy bruisability, fever.
	>40 kg	400 mg			1200 mg	Enzyme induction requires reestablishing blood levels after several weeks		Avoid during first trimester; associated with neural tube defects

(continued)

TABLE 25.1 *Treatment Guidelines for Mood Stabilizers in Children and Adolescents (continued)*

Medication	Initial Daily Dose (given bid or tid)		Titration	Half-life (hours)	Target Dose (daily)	Desired Serum Level	Laboratory Testing	Side Effects
Gabapentin	>40 kg	300 mg tid	Every 5 days	7–12	900–1800 mg	3.5–10 mL/L/day	Creatinine clearance in patients with impaired renal function	Somnolence, dizziness, ataxia, fatigue, and nystagmus Discontinuation of gabapentin and/or addition of an alternative anticonvulsant drug to existing therapy should be done gradually over a minimum of 1 week
Lamotrigine	>40 kg	25 mg	Every 15 days	32	400 mg	Currently not approved for youth under age 16 years	CBC, liver function tests	Skin rashes in 1/50–1/100 children vs. 1/1000 adults; Stevens-Johnson syndrome with rapid titration Dizziness, ataxia, somnolence, headache, diplopia, blurred vision, nausea, and vomiting
Topiramate	>40 kg	12.5–25 mg	Every 7 days	18–24	150 mg/day	Used in combination with other anticonvulsant agents for management of partial seizures in adults and children	Inducer of CYP3A If CBZ added, clearance of topiramate is decreased by 50% Topiramate will also decrease oral contraceptive levels with resultant effects	Weight loss, word-finding difficulties; poor concentration; fatigue, emotional lability

BUN, blood urea nitrogen; CBC, complete blood cell count; CBZ, carbamazepine; DVP, divalproex sodium; EKG, electrocardiogram; SIADH, syndrome of inappropriate secretion of antidiuretic hormone; TSH, thyroid-stimulating hormone.

tion between dosage and plasma concentrations of CBZ in children (AHFS, 2000). Carbamazepine has linear kinetics so that a dosage increase will result in a predicted increase in serum blood levels (Trimble and Thompson, 1984). In the course of a few weeks CBZ is expected to autoinduce its cytochrome-metabolizing enzymes in the liver (Cepelak et al., 1998), mainly CYP3A4 (Ketter et al., 1995), resulting in decreased serum level.

Absorption

Carbamazepine is slowly absorbed from the GI tract, and peak plasma concentrations are achieved in 2–8

hours following oral administration. Following chronic oral administration of CBZ extended-release tablets, peak plasma concentrations are reached in 3–12 hours (AHFS, 2000). Steady-state plasma CBZ concentrations of conventional tablets every 6 hours are comparable to those achieved following oral administration of CBZ extended-release tablets every 12 hours. A similar profile can be achieved when the extended-release capsules of CBZ (Carbatrol) are broken and the beads sprinkled over food prior to administration (AHFS, 2000). This may be a particularly useful strategy with children who prefer not taking capsules by mouth.

Distribution

Carbamazepine is widely distributed in the cerebrospinal fluid (CSF), bile, and saliva (AHFS, 2000). Plasma concentrations for anticonvulsant effect are in the range of 4–14 μg/mL. Carbamazepine, like DVP, is highly bound to protein (over 90%). At plasma concentrations of 1–50 μg/mL, 75%–90% of the drug is bound to plasma proteins (Trimble and Thompson, 1984). When protein-binding capacity is altered, marked changes in the free fractions can happen. Carbamazepine rapidly crosses the placenta, accumulates in fetal tissues, and is distributed in breast milk (AHFS, 2000).

Elimination

Autoinduction of its own metabolism is usually completed after 3–5 weeks (AHFS, 2000). The plasma half-life generally ranges from 25 to 65 hours initially and from 12 to 17 hours with multiple dosing. Carbamazepine may accelerate the metabolism of other concomitantly administered drugs metabolized by the CYP3A4 system. A major metabolic pathway appears to be oxidation by microsomal enzymes of the CYP3A4 system to form carbamazepine 10,11-epoxide (CBZ-E) (AHFS, 2000). CBZ-E has been implicated in some (Weaver et al., 1988) but not all studies (Semah et al., 1994) as contributing to adverse neurologic and toxic effects of the drug. Data also suggest that there is a block in the biotransformation from CBZ-E to *trans*-10,11-dihydroxy-10,11-dihydro-carbamazepine (CBZ-H) in pediatric patients taking CBZ + DVP, presumably caused by the inhibition effect of DVP on epoxide hydrolase (Liu et al., 1994).

Side Effects

Carbamazepine has been shown to be better tolerated as long-term monotherapy than DVP in children with epilepsy or febrile convulsions (Herranz et al., 1988). Nevertheless, a comparison of the adverse effect profile in the Kowatch sample (Kowatch et al., 2000) shows that nausea (46%), rash (8%), and dizziness (8%) were more prevalent in youngsters taking CBZ, compared to children on DVP, who experienced overall less nausea (20%), rash (0%), and dizziness (0%).

Neurotoxicity

Neurological side effects are considered the most common potential adverse effects for CBZ (Seetharam and Pellock, 1991). Diplopia is a common side effect of CBZ that often remits spontaneously or after the dosage is decreased (Menkes, 1999). Glare sensitivity may be the chief complaint from children treated with CBZ, and the clinician should develop office-screening methods to improve the detection of this potential side effect. Carbamazepine can exacerbate seizures (Parmeggiani et al., 1998) and/or worsen the electroencephalogram (EEG) (Pleak et al., 1988), or precipitate status epilepticus (Menkes, 1999). After CBZ withdrawal, clinical and EEG improvement may be evident in a few days (Parmeggiani et al., 1998). The underlying pathogenetic mechanism of EEG worsening with CBZ is not clearly understood. Drowsiness, vertigo, and nystagmus are also potential but transient side effects of CBZ (Menkes, 1999).

Congenital malformations: neural tube defects

Congenital malformations constitute some of the potentially most serious side effects in newborns of women taking CBZ (Kayemba Kay et al., 1997). Caution should be exercised in prescribing anticonvulsants to female adolescents. All women of childbearing age should receive a detailed history and pregnancy test, if necessary, before starting on CBZ or DVP.

Hematologic side effects

Leukopenia is a very common side effect of CBZ treatment (Pellock, 1987; Evans et al., 1989). Nonprogressive leukopenia of less than 4000/mm³ in approximately 13% of a sample of 220 children below the age of 16 years has been reported (Pellock, 1987). Spontaneous reversal of blood counts was seen in 75% of the children. Rarely, CBZ-induced leukopenia progresses to agranulocytosis or aplastic anemia, which is a medical emergency (Ueda et al., 1998). Upon early detection the clinician should monitor the patient for bruising, bleeding, sore throat, fever, lethargy, and mouth ulcers accompanied by a precipitous drop in white blood cell count, since death has been reported in 1/50,000 cases (Trimble, 1990). Blood counts should be monitored at least every 6 months during treatment with CBZ (AHFS, 2000). Carbamazepine-induced thrombocytopenia is often transient and, although dose related (Barratt, 1993) and perhaps autoimmune (Menkes, 1999), it may not require reduction or discontinuation of the drug (Barratt, 1993). The overall rate of blood dyscrasias was 3–4/100,000 prescriptions in a recent cohort study (Blackburn et al., 1998) investigating the frequency of blood dyscrasias in a total of 29,357 patients, ages 10–74 years.

Liver toxicity

Liver toxicity is a rare side effect of CBZ therapy (Trimble, 1990), although a recent study reported that 9% of children on CBZ had mildly elevated aspartate aminotransferase (Camfield and Camfield, 1985). Higher mean serum total cholesterol (TC) levels, mean low-density lipoprotein level, and mean TC/high-density lipoprotein ratio have been reported in children with epilepsy treated with CBZ, compared with controls (Sozuer et al., 1997). Conversely, an increase in serum high-density lipoproteins was reported in a smaller sample of patients treated with CBZ, and was therefore interpreted as a possible protective factor against atherosclerosis (Yalcin et al., 1997).

Skin Rashes

Rashes are relatively common with CBZ use (Pellock, 1987), in the range of 5% in a sample of children treated with CBZ (Pellock, 1987).

Overdose and toxicity

Carbamazepine toxicity is manifested by drowsiness, nausea and vomiting, gait disturbance, nystagmus, confusion, neuromuscular excitability, and seizures (Menkes, 1999). Overdose with CBZ can be lethal (Arana et al., 1986). In a retrospective study of 307 intoxicated patients, 41 (13%) had a fatal outcome (Schmidt and Schmitz-Buhl, 1995). Doses exceeding 24 g were important indicators of fatality. The management of CBZ overdose is primarily supportive, to prevent potential atrioventricular (AV) block (Arana et al., 1986), possible respiratory depression (Schmidt and Schmitz-Buhl, 1995), stupor, and coma.

Pediatric Uses

Many open and controlled trials have shown CBZ's efficacy in the acute (Brown et al., 1989) and prophylactic (Greil and Kleindienst, 1999a) treatment of adults with BD type I (Greil and Kleindienst, 1999a) and BD type II disorder (Greil and Kleindienst, 1999b). Increased severity of mania, rapid cycling, and poor response to lithium have been described as predictors of improved response to CBZ (Post et al., 1989). Carbamazepine is approved for the prophylactic treatment of partial seizures with complex symptomatology, generalized tonic–clonic (grand mal) seizures, and trigeminal neuralgia in children in the United States (AHFS, 2000). It is not approved for the treatment of psychiatric disorders in children. No controlled studies of the

treatment of pediatric mood disorders with CBZ have been reported thus far. A negative controlled study of CBZ for the treatment of CD (Cueva et al., 1996) did not replicate results from a previous case series suggesting the efficacy of CBZ in CD (Kafantaris et al., 1992). Conversely, a meta-analysis of the literature on children with attention-deficit hyperactivity disorder (ADHD) treated with CBZ (Silva et al., 1996) reported that seven open studies and three double-blind, placebo-controlled studies showed significant therapeutic responses (Silva et al., 1996). Nevertheless, CBZ is still considered to be a third- or fourth-line agent for the treatment of ADHD.

Dosage and Admnistration

There are no current FDA established indications for initiating and maintaining treatment with CBZ as a mood stabilizer in child psychiatric disorders. Generally, the guidelines established for treating epilepsy are used. It is important that the child or adolescent undergo a complete history and physical examination, as well as measurement of blood count with differential and platelet count, liver function tests, blood urea nitrogen (BUN), and creatinine analysis prior to the initiation of therapy. Adolescent female patients should be informed that anticonvulsants cross the placenta, therefore elected or inadvertant pregnancy should be discussed with their physician. Patients on CBZ may have false-negative pregnancy tests if human chorionic gonadotropin (HCG) is being assayed (Trimble and Thompson, 1984). Also, thyroid function tests (Kleiner et al., 1999) and urinary tests (i.e., false-positive ketones) may be altered. Carbamazepine is supplied in 200 mg and 100 mg (chewable) tablets and in oral suspension 100 mg/5 mL. The initial dosage for the management of seizure disorders in adults and children older than 12 years of age is 200 mg twice daily (as tablets) (AHFS, 2000). The initial oral dosage for the management of seizure disorders in children ages 6–12 years is 100 mg twice daily. For children under 6 years of age, the starting dosage should be even lower, i.e., 50 mg twice daily or 5 mg/kg daily. Dosage may be increased every 5–7 days by 100 mg using a 3- or 4-times daily divided dosing regimen until the optimum response is obtained (AHFS, 2000). Dosage should be increased to a maximum of 1000 mg/day in children younger than 15 years. In children 15 years and older, the dosage can be increased to a maximum of 1200 mg/day (AHFS, 2000). Serum levels of 4–12 μ/mL are considered therapeutic for seizure control. No equivalency has been determined for the treatment of pediatric mood disorders. The usual maintenance dosage is

10–20 mg/kg/day, administered in divided doses (bid or tid) given CBZ's short half-life after autoinduction. Carbamazepine half-lives may average 12 hours during chronic administration in adolescents on account of CBZ's autoinduction properties. Complete blood count (CBC) with differential and platelet count, BUN, creatinine, serum iron, and liver function tests, results should be obtained monthly after beginning treatment and then once every 3–6 months (Trimble and Thompson, 1984).

DIVALPROEX SODIUM

Valproic acid, valproate sodium, and (DVP) are carboxylic acid–derivative anticonvulsants. Divalproex sodium is a stable coordination compound consisting of valproic acid and valproate sodium in a 1:1 molar ratio (AHFS, 2000). It is a pro-drug of valproate, dissociating into valproate in the GI tract (AHFS, 2000), and a simple branched-chain carboxylic acid (n-dipropylacetic acid) with antiepileptic activity against a variety of types of seizures (Beydoun et al., 1997). Divalproex sodium has been approved for treating adults with simple and complex absence seizures (Mattson et al., 1992), and for mania. It has shown efficacy across a broad spectrum of BD subtypes (i.e., pure mania, mixed mania, and rapid cycling) (Pope et al., 1991; Bowden et al., 1994).

Mechanism of Action

Hypotheses about mechanisms of action include its enhancement of GABA accumulation (Loscher, 1993) in several cerebral regions (Wolf et al., 1994; Loscher et al., 1995), and its interaction with voltage-sensitive sodium channels (Macdonald and Kelly, 1994). Recent studies show that DVP may ultimately regulate the expression of subsets of genes via its effects on intranuclear transcription factors, i.e., DNA-binding proteins (Chen et al., 1999b). Divalproex sodium has also been shown to play a role in the regulation of calcium-calmodulin–dependent protein kinase activity, i.e., glycogen synthase kinase-3 β, a kinase that regulates various cytoskeletal processes (Chen et al., 1999a).

Pharmacokinetics

Absorption

Following oral administration of DVP tablets, DVP dissociates into valproate, which is then absorbed (AHFS, 2000). The bioavailability (delayed by food) of the DVP enteric-coated capsule is 90% with peak levels occurring in 3 hours after ingestion (Wilder et al., 1983). The relationship between dosage and total DVP concentration is nonlinear because of saturable protein binding (AHFS, 2000).

Distribution

The distribution of DVP appears to be restricted to plasma and rapidly exchangeable extracellular water (AHFS, 2000). The volume of distribution is 0.26 L/kg in children and 0.19 L/kg in adults (AHFS, 2000). The half-life is 7.2 ± 2.3 hours in children and 13.9 ± 3.4 hours in (healthy) adults (Levy et al., 1984). Valproic acid has been detected in CSF (approximately 10% of serum concentrations) and milk (about 1%–10% of plasma concentrations). The drug crosses the placenta. Valproic acid may displace other drugs from protein-binding sites.

Elimination

Valproic acid is eliminated by first-order kinetics and has an elimination half-life of 5–20 hours (average, 10.6 hours). Pediatric patients (3 months to 10 years) have a 50% higher clearance of the drug expressed by weight (i.e., mL/min/kg); over the age of 10 years, pharmacokinetic parameters of valproic acid approximate those in adults (Cloyd et al., 1993). Valproic acid is metabolized principally in the liver by β (over 40%) and ω oxidation (up to 15%–20%). Thirty through 50% of an administered dose is excreted as glucuronide conjugates (Cloyd et al., 1993).

Side Effects

High plasma levels of DVP (80–150 μg/mL; 555–1,040 μmol/L) are expected to produce significantly more frequent tremors, thrombocytopenia, alopecia, asthenia, diarrhea, vomiting, and anorexia, compared to low serum levels (25–50 μm/mL; 175–345 μmol/L), as shown in a multicenter trial of DVP monotherapy in patients with poorly controlled partial epilepsy (Beydoun et al., 1997).

Gastrointestinal effects

The most frequent adverse effects of DVP are nausea, vomiting, and indigestion (AHFS, 2000). These adverse effects are usually transient and can be minimized by administering the drug with meals. Increased appetite has been reported in up to 6% of patients and weight gain in up to 8% of patients treated with DVP. Between

1% and 5% of patients receiving valproic acid in clinical trials experienced pancreatitis, anorexia with weight loss, abdominal pain, dyspepsia, diarrhea, and constipation (AHFS, 2000). Nausea, stomach cramps, and diarrhea were among the most frequent adverse effects reported in a study of adults with rapid-cycling BD treated with DVP (Calabrese et al., 1992).

Increased appetite and weight gain

Increased appetite may be a significant side effect of DVP, particularly for responders (Menkes, 1999) who may be receiving enteric-coated medication (Bourgeois, 1988). An increase in relative weight was seen in girls treated with DVP compared to controls (Rattya et al., 1999). Conversely, patients taking CBZ and controls had similar weights. Neither DVP nor CBZ affected fasting serum insulin during the period of exposure (Rattya et al., 1999). This study suggests that DVP-related weight gain seen prepubertally in girls with epilepsy may not be associated with hyperinsulinemia (Rattya et al., 1999).

Nervous system effects

Divalproex sodium reportedly has minimal neurological adverse effects (sedation, ataxia, impairment of cognitive function) compared with other antiepileptic drugs (Davis et al., 1994). Sedation is considered to be a common potential side effect of DVP therapy. In a study of anticonvulsants in children with BD (Kowatch et al., 2000), sedation occurred as a common side effect among more children taking DVP (20%) than those taking CBZ (15%). Tremor can also constitute a side effect of DVP therapy in adults with complex partial seizures or generalized tonic–clonic seizures (Mattson et al., 1992). This appears to be dose related and may respond to a lowering of the dosage. Neural tube defects, predominantly spina bifida, at a risk of 1% to 2%, is potentially the most serious neurological side effect associated with maternal use of DVP (Davis et al., 1994). The coadministration of DVP and clonazepam can precipitate status epilepticus (Trimble, 1990).

Liver toxicity

Transient and nonprogressive DVP dose-related increases in liver function tests (Devilat and Blumel, 1991) have been described in juvenile patients treated with this agent (Menkes, 1999). Dose reduction is often therapeutic. Rare, idiosyncratic fatal hepatotoxicity associated with DVP appears to be unrelated to drug dosage (Dreifuss and Langer, 1987). During the years 1987 to 1993, 29/1,000,000 patients developed fatal hepatotoxicity (Bryant and Dreifuss, 1996). Jaundice, vomiting, and increased seizures were some of the most common presenting signs (Bryant and Dreifuss, 1996). The incidence of fatal hepatic failure is highest in patients younger than 2 years old receiving DVP as polytherapy (1:600) (Bryant and Dreifuss, 1996) and in children under the age of 3 years with mental retardation receiving polytherapy, or who have developmental delay (Appleton et al., 1990). The pathogenesis may be related to the accumulation of a toxic metabolite of DVP impairing fatty acid oxidation (Appleton et al., 1990). A panel of experts has recommended therapeutic oral L-carnitine supplementation for this group in a dosage of 100 mg/kg/day, up to a maximum of 2 g/day (De Vivo et al., 1998).

Endocrine and metabolic effects

Hyperandrogenism and chronic anovulation in the absence of identifiable adrenal or pituitary pathology characterize the syndrome of polycystic ovaries (PCO), which affects 2%–22% of women in the general population (Chappell et al., 1999). In a sample of 98 women with epilepsy (mean age 33), Isojarvi and colleagues (1998) found that 12 of 29 women (43%) taking DVP alone and 11 out of 49 (22%) taking CBZ had PCO, diagnosed with vaginal ultrasonographies and serum hormone concentrations. Eighty percent of the DVP group had started treatment prior to age 20. The association of obesity and hyperinsulinemia with possible DVP-related PCO was later postulated by this group (Isojarvi et al., 1998) and others (Eberle, 1998; Irwin and Masand, 1998). Comparable reports have not appeared in the psychiatric literature. A recent review (Murialdo et al., 1997) shows that the prevalence of PCO (16.9%) in 101 women with epilepsy (between 16 and 50 years of age) is not higher than that in the general population, lending support to Isojarvi's data. Although there are no data demonstrating that PCO occurs in women taking DVP for BD (Rasgon et al., 2000), female adolescent patients taking DVP should be carefully monitored for early signs of menstrual irregularities, hirsutism, acne, alopecia, and changes in body mass index.

Alopecia

Recent reports recognize pediatric alopecia as one of the more common dose-related side effects specific to DVP (Devilat and Blumel, 1991). It usually does not abate with continued treatment but may respond to a lowering of the dosage. Symptomatic management of alopecia includes trace mineral supplementation (i.e., zinc and multivitamins), treatment with minoxidil, and hair replacement pieces (McKinney et al., 1996).

Hematologic effects

Some (Kis et al., 1999; Verrotti et al., 1999), but not all (Tanindi et al., 1996), studies show that DVP may prolong bleeding time in pediatric patients. The mechanism of the DVP-induced platelet dysfunction has not yet been elucidated. Inhibition of the secondary phase of platelet aggregation (Verrotti et al., 1999) and the platelet arachidonate cascade (Kis et al., 1999) have been postulated as potential mechanisms contributing to the platelet-function alterations caused by DVP. Drug discontinuation may not be necessary (Kis et al., 1999).

Unusual side effects

Withdrawal seizures can occur in patients without a past history of seizure disorder (Menkes, 1999). They are considered equally rare with DVP and CBZ treatment (Duncan et al., 1990). Pancreatitis (Bourgeois, 1988) and hyperglycinemia (Mortensen et al., 1980), are also considered unusual potential side effects of DVP therapy (AHFS, 2000).

Toxicity

Divalproex sodium toxicity is manifested by drowsiness, weakness, incoordination, and confusion (Menkes, 1999) Treatment is supportive, requiring hospitalization.

Pediatric Uses

Bipolar disorder

Divalproex sodium has been reported to have acute antimanic properties (Bowden et al., 1994) in at least six controlled studies of adults with BD (Post et al., 1996). There is a paucity of controlled data for the use of DVP in children with psychiatric disorders. Case series (Papatheodorou et al., 1993, 1995) and one controlled study (Kowatch et al., 2000) suggest that DVP may be effective and well tolerated in acutely manic adolescents. Preliminary uncontrolled studies also suggest that DVP may play a role in the management of behavioral dyscontrol among adults

(Sovner, 1991) and adolescents (Kastner and Friedman, 1992) with comorbid BD and mental retardation and adolescents with impulsive–aggressive behavior (i.e., chronic temper outbursts and mood lability) (Donovan et al., 1997). Kowatch and colleagues (2000) recently completed an open randomized trial of mood stabilizers in children with type I and type II BD and found no significant differences between the groups at the completion of the study. Using a $\geq$ $\geq$ 50% change from baseline to exit in the Young Mania Rating Scale (YMRS) (Young et al., 1978) scores to define response, the response rates were as follows: DVP 53%; lithium 38%; and CBZ 38% $\chi^2 = 0.85$, $p = 0.60$) (Kowatch et al., 2000). However, the reported effect size of 1.63 for DVP, 1.06 for lithium, and 1.00 for CBZ suggested better efficacy for DVP than for the other two mood stabilizers.

Dosage

Valproic acid is supplied as DVP delayed-release 125, 250, 500 mg tablets, DVP-coated particles in 125 mg capsules (sprinkles) that may swallowed with soft food; valproic acid 250 mg capsules, valproic acid syrup (250 mg/ 5 mL), and sodium valproic acid solution for intravenous (IV) infusion (Depacon) (100 mg/mL) (AHFS, 2000). Evidence from studies in adults with BD suggests that the antimanic activity of DVP becomes most pronounced after achieving serum concentrations of 45 µg/mL or greater (Bowden et al., 1996). The initial oral dosage for treatment of mania in adolescents is 15 mg/kg/day in divided doses (bid) (Kowatch et al., 2000). The initial dosage can be increased every 3 days by 10 mg/kg/day and titrated upward (or downward) on the basis of clinical response and side effects. The maximum daily dose is 60 mg/kg/day. A plasma level should be obtained 5–7 days after the acute dosage is introduced to achieve therapeutic levels in the range of 50–125 µg/mL. Liver enzymes should be measured at baseline, every 3 months during the first semester, and every 6 months thereafter. Liver function test results and CBC should be obtained monthly for the first 2 months of therapy and then every 4–6 months.

NEW (THIRD-GENERATION) ANTICONVULSANTS

Several new drugs have been recently approved by the FDA for the control of seizures (Curry and Kulling, 1998). Three of these, gabapentin, lamotrigine, and topiramate, are used as add-on therapy for partial seizures in children above 12 years of age.

LAMOTRIGINE

Lamotrigine is a phenyltriazine anticonvulsant agent (Brodie and Yuen, 1997). The drug differs structurally from other currently available anticonvulsant agents. Initial studies suggest that lamotrigine, a sodium channel blocker (Bowden et al., 1999; Suppes et al., 1999), may have a bimodal spectrum of efficacy in the treatment of BD, especially in mixed phases of BD (Calabrese et al., 1998) and rapid cycling bipolar illness (Fatemi et al., 1997). Lamotrigine is similar to phenytoin and carbamazepine in some electrophysiologic properties and seizure-related pharmacologic properties (Leach, 1991).

Mechanisms of Action

Animal studies indicate that lamotrigine may stabilize neuronal membranes (and be effective in the management of tonic–clonic and partial seizures or absence (petit mal) seizures) by blocking voltage-sensitive sodium channels (Macdonald and Kelly, 1994; Culy and Goa, 2000). It may also inhibit the presynaptic excitatory release of glutamate and aspartate, block high-voltage activated N- and P-type calcium channels (Grunze et al., 1998), block presynaptic serotonin reuptake, and prevent amygdala and cortical kindling (Frye et al., 2000). These properties, particularly inhibition of presynaptic aspartate and glutamate release and serotonin reuptake, have been proposed to be related to lamotrigine's anticonvulsant and antidepressant action (Tekin et al., 1998).

Pharmacokinetics

Lamotrigine is metabolized by glucuronidation, possibly by the UGT 1A4 system. As such, it is vulnerable to other UGT inducers—oral contraceptives, phenytoin, carbamazepine, phenobarbital and primidone, and to a UGT inhibitor, valproate (Hachad et al., 2002).

Because of the possibility of increased seizure frequency, discontinuance of lamotrigine should be done gradually over a period of 2 weeks. Addition of DVP to lamotrigine therapy reduces lamotrigine clearance and increases steady-state plasma lamotrigine concentrations by 50% (AHFS, 2000). Conversely, steady-state plasma concentrations of lamotrigine are decreased by about 40% when CBZ is added to lamotrigine therapy.

Side Effects

Lamotrigine is generally well tolerated (Garnett, 1997) The most common adverse effects associated with lamotrigine as monotherapy in controlled clinical trial were generally minor and most frequently CNS related (e.g., ataxia, dizziness, diplopia, headache) (Messenheimer et al., 1994). A skin rash appears to be its most concerning side effect, especially with rapid dose elevations (Ramsay et al., 1991), requiring drug discontinuation in 7.4% of children and adolescents (Wallace, 1994).

Nervous system effects

Nervous system effects were among the most frequent adverse effects reported in patients receiving lamotrigine as adjunctive therapy in controlled clinical trials (Matsuo et al., 1993). The frequency of dizziness and ataxia and the rate of discontinuance of lamotrigine because of these adverse effects were dose related in clinical trials; in a dose–response study, dizziness occurred in 31% and 27% of patients receiving lamotrigine at 500 mg/day, and 300 mg/day (Rambeck et al., 1996).

Dermatologic and sensitivity reactions

Cases of Stevens-Johnson syndrome, a potentially lethal condition, associated with the use of lamotrigine have been reported (Messenheimer et al., 1998). The incidence of cases with this syndrome is 0.1% for adult patients and 0.5% for pediatric patients (Messenheimer et al., 1998). Most cases of rash associated with lamotrigine therapy seem to be associated with high plasma concentrations of the drug during the initial weeks of therapy or during concomitant DVP therapy (Messenheimer et al., 1998). Valproic acid can decrease clearance and increase plasma concentrations of lamotrigine more than twofold. Rash usually appears within 2 to 8 weeks of initiation of lamotrigine therapy. In clinical trials, 1% of patients receiving a drug regimen concomitantly with valproic acid experienced a rash requiring hospitalization, while 0.16% of patients receiving a drug regimen of lamotrigine without valproic acid were hospitalized because of rash (Messenheimer et al., 1998). The incidence of severe rash associated with lamotrigine also appears to be higher in pediatric patients than in adults (Messenheimer et al., 2000). Rashes severe enough to cause hospitalization, including Stevens-Johnson syndrome and toxic epidermal necrolysis, occurred in 0.3% of adult patients receiving lamotrigine as adjunctive therapy in controlled and uncontrolled clinical trials and in about 1% of pediatric patients receiving the drug in clinical trials (Messenheimer et al., 1998). Early signs of a possible hypersensitivity reaction should prompt immediate evaluation of the patient.

Gastrointestinal effects

Nausea was the most frequent adverse GI effect in controlled clinical trials (Rambeck et al., 1996). The frequency of nausea and vomiting appears to be dose related.

Pediatric Uses

Lamotrigine is used either in combination with other anticonvulsant agents or as monotherapy in the management of partial seizures in adults. Safety and efficacy of lamotrigine for uses other than the management of Lennox-Gastaut syndrome in children younger than 16 years of age have not been established (AHFS, 2000). Patients who weigh less than 17 kg (37 lbs) should not receive lamotrigine, since only whole tablets of the drug should be administered, and the lowest strength available (5 mg) would exceed the recommended initial dose for such patients (AHFS, 2000).

In a recent pilot study, 16 out of 22 (72%) adolescents with BD treated with additional lamotrigine during their depressed phase responded to treatment by the end of week 4; this suggests that lamotrigine might be useful in adolescent bipolar depression. (Kusumakar and Yathan, 1997).

GABAPENTIN

Gabapentin is used in combination with other anticonvulsant agents in the management of partial seizures (Bruni, 1998) with or without secondary generalization (Morris, 1999). A few (McElroy et al., 1997; Knoll et al., 1998), but not all (Dimond et al., 1996), preliminary reports suggested that gabapentin may have antimanic efficacy in adults with BD.

Mechanism of Action

Although gabapentin is structurally related to GABA (AHFS, 2000), the drug has no direct GABA-mimetic action (Kelly, 1998) and its precise mechanism of action has not been elucidated (Taylor et al., 1998). Gabapentin has no affinity for binding sites on common neuroreceptors (e.g., benzodiazepine, glutamate, histamine) or ion channels (AHFS, 2000).

Pharmacokinetics

Gabapentin does not bind to plasma proteins, is not appreciably metabolized, nor induces hepatic enzyme activity (AHFS, 2000) Consequently, it does not appear to alter the pharmacokinetics of commonly used anticonvulsant drugs or oral contraceptives (Ketter et al., 1999).

Side Effects

Gabapentin is generally well tolerated in adult patients, and adverse effects of the drug are usually mild to moderate in severity (AHFS, 2000). The most frequent adverse effects of gabapentin as adjunctive therapy are somnolence, dizziness, and asthenia (Bruni, 1998).

Pediatric Uses

The safety and efficacy of gabapentin as adjunctive therapy to CBZ and/or phenytoin has been assessed in adults, adolescents (Bruni, 1998), and children (Khurana et al., 1996) with partial seizures. A decrease of 50% or more in frequency of complex partial + secondary generalized seizures was reported in 71% of patients on a mean maintenance dose of gabapentin of 1600 mg/day (Bruni, 1998). It has also been used in the treatment of spasticity in adolescents with multiple sclerosis (Cutter et al., 2000) and in adults and adolescents with neuropathic pain (Rosenberg et al., 1997). A retrospective review of adult patients with BD or unipolar MDD found only moderate to marked effectiveness in 30% (15/50) of patients (Ghaemi et al., 1998). Likewise, a well-designed double-blind, randomized, crossover, placebo-controlled study of lamotrigine and gabapentin monotherapy in refractory mood disorders suggested clinical efficacy for lamotrigine but not for gabapentin in the treatment of 31 adult patients with refractory bipolar and unipolar mood disorders (Frye et al., 2000). The mean dosage at week 6 was 3987 ± 856 mg for gabapentin (Frye et al., 2000).

At the time of this publication, only one case of a manic adolescent being responsive to gabapentin for the treatment of mania has been reported (Soutullo et al., 1998). Conversely, several cases of aggressive behavior associated with gabapentin in children with seizures have been reported (Wolf et al., 1995, Khurana et al., 1996; Lee et al., 1996; Tallian et al., 1996) making the use of gabapentin in pediatric mood or anxiety disorders empiric and inconclusive. A careful evaluation of the risk/benefit ratio should precede the consideration of gabapentin in adolescents older than 12 years of age with severe bipolar disorder, refractory to all interventions.

TOPIRAMATE

Topiramate, a sulfamate-substituted derivative of the monosaccharide *d*-fructose, is an anticonvulsant agent (AHFS, 2000). The spectrum of topiramate's anticonvulsant activity resembles that of CBZ and phenytoin (Shank et al., 2000). Topiramate has shown preliminary antimanic (McElroy et al., 2000) and possibly antidepressant efficacy in treatment-refractory, manic patients with BD type I (Calabrese et al., 1998).

Mechanism of Action

Although the precise mechanism of action of topiramate is unknown, the drug has demonstrated properties in blocking sodium channels (Zona et al., 1997), enhancing the inhibitory action of GABA (Petroff et al., 1999), and attenuating kainate-induced responses (Gibbs et al., 2000). Topiramate appears to enhance the activity of the inhibitory neurotransmitter GABA at a nonbenzodiazepine site on $GABA_A$ receptors (Petroff et al., 1999). Topiramate weakly inhibits carbonic anhydrase CA-II and CA-IV isoenzymes and other carbonic anhydrase inhibitors (Dodgson et al., 2000), although this effect is not thought to contribute substantially to the anticonvulsant activity of topiramate (AHFS, 2000). Like other carbonic anhydrase inhibitors (e.g., acetazolamide, dichlorphenamide), topiramate may promote the formation of renal calculi (Reife et al., 2000).

Pharmacokinetics

The pharmacokinetics of topiramate are linear with peak plasma concentrations (occurring in about 2 hours) of 25 μM after 400 mg daily (Shank et al., 2000). Topiramate is poorly bound to plasma proteins (15%) and it binds to erythrocytes. In rats the maximal concentration in the brain when administered at 10 mg/kg was 10 μM (Shank et al., 2000). It is not extensively metabolized in humans and is eliminated (70%) unchanged in urine. Six minor metabolites have been identified, none with anticonvulsant activity. The average elimination half-life is 21 hours (Shank et al., 2000).

Side Effects

Its efficacy as an adjunctive medication in children with partial-onset seizures studied in a randomized double-blind, placebo-controlled trial showed only mild or moderate unspecific side effects (Glauser et al., 2000). Somnolence and anorexia were the most frequent CNS-related side effects in a recent open, add-on pilot study of topiramate in children with Lennox-Gastaut syndrome (age ranging from 4 to 14 years) (Guerreiro et al., 1999). The clinical effectiveness and possible weight loss potential of topiramate in adult manic and hypomanic patients may be considered by some clinicians to be a potential beneficial side effects in adolescents who discontinue mood stabilizers because of increased weight. A recent randomized study has suggested that topiramate may have cognitive side effects (Martin et al., 1999), i.e., declines on measures of attention and word retrieval difficulties, which would require baseline and follow-up monitoring in pediatric patients.

Pediatric Uses

The efficacy of topiramate as adjunctive therapy in pediatric patients with Lennox-Gastaut syndrome was shown in open-label treatment (Glauser et al., 2000). The Stanley Foundation Bipolar Outcome Network (SFBN) (McElroy et al., 2000) recently evaluated the clinical effectiveness of topiramate in 56 bipolar manic/hypomanic outpatients who completed a minimum of 2 weeks of adjunctive topiramate treatment. Thirty patients had manic, mixed, or cycling symptoms, 11 had depressed symptoms, and 13 were euthymic at the time topiramate was begun (McElroy et al., 2000). Improvement in 50% of the initially hypomanic/manic and depressed patients at 90 days of treatment at a mean dose of 189 ± 117 mg was reported. Topiramate adjunctive treatment was associated with a mean weight loss from 1 month to last evaluation of 11 ± 14 pounds. Similar preliminary results were reported by Chengappa et al. (1999), who treated 18 adult refractory patients with BD type I, with topiramate initiated at 25 mg/day, and increased by 25 mg every 3–7 days to a target dose between 100 and 300 mg/day (Chengappa et al., 1999). By week 5, 60% of the subjects were considered responders, i.e., had a 50% reduction on YMRS. All patients lost a mean of 9.4 lbs.; six patients experienced transient paresthesias, and two had transient "word-finding difficulties" (Chengappa et al., 1999). To date, no studies of children with mood disorders treated with topiramate have been published.

SUMMARY

The use of lamotrigine, gabapentin, or topiramate in children (especially those younger than 16 years of age) cannot be endorsed at the present time as first-line therapy until additional safety and efficacy data are available. However, with careful evaluation of the risk/benefit ratio, they could be considered in adolescents older than 16 years of age with BD, refractory to other standard interventions.

Diagnostic boundaries in juvenile-onset BD need to be defined, since children with hypomania or manic-like symptoms may be increasingly treated with mood stabilizers. In parallel, this would require more complex algorithms because very few controlled trials have been reported (Walkup, 1995). In contrast to the studies of adults reported in the literature, the pharmacological treatment of childhood bipolarity with anticonvulsants remains an understudied area. Carbamazepine appears to be less efficacious than valproate in adult rapid cycling, yet no studies have identified predictors of treatment response to CBZ or any other mood stabilizer (besides lithium) in a pediatric population.

REFERENCES

AHFS (American Hospital Formulary Service) (2000) Bethesda, American Society of Health System Pharmacists, Inc.; 2000;

AHFS (American Hospital Formulary Service) (2000) *AHFS Drug Information.* Bethesda, MD: American Society of Health System Pharmacists, pp. 1549–1553, 1958–2007.

Appleton, R.E., Farrell, K., Applegarth, D.A., Dimmick, J.E., Wong, L.T., Davidson, A.G. (1990) The high incidence of valproate hepatotoxicity in infants may relate to familial metabolic defects. *Can J Neurol Sci* 17:145–148.

Arana, G.W., Goff, D.C., Friedman, H., Ornsteen, M., Greenblatt, D.J., Black, B., and Shader, R.I. (1986) Does carbamazepine-induced reduction of plasma haloperidol levels worsen psychotic symptoms? *Am J Psychiatry* 143:650–651.

Atack, J.R., Broughton, H.B., and Pollack, S.J. (1995) "Inositol monophosphatase—a putative target for Li+ in the treatment of bipolar disorder." *Trends Neurosci,* 18:343–349.

Baptista, T.J., Hernandez, L., Burguera, J.L., Burguera, M., and Hoebel, B.G. (1990) Chronic lithium administration enhances serotonin release in the lateral hypothalamus but not in the hippocampus in rats. A microdialysis study. *J Neural Transm Gen Sect* 82:31–41.

Barratt, E.S. (1993) The use of anticonvulsants in aggression and violence. *Psychopharmacol Bull* 29:75–81.

Berridge, M.J., Downes, C.P., and Hanley, M.R. (1982) Lithium amplifies agonist-dependent phosphatidylinositol responses in brain and salivary glands. *Biochem J* 206:587–595.

Beydoun, A., Sackellares, J.C., and Shu, V. (1997) Safety and efficacy of divalproex sodium monotherapy in partial epilepsy: a double-blind, concentration–response design clinical trial. Depakote Monotherapy for Partial Seizures Study Group. *Neurology* 48: 182–188.

Biederman, J., Mick, E., Bostic, J.Q., Prince, J., Daly, J., Wilens, T.E., Spencer, T., Garcia-Jetton, J., Russell, R., Wozniak, J., and Faraone, S.V. (1998) The naturalistic course of pharmacologic treatment of children with maniclike symptoms: a systematic chart review. *J Clin Psychiatry* 59:628–637; quiz 38.

Blackburn, S.C., Oliart, A.D., Garcia Rodriguez, L.A., and Perez Gutthann, S. (1998) "Antiepileptics and blood dyscrasias: a cohort study. *Pharmacotherapy* 18:1277–1283.

Bourgeois, B.F. (1988) Pharmacologic interactions between valproate and other drugs. *Am J Med* 84:29–33.

Bowden, C.L., Brugger, A.M., Swann, A.C., Calabrese, J.R., Janicak, P.G., Petty, F., Dilsaver, S.C., Davis, J.M., Rush, A.J., Small, J.G., et al. (1994) Efficacy of divalproex vs lithium and placebo in the treatment of mania. The Depakote Mania Study Group JAMA 271:918–924 [published erratum appears in *JAMA* 1994; 271(23):1830 (see comments)].

Bowden, C.L., Janicak, P.G., Orsulak, P., Swann, A.C., Davis, J.M., Calabrese, J.R., Goodnick, P., Small, J.G., Rush, A.J., Kimmel, S.E., Risch, S.C., and Morris, D.D. (1996) Relation of serum valproate concentration to response in mania. *Am J Psychiatry* 153:765–770.

Bowden, C.L., Mitchell, P., and Suppes, T. (1999) Lamotrigine in the treatment of bipolar depression. *Eur Neuropsychopharmacol* 9 (Suppl 4): S113–S117.

Brodie, M.J. and Yuen, A.W. (1997) Lamotrigine substitution study: evidence for synergism with sodium valproate? 105 Study Group. *Epilepsy Res* 26:423–432.

Brown, D., Silverstone, T., and Cookson, J. (1989) Carbamazepine compared to haloperidol in acute mania. *Int Clin Psychopharmacol* 4:229–238.

Bruni, J. (1998) Outcome evaluation of gabapentin as add-on therapy for partial seizures. Study Investigators Group. Neurontin evaluation of outcomes in neurological practice. *Can J Neurol Sci* 25:134–140.

Bryant, A.E., 3rd and Dreifuss, F.E. (1996) Valproic acid hepatic fatalities. III. U.S. experience since 1986 [see comments]. *Neurology* 46:465–469.

Cade, J.F. (1978) Lithium—past, present and future. In: Johnson, F.N. and Johnson, S, ed. *Lithium in Medical Practice.* Lancaster, UK: MTP Press pp. 5–16. 1978.

Calabrese, J.R., Markovitz, P.J., Kimmel, S.E., and Wagner, S.C. (1992) Spectrum of efficacy of valproate in 78 rapid-cycling bipolar patients. *J Clin Psychopharmacol* 12:53S–56S.

Calabrese, J.R., Rapport, D.J., Shelton, M.D., Kujawa, M., and Kimmel, S.E. (1998) Clinical studies on the use of lamotrigine in bipolar disorder. *Neuropsychobiology* 38:185–191.

Camfield, P.R. and Camfield, C.S. (1985) Serum concentrations of carbamazepine [letter]. *J Pediatr* 107:826–827.

Campbell, M., Adams, P.B., Small, A.M., Kafantaris, V., Silva, R.R., Shell, J., Perry, R., and Overall, J.E. (1995) Lithium in hospitalized aggressive children with conduct disorder: a double-blind and placebo-controlled study. *J Am Acad Child Adolesc Psychiatry* 34:445–453. [published erratum appears in *J Am Acad Child Adolesc Psychiatry* 1995; 34(5):694]."

Cepelak, I., Zanic Grubisic, T., Mandusic, A., Rekic, B., and Lenicek, J. (1998) Valproate and carbamazepine comedication changes hepatic enzyme activities in sera of epileptic children. *Clin Chim Acta* 276:121–127.

Chappell, K.A., Markowitz, J.S., and Jackson, C.W. (1999) Is valproate pharmacotherapy associated with polycystic ovaries? *Ann Pharmacother* 33:1211–1216.

Chen, G., Huang, L.D., Jiang, Y.M., and Manji, H.K. (1999a) The mood-stabilizing agent valproate inhibits the activity of glycogen synthase kinase-3. *J Neurochem* 72:1327–1330.

Chen, G., Yuan, P.X., Jiang, Y.M., Huang, L.D., and Manji, H.K. (1999b) Valproate robustly enhances AP-1 mediated gene expression. *Brain Res Mol Brain Res* 64:52–58.

Chengappa, R.N., Rathore, D., Levine, J. Atzert, R., Solail Parepally, H., and Levin, H. (1999) Topiramate as add-on treatment for patients with bipolar disorder. *Bipolar Disord* 1:42–53.

Cloyd, J.C., Fischer, J.H., Kriel, R.L., and Kraus, D.M. (1993) Valproic acid pharmacokinetics in children. IV. Effects of age and antiepileptic drugs on protein binding and intrinsic clearance. *Clin Pharmacol Ther* 53:22–29.

Cooper, T.B., and Simpson, G.M. (1976) The 24-hour lithium level as a prognosticator of dosage requirements: a 2-year follow-up study. *Am J Psychiatry* 133:440–443.

Cueva, J.E., Overall, J.E., Small, A.M., Armenteros, J.L., Perry, R., and Campbell, M. (1996) Carbamazepine in aggressive children with conduct disorder: a double-blind and placebo-controlled study. *J Am Acad Child Adolesc Psychiatry* 35:480–490.

Culy, C.R. and Goa, K.L. (2000) Lamotrigine. A review of its use in childhood epilepsy. *Paediatr Drugs* 2:299–330.

Curry, W.J. and Kulling, D.L. (1998) Newer antiepileptic drugs: gabapentin, lamotrigine, felbamate, topiramate and fosphenytoin. *Am Fam Physician* 57:513–520.

Cutter, N.C., Scott, D.D., Johnson, J.C., and Whiteneck, G. (2000) Gabapentin effect on spasticity in multiple sclerosis: a placebo-controlled, randomized trial. *Arch Phys Med Rehabil* 81:164–169.

Davis, R., Peters, D.H., and McTavish, D. (1994) Valproic acid. A reappraisal of its pharmacological properties and clinical efficacy in epilepsy. *Drugs* 47:332–372.

Devilat, M., and Blumel, J.E. Adverse effects of valproic acid in epileptic infants and adolescents [in Spanish]. *Rev Chil Pediatr* 62:362–366.

De Vivo, D.C., Bohan, T.P., Coulter, D.L., Dreifuss, F.E., Greenwood, R.S., Nordli, D.R., Jr., Shields, W.D., Stafstrom, C.E., and Tein, I. (1998) L-carnitine supplementation in childhood epilepsy: current perspectives. *Epilepsia* 39:1216–1225.

Dimond, K.R., Pande, A.C., Lamoreaux, L., and Pierce, M.W. (1996) Effect of gabapentin (Neurontin) [corrected] on mood and well-being in patients with epilepsy. *Progress in Neuropsychopharmacol Biol Psychiatry* 20:407–17. [published erratum appears in *Prog Neuropsychopharmacol Biol Psychiatry* 1996; 20(6):1081].

Dodgson, S.J., Shank, R.P., and Maryanoff, B.E. (2000) Topiramate as an inhibitor of carbonic anhydrase isoenzymes. *Epilepsia* 41: S35–S39.

Donovan, S.J., Susser, E.S., Nunes, E.V., Stewart, J.W., Quitkin, F.M., and Klein, D.F. (1997) Divalproex treatment of disruptive adolescents: a report of 10 cases. *J Clin Psychiatry* 58:12–15.

Dreifuss, F.E. and Langer, D.H. (1987) Hepatic considerations in the use of antiepileptic drugs. *Epilepsia* 28: S23–S29.

Duncan, J.S., Shorvon, S.D., and Trimble, M.R. (1990) Effects of removal of phenytoin, carbamazepine, and valproate on cognitive function. *Epilepsia* 31:584–591.

Dunn, R.T., Frye, M.S., Kimbrell, T.A., Denicoff, K.D., Leverich, G.S. and Post, R.M. (1998) The efficacy and use of anticonvulsants in mood disorders. *Clin Neuropharmacol* 21:215–235.

Eberle, A.J. (1998) Valproate and polycystic ovaries [letter] [see comments]. *J Am Acad Child Adolesc Psychiatry* 37:1009.

Evans, O.B., Gay, H., Swisher, A., and Parks, B. (1989) Hematologic monitoring in children with epilepsy treated with carbamazepine. *J Child Neurol* 4:286–290.

Fatemi, S.H., Rapport, D.J., Calabrese, J.R., and Thuras, P. (1997) Lamotrigine in rapid-cycling bipolar disorder. *Clin Psychiatry* 58: 522–527.

Fava, M. (1997) Psychopharmacologic treatment of pathologic aggression. *Psychiatr Clin North Am* 20:427–451.

Feldman, R.S., Meyer, J.S., and Quenzer, L.F., (1997) *Principles of Neuropsychopharmacology.* Sunderland, MA: Sinauer Associates, pp. xvii, 20, 84, 909.

Flockhart, D.A. and Oesterheld, J.R. (2000) Cytochrome P450–mediated drug interactions. *Child Adolesc Psychiatr Clin North Am* 9:43–76.

Frye, M.A., Ketter, T.A., Kimbrell, T.A., Dunn, R.T., Speer, A.M., Osuch, E.A., Luckenbaugh, D.A., Cora-Ocatelli, G., Leverich, G.S., and Post, R.M. (2000) A placebo-controlled study of lamotrigine and gabapentin monotherapy in refractory mood disorders. *J Clin Psychopharmacol* 20:607–614.

Garnett, W.R. (1997) Lamotrigine: pharmacokinetics. *J Child Neurol* 12 (Suppl 1):S10–S15.

Gelenberg, A.J., Kane, J.M., Keller, M.B., Lavori, P., Rosenbaum, J.F., Cole, K., and Lavelle, J. (1998) Comparison of standard and low serum levels of lithium for maintenance treatment of bipolar disorder. *N Engl J Med* 321:1489–1493.

Geller, B., Cooper, T.B., Sun, K., Zimerman, B., Frazier, J., Williams, M., and Heath, J. (1998a) Double-blind and placebo-controlled study of lithium for adolescent bipolar disorders with secondary substance dependency. *J Am Acad Child Adoles Psychiatry* 37: 171–178.

Geller, B., Cooper, T.B., Zimerman, B., Frazier, J., Williams, M., Heath, J., and Warner, K. (1998b) Lithium for prepubertal depressed children with family history predictors of future bipolarity: a double-blind, placebo-controlled study. *J Affect Disord* 51: 165–175.

Geller, B. and Fetner, H.H. (1989a) Children's 24-hour serum lithium level after a single dose predicts initial dose and steady-state plasma level [letter]. *J Clin Psychopharmacol* 9:155.

Geller, B. and Fetner, H.H. (1989b) Use of pillminders to dispense research medication [letter]. *J Clin Psychopharmacol* 9: 72–73.

Ghaemi, S.N., Katzow, J.J., Desai, S.P., and Goodwin, F.K. (1998) Gabapentin treatment of mood disorders: a preliminary study. *J Clin Psychiatry* 59:426–469.

Gibbs, J.W., Sombati, S., DeLorenzo, R.J., and Coulter, D.A. (2000) Cellular actions of topiramate: blockade of kainate-evoked inward currents in cultured hippocampal neurons. *Epilepsia* 41: S10–S16.

Glauser, T.A., Levisohn, P.M., Ritter, F., and Sachdeo, R.C. (2000) Topiramate in Lennox-Gastaut syndrome: open-label treatment of patients completing a randomized controlled trial. Topiramate YL Study Group. *Epilepsia* 41: S86–S90.

Goode, D.L., Newton, D.W., Ueda, C.T., Wilson, J.E., Wulf, B.G., and Kafonek, D. (1984) Effect of antacid on the bioavailabiity of lithium carbonate. *Clin Pharmacol* 3:284–287.

Granger, P., Biton, B., Faure, C., Vige, X., Depoortere, H., Graham, D., Langer, S.Z., Scatton, B., and Avenet, P. (1995) Modulation of the gamma-aminobutyric acid type A receptor by the antiepileptic drugs carbamazepine and phenytoin. *Mol Pharmacol* 47: 1189–1196.

Greil, W., and Kleindienst, N. (1999a) The comparative prophylactic efficacy of lithium and carbamazepine in patients with bipolar I disorder. *Int Clin Psychopharmacol* 14:277–281.

Greil, W., and Kleindienst, N. (1999b) Lithium versus carbamazepine in the maintenance treatment of bipolar II disorder and bipolar disorder not otherwise specified. *Int Clin Psychopharmacol* 14: 283–285.

Groh, C. (1976) The psychotropic effect of Tegretol in non-epileptic children, with particular reference to the drug's indications. In:

Birkmayer, W., ed. *Epileptic Seizures—Behaviour—Pain.* Baltimore: University Park Press, pp. 259–263.

Grunze, H., von Wegerer, J., Greene, R.W., and Walden, J. (1998) Modulation of calcium and potassium currents by lamotrigine. *Neuropsychobiology* 38:131–138.

Guerreiro, M.M., Manreza, M.L., Scotoni, A.E., Silva, E.A., Guerreiro, C.A., Souza, E.A., Ferreira, V.B., Reed, U.C., Diament, A., Trefiglio, R., Chiu, H.C., and Bacaltchuk, J. (1999) A pilot study of topiramate in children with Lennox-Gastaut syndrome. *Arq Neuropsiquiatr* 57:167–175.

Hachad, H., Ragueneau-Majlessi, I., and Levy, R.H. (2002) New antiepileptic drugs: review on drug interactions. *Drug Monit* 24: 91–103.

Hagino, O.R., Weller, E.B., Weller, R.A., Washing, D., Fristad, M.A., and Kontras, S.B. Untoward effects of lithium treatment in children aged four through six years. *J Am Acad Child Adolesc Psychiatry* 34:1584–1590.

Hardy, B.G., Shulman, K.I., Mackenzie, S.E., Kutcher, S.P., and Silverberg, J.D. (1987) Pharmacokinetics of lithium in the elderly. *J Clin Psychopharmacol* 7:153–158.

Herranz, J.L., Armijo, J.A., and Arteaga, R. (1988) Clinical side effects of phenobarbital, primidone, phenytoin, carbamazepine, and valproate during monotherapy in children. *Epilepsia* 29:794–804.

Hough, C.J., Irwin, R.P., Gao, X.M., Rogawski, M.A., and Chuang, D.M. (1996) Carbamazepine inhibition of N-methyl-D-aspartate-evoked calcium influx in rat cerebellar granule cells. *J Pharmacol Exp Ther* 276:143–149.

Irwin, M. and Masand, P. (1998) "Valproate and polycystic ovaries [letter; comment]. *J Am Acad Child Adolesc Psychiatry* 37:9–10.

Isojarvi, J.I., Rattya, J., Myllyla, V.V., Knip, M., Koivunen, R., Pakarinen, A.J., Tekay, A., and Tapanainen, J.S. (1998) Valproate, lamotrigine, and insulin-mediated risks in women with epilepsy. *Ann Neurol* 43:446–451.

Jensen, J.B., and Mork, A. (1997) Altered protein phosphorylation in the rat brain following chronic lithium and carbamazepine treatments. *Eur Neuropsychopharmacol* 7:173–179.

Jermain, D.M., Crismon, M.L., and Martin, E.S. Population pharmacokinetics of lithium. *Clin Pharmacol* 10:376–381.

Kafantaris, V., Campbell, M., Padron-Gayol, M.V., Small, A.M., Locascio, J.J., and Rosenberg, C.R. (1992) Carbamazepine in hospitalized aggressive conduct disorder children: an open pilot study. *Psychopharmacol Bull* 28:193–199. [published erratum appears in *Psychopharmacol Bull* 1992;28(3):220].

Kastner, T., and Friedman, D.L. (1992) Verapamil and valproic acid treatment of prolonged mania. *J Am Acad Child Adolesc Psychiatry* 31:271–275.

Kawata, H. (1979) Contractility of the frog ventricular myocardium in sodium-free lithium solution. *Jpn J Physiol* 29:609–625.

Kayemba Kay, S.S., Beust, M., Aboulghit, H., Voisin, M., and Mourtada, A. (1997) Carbamazepine and vigabatrin in epileptic pregnant woman and side effects in the newborn infant. [in French]. *Arch Pediatr* 4:975–978.

Kelly, K.M. (1998) Gabapentin. Antiepileptic mechanism of action. *Neuropsychobiology* 38:139–44.

Ketter, T.A., Frye, M.A., Cora-Locatelli, G., Kimbrell, T.A., and Post, R.M. (1999) Metabolism and excretion of mood stabilizers and new anticonvulsants. *Cell Mol Neurobiol* 19:511–532.

Ketter, T.A., Jenkins, J.B., Schroeder, D.H., Pazzaglia, P.J., Marangell, L.B., George, M.S., Callahan, A.M., Hinton, M.L., Chao, J., and Post, R.M. (1995) Carbamazepine but not valproate induces bupropion metabolism. *J Clin Psychopharmacol* 15:327–333.

Khurana, D.S., Riviello, J., Helmers, S., Holmes, G., Anderson, J.,

and Mikati, M.A. (1996) Efficacy of gabapentin therapy in children with refractory partial seizures. *J Pediatr* 128:829–833.

Kirkwood, C.K., Wilson, S.K., Hayes, P.E., Barr, W.H., Sarkar, M.A., and Ettigi, P.G. (1994) Single-dose bioavailability of two extended-release lithium carbonate products. *Am J Hosp Pharm* 51:486–489.

Kis, B., Szupera, Z., Mezei, Z., Gecse, A., Telegdy, G., and Vecsei, L. (1999) Valproate treatment and platelet function: the role of arachidonate metabolites. *Epilepsia* 40:307–310.

Kleiner, J., Altshuler, L., Hendrick, V., and Hershman, J.M. (1999) Lithium-induced subclinical hypothyroidism: review of the literature and guidelines for treatment. *J Clin Psychiatry* 60:249–255.

Knoll, J., Stegman, K., and Suppes, T. (1998) Clinical experience using gabapentin adjunctively in patients with a history of mania or hypomania. *Affect Disord* 49:229–233.

Kowatch, R.A., Suppes, T., Carmody, T.J., Bucci, J.P., Hume, J.H., Kromelis, M., Emslie, G.J., Weinberg, W.A., and Rush, A.J. (2000) Effect size of lithium, divalproex sodium, and carbamazepine in children and adolescents with bipolar disorder. *J Am Acad Child Adolesc Psychiatry* 39:713–720.

Krachler, M., Rossipal, E., and Micetic-Turk, D. (1999) Trace element transfer from the mother to the newborn—investigations on triplets of colostrum, maternal and umbilical cord sera. *Eur J Clin Nutr* 53:486–494.

Kusumakar, V. and Yatham, L.N. (1997) An open study of lamotrigine in refractory bipolar depression. *Psychiatry Res* 72:145–148.

Lee, D.O., Steingard, R.J., Cesena, M., Helmers, S.L., Riviello, J.J., and Mikati, M.A. (1996) Behavioral side effects of gabapentin in children. *Epilepsia* 37 :87–90.

Lenox, R.H. and Hahn, C.G. (2000) Overview of the mechanism of action of lithium in the brain: fifty-year update. *J Clin Psychiatry* 61:5–15.

Levy, R.H., Moreland, T.A., Morselli, P.L., Guyot, M., Brachet-Liermain, A., and Loiseau, P. (1984) Carbamazepine/valproic acid interaction in man and rhesus monkey. *Epilepsia* 25:338–345.

Liu, H. and Delgado, M.R. (1994) The influence of polytherapy on the relationships between serum carbamazepine and its metabolites in epileptic children. *Epilepsy Res* 17:257–269.

Loscher, W. (1993) In vivo administration of valproate reduces the nerve terminal (synaptosomal) activity of GABA aminotransferase in discrete brain areas of rats. *Neurosci Lett* 160:177–80.

Loscher, W., Rohlfs, A., and Rundfeldt, C. (1995) Reduction in firing rate of substantia nigra pars reticulata neurons by valproate: influence of different types of anesthesia in rats. *Brain Res* 702: 133–44.

Macdonald, R.L. and Kelly, K.M. (1994) Mechanisms of action of currently prescribed and newly developed antiepileptic drugs. *Epilepsia* 35 (Suppl 4): S41–S50.

Malone, R.P., Delaney, M.A., Luebbert, J.F., Cater, J., and Campbell, M. (2000) A double-blind placebo-controlled study of lithium in hospitalized aggressive children and adolescents with conduct disorder. *Arch Gen Psychiatry* 57:649–654.

Manji, H.K., Bersudsky, Y., Chen, G., Belmaker, R.H., and Potter, W.Z. (1996) Modulation of protein kinase C isozymes and substrates by lithium: the role of myo-inositol. *Neuropsychopharmacology* 15:370–381.

Martin, R., Kuzniecky, R., Ho, S., Hetherington, H., Pan, J., Sinclair, K., Gilliam, F., and Faught, E. (1999) Cognitive effects of topiramate, gabapentin, and lamotrigine in healthy young adults. *Neurology* 52:321–327.

Matsuo, F., Bergen, D., Faught, E., Messenheimer, J.A., Dren, A.T., Rudd, G.D., and Lineberry, C.G. (1993) Placebo-controlled study of the efficacy and safety of lamotrigine in patients with partial seizures. U.S. Lamotrigine Protocol 0.5 Clinical Trial Group. *Neurology* 43:2284–2291.

Mattson, R.H., Cramer, J.A., and Collins, J.F. (1992) A comparison of valproate with carbamazepine for the treatment of complex partial seizures and secondarily generalized tonic-clonic seizures in adults. The Department of Veterans Affairs Epilepsy Cooperative Study No. 264 Group [see comments]. *N Engl J Med* 327: 765–771.

McElroy, S.L., Soutullo, C.A., Keck, P.E., Jr., and Kmetz, G.F. (1997) A pilot trial of adjunctive gabapentin in the treatment of bipolar disorder." *Ann Clin Psychiatry* 9:99–103.

McElroy, S.L., Suppes, T., Keck, P.E., Frye, M.A., Denicoff, K.D., Altshuler, L.L., Brown, E.S., Nolen, W.A., Kupka, R.W., Rochussen, J., Leverich, G.S., and Post, R.M. (2000) Open-label adjunctive topiramate in the treatment of bipolar disorders. *Biol Psychiatry* 47:1025–1033.

McKinney, P.A., Finkenbine, R.D., and DeVane, C.L. (1996) Alopecia and mood stabilizer therapy. *Ann Clin Psychiatry* 8:183–185.

Menkes, D.L. (1999) Images in neurology. The cutaneous stigmata of Fabry disease: an X-linked phakomatosis associated with central and peripheral nervous system dysfunction. *Arch Neurol* 56: 487.

Messenheimer, J., Mullens, E.L., Giorgi, L., and Young, F. (1998) Safety review of adult clinical trial experience with lamotrigine. *Drug Saf* 18:281–296.

Messenheimer, J., Ramsay, R.E., Willmore, L.J., Leroy, R.F., Zielinski, J.J., Mattson, R., Pellock, J.M., Valakas, A.M., Womble, G., and Risner, M. (1994) Lamotrigine therapy for partial seizures: a multicenter, placebo-controlled, double-blind, cross-over trial. *Epilepsia* 35:113–21.

Messenheimer, J.A., Giorgi, L., and Risner, M.E. (2000) The tolerability of lamotrigine in children. *Drug Saf* 22:303–312.

Mork, A. (1993) Actions of lithium on the cyclic AMP signalling system in various regions of the brain—possible relations to its psychotropic actions. A study on the adenylate cyclase in rat cerebral cortex, corpus striatum and hippocampus. *Pharmacol Toxicol* 73:1–47.

Morris, G.L. (1999) Gabapentin. *Epilepsia* 40:S63–S70.

Mortensen, P.B., Kolvraa, S. and Christensen, E. (1980) Inhibition of the glycine cleavage system: hyperglycmemia and hyperglycinuria caused by valproic acid. *Epilepsia* 21:563–569.

Murialdo, G., Galimberti, C.A., Magri, F., Sampaolo, P., Copello, F., Gianelli, M.V., Gazzerro, E., Rollero, A., Deagatone, C., Manni, R., Ferrari, E., Polleri, A., and Tartara, A. (1997) Menstrual cycle and ovary alterations in women with epilepsy on antiepileptic therapy. *J Endocrinol Invest* 20 :519–526.

Papatheodorou, G. and Kutcher, S.P. (1993) Divalproex sodium treatment in late adolescent and young adult acute mania. *Psychopharmacol Bull* and 29:213–219.

Papatheodorou, G., Kutcher, S.P., Katic, M., and Szalai, J.P. (1995) The efficacy and safety of divalproex sodium in the treatment of acute mania in adolescents and young adults: an open clinical trial. *J Clini Psychopharmacol* 15:110–116.

Parmeggiani, A., Fraticelli, E., and Rossi, P.G. (1998) Exacerbation of epileptic seizures by carbamazepine: report of 10 cases. *Seizure* 7:479–483.

Pellock, J.M. (1987) Carbamazepine side effects in children and adults. *Epilepsia* 28:S64–S70.

Petroff, O.A., Hyder, F., Mattson, R.H., and Rothman, D.L. (1999) Topiramate increases brain GABA, homocarnosine, and pyrroli-

dinone in patients with epilepsy. *Neurology* 52:473–478.

Pleak, R.R., Birmaher, B., Gavrilescu, A., Abichandani, C., and Williams, D.T. (1988) Mania and neuropsychiatric excitation following carbamazepine. *J Am Acad Child Adolesc Psychiatry* 27:500–503.

Pope, H.G., Jr., McElroy, S.L., Keck, P.E., Jr., and Hudson, J.I. (1991) Valproate in the treatment of acute mania. A placebo-controlled study. *Arch Gen Psychiatry* 48:62–68.

Post, R.M., Denicoff, K.D., Frye, M.A., Dunn, R.T., Leverich, G.S., Osuch, E., and Speer, A. (1998a) A history of the use of anticonvulsants as mood stabilizers in the last two decades of the 20th century. *Neuropsychobiology* 38:152–66.

Post, R.M., Denicoff, K.D., Frye, M.A., and Leverich, G.S. (1997) Algorithms for bipolar mania. *Mod Probl Pharmacopsychiatry* 25:114–45.

Post, R.M., Frye, M.A., Denicoff, K.D., Leverich, G.S., Kimbrell, T.A., and Dunn, R.T. (1998b) Beyond lithium in the treatment of bipolar illness. *Neuropsychopharmacology* 19:206–219.

Post, R.M., Ketter, T.A., Denicoff, K., Pazzaglia, P.J., Leverich, G.S., Marangell, L.B., Callahan, A.M., George, M.S., and Frye, M.A. (1996) The place of anticonvulsant therapy in bipolar illness. *Psychopharmacology (Berl)* 128:115–29.

Post, R.M., Rubinow, D.R., Uhde, T.W., Roy-Byrne, P.P., Linnoila, M., Rosoff, A., and Cowdry, R. (1989) Dysphoric mania. Clinical and biological correlates. *Arch Gen Psychiatry* 46:353–358.

Puig-Antich, J. (1986) Biological factors in prepubertal major depression. *Pediatr Ann* 15:867–874.

Rambeck, B., Specht, U., and Wolf, P. (1996) Pharmacokinetic interactions of the new antiepileptic drugs. *Clin Pharmacokinet* 31 : 309–324.

Ramsay, R.E., Pellock, J.M., Garnett, W.R., Sanchez, R.M., Valakas, A.M., Wargin, W.A., Lai, A.A., Hubbell, J., Chern, W.H., Allsup, T., et al. (1991) Pharmacokinetics and safety of lamotrigine (Lamictal) in patients with epilepsy. *Epilepsy Res* 10:191–200.

Rasgon, N.L., Altshuler, L.L., Gudeman, D., Burt, V.K., Tanavoli, S., Hendrick, V., and Korenman, S. (2000) Medication status and polycystic ovary syndrome in women with bipolar disorder: a preliminary report. *J Clin Psychiatry* 61:173–178.

Rattya, J., Vainionpaa, L., Knip, M., Lanning, P., and Isojarvi, J.I. (1999) The effects of valproate, carbamazepine, and oxcarbazepine on growth and sexual maturation in girls with epilepsy. *Pediatrics* 103:588–593.

Reife, R., Pledger, G., and Wu, S.C. (2000) Topiramate as add-on therapy: pooled analysis of randomized controlled trials in adults. *Epilepsia* 41:S66–S71.

Rifkin, A., Karajgi, B., Dicker, R., Perl, E., Boppana, V., Hasan, N., and Pollack, S. (1997) Lithium treatment of conduct disorders in adolescents. *Am J Psychiatry* 154:554–555.

Rosenberg, J.M., Harrell, C., Ristic, H., Werner, R.A., and de Rosayro, A.M. (1997) The effect of gabapentin on neuropathic pain. *Clin J Pain* 13:251–255.

Schmidt, S. and Schmitz-Buhl, M. (1995) Signs and symptoms of carbamazepine overdose. *J Neurol* 242:169–173.

Seetharam, M.N. and Pellock, J.M. (1991) Risk–benefit assessment of carbamazepine in children. *Drug Saf* 6:148–158.

Semah, F., Gimenez, F., Longer, E., Laplane, D., Thuillier, A., and Baulac, M., (1994) Carbamazepine and its epoxide: an open study of efficacy and side effects after carbamazepine dose increment in refractory partial epilepsy. *Ther Drug Monit* 16:537–340.

Shank, R.P., Gardocki, J.F., Streeter, A.J., and Maryanoff, B.E. (2000) An overview of the preclinical aspects of topiramate: pharmacology, pharmacokinetics, and mechanism of action. *Epilepsia* 41: S3–S9.

Silva, R.R., Munoz, D.M., and Alpert, M. (1996) Carbamazepine use in children and adolescents with features of attention-deficit hyperactivity disorder: a meta-analysis. *J Am Acad Child Adolesc Psychiatry* 35:352–358.

Soares, J.C., Chen, G., Dippold, C.S., Wells, K.F., Frank, E., Kupfer, D.J., Manji, H.K., and Mallinger, A.G. (2000) Concurrent measures of protein kinase C and phosphoinositides in lithium-treated bipolar patients and healthy individuals: a preliminary study. *Psychiatry Res* 95:109–118.

Soutullo, C.A., Casuto, L.S., and Keck, P.E., Jr. (1998) Gabapentin in the treatment of adolescent mania: a case report. *J Child Adolesc Psychopharmacol* 8:81–85.

Sovner, R. (1991) Divalproex-responsive rapid cycling bipolar disorder in a patient with Down's syndrome: implications for the Down's syndrome–mania hypothesis. *J Ment Defic Res* 35:171–173.

Sozuer, D.T., Atakil, D., Dogu, O., Baybas, S., and Arpaci, B. (1997) Serum lipids in epileptic children treated with carbamazepine and valproate. *Eur J Pediatr* 156:565–567.

Stone, K.A. (1999) Lithium-induced nephrogenic diabetes insipidus. *J Am Board Fam Pract* 12:43–47.

Strober, M., Morrell, W., Lampert, C., and Burroughs, J. (1990) Relapse following discontinuation of lithium maintenance therapy in adolescents with bipolar I illness: a naturalistic study. *Am J Psychiatry* 147:457–461.

Suppes, T., Brown, E.S., McElroy, S.L., Keck, P.E., Jr., Nolen, W., Kupka, R., Frye, M., Denicoff, K.D., Altshuler, L., Leverich, G.S., and Post, R.M. (1999) Lamotrigine for the treatment of bipolar disorder: a clinical case series. *J Affect Disord* 53:95–98.

Tallian, K.B., Nahata, M.C., Lo, W., and Tsao, C.Y. (1996) Gabapentin associated with aggressive behavior in pediatric patients with seizures. *Epilepsia* 37:501–502.

Tanindi, S., Akin, R., Koseoglu, V., Kurekci, A.E., Gokcay, E., and Ozcan, O. (1996) The platelet aggregation in children with epilepsy receiving valproic acid. *Thromb Res* 81:471–476.

Taylor, C.P., Gee, N.S., Su, T.Z., Kocsis, J.D., Welty, D.F., Brown, J.P., Dooley, D.J., Boden, P., and Singh, L. (1998) A summary of mechanistic hypotheses of gabapentin pharmacology. *Epilepsy Res* 29:233–249.

Tekin, S., Aykut-Bingol, C., Tanridag, T., and Aktan, S. (1998) Antiglutamatergic therapy in Alzheimer's disease—effects of lamotrigine. Short communication. *J Neural Transm* 105:295–303.

Trimble, M.R. (1990) Antiepileptic drugs, cognitive function, and behavior in children: evidence from recent studies. *Epilepsia* 31:S30–S34.

Trimble, M.R. and Cull, C. (1988) Children of school age: the influence of antiepileptic drugs on behavior and intellect. *Epilepsia* 29:S15–S19.

Trimble, M.R. and Thompson, P.J. (1984) Sodium valproate and cognitive function. *Epilepsia* 25:S60–S64.

Tyrer, S.P., Peat, M.A., Minty, P.S., Luchini, A., Glud, V., and Amdisen, A. (1982) Bioavailability of lithium carbonate and lithium citrate: a comparison of two controlled-release preparations. *Pharmatherapeutica* 3:243–246.

Ueda, D., Sato, T., and Hatakeyama, N. (1998) Carbamazepine-induced immune thrombocytopenia in a 12-year-old female. *Acta Haematol* 100:104–105.

Van Calker, D., Steber, R., Klotz, K.N., and Greil, W. (1991) Carbamazepine distinguishes between adenosine receptors that mediate different second messenger responses. *Eur J Pharmacol* 206:285–290.

van der Velde CD, Gordon MW (1969), Manic-depressive illness, diabetes mellitus, and lithium carbonate. *Arch Gen Psychiatry* 21:478–485.

Verrotti, A., Greco, R., Matera, V., Altobelli, E., Morgese, G., and Chiarelli, F. (1999) Platelet count and function in children receiving sodium valproate. *Pediatr Neurol* 21:611–614.

Vitiello, B., Behar, D., Malone, R., Delaney, M.A., Ryan, P.J., and Simpson, G.M. (1988) Pharmacokinetics of lithium carbonate in children. *J Clin Psychopharmacol* 8:355–359.

Vitiello, B. and Jensen, P.S. (1995) Developmental perspectives in pediatric psychopharmacology. *Psychopharmacol Bull* 31:75–81.

Wallace, S.J. (1994) Lamotrigine—a clinical overview. *Seizure* 3 (Suppl A):47–51.

Weaver, D.F., Camfield, P., and Fraser, A. (1988) Massive carbamazepine overdose: clinical and pharmacologic observations in five episodes. *Neurology* 38:755–759.

Weller, E.B., Weller, R.A. and Fristad, M.A. (1986) Lithium dosage guide for prepubertal children: a preliminary report." *J Am Acad Child Psychiatry* 25:92–95.

Wilder, B.J., Karas, B.J., Penry, J.K., and Asconape, J. (1983) Gastrointestinal tolerance of divalproex sodium. *Neurology* 33:808–811.

Wolf, R. and Tscherne, U. (1994) Valproate effect on gamma-aminobutyric acid release in pars reticulata of substantia nigra: combination of push-pull perfusion and fluorescence histochemistry. *Epilepsia* 35:226–233.

Wolf, S.M., Shinnar, S., Kang, H., Gil, K.B., and Moshe, S.L. (1995) Gabapentin toxicity in children manifesting as behavioral changes. *Epilepsia* 36:1203–1205.

Yalcin, E., Hassanzadeh, A., and Mawlud, K. (1997) The effects of long-term anticonvulsive treatment on serum lipid profile. *Acta Paediatr Jpn* 39:342–345.

Young, R.C., Biggs, J.T., Ziegler, VE, et al. (1978) A rating scale for mania: reliability, validity, and sensitivity. *Br J Psychiatry* 133:429–435.

Zona, C., Ciotti, M.T., and Avoli, M. (1997) Topiramate attenuates voltage-gated sodium currents in rat cerebellar granule cells. *Neurosci Lett* 231:123–126.

26 | Antipsychotic agents: traditional and atypical

ROBERT L. FINDLING, NORA K. McNAMARA, AND BARBARA L. GRACIOUS

Drugs that are marketed for the treatment of psychotic disorders in adults, the antipsychotics, are prescribed for a range of problems in children and adolescents. At present, 15 medications are marketed as antipsychotics in the United States. These agents come from several different classes of chemical compounds (Table 26.1).

In addition, there are several drugs that are related to the antipsychotics that may also be prescribed to youths for other conditions. These include the antidepressant amoxapine and the preanesthetic droperidol. Metoclopramide and prochlorperazine are related agents that are marketed for their effects on the gastrointestinal system.

The modern era for the somatic treatment of psychotic disorders began in the 1950s with the finding that chlorpromazine was an effective treatment for patients with schizophrenia. Numerous other antipsychotics were subsequently released as treatments for adults suffering from psychosis. However, the first generation of antipsychotics, otherwise known as *typical* antipsychotics or *neuroleptics* has several pivotal shortcomings. The first has to do with a group of neurological side effects known as the *extrapyramidal side effects* (EPS). The other major problem with these agents is that approximately 20% of adults with schizophrenia are not responsive to typical antipsychotics. This is a particularly important consideration for clinicians treating young people, for it appears that earlier age at onset is associated with a higher risk for neuroleptic-resistant schizophrenia (Meltzer et al., 1997). To address the needs of the neuroleptic-resistant patients and to improve the tolerability of the antipsychotics, new drugs were developed.

Five newer, *atypical* antipsychotics are currently marketed in the United States (Table 26.1). What makes these agents atypical is their reduced propensity to cause EPS and their improved effectiveness in the treatment of negative symptoms of schizophrenia when compared to typical antipsychotics (Shen, 1999a). As a group, the atypical antipsychotics also appear to be associated with more modest degrees of medication-induced hyperprolactinemia when compared to the neuroleptics.

Clozapine was the first atypical antipsychotic released in the United States. However, clozapine is associated with the risk of leukopenia and, potentially, lethal agranulocytosis. Because of these concerns, hematological monitoring during clozapine pharmacotherapy is required (Alphs and Anand, 1999). Due to these hematological risks, clozapine is indicated only for patients with treatment-resistant schizophrenia. The other atypical antipsychotics, risperidone, olanzapine, quetiapine, and ziprasidone, that are marketed in the United States can be used as first-line treatments for adults with schizophrenia.

Other than conceptualizing antipsychotics as either typical or atypical, these agents can also be considered in subgroups on the basis of their relative potencies. As can be seen in Table 26.1, the maximum recommended total daily doses for antipsychotics vary to a significant degree. Agents that are given in smaller total daily doses are considered high-potency drugs. Similarly, there are medium and low potency agents. As a general rule, side effects associated with dopamine type 2 receptor blockade (such as EPS and hyperprolactinemia, see Extrapyramidal Side Effects, and Endocrine, below) increase with increasing potency. The risk of sedation, hypotension, and anticholinergic side effects are greater for low-potency drugs. However, it should be remembered that antipsychotics considered to be atypical have a reduced propensity for causing EPS when compared to typical agents of similar potency.

The purpose of this chapter is to provide the reader with an overview of the pharmacology of the antipsy-

TABLE 26.1 *Antipsychotic and Related Medications Studied in Children and Adolescents*

Generic Name	Chemical Class	Dose Range (mg/day)	Potency	Approximate Dose Equivalents (mg)	Neuropsychiatric Disorder(s) Studied	Key References
Atypical antipsychotics						
Clozapine	Dibenzodiazepine	25–900	Low	100	Treatment-resistant illnesses Schizophrenia[a] Bipolar disorder Autistic disorder	Kumra et al., 1996 Kowatch et al., 1995 Zuddas et al., 1996
Olanzapine	Thienobenzodiazepine	5–20	Medium	5	Bipolar disorder PDD Schizophrenia	Frazier et al., 2000 Potenza et al., 1999 Kumra et al., 1998
Quetiapine	Dibenzothiazepine	25–750	Low	100	Psychotic disorders	McConville et al., 2000
Risperidone	Benzisoxazole	0.25–10	High	2	Bipolar disorder Conduct disorder[a] PDD Psychotic disorders Tic disorders	Frazier et al., 1999 Findling et al., 2000a McDougle et al., 1997 Armenteros et al., 1997 Lombroso et al., 1995
Ziprasidone	Benzisothiazolyl	25–160	Medium	20	Tic disorders	Salke et al., 2000a
Typical antipsychotics						
Chlorpromazine	Phenothiazine	10–1000	Low	100	Conduct disorder	Campbell et al., 1982
Fluphenazine	Phenothiazine	0.25–10	High	1.5	PDD Tic disorders	Joshi et al., 1988 Goetz et al., 1984
Haloperidol	Butyrophenone	0.25–15	High	2	Autistic disorder[a] Conduct disorder[a] Schizophrenia[a] Tic disorders[a]	Anderson et al., 1984 Campbell et al., 1984 Spencer and Campbell, 1984 Shapiro et al., 1989
Loxapine	Dibenzoxazepine	5–100	Medium	10	Schizophrenia[a]	Pool et al., 1976
Mesoridazine	Phenothiazine	10–400	Low	50	Personality disorders	Barnes, 1977
Molindone	Dihydroindolone	5–225	Medium	10	Conduct disorder[a]	Greenhill et al., 1985
Perphenazine	Phenothiazine	2–64	Medium	8	No studies available	
Pimozide	Diphenylbutylpiperidine	0.5–10	High	2	Tourette's syndrome[a]	Sallee et al., 1987
Thioridazine	Phenothiazine	10–800	Low	100	Conduct disorder[a] Schizophrenia[a]	Greenhill et al., 1985 Realmuto et al., 1984
Thiothixene	Thioxanthene	1–60	High	5	Schizophrenia[a]	Realmuto et al., 1984
Trifluoperazine	Phenothiazine	1–40	High	5	PDD	Fish et al., 1966

PDD, pervasive developmental disorder.

[a]Use supported by data from one or more randomized clinical trials.

chotic medications. Although the use of these agents in specific conditions will not be considered in detail (as that topic will be discussed in Section III-B of this book), important clinical issues specific to the use of antipsychotics will be reviewed.

MECHANISM OF DRUG ACTION

The clinical effects of the antipsychotic agents are related to their affinity for a variety of receptors in the central nervous system. These include dopamine, muscarinic, α-adrenergic, and histamine receptors. In addition, unlike the neuroleptics, atypical antipsychotics also affect serotonergic neural transmission. This pharmacological property is important in determining what makes an atypical antipsychotic atypical. Currently, the effects of antipsychotic-related receptor blockade on neural transmission have only been partially elucidated.

Dopamine

At present, five types of dopamine receptors have been identified. An important overarching principle is that all antipsychotics block dopamine type-2 (D_2) receptors in the central nervous system. It has been shown that an antipsychotic compound's affinity for D_2 receptors is proportional to the drug's potency in reducing the positive symptoms of schizophrenia. Agents with the greatest D_2 receptor binding affinity are the most potent (Peroutka and Snyder, 1980). The modulation of the mesolimbic dopaminergic system is the likely pharmacological mechanism that leads to reduction in the positive symptoms of schizophrenia. In addition, there is evidence that EPS may be due to D_2 receptor blockade in the nigrostriatal dopamine system. This is based on the finding that antipsychotic agents with greater D_2 receptor affinity have a greater propensity for causing some forms of EPS (Sekine et al., 1999). The prolactin elevation that has been observed during antipsychotic pharmacotherapy also appears to be caused by blockade of D_2 receptors in the neurohypophysis (Nordström and Farde, 1998; Table 26.2.)

It should be noted that other D_2-like receptors (D_3, D_4) have recently been discovered. Investigators have begun to examine what effect, if any, modulations in neural transmission mediated through the D_3 and D_4 receptors might have (Wilson et al., 1998; Schwartz et al., 2000). Besides the D_2 group of dopamine receptors, there is a D_1 type of dopamine receptor that includes both D_1 and D_5 receptors. Although it appears that D_1 receptor blockade may not be related to the reductions in the positive symptoms of psychosis, it has been hypothesized that agents that block D_1 receptors might have salutary cognitive effects for patients with schizophrenia (Ahlenius, 1999).

Serotonin

Although the traditional neuroleptics do not bind to serotonin (5-MT) receptors with significant affinity, all of the atypical antipsychotics do. This observation has led to the hypothesis that 5-HT receptor blockade is an essential feature of the atypical antipsychotic drugs (Lieberman et al., 1998). Currently, more than a dozen 5-HT receptors have been identified.

5-HT_{2A} receptor blockade appears to be responsible for the reduced propensity of atypical antipsychotics to cause EPS. It has also been suggested that 5-HT_{2A} receptor blockade may explain, in part, why atypical antipsychotics are more effective than traditional neuroleptics in reducing the negative symptoms of schizophrenia (Richelson, 1999). Despite the apparent advantages of atypical antipsychotics when compared to neuroleptics, the weight gain associated with the atypical agents that are currently marketed can be quite problematic for some patients. 5HT_{2c} receptor blockade may contribute to the weight gain associated with atypical antipsychotics (Tecott et al., 1995; Lader, 1999; Table 26.2). As there are many more 5-HT receptors than the two mentioned above, it has yet to be determined whether the other 5-HT receptors have a role in the pharmacological properties of the atypical antipsychotics (Meltzer, 1999).

Muscarinic

There are at least five types of muscarinic cholinergic receptors in the central nervous system. Chlorpromazine, clozapine, olanzapine, and thioridazine have the greatest affinity for muscarinic receptors. Agents that block muscarinic cholinergic receptors have a reduced risk for causing EPS. However, agents with anticholinergic effects are also associated with other adverse events, including blurred vision, cognitive dysfunction, constipation, acute onset or exacerbation of narrow-angle glaucoma, sinus tachycardia, urinary retention, and xerostomia (dry mouth) (Table 26.2). It has also been suggested that muscaric cholinergic receptor agonism leads to sialorrhea that can be seen during clozapine treatment. In addition, it is possible that modulation of the cholinergic neural transmission system might also be associated with reductions in psychotic symptomatology (Tandon, 1999; Shannon et al., 2000).

α-Adrenergic

There are two classes of α-adrenergic receptors, α_1 and α_2. Agents with the greatest affinity for α_1 blockade are chlorpromazine, thioridazine, and risperidone. There are no known beneficial effects associated with α_1-adrenergic receptor antagonism. However, α_1-adrenergic receptor blockade can lead to hypotension, dizziness, and reflex tachycardia (Table 26.2). α_2 Blockade is modest for most agents except for risperidone and clozapine. As with α_1 receptors, there are no benefits that have yet to be associated with α_2 receptor

TABLE 26.2 *Summary of Antipsychotic-Related Side Effects*

Organ System	Side Effect	CNS Receptor(s) Responsible	Recommended Routine Safety Monitoring
Cardiovascular	Dizziness, hypotension, QTc interval prolongation, tachycardia	α_1-adrenergic, muscarinic	Careful medical history and physical examination Electrocardiogram at baseline and at therapeutic dosage Blood pressure and pulse monitored at baseline and after dosage increases
Dermatological	Allergic reactions, alopecia, photosensitivity, skin discoloration	N/A	Use sunblock, limit sun exposure
Endocrine	Prolactin elevation	Dopamine 2	Obtain prolactin level for patients with breast enlargement, menstrual abnormalities, or gynecomastia
Gastrointestinal	Constipation, jaundice, steatohepatitis, weight gain	Histamine, muscarinic	Measure weight at every visit Check transaminases at baseline and yearly (more frequently if significant weight gain)
General	Thermoregulatory dysfunction	Dopamine 2	Prevent excessive exercise or exposure to temperature extremes
Hematological	Agranulocytosis, leukopenia, neutropenia	N/A	Complete blood count with differential at baseline and if symptoms of infection, pallor, or bruising develop shortly after treatment initiation White blood counts weekly for 6 months, then every other week thereafter if treated with clozapine
Neurological	Extrapyramidal side effects, sedation, seizures	Dopamine 2, histamine	Examine for Parkinsonism, akathisia, and abnormal involuntary movements at each visit Baseline electroencephalogram if treated with clozapine.
Ocular	Acute angle closure, blurred vision, cataracts, keratopathy, pigment deposits	Muscarinic	Routine eye examinations Every-6-month eye examination for cataracts if treated with quetiapine
Oral	Dry mouth, cavities	Muscarinic	Routine dental care
Sexual	Anorgasmia, ejaculatory dysfunction, impotence, priapism, reduced libido	Dopamine 2	Consider sexual dysfunction if poor compliance
Urological	Urinary retention	Muscarinic	Inquire about urinary history

N/A, not applicable.

antagonism. However, unlike α_1 receptor blockade there do not appear to be any side effects associated with α_2 receptor blockade (Richelson, 1999).

Histaminergic

Three types of histamine (H) receptors have been isolated. At present, it appears that H_1 receptor blockade

by antipsychotic agents may be responsible for some of the sedation and weight gain caused by these drugs (Sekine et al., 1999).

Summary

In short, there are five groups of receptors in the central nervous system that appear to explain some of the clinical effects of the antipsychotics. However, more needs to be learned about the receptor pharmacology of antipsychotics. It is possible that with increased understanding of how neural transmission is modulated through neural receptors, significant insights about the pharmacodynamics of the available antipsychotics can be gained. Perhaps even more importantly, as more is learned about the central nervous system, new targets for subsequent antipsychotic drug development may become established.

PHARMACOKINETICS AND DRUG METABOLISM

Most of what is known about the pharmacokinetics of antipsychotics comes from studies in adults. These have been extensively summarized elsewhere (Javaid, 1994; Fang and Gorrod, 1999). In brief, the antipsychotics are agents with complex metabolism. They are lipophilic drugs that are well absorbed when given orally and undergo an extensive amount of presystemic biotransformation. These drugs are extensively bound to plasma proteins and tissues, have large volumes of distribution, and are eliminated through hepatic metabolism. There are large interindividual differences in the pharmacokinetics and bioavailability of these compounds in adults as well as in young people. Many antipsychotics have active metabolites that can lead to either adverse events or contribute to salutary effects. At present, therapeutic blood levels have not been definitively determined for any of these agents.

Pharmacokinetic Studies

Knowledge about a drug's pharmacokinetics can inform a rational dosing strategy for that compound. However, the pharmacokinetics of any given medication may change over the first two decades of life. Therefore, what is known about the pharmacokinetics of a drug in adults may not necessarily be applicable to children or adolescents. Unfortunately, there have been only a few studies that have examined the pharmacokinetics of antipsychotics in young people.

The work that has been done with chlorpromazine, haloperidol, and pimozide suggests that these drugs are metabolized more rapidly in children than in adults (Morselli et al., 1982; Sallee et al., 1987; Furlanut et al., 1990). In addition, it appears that larger doses of chlorpromazine and haloperidol per body weight are needed in young people to achieve the same plasma concentrations as those in adults (Morselli et al., 1979; Rivera-Calimlim et al., 1979).

As far as the atypical antipsychotics are concerned,

there is evidence to suggest that plasma concentrations of clozapine are directly correlated with the clinical response noted when adolescents with treatment-resistant childhood-onset schizophrenia are prescribed this medication (Piscitelli et al., 1994). There are data to suggest that risperidone is metabolized more rapidly in young children than in adults (Casaer et al., 1994). In adolescents, it appears that the pharmacokinetics of olanzapine and quetiapine are similar to those observed in adults (Grothe et al., 2000; McConville et al., 2000). In addition, it has been reported that the pharmacokinetics of ziprasidone are similar in children, adolescents, and adults (Sallee et al., 2000b).

Drug–Drug Interactions

Numerous drug–drug interactions have been reported with the antipsychotic agents. These may be mediated through pharmacodynamic effects. For example, antipsychotics that block α_1-adrenergic receptors may potentiate the antihypertensive effects of prazosin, labetalol, and some other antihypertensive agents. Conversely, antipsychotics associated with α_2-adrenergic receptor blockade may interfere with the antihypertensive effects of clonidine and methyldopa (Richelson, 1999).

In addition, concomitant use of a variety of different medications can lead to cumulative side effects. For example, several antipsychotics (most notably, thioridazine, pimozide, and ziprasidone) can prolong the QTc interval on the electrocardiogram (EKG). This is a very important consideration because excessive QTc prolongation can lead to fatal dysrhythmias (see Cardiovascular Effects, below). As additive effects on the QTc interval can occur when more than one drug that prolongs QTc is prescribed, the coadministration of two agents that prolong the QT interval is contraindicated (Gutgesell et al., 1999).

Finally, pharmacokinetic interactions can lead to changes in drug absorption, distribution, metabolism, or excretion. These drug–drug interactions have been summarized elsewhere (Ten Eick et al., 1998; Fang and Gorrod, 1999). Probably the most important drug interactions that may occur with the antipsychotics are those that are related to changes in medication pharmacokinetics and metabolism. It should be noted, however that even when drug–drug interactions occur due to changes in medication biodisposition, the mechanisms that underlie these phenomena are not always readily apparent (Carrillo et al., 1999).

Clinicians should become familiar with drugs that have the cytochrome P450 (CYP) enzyme system involved in their metabolism because the CYP family of enzymes plays a prominent role in the biodisposition

TABLE 26.3 *Summary of Antipsychotics That Are Substrates of the Cytochrome P450 (CYP) Family of Enzymes*

Antipsychotic Substrate	Cytochrome P450 Isozyme(s)
Chlorpromazine	CYP2D6
Clozapine	CYP1A2, CYP2D6, CYP3A4
Fluphenazine	CPY2D6
Haloperidol	CYP2D6, CYP3A4
Olanzapine	CYP1A2, CYP2D6
Perphenazine	CYP2D6
Pimozide	CYP3A4, CYP1A2
Quetiapine	CYP3A4
Risperidone	CYP2D6, CYP3A4
Thioridazine	CYP2D6
Thiothixene	CYP2D6
Ziprasidone	CYP3A4

and drug–drug interactions for many agents. Several antipsychotics have been shown to be substrates of this group of drug-metabolizing cytochromes (Table 26.3).

CYP1A2 appears to play a prominent role in the metabolism of olanzapine (Ring et al., 1996) and clozapine (Buur-Rasmussen and Brøsen, 1999). This CYP isoform is also involved in the biotransformation of pimozide (Desta et al., 1998). As clozapine, olanzapine, and pimozide are substrates for CYP1A2, cigarette smoking, which induces CYP1A2 activity, may reduce blood levels of these agents. Conversely, inhibitors of this isoform (such as fluvoxamine) can lead to increases in drug levels (Ten Eick et al., 1998).

There are four antipsychotics that are substrates for CYP3A4: clozapine (Shen, 1999b), haloperidol (Fang et al., 1997), pimozide (Desta et al., 1998), and ziprasidone (Prakash et al., 2000). Concomitant administration of carbamazepine, one of several CYP3A4 inducers, may lead to reduced levels of these antipsychotics and of clozapine. There are numerous CYP3A4 inhibitors, including erythromycin, clarithromycin, nefazodone, ketoconazole, and grapefruit juice. Combination treatment with any of these inhibitory agents may lead to increased drug exposure. This is particularly an important issue for patients taking pimozide, as these children may develop a life-threatening dysrhythmia as a result of a CYP3A4-mediated drug–drug interaction (Ketter et al., 1995; Dresser et al., 2000).

The CYP2D6 isozyme is involved in the metabolism of numerous classes of drugs. Of particular importance is the fact that CYP2D6 exhibits genetic polymor-

phisms that influence enzyme activity. Thus, people can be categorized as poor, extensive, and ultra-rapid metabolizers with respect to CYP2D6. As phenotypic differences in the pharmacokinetics of some antidepressants have been identified in children and adolescents (Findling et al., 1999, 2000a), phenotypic differences in pharmacokinetics with respect to CYP2D6 can also be assumed.

There are several antipsychotics that are substrates to CYP2D6 (von Bahr et al., 1991; Jerling et al., 1996; Ring et al., 1996; (Fang and Gorrod, 1999; Flockhart and Oesterheld, 2000); (Table 26.3). Moreover, several antipsychotics may act as inhibitors of CYP2D6-mediated biotransformation. These include thioridazine, chlorpromazine, haloperidol, fluphenazine, and pimozide (Desta et al., 1998; Shin et al., 1999). Of particular salience is the fact that the serotonin selective reuptake inhibitors (SSRIs) fluoxetine and paroxetine are metabolized to a significant extent by this isoenzyme.

ADVERSE EFFECTS

Although these agents are commonly used, they are associated with a wide range of side effects (Table 26.2). For this reason, it is essential for the prescribing clinician to be familiar with the adverse events that can occur in a child who is being treated with one of these drugs.

Extrapyramidal Side Effects

When considering the adverse events associated with the antipsychotic medications, the most important group of side effects to consider is the EPS, which occur as a result of D_2 receptor blockade. Because EPS can negatively influence the tolerability and acceptability of drug therapy, these neurological events can limit the effectiveness of neuroleptics in patients of all ages. Moreover, younger patients appear to be at particularly at high risk of developing EPS (Keepers et al., 1983). Thus careful monitoring for EPS in children and adolescents is warranted. As noted above, a major driving force for the recent development and release of new antipsychotics was the hope of finding effective drugs with an improved EPS profile over that of older agents.

The most common forms of EPS that occur early in the course of treatment include acute dystonic reactions (ADRs), drug-induced Parkinsonism, and akathisia. The ADRs are involuntary muscle spasms or contractions. An ADR typically involves muscles in the neck and/or the extraocular muscles, and can be painful and distressing. In addition, acute laryngeal spasm, an uncommon form of ADR, can lead to respiratory compromise.

Akathisia is an EPS that is characterized by a sense of restlessness and/or a need to move. This side effect may be difficult to distinguish from increased agitation because of the primary diagnosis being treated. Akathisia may be very uncomfortable. It is associated with a high rate of noncompliance in adults and increased risk for suicide. Drug-induced parkinsonism is another EPS that can occur during the initial stages of antipsychotic therapy. This side effect can make the patient look medicated. The *negative* symptoms of a psychotic illness and depression are part of the differential diagnosis of antipsychotic-related Parkinsonism (Hansen et al., 1997; Arana, 2000). Perioral tremor (otherwise know as the *rabbit syndrome*) is an uncommon form of EPS that may also occur. Its onset is typically later than that of other EPS (Jus et al., 1972).

Tardive dyskinesia is a potentially irreversible movement disorder characterized by choreoathetoid movements. The possibility of a primary neurological disorder should be considered when a patient being treated with an antipsychotic develops involuntary movements. It should also be noted that patients might develop transient withdrawal dyskinesias as the dosage of neuroleptics is lowered or discontinued (Campbell et al., 1999). It appears that withdrawal dyskinesias are more common in children than adults.

There are several approaches to the treatment of EPS. One is to prevent them from happening at all. This can be done by prescribing a medication with a low propensity for leading to EPS (such as an atypical antipsychotic or a low-potency neuroleptic) or using higher-potency neuroleptics at low doses. However, when EPS do develop, besides trying to lower the dosage of the offending drug, pharmacological interventions can also be used. If a patient develops an ADR, anticholinergic agents such as diphenhydramine or benztropine can be administered intramuscularly. The recurrence of ADRs may then be prevented by treatment with oral benztropine or oral trihexyphenidyl. Akathisia may either be treated with the beta blocker propranolol, an oral anticholinergic agent (such as benztropine, diphenhydramine, or trihexyphenidyl), or clonazepam. Either an anticholinergic agent or amantadine (which acts as a dopamine agonist) may be used for drug-induced parkinsonism (Findling et al. 1998).

Neuroleptic malignant syndrome (NMS) is a rare, medication-induced syndrome that may be due to dopamine receptor blockade in the basal ganglia. An altered level of consciousness, autonomic instability, hyperthermia, and severe muscular rigidity typically characterize NMS. Laboratory studies show increased levels of creatinine phosphokinase as well as leukocytosis. Besides discontinuation of the causal agent, treatment for NMS generally consists of supportive treatments as well as the consideration of use of the dopamine agonists (such as bromocriptine) and dantrolene to address muscular rigidity (Silva et al., 1999). Quite separate from NMS, it should be remembered that treatment with antipsychotics might impair the body's ability to regulate temperature. This is likely due to disruption of thermoregulatory circuits in the hypothalamus from dopamine receptor blockade. Therefore, patients treated with neuroleptics may be at higher risk for developing heatstroke (Lazarus, 1989).

Seizures

Seizures are generally uncommon, but can occur during antipsychotic pharmacotherapy, because some of these agents may lower the seizure threshold. Unless there is a prior history of an abnormal electroencephalogram (EEG), epilepsy, or other neurological disorder, antipsychotics are not generally associated with a high risk of seizures. However, clozapine is an exception. Clozapine administration leads to EEG changes and seizures more frequently than the other antipsychotics. Clozapine-induced seizures are more prevalent at higher doses (Devinsky et al., 1991). Evidence from several clinical trials suggests that children and adolescents may be particularly prone to these clozapine-related neurological events (Findling et al., 2000b).

Weight Gain

It appears that H_1 and $5\text{-}HT_{2c}$ receptor blockade contributes to the weight gain seen during antipsychotic therapy. There is preliminary evidence to suggest that risperidone is associated with a greater amount of weight gain than that with typical antipsychotics in this age group (Kelly et al., 1998). At present there are no methodologically rigorous studies that have compared the relative ability of different atypical antipsychotics to cause weight gain in pediatric patients. When compared to adults, drug-induced weight gain appears to be more problematic in children and adolescents.

Liver Dysfunction

Cholestatic jaundice can occur during treatment with antipsychotics, and is most often reported in chlorpromazine-treated patients (Hansen et al., 1997). Elevations in liver transaminases have also been observed in a few cases of children treated with risperidone (Kumra et al., 1997). This risperidone-associated adverse effect may not be due to the direct effect of the medication per se, but may be secondary to the marked weight gain that can occur in some patients treated with antipsychotics (Szigethy et al., 1999).

Sedation

Besides weight gain, probably the most common side effect from antipsychotics in young people is sedation. Histamine receptor blockade appears to mediate this side effect. Excessive sleepiness can interfere with a youth's academic performance, cause sluggishness, and cause a child to appear drugged to their peers and family.

Anticholinergia

As noted above, several antipsychotics have prominent anticholinergic effects. Side effects due to anticholinergia may include dry mouth, blurred vision, constipation, urinary retention, and tachycardia.

Cardiovascular Effects

Antipsychotic agents may have several cardiovascular effects. Medication-induced hypotension is generally more problematic with lower-potency neuroleptics than with other antipsychotics and appears to be mediated through α_1-adrenergic blockade. Besides increases in heart rate that may be the result of hypotension, antipsychotics with appreciable anticholinergic effects (see Clinical Implications, below) can lead to tachycardia (Gutgesell et al., 1999).

Of greatest concern is that some antipsychotics may cause QTc prolongation due to quinidine-like effects. This is a particularly important consideration because QTc prolongation may lead to a fatal dysrhythmia. Numerous antipsychotics and related compounds have been reported to increase QTc intervals (Cavero et al., 2000; Welch and Chue, 2000). Although the risk of EKG changes with pimozide has been noted for years (Opler and Feinberg, 1991), recent evidence suggests that two older compounds, droperidol and thioridazine, may also be associated with a particularly high risk of dose-related QTc changes (Reilly et al., 2000).

Because thioridazine has been shown to prolong the QTc, significant labeling changes have recently been made for this drug. First, a boxed warning has been added to the package insert. In addition, although thioridazine was once considered a first-line drug, it is now only indicated for use in patients with schizophrenia who do not respond to treatment with another antipsychotic. As thioridazine is a substrate of CYP2D6, the use of thioridazine in patients who are poor metabolizers or who are receiving drugs that inhibit CYP2D6 is now contraindicated.

Endocrine

Treatment with antipsychotic agents can lead to increases in plasma prolactin due to D_2 receptor blockade in the neurohypophysis. Although atypical antipsychotics may have a reduced propensity for increasing plasma prolactin levels, it appears that clozapine and quetiapine are associated with the smallest risk of drug-induced prolactin elevations (Wudarsky et al., 1999; McConville et al., 2000). Amenorrehea, galactorrhea, menstrual changes, breast enlargement, sexual dysfunction, and gynecomastia are associated with hyperprolactinemia (Lader, 1999). In addition, the consequences of long-term exposure to increased prolactin levels in children have yet to be explored.

Sexual Side Effects

In addition to the sexual side effects that can occur as a direct result of hyperprolactinemia, other sexual side effects may occur as well. These include ejaculatory difficulties, impotence, anorgasmia, priapism, and reduced libido (Hansen et al., 1997; Arana, 2000).

Dermatological Effects

A variety of relatively uncommon dermatological side effects have been noted to be associated with antipsychotic agents. These include maculopapular rashes, urticaria, and erythema multiforme (Arana, 2000). Photosensitivity and skin pigmentation can also occur during treatment with these drugs. Although skin pigmentation has been most frequently reported with chlorpromazine, this can occur with thioridazine and trifluoperazine (Harth and Rapoport, 1996). In addition, treatment-induced alopecia has been reported for haloperidol, olanzapine, and risperidone (Mercke et al., 2000).

Ophthalmologic Effects

Acute angle closure and difficulty with accommodation can occur from the anticholinergic effects of antipsychotic agents. In addition, pigment deposits may develop in the cornea and lens. Pigmentary retinopathy has been reported with thioridazine. Keratopathy and corneal edema may occur occasionally during pharmacotherapy with chlorpromazine and fluphenazine

(Gualtieri et al., 1982; Oshika, 1995; Hansen et al., 1997). Quetiapine was reported to be associated with the development of cataracts in canine studies. For this reason, regular ophthalmic examinations are suggested for patients receiving this drug so that the possibility of cataract formation can be assessed (see Clinical Implications, below). At present, there have been no reports of a link between cataract development and quetiapine therapy in humans (Garver, 2000).

Hematological Effects

Decreases in the white blood cell count or other blood dyscrasias can occur during treatment with any antipsychotic (Lader, 1999). When they occur, these hematological changes usually emerge during the first 2 months of drug therapy (Arana, 2000). In most cases they are generally not clinically significant. Of particular note is the well-established risk of potentially fatal agranulocytosis associated with clozapine (Alphs and Anand, 1999). Unlike the adult population, children do not appear to be at increased risk for developing clozapine-related hematological side effects. Rarely, agranulocytosis can occur when other antipsychotics are prescribed (Marcus and Mulvihill, 1978; Arana, 2000). Given the available data, it appears that children who receive clozapine should receive the same hematological monitoring as recommended for adults.

CLINICAL IMPLICATIONS

The antipsychotics are prescribed to children and adolescents for a range of symptoms and neuropsychiatric disorders (Kaplan et al., 1994; Kaplan and Busner, 1997; Findling et al., 1998). In pediatric settings, antipsychotics and related drugs may also be used as either antiemetics or preanesthetics (Findling et al., 1998; Campbell et al., 1999). Although there is a wide range of clinical applications, efficacy and safety data for these agents in neuropsychiatric conditions are sparse (Table 26.1).

However, as noted above, these drugs can lead to problematic side effects. For this reason, the most important overarching strategy when prescribing antipsychotic medications to young people is to minimize the risks associated with these agents.

The difficulties that are generally most problematic during the initial phase of antipsychotic treatment of young people are the EPS and sedation. These adverse events often lead to significant management difficulties for the clinician, but also likely lead to reduced acceptability and compliance with treatment. Concerns

by clinicians, patients, and their families can lead to reluctance to use these agents in young people. In hopes of minimizing the risks associated with EPS, first-line atypical antipsychotics (risperidone, olanzapine, and quetiapine) can be prescribed.

Although the atypical antipsychotics may be associated with a reduced propensity for causing EPS in young people, EPS (including tardive dyskinesia) can occur when a youth is prescribed a first-line atypical antipsychotic. It appears that a rapid dose escalation is associated with a higher risk of acute EPS. In addition, the likelihood of other medication-related side effects increases when higher doses of medications are employed. Therefore, the principle of start low and go slow applies when initiating antipsychotic pharmacotherapy in a child or teenager. On the basis of available data, target doses of antipsychotics for adolescents with psychotic disorders appear similar to those used in adults. Children with psychosis and adolescents with other conditions generally appear to achieve optimal benefit from lower doses of medication.

It is recommended that neurological side effects be monitored carefully throughout the course of antipsychotic treatment. Rating scales can assist in monitoring for EPS and the involuntary movements seen in tardive dyskinesia. These include the Neurological Rating Scale (Simpson and Angus, 1970), the Barnes Akathisia Scale (Barnes, 1989), and the Abnormal Involuntary Movement Scale ([AIMS] National Institute of Mental Health, 1985).

In addition to neurological side effects, concerns about weight gain have also been an important therapeutic issue, particularly for the atypical agents (Martin et al., 2000). As obesity during childhood is known to be associated with a variety of general medical problems, careful monitoring of a patient's weight is essential.

If significant weight gain does occur during antipsychotic pharmacotherapy, a change in the prescribed medication may be considered. As molindone appears to be associated with a reduced propensity for weight gain in adults, this drug may be useful for children and adolescents who gain an inordinate amount of weight while being treated with other antipsychotics. Ziprasidone does not appear to be associated with significant amounts of weight gain in children treated for tic disorders (Sallee et al., 2000a). It remains to be seen whether ziprasidone will prove to be a viable treatment alternative for young patients who experience a significant amount of weight gain.

Because many antipsychotic agents can lead to either hypotension, tachycardia, or prolongation of the QTc interval on the EKG, it has been recommended that cardiovascular monitoring be employed when neuroleptic agents are prescribed to young people (Gutgesell et al., 1999). Because the atypical antipsychotic agents are being prescribed more frequently to young people, other monitoring strategies are also called for until more is known about the use of these medications in pediatric populations (Table 26.2). For example, it appears that children and adolescents are at particularly high risk for EEG changes and/or seizures during clozapine treatment. For this reason, an EEG should be obtained prior to initiating clozapine pharmacotherapy. A follow-up EEG is recommended if a seizure either occurs or is suspected or if the patient being prescribed clozapine exhibits an acute change in behavior. Because clozapine-induced seizures appear to be dose related and possibly related to rapid dosage increases, a gradual upward titration with this drug is particularly recommended. Should a patient develop clozapine-induced seizures or experience acute behavioral changes with epileptiform activity on an EEG, adjunctive treatment with divalproex sodium may be helpful. Anticonvulsant prophylaxis is not generally recommended.

As a general rule, ophthalmologic side effects do not appear to occur commonly in children treated with antipsychotics. Although a causal relationship between cataract formation and quetiapine treatment has not been demonstrated in adults, quetiapine administration has been noted in canine studies to lead to cataract formation. For this reason, extra ophthalmologic monitoring during chronic quetiapine treatment is recommended.

CONCLUSIONS

The antipsychotics are a group of drugs used for a range of disorders and target symptoms in children and adolescents. Despite the fact they have not been extensively studied in young people, child and adolescent psychiatrists appear to be prescribing the newer atypical antipsychotic agents more frequently than the older antipsychotics. This phenomenon is likely due to the fact that the atypical agents generally appear to have a superior side effect profile. However, it should be noted that these drugs might lead to a variety of side effects. In addition, it should be remembered that significant drug–drug interactions could occur with these drugs. For these reasons, antipsychotics should be used judiciously for well-defined target symptoms.

ACKNOWLEDGMENTS
A Clinical Research Center Grant from the Stanley Foundation supported this work. The authors' research on this topic is funded in part by Abbott, AstraZeneca, Bristol-Myers Squibb, Janssen, Lilly, and Pfizer.

REFERENCES

Ahlenius, S. (1999) Clozapine: dopamine D_1 receptor agonism in the prefrontal cortex as the code to decipher a Rosetta Stone of antipsychotic drugs. *Pharmacology Toxicol* 84:193–196.

Alphs, L.D. and Anand, R. (1999) Clozapine: the commitment to patient safety. *J Clin Psychiatry* 60(Suppl 12):39–42.

Anderson, L.T., Campbell, M., Grega, D.M., Perry, R., Small, A.M., and Green, W.H. (1984) Haloperidol in the treatment of infantile autism: effects on learning and behavioral symptoms. *Am J Psychiatry* 141:1195–1202.

Arana, G.W. (2000) An overview of side effects caused by typical antipsychotics. *J Clin Psychiatry* 61(Suppl 8):5–11.

Armenteros, J.L., Whitaker, A.H., Welikson, M., Stedge, D.J., and Gorman, J. (1997) Risperidone in adolescents with schizophrenia: an open pilot study. *J Am Acad Child Adolesc Psychiatry* 36:694–700.

Barnes, R.J. (1977) Mesoridazine (Serentil) in personality disorders: a controlled trial in adolescent patients. *Dis Nerv System* 28:258–264.

Barnes, T. (1989) A rating scale for drug-induced akathisia. *Br J Psychiatry* 154:672–676.

Buur-Rasmussen, B. and Brøsen, K. (1999) Cytochrome P450 and therapeutic drug monitoring with respect to clozapine. *Eur Neuropsychopharmacol* 9:453–459.

Campbell, M., Cohen, I.L., and Small, A.M. (1982) Drugs in aggressive behavior. *J Am Acad Child Psychiatry* 21:107–117.

Campbell, M., Rapoport, J.L., and Simpson, G.M. (1999) Antipsychotics in children and adolescents. *J Am Acad Child Adolesc Psychiatry* 38:537–545.

Campbell, M., Small, A.M., Green, W.H., Jennings, S.J., Perry, R., Bennett, W.G., and Anderson, L. (1984) Behavioral efficacy of haloperidol and lithium carbonate. A comparison in hospitalized aggressive children with conduct disorder. *Arch Gen Psychiatry* 41:650–656.

Carrillo, J.A., Ramos, S.I., Herraiz, A.G., Llerena, A., Agundez, J.A., Berecz, R., Duran, M., and Benítez, J. (1999) Pharmacokinetic interaction of fluvoxamine and thioridazine in schizophrenic patients. *J Clin Psychopharmacol* 19:494–499.

Casaer, P., Walleghem, D., Vandenbussche, I., Huang, M.-L., and DeSmedt, G. (1994) Pharmacokinetics and safety of risperidone in autistic children [abstract]. *Pediatr Neurol* 11:89.

Cavero, I., Mestre, M., Guillon, J.-M., and Crumb, W. (2000) Drugs that prolong QT interval as an unwanted effect: assessing their likelihood of inducing hazardous cardiac dysrhythmias. *Expert Opin Pharmacother* 1:947–973.

Desta, Z., Kerbusch, T., Soukhova, N., Richard, E., Ko, J.W., and Flockhart, D.A. (1998) Identification and characterization of human cytochrome P450 isoforms interacting with pimozide. *J Pharmacol Exp Ther* 285:428–437.

Devinsky, O., Honigfeld, G., and Patin, J. (1991) Clozapine-related seizures. *Neurology* 41:369–371.

Dresser, G.K., Spence, J.D., and Bailey, D.G. (2000) Pharmacokinetic–pharmacodynamic consequences and clinical relevance of cytochrome P450 3A4 inhibition. *Clin Pharmacokinet* 38:41–57.

Fang, J., Baker, G.B., Silverstone, P.H., and Coutts, R.T. (1997) Involvement of CYP3A4 and CYP2D6 in the metabolism of haloperidol. *Cell Mol Neurobiol* 17:227–233.

Fang, J. and Gorrod, J.W. (1999) Metabolism, pharmacogenetics, and metabolic drug–drug interactions of antipsychotic drugs. *Cell Mol Neurobiol* 19:491–510.

Findling, R.L., McNamara, N.K., Branicky, L.A., Schluchter, M.D., Lemon, E., and Blumer, J.L. (2000a) A double-blind pilot study of risperidone in conduct disorder. *J Am Acad Child Adolesc Psychiatry* 39:509–516.

Findling, R.L., McNamara, N.K., and Gracious, B.L. (2000b) Paediatric uses of atypical antipsychotics. *Expert Opin Pharmacother* 1:935–945.

Findling, R.L., Schulz, S.C., Reed, M.D., and Blumer, J.L. (1998) The antipsychotics. A pediatric perspective. *Pediatr Clin North Am* 45:1205–1232.

Fish B., Shapiro T., and Campbell M. (1966) Long-term prognosis and the response of schizophrenic children to drug therapy: a controlled study of trifluoperazine. *Am J Psychiatry* 123:32–39.

Flockhart, D.A. and Oesterheld, J.R. (2000) Cytochrome P450–mediated drug interactions. *Child Adolesc Psychiatr Clin North Am* 9:43–76.

Frazier, J.A., Biederman, J., Jacobs, T.G., Tohen, M.F., Toma, V., Feldman, P.D., Rater, M.A., Tarazi, R.A., Kim, G.A., Garfield, S.B., Gonzalez-Heydrich, J., and Nowlin, Z.M. (2000) Olanzapine in the treatment of bipolar disorder in juveniles. Presented at the American Psychiatric Association Annual Meeting, Chicago, Illinois, May 2000.

Frazier, J.A., Meyer, M.C., Biederman, J., Wozniak, J., Wilens, T.E., Spencer, T.J., Kim, G.S., and Shapiro, S. (1999) Risperidone treatment for juvenile bipolar disorder: a retrospective chart review. *J Am Acad Child Adolesc Psychiatry* 38:960–965.

Furlanut, M., Benetello, P., Baraldo, M., Zara, G., Montanari, G., and Donzelli, F. (1990) Chlorpromazine disposition in relation to age in children. *Clin Pharmacokinet* 18:329–331.

Garver, D.L. (2000) Review of quetiapine side effects. *J Clin Psychiatry* 61(Suppl 8):31–33.

Goetz, C.G., Tanner, C.M., and Klawans, H.L. (1984) Fluphenazine and multifocal tic disorders. *Arch Neurol* 41:271–272.

Greenhill, L.L., Solomon, M., Pleak, R., and Ambrosini, P. (1985) Molindone hydrochloride treatment of hospitalized children with conduct disorder. *J Clin Psychiatry* 46(8, Sec.2):20–25.

Grothe, D.R., Calis, K.A., Jacobsen, L., Kumra, S., DeVane, C.L., Rapoport, J.L., Bergstrom, R.F., and Kurtz, D.L. (2000) Olanzapine pharmacokinetics in pediatric and adolescent inpatients with childhood-onset schizophrenia. *J Clin Psychopharmacol* 20:220–225.

Gualtieri, C.T., Lefler, W.H., Guimond, M., and Staye, J.I. (1982) Corneal and lenticular opacities in mentally retarded young adults treated with thioridazine and chlorpromazine. *Am J Psychiatry* 139:1178–1180.

Gutgesell, H., Atkins, D., Barst, R., Buck, M., Franklin, W., Humes, R., Ringel, R., Shaddy, R., and Taubert, K.A. (1999) AHA Scientific Statement: Cardiovascular monitoring of children and adolescents receiving psychotropic drugs. *J Am Acad Child Adolesc Psychiatry* 38:1047–1050.

Hansen, T.E., Casey, D.E., and Hoffman, W.F. (1997) Neuroleptic intolerance. *Schizophr Bull* 23:567–582.

Harth, Y. and Rapoport, M. (1996) Photosensitivity associated with antipsychotics, antidepressants and anxiolytics. *Drug Saf* 14:252–259.

Javaid, J.I. (1994) Clinical pharmacokinetics of antipsychotics. *J Clin Pharmacol* 34:286–295.

Jerling, M., Dahl, M.-L., °Aberg-Wistedt, A., Liljenberg, B., Landell, N.-E., Bertilsson, L., and Sjöqvist, F. (1996) The CYP2D6 genotype predicts the oral clearance of the neuroleptic agents perphenazine and zuclopenthixol. *Clin Pharmacol Ther* 59:423–428.

Joshi, P.T., Capozzoli, J.A., and Coyle, J.T. (1988) Low-dose neuroleptic therapy for children with childhood-onset pervasive developmental disorder. *Am J Psychiatry* 145:335–336.

Jus, K., Villeneuve, A., and Jus, A. (1972) Tardive dyskinesia and the rabbit syndrome during wakefulness and sleep. *Am J Psychiatry* 129:143.

Kaplan, S.L. and Busner, J. (1997) Prescribing practices of inpatient child psychiatrists under three auspices of care. *J Child Adolesc Psychopharmacol* 7:275–286.

Kaplan, S.L., Simms, R.M., and Busner, J. (1994) Prescribing practices of outpatient child psychiatrists. *J Am Acad Child Adolesc Psychiatry* 33:35–44.

Keepers, G.A., Clappison, V.J., and Casey, D.E. (1983) Initial anticholinergic prophylaxis for neuroleptic-induced extrapyramidal syndromes. *Arch Gen Psychiatry* 40:1113–1117.

Kelly, D.L., Conley, R.R., Love, R.C., Horn, D.S., and Ushchak, C.M. (1998) Weight gain in adolescents treated with risperidone and conventional antipsychotics over six months. *J Child Adolesc Psychopharmacol* 8:151–159.

Ketter, T.A., Flockhart, D.A., Post, R.M., Denicoff, K., Pazzaglia, P.J., Marangell, L.B., George, M.S., and Callahan, A.M. (1995) The emerging role of cytochrome P450 3A in psychopharmacology. *J Clin Psychopharmacol* 15:387–398.

Kowatch, R.A., Suppes, T., Gilfillan, S.K., Fuentes, R.M., Brannemann, B.D., and Emslie, G.J. (1995) Clozapine treatment of children and adolescents with bipolar disorder and schizophrenia: a clinical case series. *J Child Adolesc Psychopharmacol* 5:241–253.

Kumra, S., Frazier, J.A., Jacobsen, L.K., McKenna, K., Gordon, C.T., Lenane, M.C., Hamburger, S.D., Smith, A.K., Albus, K.E., Alaghband-Rad, J., and Rapoport, J.L. (1996). Childhood-onset schizophrenia. A double-blind clozapine-haloperidol comparison. *Arch Gen Psychiatry* 53:1090–1097.

Kumra, S., Herion, D., Jacobsen, L.K., Briguglia, C., and Grothe, D. (1997) Case study: risperidone-induced hepatotoxicity in pediatric patients. *J Am Acad Child Adolesc Psychiatry* 35:701–705.

Kumra S., Jacobsen, L.K., Lenane, M., Karp, B.I., Frazier, J.A., Smith, A.K., Bedwell, J., Lee, P., Malanga, C.J., Hamburger, S., and Rapoport, J.L. (1998) Childhood-onset schizophrenia: an open-label study of olanzapine in adolescents. *J Am Acad Child Adolesc Psychiatry* 37:377–385.

Lader, M. (1999) Some adverse effects of antipsychotics: prevention and treatment. *J Clin Psychiatry* 60(Suppl 12):18–21.

Lazarus, A. (1989) Differentiating neuroleptic-related heatstroke from neuroleptic malignant syndrome. *Psychosomatics* 30:454–456.

Lieberman, J.A., Mailman, R.B., Duncan, G., Sikich, L., Chakos, M., Nichols, D.E., and Kraus, J.E. (1998) Serotonergic basis of antipsychotic drug effects in schizophrenia. *Biol Psychiatry* 44:1099–1117.

Lombroso, P.J., Scahill, L., King, R.A., Lynch, K.A., Chappell, P.B., B.S., McDougle, C.J., and Leckman, J.F. (1995) Risperidone treatment of children and adolescents with chronic tic dic disorders: a preliminary report. *J Am Acad Child Adolesc Psychiatry* 34:1147–1152.

Marcus, J. and Mulvihill, F.J. (1978) Agranulocytosis and chlorpromazine. *J Clin Psychiatry* 39:784–786.

Martin, A., Landau, J., Leebens, P., Ulizio, K., Cicchetti, D., Scahill, L., and Leckman, J.F. (2000) Risperidone-associated weight gain in children and adolescents: a retrospective chart review. *J Child Adolesc Psychopharmacol* 10:235–244.

McConville, B.J., Arvanitis, L.A., Thyrum, P.T., Yeh, C., Wilkinson, L.A., Chaney, R.O., Foster, K.D., Sorter, M.T., Friedman, L.M., Brown, K.L., and Heubi, J.E. (2000) Pharmacokinetics, tolerability, and clinical effectiveness of quetiapine fumarate: an open-label trial in adolescents with psychotic disorders. *J Clin Psychiatry* 61:252–260.

McDougle, C.J., Holmes, J.P., Bronson, M.R., Anderson, G.M., Volkmar, F.R., Price, L.H., and Cohen, D.J. (1997) Risperidone treatment of children and adolescents with pervasive developmental disorders: a prospective, open-label study. *J Am Acad Child Adolesc Psychiatry* 36:685–693.

Meltzer, H.Y. (1999) The role of serotonin in antipsychotic drug action. *Neuropsychopharmacology* 21:106S-115S.

Meltzer, H.Y., Rabinowitz, J., Lee, M.A., Cola, P.A., Ranjan, R., Findling, R.L., and Thompson, P.A. (1997) Age at onset and gender of schizophrenic patients in relation to neuroleptic resistance. *Am J Psychiatry* 154:475–482.

Mercke, Y., Sheng, H., Khan, T., and Lippmann, S. (2000) Hair loss in psychopharmacology. *Ann Clin Psychiatry* 12:35–42.

Morselli, P.L., Bianchetti, G., and Dugas, M. (1982) Haloperidol plasma level monitoring in neuropsychiatric patients. *Ther Drug Monit* 4:51–58.

Morselli, P.L., Bianchetti, G., Durand, G., LeHeuzey, M.F., Zarifian, E., and Dugas, M. (1979) Haloperidol plasma level monitoring in pediatric patients. *Ther Drug Monit* 1:35–46.

National Institute for Mental Health. (1985) Abnormal Involuntary Movement Scale (AIMS). *Psychopharmacol Bull* 21:1077–1080.

Nordström, A.-L. and Farde, L. (1998) Plasma prolactin and central D_2 receptor occupancy in antipsychotic drug-treated patients. *J Clin Psychopharmacol* 18:305–310.

Opler, L.A. and Feinberg, S.S. (1991) The role of pimozide in clinical psychiatry: a review. *J Clin Psychiatry* 52:221–233.

Oshika, T. (1995) Ocular adverse effects of neuropsychiatric agents. *Drug Saf* 12:256–263.

Peroutka, S.J. and Snyder, S.H. (1980) Relationship of neuroleptic drug effects at brain dopamine, serotonin, α-adrenergic, and histamine receptors to clinical potency. *Am J Psychiatry* 137:1518–1522.

Physicians' Desk Reference, 54th ed.. (2000) Montvale, NJ: Medical Economics Company, Inc.

Piscitelli, S.C., Frazier, J.A., McKenna, K., Albus, K.E., Grothe, D.R., Gordon, C.T., and Rapoport, J.L. (1994) Plasma clozapine and haloperidol concentrations in adolescents with childhood-onset schizophrenia: association with response. *J Clin Psychiatry* 55:(9, Suppl B): 94–97.

Pool, D., Bloom, W., Mielke, D.H., Roniger, J.J., and Gallant, D.M. (1976) A controlled evaluation of loxitane in seventy-five adolescent schizophrenic patients. *Curr Ther Res* 19:99–104.

Potenza, M.N., Holmes, J.P. Kanes, S.J., and McDougle, C.J. (1999) Olanzapine treatment of children, adolescents and adults with pervasive developmental disorders: an open-label pilot study. *J Clin Psychopharmacol* 19:37–44.

Prakash, C., Kamel, A., Cui, D., Whalen, R.D., Miceli, J.J., and Tweedie, D. (2000) Identification of the major human liver cytochrome P450 isoform(s) responsible for the formation of ziprasidone and prediction of possible drug interactions. *Br J Clin Pharmacol* 49:35S–42S.

Realmuto, G.M., Erickson, W.D., Yellin, A.M., Hopwood, J.H., and Greenberg, L.M. (1984) Clinical comparison of thiothixene and thioridazine in schizophrenic adolescents. *Am J Psychiatry* 141:440–442.

Reilly, J.G., Ayis, S.A., Ferrier, I.N., Jones, S.J., and Thomas, S.H.L. (2000) QTc-interval abnormalities and psychotropic drug therapy in psychiatric patients. *Lancet* 355:1048–1052.

Richelson, E. (1999) Receptor pharmacology of neuroleptics: relation to clinical effects. *J Clin Psychiatry* 60(Suppl 10):5–14.

Ring, B.J., Catlow, J., Lindsay, T.J., Gillespie, T., Roskos, L.K., Cerimele, B.J., Swanson, S.P., Hamman, M.A., and Wrighton, S.A. (1996) Identification of the human cytochromes P450 responsible for the in vitro formation of the major oxidative metabolites of the antipsychotic agent olanzapine. *J Pharmacol Exp Ther* 276: 658–666.

Rivera-Calimlim, L., Griesbach, P.H., and Perlmutter, R. (1979) Plasma chlorpromazine concentrations in children with behavioral disorders and mental illness. *Clin Pharmacol Ther* 26:114–121.

Sallee, F.R., Kurlan, R., Goetz, C.G., Singer, H., Scahill, L., Law, G., Dittman, V.M., and Chappell, P.B. (2000a) Ziprasidone treatment of children and adolescents with Tourette's syndrome: a pilot study. *J Am Acad Child Adolesc Psychiatry* 39:292–299.

Sallee, F.R., Miceli, J.J., Wilner, K.D., and Robarge, L. (2000b) Pharmacokinetics of ziprasidone in children and adolescents with Tourette's syndrome. In: *New Research Abstracts from the American Psychiatric Association Annual Meeting, Chicago, IL* NR563.

Sallee, F.R., Nesbitt, L., Jackson, C., Sine, L., and Sethuraman, G. (1997) Relative efficacy of haloperidol and pimozide in children and adolescents with Tourette's disorder. *Am J Psychiatry* 154: 1057–1062.

Sallee, F.R., Pollock, B.G., Stiller, R.L., Stull, S., Everett, G., and Perel, J.M. (1987) Pharmacokinetics of pimozide in adults and children with Tourette's syndrome. *J Clin Pharmacol* 27:776–781.

Schwartz, J.-C., Diaz, J., Pilon, C., and Sokoloff, P. (2000) Possible implications of the dopamine D_3 receptor in schizophrenia and in antipsychotic drug actions. *Brain Res Rev* 31:277–287.

Sekine, Y., Rikihisa, T., Ogata, H., Echizen, H., and Arakawa, Y. (1999) Correlations between in vitro activity of antipsychotics to various central neurotransmitter receptors and clinical incidence of their adverse drug reactions. *Eur J Clin Pharmacol* 55:583–587.

Shannon, H.E., Rasmussen, K., Bymaster, F.P., Hart, J.C., Peters, S.C., Swedberg, M.D.B., Jeppesen, L., Sheardown, M.J., Sauerberg, P., and Fink-Jensen, A. (2000) Xanomeline, an M1/M4 preferring muscarinic cholinergic receptor agonist, produces antipsychotic-like activity in rats and mice. *Schizophr Res* 42: 249–259.

Shapiro, E., Shapiro, A.K., Fulop, G., Hubbard, M., Mandeli, J., Nordlie, J., and Phillips, R.A. (1989) Controlled study of haloperidol, pimozide, and placebo for the treatment of Gilles de la Tourette's syndrome. *Arch Gen Psychiatry* 46:722–730.

Shen, W.W. (1999a) A history of antipsychotic drug development. *Compr Psychiatry* 40:407–414.

Shen, W.W. (1999b) The metabolism of atypical antipsychotic drugs: an update. *Ann Clin Psychiatry* 11:145–158.

Shin, J.G., Soukhova, N., and Flockhart, D.A. (1999) Effect of antipsychotic drugs on human liver cytochrome P450 (CYP) isoforms in vitro: preferential inhibition of CYP2D6. *Drug Metab Dispos* 27:1078–1084.

Silva, R.R., Munoz, D.M., Alpert, M., Perlmutter, I.R., and Diaz, J. (1999) Neuroleptic malignant syndrome in children and adolescents. *J Am Acad Child Adolesc Psychiatry* 38:187–194.

Simpson, G.M. and Angus, J.W. (1970) A rating scale for extrapyramidal side effects. *Acta Psychiatr Scand Suppl* 212:11–19.

Spencer, E.K., and Campbell, M. (1994) Children with schizophrenia: diagnosis, phenomenology, and pharmacotherapy. *Schizophr Bull* 20:713–725.

Szigethy, E., Wiznitzer, M., Branicky, L.A., Maxwell, K., and Findling, R.L. (1999) Risperidone-induced hepatotoxicity in children and adolescents? A chart review study. *J Child Adolesc Psycho-pharmacol* 9:93–98.

Tandon, R. (1999) Cholinergic aspects of schizophrenia. *Br J Psychiatry* 174(Suppl 37):7–11.

Tecott, L.H., Sun, L.M., Akana, S.F., Strack, A.M., Lowenstein, D.H., Dallman, M.F., and Julius, D. (1995) Eating disorder and epilepsy in mice lacking 5-HT2c serotonin receptors. *Nature* 374: 542–546.

Ten Eick, A.P., Nakamura, H., and Reed, M.D. (1998) Drug-drug interactions in pediatric psychopharmacology. *Pediatr Clin North Am* 45:1233–1264.

von Bahr, C., Movin, G., Nordin, C., Liden, A., Hammarlund-Udenaes, M., Hedberg, A., Ring, H., and Sjoqvist, F. (1991) Plasma levels of thioridazine and metabolites are influenced by the debrisoquin hydroxylation phenotype. *Clin Pharmacol Ther* 49:234–240.

Welch, R. and Chue, P. (2000) Antipsychotic agents and QT changes. *J Psychiatry Neurosci* 25:154–160.

Wilson, J.M., Sanyal, S., and Van Tol, H.H.M. (1998) Dopamine D$_2$ and D$_4$ receptor ligands: relation to antipsychotic action. *Eur J Pharmacol* 351:273–286.

Wudarsky, M., Nicolson, R., Hamburger, S.D., Spechler, L., Gochman, P., Bedwell, J., Lenane, M.C., and Rapoport, J.L. (1999) Elevated prolactin in pediatric patients on typical and atypical antipsychotics. *J Child Adolesc Psychopharmacol* 9:239–245.

Zuddas, A. Ledda, M.G., Fratta, A., Muglia, P., and Cianchetti, C. (1996) Clinical effects of clozapine on autistic disorder [letter]. *Am J Psychiatry* 153:738.

27 | Anxiolytics: benzodiazepines, buspirone, and others

S H A N N O N   R .   B A R N E T T   A N D   M A R K   A .   R I D D L E

In the treatment of children and adolescents with anxiety disorders clinicians have a wide variety of pharmacologic options beyond the antidepressants (Shader and Greenblatt, 1995; Lydiard et al., 1996; Riddle et al., 1999). The benzodiazepines (BZs), with their favorable safety profile and quick onset of action, are attractive alternatives for the treatment of acute anxiety. While the clinical effectiveness of buspirone has not been proven in children, buspirone is used alone or in combination with other drugs in the treatment of anxiety disorders. The antihistamines are often used to treat insomnia and may reduce acute mild agitation. Zolpidem (Ambien) is occasionally used for its sedative properties. This chapter reviews the structure, proposed mechanisms of action, pharmacodynamic principles, and pharmacokinetic principles of these drugs.

BENZODIAZEPINES

History

During the early twentieth century the barbiturates were used in children and adolescents for their sedative and hypnotic effects; however, their safety profile and propensity to cause physical dependence led scientists in search of safer anxiolytics. The development of animal models of behavioral disorders facilitated the formulation of drugs with more specific central nervous system (CNS) effects. In 1959, chlordiazepoxide (Librium) was the first benzodiazepine (BZ) to receive a patent. It entered the market in 1960, followed by diazepam (Valium) in 1963. Today, over 35 BZs have been formulated and over 10 are available in the United States (Ballenger, 1995; Hobbs et al., 1996).

Mechanism of Action

Benzodiazepines are so named because of their core structure, a 2-amino-benzodiazepine 4-oxide, (a ben-

zene ring fused with a seven-membered 1,4 diazepine ring) (see Fig. 27.1; Ballenger, 1995; Chouinard et al., 1999). Most of the BZs include a 5-aryl substituent ring (a ring fusing R_1 and R_2, see Fig. 27.1). While all BZs have similar pharmacodynamic properties, the pharmacokinetic properties (i.e., rate of onset of action and duration of effect) differ among the BZs because each has different substituents on the diazepine ring, the benzene ring, and the 5-aryl substituent ring (Chouinard et al., 1999).

Major Effects

Benzodiazepines act throughout the CNS. Proposed relationships between site of action and effect include the following: spinal cord (muscle relaxation), brain stem (anticonvulsant effects), brain stem reticular formation (sedative effects), cerebellum (ataxia), and limbic and cortical areas (anxiolytic effects). Action outside the CNS is limited to coronary vasodilation with intravenous (IV) administration and neuromuscular blockade with very high doses of BZs.

Pharmacological Profile: Receptor Occupancy

The main action of BZs occurs at the γ-aminobuteric acid A (GABA$_A$) receptors. The GABA receptors have been classified into three subtypes, GABA$_A$, GABA$_B$, and GABA$_C$. The GABA$_B$ "slow" receptors are composed of seven transmembrane subunits that activate second messenger systems. GABA$_A$ and GABA$_C$ receptors mediate fast synaptic inhibition via transmitter-gated chloride ion channels (Chebib and Johnston, 1999). Each GABA$_A$ and GABA$_C$ receptor consists of five subunits with four transmembrane domains, which combine together to form a chloride channel (Chebib and Johnston, 1999).

GABA$_A$ receptors are activated by GABA, muscimol, and isoguvacine and are inhibited by bicuculline, ga-

A

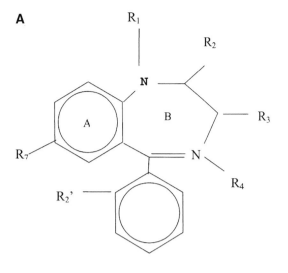

B

FIGURE 27.1. **A:** Benzodiazepine core structure. benzene ring; **B:** 1,4 diazepine ring. R_1 and R_2 often form a 5-aryl substituent.

bazine, and $(+) - \beta$-hydrastatin. Heterogeneity between $GABA_A$ receptors occurs when different subunit proteins combine to form different receptors. These subunit proteins have been classified into families according to their amino acid sequence. Identified subfamilies include six α, three β, three γ, one δ, one ε, one π, one θ and three ρ variants. Those receptors with a ρ subunit differ from other $GABA_A$ receptors because of their insensitivity to bicuculline and baclofen (Mehta and Ticku, 1999; Smith 2001). While the exact in vivo structure of the $GABA_A$ receptor is unknown, it is thought that complete BZ binding requires a γ subunit, but it is the α subunit that mediates the pharmacological effects. For example, receptors with α subunits 1, 2, 3, or 5 are sensitive to diazepam, whereas receptors with α subunit 4 or 6 are diazepam-insensitive (Hobbs et al., 1996; Smith 2001).

The BZ binding site of the $GABA_A$ receptors have been further classified into three types, ω_{1-3}, based on their location in the CNS and their ability to bind different compounds. A fourth type of BZ receptor, peripheral-type BZ receptors, occurs in the peripheral tissues as well as the CNS. The function of this type of receptor remains unknown (Lo et al., 1983; Ballenger, 1995).

The BZs predominately bind to ω_1 and ω_2 $GABA_A$ receptors. Type I (ω_1) $GABA_A$ receptors are concentrated in the cerebellum and cortical layers; they have a high affinity for triazolopyridazines and β-carbolines, and primarily occur on postsynaptic neurons. Type II (ω_2) receptors are also found in high numbers in the cortical layers, as well as in the hippocampus, striatum, and spinal cord. These receptors occur mainly on axons or terminals of the striatonigral pathways (Lo et al., 1983; Ballenger, 1995). The type III (ω_3) receptors are found mainly in the cerebellum and may play a role in alcohol-induced ataxia and incoordination (Luddens et al., 1990).

The main effects of BZs occur via positive allosteric modulation. The BZs and GABA bind to separate sites on the $GABA_A$ receptor complex. When a BZ occupies the BZ receptor, GABA's ability to open the chloride channels increases. With greater opening of the chloride channel, cellular excitability decreases (Ballenger, 1995). The final result of this decreased cellular excitability is widespread because of the extensive inhibitory role of GABA in the CNS. As a result, BZs may alter the turnover of neurotransmitters such as norepinephrine and serotonin (5-hydroxytryptamine [5-HT]).

While researchers believe that the GABAergic response is responsible for the major effects of the BZs, other mechanisms of action have been proposed. The BZs increase calcium-dependent potassium, inhibit tetrodotoxin-sensitive NA^+ channels, and antagonize cholecystokinin-induced excitation. The clinical relevance of these actions is unknown at this time (Polk, 1988; Hobbs et al., 1996).

Pharmacokinetics and Drug Disposition

Most BZs are completely absorbed from the gastrointestinal (GI) tract. The one exception is clorazepate, a pro-drug that undergoes acid hydrolysis in the stomach and is decarboxylated to form N-desmethyl-diazepam, which is then completely absorbed into the bloodstream (Bellantuono et al., 1980; Hobbs et al., 1996; Chouinard et al., 1999). In contrast, most BZs, with the exception of lorazepam and midazolam, are not consistently absorbed from intramuscular injection (Chouinard et al., 1999). Lorazepam is available as a sublingual form that reaches clinical effect at the same rate as an oral dose. In general, intravenous administration is used only for anesthesia or for the acute management of seizures. When BZs are given via this route, the onset of action is almost immediate (Chouinard et al., 1999).

The BZs are highly lipid-soluble, which not only allows them to cross the blood–brain barrier quickly but also leads to increased accumulation in obese people

(Ballenger, 1995). All of the BZs are highly bound to plasma proteins (Baldessarini, 1996; Hobbs et al., 1996).

Because all BZs are rapidly distributed to the brain, with oral dosing absorption is the rate-limiting step in the onset of action. Therefore, anything that slows gastric emptying (i.e., coadministration of an anticholinergic drug) will delay the onset of action (Chouinard et al., 1999). Diazepam and flurazepam are absorbed at a rapid rate, leading to a fast onset of action, which may lead to the feeling of a rush. In children diazepam may be absorbed in as few as 15–30 minutes. When compared to diazepam, other BZs have slower rates of absorption, and thus a slower onset of action (see Table 27.1; Lader, 1987; Baldessarini, 1996).

Because BZs are redistributed until over 95% of the drug is outside the blood circulation and the brain, it is the distribution half-life that is most important in determining the duration of action of each BZ. Unfortunately, it is the elimination half-life that is most studied and best known (see Table 27.1; Chouinard et al., 1999).

The BZs are all metabolized in the liver via the hepatic cytochrome P450 (CYP) enzymes through one or both of the following pathways: phase I oxidation and dealkylation, and/or phase II conjugation to glucuronides, sulfates, and acetylated compounds. Diazepam, chlordiazepoxide, and flurazepam all undergo both phase I and phase II metabolism. Lorazepam, lormetazepam, oxazepam, and temazepam are all metabolized by phase II alone and are better tolerated by patients with liver impairment.

Prazepam and flurazepam are almost completely converted to active metabolites before they reach the systemic circulation (Baldessarini, 1996). Other BZs are converted to active metabolites before excretion. *N*-desmethyl-diazepam (nordiazepam) is a metabolite of many BZs including diazepam, prazepam, ketazolam, and to a lesser extent, clordiazepoxide (see Table 27.1). Because nordiazepam has an elimination half-life of over 100 hours, this metabolite can accumulate over time to plasma levels that exceed those of the parent drug (Lader, 1987).

Knowing the structure of a particular BZ drug can help predict the metabolic pathway for that drug. For example, oxazepam, lorazepam, and temazepam are all 3-OH BZs and are directly conjugated (Chouinard et al., 1999). Temazepam is partly demethylated to oxazepam, but otherwise these drugs have no active metabolites (Bellantuono et al., 1980).

Clonazepam reaches a peak plasma level in 1 to 4 hours. It is metabolized by acetylation, so the half-life ranges from 20 to 80 hours and is dependent on whether a person has a rapid or slow acetylation phenotype (DeVane et al., 1991).

Choosing Among the Benzodiazepines

The drugs that have longer half-lives have the disadvantage of causing daytime drowsiness but the advantage of providing more consistent anxiolytic effects (Ballenger, 1995). Prazepam may cause less daytime drowsiness because desmethyldiazepam appears at a relatively slow rate (Greenblatt et al., 1983).

A long half-life is needed for a BZ to be effective as an anticonvulsant to avoid a withdrawal effect. Clonazepam, nitrazepam, and nordiazepam are the BZs most often used for their anticonvulsant effects, al-

TABLE 27.1 *Benzodiazepines*

Drug	Active Metabolites	Onset of Action[a]	Rate of Elimination[b]	Primary Metabolic Route
Triazolam (Halcion)	None	Short	Short	Hydroxylation
Alprazolam (Xanax)	None	Intermediate	Intermediate	Hydroxylation
Oxazepam (Serax)	None	Intermediate	Intermediate	Conjugation
Lorazepam (Ativan)	None	Intermediate	Intermediate	Conjugation
Clonazepam (Klonopin)	None	Intermediate	Long	Reduction, acetylated, and hydroxylated
Chlordiazepoxide (Librium)	Desmethyl-chlordiazepoxide Demoxepam Nordiazepam Oxazepam	Intermediate	Long	Phase I
Diazepam (Valium)	Nordiazepam	Fast	Long	Phase I

[a]Onset of action: short, <2 hours; intermediate, 1–3 hours; gradual, >3 hours.
[b]Rate of elimination: short, <6 hours; intermediate, 6–20 hours; long, >20 hours.

though patients may become tolerant to the anticonvulsant effect (Hobbs et al., 1996).

A short elimination half-life is desirable for the treatment of insomnia to minimize daytime sedation and unwanted cognitive effects. The disadvantages of BZs with short elimination half-lives include the increased severity of withdrawal symptoms with rapid discontinuation after chronic use (see below)(Hobbs et al., 1996).

Antianxiety agents, in contrast, should have a long half-life, although a long elimination half-life leads to drug accumulation and thus increases the risk of neuropsychological deficits (Hobbs et al., 1996).

Partial Benzodiazepine Agonists

Several partial BZ agonists have been described, including abecarnil, alpidem, bretazenil, and suriclone (Shader and Greenblatt, 1995). The potential advantage of a partial agonist is a comparable anxiolytic effect with less sedation. However, at this time there are limited data supporting advantages of the partial agonists. Preliminary studies have suggested that at low doses, abecarnil may have anxiolytic effects with low levels of sedation (Ballenger et al., 1991).

Drug–Drug Interactions

For most child psychiatrists, the drug interactions most frequently encountered are interactions with other psychotropics. Fluoxetine inhibits the CYP3A isozymes and thus increase the plasma concentration of the triazolobenzodiazepines (alprazolam, midazolam, and triazolam), causing increased psychomotor effects (Shader and Greenblatt, 1995). To avoid unwanted psychomotor effects, the dosage of alprazolam should be decreased when it is coadministered with fluoxetine (Chouinard et al., 1999). Nefazadone has also been shown to increase the pharmacodynamic effects of triazolam and, to a lesser extent, alprazolam (Chouinard et al., 1999).

Certain drugs interact with BZs by altering their absorption. In addition to adding to CNS depression, ethanol increases the rate of absorption of BZs (Hobbs et al., 1996). Conversely, antacids slow the absorption of BZs (Ballenger, 1995).

Cimetidine slows the metabolism of BZs. This slowing causes clinically significant increases in cognitive impairment when coadministerd with midazolam (Chouinard et al., 1999). Cimetidine increases the levels of diazepam and its metabolite, but no pharmacodynamic effects have been demonstrated (Greenblatt et al., 1984).

Like fluoxetine, erythromycin and other macrolides inhibit the CYP-3A isoenzyme and increase the levels and effects of the triazolobenzodiazepines (Shader and Greenblatt, 1995; Chouinard et al., 1999). Midazolam should be avoided or the dosage dropped by 50% in patients receiving erythromycin (Olkkola et al., 1993). Ketoconazole and itraconazole may also interact with triazolam and midazolam, and combinations of these drugs should be avoided (Varhe et al., 1994; Chouinard et al., 1999).

Tobacco and rifampin both induce hepatic enzymes, which may decrease the duration of action of the BZs. Grapefruit juice has received recent recognition as a factor in the pharmacokinetics of many drugs. Grapefruit juice slows down the GI absorption of midazolam and also decreases biotransformation, which leads to a delayed onset of effect and an increase in drowsiness (Ameer and Weintraub, 1997).

The BZs are not significant inducers of the hepatic enzymes, so the use of BZs does not alter the metabolism of the BZs or most other drugs (Chouinard et al., 1999). However, BZs have been shown to increase the half-life of digoxin (Ballenger, 1995).

Side Effects and Toxicity

The most common adverse event encountered with the BZs is sedation. The extent of sedation does not appear to differ among the BZs, although daytime drowsiness may occur more frequently with longer half-life agents as the concentration of these BZs and their metabolites gradually increases with chronic use (Greenblatt et al., 1983; Shader and Greenblatt, 1993).

Clinicians have taken advantage of the sedating effects of the BZs and used them to treat initial insomnia. However, while the reduction in sleep latency and decreased awakenings may be desirable, the BZs have other effects on sleep. There is an increase in the amount of stage 2 sleep, which leads to a longer period of sleep. There is a decreased time from the onset of spindle sleep to the first burst of rapid eye movement (REM) sleep. While the number of REM cycles increases, the cycles are shortened and the total time spent in REM sleep is decreased. The changes in sleep architecture do not appear to decrease the amount of restfulness people feel after sleeping with the aid of a BZ. Patients sometimes complain of more vivid dreams upon the onset of treatment with a BZ. In addition, discontinuation of a BZ is often followed by a period of increased REM sleep, known as *rebound*, which may be experienced as a brief period of vivid dreaming (Hobbs et al., 1996).

Adverse cognitive changes can occur with BZ use.

Anterograde amnesia is seen most commonly with IV administration of BZs, but, in a review of the literature, King (1992) concluded that all BZs have the ability to cause anterograde amnesia. The amnesia appears to be secondary to sedation, reduced attention, and reduced rehearsal. The BZs have been shown to impair the encoding of new information (Greenblatt et al., 1983; Ghoneim and Mewaldt, 1990). While child psychiatrists do not frequently encounter anterograde amnesia, the effects of the BZs on acquiring new information is relevant. Chronic use of BZs in children may adversely affect learning, although more research is required to fully understand the impact (Greenblatt et al., 1983; Ghoneim and Mewaldt, 1990). One study by Huron et al. (2002) suggests that the amount of sedation does not fully explain certain recall deficits.

Less frequently encountered side effects include reduced motor coordination, ataxia, increased reaction time, lightheadedness, vertigo, transient hypotension, lassitude, blurred vision, nausea and vomiting, epigastric distress, and drug fever (Finkle et al., 1979; Bellantuono et al., 1980; Greenblatt et al., 1983; Baldessarini, 1996; Hobbs et al., 1996). Rare side effects include failure to ovulate, impairment of sexual function, agranulocytosis, hepatic reactions, hallucinations, hypomanic behavior, paranoia, depression, suicidal ideation, and seizures in patients with epilepsy (Baldessarini, 1996; Hobbs et al., 1996).

Unless BZs are taken in combination with other drugs such as ethanol, the BZs do not appear to cause respiratory depression even at high doses. However, death can occur when BZs and ethanol are combined (Finkle et al., 1979; Hobbs et al., 1996).

In studies with children, BZs are usually well tolerated. Sedation is the most common side effect (Graae et al., 1994; AACAP, 1997). One child study with alprazolam found a decrease in cognitive efficiency in the placebo group but not in the alprazolam group (Simeon et al., 1992).

Behavioral disinhibition has been described in children taking BZs. In one case series of four children with epilepsy (ages 1.5, 4, 8, and 11 years) and no history of behavior problems, each child developed aggressive and agitated behavior on clonazepam. All four returned to baseline after discontinuation of clonazepam (Commander et al., 1991). Behavioral disinhibition has not been well studied, but the phenomenon appears to be rare (Rothschild et al., 2000). Because these drugs are sedating, clinical experience suggests that, like alcohol, any disinhibition can be overcome by increasing the dosage. Psychotic symptoms are another rare side effect in children and adolescents (AACAP, 1997).

Clinical Use in Children and Adolescents

While the BZs have been used to treat anxiety and insomnia in children, the data supporting this use are minimal (Simeon et al., 1992; Graae et al., 1994). However, multiple studies with adults demonstrate that the BZs are effective at relieving insomnia and anxiety. In children, BZs have a Federal Drug Administration (FDA)-approved indication for preanesthetic use only. However, because of their mild adverse effects, low toxicity, and long history of use, the BZs may be used effectively in children at the time of an acute stressor or before medical procedures. They may also be used for acute symptomatic relief in the treatment of anxiety disorders; however, long-term use is not generally recommended because of the potential to develop physical tolerance toward BZs as well as their sedative effects and ability to interfere with memory and learning. Long-term use may be indicated when the BZs are used in adolescents with schizophrenia, to treat patients with catatonia, and when used as an adjunctive treatment for obsessive-compulsive disorder and mania.

Pretreatment Considerations

No additional work-up, apart from what is indicated by the history and physical examination, is needed before starting BZs. However, because of the rare occurrence of disinhibition, it is important to carefully document behavior patterns for future comparison before starting a BZ (Commander et al., 1991). In the treatment of anxiety, multiple daily doses are recommended to maximize effects and minimize sedation and withdrawal. This recommendation holds true even for BZs with relatively long half-lives (Baldessarini, 1996).

Long-term Considerations

Long-term use is not recommended in most children and adolescents, but when it does occur, patients may develop tolerance to many of the side effects, particularly sedation. Tolerance does not appear to develop toward the anxiolytic effects, and the vast majority of patients do not require escalating doses once a therapeutic effect is found (Lader, 1987; Hobbs et al., 1996).

With BZ use there is no correlation between plasma level and therapeutic response or side effects, the possible exception being alprazolam. Even with alprazolam the therapeutic window of 20 to 40 ng/mL was found at 3 weeks, but had disappeared by week 8 (Greenblatt et al., 1993). Drug levels may be used when clarifying whether symptoms represent continued anxiety or, conversely, are due to side effects. Plasma levels can be helpful in determining whether a particular patient is a rapid metabolizer (Lydiard et al., 1996), although this measure is not often used in clinical practice. Suggested target levels in adults are as follows: diazepam + desmethyldiazepam, 300 to 1000 ng/mL; desmethyldiazepam alone, 600 to 1500 ng/mL; and lorazepam, 20 to 80 ng/mL (Greenblatt et al., 1993; Shader and Greenblatt, 1993).

Discontinuation

Patients usually develop physiologic dependence within the first 3 to 4 months of chronic BZ use. These patients may undergo a true withdrawal syndrome when the medication is discontinued. Symptoms occurring after discontinuation can be divided into three categories: a return of the original symptoms, a rebound effect, that includes several days when the original symptoms occur at a more severe intensity, and symptoms of physiologic withdrawal (Salzman, 1990). Common withdrawal symptoms include insomnia, trembling, sweating, palpitations, dry mouth, and hot and cold flashes. Psychiatric symptoms include anxiety, depression, and feelings of derealization. Perceptual disturbances occur infrequently, but may include a feeling of motion, strange smells, and a metallic taste. Rarely patients may develop withdrawal seizures and paranoia (Lader, 1987).

A withdrawal syndrome can occur even when the BZ was used in a therapeutic dose range (Baldessarini, 1996; Hobbs et al., 1996). Withdrawal symptoms are less severe when the BZ is tapered gradually, but patients should be educated that withdrawal symptoms are possible even with a gradual taper (Lader, 1987). When the taper is relatively fast, there is a benefit to using a BZ with a longer half-life, but with a long and gradual taper, factors such as half-life, daily dose, and years of therapy do not correlate with the degree of withdrawal symptoms (Rickels et al., 1990).

BUSPIRONE

History

Buspirone was developed in the late 1960s with the intent of developing a better neuroleptic. Clinical trials demonstrated little antipsychotic effects; however, animal models suggested some anxiolytic effects. The drug was marketed as an anxiolytic in 1986 (Cole and Yonkers, 1995; Baldessarini, 1996).

Mechanism of Action

The structure of buspirone is presented in Figure 27.2. Buspirone is the only azaspirone on the market. Other

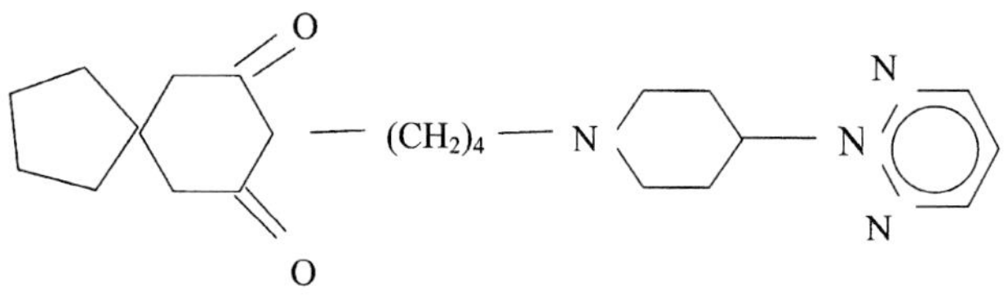

FIGURE 27.2. Structure of buspirone.

azaspirones include gepirone, ipsapione, and tandospirone. All four have serotonergic effects, but only buspirone has dopaminergic effects (Cole and Yonkers, 1995).

Pharmacologic Profile: Receptor Occupancy

Buspirone acts as an agonist of somatodendritic 5-HT$_{1A}$ autoreceptors, and has variable antagonistic effects on postsynaptic 5-HT$_{1A}$ receptors (Jann, 1988; Baldessarini, 1996; Chouinard et al., 1999). It also causes down-regulation of 5-HT$_2$ receptors (Cole and Yonkers, 1995).

In addition to the effects on seretonin, buspirone demonstrates moderate affinity for presynaptic dopamine D$_2$ receptors (Hiner et al., 1988; Hardman et al., 1996; Chouinard et al., 1999). The effect on the D$_2$ receptors allows buspirone to reverse neuroleptic-induced catalepsy (Cole and Yonkers, 1995; Baldessarini, 1996). The clinical significance of the action of buspirone on the D$_2$ autoreceptors is unknown (Jann, 1988).

All azapirones increase the turnover of both cerebral dopamine and norepinephrin. At high doses they cause a mild elevation of prolactin (Baldessarini, 1996). However, in humans, doses of 30 mg/day for 28 days led to no changes in the levels of prolactin, growth hormone, or cortisol (Jann, 1988)

Buspirone does not appear to have a major effect on the BZ–GABA–chloride ionophore complex and, if anything, has some antagonistic interactions with GABAergic transmission (although it does not induce seizures) (Jann, 1988; Baldessarini, 1996). The lack of GABAergic effects is evident in the fact that buspirone does not consistently cause sedation, it is not a muscle relaxant, it is not an anticonvulsant, and it does not relieve BZ withdrawal (Jann, 1988; Cole and Yonkers, 1995).

Buspirone does not affect either monoamine oxidase A (MAO-A) or MAO-B (Jann, 1988; Cole and Yonkers, 1995). There is also no evidence of action on the adenosine, cholinergic (mucarinic), glutamate, glycine, histamine, or opiate systems (Jann, 1988).

Pharmacokinetics and Drug Disposition

While buspirone is almost completely absorbed within 1 hour of oral administration, the oral bioavailability is reduced because of substantial first-pass metabolism (Mayol et al., 1985; Gammans et al., 1986; Jann, 1988; Chouinard et al., 1999; Mahmood and Sahajwalla, 1999). The peak plasma level of buspirone is higher in children when compared to adults (Salazar et al., 2001). Throughout the therapeutic dosing range, first-pass metabolism increases with escalation of dosage (Gammans et al., 1986). Although absorption does not change when buspirone is administered with food, first-pass metabolism is decreased, improving the oral bioavailability (Gammans et al., 1986; Jann, 1988). Once buspirone reaches the systemic circulation, it is highly protein bound (>95%) (Jann, 1988; Baldessarini, 1996; Chouinard et al., 1999).

The half-life of buspirone in healthy volunteers is 1 to 11 hours (Cole and Yonkers, 1995; Chouinard et al., 1999). Buspirone is metabolized mainly by hydroxylation to 6'OH-buspirone and by N-dealkylation to 1-pyrimidinylpiperaxine (1-PP) (Jajoo et al., 1989). There are at least seven major and five minor metabolites (Jajoo et al., 1989; Chouinard et al., 1999).

About 40% metabolism results in the formation of 1-PP (Jajoo et al., 1989). Effects of 1-PP include blocking α_{-2}-noradrenergic receptors and causing an increase in 3-methoxy-4-phenylglycol (MHPG). There are no apparent serotonergic effects (Baldessarini, 1996). There is speculation that the noradrenergic effects of 1-PP may decrease buspirone's effectiveness in the treatment of BZ withdrawal and panic attacks. If this hypothesis holds true, one would expect greater efficacy for panic attacks and BZ withdrawal with the other aspirones, none of which form 1-PP (Cole and Yonkers, 1995). An extended release preparation of buspirone has been developed that, when compared to the immediate release form, appears to have a higher bioavailability and a higher buspirone to 1-PP ratio (Sakr and Andheria, 2001).

Metabolism and clearance of buspirone is decreased with hepatic cirrhosis and renal disease (Gammans et al., 1986).

Drug Interactions

Some data suggest that buspirone increases the desmethyldiazepam metabolite of diazepam (Cole and Yonkers, 1995), although not all data support this finding (Gammans et al., 1986). Buspirone may also increase levels of haloperidol and cyclosporin-A (Cole and Yonkers, 1995).

The actions of buspirone may interact with other psychotropics. For example, there is a mild increase in blood pressure when buspirone is given with MAO inhibitors, although experts do not prohibit using this combination. There are no known cases of serotonergic syndrome with buspirone and the selective serotonin reuptake inhibitors (SSRIs) (Cole and Yonkers, 1995). Buspirone may worsen symptoms of withdrawal from benzodiazepines by facilitation of central adrenergic action (Baldessarini, 1996). Buspirone may reduce SSRI-induced sexual dysfunction (Cole and Yonkers, 1995).

Verapamil, diltiazem, erythromycin, and itraconazole all increase the plasma concentration of buspirone. The plasma concentration is decreased almost 10-fold by rifampicin. Grapefruit juice increases the overall subjective effect of the drug (Mahmood and Sahajwalla, 1999).

Side Effects and Toxicity

The most common adverse events associated with buspirone use include dizziness, headache, nausea, nervousness, lightheadedness, and agitation. These adverse effects decrease over time. Buspirone does not cause seizures or abnormal involuntary movements or impair psychomotor performance.

Most studies of buspirone in children report only mild side effects, including headache, nausea, lightheadedness, dizziness, sedation dyspepsia, and asthenia, all of which usually remit within 1 week (Kranzler, 1988; Zwier and Rao, 1994; Pfeffer et al., 1997; Riddle et al., 1999, Salazar et al., 2001). A study by Pfeffer et al. (1997) of 19 children found no significant change in pulse, blood pressure, respiration, temperature, electrocardiogram (EKG), or electroencephalogram (EEG). However, of the 25 patients who began this open-label study, 4 developed an increase in aggression and agitation and 2 developed what was termed "euphoric mania," which consisted of euphoric mood, increased impulsivity, and out-of-control behavior, all of which improved with the addition of a mood stabilizer.

Uses in Children and Adolescents

While some anecdotal evidence has suggested possible benefit from buspirone in children (Zwier and Rao, 1994), in the study by Pfeffer (1997), only 3 of the 19 children who completed the study continued on buspirone after the study. The benefits of buspirone in children with anxiety disorders continue to be unproven. However, open-label studies have demonstrated reductions in anxiety in children with pervasive developmental disorders (Buitelaar et al., 1998).

Pretreatment Considerations

No particular work-up is required before starting a child on buspirone. If liver disease is suspected, a serum level of alkaline phosphate can be obtained because decreases in clearance are directly correlated with increases in alkaline phosphate (Gammans et al., 1986).

Discontinuation

Buspirone is not associated with any withdrawal syndrome. Little is known about discontinuing the dosage, but a conservative approach would include a brief taper.

ANTIHISTAMINES

History

Bovet and Staub first described agents that block histamine with the discovery that these agents provide protection against anaphylactic shock. Pyrilamine maleate was described as a specific and effective histamine antagonist in 1944. Diphenhydramine and tripelennamine soon followed (Babe and Serafin, 1996).

Mechanism of Action

The antihistamines act as competitive inhibitors of histamine at the H_1 receptors. Diphenhydramine is an ethanolamine and hydroxyzine hydrochloride and hydroxyzine pamoate are both piperidines (Peggs et al., 1995). The structures of antihistamines resemble histamine in that many H_1 blockers contain a substituted ethylamine moity, C-C-N<. The H_1 antagonists differ from histamine by replacing the primary amino group and single aromatic ring with a tertiary amino group linked by a two- or three-atom chain to two aromatic substituents (Babe and Serafin, 1996).

The first generation H_1 blockers (including diphenhydramine and hydroxyzine) cross the blood–brain barrier. Subsequent generations of antihistamines have been developed so that they do not cross the blood–brain barrier, and therefore are not effective as sedatives or anxiolytics.

Pharmacological Profile

In medicine and pediatrics, the H_1 antagonists are most commonly used for their effects outside the CNS. Outside the CNS they act by blocking the H_1 receptors, leading to the inhibition of the following effects of histamine: smooth muscle contraction; vasoconstriction and, to a lesser degree, the vasodilator effects on en-

dothelial cells; increased capillary permeability and the formation of the edema and wheel; and the itch caused by intradermal injection of histamine. They do not block histamine-mediated gastric secretion. The first-generation H_1 antagonists also block the muscarinic receptors (Babe and Serafin, 1996).

Central Nervous System Effects

In the CNS, the histamine blockade leads to diminished alertness, slowed reaction times, and somnolence. The antihistamines should only be used as sedatives for a brief period of time because most people develop tolerance to the sedative properties within 1 week (Peggs et al., 1995). Occasionally a patient may become restless, nervous, and develop insomnia.

The antihistamines also decrease motion sickness, which is thought to be secondary to anticholinergic effects (Babe and Serafin, 1996).

Pharmacokinetics and Drug Disposition

The first-generation antihistamines include diphenhydramine and hydroxyzine. They are both well absorbed from the GI tract, and peak plasma concentrations occur within 2 to 3 hours.

The H_1 antagonists are metabolized in the liver, and the metabolites are excreted in the urine. Diphenhydramine is mainly metabolized via N-demethylation, and its primary metbolite is monodesmethyldiphenhydramine (Scavone et al., 1998). These agents are able to induce hepatic microsomal enzymes and may increase the rate of their own metabolism. The half-life of diphenhydramine is approximately 4 hours. In general, the half-life is decreased in children and increased in patients with severe liver disease (Babe and Serafin, 1996).

Drug Interactions

In vitro, diphenhydramine inhibits CYP2D6 and therefore may interact with beta-blockers, some antidepressants such as desipramine, and antipsychotics such as promethazine. In a study by Hamelin et al. (2000), diphenhydramine was found to inhibit the metabolism of metoprolol in phenotypically extensive metabolizers, but not in poor metabolizers. The effects where observed clinically as well as pharmacokinetically.

Side Effects and Toxicity

The most common side effects include sedation, dizziness, tinnitus, lassitude, incoordination, fatique, blurred vision, diplopia, euphoria, nervousness, insomnia, nausea, vomiting, constipation, diarrhea, and tremor. Anticholinergic effects include dry mouth and respiratory passages, cough, urinary retention, and dysuria. Some patients experience loss of appetite while others have an increased appetite and weight gain (Babe and Serafin, 1996). The sedating effects of the first generation antihistamines may impair learning, although a study by Bender et al. (2001) found that chronic use of diphenhydramine for the treatment of allergies did not impair childrens' ability to acquire new information.

In overdose, the antihistamines cause convulsions, hallucinations, excitement, ataxia, incoordination, and athetosis. On exam patients may exhibit fixed, dilated pupils with a flushed face, sinus tachycardia, urinary retention, dry mouth, and fever. At high doses the patient can become comatose, which is often followed by cardiorespiratory collapse and death within 2 to 18 hours (Babe and Serafin, 1996). Treatment of overdose is mainly supportive, with efforts to manage the anticolinergic effects.

Uses in Children and Adolescents

Antihistamines have been used for several decades in the treatment of anxiety in children (Lader, 1988). Prescription data show that antihistamines are widely used in pediatric psychiatric practices (Zito et al., 2000). Diphenhydramine and hydroxyzine have been reported to modify anxiety symptoms in children with various psychiatric disorders. They are mainly used as a sedative in patients with insomnia. Occasionally they are used for mild acute agitation (AACAP, 1997).

ZOLPIDEM (AMBIEN)

Zolpidem is an imidazopyridine, with a chemical structure of N,N,6-trimethyl-2-(4-methylphenyl)-imidazo[1,2-alpha]-pyridine-3-acetamine hemitartrate (Salva and Costa, 1995). This nonbenzodiazepine sedative hypnotic was first released in Europe, and then introduced in the United States in 1993 (Hobbs et al., 1996). Zolpidem has a strong sedative effect that seems to preclude its use as an anxiolytic. It has only weak anticonvulsant effects (Salva and Costa, 1995; Hobbs et al., 1996).

Zolpidem interacts with ω_1 BZ receptors, but only exhibits weak binding to the ω_2 and ω_3 subtypes. Like the BZs, zolpidem appears to potentiate GABAergic transmission (Lantry and Benfield, 1990; Salva and Costa, 1995).

Zolpidem is rapidly absorbed from the GI tract, and after first-pass metabolism has an oral bioavailability of approximately 70%. The oral bioavailivity is decreased when zolpidem is administered with food (Salva and Costa, 1995; Hobbs et al., 1996).

Zolpidem is almost fully metabolized in the liver via oxidation and hydroxylation mainly through CYP3A but also through CYP2D6. There are three major metabolites, all of which appear to be inactive. The elimination half-life of zolpidem ranges from 1.5 to 3.2 hours. The pharmacokinetics of zolpidem are not altered with chronic daily administration. The rate of clearance in children is three times faster (leading to a decrease in blood level) than that in young adults (Salva and Costa, 1995; Greenblatt et al., 1998b).

Zolpidem reaches peak plasma concentrations between 0.75 and 2.6 hours after a dose. In the plasma, it is approximately 92% protein bound. The drug is slightly lipophilic, leading to higher concentrations in glandular tissues and fats, and lower concentrations in the CNS (Salva and Costa, 1995).

Because zolpidem is metabolized by CYP3A, elimination may be slowed by inhibitors of CYP3A. A study by Greenblatt et al. (1998b), demonstrated that ketoconazole, but not itraconazole or fluconazol, impairs clearance of zolpidem to an extent that it has clinical effects. The clinical use of zolpidem is reserved mainly for its sedative effects. Zolpidem reduces sleep latency and prolongs total sleep time in patients with insomnia without exhibiting much effect on the sleep architecture of normal subjects. In addition, after short-term use, there is no rebound insomnia or other withdrawal reactions. Finally, tolerance does not appear to develop toward the sedating effects (Lantry and Benfield, 1990; Salva and Costa, 1995; Hobbs et al., 1996) although there have been four case reports of zolpidem dependence (Madrak and Rosenberg, 2001).

The most frequent side effects with zolpidem include dizziness, lightheadedness, somnolence, headache, and GI upset. The rates of daytime sedation and amnesia are low. There may be some anterograde amnesia when administered as a preanesthetic, but when given for nighttime sedation, there are usually no morning memory deficits (Lantry and Benfield, 1990; Salva and Costa, 1995; Hobbs et al., 1996). However, a study by Greenblatt et al. (1998a) demonstrated impaired initial learning 1½ hours after administration and impaired free recall 24 hours after dosing. Relearning at 24 hours post-dose was not affected (Greenblatt et al., 1998a).

In a study of 12 children ages 8–13, only 1 reported an adverse event, which was limited to 5 minutes of a not unpleasant feeling of movement, "as if swinging in a hammock" (Colle et al., 1991). This same study found no observed effects on nocturnal growth hormone secretion in these children, all of whom had short stature.

Clinicians should be aware of a few drug interactions with zolpidem. Flumazenil acts as an antagonist to the hypnotic effects of zolpidem. There is decreased alertness when zolpidem is combined with cimetidine. There is an increase in anterograde amnesia in volunteers treated with a combination of imipramine and zolpidem. Haloperidol, ranitidine, chlorpromazine, warfarin, and digoxin, along with cimetidine and flumazenil, do not alter the pharmacokinetics of zolpidem (Salva and Costa, 1995).

FUTURE DIRECTIONS

Zaleplon (Sonata) is a new medication that, like zolpidem, appears to act only at the ω_1 BZ site on the GABA receptor. It is absorbed and eliminated at a quicker rate than that of zolpidem (Greenblatt et al., 1998a). Early studies suggest that there is no residual sedation 5 hours after a dose is given (Walsh et al., 2000), and no significant changes in slow wave sleep (Noguchi et al., 2002).

The 2,3-benzodiazepines, tofisopam, girisopam, and nerisopam, form a second category of potential anxiolytics currently under investigation. These BZs appear to exert actions only in the basal ganglion. These agents may act in part by interaction with the opiod signal transduction. Preliminary data suggest that these agents may have anxiolytic activities with less sedation (Horvath et al., 2000). Agents that target specific alpha subunits, leading to an anxiolytic response without sedation, are in the early stages of development (Mohler et al., 2002). Antagonists of corticotropin-releasing hormone type 1 receptors are gaining interest because of their ability to block symptoms of anxiety, including behavioral, neuroendocrine, and autonomic responces, in both rats and primates who have been placed in anxiogenic situations (Habib et al., 2000; Spina et al., 2000). Also, a glutamate antagonist that is selective at the mGlu5 receptor, MPEP, demonstrates anxiolytic properties (Tatarczynska et al., 2001).

ACKNOWLEDGMENTS
We thank Raymond C. Love, Pharm.D., for his excellent feedback and David Barnett and Dorothy Barnett for their help drawing Figures 27.1 and 27.2.

REFERENCES

AACAP (American Academy of Child and Adolescent Psychiatry) (1997) Practice parameters for the assessment and treatment of children and adolescents with anxiety disorders. *J Am Acad Child Adolesc Psychiatry* 36:69S–84S.

Ameer, B. and Weintraub, R.A. (1997) Drug interactions with grapefruit juice. *Clin Pharmacokinet* 33:103–121.

Babe, K.S.J. and Serafin, W.E. (1996) Histamine, bradykinin, and their antagonists. In: Hardman, J.G., Limbird, L.E., Molinoff, P.B., Ruddon, R.W., and Gilman, A.G., eds. *Goodman and Gillman's The Pharmacological Basis of Therapeutics*, 9th ed. New York: McGraw-Hill, pp. 581–600.

Baldessarini, R.J. (1996) Drugs and the treatment of psychiatric disorders. In: Hardman, J.G., Limbird L.E., Molinoff P.B., Ruddon R.W., and Gilman A.G., eds. *Goodman and Gilman's The Pharmacological Basis of Therapeutics*, 9th ed. New York: McGraw-Hill, pp. 399–430.

Ballenger, J.C. (1995) Benzodiazepines. In: Schatzberg, A.F. and Nemeroff, C.B., eds. *The American Psychiatric Press Textbook of Psychopharmacology*, 1st ed. Washington, DC: American Psychiatric Press, pp. 215–230.

Ballenger, J.C., McDonald, S., Noyes, R., Rickels, K., Sussman, N., Woods, S., Patin, J., and Singer, J. (1991) The first double-blind, placebo-controlled trial of a partial benzodiazepine agonist abecarnil (ZK 112–119) in generalized anxiety disorder. *Psychopharmacol Bull* 27:171–179.

Bellantuono, C., Reggi, V., Tognoni, G., and Garattini, S. (1980) Benzodiazepines: clinical pharmacology and therapeutic use. *Drugs* 19:195–219

Bender, B.G., McCormick, D.R., and Milgrom, H. (2001) Children's school performance is not impaired by short-term administration of diphenhydramine or loratadine. *J Pediatr* 138:656–660.

Buitelaar, J.K., van der Gaag, R.J., and van der Hoeven, J. (1998) Buspirone in the management of anxiety and irritability in children with pervasive developmental disorder: results of an open-label study. *J Clin Psychiatry* 59:56–59.

Chebib, M. and Johnston G.A. (1999) The 'ABC' of GABA receptors: a brief review. *Clin Exp Pharmacol Physiol* 26:937–940.

Chouinard, G., Lefko-Singh, K., and Teboul, E. (1999) Metabolism of anxiolytics and hypnotics: benzodiazepines, buspirone, zoplicone, and zolpidem. *Cell Mol Neurobiol* 19:533–552.

Cole, J.O. and Yonkers, K.A. (1995) Nonbenzodiazepine anxiolytics. In: Schatzberg, A.F. and Nemeroff, C.B., eds. *The American Psychiatric Press Textbook of Psychopharmacology*. Washington, DC: American Psychiatric Press, pp. 231–244.

Colle, M., Rosenzweig, P., Bianchetti, G., Fuseau, E., Ruffie, A., Ruedas, E., and Morselli, P.L. (1991) Nocturnal profile of growth hormone secretion during sleep induced by zolpidem: a double-blind study in young adults and children. *Horm Res* 35:30–34.

Commander, M., Green, S.H., and Prendergast, M. (1991) Behavioral disturbances in children treated with clonazepam SIR [letter to the editor]. *Dev Med Child neurol* 33:362–363.

DeVane, C.L., Ware, M.R., and Lydiard, R.B. (1991) Pharmacokinetics, pharmacodynamics, and treatment issues of benzodiazepines: alprazolam, adinazolam, and clonazepam. *Psychopharmacol Bull* 27:463–473.

Finkle, B.S., McCloskey, K.L., and Goodman L.S. (1979) Diazepam and drug-associated deaths: a survey in the United States and Canada. *JAMA* 242:429–434.

Friedman, R. (1991) Possible induction of psychosis by buspirone [letter to the editor]. *Am J Psychiatry* 148:1606.

Gammans, R.E., Mayol, R.F., and Labudde, J.A. (1986) Metabolixm and disposition of buspirone. *Am J Med* 80:41–51.

Ghoneim, M.M. and Mewaldt, S.P. (1990) Benzodiazepines and human memory: a review. *Anesthsiology* 72:926–938.

Graae, F., Milner, J., Rizzotto, L., and Klein, R. (1994) Clonazepam in childhood anxiety disorders. *J Am Acad Child Adolesc Psychiatry* 33:372–376.

Greenblatt, D.J., Abernethy, D.R., Morse, D.S., Harmatz, J.S., and Shader, R.I. (1984) Clinical importance of the interaction of diazepam and cimetidine. *N Engl J Med* 310:1639–1643.

Greenblatt, D.J., Harmatz, J.S., and Shader, R.I. (1993) Plasma alprazolam concentrations: relation to efficacy and side effects in the treatment of panic disorder. *Arch Gen Psychiatry* 50:715–722.

Greenblatt, D.J., Harmatz, J.S., von Moltke, L.L., Ehrenberg, B.L., Harrel, L., Corbett, K., Counihan, M., Graf, J.A., Darwish, M., Mertzanis, P., Martin, P.T., and Cevallos, W.H. (1998a) Comparative kinetics and dynamics of zaleplon, zolpidem, and placebo. *Clin Pharmacol Ther* 64:553–61.

Greenblatt, D.J., Shader, R.I., and Abernethy, D.R. (1983) Drug therapy: current status of benzodiazepines (second of two parts). *N Engl J Med* 309:410–416.

Greenblatt, D.J., von Moltke, L.L., Harmatz, J.S., Mertzais, P., Graf, J.A., Durol, A.L., Counihan, M., Roth-Schechter, B., and Shader, R.I. (1998b) Kinetic and dynamic interaction study of zolpidem with ketoconazole, itraconazole, and fluconazole. *Clin Pharmacol Ther* 64:661–671.

Habib, K.E., Weld, K.P., Rice, K.C., Pushkas, J., Champoux, M., Listwak, S., Webster, E.L., Atkinson, A.J., Schulkin, J., Contoreggi, C., Chrousos, G.P., McCann, S.M., Suomi, S.J., Higley, J.D., and Gold, P.W. (2000) Oral administration of a corticotropin-releasing hormone receptor antagonist significantly attenuates behavioral, neruoendocrine, and autonomic responses to stress in primates. *Proc Natl Acad Sci USA* 97:6079–6084.

Hamelin, B.A., Bouayad, A., Methot, J., Jobin, J., Desgagnes, P., Poirier, P., Allaire, J., Dumesnil, J., and Turgeon, J. (2000) Significant interaction between the nonprescription antihistamine diphenhydramine and the CYP2D6 substrate metoprolol in healthy men with high or low CYP2D6 activity. *Clin Pharmacol Ther* 67:466–477.

Hardman, J.G., Limbird, L.E., Molinoff, P.B., Ruddon, R.W., and Gilman, A.G., eds. (1996) *Goddman & Gilman's The Pharmacolgical Basis of Therapeutics, 9th ed.* New York: McGraw-Hill.

Hiner, B.C., Mauk, M.D., Peroutka, S.J., and Kocsis, J.D. (1988) Buspirone, 8-OH-DPAT and ipsapirone: effects on hippocampal cerebellar and sciatic fiber excitability. *Brain Res* 461:1–9.

Hobbs, W.R., Rall, T.W., and Verdoorn, T.A. (1996) Hypnotics and sedatives; ethanol. In: Hardman, J.G., Limbird, L.E., Molinoff, P.B., Ruddon, R.W., and Gilman, A.G., eds. *Goodman & Gillman's The Pharmacological Basis of Therapeutics*, 9th ed. New York: McGraw-Hill, pp. 361–396.

Horvath, E.J., Horvath, K., Hamori, T., Fekete, M.I., Solyom, S., and Palkovits, M. (2000) Anxiolytic 2,3-benzodiazepines, their specific binding to the basal ganglia. *Prog Neurobiol* 60:309–342.

Huron, C., Giersch, A., and Danion, J.M. (2002) Lorazepam, sedation, and conscious recollection: a dose-response study with healthy volunteers. *Int Clin Psychopharmacol* 17:19–26.

Jajoo, H.K., Mayol, R.F., Labudde, J.A., and Blair, I.A. (1989) Metabolism of the antianxiety drug buspirone in human subjects. *Drug Metab Dispos* 17:634–640.

Jann, M.W. (1988) Buspirone: an update on a unique anxiolytic agent. *Pharmacotherapy* 8:100–16.

King, D.J. (1992) Benzodiazepines, amnesia and sedation: theoretical and clinical issues and controversies. *Hum Psychopharmacol* 7:79–87.

Kranzler, H.R. (1988) Use of buspirone in an adolescent with overanxious disorder. *J Am Acad Child Adolesc Psychiatry* 27:789–790.

Lader, M. (1987) Clinical pharmacology of benzodiazepines. *Annu Rev Med* 38:19–28.

Lader, M. (1988) Clinical pharmacology of non-benzodiazepine anxiolytics. *Pharmacol Biochem Behav* 29:797–798.

Lantry, H.D. and Benfield, P. (1990) Zolpidem. A review of its pharmacodynamic and pharmacokinetic properties and therapeutic potential. *Drugs* 40:291–213.

Lo, M.M.S., Niehoff, D.L., Kuhar, M.J., and Snyder, S.H. (1983) Differential localization of type I and type II benzodizepine binding sites in substantia nigra. *Nature* 306:57–60.

Luddens, H., Pritchett, D.B., Kohler, M., Killisch, I., Keinanen, K., Monyer, H., Sprengel, R., and Seeburg, P.H. (1990) Cerebellar GABA$_A$ receptor selective for a behavioural alcohol antagonist. *Nature* 346:648–651.

Lydiard, R.B., Brawman-Mintzer, O., and Ballenger, J.C. (1996) Recent developments in the psychopharmacology of anxiety disorders. *J Consult Clin Psychol* 64:660–668.

Madrak, L.N. and Rosenberg, M. (2001) Zolpidem abuse. *Am J Psychiatry* 158:1330–1331.

Mahmood, I. and Sahajwalla, C. (1999) Clinical pharmacokinetics and pharmacodynamics of buspirone, an anxiolytic drug. *Clin Pharmacokinet* 36:277–287.

Mayol, R.F., Adamson, D.S., Gammans, R.E., and LaBudde, J.A. (1985) Pharmacokinetics and disposition of 14C-buspirone HCl after intravenous and oral dosing in man. *Clin Pharmacol Ther* 37:210.

Mehta, A.K. and Ticku, M.K. (1999) An update on GABA$_A$ receptors. *Brain Res Brain Res Rev* 29:196–217.

Mohler, H., Fritschy, J.M., and Rudolph, U. (2002) A new benzodiazepine pharmacology. *J. Pharmacol Exp Ther* 300:2–8.

Noguchi, H., Kitazumi, K., Mori, M., and Shiba, T. (2002) Binding and neuropharmacological profile of zaleplon, a novel nonbenzodiazepine sedative/hypnotic. *Eur J Pharmacol* 434:21–8.

Olkkola, K.T., Aranko, K., Luurila, H., Hiller, A., Saarnivaara, L., Jaakko-Juhani, H., and Neuvonen, P.J. (1993) A potentially hazardous interaction between erythromycin and midazolam. *Clin Pharmacol Ther* 53:298–305.

Peggs, J.F., Shimp, L.A., and Opdycke, R.A. (1995) Antihistamines: the old and the new. *Am Fam Physician* 52:593–600.

Pfeffer, C.R., Jiang H., and Domeshek, L.J. (1997) Buspirone treatment of psychiatrically hospitalized prepubertal children with symptoms of anxiety and moderately severe aggression. *J Child Adolesc Psychopharmacol* 7:145–155.

Polk, P. (1988) Electrophysiology of benzodazepine receptor ligands: multiple mechanisms and sites of action. *Prog Neurobiol* 31:349–423.

Rickels, K., Case, W.G., Schweizer, E., Garcia-Espana, F., and Fridman, R. (1990) Benzodiazepine dependence: management of discontinuation. *Psychopharmacol Bull* 26:63–68.

Riddle, M.A., Bernstein, G.A., Cook, E.H., Leonard, H.L., March, J.S., and Swanson, J.M. (1999) Anxiolytics, adrenergic agents, and naltrexone. *J Am Acad Child Adolesc Psychiatry* 38:546–556.

Rothschild, A.J., Shindul-Rothschild, V.A., Murray, M., and Brewster, S. (2000) Comparison of the frequency of behavioral disinhibition on alprazolam, clonazepam, or no benzodiazepine in hospitalized psychiatric patients. *J Clin Psychopharmacol* 20:7–11.

Sakr, A. and Andheria, M. (2001) A comparative multidose pharmacokinetic study of buspirone extended-release tablets with a reference immediate-release product. *J Clin Pharmacol* 41:886–894.

Salazar, D.E., Frackiewicz, E.J., Dockens, R., Kollia, G., Fulmor, I.E.,

Tigel, P.D., Uderman, H.D., Shiovitz, T.M., Sramek, J.J., and Cutler, N.R. (2001) Pharmacokinetics and tolerability of buspirone during oral administration to children and adolescents with anxiety disorder and normal healthy adults. *J Clin Pharmacol* 41: 1351–1358.

Salva, P. and Costa, J. (1995) Clinical pharmacokinetics and pharmacodynamics of zolpidem. *Clin Pharmacokinet* 29:142–153.

Salzman, C. (1990) Benzodiazepine dependency: summary of the APA task force on benzodiazepines. *Psychopharmacol Bull* 26: 61–62.

Scavone, J.M., Greenblatt, D.J., Harmatz, J.S., Engelhardt, N., and Shader, R.I. (1998) Pharmacokinetics and pharmacodynamics of diphenhydramine 25 mg in young and elderly volunteers. *J Clin Pharmacol* 38:603–609.

Shader, R.I. and Greenblatt, D.J. (1993) Use of benzodiazepines in anxiety disorders. *N Engl J Med* 328:1398–1405.

Shader, R.I. and Greenblatt, D.J. (1995) The pharmacotherapy of acute anxiety. In: Bloom, F.E. and Kupfer, D.J., eds. *Psychopharmacology: The Fourth Generation of Progress*. New York: Raven Press, pp. 1341–1348.

Simeon, J.G., Ferguson, H.B., Knott, V., Roberts, N., Gauthier, B., DuBois, C., and Wiggins, D. (1992) Clinical, cognitive, and neurophysiological effects of alprazolam in children and adolescents with overanxious and avoidant disorders. *J Am Acad Child Adolesc Psychiatry* 31:29–33.

Smith, T.A. (2001) Type A gamma-aminobutyric acid (GABAa) receptor subunits and benzodiazepine binding: significance to clinical syndromes and their treatment. *Br J Biomed Sci* 58:111–121.

Spina, M.G., Basso, A.M., Zorrilla, E.P., Heyser, C.J., Rivier, J., Vale, W., Merlo-Pich, E., and Koob, G.F. (2000) Behavioral effects of central administration of the novel CRF antagonist astiessin in rats. *Neuropsychopharmacology* 10:429–435.

Tatarczynska, E., Klodzinska, A., Chojnacka-Wojcik, E., Palucha, A., Gasparini, F., Kuhn, R., and Pilc, A. (2001) Potential anxiolytic- and antidepressant-like effects of MPEP, a potent, selective and systemically active mGlu5 receptor antagonist. *Br J Pharmacol* 132:1423–30.

Varhe, A., Olkkolam, K.T., and Neuvonen, P.J. (1994) Pharmacokinetics and drug disposion: oral triazolam is potentially hazardous to patients receiving systemic antimycotics ketoconazole or itraconazole. *Clin Pharmacol Ther* 56:601–607.

Walsh, J.K., Pollak, C.P., Scharf, M.B., Schweitzer, P.K., and Vogel, G.W. (2000) Lack of residual sedation following middle-of-the-night zaleplon administration in sleep maintenance insomnia. *Clin Neuropharmacol* 23:17–21.

Zito, J.M., Safer, D.J., dosReis, S., Gardner, J.F., Boles, M., and Lynch, F. (2000) Trends in the prescribing of psychotropic medications to preschoolers. *JAMA* 283:1025–1030.

Zwier, K.J. and Rao, U. (1994) Buspirone use in an adolescent with social phobia and mixed personality disorder (cluster A type). *J Am Acad Child Adolesc Psychiatry* 33:1007–1011.

28 | Miscellaneous compounds: beta-blockers and opiate antagonists

JAN K. BUITELAAR

BETA-BLOCKERS

Beta-blockers are medications that block β-adrenergic receptors and thereby influence the activation of centrally located systems that use norepinephrine and epinephrine as a neurotransmitter, as well as that of the adrenergic sympathetic nervous system. Beta-blockers have long been used in general medicine. For example, by blocking β-receptors in the heart, heart rate, cardiac output, and blood pressure are decreased. This has led to clinical applications in the treatment of hypertension, angina pectoris and cardiac arrhythmias. In psychiatry, beta-blockers have been used on the basis of the hypothesis that "overarousal," i.e., overactivation of adrenergic systems, may underlie various psychiatric symptoms. Clinical indications in adult psychiatry for treatment with beta-blockers are mainly anxiety disorders with somatic manifestations such as palpitations and tremor (Neppe, 1989; Lader, 1988); prophylactic treatment of migraine (Evers, 1999), various forms of aggression and rage outbursts (Haspel, 1995; Silver et al., 1999); akathisia (Wells et al., 1991; Kurzthaler et al., 1997), and simple or drug-induced tremor (Henderson et al., 1995). A recent meta-analysis found insufficient support to recommend beta-blockers as an add-on to neuroleptics in the treatment of schizophrenia (Cheine et al., 2000). A small but controlled study in three adolescents and two adults found propranolol to be ineffective in Tourette's syndrome (Sverd et al., 1983). There are limited data on the efficacy and safety of beta-blockers in children and adolescents. Possible psychiatric indications for the use of beta-blockers in pediatric populations, namely aggression, rage outbursts, and anxiety, will be discussed here.

Mechanism of Action: Noradrenergic and Adrenergic Systems and β-Adrenoceptors

The brain's major noradrenergic site is the locus ceruleus (LC), a cell group in the central gray matter of the caudal pons. The two main ascending pathways from the LC are the central tegmental and the dorsal tegmental tracts (Grace et al., 1998). The axons of the central tegmental tract end in the hypothalamus and the limbic system and appear to play a role in sympathoregulation (Aston-Jones et al., 1986). The axons of the dorsal tegmental tract extend to the cerebellum, thalamus, limbic sysyem, hippocampus, and virtually the entire forebrain, including the neocortex. The areas to which the dorsal tegmental tract projects are known to participate in responses to fear and pain, and he involved in vigilance, cardiovascular regulation, and the mediation of motor activity (Fallon et al., 1978). Adrenergic cells in the central nervous system (CNS) are found in three brain stem groups of cells (Hokfelt et al., 1984). From these cells, projections are sent, among others, to the hypothalamus, the periventricular region, the LC, and the nuclei of visceral efferent and afferent systems. These cell groups are thought to participate in autonomic and neuroendocrine regulation.

Two main subtypes of β adrenoreceptors, β_1 and β_2, have been identified in the periphery and in the CNS (Minneman et al., 1979; Palacios and Kuhar, 1980). Both are located at postsynaptic terminals and have been cloned. In the periphery, β_1 receptors are located in myocardial tissue, and β_2 receptors are located in pulmonary bronchi and bronchioli, as well as in some blood vessels. β_1 Adrenoceptors are the major subtype throughout the brain, except for the cerebellum, where β_2 receptors are predominant. Areas that contain high concentrations of β adrenoceptors include the superficial layers of the neocortex, nucleus accumbens, substantia nigra, and subiculum (Palacios and Kuhar, 1980). Both types of β adrenoceptors are coupled to adenylate cyclase (Fallon et al., 1978). Receptor activation generates the second messenger cyclic adenosine monophosphate (cAMP) and thereby stimulates protein kinase–mediated phosphorylation processes. The density of β adrenoceptors in the CNS is a function of the availability of noradrenaline at the receptor, since treatment with antidepressants that act as noradrenergic reuptake inhibitors (e.g. desipramine) leads to down-regulation of β adrenoceptors (Sulser et al., 1984). Lesioning of serotonin (5-hydroxytryptamine [5-HT]) neurons (Janowsky et al., 1982) and hyperthyroidism (Perumal et al., 1984) are both associated with increased density of β adrenoceptors.

Pharmacology

The pharmacological properties of beta-blockers differ, depending on whether they nonselectively block both β_1 and β_2 receptors (e.g., propranolol, nadolol) or selectively block β_1 (e.g., atenolol and metoprolol) or β_2 adrenoceptors. Furthermore, some beta-blockers (e.g., pindolol) have intrinsic sympathomimetic activity by being partial agonists at the β adrenoceptor. This results in a more intrinsic sympathomimetic tone, which may protect against treatment-emergent bradycardia and hypotension. The main distinction, however, is between lipid-soluble (lipophilic) beta-blockers that easily cross the blood–brain barrier and penetrate into the CNS to exert central effects (e.g., propranolol, metoprolol, pindolol) and hydrophylic beta-blockers that only have peripheral effects (e.g., nadolol, atenolol). It is unclear, however, to what extent blockade of β adrenoceptors in the brain is essential for obtaining therapeutic effects on psychiatric symptoms such as aggression and anxiety. For example, treatment with nadolol, a nonspecific, peripherally acting beta-blocker, had effects similar to those of propranolol in the treatment of aggression (Polakoff et al., 1986; Ratey et al., 1987a, b; Connor et al., 1997). Another pharmacologic property of many beta-blockers (e.g., propranolol and pindolol) is blockade of 5-HT$_1$ receptors (Middlemiss, 1986). Beta-blockers also exert an inhibiting influence on glycogenolysis and can induce hypoglycemia, especially in youngsters with insulin-dependent diabetes.

The emphasis in this chapter will be on propranolol as the prototypical beta-blocker that has been most often used for psychiatric indications. Propranolol is almost completely and rapidly absorbed after oral administration, but most of an orally administered dose is metabolized by the liver during its first pass through the portal circulation. Thus, only one-third of the original oral dose reaches the systemic circulation. Interindividual variability is quite substantial with regard to the first-pass effect. As a consequence, an up to 20-fold variation is found after the administration of the same oral dose of propranolol in different subjects. Plasma half-life is relatively short, and varies between 3–4 hours after the first administration and 6 hours after multiple dosing and repeated administration. This implies that propranolol should be given in two or three doses per day. Propranolol is also available in a long-acting form that can be give once daily. Propranolol is 90%–95% bound to plasma proteins, but no drug interactions are attributable to displacement of the binding. Important drug interactions exist with other lipophilic medications (neuroleptics, antidepressants, benzodiazepines) because of competition for the cytochrome P450 enzyme system in the liver. Combining these medications with propranolol will result in higher circulating levels of both drugs, sometimes up to fivefold the original drug levels (Silber et al., 1981; Gillette and Tannery, 1994).

An example of a peripherally acting beta-blocker is nadolol. This drug has a rather long half-life of over 20 hours and may be given in one or two doses per day. It is eliminated by renal mechanisms, largely unchanged by hepatic biotransformation (Frishman, 1981). This gives nadolol the advantage over propranolol in having a much lower risk for troublesome drug–drug interactions.

Clinical Indications

Aggression, rage outbursts, and other externalizing behaviors

There has been only one relatively large double-blind, controlled study of a beta-blocker in a pediatric population (Buitelaar et al., 1996). The study included 32 children with attention, deficit hyperactivity disorder (ADHD), 7–13 years old, treated with methylphenidate (10 mg bid) or pindolol (20 mg bid) for 4 weeks in a randomized crossover trial. Forty percent ($n = 12$) of the children had comorbid conduct disorder, but subjects had not been selected particularly for the presence of aggressive symptoms. Using the Conners Parent and Teacher Rating Scales as the main outcome measures, pindolol proved to be as effective as methylphenidate in decreasing hyperactivity and aggression at home and hyperactivity at school. Pindolol, however, had less therapeutic effects than methylphenidate in improving task-related behavior during psychological testing and in affecting aggression at school (Buitelaar et al., 1996). Overall, pindolol appeared to be modestly effective in the treatment of ADHD. The frequency of side effects was similar following treatment with either drug. However, paraesthesias and nightmares, at times rather disstressing and intense, were problematic in 10% of the children treated with pindolol. One of the limitations of this study was a standard, rather than an individualized, dosage schedule. Because of this, the dosage of pindolol may have been too high for some children, with distressing side effects eclipsing treatment benefits as a result.

Support for the use of beta-blockers (mostly propranolol) in the treatment of aggression comes from a number of small, mostly open-label studies and anecdotal reports, some of which have included children and adolescents (Williams et al., 1982; Kuperman and Stewart, 1987; Sims and Galvin, 1990; Lang and Remington, 1994). Part of the population had cognitive functioning in the mentally retarded range and/or were suffering from developmental disorders (for more extensive review, see Arnold and Aman, 1991; Connor, 1993). The patient population in these studies received heterogeneous diagnoses, such as intermittent explosive disorder, episodic dyscontrol, and "organic aggressive syndrome." Target symptoms such as physical aggression, violence, rage, and self-injury that were unresponsive to more conservative treatment were reported to improve following relative high dosages of beta-blockers. On an individual basis, about 75% of the subjects showed a clinically meaningful treatment gain (Volavka, 1988). In a recent open-label study in children with heterogeneous diagnoses and overt aggression, nadolol was well tolerated and led to clinical improvements in 10/12 subjects (Connor et al., 1997).

In spite of these data, the effects of beta-blockers on aggression and rage have not been firmly established because the methodological limitations already mentioned, as well as other design failures. In most cases ongoing medication treatment (particularly neuroleptics) was continued when beta-blocker treatment was started. This may have resulted in increased plasma levels of neuroleptics, which complicates the interpretation of the study outcome. In fact, in most cases, the dosage of concomitant neuroleptic medication can be lowered during treatment with propranolol. Furthermore, many studies lacked standardized and objective methods of measuring severity of target symptoms before and after treatment.

Thus, at this stage, aggression seems to be only an eperimental indication for beta-blocker treatment, when medications higher on the treatment algorithm (e.g., conventional and newer neuroleptics, mood sta-

bilizers) have not been sufficiently effective (Connor and Steingard, 1996). At the same time, there seems to be enough evidence to warrant prospective controlled trials of beta-blockers in the treatment of severe physical and verbal aggression and self-injury in children.

Anxiety

The efficacy of beta-blockers in the symptomatic relief of anxiety in adults has been established in over a dozen controlled trials (Neppe, 1989). In a number of countries, beta-blockers have been licensed for the treatment of anxiety disorders. Somatic manifestations of anxiety such as palpitations, diaphoresis, and tremor, rather than core psychological symptoms, were particularly responsive to beta-blocker treatment. In comparative trials that included patients with severe anxiety and panic attacks, the antianxiety effect of beta-blockers was, however, somewhat less powerful than that of benzodiazepines (Lader, 1988), with the exception of a small trial that compared alprazolam to propranolol (Ravaris et al., 1991). Head-to-head comparisons of beta-blockers and selective serotonin reuptake inhibitors (SSRIs) are lacking. Performance and stress-related anxiety that may affect public performers, such as musicians or people taking an examination or giving a speech, seems to be particularly suited for beta-blocker treatment (Lader, 1988). Beta-blockers may be given on an as-required basis 1–2 hours before the stressful situation.

Controlled studies of the effects of beta-blockers on anxiety in children and adolescents are lacking. In the controlled study of children with ADHD discussed above neither pindolol nor methylphenidate was able to improve comorbid anxiety symptoms (Buitelaar et al., 1996). An open-label study suggested marked efficacy for propranolol in a dosage of 30 mg/day in 13 of 14 children with hyperventilation attacks (Joorabchi, 1977). In another study, open-label propranolol was found to be helpful in reducing the psychological and somatic symptoms of anxiety of 11 children with post-traumatic stress disorder (Famularo et al., 1988). In adult psychiatry, beta-blockers are not a treatment of first choice for anxiety, but may be used as second-line or adjunct treatment (Uhlenhuth et al., 1999). In child psychiatry, the use of beta-blockers for treating anxiety symptoms is still considered experimental.

Clinical Use

Dosage

Effective dosages of propranolol are in the range of 10–120 mg/day for younger children, and 20–300 mg/day for older subjects, usually given in two doses. The starting dosage is between 10 mg/day in younger children and 40 mg/day in older subjects (about 0.8 mg/kg/day). The dose is titrated upward by 10–20 mg every 3–4 days until the appearance of intolerable side effects (usually bradycardia) or clinical improvement. The maximum dosage is about 2.5 mg/kg/day. A response should be apparent within 4 weeks of treatment at maximum dosage. Beta-blockers should be discontinued gradually, with dose decreases of 10–20 mg every 3–4 days, to prevent rebound tachycardia. Incidental use for performance anxiety is usually in a dosage of 0.7–1.3 mg/kg, 1–2 hours before the stressor. Nadolol has been used in dosages between 30 and 220 mg/day (0.6–5.8 mg/kd/day). Nadolol was initiated with a standard dose of 10 mg bid (Connor et al., 1997).

Monitoring

Before starting beta-blockers, careful physical examination and history taking are necessary, including an electrocardiogram (EKG) to assess the presence of preexistent abnormalities of cardiac conduction, and the determination of a baseline blood glucose level. Heart rate and blood pressure need to be monitored at each medical visit and at regular times throughout treatment. It is generally recommended to hold a dose if the pulse is below 50 (adolescents and adults) or 60 (younger children), or if blood pressure drops below 90/60. At maximum dosage, EKG and blood glucose analysis should be repeated.

Side effects and toxicity

The most common side effects are Raynaud's phenomenon with cold or even cyanotic distal extremities and digits, tiredness or weakness, bradycardia, and sexual impotence. Less common side effects are depression and dysphoria, bronchoconstriction, congestive heart failure, hallucinations, hypotension, vomiting or nausea, diarrhea, insomnia and nightmares, dizziness, and hypoglycemia. When due attention is paid to contraindications and the treatment is carefully monitored, the side effects of beta-blocker treatment are generally mild.

Contraindications

Patients should be excluded from beta-blocker treatment if they have significant cardiorespiratory diseases (asthma and other pulmonary obstructive diseases, congestive heart failures, angina), insulin-dependent diabetes, severe vascular disease, renal disease, or hyperthyroidism.

Interactions

Beta-blockers interact with a large number of other medications. The combination of beta-blockers with calcium antagonists should be avoided, given the risk for hypotension and cardiac arrhythmias. Cimetidine, hydralazine, and alcohol all increase blood levels of beta-blockers, whereas rifampicin decreases their concentrations. Beta-blockers may increase blood levels of phenothiazines and other neuroleptics, clonidine, phenytoin, anesthetics, lidocaine, epinephrine, monoamine oxidase inhibitors and other antidepressants, benzodiazepines, and thyroxine. Beta-blockers decrease the effects of insulin and oral hypoglycemic agents. Smoking, oral contraceptives, carbamazepine, and nonsteroidal anti-inflammatory analgesics decrease the effects of beta-blockers (Coffey, 1990).

Overdose

The first signs of overdose of beta-blockers are bradycardia, hypotension, bronchospasm, prolongation of cardiac AV conduction time, and sedation. Among patients taking an overdose of beta-blockers, two-thirds of those who ingested > 2 gr of propranolol developed seizures (Reith et al., 1996). All patients who developed toxicity in that sample did so within 6 hours of ingestion. Following evacuation of gastric contents, severe bradycardia should be treated by intravenous injection with atropine and, if necessary, isoprenaline (a β-adrenergic agonist). In refractory cases, a pacemaker should be implanted. Hypotension should be managed with plasma substitution and intraveneous administration of isoprenaline (or another adrenergic agonist) and, in cases of insufficient response, glucagon. Close attention should be paid to the serum calcium level (Reith et al., 1996).

OPIATE ANTAGONISTS

Following the first description of endogenous opioid ligands in the mid-1970s (Hughes et al., 1975), a wide variety of endogenous peptides were identified that exert opioid activity, including enkephalins, endorphins, and dynorphins (Akil et al., 1998). The best known effects of opioids are analgesia and the induction of euphoria. In addition, opioid systems are involved in a broad spectrum of activities, including stress, tolerance, and dependence; eating and drinking, learning, memory and reward; mental illness and mood; general activity and locomotion; sex, pregnancy, and development; and social behaviors (Vaccarino and Kastin, 2000). Opioid systems contribute to the regulation of naturally reinforced behaviors (i.e., sexual behavior, feeding, drinking, and social behavior) (Rodgers and Cooper, 1988) and to the rewarding effects of artificial reinforcers, such as chemical rewards as cocaine and ethanol (van Ree et al., 1999).

The part played by endogenous opioid systems in the regulation of these various physiological and behavioral functions has led to the experimental application of opiate antagonists in psychiatric disorders. This chapter focuses on autism and self-injury, which are two potential indications for opiate antagonists in pediatric populations. In adults, treatment with opiate antagonists has shown to be useful in the relapse prevention of alcoholism as part of a comprehensive treatment approach (Anton et al., 1999, 2001).

Mechanism of Action: Opioid Systems and Receptors

Endogenous opioid peptides are derived from three distinct precursor molecules, which are the primary products of three separate genes (Simon and Hiller, 2001). The precursor proteins pro-opiomelanocortin (POMC), pro-enkephalin (ProEnk), and pro-dynorphin (ProDyn) are post-translationally processed by proteolytic enzymes, resulting in a mixture of products that is tissue-specific. Each of the three precursors has a unique anatomical distribution throughout the CNS and the periphery (Mansour et al., 1988). In the brain, the POMC-producing neurons can be found in the arcuate nucleus of the medial basal hypothalamus and the brain stem nucleus tractus solitarius. The POMC-containing neurons of the arcuate nucleus have long projections that innervate many brain regions, including the septum, the amygdala, and the hypothalamus. In contrast to the rather limited distribution of POMC-containing neurons, the ProEnk-producing neurons are located in many neuronal systems throughout the CNS, from the cerebral cortex down to the spinal cord. Most of the brain regions that contain enkephalin cells and terminals also contain dynorphin. ProDyn is synthesized in multiple cell groups throughout the CNS, the anterior lobe of the pituitary, and in the gonadotrophs.

It is generally accepted that three major classes of opioid receptors exist. The most commonly used terminology discriminates between μ-, κ-, and δ-opioid receptors. However, after cloning of the three genes encoding opioid receptors, a new nomenclature was agreed upon: OP1 (corresponding to the δ receptor), OP2 (κ receptor) and OP3 (μ receptor) (Dhawan et al.,

1996). Autoradiography studies have shown that OP1, OP2, and OP3 binding sites are present in most regions of the CNS. The distribution is heterogeneous, such that each type has a distinct localization (Zaki et al., 1996). The OP1 binding site is particulary found in the olfactory bulb, neocortex, caudate, putamen, and nucleus accumbens. The OP2 is present in the nucleus accumbens, endopiriform nucleus, claustrum, and interpeduncular nucleus. The caudate, putamen, neocortex, thalamus, nucleus accumbens, hippocampus, and amygdala have the highest densities of OP3 sites. The cloned opioid receptors are highly homologous and belong to the family of the seven-transmembrane, G protein–coupled receptors, which upon opioid binding, inhibit the activation of second messenger systems (Standifer and Pasternak, 1997).

Pharmacology

The two opiate antagonists that have been used clinically are naloxone and naltrexone. Naloxone is a short-acting agent that can only be administered parenterally. This clearly limits the clinical use of naloxone. Following intravenous injection, naloxone is active within 1–2 minutes, its plasma half-life is about 1 hour, and its duration of action is 1–4 hours. Naltrexone is a relatively pure opioid antagonist with undetectable or minimal agonistic effects. It can be given orally and is maximally absorbed within about 1 hour. There is a large first-pass effect, in which about 95% is converted in the liver to active metabolites, which are then excreted by the kidneys. Plasma half-life of naltrexone is 4–10 hours, and that of naltrexone's major active metabolite, 6-β-naltrexol, 11–17 hours (Verebey et al., 1976). The half-life of blockade by naltrexone of OP3 (μ)-receptors in the brain ranges from 72 to 108 hours (Lee et al., 1988).

Clinical Indications

Autism

Pharmacologic interventions in the endogenous opioid system in subjects with autism are based upon the putative role of opioids in the regulation of social behavior (Benton and Brain, 1988). For example, opioids are involved in maternal–infant attachment in animal studies by influencing feelings of social comfort and blocking separation distress reactions (Panksepp et al., 1978). This led to the hypothesis that excessive activity of opioid systems in the CNS would prevent the formation of social bonding in humans and contribute to the pathogenesis and maintenance of autistic symptoms

(Panksepp, 1979). However, research on β-endorphin levels in cerebrospinal fluid (CSF) (Gillberg et al., 1985; 1990; Ross et al., 1987) and plasma (Weizman et al., 1984; 1988; Herman et al., 1986; Marchetti et al., 1990; Sandman et al., 1991; Leboyer et al., 1994; Willemsen-Swinkels et al., 1996; Tordjman et al., 1997) of subjects with autism has yielded inconsistent results and does not directly support an opioid excess hypothesis of autism. The finding that the levels of both β-endorphin and corticotropin were increased in the plasma of individuals with severe autism in the absence of changes in plasma level of cortisol most likely indicates that there is a heightened response to acute stressors rather than a chronic alteration of the basal level of functioning of these systems (Tordjman et al., 1997).

The initial reports of open-label studies of naltrexone in autism seemed to be very promising (Leboyer et al., 1988; Campbell et al., 1989; Panksepp and Lensing, 1991; Lensing et al., 1992), but results of later placebo-controlled studies were overall disappointing. The social and communicative core deficits of autism and stereotyped behaviors at group level were not ameliorated in three larger studies that included 41 children in a parallel design, and 23 and 24 children in a crossover design, respectively (Campbell et al., 1993; Willemsen-Swinkels et al., 1996; Feldman et al., 1999). The dosages administered were about 1.0 mg/kg/day. Three other placebo-controlled crossover studies used lower dosages (0.5 to 1.5 mg/kg every other day, and 0.5 mg/day) and were able to report modest improvements of autistic symptoms (Scifo et al., 1991; Leboyer et al., 1992; Bouvard et al., 1995). Higher baseline levels of β-endorphin in plasma were associated with a better treatment response, but the reduction of β-endorphin plasma levels per se was unrelated to the effect of treatment (Leboyer et al., 1992; Bouvard et al., 1995). Open-label continuation treatment for a period of 6 months in five autistic children who showed clear individual response in a placebo-controlled trial of 4 weeks did not reveal later therapeutic effects on social and communicative functioning (Willemsen-Swinkels et al., 1999). A consistent positive finding across a number of studies is that treatment with naltrexone in a dosage of about 1.0 mg/kg/day is associated with a statistically significant but clinically modest reduction of hyperactivity in both single dose (Herman et al., 1991b; Willemsen-Swinkels et al., 1995b) and subchronic (Campbell et al., 1993; Willemsen-Swinkels et al., 1996a; Kolmen et al., 1997) controlled designs. Post-hoc analysis on an individual level revealed that the largest reductions of hyperactivity were observed in children with marked social isolation, rather than in those with initial levels of severe hyperactivity

(Willemsen-Swinkels et al., 1996a). This further seems to detract from the clinical utility in prescribing naltrexone to treat hyperactivity in subjects with autism. Although an expert has advocated that all autistic children should have a trial with naltrexone, this opinion has not met consensus within the professional community (Campbell and Harris, 1996).

Self-injury

There are two main hypotheses about the involvement of endogenous opioid systems in the maintenance of self-injurious behaviors (Sandman, 1988; Buitelaar, 1993). The *pain hypothesis* suggests that in some subjects self-injury does not induce pain because excessive basal activity of opioid systems in the CNS has led to an opioid analgesic state. The *addiction hypothesis* posits that particularly repetitive and stereotyped forms of self-injury stimulate the production and release of endogenous opioids. Therefore, chronic maintenance of self-injury may be due to addiction to endogenous opioids or to positive reinforcement by a central release of opioids triggered by the self-injurious behavior. Irrespective of which hypothesis one favors, treatment with opiate antagonists seems to be a rational approach.

The data, however, on levels of opioids in body fluids and on therapeutic effects of opiate antagonists in subjects with self-injury are complex and contradictory. A number of studies have found lower levels of β-endorphin in plasma of subjects with severe self-injury than those of normal control individuals (Weizman et al., 1988; Herman, 1990; Willemsen-Swinkels et al., 1996b). This does not necessarily refute the hypothesis of an overactive opioid system in self-injurious subjects, since there may be a negative feedback between the hypothalamus and the pituitary, which regulates the central and peripheral levels of β-endorphin. However, subjects with self-injury were reported to have higher β-endorphin levels in plasma than those of learning-disabled people without self-injury (Sandman et al., 1990). The same research group further found that β-endorphin levels in plasma of patients with self-injury were elevated within minutes after an episode of self-injury when compared to baseline and control levels. Elevated β-endorphin levels predicted a better response to treatment with a high dose (2 mg/kg) of naltrexone (Sandman et al., 1997). Another group, however, was unable to document differences in plasma β-endorphin levels between mentally retarded subjects with self-injury, those without self-injury but with stereotyped behavior patterns, and mentally retarded controls (Verhoeven et al., 1999).

On a regular basis reports have been published about

beneficial effects of opiate antagonists on the frequency of self-injury. Though therapeutic effects are claimed in about 70% of the patients, these reports are limited by the small number of subjects and mainly uncontrolled designs (for review see Willemsen-Swinkels et al., 1995a). The results of larger controlled studies are conflicting. Two placebo-controlled studies failed to establish therapeutic effects of naltrexone on self-injury (Zingarelli et al., 1992; Willemsen-Swinkels et al., 1995a), whereas other smaller controlled studies had positive findings (Sandman et al., 1993; Thompson et al., 1994). To complicate matters further, a subgroup of subjects with self-injury has been identified with decreased self-injury for a year following acute exposure to naltrexone (Sandman et al., 2000). Another subgroup showed decrease of self-injury after acute treatment with naltrexone but later increases during long-term treatment (Sandman et al., 2000).

The best conclusion that can be drawn from these data is perhaps that treatment with naltrexone may offer promise for some, but certainly not all, patients with self-injury. Treatment effects may depend on background opioid levels, dosage, and treatment regimen. Noninvasive measures that predict individual treatment response have not been established. Self-injury is a heterogeneous phenomenon from a clinical and biological perspective (Buitelaar, 1993; Willemsen-Swinkels et al., 1998). Further studies are required in this area, and and should include carefully clinically documented cases, large samples, and controlled designs. At this time, the use of naltrexone for the treatment of self-injury is to be considered experimental.

Clinical Use

Dosage

For both the treatment of autism and self-injury, dosages of naltrexone have been in the range of 0.5–2.0 mg/kg/day in single-dose and subchronic designs. In autism, some researchers have advocated the use of low dosages, i.e., 0.5 mg/kg/day or every other day (Scifo et al., 1991; Lensing et al., 1992). This approach is based on the idea that the subsequent release of opioids following a just sufficient blockade of opiate receptor systems would be associated with improvement of social and communicative behaviors (Panksepp and Lensing, 1991). Controlled data in support of this approach are lacking, however. The controlled subchronic trials with naltrexone in autism used a standard dosage of about 1.0 mg/kg/day, usually given in one early-morning dose or in two doses. In subjects with self-injury, there is some suggestion that higher

dosages, close to 2.0 mg/kg/day, are more effective than lower dosages (Sandman et al., 1993). However, in the largest controlled study in adults with self-injury, the effects of a higher dosage of 150 mg/day (about 2.5 mg/kg/day) were similar to those of a lower dosage of 50 mg/day (about 0.8 mg/kg/day) (Willemsen-Swinkels et al., 1995a). In clinical practice, it is recommended to start with a low dose of naltrexone (12.5 mg in young children, and 25 mg in older subjects) and to increase the dosage the next day to 25 or 50 mg, respectively (about 1.0 mg/kg/day). When no treatment effects are observed within about 2 weeks, dosages may be titrated upward until side effects occur or the maximum dosage of 2.0 mg/kg/day is reached. Liver function tests should be performed before treatment starts and at regular times during treatment. Self-injurious behavior is highly variable over time in some individuals: a long observation period at baseline and during treatment is thus essential in making reliable judgements about treatment benefits. In many cases, the application of single-case trial methodology merits consideration (Kazdin, 1982).

Side effects

In dose-ranging tolerance studies (0.5–2.0 mg/kg/day), mild sedation of brief duration was the only side effect (Campbell et al., 1989). The EKG parameters, liver function tests, and all other laboratory tests, body temperature, eating and sleeping patterns, and weight remained unchanged (Campbell et al., 1989; Herman et al., 1989). In the subchronic studies naltrexone was also well tolerated and no serious side effects were observed. The EKG, weight, and lab tests remained within normal limits. Excessive sedation, decreased appetite, and vomiting were reported more often following naltrexone treatment than following placebo in one study (Campbell et al., 1993), whereas no differences in side effects between naltrexone and placebo were reported in another (Willemsen-Swinkels et al., 1996a). Naltrexone has a bitter taste that has led to complaints of some children. Since this may compromise treatment compliance, neutralizing the taste by combining naltrexone with chocolate may offer a solution.

Contraindications

Before initiating treatment, careful attention should be paid to the use of any opioid analgesics, since naltrexone may provoke acute withdrawal symptoms. The main contraindications are (1) treatment with opioid analgesics, (2) opioid dependence, (3) acute opioid withdrawal, and (4) hepatitis or other forms of liver failure.

Overdose

There are no reports about toxic reactions following ingestion of an overdose of naltrexone.

REFERENCES

Akil, H., Owens, C., Gutstein, H., Taylor, L., Curran, E., and Watson, S. (1998) Endogenous opioids: overview and current issues. *Drug Alcohol Depend* 51:127–40.

Anton, R.F., Moak, D.H., Waid, L.R., Latham, P.K., Malcolm, R.J., and Dias, J.K. (1999) Naltrexone and cognitive behavioral therapy for the treatment of outpatient alcoholics: results of a placebo-controlled trial. *Am J Psychiatry* 156:1758–1764.

Anton, R.F., Moak, D.H., Latham, P.K., Waid, L.R., Malcolm, R.J., Dias, J.K., and Roberts, J.S. (2001). Posttreatment results of combining naltrexone with cognitive-behavior therapy for the treatment of alcoholism. *J Clin Psychopharmacol*, 21, 72–77.

Arnold, L.E., and Aman, M.G. (1991) Beta blockers in mental retardation and developmental disorders. *J Child Adolesc Psychopharmacol* 1:361–373.

Aston-Jones, G., Ennis, M., Pieribone, V.A., Nickell, W.T., and Shipley, M.T. (1986) The brain nucleus locus coeruleus: restricted afferent control of a broad efferent network. *Science* 234:734–737.

Benton, D. and Brain, P.F. (1988) The role of opioid mechanisms in social interaction and attachment. In: Rodgers, R.J. and Cooper, S.J., eds. *Endorphins, Opiates and Behavioural Processes.* New York: John Wiley & Sons, pp. 215–235.

Bouvard, M.P., Leboyer, M., Launay, J.M., Recasens, C., Plumet, M.H., Waller Perotte, D., Tabuteau, F., Bondoux, D., Dugas, M., Lensing, P., et al. (1995) Low-dose naltrexone effects on plasma chemistries and clinical symptoms in autism: a double-blind, placebo-controlled study. *Psychiatry Res* 58:191–201.

Buitelaar, J.K. (1993) Self-injurious behavior in retarded children, clinical phenomena and biological mechanisms. *Acta Paedopsychiatr* 56:105–111.

Buitelaar, J.K., Van der Gaag, R.J., Swaab-Barneveld, J.T., and Kuiper, M. (1996) Pindolol and methylphenidate in children with attention-deficit hyperactivity disorder. Clinical efficacy and side effects. *J Child Psychol Psychiatry* 37:587–595.

Campbell, M., Anderson, L.T., Small, A.M., Adams, P., Gonzalez, N.M., and Ernst, M. (1993) Naltrexone in autistic children—behavioral symptoms and attentional learning. *J Am Acad Child Adolesc Psychiatry* 32:1283–1291.

Campbell, M. and Harris, J.C. (1996) Resolved: autistic children should have a trial of naltrexone. *J Am Acad Child Adolesc Psychiatry* 35:246–249.

Campbell, M., Overall, J.E., Small, A.M., Sokol, M.S., Spencer, E.S., Adams, P., Foltz, R.L., Monti, K.M., Perry, R., Nobler, M., and Roberts, E. (1989) Naltrexone in autistic children: an acute open dose range tolerance trial. *J Am Acad Child Adolesc Psychiatry* 28:200–206.

Cheine, M., Ahonen, J., and Wahlbeck, K. (2000) Beta-blocker supplementation of standard drug treatment for schizophrenia. *Cochrane Database Syst Rev* 16: CD000234.

Coffey, B.J. (1990) Anxiolytics for children and adolescents. *J Child Adolesc Psychopharmacol* 1:57–83.

Connor, D.F. (1993) Beta blockers for aggression: a review of the pediatric experience. *J Child Adolesc Psychopharmacol* 3:99–114.

Connor, D.F., Ozbayrak, K.R., Benjamin, S., Ma, Y., and Fletcher, K.E. (1997) A pilot study of nadolol for overt aggression in developmentally delayed individuals. *J Am Acad Child Adolesc Psychiatry* 36:826–834.

Connor, D.F. and Steingard, R.J. (1996) A clinical approach to the pharmacotherapy of aggression in children and adolescents. *Ann N Y Acad Sci* 794:290–307.

Dhawan, B.N., Cesselin, F., Raghubir, R., Reisine, T., Bradley, P.B., Portoghese, P.S., and Hamon, M. (1996) International Union of Pharmacology. XII. Classification of opioid receptors. *Pharmacol Rev* 48:567–592.

Evers, S. (1999) Drug treatment of migraine in children: a comparative review. *Paediatr Drugs* 1:7–18.

Fallon, J.H., Koziell, D.A., and Moore, R.Y. (1978) Catecholamine innervation of the basal forebrain. II. Amygdala, suprarhinal cortex and entorhinal cortex. *J Comp Neurol* 180:509–532.

Famularo, R., Kinscherff, R., and Fenton, T. (1988) Propranolol treatment for childhood post-traumatic stress disorder, acute type. *Am J Dis Child* 142:1244–1247.

Feldman, H.M., Kolmen, B.K., and Gonzaga, A.M. (1999) Naltrexone and communication skills in young children with autism. *J Am Acad Child Adolesc Psychiatry* 38:587–593.

Frishman, W.H. (1981) Nadolol: a new β-adrenoceptor antagonist. *N Engl J Medi* 305:678–682.

Gillberg, C., Terenius, L., Hagberg, B., Witt-Engerstrom, I., and Eriksson, I. (1990) CSF β-endorphins in childhood neuropsychiatric disorders. *Brain Dev* 12:88–92.

Gillberg, C., Terenius, L., and Lonnerholm, G. (1985) Endorphin activity in childhood psychosis. Spinal fluid levels in 24 cases. *Arch Gen Psychiatry* 42:780–783.

Gillette, D.W., and Tannery, L.P. (1994) Beta blocker inhibits tricyclic metabolism. *J Am Acad Child Adolesc Psychiatry* 33: 223–234.

Grace, A.A., Gerfen, C.R., and Aston-Jones, G. (1998) Catecholamines in the central nervous system. Overview. *Adv Pharmacol* 42:655–670.

Haspel, T. (1995) Beta-blockers and the treatment of aggression. *Harv Rev Psychiatry* 2:274–281.

Henderson, J.M., Einstein, R., Jackson, D.M., Byth, K., and Morris, J.G. (1995) 'Atypical' tremor. *Eur Neurol* 35:321–326.

Herman, B.H. (1990) A possible role of proopiomelanocortin peptides in self-injurious behavior. *Prog Neuropsychopharmacol Biol Psychiatry* 14: S109–S139.

Herman, B.H., Asleson, G.S., Borghese, I.F., Chatoor, I., Powell, A., Papero, P., Allen, R.P., and McNulty, G. (1991) Acute naltrexone in autism: selective decreases in hyperactivity. In: *Proceedings of the 38th Annual Meeting of the American Academy of Child and Adolescent Psychiatry.* San Francisco: AACAP.

Herman, B.H., Hammock, M.K., Arthur-Smith, A., Egan, J., Chatoor, I., Zelnik, N., Corradine, M., Appelgate, K., Boecks, R., and Sharp, S.D. (1986) Role of opioid peptides in autism: effects of acute administration of naltrexone [abstract]. *Soc Neurosci Abstr* 12:320.

Herman, B.H., Hammock, M.K., Arthur-Smith, A., Kuehl, K., and Appelgate, K. (1989) Effects of acute administration of naltrexone on cardiovascular function, body temperature, body weight and serum concentrations of liver enzymes in autistic children. *Dev Pharmacol Ther* 12:118–27.

Hokfelt, T., Johansson, O., and Goldstein, M. (1984) Chemical anatomy of the brain. *Science* 225:1326–1334.

Hughes, J., Smith, T.W., Kosterlitz, H.W., Fothergill, L.A., Morgan,

B.A., and Morris, H.R. (1975) Identification of two related pentapeptides from the brain with potent opiate agonist activity. *Nature* 258:577–580.

Janowsky, A., Okada, F., Manier, D.H., Applegate, C.D., Sulser, F., and Steranka, L.R. (1982) Role of serotonergic input in the regulation of the β-adrenergic receptor–coupled adenylate cyclase system. *Science* 218:900–901.

Joorabchi, B. (1977) Expressions of the hyperventilation syndrome in childhood: studies in management, including an evaluation of the effectiveness of propranolol. *Clin Pediatr (Phila)* 16:1110–1115.

Kazdin, A.E. (1982) *Single-Case Research Designs. Methods for Clinical and Applied Settings*. New York: Oxford University Press.

Kolmen, B.K., Feldman, H.M., Handen, B.L., and Janosky, J.E. (1997) Naltrexone in young autistic children: replication study and learning measures. *J Am Acad Child Adolesc Psychiatry* 36:1570–1578.

Kuperman, S. and Stewart, M.A. (1987) Use of propranolol to decrease aggressive outbursts in younger patients. *Psychosomatics* 28:315–319.

Kurzthaler, I., Hummer, M., Kohl, C., Miller, C., and Fleischhacker, W.W. (1997) Propranolol treatment of olanzapine-induced akathisia. *Am J Psychiatry* 154:1316.

Lader, M. (1988) Bèta-adrenoreceptor antagonists in neuropsychiatry: an update. *J Clin Psychiatry* 49:213–223.

Lang, C. and Remington, D. (1994) Treatment with propranolol of severe self-injurious behavior in a blind, deaf, retarded adolescent. *J Am Acad Child Adolesc Psychiatry* 33:265–269.

Leboyer, M., Bouvard, M.P., and Dugas, M. (1988) Effects of naltrexone on infantile autism [letter]. *Lancet* 1:715.

Leboyer, M., Bouvard, M.P., Launay, J., Tabuteau, F., Waller, D., Dugas, M., Kerdelhue, B., Lensing, P., and Panksepp, J. (1992) Brief report: a double-blind study of naltrexone in infantile autism. *J Autism Dev Disord* 22:309–319.

Leboyer, M., Bouvard, M.P., Recasens, C., Philippe, A., Guilloudbataille, M., Bondoux, D., Tabuteau, F., Dugas, M., Panksepp, J., and Launay, J.M. (1994) Difference between plasma N- and C-terminally directed β-endorphin immunoreactivity in infantile autism. *Am J Psychiatry* 151:1797–1801.

Lee, M.C., Wagner, H.N., Jr., Tanada, S., Frost, J.J., Bice, A.N., and Dannals, R.F. (1988) Duration of occupancy of opiate receptors by naltrexone. *J Nucl Med* 29:1207–1211.

Lensing, P., Klingler, D., Lampl, C., Leboyer, M., Bouvard, M., Plumet, M.H., and Panksepp, J. (1992) Naltrexone open trial with a 5-year-old-boy. A social rebound reaction. *Acta Paedopsychiatr* 55:169–173.

Mansour, A., Khachaturian, H., Lewis, M.E., Akil, H., and Watson, S.J. (1988) Anatomy of CNS opioid receptors. *Trends Neurosci* 11:308–314.

Marchetti, B., Scifo, R., Batticane, N., and Scapagnini, U. (1990) Immunological significance of opioid peptide dysfunction in infantile autism. *Brain Dysfunction* 3:346–354.

Middlemiss, D.N. (1986) Blockade of the central 5-HT autoreceptor by β-adrenoceptor antagonists. *Eur J Pharmacol* 120:51–56.

Minneman, K.P., Dibner, M.D., Wolfe, B.B., and Molinoff, P.B. (1979) β₁- and β₂-Adrenergic receptors in rat cerebral cortex are independently regulated. *Science* 204:866–868.

Neppe, V.M. (1989) *Innovative Psychopharmacotherapy*. New York: Raven Press.

Palacios, J.M. and Kuhar, M.J. (1980) Beta-adrenergic-receptor localization by light microscopic autoradiography. *Science* 208:1378–1380.

Panksepp, J. (1979) A neurochemical theory of autism. *Trends Neurosci* 2:174–177.

Panksepp, J., Herman, B., Connor, R., Bishop, P., and Scott, J.P. (1978) The biology of social attachments: opiates alleviate separation distress. *Biol Psychiatry* 13:607–618.

Panksepp, J. and Lensing, P. (1991) Brief report: a synopsis of an open trial of naltrexone treatment of autism with four children. *J Autism Dev Disord* 21:243–249.

Perumal, A.S., Halbreich, U., and Barkai, A.I. (1984) Modification of β-adrenergic receptor binding in rat brain following thyroxine administration. *Neurosci Lett* 48:217–221.

Polakoff, S., Sorgi, P., and Ratey, J.J. (1986) The treatment of impulsive and aggressive behaviors with nadolol. *J Clin Psychopharmacol* 6:125–126.

Ratey, J.J., Bemporad, J., Sorgi, P., Bick, P., Polakoff, S., O'Driscoll, G., and Mikkelsen, E. (1987a) Brief report: open trial effects of beta-blockers on speech and social behaviors in 8 autistic adults. *J Autism Dev Disord* 17:439–446.

Ratey, J.J., Mikkelsen, E., Sorgi, P., Zuckerman, S., Polakoff, S., Bemporad, J., Bick, P., and Kadish.W. (1987b) Autism: the treatment of aggressive behaviors. *J Clin Psychopharmacol* 7:35–41.

Ravaris, C.L., Friedman, M.J., Hauri, P.J., and McHugo, G.J. (1991) A controlled study of alprazolam and propranolol in panic-disordered and agoraphobic outpatients. *J Clin Psychopharmacol* 11:344–350.

Reith, D.M., Dawson, A.H., Epid, D., Whyte, I.M., Buckley, N.A., and Sayer, G.P. (1996) Relative toxicity of beta blockers in overdose. *J Toxicol Clin Toxicol* 34:273–278.

Rodgers, R.J. and Cooper, S.J. (1988) *Endorphins, Opiates and Behavioural Processes*. Chichester: John Wiley & Sons.

Ross, D.L., Klykylo, W.M., and Hitzemann, R. (1987) Reduction of elevated CSF β-endorphin by fenfluramine in infantile autism. *Pediatr Neurol* 3:83–86.

Sandman, C.A. (1988) Beta-endorphin disregulation in autistic and self-injurious behavior: a neurodevelopmental hypothesis. *Synapse* 2:193–199.

Sandman, C.A., Barron, J.L., Chicz DeMet, A., and DeMet, E.M. (1990) Plasma β-endorphin levels in patients with self-injurious behavior and stereotypy. *Am J Ment Retard* 95:84–92.

Sandman, C.A., Barron, J.L., Chicz-DeMet, A., and DeMet, E.M. (1991) Brief report: plasma β-endorphin and cortisol levels in autistic patients. *J Autism Dev Disord* 21:83–87.

Sandman, C.A., Hetrick, W.P., and Taylor, D.V. (1993) Naltrexone reduces self-injury and improves learning. *Exp Clin Psychopharmacol* 1:1–17.

Sandman, C.A., Hetrick, W., Taylor, D.V., and Chicz DeMet, A. (1997) Dissociation of POMC peptides after self-injury predicts responses to centrally acting opiate blockers. *Am J Ment Retard* 102:182–199.

Sandman, C.A., Hetrick, W., Taylor, D.V., Marion, S.D., Touchette, P., Barron, J.L., Martinezzi, V., Steinberg, R.M., and Crinella, F.M. (2000) Long-term effects of naltrexone on self-injurious behavior. *Am J Ment Retard* 105:103–117.

Scifo, R., Batticane, N., Quattropani, M.C., Spoto, G., and Marchetti, B. (1991) A double-blind trial with naltrexone in autism. In: *Proceedings of OASI Conference* (unpublished paper).

Silber, B., Mico, B.A., Ortiz de Montellano, P.R., Dols, D.M., and Riegelman, S. (1981) In vivo effects of the cytochrome P-450 suicide substrate 2-isopropyl-4-pentenamide (allylisopropylacetamide) on the disposition and metabolic pattern of propranolol. *J Pharmacol Exp Ther* 219:125–133.

Silver, J.M., Yudofsky, S.C., Slater, J.A., Gold, R.K., Stryer, B.L., Williams, D.T., Wolland, H., and Endicott, J. (1999) Propranolol treatment of chronically hospitalized aggressive patients. *J Neuropsychiatry Clin Neurosci* 11:328–335.

Simon, E.J. and Hiller, J.M. (2001) Opioid peptides and opioid receptors. In: Siegel, G.J., Agranoff, B.W., Albers, R.W., and Molinoff, P.B., eds. *Basic Neurochemistry: Molecular, Cellular, and Medical Aspects.* New York: Raven Press, (pp. 321–339).

Sims, J. and Galvin, M.R. (1990) Pediatric psychopharmacologic use of propranolol. *J Child Adolesc Psychiatr Ment Health Nurs* 3: 18–24.

Standifer, K.M. and Pasternak, G.W. (1997) G proteins and opioid receptor-mediated signalling. *Cell Signal* 9:237–248.

Sulser, F., Gillespie, D.D., Mishra, R., and Manier, D.H. (1984) Desensitization by antidepressants of central norepinephrine receptor systems coupled to adenylate cyclase. *Ann N Y Acad Sci* 430: 91–101.

Sverd, J., Cohen, S., and Camp, J.A. (1983) Brief report: effect of propranolol in Tourette syndrome. *J Autism Dev Disord* 13:207–213.

Thompson, T., Hackenberg, T., Cerutti, D., Baker, D., and Axtell, S. (1994) Opioid antagonist effects on self-injury in adults with mental retardation: response form and location as determinants of medication effects. *Am J Ment Retard* 99:85–102.

Tordjman, S., Anderson, G.M., McBride, P.A., Hertzig, M.E., Snow, M.E., Hall, L.M., Thompson, S.M., Ferrari, P., and Cohen, D.J. (1997) Plasma β-endorphin, adrenocorticotropic hormone, and cortisol in autism. *J Child Psychol Psychiatry* 38:705–715.

Uhlenhuth, E.H., Balter, M.B., Ban, T.A., and Yang, K. (1999) International study of expert judgment on therapeutic use of benzodiazepines and other psychotherapeutic medications: VI. Trends in recommendations for the pharmacotherapy of anxiety disorders, 1992–1997. *Depres Anxiety* 9:107–116.

Vaccarino, A.L. and Kastin, A.J. (2000) Endogenous opiates: 1999. *Peptides* 21:1975–2034.

van Ree, J.M., Gerrits, M.A., and Vanderschuren, L.J. (1999) Opioids, reward and addiction: an encounter of biology, psychology, and medicine. *Pharmacol Rev* 51:341–396.

Verebey, K., Volavka, J., Mule, S.J., and Resnick, R.B. (1976) Naltrexone: disposition, metabolism, and effects after acute and chronic dosing. *Clin Pharmacol Ther* 20:315–328.

Verhoeven, W.M., Tuinier, S., van den Berg, Y.W., Coppus, A.M., Fekkes, D., Pepplinkhuizen, L., and Thijssen, J.H. (1999) Stress and self-injurious behavior; hormonal and serotonergic parameters in mentally retarded subjects. *Pharmacopsychiatry* 32:13–20.

Volavka, J. (1988) Can aggressive behavior in humans be modified by beta blockers? *Postgrad Med* Special issue 2:163–168.

Weizman, R., Gil-ad, I., Dick, J., Tyano, S., Szekely, G.A., and Laron, Z. (1988) Low plasma immunoreactive β-endorphin levels in autism. *J Am Acad Child Adolesc Psychiatry* 27:430–433.

Weizman, R., Weizman, A., Tyano, A., Szekely, B., Weissman, B.A., and Sarne, Y. (1984) Humoral-endorphin blood levels in autistic, schizophrenic and healthy subjects. *Psychopharmacology* 82: 368–370.

Wells, B.G., Cold, J.A., Marken, P.A., Brown, C.S., Chu, C.C., Johnson, R.P., Nasdahl, C.S., Ayubi, M.A., Knott, D.H., and Arheart, K.L. (1991) A placebo-controlled trial of nadolol in the treatment of neuroleptic-induced akathisia. *J Clin Psychiatry* 52:255–260.

Willemsen-Swinkels, S.H.N., Buitelaar, J.K., Dekker, M., and Van Engeland, H. (1998) Subtyping stereotypic behavior in children: the association between stereotypic behavior, mood and heart rate. *J Autism Dev Disord* 28:547–557.

Willemsen-Swinkels, S.H.N., Buitelaar, J.K., Nijhof, G., and Van Engeland, H. (1995a) Failure of naltrexone hydrochloride to reduce self-injurious and autistic behavior in mentally retarded adults. Double-blind placebo-controlled studies. *Arch Gen Psychiatry* 52:766–773.

Willemsen-Swinkels, S.H.N., Buitelaar, J.K., Van Berckelaer-Onnes, I.A., and Van Engeland, H. (1999) Six-month continuation treatment of naltrexone-responsive children with autism: an open-label case-control design. *J Autism Dev Disord* 29:167–169.

Willemsen-Swinkels, S.H.N., Buitelaar, J.K., and Van Engeland, H. (1996a) The effects of chronic naltrexone treatment in young autistic children: a double-blind placebo-controlled crossover study. *Biol Psychiatry* 39:1023–1031.

Willemsen-Swinkels, S.H.N., Buitelaar, J.K., Weijnen, F.G., Thijssen, J.H.H., and Van Engeland, H. (1996b) Plasma β-endorphin concentrations in people with learning disability and self-injurious and/or autistic behaviour. *Br J Psychiatry* 168:105–109.

Willemsen-Swinkels, S.H.N., Buitelaar, J.K., Weijnen, F.G., and Van Engeland, H. (1995c) Placebo-controlled acute dosage naltrexone study in young autistic children. *Psychiatr Res* 58:203–215.

Williams, D.T., Mehl, R., Yudofsky, S., Adams, D., and Roseman, B. (1982) The effect of propranolol on uncontrolled rage outbursts in children and adolescents with organic brain dysfunction. *J Am Acad Child Psychiatry* 21:129–35.

Zaki, P.A., Bilsky, E.J., Vanderah, T.W., Lai, J., Evans, C.J., and Porreca, F. (1996) Opioid receptor types and subtypes: the delta receptor as a model. *Annu Rev Pharmacol Toxicol* 36: 379–401.

Zingarelli, G., Ellman, G., Hom, A., Wymore, M., Heidorn, S., and Chicz DeMet, A. (1992) Clinical effects of naltrexone on autistic behavior. *Am J Ment Retard* 97:57–63.

OTHER SOMATIC INTERVENTIONS

29 | Complementary and alternative medicine in pediatric psychopharmacology

JOSEPH M. REY, GARRY WALTER, AND JOSEPH P. HORRIGAN

Alternative medicine refers to a group of treatments that exist largely outside the institutions where mainstream health care is provided (Zolman and Vickers, 1999). The boundary between these practices and traditional medicine has become progressively blurred because of some physicians using alternative treatments in their practice and to their inclusion in health insurance packages. Many universities now offer courses on alternative medicine and scientific methods (e.g., randomized, placebo-controlled trials) are beginning to be used to test the efficacy of these treatments. Alternative medicine is increasingly seen as complementing mainstream practices and is often referred to as *complementary and alternative medicine* (CAM). For example, the National Institutes of Health (NIH) in the United States include the National Center for Complimentary and Alternative Medicine, which conducts and supports basic and applied research in this field. Complementary and alternative medicine comprises a wide range of treatments as disparate as acupuncture, yoga, herbal medicine, homoeopathy, and reflexology. This chapter will focus on the herbal remedies or "dietary supplements," particularly St. John's wort, that are more relevant to clinical practice and research.

EXTENT OF USE OF COMPLEMENTARY AND ALTERNATIVE MEDICINE

Alternative remedies are consumed extensively and their use is increasing. For example, a telephone survey of over 2000 persons in the United States in 1997 found that there had been a 45% increase in use from 1990 (Eisenberg et al., 1993, 1998). Furthermore, fewer than 40% of the participants had discussed the use of alternative therapy with their physician and al-most one half had used CAM without any form of medical supervision (Eisenberg et al., 1993, 1998). A large South Australian study found that almost half of that state's population used alternative medicines and that a fifth consulted alternative practitioners (MacLennan et al., 1996). There are data suggesting that persons with a mental disorder have higher rates of use of CAM. For example, a national survey in the United States found that 21% of respondents who used CAM met diagnostic criteria for one or more mental disorders, compared to 13% for respondents who did not use CAM (Unutzer et al., 2000). In another study (Druss and Rosenheck, 2000), 10% of persons reporting a mental condition had made a complementary visit and about half of these people (4.5%) had made the visit to treat the mental condition. Many people from advanced Western countries have considerable trust in the effectiveness of dietary supplements. More than half (57%) of an Australian community sample believed that vitamins, minerals, tonics, or herbal medicines were helpful in the treatment of schizophrenia and depression. Only 3% believed they were harmful. By comparison, the figures for antidepressants were 29% helpful and 42% harmful (Jorm et al., 1997).

Complementary and alternative medicine is often used in children (Sawyer et al., 1994; Andrews et al., 1998; Ernst, 1999). Regrettably, there are negligible data about the use of CAM among young people with mental health problems. An Australian survey that collected data in 1998 from a representative sample of 3597 children aged 6–17 years, reported that seven children (0.02%) were using herbal remedies—compared with 2.4% who were taking psychotropic drugs (Sawyer et al., in press). For a 1-month period in early 1998, parents of children who visited a clinic were asked to complete a brief questionnaire regarding

CAM. Data about 145 boys and 35 girls, with a mean age of 10 years, were obtained. The most popular form of alternative therapy was vitamins, minerals, and antioxidants (51%), followed by nutritional supplements (14%), herbs and botanical medicines (11%), massage (9%), chiropractic (4%), homeopathy (4%), and acupuncture (2%). (Horrigan et al., 1998). An anecdotal report described the use of St. John's wort by four teenagers who were under psychiatric care (Walter and Rey, 1999). Three of the patients had been reluctant to reveal this to their psychiatrist, believing the doctor had no interest in alternative medicine or would disapprove of it.

ATTITUDES OF MENTAL HEALTH PROFESSIONALS TOWARD COMPLEMENTARY AND ALTERNATIVE MEDICINE

The experiences and attitudes of mental health professionals about alternative treatments are important because the use of CAM has implications for psychiatry in several domains, including drug interactions (in the case of biologically active substances), compliance with "conventional" treatments, and patients' attitudes towards health professionals. Furthermore, psychiatrists may be a source of information about effectiveness and adverse events associated with alternative treatments. A survey conducted in 1999 of all members of the Royal Australian and New Zealand College of Psychiatrists found that a quarter of respondents had recommended St. John's wort to patients. The vast majority (86%) believed that psychiatrists should be taught about alternative treatments and 39% had used herbal remedies themselves. However, only a minority (38%) routinely asked patients if they used alternative remedies. This suggests that Australian psychiatrists (and probably psychiatrists in general) are open-minded about CAM but feel they do not have enough knowledge and experience about it (Walter et al., 2000).

REGULATORY AND ETHICAL ISSUES

A *dietary supplement* is any product taken by mouth that contains a so-called dietary ingredient and whose label clearly states that it is a dietary supplement. The dietary ingredients in dietary supplements may include vitamins, minerals, herbs, and amino acids as well as substances such as enzymes, organ tissues, metabolites, extracts, or concentrates. Dietary supplements can be found in many forms, such as tablets, capsules, liquids, or powders.

In the United States, nutritional supplements are not subject to regulation by the federal government (e.g., by the Food and Drug Administration) in the same manner as prescription drugs. This state of affairs was precipitated by the Dietary Supplement Health and Education Act of 1994, which classified agents such as pyridoxine, St. John's wort, and flax seed oil as food products in the wake of strong lobbying by the manufacturers of these supplements (Bull, 1999). In Australia, the Register of Therapeutic Goods currently categorizes most herbal preparations as "listed drugs," which are subject to fewer checks than "registered [prescription] drugs." Continental Europe has a more established tradition of herbal use for medicinal purposes, including in pediatric populations. For instance, the curriculum in many European medical schools incorporates formal training in the use of these agents. In 1976, the German government passed legislation that required that botanical medicines be reviewed in a formal manner for safety and efficacy. In 1978, the so-called Commission E was established in Germany to accomplish this task. Subsequently, this commission has published more than 300 monographs on solitary and fixed combinations of botanical products (herbs). These monographs are available in English translation (www.herbalgram.org/browse.php/commission_e). The content includes a review of the specific composition of botanical products, their uses, contraindications, side effects, drug interactions, dosages, modes of administration, and their actions.

As a result of the lower standards required, there are concerns about the fidelity of botanical and nutritional products. These are now causing growing unease among consumers and professionals. Apart from having to satisfy less rigorous efficacy and safety criteria than prescription drugs, herbal remedies and dietary supplements lack standardized preparation and are more prone to contamination, substitution, adulteration, incorrect packaging, wrong dosage, and inappropriate labeling and advertising (Drew and Myers, 1997). For example, in the case of St. John's wort there is presently no way of knowing that the correct species of *Hypericum* is used, that the plant is harvested at the right time of year, that appropriate plant parts are chosen, dried, and stored properly, and that the extraction process is uniform. All of these factors are believed to affect biological activity. In conjunction with this, there are wide variations in the degree of quality control that is exercised after manufacturing. For instance, fatty acid nutritional supplements as well as probiotics (e.g., acidophilus) can denature if stored for any length of time above common room temperatures. This fact is rarely appreciated by wholesale and retail outlets that may use nonrefrigerated storage facilities for their products. As a consequence, products purchased directly off the retail shelf may have markedly diminished activity.

Several recent events illustrate the dangers inherent in the current regulatory system. A Chinese herbal remedy contaminated with *Aristolochia fangchi* was widely used for weight reduction in Belgium and other European countries in the early 1990s. It was found later that many consumers (up to 40%) who had taken the herbs had developed chronic renal disease and at least 18 were diagnosed with cancer of the urinary tract (Vanherweghem et al., 1993; Nortier et al., 2000). Another example is the eosinophilia-myalgia syndrome (EMS). An epidemic was first recognized in 1989 in New Mexico (Hertzman et al., 1990) but many cases were subsequently identified throughout the United States. A number of them were patients being treated by psychiatrists (Sullivan et al., 1996). This syndrome is a serious illness with a high mortality rate. Contaminated tryptophan, an essential amino acid, produced by one manufacturer was shown to be the cause. Although the precise nature of the contaminant is not yet known, EMS is very similar to the toxic oil syndrome, an epidemic that affected more than 20,000 individuals who consumed contaminated oil in Spain during 1981. The toxic oil syndrome was caused by rapeseed oil denatured with aniline.

Underreporting of adverse events of medication is a global phenomenon. It applies to prescription and over-the-counter medicines and undoubtedly the same is likely to be true for CAM treatments. However, manufacturers of alternative treatments do not provide ongoing monitoring of the safety of their products that is comparable to that of pharmaceutical companies.

LIABILITY

Medical malpractice liability exists for treatment with CAM, particularly if clinicians recommend that patients take a supplement that is inferior in quality and, as a consequence, harmful. The same holds true if physicians direct patients to a negligent CAM practitioner. The referring clinician may be vicariously liable. The risk of negligence is especially keen if clinicians refer patients for a particular type of alternative therapy that

they know, or *should know*, offers no practical benefit (Studdert et al., 1998). Furthermore, there is increasing concern that clinicians may be at risk if they simply fail to inquire about patients' use of nutritional supplements, given the high prevalence of such use (Eisenberg et al., 1993; Druss and Rosenheck 2000).

From a practical viewpoint, clinicians interested in these products must acquaint themselves with the range available as well as the quality standards that are applied by the various manufacturers and wholesalers or retailers. This can be a daunting task, as information of this sort is not readily available. Nonpartisan, independent Internet sites may assist in this task (e.g., www.supplementwatch.com). The Office of Dietary Supplements at the NIH (http://odp.od.nih.gov/databases/ibids.html) and the University of Pittsburgh (www.pitt.edu/~cbw/database.html) have highly informative sites. It is also encouraging that there have been an increasing number of reports, reviews (e.g., Ernst et al., 1998; Wong et al., 1998), and books (eg., Muskin, 2000) on alternative treatments in the medical literature, which may assist clinicians. Table 29.1 summarizes the issues to keep in mind to minimize the risk of mishaps.

TABLE 29.1 *Issues to Consider and Discuss with Patients or Parents in Relation to Herbal Treatments and Dietary Supplements*

- Ask all patients and parents about use of herbal treatments and dietary supplements. Use of these agents should be documented in the medical record.
- An accurate diagnosis and discussion of proven treatment options are essential prior to the patient or parent considering alternative remedies.
- Patients and parents need to be advised through appropriate examples of the following:
  "Natural" does not necessarily mean safe.
  Lack of standardization or inadequate storage of preparations may result in variability in efficacy.
  Lack of quality control may result in contamination during manufacture or misidentification of plant species.
  Herbal–pharmaceutical interactions can occur, therefore avoid combining them.
  Herbal treatments should not be used during pregnancy or lactation or if the patient is contemplating pregnancy, because of the lack of data about safety.
  Larger than recommended dosages should not be used.
  Herbal treatments should not be used for long periods unless they are proving to be effective and there is reliable evidence about long-term safety.
- Inquire about adverse events and document them. Emerging side effects may require discontinuation.

Modified from Cirigliano and Sun (1998)

ST. JOHN'S WORT (*HYPERICUM*)

Hypericum perforatum, more commonly known as *Hypericum* or St. John's wort, is used widely because of the perception that it is a safer, "natural" antidepressant. In Germany, *Hypericum* is used more extensively than conventional antidepressants for treating depression. Because St. John's wort has been attracting increasing media attention worldwide, consumption of this herb is likely to become more prevalent.

Botany

The genus *Hypericum* contains more than 300 species. *Hypericum perforatum* is the one most often used in herbal remedies. It is an upright bush, growing to a metre tall, with oblong, perforated leaves and bright yellow flowers. The leaves are dotted with translucent glands. There are many explanations for the appellation *St. John's wort* (*wort* means "plant" in Old English); one is that the plant was named after St. John the Baptist because the flowers were said to bloom on the anniversary of his execution. St. John's wort is native to Europe, Asia, and Africa. *Hypericum perforatum* was introduced by European migrants to North America where it grows wild, particularly in Oregon and the Pacific Northwest ("klamath weed"). In Australia, introduction has been traced to Victoria during a gold boom in the 1880s, when a German woman imported seed of the plant and established it for medicinal purposes. It soon overran her garden and spread. St. John's wort was subsequently declared a noxious weed and there are now laws requiring its eradication from rural pastures (Rey and Walter, 1998). Among other names, St. John's Wort is known as *corazoncillo* in Spain, *Johanniskraut* in Germany, *millepertuis* in France, *perforata* in Italy, and *quiang ceng lou* in China.

Active Constituents and Mechanism of Action

Many constituents with potential biological activity have been extracted from the flowers and leaves, the parts of the plant used for medicinal purposes. These include naphthodianthrones, flavonoids, phloroglucinols, and xanthones. Hypericin, one of the naphthodianthrones, has traditionally been considered the main active ingredient, but it is not known whether this is the compound with antidepressant activity. Recent data suggest that a component called *hyperforin* may be more important than hypericin for the antidepressant activity.

The exact mechanism of action of St. John's wort remains obscure. Substances contained in *Hypericum* extracts have been found to interact with a number of neurotransmitter systems implicated in depression and in psychiatric illness generally. St. John's wort inhibits uptake of serotonin, noradrenaline, and dopamine, although these effects seem weak. Crude extracts of St. John's wort have a potent affinity for γ-aminobutyric acid (GABA) receptors. In vitro studies show that *Hypericum* inhibits monoamine oxidase (MAO) but there is little evidence of MAO activity in humans at therapeutic doses and no reports of hypertensive crises in individuals using St. John's wort. It has also been postulated that the antidepressant activity of St. John's wort may be due to its effect on interleukin-6 (Thiele et al., 1994; Cott, 1995; Yu, 2000).

Evidence of Effectiveness

Contrary to the situation with most alternative treatments, there is a growing body of research about the efficacy of St. John's wort in treating depression. At the time of writing, however, there were no controlled trials of children and adolescents.

Studies involving adults have been the object of several meta-analyses (e.g., Linde et al. 1996; Gaster and Holroyd, 2000). A recent systematic review (Gaster and Holroyd, 2000) identified eight controlled trials of good methodological quality published between 1980 and 1998. Participants ranged from 19 to 75 years of age (average 47 years). The four trials testing St. John's wort extract against placebo (with a total of 364 participants) found that St. John's wort was superior. Across studies, 69% of participants in the St. John's wort groups were considered responders, compared with 29% in the placebo groups. Four trials that tested St. John's wort against an antidepressant showed broadly similar efficacy with both. These trials, however, had significant limitations. Most notably, the comparison drug was a tricyclic antidepressant and the dosage of the tricyclic was probably too low to achieve antidepressant effect.

A multicenter trial comparing more appropriate doses of imipramine (75 mg twice daily, N = 167) and St. John's wort extract (250 mg twice daily standardized to 0.2% hypericin, N = 157) showed no difference in efficacy after 6 weeks of treatment. However, St. John's wort seemed to reduce anxiety symptoms more often than imipramine and was better tolerated (Woelk, 2000). A study including 240 participants compared St. John's wort with fluoxetine in mild to moderate depression and also concluded that efficacy of both treatments was comparable (Schrader, 2000). These results have been replicated in a smaller trial using sertraline as the comparison treatment (Brenner et al., 2000). Contrary to these reports, a multicenter, randomized, placebo-controlled trial of St. John's wort extract in 200 participants with major depressive disorder conducted in the United States concluded that St. John's wort was not effective for treatment of major depression (Shelton et al., 2001). Another multicentre trial conducted in the United States compared the effectiveness of *Hypericum* (900–1500 mg, 113 participants) with sertraline (50–100 mg, 109 participants) and placebo (116 participants) in the treatment of outpatients meeting criteria from DSM-IV major depressive disorder. Neither *Hypericum* nor sertraline were superior to placebo at 8 weeks although there were more partial responders to sertraline (24%) than to *Hypericum* (14%) or placebo (11%) (*Hypericum* Depression Trial Study Group, 2002).

In summary, there is evidence that *Hypericum* is effective in the treatment of adults with depression of mild to moderate severity. It appears also that patients tolerate St. John's wort well. Nevertheless, there are no reports involving children and adolescents. Until such data become available it cannot be concluded whether St. John's wort is effective in this age group.

Pharmacokinetics and Drug Disposition

It is not possible to discuss pharmacokinetics when the active compound or compounds of St. John's wort are not known. The half-life of hypericin and hyperforin have been estimated at between 6 and 9 hours, with peak plasma concentrations at about 2–3 hours after administration. Some of the ingredients of *Hypericum* extracts are metabolized in the liver.

Safety

There is a belief among many that "mother nature" is nurturing and harmless; hence, the mistaken conviction that herbal treatments, being natural, are safe. The evidence from controlled trials suggests that St. John's wort is a well-tolerated treatment (Gaster and Holroyd, 2000; Woelk, 2000; Shelton et al., 2001). However, adverse events related to St. Jonh's wort have been underreported (Rey and Walter, 1998; Ernst, 1999b). For example, the Australian Drug Reactions Advisory Committee received 12 reports involving *Hypericum* prior to January 2000. Conversely, a survey conducted in July 1999 of all the members of the Royal Australian and New Zealand College of Psychiatrists showed that 80% had patients who used St. John's wort. Twenty eighty percent had noticed side effects in their patients that they attributed to St. John's wort or to interactions between this herb and other psychotropics (Walter et al., 2000). These data indicate a discrepancy between responses by the psychiatrists and the number of reports to the Australian Drug Reactions Advisory Committee. Data from both sources are anecdotal and a cause–effect relationship cannot be established. Furthermore, *Hypericum* preparations often contain several ingredients. Nevertheless, this information suggests that underestimation of adverse events is likely. *Hypericum* might not be as safe as the literature led us to believe, for the above data contrast with the few unwanted events reported in treatment studies (Linde et al., 1996; Gaster and Holroyd, 2000; Woelk, 2000). Rates of side effects among individuals enrolled in trials may be lower because of participant selection and the use of a single medicine. Persons not enrolled in trials may combine St. John's wort and prescribed or over-the-counter medications more often. Thus clinical trials are limited in establishing the safety profile of a treatment. The more common side effects will generally be detected but the rarer, idiosyncratic, and often serious adverse events and drug interactions are less likely to be discovered during trials. Alternative and mainstream practitioners may also be less inclined to report adverse events associated with herbal remedies. Therefore, underestimation of unwanted events associated with St. John's wort needs to be kept in mind.

Side Effects

Rates of side effects with placebo and St. John's wort in placebo-controlled trials are comparable (Linde et al., 1996; Gaster and Holroyd, 2000). Fewer than 2% of patients in studies have stopped taking St. John's wort. In an open trial of 3250 patients taking *Hypericum*, side effects were reported by 2.4% of subjects. The most commonly noted side effects were gastrointestinal symptoms (0.6%), allergic reactions (0.5%), fatigue (0.4%), and restlessness (0.3%). Other adverse reactions reported were emotional vulnerability, pruritus, weight gain, and dizziness (Woelk, 1994). Headaches also seem to be common (Shelton et al., 2001). St. John's wort has been shown to have uterotonic action. This would make it unadvisable during pregnancy. Manic switch or manic symptoms can occur.

Severe phototoxicity has been reported in cattle and sheep grazing on the plant (the veterinary term is *hypericism*) but not in humans taking therapeutic doses. However, photosensitivity does appear to be a problem

(Bove, 1998, Walter et al., 2000). People using St. John's wort should take extra care if they go out in the sunshine and avoid sun bathing. This can be difficult for children and adolescents. Furthermore, concerns have been raised that St. John's wort and bright light may lead to the development of cataracts (Schey et al., 2000). In this context, the combination of St. John's wort and light-box therapy in patients with seasonal affective disorder could be hazardous.

Drug Interactions

Hypericum extracts can have clinically significant interactions with prescribed medications (Rey and Walter, 1998; Ernst, 1999b; Piscitelli et al., 2000; Walter et al., 2000). The more important interactions known are presented in Table 29.2. There is limited information about the mechanisms involved. The more common view is that St. John's wort extracts activate the

TABLE 29.2 *Reported Clinically Significant Interactions of St. John's Wort (SJW) with Prescription Drugs*

Interacting Agent	Mechanism of Interaction	Clinical Effect/Presentation	Management/Comments
SSRIs and similar drugs (e.g., citalopram, fluoxetine, fluvoxamine, paroxetine, sertraline)	Stimulation of 5-HT receptors	Increased serotonergic effects and increased likelihood of adverse reactions (e.g., serotonergic syndrome)	Avoid concurrent use
Oral contraceptives	Probable induction of cytochrome P450 metabolic pathway	Reduced blood levels with risk of breakthrough bleeding Possible failure to prevent conception	Weigh benefits of continuing use of SJW and possibly reduced contraceptive effect
Anticonvulsants (e.g., carbamazepine, phenytoin)	Probable induction of cytochrome P450 metabolic pathway	Reduced blood levels Lowered anticonvulsant action	Monitor anticonvulsant levels and stop SJW Readjust dose if required
Cyclosporin, tacrolimus	Probable induction of cytochrome P450 metabolic pathway	Reduced blood levels Risk of rejection of transplant	Monitor cyclosporine levels and stop SJW Readjust dose of cyclosporine if required
Warfarin	Probable induction of cytochrome P450 metabolic pathway	Reduced blood levels Reduced anticoagulant effect	Check prothronbin time and stop SJW Monitor prothronbin time closely and readjust dose of warfarin if necessary
Theophylline	Probable induction of cytochrome P450 metabolic pathway	Reduced blood levels and bronchodilator action	Monitor theophyline levels and stop SJW Readjust theophyline dose if required
Digoxin	Probable induction of cytochrome P450 and P-glycoprotein metabolic pathways	Reduced blood levels and effectiveness Toxicity upon cessation of SJW	Monitor digoxin levels closely and stop SJW Readjust dose of digoxin if necessary
HIV protease inhibitors (e.g., indinavir, nelfinavir, ritonavir)	Probable induction of cytochrome P450 metabolic pathway and P-glycoprotein	Reduced blood levels with possible loss of HIV suppression Resistance	Measure HIV RNA viral load and stop SJW
HIV non-nucleoside reverse transcriptase inhibitors (e.g., efavirenz, nevirapine)	Probable induction of cytochrome P450 metabolic pathway and P-glycoprotein	Reduced blood levels with possible loss of HIV suppression Resistance	Measure HIV RNA viral load and stop SJW
Triptans (e.g., sumatripan, naratripan, zolmitriptan)	Stimulation of 5-HT receptors	Increased serotonergic effects and increased likelihood of adverse reactions	Weigh benefits of continuing use of SJW against potential for adverse events

cytochrome P450 (CYP) system, mostly CYP3A4 (Ernst, 1999b; Moore et al., 2000). There is evidence that a reporter construct derived from the CYP3A promoter is activated by St. John's wort via the steroid X receptor, which induces hepatic CYP gene expression. The induction is dose-dependent and of comparable magnitude to the effects of rifampicin, a known CYP3A activator. Hyperforin, and not hypericin, seems to be the constituent that mediates this activation (Wentworth et al., 2000). Because CYP3A4 is involved in the oxidative metabolism of more than half of all drugs, there are potential interactions with more medications than has been realized (see Chapter 5).

Hypericum has been found to also interact with drugs metabolized via other pathways. For example, it decreases serum levels of digoxin, which is metabolized via the P-glycoprotein drug transporter, and reduces levels of theophylline and warfarin, which are metabolized via CYP1A2 and CYP2C9 pathways, respectively. It is possible that St. John's wort might also induce those enzymes via the steroid X receptor (Wentworth et al., 2000).

It is of note that *Hypericum*, often described as "the natural Prozac," has the opposite effect of fluoxetine—and selective serotonin reuptake inhibitors (SSRIs) in general—on the CYP system. Fluoxetine inhibits several CYP isoenzymes, potentially resulting in increased blood levels of drugs metabolized through this pathway (See Chapter 22).

Serotonin syndrome (Sternbach, 1991) has been reported when St. John's wort is used concurrently with other serotonergic drugs. This syndrome is believed to be due to an excess stimulation of the $5\text{-}HT_{1A}$ receptor, probably as a result of the serotonergic activity of St. John's wort compounds.

Clinical Uses in Children and Adolescents

There is no empirical evidence available for clinical use in children and adolescents. Yet, *Hypericum* seems to be used for the treatment of mild to moderate depression in the young (Walter et al., 2000). St. John's wort should be avoided in young patients with severe depression and bipolar disorder (given the lack of adult data about effectiveness and risk of manic induction, respectively) and in those who have significant suicide risk. Treatments of proven efficacy (e.g., SSRIs, mood stabilisers) should be preferred in these cases. However, St. John's wort may be considered in cases of unipolar depression where conventional treatments have failed and prior to the use of combinations of drugs that have an increased risk of side effects and whose efficacy has not been demonstrated.

The principles outlined in Table 29.1 should be followed prior to initiating treatment. In particular, patients and parents ought to be informed of other treatment options, along with their potential benefits and risks. For example, St. John's wort is contraindicated in pregnant or sexually active adolescents (there is a risk of miscarriage and lack of teratogenic effect is not established). Cost of treatment should be discussed as well. *Hypericum* should not be used concurrently with other medications, particularly SSRIs, given the risk of drug interactions (see Table 29.2). Monitoring should be the same as for antidepressant drugs and should include systematic inquiry about side effects, adherence to treatment, and symptom improvement.

Preparations, Dosage, and Administration

St. John's wort is available as tablets, capsules, drops, and teas. Many brands exist and *Hypericum* is widely available in health food stores or through the Internet. There is an oil form for external use but this has no place in treating depression. Many St. John's wort preparations have other ingredients and should be avoided.

The adult dosage of St John's wort traditionally recommended for treating depression is 300 mg of plant extract orally three times daily (plant extracts are usually standardised to 0.3% hypericin). There are no data about optimal dosage in young people. Clinicians often start with half the adult dose and increase the amount up to 300 mg three times daily after 3 or 4 weeks if the herb is well tolerated and there is no improvement. Clinical experience shows this regime results in few unwanted effects in the young.

It is important to note that amounts used vary considerably and there are no systematic studies on the minimum therapeutic dosage. Furthermore, the quantity of active substances can change depending on factors such as the extraction process, season, and plant part used. Quality control studies show that the amount of active ingredients (e.g., hypericin) is often very different from those advertised in the label.

As with prescription antidepressants, there is a 2- or 3-week lag in onset of action. If side effects are marked, or if at 6 to 8 weeks *Hypericum* is deemed to be ineffective, the patient can be weaned off and another treatment considered. Unfortunately, there are no data about washout periods following discontinuation of St. John's wort. A conservative approach is to wait 2 weeks after ceasing St. John's wort before commencing another agent.

There is little information about long-term use in adults and no data on such use in children. Given the similarities between *Hypericum* and other antidepressants, it would be wise to continue treatment for 6 to 12 months in cases of good response and tolerance. There is no evidence on the role of St. John's wort in preventing recurrence or in cases with recurrent depression. When discontinuing treatment, the dosage should be reduced gradually to avoid withdrawal symptoms, which have been described in some cases (Beckman et al., 2000).

Other Uses

St. John's wort has been used to treat a wide range of ailments for more than 2000 years, and is said to have been prescribed by Hippocrates himself. Apart from depression, St. John's wort is being promoted or used as a treatment for attention-deficit hyperactivity disorder (ADHD), anxiety, stress, obsessive-compulsive disorder, sleep problems, nocturnal enuresis, bacterial and viral infections such as HIV-AIDS, respiratory conditions, peptic ulceration, inflammatory arthritis, cancer, and skin wounds (Rey and Walter, 1998; Walter et al., 2000). It is also said to increase libido, an application dating from the Middle Ages (Fletcher, 1996). No empirical evidence is currently available to support any of these uses.

ESSENTIAL FATTY ACIDS

The psychiatric community, the lay press, and ads on the Internet have drawn attention to the role of essential fatty acids (EFAs) on neural development and on the treatment of mental illness. The EFAs are often referred to as omega-3 and omega-6 fatty acids, and include fish oil, flax seed oil, and evening primrose oil supplements.

The central nervous system (CNS) is second only to adipose tissue in terms of lipid concentration. Neuronal membranes are composed of phospholipids that are particularly dense in long-chain polyunsaturated fatty acids of the omega-3 and omega-6 families. Omega-3 and omega-6 fatty acids are termed *essential* given that the body does not manufacture them and they must be acquired through dietary intake. The most common omega-3 derived from dietary sources is α-linolenic acid, while linoleic acid is the most common omega-6 fatty acid.

It has been known for some time that humans are prone to deficiencies in EFAs. Various disease states can occur in the wake of this, affecting virtually all organ systems (Simopoulos, 1991). A pertinent example for child psychiatrists is the higher rate of reading disabilities and visual problems in children with a history of preterm deliveries. These phenomena have been linked to critically low lipid depots (particularly involving the omega-3 family) in the CNS at the time of delivery (Lutz, 1998). The EFAs seem to play an important role in the regulation of membrane activity in neurones. Rats deficient in EFAs show impaired learning, attention, and behavior (Yehuda et al., 1997). The EFAs may also enhance normal development (Scott et al., 1998; Birch et al., 2000). Certain populations appear to be more prone to deficiencies of EFAs, including children from lower socioeconomic strata as well as children who are administered strict vegetarian diets by their parents (Krajcovicova-Kudlackova et al., 1997). The increasingly popular low-fat diets may not serve children well if proper intake of EFAs is not assured.

There are reports of an association between low fish consumption and increased prevalence of depression (Hibbelin, 1998). Some studies have found a reduced level of omega-3 fatty acids in depressed patients. It has also been speculated that EFAs have a role in the causation of schizophrenia and, more recently, ADHD and behavioral problems (Stevens et al., 1996; Burgess et al., 2000).

Although this is an area in which research is burgeoning, definite evidence of the effectiveness of EFAs in the treatment of mental disorders is lacking. There are some controlled trials of varying methodological quality in adult patients with schizophrenia, and unipolar and bipolar depression, with conflicting results (Fenton et al., 2000; Maidment, 2000). The most encouraging trial is a preliminary study of 30 patients with bipolar disorder. It found that EFAs concurrent with mood stabilizers reduced the rate of recurrence of episodes (Stoll et al., 1999).

Controlled studies involving lipid manipulation in children date back to the 1920s, when the ketogenic diet was pioneered to control treatment-resistant seizures in select pediatric populations (Freeman et al., 1998). However, no controlled evidence is available in children with depression, bipolar disorder, behavioral problems, or ADHD. In the absence of definite empirical data about effectiveness, treatment with EFA supplements should be considered unproven and patients ought to be advised accordingly.

Commercial products that contain high levels of omega-3 fatty acids include marine fish oils and flax seed oil, while evening primrose oil contains a higher proportion of omega-6 fatty acids. During processing and storage, these products must be kept in conditions that avoid excess light, heat, and air exposure to prevent oxidation and subsequent rancidity. In addition, there have been concerns about the safety of some products. For instance, organochlorine residues have been found in fish oils sold as dietary supplements in the United States (Jacobs et al., 1998).

The type of fatty acid employed may be a critical factor in the efficacy (or lack thereof). Omega-6 supplementation may have less impact than omega-3 administration (Hodge et al., 1998). Typical dosing strategies are similar for both children and adults, namely from 3 to 10 g of refrigerated fish oil or 3 tablespoons of refrigerated flax seed oil per day, split into multiple administration times (e.g. three times per day).

The EFAs are generally regarded as safe unless consumed in very large quantities. Belching, mild nausea, exacerbation of asthma in aspirin-sensitive patients and a rise in glucose in individuals with non–insulin-dependent diabetes are some of the side effects reported. The EFAs should be used with caution by patients taking anticoagulants or suffering from hemophilia (Fenton et al., 2000).

VALERIAN

Of about 200 species of the genus *Valeriana*, *Valeriana officinalis* is the one most commonly used medicinally (Plushner, 2000). The parts of this plant that are used for this purpose are the dried rhizomes and roots.

As with studies of many other herbs and nutritional supplements, interpretation of clinical trials of valerian is hampered by small sample sizes, suboptimal study design, lack of specified inclusion and exclusion criteria, and unknown composition of valerian extract (Plushner, 2000). Furthermore, none of the trials have included children or teenagers. Nevertheless, several studies have showed a mild hypnotic action in persons with insomnia and in normal sleepers, as well as a mild sedative effect (Leathwood and Chauffard, 1983, 1985; Balderer and Borbely, 1985). One report has described an anxiolytic effect (Kohnen and Oswald, 1988). There are suggestions that valerian may have beneficial effects on sleep latency, frequency of waking, nighttime motor activity, and overall sleep quality.

The mechanism of action of valerian is unknown. Possible mechanisms include affinity for $GABA_A$ and 5-HT_A receptors, inhibition of GABA catabolism, and targeting of adenosine receptors (Riedel et al., 1982; Holzl and Godau, 1989; Wong, et al., 1998).

In adults, the dosage for valerian ranges from 2 to 3 g given three times a day or at bedtime (Wong, 1998). There are no data about dosage in children. Although

side effects are generally minimal, dystonia and hepatitis have been reported (Bos et al., 1997; Muskin, 2000, p. 21) However, in these cases a mixture of valerian and other substances had been used.

KAVA

Kava has long been a ceremonial and social drink in Fiji, Samoa, and Tonga; in these countries it has also been used as an analgesic, to induce relaxation and sleep, and to counteract fatigue (Muskin, 2000, p. 18; Pittler and Ernst, 2000). More recently, kava has emerged as a popular botanical therapy in adult populations. In 1998, kava was among the top-selling herbs in the United States, with an annual turnover of approximately $8 million and a growth rate of 473% (Pittler and Ernst, 2000). Kava is the beverage prepared from the rhizome of the oceanic kava plant (*Piper methysticum*).

Kavapyrones seem to be the therapeutically active constituents. Kava appears to influence a number of monoamine, amino acid, and neuropeptide transmitters in the CNS. Animal studies suggest that kava activates mesolimbic dopaminergic neurons (e.g., in the nucleus accumbens) while also altering 5-HT levels in various brain regions (Baum et al., 1998). Kava may also act as a reversible MAO inhibitor and a noradrenergic reuptake inhibitor (Uebelhack et al., 1998).

A recent meta-analysis identified seven double-blind, placebo-controlled studies of acceptable quality (Pittler and Ernst, 2000). The review concluded that compared with placebo, kava extract is an effective symptomatic treatment for anxiety. There are no published reports concerning its usefulness in children.

There appears to be little difference between benzodiazepines and kava extract in anxiolytic activity. However, kava extracts seem to have fewer side effects. Two studies with more than 3000 patients each found unwanted events in about 2% of patients during treatment with kava extract. The more frequently reported side effects were gastrointestinal complaints, allergic skin reactions, headache, and photosensitivity (Pittler and Ernst, 2000). There have been isolated reports of hepatotoxicity and acute liver failure (Escher et al., 2001). Kava may potentiate the sedative effects of other medications including barbiturates and benzodiazepines. Kava can also cause behavioral disinhibition in a minority of individuals, including children. The most common problem, which is usually associated with persistent and excessive usage, is a scaly skin rash called "kava dermopathy," which is reversible.

The onset of the anxiolytic action of kava may be delayed as long as 8 weeks, thus limiting its potential as an acute pharmacotherapeutic agent (Volz and Kieser, 1997). The published studies in adult populations describe dosages in the range of 100 mg twice daily of the 70% kavalactone standardized product (Wong et al., 1998). No specific guidelines are available concerning pediatric dosing.

CONCLUSION

Clinicians should be aware that many of their patients may be taking alternative treatments either via self-care or prescribed by CAM practitioners. Inquiring about this should be routine because of potential side effects and drug interactions. A working knowledge of CAM treatments will allow child psychiatrists to give parents and patients advice about safety and effectiveness. Use of St. John's wort in children with unipolar depression may at times be appropriate, particularly in cases where more standard treatments are contraindicated or have failed. However, it should be used cautiously and with an appropriate explanation of its risks and benefits, as a competent clinician would do for any treatment. Use of St. John's wort for other conditions is not currently recommended given the lack of evidence for efficacy. Kava extracts may be used for anxiety, with similar provisos. There are much fewer data about the efficacy and safety of other dietary supplements and their use cannot be supported at this point.

REFERENCES

Andrews, L., Lokuge, S., Sawyer M., Lillywhite, L., Kennedy, D., and Martin J. (1998) The use of alternative therapies by children with asthma: a brief report. *Paediatr Child Health* 34:131–134.

Balderer, G. and Borbely, A.A. (1985) Effect of valerian on human sleep. *Psychopharmacology* 87:406–409.

Baum, S.S., Hill, R., and Rommelspacher, H. (1998) Effect of kava extract and individual kavapyrones on neurotransmitter levels in the nucleus accumbens of rats. *Prog Neuropsychopharmacol Biol Psychiatry* 22:1105–1120.

Beckman, S.E., Sommi, R.W., and Switzer, J. (2000) Consumer use of St. John's wort: a survey on effectiveness, safety and tolerability. *Pharmacotherapy* 20:568–574.

Birch, E.E., Garfield, S., Hoffman, D.R., Uauy, R., and Birch, D.G. (2000) A randomized controlled trial of early dietary supply of long-chain polyunsaturated fatty acids and mental development in term infants. *Dev Med Child Neurol* 42:174–181.

Bos, R., Woerdenbag, H.J., De Smet, P., and Scheffer, J.J.C. (1997) *Valeriana* species. In: De Smet, P., ed. *Adverse Effects of Herbal Drugs*. Berlin: Springer-Verlag.

Bove, G.M. (1998) Acute neuropathy after exposure to sun in a patient treated with St. John's wort. *Lancet* 352:1121–1122.

Brenner, R., Azbel, V., Madhusoodam, S., and Pawlowska, M. (2000)

Comparison of an extract of *Hypericum* (LI 160) and sertraline in the treatment of depression: a double-blind randomized pilot study. *Clin Ther* 22:411–419.

Bull, J.C. (1999) Dietary supplements: current FDA activities. *J Am Med Wom Assoc* 54:199–200.

Burgess, J.R., Stevens, L., Zhang, W., and Peck, L. (2000) Long-chain polyunsaturated fatty acids in children with attention-deficit hyperactivity disorder. *Am J Clin Nutr* 71(1 Suppl):327S–330S.

Cirigliano, M. and Sun, A. (1998) Advising patients about herbal therapies. *JAMA* 280:1565–1566.

Cott, J. (1995) Natural product formulations available in Europe for psychotropic indications. *Psychopharmacol Bull* 31:745–751.

Drew, A.K. and Myers, S.P. (1997) Safety issues in herbal medicine: implications for the health professions. *Med J Aust* 166:538–541.

Druss, B.G. and Rosenheck, R.A. (2000) Use of practitioner-based complementary therapies by persons reporting mental conditions in the United States. *Arch Gen Psychiatry* 57:708–714.

Eisenberg, D.M., Davis, R.B., and Ettner, S.L. (1998) Trends in alternative medicine use in the United States, 1990–1997: results of a follow-up national survey. *JAMA* 280:1569–1575.

Eisenberg, D.M., Kessler, R.C., Foster, C., Norlock, F.E., Calkins, D.R., and Delbanco, T.L. (1993) Unconventional medicine in the United States: prevalence, costs, and patterns of use. *N Engl J Med* 328:246–252.

Ernst, E. (1999a) Prevalence of complementary/alternative medicine for children: a systematic review. *Eur J Pediatr* 158:7–11.

Ernst, E. (1999b) Second thoughts about safety of St. John's wort. *Lancet* 354:2014–2016.

Ernst, E., Rand, J.I., and Stevinson, C. (1998) Complementary therapies for depression: an overview. *Arch Gen Psychiatry* 55:1026–1032.

Escher, M., Desmeules, J., Giostra, E., and Mentha, G. (2001) Hepatitis associated with kava, a herbal remedy for anxiety. *BMJ* 322:139.

Fenton, W.S., Hibbeln, J., and Knable, M. (2000) Essential fatty acids, lipid membrane abnormalities, and the diagnosis and treatment of schizophrenia *Bio Psychiatry* 47:8–21.

Fletcher, K. (1996) *Themes for Herbal Gardens*. Ringwood, Victoria: Viking, p. 16.

Freeman, J.M., Vining, E.P., Pillas, D.J., Pyzik, P.L., Casey, J.C., and Kelly, L.M. (1998) The efficacy of the ketogenic diet—1998: a prospective evaluation of intervention in 150 children. *Pediatrics* 102:1358–1363.

Gaster, B. and Holroyd, J. (2000) St. John's wort for depression: a systematic review. *Arch Intern Med* 160:152–156.

Hertzman, P.A., Blevins, W.L., Mayer, J., Greenfield, B., Ting, M., and Gleich, G.J. (1990) Association of the eosinophilia-myalgia syndrome with the ingestion of tryptophan. *N Engl J Med* 322:869–873.

Hibbelin, J.R. (1998) Fish consumption and major depression. *Lancet* 351:1213.

Hodge, L., Salome, C.M., Hughes, J.M., Liu-Brennan, D., Rimmer, J., Allman, M., Pang, D., Armour, C., and Woolcock, A.J. (1998) Effect of dietary intake of omega-3 and omega-6 fatty acids on severity of asthma in children. *Eur Respir J* 11:361–365.

Holzl, J. and Godau, P. (1989) Receptor binding studies with *Valeriana officinalis* on the benzodiazepine receptor. *Planta Med* 55:642.

Horrigan, J.P., Sikich, L., Courvoisie, H.E., and Barnhill, L.J. (1998) Alternative therapies in the child psychiatric clinic. *J Child Adolesc Psychopharmacol* 8:249–250.

Hypericum Depression Trial Study Group (2002) Effect of *Hyperi-*

cum perforatum (St. John's wort) in major depressive disorder. *JAMA* 287:1807–1814.

Jacobs, M.N., Santillo, D., Johnston, P.A., Wyatt, C.L., and French, M.C. (1998) Organochlorine residues in fish oil dietary supplements: comparison with industrial grade oils. *Chemosphere* 37: 1709–1721.

Jorm, A.F., Korten, A.E., Jacomb, P.A., Christensen, H., Rodgers, B., and Pollitt P. Mental health literacy: a survey of the public's ability to recognise mental disorders and their beliefs about the effectiveness of treatment. *Med J Aust* 166:182–186.

Kohnen, R. and Oswald, W.D. (1988) The effects of valerian, propanolol and their combination on activation, performance and mood of healthy volunteers under social stress conditions. *Pharmacopsychiatry* 21:447–448.

Krajcovicova-Kudlackova, M., Simoncic, R., Bederova, A., and Klvanova, J. (1997) Plasma fatty acid profile and alternative nutrition. *Ann Nutr Metab* 41:365–370.

Leathwood, P.D. and Chauffard, F. (1983) Quantifying the effects of mild sedatives. *J Psychiatr Res* 17:115–122.

Leathwood, P.D. and Chauffard, F. (1985) Aqueous extract of valerian reduces latency to fall asleep in man. *Planta Med* 51:144–148.

Linde, K., Ramirez, G., Mulrow, C.D., Pauls, A., Weidenhammer, W., and Melchart, D. (1996) St. John's wort for depression: an overview and meta-analysis of randomised clinical trials. *BMJ* 313:253–258.

Lutz, M. (1998) Diet as a determinant of central nervous system development: role of essential fatty acids. *Arch Latinoam Nutr* 48:29–34.

MacLennan, A.H., Wilson, D.H., and Taylor, A.W. (1996) Prevalence and cost of alternative medicine in Australia. *Lancet* 347: 569–573.

Maidment, I.D. (2000) Are fish oils an effective therapy in mental illness—an analysis of the data. Acta Psychiatr Scand 102:3–11.

Moore, L.B., Goodwin, B., Jones, S.A., Wisely, G.B., Serabjit-Singh, C.J., Willson, T.M., Collins, J.L., and Kliewer, S.A. (2000) St. John's wort induces hepatic metabolism through activation of the pregnane X receptor. *Proc Nat Acad Sci USA* 97:7500–7502.

Muskin, P.R. (2000) *Complementary and Alternative Medicine and Psychiatry*. Washington, DC: American Psychiatric Press.

Nortier, J.L., Martinez, M.C., Schmeiser, H.H., Arlt, V.M., Bieler, C.A., Petein, M., Depierreux, M.F., De Pauw, L., Abramowicz, D., Vereerstraeten, P., and Vanherweghem, J.L. (2000) Urothelial carcinoma associated with the use of a chinese herb (Aristolochia fangchi). *New Engl J Med* 342:1686–1692.

Piscitelly, S.C., Burstein, A.H., Chaitt, D., Alfaro, R.M., and Falloon, J. (2000) Indinavir concentrations and St. John's wort. *Lancet* 355:547–548.

Pittler, M.H. and Ernst, E. (2000) Efficacy of kava extract for treating anxiety: systematic review and meta-analysis. *J Clin Psychopharmacal* 20:84–89.

Plushner, S.L. (2000) Valerian: *Valeriana officinalis*. *Am J Health Syst Pharm* 57:328–335

Rey, J.M. and Walter, G. (1998) *Hypericum perforatum* (St. John's wort) in depression: pest or blessing? *Med J Aust* 169:583–586.

Riedel, E., Hansel, R., and Ehrke, G. (1982) inhibition of GABA catabolism by valerenic acid derivatives. *Planta Med* 46:219–220.

Sawyer, M.G., Gannoni, A.F., Toogood, I.R., Antoniou, G., and Rice, M. (1994) The use of alternative therapies by children with cancer. *Med J Aust* 160:320–322.

Sawyer, M.G., Rey, J.M., Graetz, B., Clark, J.J., and Baghurst, P.A. (2002) Use of medication by young people with attention-deficit/hyperactivity disorder. *Med J Aust*. (in press)

Schey, K.L., Patat, S., Chignell, C.F., Datillo, M., Wang, R.H., and Roberts, J.E. (2000) Photooxidation of lens alpha-crystallin by hypericin (active ingredient in St. John's wort). *Photochem Photobiol* 72:200–2003.

Schrader, E. (2000) Equivalence of St. John's wort extract (Ze 117) and fluoxetine: a randomized, controlled study in mild-moderate depression. *Int Clin Psychopharmacol* 15:61–68.

Scott, D.T., Janowsky, J.S., Carroll, R.E., Taylor, J.A., Auestad, N., and Montalto, M.B. (1998) Formula supplementation with long-chain polyunsaturated fatty acids: are there developmental benefits? *Pediatrics* 102:E59.

Shelton, R.C., Keller, M.B., Gelenberg, A., Dunner, D.L., Hirschfeld, R., Thase, M.E., Russell, J., Lydiard, R.B., Crits-Cristoph, P., Gallop, R., Todd, L., Hellerstein, D., Goodnick, P., Keitner, G., Stahl, S.M., and Halbreich, U. (2001) Effectiveness of St. John's wort in major depression: a randomized controlled trial. *JAMA* 285: 1978–1986.

Simopoulos, A.P. (1991) Omega-3 fatty acids in health and disease and in growth and development. *Am J Clin Nutr* 54:438–463.

Sternbach, H. (1991) The serotonin syndrome. *Am J Psychiatry* 148: 705–713.

Stevens, L.J., Zentall, S.S., Abate, M.L., Kuczek, T., and Burgess, J.R. (1996) Omega-3 fatty acids in boys with behavior, learning, and health problems. *Physiol Behav* 59:915–920.

Stoll, A.L., Severus, W.E., Freeman, M.P., Rueter, S., Zboyan, H.A., Diamond, E., Cress, K.K., and Marangell, L.B. (1999) Omega 3 fatty acids in bipolar disorder: a preliminary double-blind, placebo-controlled trial. *Arch Gen Psychiatry* 56:407–412.

Studdert, D.M., Eisenberg, D.M., Miller, F.H., Curto, D.A., Kaptchuk, T.J., and Brennan, T.A. (1998) Medical malpractice implications of alternative medicine. *JAMA* 280:1610–1615.

Sullivan, E.A., Kamb, M.L., Jones, J.L., Meyer, P., Philen, R.M., Falk, H., and Sinks, T. (1996) The natural history of eosinophilia-myalgia syndrome in a tryptophan-exposed cohort in South Carolina. *Arch Intern Med* 156:973–975.

Thiele, B., Brink, I., and Ploch, M. (1994) Modulation of cytokine expression by *Hypericum* extract. *J Geriatr Psychiatry Neurol* 7 (Suppl 1):S60–S62.

Uebelhack, R., Franke, L., and Schewe, H.J. (1998) Inhibition of platelet MAO-B by kava pyrone–enriched extract from *Piper methysticum Forster* (kava-kava). *Pharmacopsychiatry* 31:187–192.

Unutzer, J., Klap, R., Sturm, R., Young, A.S., Marmon, T., Shatkin, J., and Wells, K.B. (2000) Mental disorders and use of alternative medicine: results from a national survey. *Am J Psychiatry* 157: 1851–1857.

Vanherweghem, J.L., Depierreux M., Tielemans, C., Abramowicz, D., Dratwa, M., Jadoul, M., Richard, C., Vandervelde, D., Verbeelen, D., and Vanhaelen-Fastre, R. (1993) Rapidly progressive interstitial renal fibrosis in young women: association with slimming regimen including Chinese herbs. *Lancet* 341:387–391.

Volz, H.P. and Kieser, M. (1997) Kava-kava extract WS 1490 versus placebo in anxiety disorders—a randomized placebo-controlled 25-week outpatient trial. *Pharmacopsychiatry* 30:1–5.

Walter, G. and Rey, J.M. (1999) Use of St. John's wort by adolescents receiving treatment for a psychiatric disorder. *J Child Adolesc Psychopharmacol* 9:307–311.

Walter, G., Rey, J.M., and Harding, A. (2000) Psychiatrists' experience and views regarding St. John's wort and "alternative" treatments. *Aust N Z J Psychiatry* 34:992–996.

Wentworth, J.M., Agostini, M., Love, J., Schwabe, J.W., and Chatterjee, V.K. (2000) St. John's wort, a herbal antidepressant, activates the steroid X receptor. *J Endocrinol* 166:R11–R16.

Woelk, H. (1994) Benefits and risks of the *Hypericum* extract L1
160: drug monitoring study with 3250 patients. *J Geriatr Psy-chiatry Neurol* 7 (Suppl 1):S34–S38.

Woelk, H. (2000) Comparison of St. John's wort and imipramine for
treating depression: randomised controlled trial. *BMJ* 321:536–539.

Wong, A.H.C., Smith, M., and Boon, H.S. (1998) Herbal remedies
in psychiatric practice. *Arch Gen Psychiatry* 55:1033–1044.

Yehuda, S., Rabinovitz, S., and Mostofsky, D. (1997) Effects of es-sential fatty acid preparation (SR-3) on brain lipids, biochemistry,
and behavioural and cognitive functions. In Yehuda, S. and Mos-tofsky, D., eds. *Handbook of Essential Fatty Acid Biology, Bio-chemistry, Physiology, and Behavioural Neurobiology.* Totowa,
NJ: Humana Press, pp. 427–452.

Yu, P.H. (2000) Effect of *Hypericum perforatum* extract on serotonin
turnover in the mouse brain. *Pharmacopsychiatry* 33:60–65.

Zollman, C. and Vickers, A. (1999) What is complementary medi-cine? *BMJ* 319:693–696.

30 Electroconvulsive therapy and transcranial magnetic stimulation

GARRY WALTER, JOSEPH M. REY, AND NEERA GHAZIUDDIN

Electroconvulsive therapy (ECT) is a treatment that involves the production of a seizure through the brief passage of an electric current through the brain, via electrodes placed on the scalp. ECT in young persons remains an uncommon treatment that is usually administered as a last resort. However, the subject is attracting increasing attention because of its effectiveness in some severe illnesses (e.g., psychotic depression, mania, catatonia) and because of lay concerns about its use in the young. This chapter examines the treatment's history, effectiveness and indications, adverse events, mode of administration (including legislative and ethical issues), and attitudes towards its use. We also describe the novel treatment of transcranial magnetic stimulation (TMS) and its potential usefulness in the treatment of children and adolescents.

HISTORY

Electroconvulsive therapy was first administered in 1938 to a 39-year-old man with schizophrenia (Abrams, 1997). When the treatment was first given to a child or adolescent is less clear (Rey and Walter, 1997). The earliest ECT studies, in 1938, 1939, and 1940, make no reference to treatment of children or adolescents. Similarly, the memoirs of the first generation of ECT exponents—Bini, Cerletti, Kalinowski, Accornero, and Fleischer—do not mention the treatment's application in the young. Because chemically induced seizures were extensively used in young persons with mental illnesses at the time ECT emerged, it might be assumed that ECT was soon applied to the young.

The first published account was from France. In 1942, during the German occupation, Georges Heuyer and colleagues reported the positive effects of ECT in two adolescents (Heuyer et al., 1942). The next year the same group described ECT treatment in 40 children and adolescents (Heuyer et al., 1943). They reported

that ECT was most useful in those with melancholia, less effective in mania, and not helpful in treating schizophrenia. Furthermore, ECT was described as a safe treatment in this age group.

It is not surprising that ECT soon became popular in treating children and adolescents with mental illness; in the 1940s effective treatments for mental disorders in this age group were few. For example, in 1947 Lauretta Bender reported on ECT use at Bellevue Hospital in New York in 98 children under the age of 12 years (Bender, 1947). The children were described as suffering from "childhood schizophrenia." However, looking at the clinical descriptions, today they would probably be given diagnoses of disruptive behavior disorder or developmental disorder. Bender reported beneficial effects of ECT in all but two or three of the children, while conceding that remissions "such as are seen in adults occurred in only a few."

Despite the early encouraging results described above, the use of ECT in minors then diminished. A constellation of factors may be implicated, including concerns about possible harmful effects (such as how ECT might impair brain development), the advent of psychotropic drugs, the antipsychiatry movement, and negative media depictions of the treatment (Bauer, 1976; Perkins and Tanaka, 1979). ECT in children and adolescents became a controversial treatment of last resort in most countries. There have been attempts in England to prohibit ECT for this age group (Baker, 1994), while ECT has been outlawed for people below 16 years in several states in the United States.

In the 1990s the psychiatric profession attempted to delineate the indications for ECT in minors and the way the treatment should be administered. For example, the American Psychiatric Association (APA) in 1990 (American Psychiatric Association, 1990) and Royal College of Psychiatrists in 1995 (Freeman, 1995) devoted special sections to the use of ECT in the young in their ECT guidelines. In 1999, the Royal Australian and New Zealand College of Psychiatrists (Royal Australian and New Zealand College of Psychiatrists, 1999) did the same. The American Academy of Child and Adolescent Psychiatry is currently preparing practice parameters for ECT use in adolescents (Ghaziuddin et al., in preparation).

Despite the long history of ECT use in young persons, published studies have been few and of poor quality. A recent review (Rey and Walter, 1997) found that, of 60 published accounts, there were no controlled or whole population studies on the topic, that almost half the reports provided no diagnosis or insufficient information to make a diagnosis, that unwanted effects were usually not commented upon, and that information about outcome was often deficient. Studies published after 1980 were found to be of better quality than those published earlier.

EVIDENCE OF EFFECTIVENESS

Given the infrequent use of ECT in the young and ethical concerns about sham-ECT in minors, it is unlikely that controlled trials will ever take place. Therefore, clinical decision making relies on evidence of a lower level of quality. The few existing data refer to adolescents, since ECT is used very rarely in prepubertal children. For example, Walter and Rey (1997) reported on the effectiveness of ECT in all patients younger than 19 years who had received this treatment between 1990 and 1996 in the Australian State of New South Wales (*n* = 42). The youngest was 14 years of age. They concluded that a marked improvement or resolution of symptoms occurred in half of the adolescents who had completed the course of ECT, irrespective of gender. Those with mood disorders derived the most benefit, while those with comorbid personality disorders showed a poorer response. The systematic review mentioned above that included most of the cases published over more than 50 years concluded that effectiveness of ECT in adolescents was similar to that in adults (Rey and Walter, 1997; Walter et al., 1999). Electroconvulsive therapy was particularly effective (about 80% response) in bipolar disorder, either depression or mania, and psychotic depression. The rate of response in adolescents with major depression was 64%, and for schizophrenia, 42% (Table 30.1). Rates of response for adults have been estimated at 70% for major depression, 80% for mania, and 80% for schizophrenia (Isenberg and Zorumski, 2000). However, the stated rates for the young might underestimate the efficacy of ECT because they are based on the most severe cases. Prior to receiving ECT, almost all young

TABLE 30.1 *Response to ECT in Patients Younger Than 19 Years Reported in the Literature up to 1998, According to Diagnosis*

Diagnosis	Adolescents (n = 224) Who Showed Remission or Marked Improvement of Symptoms after ECT Treatment (%)
Depression	67
Major depression	64
Psychotic depression	71
Manic episode	79
Bipolar disorder	71
Schizophrenia	42
Schizoaffective	67
Catatonia	72
Neuroleptic malignant syndrome	50
Other disorders	14
Total	57

Reproduced with permission from Walter et al. (1999)

patients had been refractory to other treatments. Prior failure to respond to antidepressant drugs seems to also reduce the likelihood of responding to ECT (Prudic et al., 1996).

CLINICAL USES

The primary indication for ECT in adolescents is the short-term treatment of mood symptoms, depressive or manic (Walter et al., 1999). Mood symptoms in the course of major depression, psychotic depression, bipolar disorder, organic mood disorders, schizophrenia, and schizoaffective disorder respond well to ECT. Psychotic symptoms in mood disorders also respond well to ECT whereas the effectiveness of ECT in the treatment of psychotic symptoms in schizophrenia is doubtful. There are suggestions that other uncommon clinical conditions in adolescents such as catatonia and neuroleptic malignant syndrome also benefit from ECT. The effectiveness of ECT seems to lessen when there is a comorbid personality disorder or drug and/or alcohol problems. There are very few data about usefulness on prepubertal children.

In adolescents, ECT is mainly used as a treatment of last resort. Given its effectiveness and, as shall be discussed, relative safety, the degree to which clinicians should wait before considering ECT is a vexed issue, particularly in severely depressed adolescents. Many of these patients often receive several trials of medication or combinations of drugs, develop side effects, and suffer considerable impairment. In these situations, if improvement does not occur after two or three medication trials, ECT should probably be considered.

ADVERSE EVENTS

In adolescents, as in adults, ECT is generally well tolerated. In only a few young patients reported in the literature has ECT been discontinued because of side effects (Rey and Walter, 1997). It should be noted that much of the data about adverse events of ECT in adolescents are based on ECT practice that is becoming superseded (e.g., ECT without seizure threshold determination and without electroencephalographic [EEG] monitoring). Nevertheless, side effects are usually mild and transient and include headache (rates in more recent studies range from 42% [Cohen et al., 1997] to 80% [Ghaziuddin et al., 1996]), nausea or vomiting (2% [Kutcher and Robertson, 1995] to 64% [Ghaziuddin et al., 1996]), generalized muscle aches, subjective memory problems (9% [Kutcher and Robertson, 199] to 52% [Cohen et al., 1997]), and confusion (0% [Ghaziuddin et al., 1996] to 18% [Walter and Rey, 1997]). Manic switch, hemifacial flushing, and sinus tachycardia have also been reported but are uncommon.

There have been no fatalities attributable to ECT that have been described in young persons. There is an account of a 16-year-old girl who had eight ECTs and died of cardiac failure 10 days after the last treatment (Kish et al., 1990). However, her death is likely to have been due to the continued administration of neuroleptic medication in spite of her neuroleptic malignant syndrome.

Three areas that warrant special examination in relation to the safety of ECT are prolonged ECT seizures, cognitive effects, and the potential consequences of the treatment on the developing brain.

Prolonged Seizures

Guttmacher and Cretella (1988) have suggested that young persons have increased rates of prolonged ECT seizures compared to adults. Duration of more than 3 minutes is the criterion for prolonged seizures according to the American Psychiatric Association (1990). However, there is evidence that challenges Guttmacher and Cretella's viewpoint. For example, in a series of 42 adolescents who received 49 courses of ECT, seizures lasting longer than 3 minutes by motor and/or EEG criteria occurred in 2 (0.4%) of the 450 treatments (Walter and Rey, 1997). Such rates are similar to those found in adults. Nevertheless, debate about comparative rates of prolonged seizures—in both young and adult patients—is complicated by a lack of information about seizure length in many of the studies of minors, lack of consensus about rates of prolonged seizures in adults, and lack of uniform definition for prolonged seizures (Walter and Rey, 1998). When prolonged seizures do occur in young patients having ECT, they are more likely to take place in the first part of the ECT course (Walter and Rey, 1997).

Post-ECT (or "tardive") seizures have been described in young recipients of ECT but these are rare. Both Schneekloth et al. (1993) and Ghaziuddin et al. (1996) reported a single spontaneous seizure in their series.

Psychometric Studies

Regrettably, most studies that have formally assessed cognitive effects of ECT in young persons were conducted in the 1940s and 1950s, before the treatment technique was refined. It is noteworthy, however, that these early studies found no enduring ill effects. For example, in 1947 Bender reported no decline in IQ immediately after ECT and "at intervals thereafter" (Bender, 1947). That same year, Des Laurieres and Halpern (1947) found that, following ECT, young patients showed a slight increase in IQ and "greater ability to concentrate" but no change in reasoning and judgement. The next decade, Gurevitz and Helme (1954) noted that "intellectual efficiency" was reduced immediately after a course of treatment but recovered at follow-up 5–27 months later. Recent studies have not detected long-term cognitive effects following ECT. For example, Cohen et al. (2000) compared 10 subjects treated in adolescence with bilateral ECT, with controls matched for age, gender, and diagnosis. Evaluation (on average) 3.5 years after the last treatment revealed no significant group differences on tests of short-term memory, attention, new learning and objective memory scores. Ghaziuddin et al. (1996, 2000) compared pre- and post-ECT cognition among 16 adolescents. At the first post-ECT testing (about 1 week following the last treatment), there was deterioration in attention, concentration, verbal and visual delayed recall, and verbal fluency. However, these functions recovered completely by the second testing (about 8 months after the last ECT treatment).

The findings of Cohen et al. (2000) and Ghaziuddin et al. (2000) notwithstanding, there are considerable data from adult studies showing that ECT can cause mild cognitive deficits. The most persistent adverse effect is retrograde amnesia. Shortly after ECT, most patients have gaps in their memory for events that occurred close in time to the course of ECT, but amnesia may extend back several months or years. Retrograde amnesia usually improves during the first few months after ECT. Nonetheless, recovery is incomplete for some patients who may show permanent memory loss for some events that occurred close in time to the treatment (Lisanby et al., 2000). Cognitive deficits are lower with unilateral than with bilateral ECT. In the case of right unilateral ECT, cognitive side effects increase as the stimulus dose increases relative to initial seizure threshold (McCall et al., 2000). The amnestic effects of ECT are greater and more persistent on knowledge about the world than on knowledge about the self, on recent (close to the time ECT was administered) then on remote events, and on less salient events. Bilateral ECT produces more profound amnestic effects than right unilateral ECT, particularly for memory of impersonal events (Lisanby et al., 2000). It remains to be seen whether these unwanted effects are less pronounced for young people.

ECT and Brain Development

The concern that ECT may impair brain development is not uncommonly harbored by professionals, adolescents who received ECT, and their parents (38% of recipients and 18% of parents [Walter et al., 1999a,b]). There are currently no specific data to suggest that ECT damages a young person's brain or adversely affects brain development. However, there are no studies that have specifically addressed this topic. Early publications in which young patients received large numbers of treatments, e.g., up to 200 (Bauer, 1976), and/or very frequent treatments, e.g., 15 treatments in 3 days (Heuyer et al., 1948), reported no long-term problems in this regard. In adults, ECT does not appear to be associated with structural brain damage (Devanand et al., 1994; Devanand, 1995). However, this finding cannot be easily extrapolated to the young because of differences between the adolescent and adult brain. Recent research in humans and mice (Vaccarino et al., 2000; Rapoport et al., 2001; see Chapter 1 in this volume) indicates that adolescence is a period of active development in brain neurobiology

PROCEDURE

Legal and Ethical Aspects

The most important legal aspect of ECT in minors pertains to informed consent, which is an essential consideration before the treatment is administered. Whenever possible, the rationale for ECT, alternatives to ECT, and the natural course of illness without treatment should be explained to adolescents and their families. State and institutional guidelines, the patient's age, and the recommendations of an independent psychiatrist may also determine whether a young person receives ECT. It is important that clinicians be knowledgeable and compliant with institutional guidelines and legal requirements.

Psychiatrists who use ECT or refer adolescents for ECT should be familiar with all aspects of the treatment. For example, several states in the United States have age-related prohibitions for the use of ECT. It is not permitted in Texas and Colorado in persons under 16 years of age, in Tennessee for those under 14 years, and in California for those under 12. Most states require independent assessment of children and juveniles by one or more child and adolescent psychiatrists before ECT may be administered. This assessment must be conducted by psychiatrists not involved in the treatment of the patient. There are some noteworthy problems with the second opinion or independent assessment requirement, given a lack of knowledge about or experience with the treatment among many child psychiatrists (Parmar, 1993; Walter et al., 1997; Ghaziuddin et al., 2001).

In some countries, legal consent for ECT may be given by a parent or a legal guardian. However, every effort should be made to obtain the informed assent of a minor. Although informed consent from adolescents may be complicated by lack of maturity and presence of severe psychiatric symptoms, the principles of informed consent are similar to those applicable to adult patients. Beneficence and autonomy are important concepts of medical ethics which should be incorporated in the consent for ECT. *Autonomy* is a patient's right to choose a course of action under his or her free will; *beneficence* is the expected positive outcome. A psychiatrist is likely to face a difficult decision when the patient's exercise of autonomy may be discordant with beneficence. However, it is useful to regard informed consent as a process rather than a moment in time. For example, adolescents unwilling to give consent early during treatment may change their mind later as symptoms do not improve or because of side effects of medication. A detailed explanation of the procedure, particularly with the assistance of audiovisual aids, is often helpful.

Krener and Mancina (1994) described five philosophical and "tactical" questions relevant to treating children and adolescents. Although these issues were described in the context of the use of psychotropic drugs, they are equally applicable to ECT. These include (1) the rights of the child; (2) the child's relationship to the adults responsible for his or her care; (3) the child's developmental capacity to understand the treatment; (4) the process of consent as it unfolds within the treatment alliance; and (5) the potential for coercion of the minor, either by the adults in the environment or by the treatment process itself. Additionally, all ethical concerns for ECT should consider a patient's right to refuse, as well as to receive, an effective treatment.

Psychiatric and Medical Assessment

A comprehensive psychiatric history and psychiatric diagnosis according to a major classification system such as the *Diagnostic and Statistical Manual, 4th ed.* (DSM-IV) or *International Classification of Diseases, 10th ed.* (ICD-10) is needed for all patients. A structured diagnostic interview may be helpful for some cases. The mortality rate associated with ECT in adults is approximately the same as that for anesthesia alone, about 1 death per 10,000 patients treated (or per 40,000 ECT treatments).

Cardiovascular complications, arrythmias, myocardial infarction, congestive heart failure, and cardiac arrest are the most common causes of peri-ECT mortality (Abrams, 1997). The aim of the pre-ECT medical assessment is to detect any medical condition that may increase the risk for anesthesia or for the procedure itself. Although no ECT-related death has been reported for adolescents, the total experience with ECT in this population is very limited and lack of fatalities does not necessarily imply absence of risk for this age group. Nevertheless, it can be expected that adult and particularly elderly patients will have higher mortality rates due to the increased likelihood of physical ill health. Patients considered at high risk may include those with significant arrhythmias, severe valvular disease, unstable coronary syndrome, and decompensated congestive cardiac failure. The American College of Cardiology and American Heart Association (1996) have published guidelines to evaluate patients with cardiovascular disease who are undergoing noncardiac procedures. These guidelines should be followed for all adolescents with underlying cardiovascular pathology.

Medical history and a physical examination should be completed for every patient. Given the physiological changes during ECT, the physical examination should include assessment of the airway, cardiovascular, pulmonary, and central nervous systems. Laboratory examinations may include a blood count, liver and thyroid function tests, urine analysis, and electrocardiogram (EKG). Other investigations such as skeletal X-ray, completed tomographic (CT) scan of the head, or magnetic resonance imaging (MRI) may be indicated on a case-by-case basis.

Concurrent Medications

Generally, most psychotropic medications are discontinued prior to ECT to minimize the chance of adverse events. However, this practice is currently under review as concomitant use of psychotropics may improve efficacy and prevent relapse. Adverse reactions with concomitant psychotropic use may include potentiation of barbiturate and succinylcholine with lithium (Hill et al., 1997), organic brain syndrome with lithium (Penny et al., 1990), and prolonged seizures with the concomitant use of trazadone or fluoxetine (Carcacci and Decina, 1991; Lanes and Ravaris, 1993; Gamage and Plant, 1995). Tricyclic antidepressants (TCAs) and monoamine oxydase inhibitors (MAOIs) are generally discontinued prior to treatment, although some studies have failed to find any complications (Azar and Lear 1984). Benzodiazepines have anticonvulsant properties, can shorten seizure duration (Gassy and Rey, 1990), and possibly decrease treatment effectiveness. Benzodiazepines should be avoided whenever possible and should be tapered off before ECT. If they are required, a short-acting benzodiazepine (temazepam, oxazepam) can be considered, but should not be administered shortly before treatment.

Anesthesia

Anesthesia should be administered by an appropriately qualified professional. After an overnight fast, the adolescent having ECT wears loose-fitting clothes, and is accompanied by a staff member to the treatment area. The most commonly used anesthetic agent is methohexital (0.75 to 1 mg/kg), which is a short-acting barbiturate. The most commonly used muscle relaxant is succinylcholine, at 0.5 to 1 mg/kg. Both agents are rapidly metabolized and the total duration of anesthesia varies between 3 and 10 minutes. The muscle relaxant is administered when the patient is well sedated. Alternatives for succinylcholine are atracurium, mivacurium, and glycopyrrolate. The cardiovascular responses during ECT consist of an initial parasympathetic outflow accompanied by bradycardia and asystole. This is followed by sympathetic outflow with tachycardia, dysrrythmias, and hypertension (Gaines and Rees, 1992). An anticholinergic agent such as atropine may be used in some cases to minimize the excessive vagal activity, which induces bradycardia, and to reduce secretions in the airways (Gaines and Rees, 1992). However, premedication with atropine or glycopyrrolate is mandatory if the seizure threshold is being determined using the dose titration method (titrating the electrical dose according to the individual patient). It has also been suggested that one of these agents must be administered before the first treatment with right unilateral electrode placement, when seizure threshold is unknown and the patient is likely to receive more than one stimulus. Prior to the administration of anesthesia and throughout the procedure, airway patency should be maintained and the patient adequately ventilated. Just prior to administering the anaesthetic and the muscle relaxant, the patient is asked to breathe 100% oxygen. This diminishes the memory loss associated with ECT.

Administration

Electroconvulsive therapy is generally given two or three times a week. In adult patients, there is no difference in outcome between the two schedules. Rate of response may be more rapid with thrice-weekly ECT, but this regimen may also be associated with greater cognitive impairment (Shapira et al., 1998).

The ECT unit should be staffed by experienced professionals trained in the use of the procedure and in the care of an unconscious patient, including measures for intravenous access, monitoring of blood pressure, pulse oximetry, and EKG (Gaines and Rees, 1992). The ECT team usually includes a psychiatrist, an anesthesiologist, and a nurse.

Among adult patients, electrical variables used for ECT have been extensively studied. These variables have not received systematic scrutiny in the adolescent age group. Until controlled studies can identify the optimum parameters for adolescents, the practice of ECT for young patients is based on adult data and clinical experience. The goal of the procedure is the induction of a seizure that lasts 25–30 seconds, and is associated with minimum side effects. All ECT devices available in the United States deliver brief-pulse electricity. Other features of the electrical current include wave frequency of 30 to 70 cycles per second, pulse width of 0.5 to 2.0 milliseconds, and a total charge between 32 to 576 millicoulombs. The overall aim is to select an electrical charge, by adjusting one or more variables, that would result in a seizure of adequate duration (a seizure lasting at least 20–25 seconds).

Electroconvulsive therapy may be administered using unilateral or bilateral electrode placement. Either mode requires consideration of seizure threshold. Several studies involving adults have shown that neither age nor other demographic variables are good predictors of seizure threshold (Coffey et al., 1995; Enns and Karvelas, 1995). Knowledge of seizure threshold may be especially pertinent for unilateral electrode placement as this mode has been found to be less effective (when low dose is used) than bilateral electrode placement. Sackeim et al. (1993) noted that, in adults, the response rate following low-dose unilateral ECT was lower than that following either high-dose unilateral or low-dose bilateral treatment. Further research has confirmed that right unilateral ECT at high dosage is as effective as bilateral ECT, but produces less severe and persistent cognitive effects (Sackeim et al., 2000). Since there are no studies regarding the best electrode placement for adolescents, based on the existing literature and experience, low-dose unilateral treatment is likely to be ineffective and should not be used. Treatment may generally be started with moderately suprathreshold unilateral placement; where urgency of response is paramount, treatment may be commenced with bilateral electrode placement.

Stimulus pulse width may vary from 0.5 to 2.0 milliseconds. A recent study compared 0.5 msecond pulse width to 1.0 mseconds; the shorter pulse width was found to be more efficient in inducing a seizure of adequate duration and less likely to result in a failed or an abortive seizure, and the associated peak heart rate was lower (Swartz and Manly, 2000). The authors also found that the pulse frequency (30 Hz vs. 60 Hz) did not influence the outcome. They concluded that a shorter pulse width was more efficient than a wider pulse width. Since data regarding pulse width are based on ETC in adults, until similar studies are conducted in adolescents, a shorter pulse width is preferable for adolescents.

For all juveniles, there should be EEG monitoring during ECT and recording of seizure length by both direct observation of the motor fit and by the EEG. Prolonged seizures should be terminated by means of diazepam or further general anesthetic.

Assessment of Progress and Side Effects

Improvement can be determined by regular clinical assessment, patient self-report, and weekly use of subjective and objective symptom measures. It can commence very early in the ECT course. ECT should be continued until the patient no longer seems to be improving. The usual number of treatments required by young persons is similar to that required by adults (a mean of 6–12). Assessment of unwanted events should be made following each ECT administration by systematic inquiry of the common side effects or by use of specially developed scales such as the Columbia ECT Subjective Side Effects Schedule (Sackeim et al., 1987). Where possible, neuropsychological assessment should be performed prior to onset of treatment and 6 months after completion of ECT; a minimum battery should comprise the Wechsler Intelligence Scale for children, Children's Memory Scale, and Wechsler Individual Achievement Test.

VIEWS OF HEALTH PROFESSIONALS, PATIENTS AND PARENTS

Few treatments have engendered such strong and passionate views as the use of ECT in young persons. Opponents have asserted that ECT should not be used in this age group because it is far too costly in human terms and that ECT administration to one child or adolescent per year is one too many (Walter et al., 1999a). Conversely, ECT in young persons has been considered life-saving. However, views about ECT in adolescents have only recently been systematically studied.

There have been three studies of professional experience of and attitudes on ECT, conducted in the United Kingdom (Parmar, 1993), Australia and New Zealand (Walter et al., 1997) and the United States (Ghaziuddin et al., 2001). All studies showed significant deficits in knowledge about ECT in the young and strong views about the subject. For example, in the survey of all child psychiatrists in Australia and New Zealand, 40% of respondents rated their knowledge about ECT in the young as nil or negligible; 39% of respondents believed that ECT was unsafe in children, compared to 17% for adolescents and 3% for adults. Findings were similar in a study of randomly selected child and adolescent psychiatrists and psychologists in the United States. The vast majority of respondents (93%) stated that they possessed little knowledge about the use of ECT in children and adolescents, and that this treatment was less safe in young persons, than in adults.

Arguably more important than the views of mental health professionals about this subject are the opinions of adolescent patients who received ECT and their parents. Data are available from Australia and France (Walter et al., 1999a, b; Taieb et al., 2000). In the Australian study (Walter et al., 1999a), the vast majority of patients considered ECT a legitimate treatment and, if medically indicated, would have ECT again and would recommend it to others. Approximately three-quarters believed their psychiatric illness was worse than either ECT or pharmacotherapy. Their parents' opinions about ECT were also favorable (Walter et al., 1999b). The findings from France (Taieb et al., 2000) were similar; for example, all patients and parents regarded ECT as a very helpful treatment and disagreed with the statement "ECT is dangerous and should not be used."

LAY ATTITUDES

Unfortunately, there are no systematic data about lay attitudes towards ECT in children and adolescents. Not surprisingly, however, the limited information from various media suggest that there is antipathy towards convulsive therapy in this age group. Two movies, *Ordinary People* (1980) and *Return to Oz* (1985), have made negative references to the treatment in young persons (Walter, 1998). For example, *Ordinary People* is often championed (e.g., Schneider, 1987) as one of the motion picture industry's more sympathetic representations of psychiatry, yet ECT is devalued in the film. On being informed that Conrad (played by Timothy Hutton) had ECT in adolescence, Conrad's swim coach castigated him and the treatment: "I would never have let them put electricity in my head." Similarly, the deliberately arresting headline in an Australian newspaper, "Shock therapy for kids" (*The Sun-Herald,* July 13, 1997), which heralded a story that had nothing to do with ECT, also captures the popular sentiment.

TRANSCRANIAL MAGNETIC STIMULATION

Transcranial magnetic stimulation (TMS) is a novel treatment for psychiatric illness (George et al., 1999; Pridmore and Belmaker, 1999). In the procedure, a current is passed around an insulated coil held in contact with the patient's head, causing a magnetic field to pass into the first few millimeters of cortex. Unlike ECT, a specific area of the brain is stimulated, the procedure does not require a general anesthetic, and a seizure does not occur.

Several studies have been conducted in adults, particularly in patients with depression, which suggest that TMS may be beneficial, has few adverse events, and appears to be acceptable to recipients (Pascual-Leone et al., 1996; George et al., 1997; Wasserman, 1998; Klein et al., 1999; Walter et al., 2001a). Transcranial magnetic stimulation has been used in young persons—aged 7 months to 18 years—as an investigative tool to examine maturation and plasticity of the corticospinal tract (e.g., Pascual-Leone et al., 1992; Rossini et al., 1992; Heinen et al., 1998; Reitz and Muller, 1998; Mayston et al., 1999), but there is only one published account relating to its use as a treatment for psychiatric disorders in the young (Walter et al., 2001b). The outcome of seven patients, aged 16 to 18 years, treated with TMS suggests that this treatment is well tolerated and of some benefit (Walter et al., 2001b). Three of the patients had unipolar depression, three had schizophrenia, and one had bipolar disorder. Five of the seven patients had improved by the conclusion of the TMS course. The only adverse event reported was headache in one patient. It is clear that it is much too early to conclude whether TMS is effective in the treatment of mental disorders in both adults and young persons but, given the encouraging reports, further trials in young people to investigate the effectiveness and safety of TMS are warranted.

CONCLUSION

All physical treatments in child psychiatry have been regarded with caution by sections of the profession and community more generally. Throughout its history, ECT has engendered particularly strong views. Transcranial magnetic stimulation remains too new a treatment to have attracted passionate comment. Although controlled trials are lacking and further studies of side effects are needed, the available evidence suggests that ECT in young people is effective, safe, and acceptable to patients and families. Despite major advances in pediatric psychopharmacology, there will be occasions in which ECT will be the best treatment option.

REFERENCES

Abrams, R. (1997). *Electroconvulsive Therapy*. NY: Oxford University Press.

American College of Cardiology/American Heart Association Task Force (1996) ACC/AHA guidelines for perioperative cardiovascular evaluation for noncardiac surgery. *Circulation* 93:1278–1317.

American Psychiatric Association (1990) *Electroconvulsive Therapy: Recommendations for Treatment, Training and Privileging*. Washington, DC: American Psychiatric Association.

Azar, I. and Lear, E. (1984) Cardiovascular effects of ECT in patients taking trycyclic antidepressants. *Anesth Analg* 63:1139–1144.

Baker, T. (1994) ECT and young minds. *Lancet* 345:65.

Bauer, W. (1976) Treatment of a 15-year-old hebephrenic girl in community hospital. *Dis Nerv Syst* 37:474–476.

Bender, L. (1947) One hundred cases of childhood schizophrenia treated with electric shock. *Trans Am Neurol Soc* 72:165–169.

Caracci, G. and Decina, P. (1991) Fluoxetine and prolonged seizure. *Convulsive Ther* 7:145–147.

Coffey, C.E., Lucke, J., Weiner, R.D., Krystal, A.D., and Aque, M. (1995) Seizure threshold in electroconvulsive therapy: initial seizure threshold. *Biol Psychiatry* 37:713–720.

Cohen, D., Paillere-Martinot, M.L., and Basquin, M. (1997) Use of electroconvulsive therapy in adolescents. *Convulsive Ther* 13:25–31.

Cohen, D., Taieb, O., Benoit, N., Chevret, S., Corcos, M., Fossati, P., Jeammet, P., Allilaire, J.F., and Basquin, M. (2000) Absence of cognitive impairment at long-term follow-up in adolescents treated with ECT for severe mood disorders. *Am J Psychiatry* 157:460–462.

Des Lauriers, A. and Halpern, F. (1947) Psychological tests in childhood schizophrenia. *Am J Orthopsychiatry* 17:57–67.

Devanand, D.P. (1995) Does electroconvulsive therapy damage brain cells? *Semin Neurol* 15:351–357.

Devanand, D.P., Dwork, A.J., Hutchinson, E.R., Bolwig, T.G., and Sackeim, H.A. (1994) Does ECT alter brain structure? *Am J Psychiatry* 151:957–970.

Enns, N. and Karvelas, L. (1995) Electrical dose titration for electroconvulsive therapy: a comparison with dose prediction methods. *Convulsive Ther* 11:86–93.

Freeman, C.P. (1995) ECT in those under 18 years old. In; Freeman, C.P., ed., *The ECT Handbook*. London: Royal College of Psychiatrists, pp. 18–21.

Gaines, G.Y. and Rees, D.I. (1992) Anesthetic considerations for electroconvulsive therapy. *South Med J* 85:469–482.

Gamage, C.A. and Plant, L.D. (1995) Fluoxetine, electroconvulsive therapy, and prolonged seizures. *J Psychosoc Nurs Ment Health Servi* 33(2):24–26.

Gassy, J.E. and Rey, J.M. (1990) A survey of ECT in a general hospital psychiatry unit. *Aust N Z J Psychiatry* 24:385–390.

George, M.S., Lisanby, S.H., and Sackeim, H.A. (1999) Transcranial magnetic stimulation: applications in neuropsychiatry. *Arch Gen Psychiatry* 56:300–311.

George, M.S., Wasserman, E.M., Williams, W.E., Danielson, A.L., Greenberg, B.D., Hallett, M., and Post, R.M. (1997) Mood improvements following daily left prefrontal repetitive transcranial magnetic stimulation in patients with depression: a placebo-controlled crossover trial. *Am J Psychiatry* 154:1752–1756.

Ghaziuddin, N., Kaza, M., Ghazi, N., King, C., Walter, G., and Rey, J.M. (2001) Electroconvulsive therapy for minors: experiences and attitudes of child psychiatrists and psychologists. *J ECT* 17:109–117.

Ghaziuddin, N., King, C.A., Naylor, M.W., Ghaziuddin, M., Chaudhary, N., Giordani, B., Dequardo, J.R., Tandon, R., and Greden, J. (1996) Electroconvulsive treatment in adolescents with pharmacotherapy-refractory depression. *J Child Adolesc Psychopharmacol* 6:259–271.

Ghaziuddin, N., Laughrin, D., and Giordani, B. (2000) Cognitive side effects of electroconvulsive therapy in adolescents. *J Child Adolesc Psychopharmacol* 10:269–276.

Gurevitz, S. and Helme, W.H. (1954) Effects of electroconvulsive therapy on personality and intellectual functioning of the schizophrenic child. *J Nerv Ment Dis* 120:213–226.

Guttmacher, L.B. and Cretella, H. (1988) Electroconvulsive therapy in one child and three adolescents. *J Clin Psychiatry* 49:20–23.

Heinen, F., Glocker, F.X., Fietzek, U., Meyer, B.U., Lucking, C.H., and Korinthenberg, R. (1998) Absence of transcallosal inhibition following focal magnetic stimulation in preschool children. *Ann Neurol* 43:608–612.

Heuyer, G., Bour, and Feld, (1942) Electro-choc chez les adolescents. *Ann Med Psychol (Paris)* 2:75–84.

Heuyer, G, Bour, and Leroy, R. (1943) L'electrochoc chez les enfants. *Ann Med Psychol (Paris)* 2:402–407.

Heuyer, G., Lebovici, S., and Amado, G. (1948) Les electrochocs en sommation. *Ann Med Psychol (Paris)* 1:205–208.

Hill, M.A., Courvoisie, H., Dawkins, K., Nofal, P., and Thomas, B. (1997) ECT for the treatment of intractable mania in two prepubertal male children. *Convulsive Ther* 13:74–82.

Isenberg, K.E and Zorumski, C.F (2000) Electroconvulsive therapy. In: Sadock, B.J. and Sadock, V.A., eds. *Kaplan & Sadock's Comprehensive Textbook of Psychiatry, 7th ed.* Philadelphia, PA: Lippincott, Williams & Wilkins, pp. 2503–2515.

Jha, A.K., Stein, G.S., and Fenwick, P. (1996). Negative interaction between lithium and electroconvulsive therapy: a case–control study. *Br J Psychiatry* 168:241–243.

Kish, S.J., Kleinert, R., Minauf, M., Gilbert, J., Walter, G.F., Slimovitch, C., Maurer, E., Rezvani, Y., Myers, R., and Hornykiewicz, O. (1990) Brain neurotransmitter changes in three patients who had a fatal hyperthermia syndrome. *Am J Psychiatry* 147:1358–1363.

Klein, E., Kreinin, I., Christyakov, A., Koren, D., Mecz, L., Marmur, S., Ben-Shachar, D., and Feinsod, M. (1999) Therapeutic efficacy of right prefrontal slow repetitive transcranial magnetic stimulation in major depression: a double blind controlled study. *Arch Gen Psychiatry* 56:315–320.

Krener, K.P. and Mancina, R.A. (1994) Informed consent or informed coercion? Decision-making in pediatric psychopharmacology. *J Child Adolesc Psychopharmacol* 4:183–200.

Kutcher, S. and Robertson, H.A. (1995) Electroconvulsive therapy in treatment resistant bipolar youth. *J Child Adolesc Psychopharmacol* 5:167–175.

Lanes, T. and Ravaris, C.L. (1993) Prolonged ECT seizure duration in a patient taking trazodone. *Am J Psychiatry* 150:525.

Lisanby, S.H., Maddox, J.H., Prudic, J., Devanand, D.P., and Sackeim, H.A. (2000) The effects of electroconvulsive therapy on memory of autobiographical and public events. *Arch Gen Psychiatry* 57:581–590.

McArthur, J. (1997) Shock therapy for kids. *The Sun-Herald*, Sydney July 13:7.

McCall, W.V., Reboussin, D.M., Weiner, R.D., and Sackeim, H.A. (2000) Titrated moderately spuprathreshold vs fixed high-dose right unilateral eclectroconvulsive therapy. *Arch Gen Psychiatry* 57:438–444.

Mayston, M.J., Harrison, L.M., and Stephens, J.A. (1999) A neurophysiological study of mirror movements in adults and children. *Ann Neurol* 45:583–594.

Parmar, R. (1993) Attitudes of child psychiatrists to electroconvulsive therapy. *Psychiatri Bull* 17:12–13.

Pascual-Leone, A., Chugani, H.T., Cohen, L.G., Brasil-Neto, J., Valls-Solé, J., Wassermann, E.W., and Hallett, M. (1992) Reorganization of human motor pathways following hemispherectomy. *Ann Neurol* 32:261.

Pascual-Leone, A., Rubio, B., Pallardo, F., and Catala, M.D. (1996) Rapid-rate trancranial magnetic stimulation of left dorsolateral prefrontal cortex in drug-resistant major depression. *Lancet* 348:233–237.

Penny, J., Dinwiddie, S.H., Zorumski, C.F., and Wetzel, R.D. (1990) Concurrent and close temporal administration of lithium and ECT. *Convulsive Ther* 6:139–145.

Perkins, I.H. and Tanaka, K. (1979) The controversy that will not die is the treatment that can and does save lives: electroconvulsive therapy. *Adolescence* 14:607–616.

Pridmore, S. and Belmaker, R. (1999) Transcranial magnetic stimulation in the treatment of psychiatric disorders. *Psychiatry Clini Neurosci* 53:541–548.

Prudic, J., Haskett, R.F., Mulsant, B., Malone, K.M., Pettinati, H.M., Stephens, S., Greenberg, R., Rifas, S.L., and Sackeim, H.A. (1996) Resistance to antidepressant medications and short-term clinical response to ECT. *Am J Psychiatry* 153:985–992.

Rapoport, J.L., Castellanos, X., Gogate, N., Janson, K., Kohler, S., and Nelson, P. (2001) Imaging normal and abnormal brain development—new perspectives for child psychiatry. *Aust N Z J Psychiatry* 35:272–281.

Reitz, M. and Muller, K. (1998) Differences between 'congenital mirror movements' and 'associated movements' in normal children: a neurophysiological case study. *Neurosci Lett* 256:69–72.

Rey, J.M. and Walter, G. (1997) Half a century of ECT use in young people. *Am J Psychiatry* 154:595–602.

Rossini, P.M., Desiato, M.T., and Caramia, M.D. (1992) Age-related changes of motor evoked potentials in healthy humans: noninvasive evaluation of central and peripheral motor tracts excitability and conductivity. *Brain Res* 593:14–9.

Royal Australian and New Zealand College of Psychiatrists (1999) ECT Guidelines. Royal Australian and New Zealand College of Psychiatrists, Melbourne.

Sackeim, H.A., Prudic, J., Devanand, D.P., Kiersky, JE., Fitzimons., L., Moody, B.J., McElhiney, M.C., Coleman, E.Z., and Settembrino, J.M. (1993). Effects of stimulus intensity and electrode placement on the efficacy and cognitive effects of electroconvulsive therapy. *N Engl J Med* 328:839–846.

Sackeim, H.A., Prudic, J., Devanand, D.P., Nobler, M.S., Lisanby, S.H., Peyser, S., Fitzsimons, L., Moody, B.J., and Clark, J. (2000) A prospective, randomized, double-blind comparison of bilateral and right unilateral electroconvulsive therapy at different stimulus intensities. *Arch Gen Psychiatry* 57:425–434.

Sackeim, H.A., Ross, F.R., Hopkins, N., Calev, L., and Devanand, D.P. (1987) Subjective side effects acutely following ECT: associations with treatment modality and clinical response. *Convulsive Ther* 3:100–110.

Schneekloth, T.D., Rummans, T.A., and Logan, K.M. (1993) Electroconvulsive therapy in adolescents. *Convulsive Ther* 9:159–166.

Schneider, I. (1987) Theory and practice of movie psychiatry. *Am J Psychiatry* 144:996–1002.

Shapira, B., Tubi, N., Dexler, H., Lidsky D., Calev, A., and Lerer B. (1998) Cost and benefit in the choice of ECT schedule: twice weekly versus three times weekly ECT. *Br J Psychiatry* 172:44–48.

Swartz, C.M., and Manly, D.T. (2000) Efficiency of the stimulus characteristics of ECT. *Am J Psychiatry* 157:9;1504–1506.

Taieb, O., Cohen, D., Mazet, P., and Flament, M., (2000) Adolescents' experiences with ECT. *J Am Acad Child Adolesc Psychiatry* 39:943–944.

Vaccarino, F.M., Rapoport, J.L., and Benes, F.M. (2000) Brain neurobiology during adolescence. Presented at the 47th Annual Meeting, American Academy of Child and Adolescent Psychiatry, New York, NY.

Walter, G. (1998) The portrayal of ECT in movies from Australia and New Zealand. *J ECT* 14:56–60.

Walter, G., Koster, K., and Rey, J.M. (1999a) ECT in adolescents: experience, knowledge and attitudes of recipients. *J Am Acad Child Adolesc Psychiatry* 38:594–599.

Walter, G., Koster, K., and Rey, J.M. (1999b) Views of treatment among parents of adolescents who received electroconvulsive therapy. *Psychiatr Serv* 50:701–702.

Walter, G., Martin, J., Kirkby, K., and Pridmore, S. (2001a) Transcranial magnetic stimulation: experience, knowledge and attitudes of recipients. *Aust N Z J Psychiatry* 35:58–61.

Walter, G., and Rey, J.M. (1997) An epidemiological study on the use of ECT in adolescents. *J Am Acad Child Adolesc Psychiatry* 36:809–815.

Walter, G., and Rey, J.M. (1998) Prolonged seizures in the young. *J ECT*, 14:121–123.

Walter, G., Rey, J.M., and Mitchell, P. (1999) Practitioner review: electrconvulsive therapy in adolescents. *J Child Psychol Psychiatry Allied Disciplines* 40:325–334.

Walter, G., Rey, J.M., and Starling, J. (1997) Experience, knowledge and attitudes of child psychiatrists regarding ECT in the young. *Aust N Z J Psychiatry* 1:676–681.

Walter, G., Tormos, J.M., Israel, J.A., and Pascual-Leone A. (2001b) Transcranial magnetic stimulation in young persons: a review of known cases. *J Child Adolesc Psychopharmacol* 11:69–76.

Wasserman, E.M. (1998) Risk and safety of repetitive transcranial magnetic stimulation: report and suggested guidelines from the International Workshop on the Safety of Repetitive Transcranial Magnetic Stimulation, June 5–7, 1996. *Electroencephalogr Clin Neurophysiol* 108:1–16.

III | ASSESSMENT AND TREATMENT

This can serve as the mantra for our approach to clinical care. For any illness that cannot be cured—and even for those that can but where the treatment is painful or prolonged—a major responsibility of the clinician is to help maintain the child's development on course. This means keeping the clinical eye on the child, not the symptoms.

J.F. Leckman and D.J. Cohen (1999)
Tourette's Syndrome—Tics, Obsessions,
Compulsions. Developmental Psychopathology
and Clinical Care, p. 14

GENERAL *Principles*, the first part of the volume's third and longest section, provides principles that are broadly applicable across disorders and clinical settings. An initial chapter summarizes the overall clinical evaluative process, and is followed by one that culls together the diagnostic instruments and rating scales most commonly used in practice and research. The third chapter describes the importance of attending to the child's inner world of perceptions and feelings during treatment, and serves as a reminder of the "conceptual multilingualism" that is essential for the contemporary practice of child psychiatry. A final, integrative chapter address the combination of pharmacotherapy with other psychotherapeutic modalities, and formally introduces key concepts of evidence-based medical practice to pediatric psychopharmacology.

Ten chapters comprise the middle part, *Specific Disorders and Syndromes*, which is organized to complement the parallel chapters in the *Development Psychopathology* part of the book's first section. The available evidence base for each of the diagnostic categories is reviewed in detail here, and disorder-specific clinical paradigms and relevant algorithms are proposed. Particular attention is given to assessment and evaluation, measurement of symptomatic change, and considerations pertinent to psychiatric comorbidity, partial treatment response or failure, and the role of combined non-medication interventions.

A third part, *Special Clinical Populations*, is devoted to those children and adolescents with comorbid conditions who deserve particular clinical attention and expertise. Chapters address the needs of youths with substance abuse, mental retardation, or medical illness. Two last chapters focus on the youngest of the young: those infants exposed in utero to psychotropic medications, and those preschoolers for whom recent epidemiological studies suggest medications are being prescribed with increasing (and at times alarming) frequency.

A fourth and final part, *Other Areas of Clinical Concern*, addresses the pharmacological management of aggressive or agitated children, and those with the elimination disorders enuresis or encopresis.

31 | Clinical assessment of children and adolescents treated pharmacologically

ROBERT L. HENDREN AND STEPHANIE HAMARMAN

As many as 10% of children have a medication-responsive psychiatric disorder (Riddle et al., 1998) and there has been a dramatic increase in the use of psychotropic medication to treat mental disorders in youth (Rappley et al., 1999). Multiple factors account for this increase, including scientific advances in fields such as epidemiology, nosology, neuroscience, drug development, and clinical measurements, and efforts to educate the public about the benefits of early, effective treatment. Despite large gaps between research and practice, many medications are used in children on the basis of a small amount of scientific data. Factors that contribute to this situation are societal desires for rapid, effective treatment, acceptance of medication as a therapeutic modality, and a reimbursement climate in which there is increased pressure for brief treatment. Clearly there is a need to balance clinical and administrative pressures with a resort to treatment based on the best available data.

The aims of this chapter are to (1) describe a contemporary approach to assessment for pharmacotherapy; (2) describe clinical principles of pediatric psychopharmacology; (3) describe clinical decision making in pediatric psychopharmacology; and (4) describe current approaches to the medical monitoring of children treated with psychotropic medications.

Several principles organize the approach described in this chapter. The first is that children are developmentally different from adults. This has implications for diagnosis, choice of medication and dosing, and forming a therapeutic alliance. Second, there are fundamental limitations in the nosology of childhood mental disorders due to the developmental trajectory of disorders and to symptom overlap and comorbidity. Thus, treatment should focus on target symptoms rather than solely on diagnoses. In addition, pharmacological treatment should be based on available data that support a match between identified target symptoms and the medication selected according to the likelihood it will improve the target symptom.

A third principle of this chapter is that the assessment process in child psychiatry has unique challenges, including the use and consideration of multiple informants and the developmental level of the child. These challenges lead to the fourth principle, which is that successful treatment requires education and collaboration with the family and others involved with the child. Treatment of developmental neurobiology affects the environment that surrounds the child, and treatment of the surrounding environment in turn affects developmental neurobiology. This interaction implies that early and effective intervention can alter the developmental trajectory of a child with a mental disorder.

SOURCES OF INFORMATION

Information from and about multiple sources—family, school, and peers—needs to be integrated in the assessment of the child. The use of rating scales described in Chapter 32 can help organize and quantify across settings the symptoms described by these informants.

The reason for the referral, as well as the person(s) referring the child, determines the social context of the identified problem. Pre-interview screening can help provide preliminary background information in a time-efficient manner and define the context for the referral. Figure 31.1 contains highlights from a developmental history questionnaire that can be used as a template or be adapted and modified to individual practice settings and needs. This type of questionnaire should be sent

FIGURE 31.1 *Developmental History Questionnaire.*

Child's Name: _____

Date: _____

Date of Birth: _____

A. Demographic Information

1. Parent/Guardians:
2. Who currently lives in this child's home? Please include yourself:
   Name: Date of birth: Relationship to child:
3. List family members (siblings, parents) living outside of this child's home:
   Name: Date of birth: Relationship to Child:
4. Is this child or family currently involved with protective services?   ___ No   ___Yes
5. Adoptive status: ___ No   ___ Yes
6. Is anyone else in the family adopted? ___ No   ___ Yes—whom?
7. Parent/Guardian Information
   Name: Address:
   Education: Occupation:
   Hours: Phone:
8. Household income: (yearly/approximate)
   a. ___ under $20,000   b. ___ $20,000–35,000   c. ___ $35,000–50,000   d. $50,000–65,000   e. ___$65,000–80,000
   f. ___ $80,000–100,000   g. ___ Over $100,000   h. ___ Prefer not to answer
9. Language (s) spoken at home:_____
10. Ethnicity of caregivers:
    a. ___ African-American   b. ___ Latino/Hispanic   c. ___ Asian-American   d. ___ Caucasian
    e. ___ Asian-Indian   f. ___
    Other: _____
11. Religion:
    a. ___ Catholic   b. ___ Protestant   c. ___ Jewish
    d. ___ Muslim   e. ___ Other: _____
12. Current grade in school: ___
13. School and address
14. Current teacher: _____School phone number: _____
15. Is this child classified as having special educational needs?   ___ No   ___ Yes–Classification/diagnosis: _____
16. Child study team case manager:
    Name: _____ Phone: _____
17. Referral source:

B. Presenting Problems

1. Why are you bringing this child to treatment at this time?
   What is the main concern?
2. What is the history of the problem?
3. What do you expect from treatment?
4. Are you willing to be involved in this child's treatment?
   ___ Yes   ___ No
5. Please check all current concerns that you have for this child:
   a. ___ Relationship problems at home
   b. ___ Has no friends
   c. ___ Withdrawn/unresponsive
   d. ___ School problems
   e. ___ "Weird" thoughts; believes he/she has unusual ability or power
   f. ___ Fears without reason that others are out to get him/her
   g. ___ Thinks about/talks about the same thing most of the time; excessively preoccupied
   h. ___ Confusion; doesn't know what is happening around him/her
   i. ___ Can't pay attention, gets sidetracked
   j. ___ Often depressed or sad
   k. ___ Loss of interest in things previously enjoyed
   l. ___ Frightened, nervous, upset easily, and often angry or irritable
   m. ___ Cries excessively
   n. ___ Victim of sexual abuse, current or past
   o. ___ Victim of physical abuse, current or past
   p. ___ Bullies others
   q. ___ Oppositional
   r. ___ Does behaviors over and over and can't stop self

(continued)

FIGURE 31.1 *Developmental History Questionnaire (continued)*.

s. ___ Overactive
t. ___ Runaway behavior
u. ___ Destroys property
v. ___ Sets fires
w. ___ Sexual offenses (inappropriate touching of another person)
x. ___ Cruel to animals
y. ___ Steals
z. ___ Chronic lying
aa. ___ Police involved
bb. ___ Involved in gang or gang activity
cc. ___ Expressed thoughts about killing self
dd. ___ Made an attempt or gesture to seriously injure or kill self this past year
ee. ___ Plans to harm others or threatens others
ff. ___ Seriously injured someone
gg. ___ Child has access to firearms
hh. ___ You or others suspect that this child currently uses alcohol or drugs
What substances do you suspect or know that this child has used:
   a. ___ Cigarettes   b. ___ Alcohol   c. ___ Marijuana   d. ___ Cocaine   e. ___ Heroin   f. ___ Other
6. Recent Stressors in the Family
   a. ___ Drug abuse
   b. ___ Alcohol abuse
   c. ___ Money problems
   d. ___ Change of residence
   e. ___ Change in caregiver's employment
   f. ___ Loss of job for parent or guardian
   g. ___ New school, change in school
   h. ___ Child has seen others get hurt, beat up
   i. ___ Physical illness in family member
   j. ___ Parent or guardian in prison/jail
   k. ___ Homeless/no long-term home
   l. ___ Legal problems
   m. ___ Couple/marital problems
   n. ___ Separation
   o. ___ Divorce
   p. ___ Remarriage
   q. ___ Domestic violence
   r. ___ Birth of family member
   s. ___ Child recently hospitalized
   t. ___ Friend died or tried to kill self
   u. ___ Death of family member/significant other
   v. ___ Other

C. Prenatal and Neonatal History
1. When you (or biological mother) were pregnant with this child, were you under the care of a physician? ___ yes   ___ no
2. This child was pregnancy number   ___ 1   ___ 2   ___ 3   ___ 4   ___ 5   ___ 6   ___ other
3. Length of pregnancy: ___months
4. During the pregnancy, did you experience:

	Yes	No	When
a. Anemia	___	___	___
b. High blood pressure	___	___	___
c. Gestational diabetes	___	___	___
d. Vaginal bleeding	___	___	___
e. Toxemia	___	___	___
f. Swollen ankles	___	___	___
g. Flu or virus	___	___	___
h. German measles	___	___	___
i. Accident or injury	___	___	___
j. Emotional problems	___	___	___
k. Risk of miscarriage	___	___	___
l. Other _____			

(continued)

FIGURE 31.1 *Developmental History Questionnaire (continued).*

5. Did you take medication during pregnancy? ___ No ___ Yes
   Please describe what type and when: _____
6. Was the child active in utero? ___ Yes ___ No
7. Did you use drugs or drink alcohol during this pregnancy?
   ___ No ___ Yes
   Please describe what type and when: _____
8. Did you have a cesarean section? ___ No ___ Yes
9. Was this delivery unusual in any way? ___ No ___ Yes
   Please describe: _____
10. Birth weight: _____
11. Was this child healthy at birth? ___ Yes ___ No
    Please describe: _____
12. In the first few days after birth, did this baby experience any of the following:
    a. ___ Yellow jaundice
    b. ___ Breathing problems
    c. ___ Convulsions
    d. ___ Infection
    e. ___ Receive medication
    f. ___ Blood transfusion
    g. ___ Incubator time
    h. ___ Special nursing care
13. Did mother and baby leave the hospital together? ___ Yes ___ No
14. How long after birth?   Mother _____   Baby _____

D. Developmental History
1. During the first 12 months, was this child:
   a. ___ Overactive, in constant motion?   b. ___ Difficult to put on a schedule?   c. ___ Difficult to feed?   d. ___ Difficult to put to sleep?   e. b___ Colicky?
2. What was this baby's activity level? ___ High ___ Average ___ Low
3. At what approximate age did this child:
   a. Sit without help _____
   b. Crawl _____
   c. Walk alone _____
   d. Eat solid food _____
   e. Feed self _____
   f. Say single word (e.g., mama, dada) _____
   g. Talk in two-word sentences _____
   h. Gain bowel control _____
   i. Stay dry (day) _____
   j. Stay dry (night) _____
   k. Smile when played with _____
   l. Learn simple games (e.g., peek-a-boo) _____
   m. Show shyness with strangers _____

E. History of General Behaviors and Personality Traits: Check Characteristics That Describe This Child in the Past and/or Present
1. ___ Shy or timid
2. ___ Disliked attention
3. ___ Unfriendly
4. ___ Unaffectionate
5. ___ Stubborn
6. ___ More interested in things than people
7. ___ Eating difficulties
8. ___ Temper tantrums
9. ___ Destroyed toys more than normal
10. ___ Right-handed
11. ___ Left-handed
12. ___ Poor gross motor coordination
13. ___ Poor fine motor coordination
14. ___ Falling spells
15. ___ Daredevil behavior

(continued)

FIGURE 31.1 *Developmental History Questionnaire (continued).*

16. ___ Unusual fears
17. ___ Rocking
18. ___ Head banging
19. ___ Blank spells
20. ___ Distractible
21. ___ Short attention span
22. ___ Impulsive
23. Intensity of expression of mood: ___ High   ___ Moderate   ___ Low
24. General mood: ___ Positive   ___ Negative
25. Response to new things: ___ Withdraw   ___ Approach
26. Time for adaptation to change: ___ Short   ___ Moderate   ___ Long
27. Nature of school experience: Check if positive or negative

	Positive	Negative
Preschool	___	___
Kindergarten	___	___
Grammar	___	___
High school	___	___

F. Medical History
1. ___ Allergies, describe: _____
2. ___ Takes nonpsychiatric medicine
   a. Medication 1: type and dose: _____
   b. Prescribed by: _____
   c. Medication 2: type and dose: _____
   d. Prescribed by: _____
   e. Medication 3: type and dose: _____
   f. Prescribed by: _____
3. ___ Serious infections disease
4. ___ Diabetes
5. ___ Thyriod problem
6. ___ Cardiovascular problems
7. ___ Seixure disorder
8. ___ Head injury
9. ___ Medical hospitalizations, specify dates and reason: _____
10. ___ Complains of stomach aches
11. ___ Can't get to sleep
12. ___ Can't stay asleep, wakes up a lot
13. ___ Wets the bed at night or clothing during the day
14. ___ Soils his/her pants in bed or during the day
15. ___ Often complains of body pains or being sick
16. ___ Weight change (more than 10% of body weight)
17. ___ Speech problems, specify: _____
18. ___ Hearing difficulty, specify: _____
19. ___ Frequent ear infections
20. ___ Vision problem, specify: _____
21. ___ Serious accident or injury, specify: _____
22. ___ Major surgery, specify date and type: _____
23. ___ Asthma-breathing attacks
24. ___ Dental problems
25. ___ Other, specify: _____
26. ___ Are your child's immunizations up to date?   ___ Yes   ___ No
27. ___ Name of child's physician: _____
28. ___ Phone number of child's physician: _____
29. ___ Date of last doctor's physical examination and results: _____
G. Past Psychiatric Illness and Treatment
1. ___ Child received outpatient counseling
   a. Diagnosis: _____
   b. Dates of treatment: _____
   c. Name, phone number of previous or current counselors: _____

(continued)

FIGURE 31.1 *Developmental History Questionnaire (continued).*

2. ___ Sibling, parent, or immediate family member of child received outpatient counseling
3. ___ Child was hospitalized in psychiatric setting
4. ___ Child is currently prescribed psychiatric medication
   a. Medication 1: type and dose: _____
   b. Prescribed by: _____
   c. Medication 2: type and dose: _____
   d. Prescribed by: _____
   e. Medication 3: type and dose: _____
   f. Prescribed by: _____
5. ___ Child was prescribed psychiatric medication in the past
   a. Medication 1: type and dose: _____
   b. Prescribed by: _____
   c. Medication 2: type and dose: _____
   d. Prescribed by: _____

H. **Family History**
1. Mother
   a. ___ Deceased   b. ___ Living   c. ___ Unknown
   d. Cause of death, if known:
2. Father
   a. ___ Deceased   b. ___ Living   c. ___ Unknown
   d. Cause of death, if known:
3. Check below if any family members have experienced the following (indicate which relative, including child's parents, brothers, sisters, aunts, uncles, cousins, and grandparents):
   a. Developmental disability: _____
   b. Physical disability: _____
   c. Depression: _____
   d. Anxiety: _____
   e. Mental illness: _____
   f. Alcohol or drug addiction: _____
   g. Learning problem: _____
   h. Other: _____

I. **Strengths**
1. What are this child's strengths?
   a. ___ Manages emotions well   e. ___ Motivated   i. ___ Intelligent
   b. ___ Self-disciplined   f. ___ Interpersonal skills j. ___ Insightful
   c. ___ Articulate   g. ___ Wants to please others k. ___ Plays sports
   d. ___ Does well in school   h. ___ Entertains self   l. ___ Other
2. Additional Comments:

to parents to complete and return before the first interview.

CLINICAL INTERVIEW

An initial joint interview that includes the child or adolescent and the parent(s) should establish the chief complaint and begin to define the target symptoms for intervention. It is useful to know if the family cannot define the problem together, as this suggests that communication among them about their concerns is indirect or unclear. If the youngster refuses to cooperate with the joint interview, he or she might be seen alone to determine if an alliance can be established in the absence of the parents. Parents might be seen alone if they indicate that there is sensitive information that they prefer to share in private.

The interview might start by asking the child if he or she knows why this appointment has been scheduled. Family members can be asked to join in as the problem begins to be defined. Everyone's perceptions are important for determining the family context of the target symptoms. The definition of these target symptoms builds the therapeutic alliance and identifies for everyone the symptoms that are the focus of potential change.

Symptoms should be carefully characterized over time. Those of particular relevance to the psychopharmacology assessment include inattention and distractibility, impulsivity, affect expression and regulation, anxiety, aggression, thought disorganization, and language, cognitive, and social skills. It is possible that a particular symptom is part of several diagnostic categories, so it should be carefully delineated. For instance, inattention can be thought to be the hallmark of attention-deficit hyperactivity disorder (ADHD), but it can also be an early symptom of schizophrenia or bipolar disorder, or can be confused with the difficulty in shifting attention seen in children with pervasive developmental disorders. It can also be the result of anxiety in post-traumatic stress disorder (PTSD) or be related to concentration difficulties seen in depressive disorders.

DEVELOPMENTAL AND FAMILY HISTORY

Additional information from the parent(s) or primary care taker(s) should include the child's medical and developmental history and the family's history of mental disorders and stressors. Reports of the direct observation of the youngster's behavior from the parent(s) or primary caretaker(s), school personnel, and others who have had contact with the child can help guide the definition of the most pressing target symptoms.

A targeted biopsychosocial developmental history from key informants should be included in the initial assessment. In addition to the information contained in Figure 31.1, a history of stress and trauma should also be gathered. In children and adolescents this includes caretaker absence, neglect, physical, sexual, and emotional abuse, as well as transfer to a foster home, divorce, or psychiatric disorder in a close family member.

Signs and symptoms of neurodevelopmental instability can be identified from the history of attainment of milestones, and so help identify a vulnerability to mental disorders. These signs include physical anomalies (Green et al., 1994), neurologic soft signs (Pine et al., 1997), and poor coordination or integration difficulties, as well as temperament and personality traits, all of which can be identified during the course of development. It is important to know if symptoms are present across settings or are restricted to certain situations.

Children with internalizing disorders such as depression and anxiety are often the best informants about their affective states. However, if children experience depressed or anxious mood as their normal state, no baseline frame of reference is available for comparison. Children and adolescents with externalizing disorders such as ADHD and conduct disorder are often poor informants and may be minimally cooperative with the interview. Since they often deny the existence of a problem and blame others, reports from other informants (parent, school) are essential.

Parents and children often do not agree on the presence of diagnostic conditions, regardless of diagnostic type (Jensen et al., 1999). While agreement between adolescent report and parent report of psychiatric di-

agnostic data is shown to be good for conduct disorder, ADHD, and oppositional defiant disorder (ODD), it is poor for major depression, dysthymia, and anxiety disorders, other than separation anxiety disorder (Cantwell et al., 1997).

A family history of mental disorders should be gathered, but the identification of mental disorders in family members becomes less reliable when it moves beyond the person directly interviewed. Family history can be useful in narrowing the differential diagnosis and in interpreting potential comorbidity. For instance, consideration of the potential contribution of depression or hypomania to ADHD can be aided if there is a family history of affective disorder. A family history of certain disorders such as tics may also be helpful in selecting and monitoring medications.

Significant medical conditions, including head trauma, metabolic disorders, and neurologic conditions, should be identified. Eating and sleeping patterns are important to identify over time to know if these relate to the present condition and to know if medications affected them. Information about potential drug sensitivities or interactions may be obtained from a medication history that includes antibiotics commonly used, cold preparations, vitamins, health supplements, and present and past psychotropic medications. It is important to find out about previous medication trials: what was tried, what worked, what did not work, and why.

Developmental norms are important to consider in evaluating potential medication effects and side effects. Neurotransmitter and other neurochemical levels fluctuate throughout development and can result in variable medication response at different times. Behavioral toxicity from medication can include negative effects on mood, behavior, or learning, and often develops before physical side effects are observed, especially in younger children (Campbell et al., 1985). These side effects may be the result of an interaction of the particular drug and the child's stage of physical, cognitive, or emotional development (Dulcan et al., 1988).

MENTAL STATUS EXAMINATION

Essential elements of the mental status examination for children are described below, with a nonexhaustive list of examples.

Appearance. Eye contact and clothing are important to observe. Physical anomalies, dysmorphic facial features, or suggestions of a genetic or neurodevelopmental condition are also important to identify.

Behavior. Activity level, restlessness, distractibility, behavioral inhibition, expressions of anxiety, engagement with the parents and with the interviewer, and evidence of medication side effects should be observed. Increased activity level could be a symptom of anxiety, ADHD, or mania. Particular rating scales may be useful, as discussed in Chapter 32 of this text.

Affect. Expressed affect should be characterized and questioned. Depression may be confused with shyness at first. A blunted or constricted affect could be a symptom of depression, demoralization, or schizophrenia, or be a side effect of medication. Bored affect in children is often a symptom of depression.

Language and speech. Speech spontaneity, articulation, vocabulary, and prosody should be noted. Pedantic speech may be a symptom of Asperger's disorder or of a nonverbal learning disorder. Diminished speech may be the result of depression or autism. Excessive speech may be the result of anxiety, ADHD, or hypomania. Unusual speech may be an early sign of neurodevelopmental vulnerability to psychosis. Slurred speech may be evidence of a neurologic abnormality or a medication side effect.

Social relatedness. Nonverbal communication, eye contact, evidence of social reciprocity such as the ability to have a conversation with appropriate interchange, and play (symbolic, imaginative, or repetitive) furnish data to assess social relatedness. Recognition of boundaries and the emotional state of others are important to observe.

Thought process. How do the child's thoughts connect? A child in the preoperational stage can have illogical, magical thinking that may not be normal for a child in middle childhood.

Thought content. Patterns in a child's thinking may include suicidality, homicidality, paranoia, delusions, preoccupations, anxieties, and themes emerging from a disorganized thinking pattern.

Alertness. Alertness involves attention, the ability to shift sets, and concentration, and cognitive abilities. Somnolence could be a symptom of a disorder such as depression or a medication side effect.

Estimation of intellect, judgement, and insight. Developmental norms should be used to estimate age-appropriate executive functions and intellectual abilities.

Playing with younger children in addition to talking with them often helps the clinician to understand the nature of their inner world and to determine their developmental level. Watching the child play with toys in the office while interviewing the parents is a time-efficient way of indirectly observing the child play and observing interactions with parents.

THERAPEUTIC ALLIANCE

The initial assessment begins to establish the therapeutic alliance between the physician and the family. A working partnership with the parents and with the youngster is essential for comprehensive treatment and for compliance. The physician should be a collaborator with the child and family to empower them to effect improvements in their lives. Within this therapeutic alliance, the psychological "power" of medication treatment needs to be considered (see Chapter 33) to avoid the pitfall of assuming that medication *alone* will independently transform the identified problems.

The Multimodal Treatment of ADHD (MTA) Study, a large, multisite study of ADHD treatment (MTA Cooperative Group, 1999), highlights the importance of this therapeutic alliance. When outcome was measured only in terms of the child's inattention, stimulant medication alone did as well as medication plus psychosocial treatment. However, the combination of medication and psychotherapy had the best outcome in parent satisfaction and in reducing disruptive behaviors (Hinshaw et al., 2000), which are important factors in longer-term compliance with treatment and outcome.

DECISION MAKING

The diagnostic formulation should include an integrated biopsychosocial and developmental understanding of the etiology of the child's disorder in the context of the family. This should lead to an integrated treatment plan, including medication management when appropriate, that addresses each aspect of the overall formulation. Key symptoms should be identified, with consideration given to primary and comorbid diagnoses. Additional information needed to elucidate the diagnosis and treatment plan should be identified.

A complete medical history and physical examination by a pediatrician or primary care provider should have been completed since the onset of symptoms or within the past year. Chronic medical illnesses such as asthma, cancer, diabetes mellitus, and neurologic disorders increase the risk for psychiatric disorders, particularly if physical disabilities result (Knapp and Harris, 1988). Somatization in children and adolescents is associated with mental disorders, especially anxiety and depressive disorders (Campo and Fritsch, 1994).

Neurological consultation or testing (EEG, CT, MRI) is indicated if focal neurological signs and symptoms are present, or if the history suggests seizures, regression, or decline in cognitive or physical functioning, or sequelae from brain injury (Dulcan and Martin, 2000). While it is likely that some day brain neuroimaging procedures will help with the differential diagnosis of mental disorders, it is not yet a clinical diagnostic instrument (Hendren et al., 2000).

Laboratory testing will depend on the medical condition, the psychiatric condition, and the drug therapy being considered. Liver function tests, complete blood cell count (CBC) with differential, and urine toxicology (to rule out substance abuse) are often obtained when using neuroleptics or mood stabilizers. Baseline drug screening is of particular value in the assessment of adolescents when there is (1) a high index of suspicion of substance abuse, (2) breakthrough mood or psychotic symptoms in the presence of adequate pharmacological management, and (3) inadequate response to trials of optimal pharmacological treatments (Kutcher, 1997).

Pregnancy testing in females of childbearing potential should be routinely obtained. Lead levels should be obtained in the evaluation of behavior disorders if lead toxicity is a possibility (Burns et al., 1999). If tricyclic antidepressants (TCAs) or antipsychotic agents are contemplated, a baseline electrocardiogram (EKG) is recommended, and is essential during follow-up and maintenance at higher dosages. The need for EKG monitoring when using α-adrenergic agonists such as clonidine is controversial; (the American Academy of Child and Adolescent Psychiatry (AACAP) Practice Parameters recommend a baseline EKG (Dulcan, 1997), but the American Heart Association Scientific Statement says it is not necessary (Gutgesell et al., 1999).

It would be helpful if there were a peripheral measure of neurotransmitter function that could be used to guide medication selection and dosing, but unfortunately this has not yet been developed. Some measures can be obtained from the cerebro spinal fluid, but even these levels have not been established as a guide to treatment. Peripheral measures or related measures of neuroendocrine function (Birmaher et al., 2000) may some day be useful guides. Likewise, pharmacogenetics may help select the most appropriate medication and dosage (Anderson and Cook, 2000, Chapter 7 in this volume).

The child's teacher can provide valuable information about the child and the family. Teachers may be given checklists to complete. Information from school records, including grades, attendance, scholastic achievement, and psychological testing, can all provide additional diagnostic information.

It is important to consider learning and language disabilities in the etiology of mental disorders and in the differential diagnosis. Psychological evaluation may pinpoint deficits susceptible to educational intervention. Identification and treatment of receptive and expressive language disabilities should be considered in the formulation. If cognitive impairment or head injury is suspected, referral to a neuropsychologist may help delineate the nature and extent of this deficit.

IDENTIFICATION OF PROBLEM HIERARCHY

The initial treatment plan should identify (1) target symptoms, (2) baseline impairment, preferably with quantitative rating scales; (3) comorbid psychiatric conditions that should be monitored and treated; and (4) a problem hierarchy based on target symptoms that are the most troubling and the most likely to respond to medication. These include inattention and distractibility, impulsivity, depression, affective instability, anxiety, thought disorganization, and non-premeditated (affective) aggression. Improvement in these symptoms may benefit from the consideration of more complex behaviors such as social skills, school performance, behavioral inhibition, and communication, but it is important to break these complex behaviors into a prioritized problem hierarchy when selecting a medication and measuring an outcome.

Once the family and the physician agree to use a pharmacological intervention to treat the child's disorder, the identified target symptoms should be reviewed and the medication options to treat these symptoms described. The prioritized problem list should be matched with appropriate interventions based on evidence from the research literature regarding the potential of the medication to benefit the target symptoms, as well as its side effects. The experience of the child or family members with other medication treatments, ease of administration, and length of time for treatment response should also be considered.

The treatment plan should be multimodal, including psychosocial and psychoeducational interventions as well as medication. Treatment alternatives should be described and the advantages and disadvantages of each discussed. Parents should understand that even if medication helps some biologically determined symptoms, the disorder might have caused psychological, interpersonal, or social difficulties that require other concomitant therapeutic interventions. This might include behavior modification, parent management training, social skills training, family therapy, group therapy, or individual psychotherapy. Explanations should be in language the child and parents can understand.

CLINICAL MANAGEMENT

The meaning of the psychiatric illness to the child and his or her family should be considered. Denial and confusion about the illness may not be expressed directly. Specific points for medication education include (1) the reasons for medications being used, (2) the goals of medication and when they might be achieved; (3) the common side effects and when they will emerge; (4) the rare side effects and when they might emerge; (5) the activities, foods, drinks, and other medications that are contraindicated or require caution; (6) recommended parental response to potential side effects; and (7) duration of treatment (Kutcher, 1997).

Both verbal and written information should be included as part of the patient and family education. A written set of instructions about taking medications with dates, times, and doses is often helpful. In addition to reading materials provided by the physician or nurse, the patient and family should be encouraged to read about and research the illness and treatment. This collaboration facilitates active learning and helps ensure compliance by giving the patient and family autonomy and control over the treatment.

Some causes for resistance to medication include unsatisfactory prior experience, the belief that behavior, mood, and cognitive problems should not be treated with drugs, and general misinformation. Typical concerns are that the medicine will make the child a "different person" or that the child will become addicted to the medication. The physician might emphasize that the medication is being used to treat an illness that interferes with the child expressing the best parts of him or herself, not to change the child's underlying personality. Side effects that seem to change the child's personality in negative ways require treatment modification. The long-term effects of the medication should also be discussed.

The ongoing treatment plan should (1) monitor target symptoms; (2) evaluate efficacy and need for additional interventions; (3) include ongoing, supportive contact with the family, school, and patient; (4) continue psychoeducation; and (5) suggest school and/or educational interventions (see Table 31.1).

TABLE 31.1 *Key Elements in the Treatment Plan and Follow-Up Visits*

1. Target symptoms—inattention, impulsivity, affect, anxiety, aggression, cognitive disorganization
2. Baseline impairment—developmental instability, family dysfunction, medical condition, mental status abnormalities, therapeutic alliance
3. Comorbid conditions
4. Prioritized treatment modalities—pharmacologic, psychosocial, psychoeducational
5. Plan to monitor target symptoms and effectiveness
6. Plan to add other necessary interventions
7. Plan to contact family and school
8. Psychoeducation
9. School interventions
10. Evaluation of outcomes
11. Review of side effects
12. Compliance issues
13. Emerging concerns and life events

EVALUATION OF OUTCOMES

For each targeted symptom, symptom-rating scales can be utilized before treatment and at appropriate intervals after treatment is initiated. Whenever possible, it is helpful to combine self-report measure(s) with observer report measure(s).

It is useful to identify (1) common, mild side effects that often go away, (2) troubling but not serious side effects, and (3) serious, adverse side effects that should be brought to the timely attention of the physician. Mild side effects such as sweating, gastrointestinal upset, stomachache, and headache may not be the most worrisome or dangerous from a medical perspective, but they often lead to noncompliance. Troubling side effects such as dystonia from neuroleptics, behavioral activation from selective serotonin reuptake inhibitors (SSRIs), sleep disturbance, or anorexia from stimulants, and weight gain from atypical neuroleptics should be discussed when choosing a medication with the family. These side effects may cause physiologic changes in body functioning, but usually do not lead to immediate negative consequences. Strategies for dealing with these side effects are to (1) adjust the dose, (2) change the time of administration, or (3) use another or an additional medication.

More problematic behavioral or physical side effects such as arrhythmia, prolonged QTc interval, seizures, liver failure, or orthostatic hypotension are described in the relevant chapters in this text. The acute effects from certain medications, such as neuroleptic malignant syndrome, acute dystonia, tricyclic antidepressant (TCA)-induced cardiac arrhythmia, or clozapine-induced seizures or agranulocytosis may be life threatening and often require immediate medical intervention and/or discontinuation of the culprit medication.

It is important to inform the child and family of the expected length of treatment time before they will be likely to observe symptomatic improvement. This discussion should include the decision-making process for determining the duration of the medication trial before trying another one if unsuccessful, and the considerations for eventual treatment discontinuation. Side effects from abrupt discontinuation should also be covered.

COMPLIANCE ISSUES

Noncompliance with medication treatment can be multidetermined in children and adolescents and occurs more frequently than physicians recognize. A recent study found that only 38% of adolescents were compliant with medication treatment 14 months after inpatient hospitalization (Lloyd et al., 1998), despite a relatively low level (23%) of side effects.

Potential reasons for noncompliance include resistance to taking medication in either the child, the parent, or both; incomplete or poorly understood directions for taking the medication; and poor organization of medication administration. In addition, parents or legal guardians may be resistant to treatment if they feel pressured to have the evaluation and treatment provided by outside agencies such as the school, child protective services, or the legal system.

Developing a schedule for taking medication is often helpful in improving compliance. The actual medication preparation (e.g., liquid or tablet) may likewise affect compliance. Children suffering from ADHD and depression may forget to take their medication; other children may actively resist. A strong therapeutic alliance has a positive effect on compliance. Active participation and collaboration from parents and the youngster to identify target symptoms and select the medication improves the therapeutic alliance. Respect for the youngster's autonomy and control over their mind and body also improves the alliance.

INFORMED CONSENT AND CONFIDENTIALITY

The risks, benefits, and alternatives to treatment should be fully explained to the parent and the young person,

and this discussion should be documented in the medical record. Since the Food and Drug Administration (FDA) has not approved many of the medications used to treat children and adolescents, they are often used off label. The implications of this and the published experience with the medication should be discussed to provide a fully informed consent. Consent is not a one-time occurrence, and patient and parent education about the prescribed medication(s) is an ongoing process. A developmentally adjusted assent should be obtained from the child.

If the child's parents are divorced, or if social services are involved with a child, the physician must find out who can give consent to treatment. Social service involvement may mean that the state has legal custody and an assigned social worker may act as the legal guardian. For divorced parents, sole or joint custody should be determined not only for residential status but also for medical decision making. Ideally, both parents should be involved in the consent process to gain their joint support and to avoid a potential sabotage on the part of an excluded parent.

Confidentiality about information shared during the interview should be addressed, particularly with adolescents. The adolescent might be told that all information arising from the therapeutic interaction will remain confidential except for that which may lead to significant harm to the youth or to others. Such exceptions include suicidality, substance abuse, and serious criminal activity. Adolescents should be assured that if the physician believes that certain issues require parental awareness, these would be discussed with the adolescent first, before the parents are alerted, except in an emergency situation. The adolescent might be offered the option of sharing the information with the parents along with the physician.

PSYCHOPHARMACOLOGY FOLLOW-UP VISITS

Key elements to be covered in the medication follow-up visit include (1) a change in target symptoms from baseline, (2) a review of side effects, (3) compliance and resistance, and (4) discussion of the concerns of the child and the parents (see Table 31.1). The medication follow-up visit also includes dosage adjustment and laboratory monitoring. Guidelines for specific disorders and medications are contained in the relevant chapters in this text.

Continued education about the disorder being treated, the treatment plan, including duration of treatment, use of concomitant medications, prognosis, and long-term issues regarding medications are all important. The physician should also learn something about the child's and family's functioning, stress, and significant events.

Once the target dosing has been reached, the dosage should be maintained at that level for a reasonable length of time, provided that side effects are tolerable. The temptation to increase the dosage of a medication too quickly or if the child shows an initial response followed by a plateau period should be carefully considered.

Ascertainment of treatment-emergent side effects requires a baseline symptom assessment before treatment is begun and at regular intervals thereafter. An ideal way to monitor side effects is to use medication-specific side effect scales that are designed for a particular drug class. These combine physical and behavioral symptoms with information obtained from the medical evaluation of the patient. Rating scales may help differentiate treatment-emergent side effects from an exacerbation of a symptom present at baseline, or from other causes of physical or behavioral symptoms. They may also help the family and the child accurately identify and label these side effects and then discuss them with the physician.

Medication management provides the opportunity to develop a relationship with the child and the family. Asking about medication benefits and side effects in the context of academics, sports, team activities, friends, and overall functioning gives youths an opportunity to talk about how the disorder and the medication are affecting their life, what is important in their life, and what they wish it could be like. Phone calls and e-mail can help with medication monitoring, but face-to-face contacts provide a more comprehensive treatment relationship.

SUMMARY AND CONCLUSION

Assessment and decision making in pediatric psychopharmacology involve a unique approach that takes into account development, the psychosocial context, and the limitations in diagnostic precision, efficacy, and effectiveness research that characterize childhood mental disorders. Successful treatment requires education and collaboration with the family. The decision-making process consists of the identification of a problem hierarchy and matching target symptoms with interventions. Clinical management includes psychoeducation, evaluation of outcomes, including therapeutic effects and side effects, and appropriate modification of a collaborative treatment plan. Pressures for short visits need not preclude the therapeutic interaction between the physician and the family.

REFERENCES

Anderson, G.M. and Cook, E.H. (2000) Pharmacogenetics: promise and potential in child and adolescent psychiatry in *Psychopharmacol Child Adolesc Psychiatr Clin North Am* 9(1):23–39.

Birmaher, B., Dahl, R.E., Williamson, D.E., Perel, J.M., Brant. D.A., Axelson, D.A., Kaufman. J., Don, L.D., and Still, S. (2000) Growth hormone secretion in children and adolescents at high risk for major depressive disorder. *Arch Gen Psychiatry* 57:867–872.

Burns, J.M., Baghurst, P.A., Sawyer, M.G., McMichael, A.J., and Tong, S.L. (1999) Lifetime low-level exposure to environmental lead and children's emotional and behavioral development at ages 11–13 years. The Port Pirie Cohort Study. *Am J Epidemiol* 149:740–749.

Campbell, M., Green, W.H., and Deitsch, S.I., eds. (1985) *Child and Adolescent Psychopharmacology*. Beverly Hills, CA: Sage.

Campo, J. and Fritsch, S. (1994) Somatization in children and adolescents. *J Am Acad Child Adolesc Psychiatry* 33:1223–1235.

Cantwell, D., Lewinsohn, P., Rohde, P., and Seeby, J. (1997) Correspondence between adolescent report and parent report of psychiatric diagnostic data. *J Am Acad Child Adolesc Psychiatry* 36:610–619.

Dulcan, M. (1997) Practice parameters for the assessment and treatment of children, adolescents, and adults with attention deficit hyperactivity disorder. *J Am Acad Child Adolesc Psychiatry* 36:85S–121S.

Dulcan, M., Bregman, J., Weller, E., and Weller, R. (1998) Treatment of childhood and adolescent disorders. In: Schatzberg, A.F., and Nemeroff, C.B., ed. American Psychiatric Press *Textbook of Psychopharmacology*, 2nd ed. Washington, DC: American Psychiatric Press, p. 805.

Dulcan, M.K. and Martin, D.R. (2000) *Concise Guide to Child and Adolescent Psychiatry, 2nd ed.*, Washington, DC, American Psychiatric Press.

Green, M.F., Satz, P., and Christenson, C. (1994) Minor physical anomalies in schizophrenic patients, bipolar patients, and their siblings. *Schizophr Bull* 20:433–440.

Gutgesell, H., Atkins, D., Barst, R., Buck, M., Franklin, W., Humes, R., Ringel, R., Shaddy, R., and Taubert, K.A. (1999) AHA Scientific Statement: cardiovascular monitoring of children and adolescents receiving psychotropic drugs. *J Am Acad Child Adolesc Psychiatry* 38:1047–1050.

Hendren, R.L., DeBacker, I., and Pandina, G. (2000) Review of neuroimaging studies of child and adolescent psychiatric disorders from the past ten years. *J Am Acad Child Adolesc Psychiatry* 39:815–828.

Hinshaw, S.P., Ownes, E.B., Wells, K.C., Kraemer, H.C., Abikoff, H.B., Arnold, L.E., Connors, C.K., Elliott, G., Greenhill, L.L., Hechtman, L., Hoza, B., Jensen, P.S., March, J.S., Newcorn, J.H., Pelham, W.E., Swanson, J.M., Vitiello, B., and Wigal, T. (2000) Family processes and treatment outcome in the MTA: negative/ineffective parenting practices in relation to multimodal treatment. *J Abnorm Child Psychol* 28:555–568.

Jensen, P., Rubo-Stipec, M., Canino, G., Bird, H., Dulcan, M.K., Schwab-Stone, M., and Lahey, B. (1999) Parent and child contributions to diagnosis of mental disorder: are both informants always necessary? *J Am Acad Child Adolesc Psychiatry* 38:1569–1579.

Knapp, P.K. and Harris, E. (1988) American Academy of Child and Adolescent Psychiatry work group on quality issues practice parameters for consultation liaison. *J Am Acad Child Adolesc Psychiatry* 37:139–146.

Kutcher, S.P. (1997) *Child and Adolescent Psychopharmacology.* Philadelphia: W.B. Saunders.

Lloyd, A., Horan, W., Borgaro, S.R., Stokes, J.M., Pogge, D.L., and Harvey, P.D. (1998) Predictors of medication compliance after hospital discharge in adolescent psychiatric patients. *J Child Adolesc Psychopharmacol* 8:133–41.

MTA Cooperative Group (1999) Moderators and mediators of treatment response for children with ADHD: the MTA Study. *Arch Gen Psychiatry* 56:1088–1096.

Pine, D.S., Shaffer, D., and Schonfeld, I.S. (1997) Minor physical anomalies: modifiers of environmental risks for psychiatric impairment. *J Am Acad Child Adolesc Psychiatry* 36:395–403.

Rappley, M.D., Mullan, P.B., Alvarez, F.J., Eneli, I.U., Wang, J., and Gardiner, J.C. (1999) Diagnosis of attention-deficit/hyperactivity disorder and use of psychotropic medication in very young children. *Arch Pediatr Adolesc Med* 153:1039–1045.

Riddle, M.A., Labellarte, M.J., and Walkup, J.T. (1998) Pediatric psychopharmacology: problems and prospects. *J Child Adolesc Psychopharmacol* 8:87–97.

Waldrop, M.F. and Halverson, C.F.J. (1971) Minor physical anomalies and hyperactive behavior in young children. In: Hellumuth, J. ed. *Exceptional Infant: Studies of Abnormalities*, Vol II. New York, Brunner/Mazel, pp. 343–380.

32 | Clinical instruments and scales in pediatric psychopharmacology

L. EUGENE ARNOLD AND MICHAEL G. AMAN

GENERAL PRINCIPLES

This review of instruments for assessing psychopathology in toddlers, children, and adolescents is not intended to be comprehensive. For readers seeking more details, we recommend an extensive textbook, the *Handbook of Psychiatric Measures,* (Rush et al., 2000), a detailed chapter (Aman and Pearson, 1999), and the disorder-specific chapters in Part III-B of this volume. Before describing specific instrument options, we summarize some basic principles that are applicable in clinical practice and in research on psychoactive medication. Although we use attention-deficit hyperactivity disorder (ADHD) as a frequent example, the principles are generally applicable to assessment of most disorders.

Informants

Scales and other instruments do not measure in a vacuum. One of the factors affecting reliability and validity of assessment is the informant—the person who fills out the scale, provides ratings, or provides information to the person filling out a questionnaire, scale, or other instrument. Most informants, especially in the context of child psychopathology, do not have full information, but some may be better informed than others about specific issues. For example, a teacher is usually the best informant for rating a child's sustained attention while the parent is usually a better informant about a young child's anxiety or sleep disturbance; the older child may be best for anxiety; and the adolescent may be the best informant for conduct disorder symptoms or substance use (Table 32.1). A young child is of limited use as an informant for certain disorders; for example, young children are often oblivious to ADHD symptoms. For some disorders, such as psychosis or severe major mood disorder, the clinician's examination and observation may be the best "informant."

Multiple informants

Any single informant has limitations of either opportunity to observe (e.g., separate home and school settings; limited time sample for clinician observation), insight (e.g, young children or patients with mental retardation), or nondefensive willingness to disclose (child or parent especially, but potentially also teacher). Therefore it is common to resort to multiple informants for important parameters. For example, the accepted practice in monitoring treatment of ADHD is to obtain both parent and teacher ratings because their observations are complementary, covering different times of day and different activities as well as different time-dependent side effects and time–action effects. The two ratings are complementary, not necessarily correlated. Even though they correlate in many studies at only about $r = 0.3$, they each contribute essential information, and usually reflect change in the same direction (see Scale Sums, Composites, and Averages, below). For disorders such as ADHD, in which the diagnostic criteria specify impairing symptoms in more than one setting, it becomes crucial to obtain information from more than one setting in monitoring response to treatment. For children in upper grades (with class changing), it may be necessary to obtain ratings from several teachers to cover the school day (and manage time–action effects of medication) or ask a school counsellor to synthesize ratings from several teachers.

Baseline Data

This self-evident axiom will be briefly stated because it is sometimes forgotten in busy clinical practice: baseline ratings or other data must be obtained prior to starting treatment for any instruments one plans to use as a monitoring tool. This is the only way one can know whether a given rating represents great improve-

TABLE 32.1 *Priority of Informants for Diagnosis and Treatment Monitoring of Disorders in Psychopharmacology of Children and Adolescents*

Disorder	Young Child	Adolescent
Attention-deficit hyperactivity disorder	1. Teacher and parent 2. Sitter, after-school program (day-care) director, scout leader, coach, bus driver	1. Teacher(s) and parent 2. Coach, employer, bus driver, cafeteria staff 3. Adolescent
Anxiety	1. Parent 2. Teacher, sitter, after-school program director, others 3. Child	1. Adolescent 2. Parent 3. Teacher, coach, others
Conduct disorder	1. Parent 2. Teacher, sitter, coach, scout leader, bus driver 3. Child	1. Adolescent 2. Parent, teacher
Depression	1. Child 2. Parent 3. Teacher, sitter, day-care director, coach, scout leader	1. Adolescent 2. Parent 3. Teacher, coach, employer
Eating disorder	1. Parent 2. Teacher, sitter, after-school program director, cafeteria staff 3. Child	1. Parent 2. Adolescent 3. Teacher, cafeteria staff
Enuresis	1. Parent and child	1. Adolescent 2. Parent
Mania/bipolar disorder	1. Parent and teacher 2. Sitter, after-school director, coach, scout leader, bus driver. 3. Child	1. Parent and teacher 2. Adolescent 3. Coach, employer
Oppositional-defiant disorder	1. Parent and teacher 2. Sitter, after-school director, coach, scout leader	1. Parent 2. Teacher 3. Employer, coach 4. Adolescent
Obsessive-compulsive disorder	1. Parent 2. Child and teacher 3. Sitter, after-school program director, coach, scout leader	1. Adolescent 2. Parent and teacher 3. Coach, employer
Pervasive developmental disorder, severe with pharmacological target symptoms	1. Parent 2. Teacher 3. Drivers, other caregivers 4. Child, if he or she communicates	1. Parent 2. Teacher 3. Adolescent, if he or she communicates 4. Drivers, other caregivers
Post-traumatic stress disorder	1. Parent 2. Child 3. Teacher, sitter, other caregiver	1. Adolescent 2. Parent 3. Teacher, coach, employer
Psychosis	1. Child 2. Parent and teacher 3. Other observers	1. Adolescent 2. Parent, teacher, others
Substance use	1. Child 2. Teacher, Parent	1. Adolescent 2. Sibling 3. Parent, teacher, coach
Tics/Tourette's syndrome	1. Parent, child, teacher 2. Others	1. Adolescent 2. Parent, teacher, others

Within each cell, informants are listed in approximate order of importance and /or desirability. *Parent* should be understood broadly as primary caregiver(s), including residential center staff. Prepubertal children phase into the adolescent priorities about ages 10–12 years (transition from concrete operations to formal operations). For patients with mental retardation or pervasive developmental disorder, mental age and communication ability must be considered.

ment, small improvement, no change, or worsening. A corollary is that the baseline data should be obtained from the same informants who will provide the subsequent monitoring information. This is necessary because of the rater-variance problem mentioned above, but it may not always be possible in long-term follow-up, as some informants (notably teachers) change over time. In the case of unavoidably changing informants, the new informants' ratings should not be individually compared to the previous ones for clinical management purposes, but should be evaluated de novo in their own right. In research, by contrast, group means can be compared between old and new teachers as long as there is a comparison control group.

Rating attenuation

Some time ago, investigators noted that parent and teacher ratings often decline or attenuate (improve) after the first rating is performed. This phenomenon occurs even without any form of treatment. It appears to be due to regression to the mean, as such research (and clinical) samples are usually selected because they deviate markedly from the norm on the scale in question. The easiest way to avoid such a spontaneous rating reduction is to repeat the rating before starting treatment, if time and circumstances allow. The clinician or investigator would ordinarily either use the second rating as the "true" baseline assessment or average the two ratings to obtain a more reliable baseline. If this is not possible, it is important to remember that some rating change can be due to attenuation rather than to a pharmacological effect.

Ease of Repeated Collection and Usage

In choosing an instrument to monitor treatment results, the feasibility of assessment burden for repeated collection must be considered. One consideration is the length. For clinical use without compensation, a regular classroom teacher should not be expected to spend more than 5 minutes on a repeated basis unless there is some necessitating special complication that the clinician has explained to the teacher. Teachers in special small classes can be expected to give a little more time. Parents in general are willing to spend more time on ratings than teachers, and can often fill out forms in the waiting room without costing them additional time. But even here, more than 2–5 pages on a repeated basis easily becomes a mechanical chore without considered thought. The clinician and staff time required to score and digest data is another consideration. Six pages of ratings do not make sense for clinical practice

if the clinician only has time to digest two pages. To ensure quality, timeliness, completeness, and usability of data collected, less is often more. Another consideration in ease of collection is the modality or procedure used. Assessments that require going to a special place or providing information in a certain way add to informant burden and may result in missed collections. Ideally, the informant should be offered a choice of phone, fax, mail, or e-mail (or in the case of teachers, sending information with the patient's parent). For clinical purposes, the informant could even be offered a choice of instrument from a short preselected list relevant to the targets being monitored. For example, a teacher reporting on a child with ADHD could use either the Conners 10-item scale, the ADHD Checklist, a list of *Diagnostic and Statistical Manual* [DSM] symptoms on a 0–3 metric), behavior counts, or daily report card scores; all of these provide usable information as long as the baseline is established pretreatment. For other disorders, of course, different instruments would be on the short list.

Reliability and Validity

In addition to having intuitive clinical relevance, instruments should be reliable and valid for the disorder or symptoms being diagnosed or monitored. Most published instruments are normed with information about reliability and validity. *Reliability* is how consistent the instrument is from one administration to another and from one rater to another. Generally, reliabilities above 70% (i.e., 70% or more agreement between raters observing the same phenomenon and/or 70% agreement from one administration to another without actual change in clinical status) are considered acceptable.

Validity is how well the instrument actually measures what it is supposed to measure. This has two aspects—sensitivity (picking up the problems) and specificity (picking up only actual problems). For diagnostic or categorical screening instruments, *sensitivity* means that if there really is a case (as determined by expert clinicians or some other standard), the instrument will detect it, avoiding false negatives. For example, if sensitivity is 0.9, 90% of the actual cases will be picked up, and there will be a false-negative rate of 10% of the actual cases. *Specificity* for a diagnostic instrument means that a person who does not have the disorder will not be diagnosed, thus false positives are avoided. If specificity is 0.85, 85% of those who do not have the disorder will not be diagnosed, and there will be a false-positive rate of 15%. Thus an instrument with 90% sensitivity and 85% specificity, when used on a population with a 40% rate of the problem being screened for, would correctly identify 36% (90% × 40%) as having the problem and 51% (85% × 60%) as not having the problem (87% correct classification), and would incorrectly identify 4% (10% × 40%) as not having the problem who actually do have it and 9% (15% × 60%) as having the problem who do not have it. The practical implication is that in screening a sample of 100, 36 true cases and 51 non-cases would be correctly classified, 4 cases would be missed, and 9 "cases" would need a work-up to establish that they do not really have the condition.

Mathematical caution

Instrument users must beware of a mathematical quirk in which an instrument with good specificity and sensitivity applied to a population with a low base rate of the disorder (e.g., 5% or less) may result in more false positives than valid diagnoses. For example, with a 5% population rate, an instrument with 100% sensitivity and 90% specificity (both outstanding) would correctly identify 5% as having the disorder and incorrectly identify 9.5% as having the disorder. Thus 14.5% would be identified as having the disorder, almost two-thirds of whom (9.5/14.5%) would be false positives. If the base rate is 1%, an instrument could have 100% sensitivity and 98% specificity (almost unheard of instrument perfection) and still identify almost twice as many false positives as true positives. This low base–rate phenomenon is mainly a problem in epidemiological or screening programs. In clinical populations the base rate of actual disorder is usually high enough to minimize this mathematical quirk.

Predictive power

Such considerations have led to development of the concept of predictive power, which is more directly useful in evaluating the results from a screening instrument. *Positive predictive power* is the probability that a child identified by the instrument as having the disorder or symptom actually does have it, and *negative predictive power* is the probability that a child identified as not having the disorder or symptom actually does not have it. In some ways, predictive power is the converse of specificity and sensitivity, but it usually also depends on the base rate. If sensitivity is 100% then the negative predictive power would be 100%. If specificity is 100%, then positive predictive power is 100%. But when sensitivity and specificity are less than 100% (the usual situation), the base rate enters into the calculation. With 90% sensitivity, 90% specificity, and a 5% base rate, there are 4.5% true positives, 85.5%

true negatives, 9.5% false positives, and 0.5% false negatives, making 14% total positives and 86% total negatives. In such a case, positive predictive power would be 4.5%/14% (4.5% true positives divided by all identified positives) = 35.1%; and negative predictive power would be 85.5%/86% (85.5% true negatives divided by all negatives) = 99.4%. Such low levels of confidence in positive identifications, even under conditions of psychometric robustness, underscore the wisdom of not basing a diagnosis (especially a rare one, such as psychosis) on an instrument alone, although the instrument can conveniently gather data for clinical evaluation or judgment. Even in a clinical population with a suspected base rate of 60%, an instrument with 80% sensitivity and specificity would yield 48% true positives, 12% false negatives, 32% true negatives, and 8% false positives, making positive predictive power of 48/56 = 85.7% and negative predictive power of 32/44 = 72.7%. These may be acceptable error rates for scientific group-analysis purposes, but they indicate caution in application to individual patients.

Face validity and content validity

Some instruments are said to have *face validity*—common-sense validity that is so obvious and self-evident that it doesn't need psychometric demonstration. For example, a scale made up of the symptoms of a disorder in lay language might be considered face-valid for those symptoms: if a child is rated as having "very much" of a problem sustaining attention, it is likely that he or she has a problem sustaining attention, one of the symptoms of ADHD. This, of course, assumes that the rater understands the words of the scale in the same way as the clinician and scale designer (see next section). A formal refinement is *content validity*, in which a panel of expert judges rates the items for their relevance to the construct being measured.

Clinical Tempering of Scores

Here is an anecdote that should be sobering for all clinical scientists. L.E.A. was using a one-sheet (both sides) scale to monitor progress of an autistic child in treatment. The scale came with an attached score sheet to which numbers were to be transposed. The child's father, of apparently normal intelligence, fluent English, and no obvious psychopathology (although of lower socioeconomic status), had filled out the instrument uneventfully twice (baseline and after 2 weeks of medicine). On the third occasion, the clinician mistakenly handed the father the score sheet rather than the questionnaire. The father studied it for awhile, then dutifully filled numbers in the blanks and handed it back. He obviously had no idea what the numbers meant, though he apparently aimed to please. Would he have had any better idea what the numbers meant if he had been given the correct form? In retrospect, it appears that the father may have had a reading disorder that he was too embarrassed to mention. The moral of this story is that clinical judgment must be used in interpreting the results of any rating obtained. It is as important to listen to narrative information as it is to score ratings—maybe more so. For example, if a teacher's report card comments and notes to parents suggest severe ADHD but she rates the child as normal on a scale, one might wonder how she feels about giving a child poor ratings. Currency of data is also an issue; clinical review should consider the date of the ratings and the time window referenced.

Categorical versus Dimensional Measures

Both categorical and dimensional measures are used for clinical care and research. Each type has its own advantages. *Categorical measures* are usually dichotomous, such as diagnosed case versus not a case or responder versus nonresponder, but can have more than one category, such as responder, placebo responder, and nonresponder. These measures generate a descriptive conclusion that is easily understood and practical, and usually suits the needs of clinical practice to determine whether or not to do something. *Dimensional*, or *continuous, measures*, such as rating scales, weight, or blood pressure, provide much more flexibility and accuracy of measurement, capturing many gradations of the variable. The individual scores distribute into a continuum with a mean and median (as well as mode, which categorical measures also have). Treatment might be defined as an attempt to move the patient from a deviant position on the continuum to one nearer the normal mean. Because of their more finely graduated accuracy, dimensional measures usually have more statistical power to detect changes than do categorical ones. A dimensional measure can be converted to a categorical measure (usually with loss of power) by applying a threshold or cutpoint, and categorical measures often have dimensional measures, such as symptom counts, embedded in them as operational criteria. Both kinds of measure are useful, and research studies usually include both.

Selection of Instrument

The following points should be considered in selecting instruments:

1. More extensive instrumentation may be appropriate for pretreatment characterization of a patient or sample than can be practically carried out for monitoring.

2. The instruments to be used for monitoring should be included in the baseline assessment.

3. Each instrument has to be appropriate for the age of the patient.

4. When multiple informants are used, it is desirable to use the same instrument for each informant, if practical, so the results can be averaged or easily compared.

5. The cost, both in dollars (for commercially sold instruments) and in clinician time, must be considered. A clinician-rated instrument is sometimes superior (for some disorders), but when a parent rating or teacher rating is as useful, it might be preferred.

6. Of course, the most basic principle is that the instrument has to be appropriate for the target clinical problems (Table 32.2).

Analyzing and Interpreting Instrument Scores: Initial Values

The most carefully chosen and diligently administered instrument can be vitiated by inadequate thought regarding proper analysis and interpretation. The issues of attenuation and regression to the mean were mentioned with regard to valid baseline scores, but they also apply to the analytic strategy and drawing of conclusions. For example, Swanson (1988) illustrated how erroneous conclusions could be drawn from superficially plausible statistical manipulations if one is unaware of a phenomenon variously called *rate dependency, law of initial values,* or *base-state dependency.* If one generates two large sets of random numbers that are putative pretest and post-test scores on the same subjects and then calculates the correlation between the first set (baseline) and the change score from baseline to post-test, one finds $r = -0.7$, a highly significant correlation entirely due to chance! Such manipulations could lead to confident but erroneous conclusions, for example, that a given treatment has a normalizing effect on all the parameters measured, or that severity moderates treatment effect (the more severe cases benefitting significantly more). Taking additional measures over time and regressing the baseline on the slope of the other measures instead of on the single post-test can reduce the chance correlation resulting from statistical regression to $r = 0.65$. The need for expert statistical consultation becomes obvious.

The intended use of the instrument must also be considered, and deviations from its natural scoring must be carefully thought out. In changing an intended dimensional instrument to categorical by collapsing

TABLE 32.2 *Assessment Instruments Specific for Disorders, Syndromes, or Symptoms*

Disorder	Instruments	Size, Description	Rater	Reference, Source
Attention-deficit hyperactivity disorder (ADHD)	ADHD Checklist, SNAP-IV	18 DSM-IV Symptoms on 0–3 metric	T,P	Swanson, 1992; ADHD.net
	Conners' Global Index	10 items 0–3 from Conners factors	T,P	Multi-Health Systems
	Iowa Conners Scale	10 items 0–3 on ADHD, aggression	T,P	Loney Mylich, 1987
	SWAN	18 DSM symptoms restated positively, 1–7 metric	T,P	Swanson, ADHD.net
	Conners-Wells Adolescent SR, HA factor	1 factor of 6 in 102-item scale		Conners and Wells, 1995
Anxiety	Revised Children's Manifest Anxiety Scale (RCMAS)	37 true–false items, 3 subscales: Physiological, Worry, Concentration	Ch, A	Reynolds and Richmond, 1985
	Multidimensional Anxiety Scale for Children (MASC)	39 items based on DSM-IV, with 4 subscales: physical symptoms, social anxiety, harm avoidance, separation/panic	Ch, A	March et al., 1999; Multi-Health Systems Gresham and Elliott, 1990; Achenbach, 1991a; b
	Internalizing factor of Social Skills Rating System (SSRS), Child Behavior Checklist (CBLL), or Teacher Report Form (TRF)		P, T	
	Childhood Anxiety Sensitivity Index	Measures patient's reaction to anxiety; 18 items, 10 minutes	Ch	Silverman et al., 1991
	Screen for Child Anxiety-Related Emotional Disorders (SCARED)	41 items	P, T	Birmaher et al, 1999
Conduct disorder (CD)	DSM-IV Aggression and Conduct D/O Rating Scale	15 DSM-IV symptoms of CD on 4-part metric	P, T	American Psychiatric Association, 1994 Rush et al., 2000;
	New York Teacher Rating Scale (NYTRS)		T	Miller and Kamboukos, 2000
	Self-report of Delinquency (SRD) or Self-report of Antisocial Behavior (SRA–younger)	Items cover overt and covert antisocial behavior	Ch, A	Elliott et al., 1985
	Child Behavior Checklist (CBCL) and Teacher Report Form (TRF)	Delinquent, aggressive subscales + externalizing factor within 112 items	P, T	Achenbach, 1991a, b
Depression	Children's Depression Inventory (CDI)	27-item depression symptoms	Ch, A	Kovacs, 1985, 1995
	Internalizing factor of Social Skills Rating System (SSRS)	Anxious/depressive symptoms subscale	P, T	Gresham and Elliott, 1990
	Children's Depression Rating Scale–Revised (CDRS-R)	Clinician rated, 17 items, 20 minutes	CI with P and Ch or A	Poznanski and Mokros, 1999

(continued)

Disorder	Instruments	Size, Description	Rater	Reference, Source
Eating disorder	Eating Disorder Inventory	91-item multidimensional		Garner et al., 1983
Enuresis	Log/calendar of dry nights	Behavior count	Ch, P	
Mania/bipolar disorder	Mania Rating Scale (MRS)	7 items rated 0–4 and 4 items rated 0–8, higher scores = more symptomatology Initially, 45–60 minutes; repeats, 10–30 minutes	Cl with Ch/A	Fristad et al., 1992, 1995
	Sleep log/calendar	Quantification of sleep deprivation	P, A	
Oppositional-defiant disorder (ODD)	SNAP-IV ODD items	8 DSM-IV ODD symptoms on 0–3 metric	P, T	Swanson, 1992; ADHD.net
	New York Teacher Rating Scale	Comprehensive list of antisocial symptoms	T	Rush et al., 2000
	Self-Report Antisocial Behavior	Overt and covert antisocial behavior	Ch	Elliott et al., 1985
Obsessive-compulsive disorder	Children's Yale-Brown Obsessive-Compulsive Scale (CY-BOCS)	2-page quantification of obsessions, compulsions, and resulting impairment (30–45 minutes; 10–20 minutes on repeat)	Cl with A or P and Ch input	Scahill et al., 1997
Pervasive developmental disorder (PDD)	Aberrant Behavior Checklist (ADB)	58 items rated 0–3, 5 subscales: irritability, lethargy, stereotypy, hyperactivity, inappropriate speech	P, T	Aman et al., 1985; Aman and Singh, 1994
	Autism Diagnostic Observation Schedule	½-hour coded observation (core symptoms of autism)	Cl observed	Lord et al., 1989
	Vineland Adaptive Behavior Scales	261 items, 4 factors: communication, daily living skills, socialization, motor; ½–1 hour	Parent	Sparrow et al., 1984
	Nisonger Child Behavior Rating Form	2 prosocial and 6 problem behavior subscales; items rated 0–3; 8–15 minutes	P, T	Aman et al., 1996; Tassé et al., 1996
	Gilliam Autism Rating Scale (GARS)	Core and comorbid symptoms	Parent	Gilliam, 1995
	Children's Yale-Brown Obsessive-Compulsive Scale, PDD Adaptation	Quantification of compulsions and ritualistic behavior that accompany the PDD and resulting impairment	Cl with P and Ch or A input	Adapted from Scahill et al., 1997, as referred to in Arnold et al., 2000
Post-traumatic stress disorder (PTSD)	PTSD Reaction Index	½-hour semistructured interview	P, or Cl with Ch	Stuber et al., 1991
	PTSD module from the DICA	½-hour structured interview		Sack et al., 1997
Psychosis	Children's version Brief Psychiatric Rating Scale (BPRS–C)	21 items rated by observation and interview	Cl with Ch	NIMH, 1985
Substance use	Self-report of Delinquency (SRD)	Includes substance use items	A	Elliott et al., 1986

(continued)

TABLE 32.2 *(continued)*

Disorder	Instruments	Size, Description	Rater	Reference, Source
Tics/Tourette's syndrome	Yale Global Tic Severity Scale	42 items rated 0–5 for 4 types tics: simple vs. complex × motor vs. phonic; 15 to 20 minutes	Cl with Ch/A	Leckman et al., 1989
Mental retardation with target psychopathology	Aberrant Behavior Checklist	58 items rated 0–3, 5 subscales: irritability, lethargy, stereotypy, hyperactivity, inappropriate speech	P, T	Aman et al., 1985; Aman and Singh, 1994
	Nisonger Child Behavior Rating Form	76 items rated 0–3; 2 prosocial and 6 problem behavior subscales; 8–15 minutes	P, T	Aman et al., 1996; Tassé et al., 1996
Preschoolers	Child Behavior Checklist/ 2–3	100 items rated 0–2, 6 subscales: social withdrawal, depressed, sleep problems, somatic problems, aggressive, destructive	P	Achenbach et al., 1992
	Preschool Behavior Questionnaire (PBQ)	30 items, 3 subscales: hostile-aggressive, anxious-fearful, hyperactive-distractible	P	Behar, 1974a, b

A, adolescent; Ch, child; Cl, clinician; HA, hyperactivity; P, parent; T, teacher. ADHD.net is the Internet address to obtain SNAP-IV and SWAN.

scores or using a cutpoint, the instrument can lose enough power to fail the experiment. Similarly, attempting a dimensional analysis of an instrument with a narrow range of scores intended for categorical use, might be inappropriate (see Clinical Global Impression, below). Using a diagnostic or screening instrument as an outcome measure generally results in poor sensitivity to treatment.

DIAGNOSTIC INSTRUMENTS

The most important diagnostic "instrument" is the operational criteria of DSM. Although these criteria change somewhat over time with successive editions and refinements, they generally crystallize the best clinical–scientific thinking at the time of publication. Therefore, they offer reasonable guidelines for the necessary clinical judgment. In fact, much of the diagnostic process is devoted to determining whether the patient's symptoms and impairment meet those criteria, as judged by a clinician. In addition to a clinician-filtered open-ended narrative approach, there are various structured or semistructured interviews to assist with organizing the information and making sure nothing is missed. These are routinely used in diagnosing for inclusion criteria in pharmacological research, and some may have utility in clinical practice. Most are available

in both a parent version (based on interview of parent) and a child version (based on interview of child/adolescent). The parent version is generally used for prepubertal children. The child version is generally valid above about age 11, at which age both versions are often used. When both are administered, an either-or algorithm is often used to combine the information: the "Or Rule" specifies that if either child or parent reports the symptom, it is counted as present.

Semi-structured interviews such as the Schedule for Affective Disorders and Schizophrenia, Kiddie version–Present & Lifetime version [K-SADS-PL] Kaufman et al., 1997) require a clinician to administer. The interviewer makes clinical diagnostic judgments as the interview progresses, and by the end of the interview has generated a rigorous, clinically informed diagnostic profile. This is essentially a quality-controlled clinical evaluation, guided "by the book." Although it is considered a superior method of diagnosis, it unfortunately takes longer than the usual clinical evaluation and takes more clinician time than structured interviews. Consequently, it is generally reserved for clinical studies in which a premium is placed on accurate diagnosis.

Highly structured (usually just called *structured*) *interviews* are designed for administration by a nonclinician research assistant or office assistant. They require clinician review for validity (mainly specificity), but make the clinician's time more efficient. They are generally acknowledged to be reasonably sensitive in picking up problems, but tend to overdiagnose some disorders, such as anxiety and psychosis, when administered by lay interviewers. The Diagnostic Interview Schedule for Children (DISC: current version, DISC-IV) is available from Columbia DISC (1999) in a DSM-IV computer-assisted version for lay administration. Although developed mainly for research use, it can also be used in clinical practice to save clinician time if an assistant is available to administer it. The Children's Interview for Psychiatric Syndromes (ChIPS; Teare et al., 1998) was specifically developed for clinical use rather than research, but can also be used for research. It is available both in paper-and-pencil and computer-assisted versions (American Psychiatric Press, 1999).

Structured and semistructured diagnostic interviews are mainly useful for diagnosis, not for monitoring treatment. The following instruments are suitable for monitoring as well as dimensional "diagnosis"—i.e., quantifying the severity of symptoms and impairment.

GLOBAL INSTRUMENTS

These instruments allow ratings of overall or global function or impairment. Most of them are usually clinician rated because it is considered necessary to have clinical judgment to integrate all the diverse sources of information (including more specific scales filled out by other informants). However, some global instruments have also been successfully filled out by parents or teachers with appropriate consultation and clarification of terms (e.g., in the highly successful Multimodal Treatment study of children with ADHD [MTA] medication maintenance algorithm for ADHD, in which parent and teacher CGIs were used along with clinician CGI to guide dosage adjustments, not as outcome data).

Clinical Global Impression

The Clinical Global Impression (CGI), Psychopharmacology Bulletin, 1985) is almost standard equipment for pharmacologicial studies, and can be adapted easily to clinical use. It can be done in about 5 minutes, requiring much more thought than writing. It has two component 7-point scales, often used together in monitoring and assessing treatment effects, but each can stand alone. The CGI-Severity (CGI-S) scale estimates the overall seriousness from 1 (essentially normal) to 7 (extremely severe), with 4, the midpoint, being moderate illness or impairment. The anchors are often re-

worded or redefined to be specific to the disorder being treated or otherwise adapted to the preference of the user. For example, to allow room for measuring variance in associated secondary symptoms that were the target of treatment, the Autism Research Units in Pediatric Psychopharmacology (RUPP) Autism Network defined uncomplicated autistic disorder as 3 ("mild"), even though autistic disorder is by definition always serious (Arnold et al., 2000).

On the 7-point CGI-Improvement (CGI-I) scale, 4 is no change, with lower numbers reflecting degrees of improvement and higher numbers degrees of worsening. Usually 1 = very much improved, 2 = much improved, and 3 = minimally improved, but again the anchors may be reworded to fit the user's need or preference A CGI-I of 1 or 2 generally demarcates a treatment "responder." It is often useful to elicit at baseline several specific target symptoms that can be monitored over time as partial input into the CGI-I rating (see Target Symptom Quantification, below).

Although the CGI-S can be used to monitor treatment clinically, e.g., to determine an appropriate titration end point such as minimal illness (CGI-S of 2), a better measure of significant improvement is the CGI-I, which was designed for that purpose and is more sensitive to treatment effect for research purposes.

The strength of the CGI and other clinician global assessments is that they provide a bottom-line appraisal. Perhaps their greatest weakness is that, without specific training and exposition of detailed anchors, a reader may not know what the rater was weighing most heavily. Thus global impressions may be ambiguous about *what* occurred while describing well its *importance*.

Columbia Impairment Scale

The Columbia Impairment Scale (CIS) (Bird and Gould, 1995) is a 17-item scale that differs from the CGI not only in length, but also in focusing on impairment of function rather than global pathology and function. It assesses how well the patient carries out daily activities appropriate for age or mental age. It can be filled out by the clinician or caregiver.

Global Assessment of Function

The Global Assessment of Function (GAF) is Axis 5 in DSM-IV multi-axial classification (American Psychiatric Association, 1994). It is similar to the Global Assessment Scale (GAS), which has separate adult and child (C-GAS: Shaffer et al., 1983) versions. The GAF has anchors with examples for both adults and children

TABLE 32.3 *Commercial and Other Sources for Scales and Other Instruments*

Aberrant Behavior Checklist: Slosson Educational Publications, P.O. Box 280, East Aurora, NY 14052 (716-652-0930).

ADHD Rating Scale: Public Domain, George DuPaul, Ph.D., College of Education, Lehigh University, 111 Research Drive, Bethlehem, PA 18015

Brief Psychiatric Rating Scale–Children's version: Public domain, *Psychopharmacology Bulletin* 1985; 21(4)

Child Behavior Checklist/2–3 (CBCL/2–3): Private, via author Thomas Achenbach, Ph.D., Department of Psychiatry, University of Vermont College of Medicine, 1 S. Prospect St., Burlington, VT 05401 (802-656-2602)

Child Behavior Checklist/4–18 (CBCL/4–18): Private, via author Thomas Achenbach, Ph.D., Department of Psychiatry, University of Vermont College of Medicine, 1 S. Prospect St., Burlington, VT 05401 (802-656-2602)

Childhood Anxiety Sensitivity Index (CASI): Private, via author W.K. Silverman, Ph.D., Department of Psychology, Florida International University, University Park, Miami, FL: also in Werry, J.S. and Aman, M.G. eds., *Practitioner's Guide to Psychoactive Drugs for Children and Adolescents.* New York: Plenum.

Children's Depression Inventory: Multi-Health Systems Inc., 908 Niagra Falls Blvd., North Tonowanda, NY 14120-2060 (www.mhs.com)

Children's Depression Rating Scale–Revised: Western Psychological Services, 12031 Wilshire Blvd., Los Angeles, CA 90025–1251 (www.wpspublish.com)

Children's Yale-Brown Obsessive-Compulsive Scale (CY-BOCS): Private; via author Larry Scahill, M.S.N., Ph.D., Yale Child Study Center, PO Box 207900, New Haven, CT 06520 (lawrence.scahill@yale.edu)

Conners' Global Index: Multi-Health Systems Inc., 908 Niagra Falls Blvd., North Tonowanda, NY 14120–2060 (www.mhs.com)

Conners-Wells Adolescent Self-Report: Multi-Health Systems Inc., 908 Niagra Falls Blvd., North Tonowanda, NY 14120–2060 (www.mhs.com)

IOWA Conners' Rating Scale: Private, via author Jan Loney, Ph.D., New York State Psychiatric Institute., Stony Brook University, Stony Brook, NY

Mania Rating Scale: Public domain, *Journal of American Academy of Child & Adolescent Psychiatry* 1992; 31: 252–257 (appendix)

Multidimensional Anxiety Scale for Children (MASC): Multi-Health Systems Inc., 908 Niagra Falls Blvd., North Tonowanda, NY 14120–2060 (www.mhs.com)

New York Teacher Rating Scale (NYTRS): Private, via author, Dr. L.S. Miller, Institute for Children at Risk, NYU Child Study Center, 550 First Avenue, New York, NY 10016 (laurie.miller.2@med.nyu.edu)

Nisonger Child Behavior Rating Form: Public domain, Michael Aman, Ph.D., The Nisonger Center, Ohio State University, 1581 Dodd Drive, Columbus, OH 43210–1257

Post-Traumatic Stress Disorder Reaction Index for Children: Private, via author, A.M. La Greca, Ph.D., Department of Psychology, 4100 Malaga Ave, Miami, FL 33133–6325

Preschool Behavior Questionnaire (PBQ): Private, via author, Dr. L.B. Behar, Learning Institute of North Carolina, Durham, NC

Revised Children's Manifest Anxiety Scale: Western Psychological Services, 12031 Wilshire Blvd., Los Angeles, CA 90025–1251 (www.wpspublish.com)

SNAP–IV: Private, via author James M. Swanson, Ph.D., Irvine Child Development Center, University of California at Irvine (download from www.ADHD.net)

Social Skills Rating System (SSRS): American Guidance Service, Inc., Publishers, Building 1, 4201 Woodland Rd., Circle Pines, MN 55014

SWAN: Private, via author, James M. Swanson, Ph.D., Irvine Child Development Center, University of California at Irvine (download from www.ADHD.net)

Teacher Report Form (TRF): Private via author, Thomas Achenbach, Ph.D., Department of Psychiatry, University of Vermont College of Medicine, 1 S. Prospect St., Burlington, VT 05401 (802-656-2602)

Yale Global Tic Severity Scale: Public domain, James Leckman, M.D., Yale Child Study Center, 230 S. Frontage Rd., P.O. Box 207900, New Haven, CT 06520

in one unified scale. There are several advantages to using this scale for monitoring treatment effects. It is already familiar to clinicians from diagnostic use, it allows direct extrapolation from experience with other age groups, it is readily interpreted by anyone who has a copy of DSM, it was designed for clinical use, it minimizes cost because there is nothing to buy, and it avoids reinventing the wheel.

Scale Sums, Composites, and Averages

With various scale data in electronic form, another option for deriving a global scale is to sum, average, or otherwise composite across all scales covering all the relevant domains. Conners et al. (2001) and Swanson et al. (2001) have illustrated how such a strategy can yield an overall outcome measure of high reliability and power. It can be especially useful to average or composite data across informants. The variance in any rating comes from two sources: child and rater. By compositing scores from two raters, the rater variance can be largely cancelled out or neutralized, leaving a stronger "signal" of the child's actual condition (Swanson et al., 2001). If the scales are on different metrics so that item means cannot be used, the individual scores can be converted to Z or T scores based on the published norms and then averaged. Although mainly a research tool, this strategy might be adaptable to a large clinical practice in which either scales are optically scanned or raters enter ratings directly into a computer. A poor person's composite can be gleaned from some single rating scales that attempt to cover many domains and provide a global summary score of the whole scale (e.g., Child Behavior Checklist, Teacher Report Form, the most recent long-version Conners scales).

SPECIFIC TAILORED ASSESSMENT: TARGET SYMPTOM QUANTIFICATION

In contrast to the global assessments above, it is sometimes desirable to focus on a few specific target symptoms that are either not covered well on the standard rating forms or may be diluted in overall ratings by the "noise" of irrelevant items (Arnold et al., 1972, 2000). The target symptoms, chosen by consensus of parent, clinician, teacher, and/or child or adolescent in consultation, are the reason for the pharmacotherapy and are of great import to the consumer. One way to carry this out is to ask each interested party to name one or two things they are most concerned about. The clinician then winnows these down to not more than three concerns. The symptoms chosen should either be selected by consensus or at least include something of concern to each party, and should be judged by the clinician as likely to show treatment changes. For example, the symptom must be frequent enough that a change could be noted within the time window of the assessment; something that occurs twice a month could not reliably show change on weekly assessments. Informants are asked to quantify the baseline rate and severity of the target symptoms; then at subsequent monitoring points, they are asked to restate the frequency and severity. This strategy is also helpful in gathering information for a CGI or GAF.

DISORDER-SPECIFIC ASSESSMENT

Table 32.2 lists representative instruments commonly used to monitor and dimensionally diagnose disorders encountered in child and adolescent psychopharmacology. Other commonly used instruments can be found in disorder-specific chapters in Section III-B of this volume. For clinical use, the longer instruments do not have to be repeated in their entirety for monitoring drug effects. It is good to administer the whole scale at baseline, but is acceptable thereafter to select the subscale, factor, module, or other item cluster that measures the treatment target(s). When titration (medication adjustment) has been completed to a satisfactory score, then the whole scale can be repeated to (1) make sure the factor score of interest comes out the same when embedded in the larger scale, and (2) to see what else may have changed. This strategy is sometimes also used for research—e.g., in the Autism RUPP risperidone trial, in which the whole Vineland Adaptive Behavior Scale (Sparrow et al., 1984) is administered at baseline and at the end, but only the Maladaptive Behavior Subscale is administered at two points between (Arnold et al., 2000). Table 32.3 lists commercial and other sources for most of the instruments in Table 32.2.

REFERENCES

Achenbach, T.M. (1991a). *Manual for the CBCL/4–18 and profile.* Department of Psychiatry, University of Vermont: Author (University of Vermont college of Medicine, I S. Prospect St., Burlington, VT 05401).

Achenbach T.M. (1991b). *Manual for the Teacher's Report Form and 1991 Profile.* Burlington, VT: Author.

Achenbach T.M. (1992). *Manual for the Child Behavior Checklist/ 2–3 and 1992 Profile.* Burlington, VT: Author.

Aman, M.G. and Pearson, D.A. (1999) Monitoring and measuring drug effects: behavioral, emotional, and cognitive effects. In: Werry, J.S. and Aman, M.G., eds. *Practitioners' Guide to Psychoactive Drugs for Children and Adolescents.* New York: Plenum, pp. 99–164.

Aman, M.G. and Singh, N.N. (1994) *Supplement to Aberrant Checklist Manual.* East Aurora, NY: Slosson Educational Publications.

Aman, M.G., Singh, N.N., Stewart, A.W., and Field, C.J. (1985) The Aberrant Behavior Checklist: a behavior rating scale for the assessment of treatment effects. *Am J Ment Defic* 89;485–491.

Aman, M.G., Tassé, M.J., Rojahn, J., and Hammer, D. (1996) The Nisonger CBRF: a child behavior rating form for children with developmental disabilities. *Res Dev Disabil,* 17, 41–57.

American Psychiatric Association (1994) *Diagnostic and Statistical Manual of Mental Disorders, 4th ed. (DSM-IV).* Washington, DC: American Psychiatric Association Press.

American Psychiatric Press (1999) Children's Interview for Psychiatric Syndromes (ChIPS). Washington, DC: American Psychiatric Press (800-368-7777; e-mail www.appi.org).

Arnold, L.E., Aman, M.G., Martin, A., Collier-Crespin, A., Vitiello, B., Tierney, E., Asarnow, R., Bell-Bradshaw, F., Freeman, B.J., Gates-Ulanet, P., Klin, A., McCracken, J.T., McDougle, C.J., McGough, J.J., Posey, D.J., Scahill, L., Swiezy, N.B., Ritz, L., and Volkmar, F. (2000) Assessment in multisite randomized clinical trials (RCTs) of patients with autistic disorder: the Autism RUPP network. *J Autism Dev Disord* 30:99–111.

Arnold, L.E., Wender, P.H., McCloskey, K., and Snyder, S. (1972) Levoamphetamine and dextroamphetamine: comparative efficacy in the hyperkinetic syndrome: assessment by target symptom. *Arch Gen Psychiatry* 27:8l6–822.

Behar I.B. and Stringfield, S. (1974a) A behavior rating scale for the preschool child. *Development Psychology, 10,* 601–610.

Behar L.B. and Stringfield, S. (1974b) *Manual for the Preschool Behavior Questionnaire.* Durham, NC: Author

Bird, H. and Gould, M. (1995). The use of diagnostic instruments and global measures of functioning in child psychiatry epidemiologic studies. In: Verhulst, F.C. and Koot, H.M. eds. *The Epidemiology of Child and Adolescent Psychophathology.* Oxford: Oxford University Press, pp. 86–103.

Birmaher, B., Brent, D.A., Chiappetta, L., Bridge, J., Monga, S., and Baugher, M. (1999) Psychometric properties of the Screen for Child Anxiety-Related Emotional Disorders (SCARED): a replication study. *J Am Acad Child Adolesc Psychiatry* 38: 1230–1236.

Columbia DISC (1998) Diagnostic Interview Schedule for Children—DSM-IV version (DISC-IV). E-mail: disc@worldnet.att.net; phone: 212-543-5948.

Conners, C.K., Epstein, J.N., March, J.S., Angold, A., Wells, K.C., Klaric, J., Swanson, J.M., Abikoff, H.B., Arnold, L.E., Elliott, G.R., Greenhill, L.L., Hechtman, L., Hinshaw, S.P., Hoza, B., Jensen, P.S., Kraemer, H.C., Newcorn, J., Pelham, W.E., Severe, J.B., Vitiello, B., and Wigal, T. (2001) Multimodal treatment of ADHD (MTA): an alternative outcome analysis *J Amer Acad Child Adolesc Psychiatry* 40:159–167.

Conners, C.K., and Wells, K. (1995) Conners-Wells Adolescent Self-Report Scale: item selection and replication of the factor structure. Unpublished.

Elliott, D.S., Huizinga, P., and Ageton, S.S. (1985) *Explaining Delinquency and Drug Use.* Thousand Oaks, CA: Sage.

Elliott, D.S., Huizinga, P., and Morse, B. (1986) Self-reported violent offending—a descriptive analysis of juvenile violent offenders and their offending careers. *J Interpers Viol* 1:472–514.

Freeman, B.J., Ritvo, E.R., Yokota, A., and Ritvo, A. (1985): A scale of rating symptoms of patients with the syndrome of autism in real life settings. *J Am Acad Child Adolesc Psychiatry* 25:130–136.

Fristad M.A., Weller, E.B., and Weller, R.A. (1992) The Mania Rating Scale: Can it be used in children? A preliminary report. *J Am Acad Child Adolesc Psychiatry* 31:252–257.

Fristad M.A., Weller, R.A., and Weller, E.B. (1995) The Mania Rating Scale: Further reliability and validity studies with children. *Ann Clin Psychiatry* 7:127–132.

Garner, D.M., Olmsted, M.P., and Polivy, J. (1983) Development and validation of a multidimensional eating disorder inventory for anorexia nervosa and bulimia. *Int J Eat Disord* 2:15–34.

Gilliam, J.S. (1995) Gilliam Autism Rating Scale. Examiner's Manual. Austin, TX: Pro-ed.

Gresham, F.M., and Elliott, S.N. (1990) *Social Skills Rating System Manual.* Circle Pines, MN: American Guidance Systems.

Kaufman, J., Birmaher, B., Brent, D., Rao, U., Flynn, C., Moreci, P., Williamson, D., and Ryan, N. (1997) Schedule for Affective Disorders and Schizophrenia for School-Age Children-Present and Lifetime Version (K-SADS-PL): initial reliability and validity data [see comments]. *J Am Acad Child Adolesc Psychiatry* 36:980–988.

Kovacs, M. (1985) The Children's Depression Inventory (CDI). *Psychopharm Bull* 21:995–998.

Kovacs, M. (1995) *Manual: The Children's Depression Inventory.* Toronto, Canada: MultiHealth Systems.

Leckman, J., Riddle, M., Hardin, M., Ort, S., Schwartz, K., Stevenson, J., and Cohen, D. (1989) The Yale Global Tic Severity Scale: initial testing of a clinician-rated scale of tic severity. *J Am Acad Child Adolesc Psychiatry* 28:566–573.

Loney, J. and Milich, R. (1982) Hyperactivity, inattention, and aggression in clinical practice. In: Wolraich, M., and Routh, D.K., eds., *Advances in Developmental and Behavioral Pediatrics* Greenwich, CT: JAI Press, pp. 113–137.

Lord, C., Rutter, M., Goode, S., Heemsbergen, J., Jordan, H., Mawhood, L., and Schopler, E. (1989). Autism diagnostic observation schedule: a standardized observation of communicative and social behavior. *J Autism Dev Disord* 19:185–212.

March, J.S., Conners, C.K., Arnold, L.E., Epstein, J., Parker, S., Hinshaw, S., Abikoff, H., Molina, B., Wells, K., Newcorn, J., Schuck, S., Pelham, W.E., and Hoza, B. (1999) The Multidimensional Anxiety Scale for Children (MASC): confirmatory factor analysis in a pediatric ADHD sample. *J Attention Disord* 3:85–90.

Miller, S. and Kamboukos, D., (2000) Symptom-specific measures for disorders usually first diagnosed in infancy, childhood or adolescence. In Rush, A.J., Pincus, H.A., First, M.B., Blacker, D., Endicott, J., Kieth, S.J., Phillips, K.A., Ryan, N.D., Smith, G.R., Tsuang, M.T., Widiger, T.A., and Zarin D.A., eds. *Handbook of Psychiatric Measures.* Washington, DC: American Psychiatric Association, 2008 pp. 325–357.

Poznansky, E. and Mokros, H.B. (1999) Children's Depression Rating Scale–Revised. Los Angeles: Western Psychological Services.

Psychopharmacology Bulletin (1985). Special feature: Rating scales and assessment instruments for use in pediatric psychopharmacology research. *Psychopharmacology Bull* 21(4).

Rush, A.J., Pincus, H.A., First, M.B., Blacker, D. Endicott, J., Kieth, S.J., Phillips, K.A., Ryan, N.D., Smith, G.R., Tsuang, M.T., Widiger, T.A., and Zarin, D.A., eds. 2000 *Handbook of Psychiatric Measures.* Washington, DC: American Psychiatric Association Press.

Reynolds, C.R. and Richmond, B.O. (1985) *Revised Children's Manifest Anxiety Scale.* Los Angeles, CA: Western Psychological Services.

Sack, W.H., Seely, J.R., and Clarke, G.N. (1997) Does PTSD transcend cultural barriers? A study from the Khmer Adolescent Refugee Report. *J Am Acad Child Adolesc Psychiatry* 36:49–54.

Scahill, L, Riddle, M.A., McSwiggin-Hardin, M., Ort, S.I., King, R.A., Goodman, W.K., Cicchetti, D., and Leckman, J.F. (1997) Children's Yale-Brown Obsessive Compulsive Scale: reliability and validity. *J Amer Acad Child Adolesc Psychiatry* 36:844–852.

Shaffer, D., Gould, M.S., Brasic, J., Ambrosini, P., Fisher, P., Bird, H., and Aluwahlia, S. (1983) A children's global assessment scale (CGAS). *Arch Gen Psychiatry* 40:1228–1231.

Silverman W.K., Fleisig, W., Rabian, B., et al. (1991) Childhood Anxiety and Sensitivity Index. *J Clin Child Psychol* 20:162–168.

Sparrow, S., Balla, D., and Cicchetti, D. Vineland Adaptive Behavior Scales: Interview Edition Survey Form. Circle Pines, MN: American Guidance Service, Inc.

Stuber, M.L., Nader, K., Yasuda, P., Pynoos, R.S., and Cohen, S. (1991) Stress responses after pediatric bone marrow transplantation. *J Am Acad Child Adolesc Psychiatry* 30:952–957.

Swanson, J.M., (1992) *School-based Assessments and Interventions for ADD Students.* Irvine, CA: K.C. Publishing.

Swanson, J.M., Kraemer, H.C., Hinshaw, S.P., Arnold, L.E., Conners, C.K., Abikoff, H.B., Clevenger, W., Davies, M., Elliott, G., Greenhill, L.L., Hechtman, L., Hoza, B., Jensen, P.S., March, J.S., Newcorn, J.H., Owens, L., Pelham, W.E., Schiller, E., Severe, J., Simpson, S., Vitiello, B., Wells, C.K., Wigal, T., and Wu, M. (2001) Clinical relevance of the primary findings of the MTA: success rates based on severity of ADHD and ODD symptoms at the end of treatment. *J Am Acad Child Adolesc Psychiatry* 40:168–179.

Tassé, M.J., Aman, M.G., Hammer, D., and Rojahn, J. (1996) The Nisonger Child Behavior Rating Form: age and gender effects and norms. *Res Dev Disabil* 17:59–75.

Teare, M., Fristad, M.A., Weller, E.B., Weller, R.A., and Salmon, P. (1998). Development and criterion validity of the Children's Interview for Psychiatric Syndromes (ChIPS). *J Child Adolesc Psychopharmacol* 8:205–211.

33 | Thinking about prescribing: the psychology of psychopharmacology

KYLE D. PRUETT AND ANDRÉS MARTIN

...the language of psychology and the language of biology involve two different levels of discourse when working with a patient (Resier, 1985; Edelson, 1984). The biopsychosocial psychiatrist must be conceptually bilingual.

Gabbard and Kay, 2001

Our patients have myriad thoughts, feelings, and wishes about the substances we prescribe for them, and about the processes we go through when prescribing them. As clinicians, we too are no less psychologically involved in these very concerns. Indeed, we often share their preoccupations and "magic bullet" fantasies of finding the perfect potion for just their problem. For all our increasing sophistication in understanding pharmacokinetics, drug–environment interaction, and symptoms as targets, we (rightly) remain as intrigued as ever by the way a particular agent works, or doesn't, in a particular patient, at any given moment in time.

Psychopharmacotherapy is the combined use of psychoactive medication and psychotherapy. Brent and Kolko (1998) define the latter as a treatment modality in which therapist and patient collaborate to ease functional psychopathological impairment through attention to (*1*) the therapeutic relationship, (*2*) the patient's behavior, thoughts, attitudes and affect (the working diagnosis), and (*3*) the social context and development (this is especially salient in the work of the child and adolescent psychiatrist).

This chapter will examine the multiple meanings of the use of medication in the wider domain of psychopharmacotherapy. Just as psychoanalysis struggled to understand the undue influence of the "gang beneath the couch," we will explore the meanings of the act of prescribing in the service of measuring and ameliorating the influence of the "gang between the prescription pad sheets." We shall examine the meaning to our patients of medication itself, the processes of prescribing, the specific context in which the prescription is written, and the influences on the prescription choice and fre-

quency of use, and then conclude with a discussion of the clinical implications of the complex act of prescribing.

The only legitimate framework for even discussing psychopharmacotherapy is not the "medcheck," but rather the therapeutic relationship itself. During the past 30 years, the therapeutic relationship has evolved from one in which medicating was initially seen as an alliance-undermining act, to one that is now a valued enhancement. Not coincidental to this change, those same three decades began with but a handful of reasonably effective agents for seriously affected children, typically used in university teaching centers, and has ended with dozens of highly effective therapeutic choices, often marketed directly to parents.

The therapeutic relationship, or more properly, the alliance, is the fundamental dimension of care. Its effectiveness as a separate therapeutic entity has been shown to correlate positively with the accuracy of the intervention itself, the fit of the theoretical approach, and the proper use of particular therapeutic techniques (Crits-Christoph et al., 1993; Luborsky et al., 1985). In other words, how clinicians are with their patients is as important as what clinicians do to, or with, their patients. Poor alliances lead to premature termination of care (Magnavita, 1993), just as good ones, in which patients feel understood, lead to far better follow-up and outcome (Zisook et al., 1978–79).

All too often, however, Blackwell's (1973) admonition prevails, and "a prescription signals the end of an interview rather than the start of an alliance." This is especially true in the child–parent–therapist triangle, where the parents' more urgent need for relief adds a magnitude of pressure to "doing something" before sufficient understanding exists. With our increasingly acute clinical populations, more attention to and understanding of alliance psychodynamics, diagnosis, and symptoms is required because of these complexities, not less.

417

THE PSYCHOLOGICAL MEANING OF MEDICATION ITSELF

An articulate 14-year-old who had initially responded well to a brief course of psychopharmacotherapy began to complain that she felt like a 'poser' on her selective serotonin reuptale inhibitor (SSRI).

I know I'm less depressed and irritable. My boyfriend says I'm easier to take, but I'm not sure this is really *me*. I feel like this poser [posing as another]. Like, every time I take my pills it reminds me that I'm this fuck-up who can't manage her feelings on her own. I hated feeling suicidal, but hey, maybe that's more me.

Although this statement was an important gateway to significant psychological work she needed to do on her core depression, it lays bare a concern so many of our patients and their parents have about the meaning of medicine as a change agent itself: Will it change me, or my, or other's, ideas of me, and not just my symptoms or behavior?

A bright 10-year-old boy had had a life-changing response to combined cognitive behavioral therapy and stimulant medication that allowed him to transfer to a better school, make new friends, and return to his beloved music classes. Still, his father, who had suffered similarly, but gone untreated as a child, was concerned that all we had done was a "naughty-ectomy, not real therapy." His son, somehow aware of his father's concerns, would occasionally taunt him: "Just call me Speedo [aware he was on a stimulant]—*I am what I take!*"

These clinical insights provide evidence of both the child and the parental concern that medication will somehow modify the child's ability to be *themselves*, as though to be otherwise were ever possible. Still, this issue needs to be addressed as part of the alliance because of the implied concern over who is in control here—the patient, the parent, the therapist, or the medicine? (Rappaport, 2000)

Locus of control, a familiar paradigm in psychology, has been usefully adopted by O'Brien and Permutter (1997) and Sprenger and Josephson (1998) to describe that particular point, or locus, in the mind of the child and the family, from which emanates the power to alleviate symptoms. External and internal forces combine to shape the final location, but the clinician is wise to remember that this is a dynamic, organic concept that evolves over the growth of the alliance.

An adopted 15-year-old boy with bipolar illness took to calling the first author "Seymour" after seeing the musical comedy *Little Shop of Horrors*. In the drama, the mutating plant becomes increasingly menacing as 'he' demands his rations from Seymour, his owner/handler. Thinly veiled by the humor and wit was a deep resentment that his medication restrained his beloved manic ebullience and "blasts of creativity." He threatened to stop his medicine on numerous occasions, announcing "I love my symptoms, doc, they make me *myself*!"

In years of therapeutic work, we have seen medications and their presumed representations shape-shift endlessly in patients' imaginations as they search for the meaning of taking pills. Medications have been depicted in both patients' and parents' dreams and daydreams as poisons, magic potions, "mind restraints" aphrodisiacs, hand cuffs, binoculars, brain "implants," and contraceptives, to mention but a few. There is no shortage of grist here for the metaphor mill, and each one is important to pursue and understand as fully as possible for investigating the psychological meaning of the medication itself in the particular therapeutic alliance at work.

As if the act of prescribing weren't complicated enough, when prescribing responsibilities are passed from one clinical setting to another, as they so often are in large clinics and teaching centers, the meaning for subsequent alliances can be increasingly complex. The "old scrip," as it was dubbed by one such 15-year-old with depressive illness, was both a souvenir of the previous idealized therapist and a troubling artifact that frustrated the new alliance (with the parents as well). Only after the proper termination and grief work were done could the old therapy be integrated into the new with less guilt and resentment.

The timing of the prescription in ongoing psychotherapeutic work is itself fraught with meaning—why now, and not before or later? Bers (2001) has detailed a single case study to highlight the importance of integrating timing considerations in terms of symptom appearance and whether they should be relieved before they are understood. Premature introduction may undermine the patient's sense that they can cope with these symptoms, without the help of chemicals. "Don't you think I can do this on my own?" asked a 13-year-old girl after we began to discuss an anxiolytic to help her manage her recurring panic attacks away from home. We examined her fantasy that the first author was giving up on her, and her ability to understand herself and her behavior by merely suggesting medication. To further make the point, she acted out sufficiently to scare her parents. Subsequently, she reengaged in psychotherapy and observed that the more aware she was of her anger, the less medication she required.

Beyond connections between timing and meaning, however, the clinician's act of prescribing is perpetually hounded by this nagging question: will the medication mean *treat* or *treatment* to my patient? Gratification and frustration are balanced and rebalanced in successful psychopharmacotherapy, but awareness of this particular paradox helps both therapist and patient avoid disorientation and therapeutic diversions (Boris, 1994).

Special Concerns in Child and Adolescent Populations

Unlike the clinician working with adults, the child's clinician needs to remain alert to changes in the meaning of the drugs to the patient as the patient moves into new developmental terrain. The radical changes in bodily preoccupation, impulsive discharge, and mood lability that occur with pubescence cast any agent that in the past may have affected weight (gain or loss), endocrine function (galactorrhea), skin appearance (acne), genital arousal or dysfunction, or mood itself into an entirely different light. What might have been acceptable effects before are now intolerable because they emerge during or simply exacerbate already exquisitely sensitive developmental tasks. This is made even more complex by the fact that nearly all side effects, from extrapyramidal side effects (EPS) to nausea, are generally less well tolerated in child populations to begin with.

Of surprising salience in the child and adolescent population are the physical properties and dosing requirements of the medications themselves, hence their augmented significance to their parents (see Table 33.1). For so many of our patients, especially the younger ones, function follows form. The prevalence of normative magical thinking makes the color, shape, printing, and form (liquid versus solid) part of the child's attitude toward the medication. For a 7-year-old boy who had trouble swallowing his badly needed neuroleptic, liquids (or "sauces" as he called them) were "for babies." He whined, pouted and regressed routinely (if calmly and comfortably) "like a baby," immediately after taking his daily doses. Another patient was happy to swallow her clonazepam, but no other solid tablet, because her first initial "K" was "cut into it for [me]." Per the report of a 6-year-old boy, the pink color of guanfacine "always tricked him to think it's peppermint candy." This cocktail of wish and suspicion, sweetened with the candy association, was sufficiently positive to help him take his medication regularly. The candy connection, however, deeply worried his mother, a former drug addict.

Methylphenidate has generated the most imagery because of its widespread use. An 8-year-old boy devised a morning ritual involving an empty prescription bottle

TABLE 33.1 *Children's Thinking About Medication*

Physical properties of the medicine itself

Form: liquid, tablet, capsule, or injectable forms may each carry different meanings—e.g., liquid is "for babies" injections are "punishments"

Size: the bigger the pill (or its milligram value), the bigger the problem (or the converse)

Labeling and printing personalized associations are made with imprinted numbers and/or letters

Color: associations with candy, poison

Timing of the doseage

Frequency: the more frequent, the more trouble, or conversely, the more they help

AM or PM: AM is for school, PM is for sleeping and/or dreaming troubles

During school: concern about stigma

Self- or parent-administered: self-administration is good, mature, whereas the parent as medicator is the doctor's agent

---

that he kept in his shoe. This reminded him when dressing to remind his mother, who "forgets half the time," to give him his morning dose. Investigation of remembering rituals helps in our understanding of deeper attitudes and ambivalence about specific drugs and their roles. But why did he choose his shoes? He thought of the answer to this: once when he heard his father describe to his grandmother how the medicine helped him "keep his feet on the ground," he thought, "just like shoes!" How did he feel about taking the medicine? He liked, as he put it, "the little mines I swallow. They have codes stamped on them for each little monster inside me that they're going to blow up today. Then I'm not such a menace!"

What he did not like, however, was the way he got his midday dose at school: "The nurse puts all our pills on her metal cart in these little cups with our names on them, and then she wheels it down the hall to our room door. Six boys and two girls go to the door and wait in line and she watches us swallow the pills—right there!—with the whole class watching! It's stupid—I feel so weird." Although we recognize this (apparently overwhelmed) nurse is not the norm, thanks to the higher level of most school nursing, his example reminds us to attend to this detail, too. Medication shouldn't and needn't mean humiliation.

The potential meanings of dosing frequency are also not wasted on children. If they find their medication helpful and given in the context of a supportive alliance, more frequent dosing can actually be reassuring.

In less positive circumstances, when the effects are more ambiguous or ambivalently experienced, more frequent dosing can be intrusive, resented, or read as a sign of being sicker. Closely tied to dose frequency is the meaning of dosage size. Older children and younger adolescents can become preoccupied with the mathematical size of the dose, assuming the smaller the decimal or dose number, the less sick they are. The converse is also true.

> A teenage girl and her therapist were on their third attempt to find a more helpful agent for her unique, elusive mixture of panic and depression. She was working hard in her psychotherapy, but told her therapist she was getting discouraged. Upon reading the label of her medication, she realized that she was getting *hundreds* of milligrams of the new drug and it was only helping a *little*. She concluded that she must be much sicker than she or the therapist thought.

Finally, the cost of medication as experienced by the family can have distinct meaning for the child or adolescent patient, because of their dependent status. When kids overhear, or directly encounter, their family's discussion about prescription costs, especially in the face of spotty coverage by hugely uneven insurance plans, the child can feel like a further burden to the family. To avoid this further complication of compliance, cost is best discussed privately and preemptively with the parents.

THE PSYCHOLOGICAL MEANING OF THE PROCESS OF MEDICATING

If *primum non nocere* is behavioral *maxim primum*, then *maxim secundum* is proffering care with reasonable confidence and hope. Freud (1905) concurred when he wrote, "State of mind in which expectation is colored by hope and faith is an effective [therapeutic] force with which we have to reckon" (p. 289). The power of this state of mind, when shared between therapist and patient, is legend in our field, because of its proven influence on the process of medicating a patient for symptom relief. It is precisely this confidence and hopeful mindset that we attempt to factor out, or in, through the use of placebo controls in carefully regulated drug trials. But the effects of this second maxim are far from understood, particularly in children.

The problem, and the intrigue, with placebos is that they work through their meaning. Though actually pharmacodynamic blanks, they have been shown to be 55%–60% as effective in analgesia as codeine and as-

pirin (Kirsch, 1997). We struggle to explain their mode of action. Cognitive neuroscientists suggest a mode of action more complex than the previously favored endorphin release theory. Expectancy theory suggests that what the brain believes about the immediate future is based on conditioning from past positive experience, mediated through immune–endocrine system interaction (Kinsbourne, 2000).

So, why the placebo's seedy and tattered reputation? Placebos muddy the waters of efficacy studies because their high rate of efficacy in any given drug trial can cast doubt over more chemically active agents that performed acceptably (Puig-Antich et al., 1987). They also carry with them the folklore of the persuasive, patent medicine–hawking "doc" who sold "effective" placebos *and* alcohol- and morphine-laced compounds (all for about the same price) to loyal, witness-bearing clientele.

A remarkable classic study highlighting the processes of medicating is the prospective trial by Park and Covi (1965). This was a small *n* study to be sure, and while no participants were children, its findings remain theoretically compelling. Fifteen "newly admitted [outpatient] neurotics aged 19–67, mean age 35, were seen in an hour-long interview for evaluation of anxiety." In a follow-up 15- to 30-minute interview, they were placed on a waiting list for intervention, and introduced in a standardized way to a *nonblind* placebo trial. They were told the placebo was "a sugar pill with no medicine in it all" that had helped people with similar conditions. Pink capsules in a tid dosage were prescribed for a week, followed by an interview and administration of a symptom checklist.

All but one patient completed the course. All but one of the completers experienced some to a lot of improvement. One-third wished to continue the placebo, refusing to transfer to an active agent, two felt "cured" and just under half of the completers believed it was a "real" drug. Half of the believers experienced side effects. To quote Schowalter (1997), "placebos can elicit (both) solace and side effects" (p. 682).

The authors concluded first that "patients can be willing to take placebo and can improve despite disclosure, and that belief in the pill as drug was not a requirement for improvement. . . . Improvement was not related to belief in the nature of the pills but did appear related to certainty of belief" (p. 344). Placebos apparently need not be "lies that heal" (Harrington, 1997).

Park and Covi (1965) also concluded that the treating doctors were "optimistic about the study, yet anxious about telling the patients that they would receive placebo. The [resulting] combination of enthusiasm and alertness must have had a strong positive impact on the patients (p. 343)." NB: placebo is Latin for "I shall please."

While ethical considerations would probably preclude a similar trial in children, it seems that the forces at work in the brief therapeutic alliance studied could be similarly cogent, if not more so, in psychopharmacotherapy with children and adolescents. Until we know more, it seems best to assume that realistic hope and confidence are powerful and useful elements of the process of medicating.

THE PSYCHOLOGICAL MEANING OF THE CONTEXT IN WHICH MEDICATION IS PRESCRIBED

There is, to paraphrase Winnicott, no such thing as a prescription—one is never written in a vacuum, devoid of relational and diagnostic context. For the vast majority of children and adolescent patients with whom we consult, the dominant context in which we prescribe is the parental one. After the age of our patients, it is *sine qua non* of what distinguishes our practices from those of our general psychiatry cousins. The parent must consent, facilitate payment and acquisition, usually physically dispense, monitor, renew, ensure compliance, deal with resistance, and often explain to the balky child yet again why they have to take those pills—all without giving a second thought to venting their own doubts about the drug's effectiveness or potential dangers.

We assume that the clinician simply cannot be optimally effective without a working alliance with the parents on behalf of their child. Furthermore, thoughtful appreciation of both parental attitudes is a prerequisite for successful medication usage. Mothers and fathers have overlapping but distinct concerns about their children's health and well-being (Pruett, 2000). Understanding both will enhance compliance. The clinician is wise to assume that parents are well down their own road of frustrated and spent solutions by the time they meet with the clinician. Such parents may feel relief when medication is suggested because of the affirmation of the seriousness and accuracy of their concern for their child's difficulties. They may also feel less judgmental and self-deprecatory about failures to date, seeing medication as a new lease on effective parenting. All such attitudes obviously are best understood in the context of the parent's relationship with each other, not simply with the child. Typically, one is more forgiving, the other more judgmental, one more optimistic, the other less hopeful, but the clinician is almost guaranteed to hear at least one "I told you it wasn't just in his head!"

Given the freedom with which general and primary care physicians are currently dispensing psychoactive medication, it is increasingly likely that parents will have had their own personal experience with mood- and behavior-altering medications. If positive, they may be more open to the idea of a trial in their child, and if negative, less so. The reverse is also seen, where the child's positive experience with medication motivates the parent to investigate their own needs, especially if there are symptom similarities—e.g., fathers of sons with successfully treated attentional and hyperactivity disorders are especially common in our experience.

Less supportive medication attitudes can foul, prevent, or unilaterally terminate an alliance. Unexamined feelings of loss and grief over having a child "so sick" as to warrant a diagnostic label and a trial of medication are common. Parents may also see this as the first leg of a lifelong journey of chronic illness. Heritability questions must be gingerly handled because of the potential to exacerbate, instead of relieve, guilt and shame in the related parent. Understanding parental attitudes is a prerequisite for discussing medication choices, potential side effects, and obtaining informed consent, especially for the frequent off-label usage of medications in children. But parental attitudes may wield their greatest influence in the matter of compliance.

For all its importance to therapeutic outcome, *compliance* remains a shadowy term. It is more often honored in the breech, and is so infrequently assessed in drug trials that we know little about it in relation to the context in which it is most active. As a clinical term defining the amount of agreement between medical advice given and a patient's subsequent behavior, it has acquired a defensively authoritarian connotation. Furthermore, partial compliance is more rule than exception. This is especially true in child and adolescent psychiatry because of exponential complications when child compliance issues are multiplied by parental compliance issues. We still know relatively little about what influences compliance positively or negatively, but parental anger, envy, ambivalence, jealousy, competitive feelings about the child–therapist alliance, disorganization, psychiatric illness, and resentment toward the child and the child's difficulties have all played clinical roles affecting compliance in our clinical work.

We are aware from compliance studies with antibiotics and insulin that the more serious a parent feels the child's illness is, and the better understanding they have of the illness itself, the stronger the treatment compliance. The clinical implications are clear: understand the parents' concerns first, educate second, and anticipate some noncompliance third. The appropriately established and maintained therapeutic alliance is just the place to repair and maintain compliance in its best sense.

What parents *do* understand about their child's diagnosis and needs warrants discussion in its own right, not simply in terms of the therapist's wish for compliance. As information washes over our patients from all directions, we are hearing increasingly sophisticated questions in our consulting rooms, especially about "chemical imbalance." Though informed patients are helpful in positive outcomes (Healy, 1997), this particular concept may be less than informative. It is a vernacular phrase of no specific meaning in the lay or professional domain, and masks multiple meanings. It can cover anything from a legitimate request for thoughtful diagnostic clarification to avoiding investigation of personal or emotional issues, or a boutique approach to wellness and personal enhancement (Parens, 1998). Valenstein's sobering discussion in *Blaming the Brain* (1998) of the scientific understanding of the role of "biochemical imbalance" in mental illness keeps us wary of prematurely attributing any shared meaning to this phrase.

Schools are the next meaningful context for the medicating therapist. It may be there that the child or adolescent's distress is most externalized, as it so often is in attentional and conduct disorders. School officials may share in the "delusion of precision" (Gutheil, 1977), perceiving drugs as specific, concrete, and targeted agents that are uniformly effective—if the therapist would but prescribe them. Schools feel mounting pressures to control the child's behavior or disruptiveness for reasons beyond concern for the well-being of the individual child: overcrowding, understaffing, new meritocracies such as mandatory testing, and pressure from other parents, to name a few. Parents may or may not cooperate with the school's concerns, facilitating or frustrating appropriate use of medication in an individual case. Unlike the school, they may feel that a different classroom, approach, or curriculum would be more effective than medication. The therapist must appreciate these larger system interactions when considering medication and dosages that will directly affect the child's academic and social life. The reverse is equally true—to *not* prescribe under such systemic pressures can be seen or experienced as not caring about, or being insensitive to, the degree of child or parental distress.

INFLUENCES ON THINKING ABOUT PRESCRIBING

As if the intramural context weren't sufficiently complex to preoccupy the competent clinician, extramural influences on the way the therapist thinks about medication and the act of prescribing are increasing exponentially. Especially poignant and distracting are the combined corporate influences of the pharmaceutical and managed-care industries. Enormously powerful real-world forces that shape the therapeutic alliance, they can be strange bedfellows to the clinician and the prescribing process, as their missions can be so disparate. Making a living while doing good would seem the common goal, yet the corporate structures and ethics that vaunt profitability over access flirts with incompatibility in the practitioner's realm of *primum non nocere*.

It is hard to exaggerate the influence of the pharmaceutical industry. In the United States alone, the industry spent $13.9 billion a year on promotion and advertising, just under one-fourth of their overall sales. Three-fourths of that total was spent on advertising campaigns in our journals, at our meetings, and through direct contact between physicians and their sales forces. This works out to be about $12,000/year, per practicing physician. The sales force is well trained, chosen for its tenacity, and supported by strong incentives. Pfizer's reputation for hiring ex-military personnel has earned it the nickname "Semper Pfizer" (Kirkpatrick, 2000). There are nearly 60,000 reps, or 1 for every 11 practicing physicians in the United States.

We see this influence starting early. Our residents meet their first drug reps in the first months of their training. Shortly thereafter, our young doctors are using logo-sporting pens, mugs, bags, and getting textbooks (logo bookplates inside) paid for. The better food consumed during residency is usually provided by drug reps at sponsored teaching lunches, begun with brief talks related to their products, in the conference rooms of most teaching hospitals. The parallel process begs description; drug rep caters to future doc in a setting that encourages doc to prescribe ("cater") reps' drugs to patients—now and, it is hoped, long into the future. Some academics have sufficient concern about the easy traffic between residents, drug reps, teaching hospitals, their research funding base, and the pharmaceutical industry that they suggest ongoing vigilance of the "pharmaceutical–academic complex" (Angell, 2000).

Established practitioners can be offered elegant dinners, theater tickets, get-aways, and sometimes cash incentives to prescribe new agents during their initial launch phase. Yes, it's a free country, but this turns out not to be a free lunch. Physicians are but human and they are influenced, and not just when they are young (Wolfe, 1996):

• The prescribing therapist is more likely to prescribe a drug over the next few days after its drug rep takes them to lunch or plies them with gifts (National Institute for Health Care Management, 2000; Orlowski and Wateska, 1992).

• Even though prescribers see themselves as intellectually independent of corporate influence, the language they use to describe a drug's properties to themselves and their patients is derived more from advertising than from the more objective scientific literature (Lexchin, 1997).

• Regardless of how physicians see themselves, their patients see them as being unduly influenced. Furthermore, patients express concern about their physicians' susceptibility to such pressure (Mainous et al., 1995).

The American Medical Association's Council on Ethical Affairs was sufficiently concerned 10 years ago about these matters to issue guidelines to discourage expensive gifts without medical purpose (Council on Ethical and Judicial Affairs, American Medical Association, 1991). These guidelines were a start in addressing this problem, and the council encourages even more vigilance now (Wazana, 2000).

Direct marketing to patients, primarily parents, has been so effective that it gives new meaning to the word *compliance*. The National Institute for Health Care Management cites $2 billion as the current direct-to-consumer (DTC) marketing tab, and sees it as closely tied to increases in prescription drug sales, including that of psychoactive drugs (National Institute for Health Care Management Report, 2000). Undoubtedly, some of the information in that marketing is sufficiently helpful to raise parents' level of concern about a child's behavior, prompting them to seek consultation earlier than later. But it has also led to the unique phenomenon of parental voicemail and e-mail requests for a specific agent to be prescribed over the phone for a child never seen by the clinician.

The other corporate influence is that of managed care. The limits on approval, duration, or nature of therapeutic contact, or covered services themselves have turned prescription writing into one of the only reliable and *reimbursable* acts therapists can perform on behalf of their patients and their livelihood. The 15-minute medication check that has been established as the industry standard of care reduces the therapeutic alliance to an encounter between a "prescriber," or "med-checker," and a consumer with a target symptom. Policy statements from the American Academy of Child and Adolescent Psychiatry "oppose the use of brief medication visits." They object to the failure to include the "role of psychosocial intervention, including psychotherapy, in the treatment plan" (American Academy of Child and Adolescent Psychiatry, 2000). Such pressures from the managed-care domain to do something "therapeutic and fast" may be at work in the startling rise of prescriptions of psychoactive medication to preschoolers (Zito et al., 2000) and possibly even the increasing trend toward polypharmacy, unheard of a decade ago.

THINKING ABOUT SPLIT TREATMENT PRESCRIBING

As reimbursement systems continue to evolve, the child psychiatrist as medication prescriber in the context of psychotherapy offered by a seperate (usually nonmedical) clinician is a phenomenon growing exponentially in number and complexity. Liability, clinical, boundary, transference–countertransference, and systems issues swirl about the axis connecting these inseparable aspects of treatment. The only way to enssure that split treaters don't split the treatment is through effective communication.

When a 13-year-old was referred for medication consult, her therapist's concerns were increasing inability to concentrate at school, inattention to her homework, increasing social isolation, and failure to appropriately plan longer-term academic projects. Stimulant medication seemed indicated and she asked to be evaluated and prescribed. In consultation with her, however, one was more impressed clinically with her thought rituals, obsessive anxiety-containing behavior patterns, and the need to have "everything just right" (which took hours) before she could even start her homework. The SSRIs seemed more appropriate than stimulants. When communicating with her therapist, at her request, to share inital impressions and to suggest that we discuss this further, she replied with additional information about a strong family history for ADD, and was reluctant to accept the initial recommendation, but agreed to talk further on the phone. Discussion led to resolution, and avoided a potentially ensnaring boundary complication for this young girl who was already sufficiently anxious and confused.

This case was time consuming, yes, but the expenditure of time was minuscule, compared to the potential sequellae of bad treatment. In our experience, the upfront commitment to clear treatment planning and diagnosis is a universally effective vaccine against collaboration dysfunction. Once in place, vigilance can be turned to the two issues that sustain competent split treatments: ongoing sharing of data between collaborating clinicians, and accurately maintained perceptions of the role of the treatment personnel.

The medicating clinician must (1) prescribe in the context of medications already being prescribed, e.g., share information with the primary care physician for potential drug interactions; (2) share with the psychotherapist attention to side effect profiles that evolve over treatment, and thus prevent misattributions by the psychotherapist of changes in sleep, sexual behavior, irritabilty, etc.; and (3) do a thorough biopsychosocial psychiatric evaluation, not simply a symptom search, thus laying a foundation for a fuller understanding of what a medication might mean psychologically to a patient in changing contexts over the course of treatment.

Ongoing regard for the differing roles of treaters cannot be overemphasized. Personal knowledge and past shared experience are a great boon, but not always possible. Sharing information about each other's practices, training, practice patterns and values can create mutual respect that protects against future conflict among practioners or splitting by more disordered patients. Will medication changes always be discussed before they are instituted, and if not when? For what kinds of shared data are fax or e-mail communications adequate? Are quantities and refills issues for a particular child and family, given their level of vigilance, compliance, and potential for misuse? These issues argue for changing the name of this phenomenon from *split* treatment to *shared* treatment.

CONCLUSIONS AND RECOMMENDATIONS

When thinking about medicating, it is the patient, not the drug, that should get our major attention. Such thinking needs to be done in the context of a therapeutic alliance, not the likelihood of reimbursement. Hence we recommend the following:

• Never prescribe for a patient whom you can't remember between medchecks. You are forgetting them because neither of you is sufficiently invested in a relationship worth remembering. This is an infrastructure of insufficient substance to support pharmacotherapy, or *any* therapy, for that matter.

• Be perpetually aware of the seductions of marketing. They *are* getting to you, and affecting your judgment about drug choice.

• Psychodynamic formulations are not a gilding of the drug treatment lily. They are necessary for making good treatment choices, evaluation, and ongoing reevaluation of drug choice and combined treatment effectiveness.

• Create and sustain all the relationships necessary to address the child's needs—with parents, teachers, principals, collaborative therapists, etc.

• Don't be intimidated by time pressures, especially in the early appointments. If you've done your diagnostic work and built your alliance accordingly, the relationship will matter more than the time spent sustaining it (Tasman et al., 2000).

• "Chemical imbalance" discussions are generally less helpful than you think, as it is so difficult to predict what this means to any given patient or their parents.

• Neither over- nor undersell any one drug as part of the treatment regimen. They each carry plenty of "magic" on their own. Tell parents and patients that there are other choices; invite them to be collaborators in psychoeducation, not just "pill poppers."

• Treat your patients as though the therapeutic relationship matters more than the pills. It usually does. How often have we looked back over cases and the improvements we could or might have attributed to meds, *if* we had chosen to prescribe them?

• How you are with your patients in your office is a model for how you would like them to be conducting their interpersonal relationships outside the office.

REFERENCES

American Academy of Child and Adolescent Psychiatry (2000) Prescribing psychoactive medications for children and adolescents. *Am Acad Child Adolesc Psychiatry News* 31(5):207.

Angell, M. (2000) Is academic medicine for sale? Editorial. *N Engl J Med* 34:20.

Bers, S. (2001) Will I Still Be Me? The Meanings of Psychotropic Medication to Western New England Psychoanalytic Society. New Haven, Jan. 27

Blackwell, B. (1973) Drug therapy: patient compliance. *N Engl J Med* 289:249–252.

Blakeslee, S. Placebos prove so powerful even experts are surprised. *The New York Times*, Science Times Supplement, October 13, 1998:4.

Boris, H. (1994) *Sleights of Mind: One and Multiples of One*. Northvale, NJ: Jason Aronson, Inc.

Brent, D.A. and Kolko, D.J. (1998) Psychotherapy: definitions, mechanisms of action, and relatioship to etiological models. *J. Abnorm Child Psycholo* 26:17–25.

Council on Ethical and Judicial Affairs, American Medical Association (1991) Gifts to physicians from indusrty. *JAMA* 261:501.

Crits-Christoph, P., Barber, J.P., and Kurcias, J.S. (1993) The accuracy of the therapist's interpretations and the development of the therapeutic alliance. *Psychother Res* 3:25–35.

Edelson, M. (1984) Hypothesis and evidence in psychoanalysis. Chicago, University of Chicago Press.

Freud, S. (1905) Psychical (or mental) treatment. In: *Standard Edition*, Vol. 7. London: Hogarth Press, 1953, pp. 283–302.

Gabbard, G.O., and Kay, J. (2001) The fate of integrated treatment: whatever happened to the biopsychosocial psychiatrist? *Am J Psychiatry* 158:1956–1963.

Gutheil, T.G. (1977) Improving patient compliance: psychodynamics in drug prescribing. *Drug Ther* 7:82–83, 87, 89–91, 95.

Gutheil, T.G. (1982) The psychology of psychopharmacology. *Bull Menninger Clin* 46:321–330.

Harrington, A. (1997) *The New York Times*, Science Times Supplement, October 13, 1998: 4.

Healy, D. (1997) *The Antidepressant Era*. Cambridge, MA: Harvard University Press.

Kinsbourne, M. Mind and Nature: essays on timer subjectivity. *J Nervous Mental Dise* 189:140–147.

Kirkpatrick, D.D. (2000) Inside the happiness business. *New York*, May 15, 2000, pp. 37–43.

Kirsch, I. (1997) Specifying nonspecifics: psychological mechanisms of placebo effects. In: Harrington, A., Ed., *The Placebo Effect: An Interdisciplinary Exploration* Cambridge, MA. Harvard University Press pp. 166–186.

Lexchin, J. (1997) What information do physicians receive from pharmaceutical respresentatives? *Can Fam Physician* 43:941–945.

Luborsky, L. McLellan, A.T., Woody, G.E., O'Brien, C.P. and Auerbach, A. (1985) Therapist success and its determinates. *Arch Gen Psychiatry* 42:602–611.

Magnavita, J.J. (1993) The evolution of short term dynamic psychotherapy: treatment of the future? *Prof Psychol Res and Pract* 24: 360–365.

Mainous, A.G, III, Houeston, W.J., and Rich, E.C. (1995) Patient perceptions of physician acceptance of gifts from the pharmaceutical industry. *Arch Fam Med* 4:335–339.

National Institute for Health Care Management Foundation (2000) Prescription drugs and mass media advertising. *New York Times*, September 20, 2000.

O'Brien, J. and Perlmutter I. (1997) The effect of medication on the process of psychotherapy. *Child Adolesc Psychiatr Clin North Am* 6:185–96.

Orlowski, J.P. and Wateska, L. (1992) The effects of pharmaceutical firm enticements on physician prescribing patterns. *Chest* 102: 270–273.

Parens, E. (1998) Is better always good? The enhancement project. *Hastings Cent Rep* 28:24B–S15.

Park, L.C. and Covi, L. (1965) Nonblind placebo trial: an exploration of neurotic patients' responses to placebo when its inert content is disclosed. *Arch Gen Psychiatry* 12:336–344.

Pruett, K.D. (2000) *Fatherneed: Why Father Care Is as Essential as Mother Care to Your Child*. New York: The Free Press

Puig-Antich, J., Perel, J.M., Lupatkin, W., Davies, M., and Goetz, D. (1987) Imipramine in prepubertal major depressive disorders. *Arch Gen Psychiatry* 44:81–89.

Rappaport, N. and Chubinsky, P. (2000) The meaning of psychotropic medications for children, adolescents, and their families. *J Am Acad Child Adolesc Psychiatry* 39:1198–1200.

Resier, M.F. (1985) Converging sectors of psychoanalysis and neurobiology: mutual challenge and opportunity. *J Am Psychoanal Assoc* 33:11:34.

Schowalter, J.E. (1989) Psychodynamics and medication. *J Am Acad Child Adolesc Psychiatry* 28:681–684.

Schowalter, J.E. (1997) Psychopharmacology: the mind–brain frontier, Paper presented at Annual Meeting of the American Academy of Child and Adolescent Psychiatry. Toronto, October 15.

Sprenger, D. and Josephson, A. (1998) Integration of parmacotherapy and family therapy in the treatment of children and adolescent. *J Am Acad Child Adolesc Psychiatry* 37:887–889.

Tasman, A., Riba, M., and Silk, K. (2000) *The doctor–patient relationship in pharmacotherapy*. New York: Guilford Press.

Valenstein, E. The Truth About Drugs and Mental Health. (1998) *Blaming the Brain*. New York: The Free Press.

Wazana, A. (2000) Physicians and the pharmaceutical industry: is a gift ever just a gift? *JAMA* 283(3).

Wolfe, S.M. (1996) Why do American drug companies spend more than $12 billion a year pushing drugs? *J Gen Intern Med* 11: 637–639.

Zisook, S., Hammond, R., Jaffe, K., et al. (1978–79) Outpatient requests, initial sessions and attrition. *Int J Psychiatry Med* 9:339–350.

Zito, J.M., Safer D.J., dosReis, S., et al (2000) Trends in prescribing of Psychotropic medications to preschoolers. *JAMA* 283:1025–30.

34 Combining pharmacotherapy and psychotherapy: an evidence-based approach

JOHN S. MARCH AND KAREN WELLS

The marriage of molecular neuroscience and cognitive psychology is driving a revolution in how we understand the diagnosis and treatment of mental illness (Kandel and Squire, 2000). It is increasingly clear that psychotropic medications work by biasing specific central nervous information processes; it is less commonly acknowledged but no less true that psychosocial treatments also have both a somatic substrate and psychosocial valence. Put simply, drugs and psychotherapy work because they act on the brain (Hyman, 2000). Hence, when selecting a treatment strategy appropriate to the needs of a specific patient, the pediatric psychopharmacologist must consider not only medication but also psychosocial treatment strategies either alone or in combination with medication.

In a perfectly evidence-based world, selecting an appropriate treatment from among the many possible options would be reasonably straightforward. In the complex world of clinical practice, choices are rarely so clear-cut. Even when a comprehensive assessment produces an unambiguous diagnosis and readily defined target symptoms, expected outcomes vary by disorder, by treatment modality, and, certainly, by factors specific to the patient, the doctor, and the setting(s) in which they live and work. Depending on theoretical underpinning and nature of the treatment, psychotherapeutic options are generally more narrowly defined than drug treatments, which often have a broader spectrum of action. Implementing two distinct treatments can be complicated when they differ in dose and the time it takes to reach a desired outcome. Doctors and patients and their families sometimes differ (and rightly so) in their preferences regarding choices among appropriate treatments. These, and other factors outlined below, complicate the choice of treatment strategy for many if not most patients.

Matching treatment(s) to clinical problems has also become more complicated (albeit also more effective) as child and adolescent psychiatry has moved away from nonspecific interventions toward problem-focused treatments keyed to specific *Diagnostic and Statistical Manual of Mental Disorders, 4th ed.* (DSM-IV) diagnoses (Kazdin, 1997). In particular, the past 40 years have seen the emergence of diverse, sophisticated, empirically supported, pharmacological (this volume) and behavioral and cognitive-behavioral therapies that cover the range of childhood-onset mental disorders (Hibbs and Jensen, 1996; Kendall, 1999). Many clinicians and researchers now believe that the combination of disorder-specific medication and cognitive behavior therapy (CBT) administered within an evidence-based, disease management model is the initial treatment of choice for many if not all children and adolescents with a major mental illness (see, for example, March et al., 1997).

In this context, it is often said that 50% of what we know about treating mentally ill children will be out of date and the other 50% will be wrong within 5 to 10 years. Sometimes it is hard to tell the two scenarios apart, but the take-home message is clear: while keeping up with a rapidly expanding evidence base is extraordinarily difficult (Sackett et al., 2000), keep up we must, since new developments point toward the improved outcomes that we and our patients desire (Barlow et al., 1999). Nowhere is this truer than when divergent treatment options—be they medication or psychosocial—are on the menu.

An empirical literature on combined treatment is just beginning to emerge. Randomized controlled trials in adults with panic disorder (Barlow et al., 2000) and major depression (Keller et al., 2000) suggest advantages for combined drug and cognitive-behavioral treatment over the respective monotherapies. Illustrating the fact that we cannot simply take for granted the assumption that two treatments are better than one, combination treatment does not appear to offer a significant advantage over CBT alone, at least in adults with obsessive-compulsive disorder (OCD) (Ed. Foa, personal communication). With the notable exception of the Multimodal Treatment Study of Children with ADHD (MTA; Arnold et al., 1997a), there are no studies in mentally ill youth that have compared single modality treatments to each other or their combination against a control condition in the same patient population though such studies are currently underway in OCD and teenage major depression.

Within a stages-of-treatment model that emphasizes the practice of evidence-based medicine (EBM), this chapter provides a conceptual framework for how best to approach combining drug and psychosocial treatments at the level of the individual patient. The reader interested in exploring EBM should begin with the text by Sackett and colleagues (1997) before moving on to the excellent "User's Guides" series in the *Journal of the American Medical Association* (JAMA) (Guyatt and Rennie, 1993). The reader interested in how best to combine specific treatments for particular disorders would be well advised to consult the American Academy of Child and Adolescent Psychiatry (AACAP) practice parameters series (Dunne, 1997), textbooks that address the relative benefits of psychosocial and medication management (Van Hasselt and Hersen, 1993; Pollack et al., 1996; Hersen and Bellack, 1999), and the few available empirically derived practice guidelines that include children and adolescents (March et al., 1997; Pliszka et al., 2000a, b; Conners et al., 2001).

COMBINING TREATMENTS IN A MEDICAL FRAMEWORK

Disease Management Model

While it will be some time before stakeholder issues yield to a unifying body of widely accepted, scientific evidence concerning the etiopathogensis and treatment of mental illness, it was clear by the late 1970s that a biopsychosocially oriented disease management model is as powerful a change strategy in psychiatry as it is in other areas of medicine (Ludwig and Othmer, 1977). More specifically, the three features of disease management model—the concept of disease and diagnosis, the concept of etiology and treatment, and the nature of the doctor–patient relationship—come into play in pe-

diatric psychiatry just as they do in the rest of medicine. Outside of psychiatry, combined treatment is the rule rather than the exception—for example, hypertension is treated with antihypertensives and weight reduction, or juvenile rheumatoid arthritis, with non-steroidal anti-inflammatory drugs (NSAIDs) and physical therapy. To take an even more specific example, the treatment of pediatric OCD can be thought of as partially analogous to the treatment of juvenile-onset diabetes, with the caveat that the target organ, the brain in the case of major mental illness, requires psychosocial interventions of much greater complexity. The treatment of diabetes and that of OCD both involve medications—insulin in diabetes and in OCD, a serotonin reuptake inhibitor. Each also involves an evidence-based psychosocial intervention that works in part by biasing the somatic substrate of the disorder toward more normal function. In diabetes, the psychosocial treatment of choice is diet and exercise, and in OCD, CBT. Depending on the presence of risk and protective factors, not every patient has the same outcome. Bright youngsters from well-adjusted two-parent families typically do better with either diabetes or OCD than those beset with tremendous psychosocial adversity. Thus, adversity when present appropriately becomes a target for intervention, usually to increase compliance with treatment for the primary illness. Finally, not everybody recovers completely even with the best of available treatment, so some interventions need to target coping with residual symptoms, such as diabetic foot care in diabetes and helping patients and their families cope skillfully with residual symptoms in OCD.

Why Combine Psychosocial and Drug Treatments?

Psychosocial treatments usually are combined with medication for one of three reasons. First, in the initial treatment of the severely ill child, two treatments provide a greater "dose" and thus, may promise a better and perhaps speedier outcome. For this reason, many patients with OCD opt for combined treatment even though CBT alone may offer equal benefit (March and Leonard, 1998). Second, comorbidity frequently but not always requires two treatments, since different targets may require different treatments. For example, treating a teen who has attention-deficit hyperactivity disorder (ADHD) and major depression with a psychostimulant and CBT is a reasonable treatment strategy (Birmaher et al., 1998). Even within a single disorder, such as ADHD, important functional outcomes may vary in response to treatment. For example, hyperactivity may be more responsive to a psychostimulant and parent–child arguing, to parent training. Third, in the face of partial response, an augmenting treatment can be added to the intitial treatment to improve the outcome in the symptom domain targeted by the initial treatment. For example, CBT can be added to a selective serotonin reuptake inhibitor (SSRI) for OCD to improve OCD-specific outcomes. In an adjunctive treatment strategy, a second treatment can be added to a first one to positively impact one or more additional outcome domains. For example, a SSRI can be added to CBT for OCD to handle comorbid depression or panic disorder.

Cognitive-Behavior Therapy in a Medical Context

Most mental health clinicians are familiar with treatments that assume that psychological distress represents the outcome of historical and current relationship problems that must be uncovered and addressed in therapy. In contrast to these more story oriented approaches to psychotherapy, CBT asks clinicians to adopt a problem-solving model in which they act as a coach to teach the patient a set of adaptive coping skills (while at the same time unlearning unskillful coping behaviors) for specific symptoms associated with distress and impairment in the present tense (March, 2000). Thus CBT, unlike most other psychotherapeutic approaches, fits beautifully into a disease management framework in which the symptoms of the illness and associated functional impairments are specifically targeted for treatment. The cornerstone of CBT is a careful functional analysis of problem behaviors that is governed by several important assumptions. First, behavior (including normal as well as problem behavior) is primarily governed by environmental contingencies (and in cognitive theory, by thoughts and emotions), such that the relationship between thoughts, feelings, and behaviors is the primary focus of assessment and treatment. Second, the antecedents and consequences of target behaviors as well as target behaviors themselves must be operationally defined and accurately measured. Third, behavior may differ across settings, so that multi-informant, multimodal, multi-domain assessment is critical. Fourth, treatment planning depends on careful assessment, including periodic reassessment of how behaviors have changed, with revision of treatment interventions as necessary. While these assumptions and procedures are not necessarily incompatible with pharmacological management, the level of specificity for functional outcomes is generally greater for CBT than for medication management. The level of monitoring for change, by contrast, should be roughly equal for both pharmacological and psychosocial interventions, as it is symptomatic change and improvement in functional outcomes that govern pa-

tient and clinician assessment of degree of improvement. Put experimentally, CBT lends itself to viewing the treatment of each patient through the lens of one of several possible single case designs, which in turn makes combining pharmacological and cognitive-behavioral interventions relatively straightforward.

Being Consciously Multidisciplinary

Although cognitive-behavioral and pharmacological treatment strategies can be readily combined, psychology and psychiatry are often at odds over stakeholder issues. The authors of this chapter believe strongly that it is not possible to practice competent and ethical psychopharmacology without the availability of empirically supported psychotherapy; similarly, it is not possible to practice competent and ethical psychotherapy without the availability of empirically supported psychopharmacology. Physicians (who typically write prescriptions) and psychologists (who, for the most part, have developed and typically are better versed in CBT) must join hands in the care of individual patients if for no other reason than to acknowledge the complexity of modern mental health care, which is beyond the capacity of any one individual to master (March et al., 1995). In this regard, the current generation of comparative treatment trials (see, for example, Jensen, 1999), nicely models both the benefits and the difficulties of multidisciplinary practice in which practitioners of both disciplines become stakeholders for the experiment (the research question) or the benefit of the individual patient (the clinical question). Without this commitment to multidisciplinary practice, we shortchange our patients.

USING EVIDENCE-BASED MEDICINE AS A FRAMEWORK FOR CONSIDERING WHETHER AND HOW TO COMBINE TREATMENTS

What is Evidence-Based Medicine?

One of the more common criticisms of an evidence-based approach to clinical practice is that clinical trials and clinical practice are only weakly related. In research language, the external validity of many efficacy studies is suspect. *External validity,* which refers to the extent to which the results of the research are generalizable to clinical populations, is often contrasted to *internal validity,* i.e., the extent to which a study is methodologically sound. Without internal validity, it is hard to argue for the external validity of a study. Many internally valid studies are not fully relevant to clinical practice because the treatments used or the nature of the patients enrolled and dissimilar to clinical practice and, thus, the results do not transfer easily to clinical practice settings. This is why the National Institute of Mental Health (NIMH) recently moved away from funding efficacy trials conducted in "relatively pure" patients toward effectiveness trials, such as the MTA, conducted in "messy" clinical samples (Norquist and Magruder, 1998). From the point of view of an individual practitioner hoping to conform to best-practice standards, it is critical therefore to decide whether and how the results of a particular study are clinically relevant. Evidence-based medicine provides a simple, straightforward framework for accomplishing this task. Not an invocation to slavish adherence to an ill-defined gold standard, EBM is simply a set of tools that allow the conscientious, explicit, and judicious use of current best evidence in making decisions about the care of the individual patient through integrating individual clinical expertise with the best available external clinical evidence from systematic research (Guyatt et al. 1993, 1994; 1999).

Steps in Evaluating the Usefulness of a Treatment Study

Whether approaching diagnosis, prognosis, or treatment, EBM always begins with selecting a specific question from among the panoply of clinically relevant questions presented by the care of a specific patient.

As summarized in Table 34.1, the first step is in eval-

TABLE 34.1 *What is a PECO?*

Term	Definition	Example
Population	What is the target population to whom the treatment is intended to generalize?	In children with ADHD, . . .
Exposure	What is the active treatment or treatments?	is bupropion . . .
Control / Comparison	What is the control (inactive) or comparison (active) condition?	better than pill PBO (a control) or treatment as usual (an active comparator) . . .
Outcome	The desired outcome (benefit) or undesired outcome (harm)	in reducing symptoms of ADHD?

uating a treatment question is to frame the question as a P-E-C-O: What is the *population*, the *exposure* to active treatment, the *control or comparison* condition and the desired *outcome*? A simple PECO might be: in children with ADHD, what is the evidence that bupropion is better than placebo in reducing symptoms of hyperactivity and impulsivity? Having framed the question as a PECO, the clinician then turns to the increasingly EBM-optimized resources available on the Internet, such as the clinical queries algorithm on PubMed. In this regard, EBM provides a clear hierarchy of search strategies that move from EBM reviews, which means that your work is already done as all the relevant literature is already summarized, to critically appraised topics (CATs), which summarize one or two relevant articles, to searching and critiquing the literature yourself. Full-text articles for many journals can be retrieved from OVID, which is available either as a subscription service or free from most academic libraries. See Sacket et al. (2000) for a more detailed discussion of search strategies and CATs.

Having identified an article that is directly relevant to the question of interest, the next step is to evaluate the article for its validity and applicability to the patient. Table 34.2 summarizes the EBM approach to reviewing an article about treatment. Four relatively easy and commonsensical steps presuppose a reasonably close reading of (1) the abstract to get an overall summary, (2) the Methods section to assess validity to identify the population studied, and (3) the Results section to understand the direction and clinical importance of the outcome. Unlike in the usual approach, the Introduction and Discussion can often be skipped, as reading them is an inefficient use of time. The four steps are as follows:

1. *Is the study valid?* Did the investigators use a randomized, controlled, blinded design in which all the patients were followed up at the end? Apart from intrinsic differences in the treatments themselves, were all the patients treated the same way? Without affirming these relatively straightforward parameters, it is impossible to know whether differences in the outcome reflect true differences in the impact of the treatments or some other characteristic of the study.

2. *What were the results?* Ideally the results should be presented both dimensionally, using normed rating scales so that the reader can judge improvement toward or into the normal range, and categorically, to allow easy calculation of magnitude of clinical improvement. If the results are presented as a change score (the mean at post-treatment minus the mean at pretreatment for each treatment group), the actual means scores for each treatment group at baseline

TABLE 34.2 *Evidence-Based Medicine Applied to Treatment*

Steps in Evaluating a Treatment Article	Main Points	Hints
Is there a clear question?	Frame the question as a PECO?	For any patient, there will be many possible questions. Hence, the astute clinician must weigh the possible questions and, having done so, chose one or two. Then, having framed the question as a PECO, the clinician must search the literature for *(1)* a systematic review; *(2)* a metanalysis; *(3)* a relevant article; or *(4)* a treatment guideline that includes the question being asked, using EBM principles to evaluate the chosen article.
Are the results of the study valid?	Randomized controlled design? Investigators blind to treatment assignment? All patients treated the same way? All patients followed up?	After reading the abstract to get the big picture, quickly review the Methods section to see if the research design meets minimal standards for interpretability.
What are the results?	Dimensional and categorical outcomes? Movement into the normal range? Comorbidity? Subgroup analyses? Is the treatment safe?	To quickly calculate an NNT, look first for categorical results for the main outcome measure in the study, then for dimensional outcomes, and finally for other outcomes besides the main ones. If the results are presented as change scores, look for the baseline mean score to see how far the patient moved toward the normal range. Use this information to establish the NNT.
How strong was the effect?	Calculate an NNT. Adjust the NNT for factors that might improve or decrease the expected response. The equivalent statistic for harm in the NNH.	While the NNT can be calculated without a calculator, confidence intervals and many other EBM statistics, while conceptually simple, are more easily done using a calculator. A widely used calculator with an EBM add-in is Syncalc (www.syncalc.com). Depending on the nature of and methods for detecting adverse event, the ratio of the NNH and NNT can be thought of as the risk/benefit ratio.
Are the results applicable to my patient?	Is my patient represented? Were the clinically important outcomes considered? How long did the treatment last? Are the treatments worth the potential benefits, harms, and costs? Can we provide the treatment? Will the patient accept the treatment?	In the Methods section, quickly scan the inclusion and exclusion criteria to see if your patient falls within the type of patient entered into the study. If necessary, adjust the NNT so that the expectations for benefit match the divergence of your patient from the average patient in the study population. Factor in your preferences and expectations and preferences of your patient and family.

EBM, evidence-based medicine; NNH, number needed to harm; NNT, number needed to treat.

should also be included so that the clinician can judge whether the amount of change moved the average patient into the normal range. If comorbidity is a factor, initial levels of comorbid symptomatology and changes in comorbidity over time should also be presented. Finally, the same questions that are asked about treat-

ment effectiveness can be asked about harm to answer the critical question: Is it safe? (Levine et al., 1994).

3. *Are the results clinically meaningful?* This is an important variable for clinicians desiring to ascertain whether the results of a clinical trial can be applied at the patient level. Traditionally in psychiatry and psy-

TABLE 34.3 *Response to Selective Serotonin Reuptake Inhibitors in Pediatric Obssessive-Compulsive Disorder*

Response to SSRI in OCD		Relative Risk Reduction (RRR)	Absolute Risk Reduction (ARR)	Number Needed to Treat (NNT)
Usual Control Event Rate (CER)	SSRI Experimental Event Rate (EER)	$\dfrac{EER - CER}{EER}$	EER − CER	1/ARR
25%	45%	$\dfrac{45\% - 25\%}{25\%} = 44\%$	45% − 25% = 20%	1/0.2 = 5 patients

Using data from March (1998a), responders were defined as having a Yale-Brown Obsessive-Compulsive Scale (YBOCS) decrease >25% from baseline to end of treatment. The 95% confidence interval (CI) on an NNT = 1/(limits on the CI of its ARR) = (3 to 14), calculated as:

$$\pm 1.96 \sqrt{\frac{CER \times (1 - CER)}{\text{\# of control pts.}} + \frac{CER \times (1 - CER)}{\text{\# of exper. pts.}}} =$$

chology (Weisz, 2000), the magnitude of the effect has been portrayed in terms of small (0.3), medium (0.5) or large (> 0.8) effect sizes in standard deviation units (Cohen, 1977). Evidence-based medicine uses a much simpler rubric, the number needed to treat, or NNT. In practice, the NNT represents the number of patients who need to be treated to produce one additional good outcome beyond that obtainable with the control or comparison condition. For example, an NNT of 10 means that you would have to treat 10 patients with the active treatment to find one that wouldn't have done just as well if assigned to the control treatment.[1] A very small NNT (that is, one that approaches 1) means that a favorable outcome occurs in nearly every patient who receives the treatment and in few patients in the comparison group. An NNT of 2 or 3 indicates that a treatment is quite effective. In contrast, NNTs above 30 or 40 fall in the realm of public health effects although they may still be considered clinically effective. Tables 34.3 and 34.4 present NNT calculations for *responders* (defined as a 25% reduction in Yale-Brown Obsessive-Compulsive Scale [Y-BOCS] score) and *excellent responders* (defined as normalization = a Y-BOCS score of <10) in children and adolescents treated with sertraline (March et al., 1998). The NNTs of 5 and 10, respectively, confirm the implications in the change in mean score in the sertraline group—namely, that an average 6-point Y-BOCS drop (a pre- to post-treatment drop from 24 to 18), which parenthetically is consistent across pediatric and adult OCD SSRI trials (Greist et al., 1995; Leonard et al., 1997), leaves most patients in the clinically ill range.

4. *Is the result applicable to my patient?* Before applying the results of this study to the care of an individual patient, it is important to understand the similarities between the research study and the particular clinical situation faced in the office. This can be accomplished quickly by asking the following questions. Is my patient represented in the research sample or were patients like mine excluded from the trial? Were the clinically important outcomes, both functional (e.g., return to school) and disorder-specific (e.g., less depression) considered? How were the outcomes measured, are they clinically meaningful, and can I apply these measures in my practice? To the extent my patient offers a better or worse prognosis that the average patient in the study, would an adjusted NNT[2] bias my choice of treatments, for example, toward combined drug and psychosocial treatment in a very ill multiply comorbid patient? Are the treatments worth the potential benefits, harms and costs? Can I and/or a colleague work

[1]Starting with a dimensional response metric, ES is the a measure of the average response in standard deviation units calculated as MC − ME/SD$_{pooled}$, where ME represents the mean of the experimental treatment, MC represents the mean of the control treatment, and SD$_{pooled}$ represents pooling of the standard deviations from within both groups at the end of treatment. Starting with a categorical response metric, NNT is a measure of the average response presented as the probability of response in single patient units. Arithmetically, the NNT is the inverse of the absolute risk reduction (1/ARR), defined as the percent response in the experimental group − the percent response in the control condition. When benefit (a positive response) rather than risk (e.g., mortality) is the outcome, the ARR is often rephrased as the absolute benefit increase (ABI). For example, if 80% of patients respond to treatment X and 30% to a PBO control condition the ABI is 50% and the NNT is 2, a very robust response. As shown in Tables 34.3 and 34.4, confidence intervals (CI) can be calculated around the NNT to estimate the precision of the treatment effect. Confidence intervals are a useful measure of the certainty that you, the clinician, can provide when informing your patient about the expected outcome of treatment. The wider the CI, the less confident you can be about predicting correctly.

[2]Modifications to the NNT can be introduced depending on the extent to which the individual patient resembles the patients assembled in the treatment study. Specifically, the NNT can be adjusted for a specific patient by estimating the patient's likelihood of change relative to the average control patient in the trial report, expressing the likelihood as a decimal fraction, *F*, and then dividing the reported NNT by *F*. For example, if your patient is judged to have half the probability of a positive response as the average control patient, then *F* = 0.5 and the NNT/*F* = twice the unadjusted NNT.

TABLE 34.4 *Excellent Response to a Selective Serotonin Reuptake Inhibitors in Pediatric Obsessive-Compulsive Disorder*

Response to SSRI in OCD		Relative Risk Reduction RRR	Absolute Risk Reduction (ARR)	Number Needed to Treat (NNT)
Usual Control Event Rate (CER)	*SSRI Experimental Event Rate (EER)*	$\dfrac{EER - CER}{EER}$	$EER - CER$	$1/ARR$
5%	15%	$\dfrac{15\% - 5\%}{5\%} = 20\%$	$15\% - 5\% = 10\%$	$1/0.1 = 10$ patients

Using data from March (1998a), excellent responders can be defined as having an end-of-treatment Yale-Brown Obsessive-Compulsive Scale (Y-BOCS) ≤ 10. The 95% confidence interval (CI) on an NNT = 1 / (limits on the CI of its ARR) = (5–55), calculated as in Table 34.3.

together to provide the treatment in our treatment setting(s)? Will the patient accept the treatment? The answers to these questions bring the research study to the level of direct patient care.

Example One: Combined Treatment for Internalizing Disorders and School Refusal

The treatment of teenagers with severe anxiety, depression, and associated school refusal provides an excellent example of how EBM can be used to guide combining medication and psychosocial treatments in clinical practice. One of the most challenging clinical problems in pediatric psychiatry, these patients present with multiple behavioral and family problems and are often, if inappropriately, thought of as treatment refractory even before treatment has begun (Bernstein et al., 1996, 1999). In a recently published study, Bernstein and colleagues (2000) asked the following question (framed as a PECO): in school-refusing teenagers with combined anxiety and depressive disorders (the population), is imipramine plus CBT (the exposure) more effective than CBT plus pill PBO (the control) in returning patients to school (the outcome) after 8 weeks of treatment? They used a balanced randomized parallel group design, complete follow-up, an intent-to-treat analysis, blind assessment, and, given pill PBO to balance the CBT-alone condition, equal treatment characteristics in each group apart from the intervention. Over 8 weeks, they found a statistically significant difference favoring combined treatment over CBT alone for depression outcomes and in returning patients to school. The magnitude and precision of the NNT (NNT = 3, CI = 1–4) for this notoriously difficult-to-treat population were quite impressive in indicating that the combination of CBT and medication is better than CBT alone for anxious depressed school refusers.

The study by Bernstein and colleagues was initiated before SSRIs came into wide use in children and adolescents. A large number of studies have shown that the tricyclic antidepressants (TCAs) are not effective on average for children and adolescents with major depression (the results of a different EBM search) and, apart from effectiveness, the TCAs are riskier and more complicated to use than the SSRIs (Leonard et al., 1997; Birmaher, 1998). Thus, we might want to ask, can we substitute an SSRI for the TCA impramine, in combination with CBT in this patient population? A recently published study from the Research Units on Pediatric Psychopharmacology (RUPP) network that compared fluvoxamine to PBO in children and adolescents with generalized, social, and separation anxiety disorders provides an unambiguous affirmative answer (RUPP Anxiety Group, 2001). With an NNT of 2 (CI=1–3) in this study, we could reasonably assume that the Bernstein findings would have been as good or even better had they used fluvoxamine, though of course there is as yet no randomized evidence pointing in that direction. Given this new evidence and substantial expert opinion favoring the SSRIs over the TCAs in this patient population (Bernstein and Shaw, 1997; March, 1999), the substitution of an SSRI for impramine seems eminently reasonable.

Example Two: Combined Treatment for Children With Attention-Deficit Hyperactivity Disorder

A very large body of literature suggests that treatment with a psychostimulant is effective for externalizing symptoms in children with ADHD (Swanson, 1993). Another large body of literature suggests that behavior therapy primarily in the form of parent training also is effective as a treatment for children with ADHD (Wells et al., 2000). Until recently, empirical support for combining behavior therapy with a psychostimulant in children with ADHD was lacking (Richters et al., 1995). Nonetheless, the combination of parent training and a psychostimulant is often recommended as the first-line treatment for ADHD by experts (Conners et al., 2001) on the following grounds.

First, exclusive treatment with stimulant medication is effective, but may not be maximally effective for core ADHD outcomes in some children. That is, many children will experience reductions in symptoms that nevertheless continue to occur at clinically significant levels. Stated differently, while many children improve substantially with pharmacotherapy, most do not reach full normalization on symptoms with stimulant treatments alone, even at very high doses. Conversely, a greater percentage of children achieve normalization with combination treatment.

Second, stimulant medication may not affect the full range of symptoms of the ADHD child with other comorbid conditions. While large improvements may be seen on the primary symptoms of the syndrome (i.e., attention, impulsivity, and activity level) as a result of drug treatment, sufficient positive effects often are not achieved on other primary or comorbid characteristics of the syndrome, such as oppositional and aggressive behavior, academic underachievement, and poor peer relationships. Because these conditions (along with family dysfunction) are robust predictors of poor long-term outcome for children with ADHD, treatment with stimulants alone may not significantly improve the outcome for these children. This body of research suggests that areas of great relevance for intervention with ADHD children may be the secondary problems of aggressive behavior (and the coercive family process associated with aggression), academic underachievement and associated school behavior problems; and peer relationships. These arenas are most amenable to psychosocial treatments. Moreover, psychosocial treatments may be the only treatment available for the minority of ADHD children who do not achieve a positive treatment effect with stimulants, for children who experience intolerable side effects; or whose parents reject the use of medication.

A final limitation of stimulant treatment alone has to do with its applicability to home behavior problems. Many pharmacotherapists limit the use of stimulants to school hours during the 9 months of the academic year, to avoid growth and appetite suppression, sleep disruption, and other undesirable side effects. This leaves parents to their own devices to manage impulsive, oppositional, and disruptive behavior in the afternoons and evenings, weekends, and summers. When no other treatment is provided, parents frequently resort to coercive, hostile, and overly punitive interactions with their children, which may exacerbate rather than improve the child's behavioral problems. This is a par-

ticularly unfortunate state of affairs given that child and parent aggression is among the best predictors of poor outcome.

For all of these reasons, we might wish to know (framed as a PECO) whether in the treatment of young children with ADHD (the population) combined treatment (the exposure) has an advantage over treatment with medication or parent training alone (the comparison condition). We also might wish to know whether this is true for core ADHD outcomes as well as for non-ADHD outcomes, such as parent–child arguing, or in subgroups of ADHD children who are diagnostically more complex, such as those with a comorbid anxiety disorder.

A search of PubMed using the "clinical queries" option and the search terms ADHD, child, and combined treatment would identify the six-site NIMH collaborative MTA study (MTA Cooperative Group, 1999a,b). The MTA study was designed to addresses a priori questions about the individual and combined effects of pharmacological and psychosocial (behavioral) treatment for children of ages 7–9 years with ADHD (Arnold et al., 1997b). Parenthetically, while other trials also might emerge, assuming that the designs and outcomes are similar, the most recent and/or most powerful study likely is sufficient to construct a CAT. Conversely, where the literature is rich in randomized evidence, an up-to-date EBM review might be the most important source of information (Guyatt et al., 1999).

The rationale and design of the MTA, which serves as a heuristically valuable example of how CBT and medication can and should be combined, have been reported elsewhere (Arnold et al., 1997b). Briefly, 579 children, ages 7 to 9, meeting dimensional criteria for hyperactivity and DSM-IV criteria for ADHD, combined subtype, were randomly assigned to an intensive behavior therapy program (Beh), a titration-adjusted optimized medication management strategy (MedMgt), an interactive combination of Beh and MedMgt (Comb) in which dose and timing of interventions were adjusted for one treatment depending on response to the other, and a comparison group that was assessed and then referred to local community care resources (CC). Children and parents received comprehensive assessments at baseline and at 3, 9, and 14 months (treatment endpoint) (Hinshaw et al., 1997). The Beh treatment consisted of 14 months of parent training with both group and individual parent sessions, 4 months of classroom behavioral management by a trained paraprofessional working with the teacher, and an intensive 8-week summer treatment program (Wells et al., 2000). Optimal medication dosage was attained by acutely titrating medication (starting with methylphenidate and moving on as needed to other drugs) and subsequently adjusting the dose, and timing of drug administration, based on teacher and parent symptom ratings over the course of the study (Greenhill et al., 1996).

As recently summarized by Jensen and colleagues (Jensen et al., 2001), the Comb and MedMgt interventions proved substantially superior to Beh and CC interventions for ADHD symptoms (MTA Cooperative Group, 1999a). Despite the fact that CC children were frequently medicated, these effects were clinically meaningful, with an NNT for Comb or MedMgt relative to CC of 2, indicating clearly that well-delivered treatment that includes medication is superior to less intensive community standard care. For other functioning domains (social skills, academics, parent–child relations, oppositional behavior, anxiety/depression), results suggested modest incremental benefits of the Comb intervention over the single-component (MedMgt, Beh) treatments and community care (MTA Cooperative Group, 1999b). Secondary analyses also revealed that Comb treatment had a significant incremental effect over MedMgt when categorical indicators of excellent response and when composite outcome measures were utilized. In addition, children with parent-defined comorbid anxiety disorders, particularly those with overlapping disruptive disorder comorbidities, showed additional benefits from including a Beh component to the interventions (March et al., 2000).

Granting defensible (Jensen, 1999) limitations in generalizibility (Boyle and Jadad, 1999), the MTA study supports the use of combined treatment for some subgroups of ADHD children for some, typically noncore, outcomes. Thus, when confronted with a complex, multiply comorbid patient or perhaps even a child with more severe ADHD where the goal is clearly normalization the clinician would be wise to recommend a combination of intensive MedMgt and, at a minimum, parent training, whereas for the uncomplicated youngster, MedMgt alone will likely suffice, at least as the initial treatment of choice.

Example 3: Managing Partial Response to a Selective Serotonin Reuptake Inhibitor in Obsessive-Compulsive Disorder

Many patients in clinical practice have already failed or had a partial response to one or more initial treatments, especially when treatment was unimodal. Though robust responses may still occur, on probabilistic grounds, such patients may be expected to have a poorer response to another unimodal treatment in the

same class. For example, an OCD patient on his third SSRI trial is likely to have as much as a threefold lower chance of responding than a treatment-naive patient (Greist et al., 1995; March et al., 1998). If a patient falls into this group, the NNT will be higher than the average research subject. Taking $F = 0.3$, the NNT for an excellent response from monotherapy with a SSRI would be 30 (or 10 divided by 0.3), illustrating the fact that repeated SSRI trials are unlikely to result in full remission of symptoms. The corresponding NNT from open trials in which CBT was added to medication is approximately 2 (March, et al., 1994; Franklin et al., 1998). Hence, if full remission is the aim, the EBM-informed clinician would likely opt for adding CBT to a SSRI early in the course of partial response instead of switching to another SSRI.

LESSONS FROM THE CLINIC

While a full discussion of treatment planning procedures is beyond the scope of this chapter (for additional discussion, see Chapters 31, 32, and 33 in this volume), several important principles merit elaboration insofar as they apply to combining drug and psychosocial interventions. The discussion here is primarily clinical in orientation. A seminal discussion of methodological issues that arise in comparative treatment trials can be found in a series of articles describing the MTA study (Arnold et al., 1997a; Hinshaw et al., 1997; Greenhill et al., 1998; Wells, in press).

Importance of Differential Therapeutics

In the context of medical treatment of psychiatric illness, *differential therapeutics*—identifying treatment interventions that are appropriate to differing treatment targets—can be seen as something like a game of pick up sticks. To function effectively, the doctor has to correctly identify the targets of treatment at the symptom level (the sticks) before sequencing a set of target-specific interventions (pick up the sticks in the proper order) to help the patient get better. Put in terms of the disease management model, current best-practice treatment requires clear specification of the behavioral/emotional syndrome (e.g., ADHD), and within the syndrome, problems (e.g., oppositional behavior), and within the problems, symptoms (e.g., won't go to bed) targeted for intervention. Both behavioral/symptomatic (doctor-assigned) and functional (usually parent and child–assigned) outcomes must be factored into the selection of psychosocial and drug treatments. Depending on the nature of the problem, some outcomes will be more easily approached with medication, others, with a psychosocial intervention. Some will require both to be successful, e.g., the treatments interact rather than simply providing an additive or complimentary impact.

Rating Scales Are the Sphygmomanometer of Psychiatry

Most children present for mental health care because of problematic behaviors either in their relationships or in the school setting. Starting with the presenting complaint, the clinicians' task is to understand these behaviors in the context of the constraints to normal development that underlie them and, in doing so, to construct a differential diagnostic hierarchy that informs a thoughtfully constructed treatment regimen. In this sense, the task of the psychiatric diagnostician is much like that of the cardiologist confronted with the patient with chest pain. Based on the presenting complaint and probabilities attending important demographic factors, the clinician identifies the most likely diagnosis, possible comorbid conditions, and the important diagnoses to rule out in the process of reaching a decision regarding differential therapeutics. Of all the assessment technologies available to us, gender-, ages-, and race-normed rating scales offer perhaps the most efficient way to collect information regarding both internalizing and externalizing behavioral disturbances at home and school. Excellent scales with good psychometric properties are now available for self-report of conduct problems (Conners, 1995), anxiety (March, 1998b) and depression (Kovacs, 1985). Besides assessing an overall construct (e.g., anxiety), child self-report also measures provide useful information at the factor (e.g., physical anxiety symptoms) and item (e.g., suffocation anxiety) level. Clinician-administered ratings scales, such as the Children's Yale-Brown Obsessive-Compulsive Scale (Scahill et al., 1997) or the Childhood Autism Rating Scale (McDougle et al., 2000), are also de rigueur for some disorders. Using reliable and valid rating scales both speeds the interview and begins a dialogue between the doctor and the patient about the patient's most troubling symptoms, thereby facilitating treatment planning. Such a procedure is consistent with medical evaluation procedures across other medical specialties, and meets goals for guidelines-based practice in managed care, irrespective of whether a disease is conceptualized categorically (e.g., schizophrenia) or dimensionally (e.g., generalized anxiety). For example, much like hypertension is the extreme of

blood pressure and presages multiple adverse medical outcomes, attention-deficit hyperactivity and anxiety disorders can be conceptualized dimensionally, with the extreme of the distribution presaging functional impairments now and in the future, rendering rating scales something like the sphygmomanometer: an essential tool for best practice.

Not All Treatments Can or Should Be Tailored

While some argue that tailored treatment is the optimum treatment for all children (Hickling and Blanchard, 1997), not all treatment interventions can be matched to specific targets, no matter how obvious such a match ought to be. For example, because behavior therapy reduces impulsivity in ADHD—a change usually attributed to medication—and psychostimulants reduce negative parent–child interactions—a change readily attributable to behavioral treatment—these two conceptually divergent treatment and outcome dimensions may not be separable when it comes to matching treatments to individual patients (Wells, in press). In another example, methylphenidate has short-term positive effects on children and adolescents with conduct disorder independent of ADHD severity (Klein et al., 1997). In this study, key aspects of antisocial behavior that seemed dependent on social relationships appeared to be treatment responsive to medication. In some domains even theoretically reasonable treatment interventions do not necessarily impact the match target outcome (Wells, in press). For example, cognitive therapy (with the exception of anger management) has not been found to be effective in controlled studies of children with ADHD despite ample evidence for cognitive deficits in children with ADHD (Abikoff, 1991). Similarly, social skills training does not appear to ameliorate peer relationship deficits unless administered within an intensive, multicomponent, behavioral treatment program (Pelham et al., 1998). Given that developmentally sensitive, face-valid interventions don't always work and that treatment effects are not always highly specific, the public health benefit of empirically validated, standardized treatment packages will likely be greater than using theoretically driven tailored treatments in most, if not all, circumstances. The exception is when a treatment component can be clearly shown to have a negative or no effect in the care of an individual child; then it should, of course, be omitted. However, there is no literature to suggest that unmatched treatment ingredients provided to mentally ill children in the context of a comprehensive treatment intervention produce negative effects. The literature simply provides no guidance on this topic.

Pay Careful Attention to Dose–Response and Time–Response Issues

When initiating pharmacological treatment, the ability to construct a dose–response curve and analyze time-action effects is critical. The dose–response curve refers to the relationship between the dose of drug and the presence of benefits and adverse effects. Establishing these relationships depends on understanding time–action parameters, namely the relationship between the timing of administration and onset of response, maximum responsiveness, and loss or offset of drug effect. Departures from a linear dose–response pattern are common, with some children showing a threshold effect (no response below a threshold level) and others, a quadratic response (linear at lower doses and degradation at higher doses). Thus, each child requires an individually constructed dose–response curve, taking into consideration the time–action effects of drug at each dose before making dosage adjustments. With a single drug treatment, many clinicians start with the lowest possible dose, working upward toward the end of the expected time–response window until benefits are maximized or the patient shows prohibitive side effects. Using this strategy, which assumes that "enough drug is enough," eliminates the possibility of undertreatment while at the same time minimizing potential adverse events.

Psychosocial treatments also exhibit distinctive dose–response and time–response characteristics. For example, the average number of weekly CBT sessions is 12–16, irrespective of treatment type, or, stated differently, the dose–and time–response parameters for expected benefit are about 16 sessions over 16 weeks with a range of 6 to 24 weeks (March, 2000). Thus, when combining drug and psychosocial treatments, it is often possible to capitalize on between–treatment differences in dose–response and time response parameters. With respect to dose–response, there is some evidence that treatments can be additive (e.g., the impact of the dose of both treatments is the same as the impact of each treatment separately added together) or multiplicative (two treatments act synergistically, e.g., the benefit of the combination is greater than the additive combination). This may be the case for OCD, where partial response to medication is the rule rather than the exception (March et al., 1997; 1998). Similarly, when combining treatments, a lower dose of one or both treatments may be necessary, with a resultant decrease in expense, inconvenience, or adverse events. For ex-

ample, the MTA study implemented a very high–dose behavioral condition—a 14-month combination of parent training, a summer treatment program, and a classroom intervention (Wells et al., 2000)—that resulted in a slightly lower methylphenidate dosage in the combined group (28 mg/day in divided doses) as compared to the medication-alone group (36 mg/day in divided doses). Even when dosage does not differ, capitalizing on differences in time–response parameters can lead to reduced patient suffering. By blocking full panic episodes and quelling anticipatory anxiety, combining clonazepam with a SSRI in the acutely separation-anxious youngster allows more rapid reintroduction to school than CBT or a SSRI alone might permit (Birmaher, et al., 1998; March, 1999). In treatment for the ADHD child, combination treatment allows for immediate relief of symptoms associated with stimulant treatment while the benefits of psychosocial treatment accumulate more slowly. Finally, even when not divergent, time–response parameters can be matched to the patient's benefit, as when the patient responding to CBT for OCD experiences maximum benefit from a SSRI just at the time he or she reaches the top of the stimulus hierarchy (March, 1998a).

Monitor Desired and Undesirable Outcomes

Once treatment has started, the clinician inevitably will need to conduct additional assessments to collect detailed data on the patient's specific symptomatology and its impact on his or her day-to-day functioning. Such data will serve as a basis for evaluating the progress and rate of treatment and, where possible, for differentiating response to behavioral as contrasted to pharmacological interventions. This is why most CBT manuals include a detailed "mapping" of triggers, responses, and problem-maintaining factors, including family, peer, and school problems, as a routine part of treatment planning. Why evaluate outcome? First, tracking of symptoms requires that the clinician periodically update the problem target list, minimizing the possibility that new or reemerging symptoms will be missed. Second, child and parent ratings allow the clinician to address discrepant views of the child's progress or differential treatment response across different settings where they exist. Third, rating scales provide a detailed view of how the child is progressing in treatment. In this regard, disorder-specific rating scales, whether standardized or tailored to the patient's problems, provide a far richer source of information than global measures, which simply involve therapist ratings of general outcome. Using OCD as an example, patient symptomatology can be tracked with the Y-BOCS symptoms checklist; OCD symptoms, with the Y-BOCS itself; specific CBT targets, with a stimulus hierarchy; and reductions in anxiety in response to successive exposure trials (e.g., habituation curves), using a fear thermometer.

Think Developmentally

As with academic skills, children normally acquire social–emotional (self and interpersonal) competencies across time. The failure to do so, relative to age-, gender-, and culture-matched peers, may reflect capacity limitations, individual difference in the rate of skill acquisition for specific competencies, environmental factors, and/or the development of a major mental illness. The task of the mental health practitioner considering how to combine drug and psychosocial treatment(s) is to understand the presenting symptoms in the context of constraints to normal development, and to devise a tailored target-specific treatment program that eliminates those constraints so that the youngster can resume a normal developmental trajectory insofar as this is possible. Depending on the nature of the symptoms and the capacity of the child and family to make use of target-specific psychosocial interventions, the blend of treatments may vary within a developmental context. For example, irrespective of medication treatment, school avoidance in a separation-anxious 6-year-old will require dyadic CBT in which control is transferred from the therapist to the parent and then to the child, whereas a school-avoidant teen with panic disorder likely will do best with individual CBT perhaps in association with behavioral family therapy (Wells, 1995; Silverman and Kurtines, 1996).

Emphasize Psychoeducation

Despite our best intentions, parents and children sometimes come away with only a limited appreciation for the complexity of their situation, as we understand it, at the end of the diagnostic process. In this context, one of the primary goals of the assessment stage is to use the diagnostic process as a vehicle for psychoeducation regarding the rationale for combining treatments. When initiating or elaborating treatment in the context of partial response, the intention must always be to implement interventions that present a logically consistent and compelling relationship between the disorder, the treatment, and the specified outcome. In particular, it is critical to keep the various treatment targets ("the nails") distinct with respect to the various treatment interventions ("the hammers") so that aspects of the symptom picture that are likely to require or respond to

a psychosocial intervention as distinct from a psychopharmacological one are kept clear. This emphasis encourages a detailed review of the indications, risks, and benefits of proposed and alternative treatments, after which parents and patient generally chose a treatment protocol consisting of a monotherapy, typically either CBT or medication, or CBT in combination with an appropriate medication intervention.

Importantly, there are a panoply of complexities in treating pediatric patients, not present with most adults, that may influence whether and how to combine treatments. For example, children with ADHD rarely seek treatment themselves. Alternatively, parents are sometimes "cornered into treatment" by pressure from school or social service agencies. Children commonly fear being labeled a "mental patient" by peers or extended family and parents often have strong preferences regarding psychosocial or psychopharmacological treatment. Thus exploring the meaning of the diagnosis and resultant medication or psychosocial interventions to the child and to his or her parents is important. Placing medication in the context of an overall treatment plan that includes psychosocial treatment may ease the route to using medications, as when the OCD patient is willing to try medication because concomitant CBT offers not only improved outcomes but also a lesser chance of relapse when medication is discontinued. Finally, despite the power of pharmacological treatments, it is clear that the outcome of major mental illness is heavily dependent on the ability of the supporting environment to facilitate access to and compliance with effective treatment. This is the opposite of biological determinism, and the savvy clinician who understands this perspective takes pains to point out that the greater the degree of Central Nervous System dysregulation, the more important skillful coping by the child and support from the child's environment become.

PRACTICE GUIDELINES

As a general rule, it is always best to use the simplest, least risky, and most cost-effective treatment intervention available within a stages-of-treatment model that addresses selection of initial treatment, the management of partial response, maintenance treatment, treatment resistance, and comorbidity. When the empirical literature and expert opinion agree regarding best practice—e.g. what treatment or combination of treatments will likely work best for most if not all patients—it usually is not acceptable to substitute a less for a more empirically supported treatment, as doing so would not be in the patient's best interest. For example, initiating treatment for newly diagnosed OCD with something other than CBT, a SSRI, or the combination of the two would be difficult to justify (March et al., 1997); (King, et al., 1998). Since doctor, family, and patient preference all come into play when choosing among these treatments, any one of the three options is acceptable as initial treatment, although the doctor ought to suggest that the probability of acute and long-term remission is greater if CBT is included in the treatment mix (March et al., 1997; King et al., 1998).

Much of the time, treatment-extant literature doesn't provide much guidance when the patient has multiple comorbidities or already has failed best-practice initial interventions. The few available comparative treatment trials that include both medication and psychotherapy all focus on acute treatment or, less commonly, the heroic management of treatment-refractory patients. This leaves out the majority of patients for whom combined treatment is appropriate if not de rigueur, namely those who are partial responders to initial treatment and/or who require a combination of treatments because of comorbidity. Furthermore, for many clinically important decisions, it is unlikely that there will ever be randomized evidence. For example, how many SSRI trials should precede a clomipramine trial in the partially responsive child with OCD? How long does one wait before adding a SSRI when treating a child with OCD who is not particularly responsive to weekly CBT?

Under conditions of uncertainty, e.g., absent data-driven agreement regarding the best practice, there is less reason to be dogmatic regarding treatment choice and more reason to weigh the available treatment options in light of doctor and patient preference. How then do we define best practice? Although the ultimate utility of treatment guidelines will depend on improving the evidence base (Weisz and Hawley, 1998), such guidelines offer one increasingly attractive option (Dunne, 1997; Frances, et al., 1998). (The experts' answers to the questions in the preceding paragraph are 2 or 3 and 4 to 6 weeks, respectively [March et al., 1997].) Within the EBM framework, guidelines are defined as systematically developed statements to assist the practitioner and patient in making decisions about appropriate health care for specific clinical circumstances (Sackett et al., 2000). In contrast to unsystematic clinical reviews, which typically focus on a content area rather than on a specific clinical question or set of questions linked to clinical decision nodes, a systematically assembled guideline begins with a clear question (e.g., what CBT components are effective as initial treatment for the depressed teenager?) or set of decision nodes (e.g., specification of best-practice treat-

ment for OCD in a stages-of-treatment model), has an explicit search strategy, specifies criteria for evaluating the evidence, provides a clear statement of real or potential biases in interpretation of the review, and concludes with a recommendation for how to use the guideline in making decisions about the care of individual patients. As a result, an empirically based guideline provides expert consultation (without the expert) regarding best-practice options "at the bedside." Note that consultation in a subspecialty clinic may be the recommended option—for example, when a patient fails standard interventions for ADHD in the primary care setting (Conners et al., 2001).

Guidelines of varying quality are available, and more are under development as the idea of "care maps" gains increasing credence in psychiatric practice as it has in pediatrics (Bergman, 1999). The AACAP practice parameters, which tend to focus on content surveys for initial treatment, are perhaps the best known to child and adolescent psychiatrists (Dunne, 1997); similar efforts are underway in psychology (Weisz and Hawley, 1998); (Ammerman, et al., 1999; Weisz, 2000). Empirically based guidelines that systematically poll the experts and employ a stages-of-treatment framework are available for ADHD (Pliszka et al., 2000a,b); (Conners et al., 2001) and OCD (March et al., 1997). The Expert Consensus Guidelines for OCD (March et al., 1997), which heavily influenced the AACAP Practice Parameters on OCD (King et al., 1998), provides an excellent example of a comprehensive guideline that includes both psychosocial and medication management within the context of a stages-of-treatment model. (The full guideline is available for downloading at http://www.psychguides.com.) As shown in Figure 34.1, which presents the guideline in flowchart format, the experts (an even mixture of psychiatrists and psychologists) recommend starting with CBT or CBT plus a SSRI, depending on severity and pattern of comorbidity; both recommend that patients started on SSRI monotherapy who are partial responders have their treatment augmented with CBT. Thus, experts generally consider CBT a first-line augmentation strategy and medication augmentation a second-line option. Options for treatment-resistant OCD include high (intensive) dosing strategies for both CBT and medications, aggressive polypharmacy, and, in some cases, neurosurgery. Maintenance treatment recommendations depend on severity of symptoms, residual symptoms, and previous relapse history, all of which bias toward longer treatment even in the presence of CBT, which is generally believed to be of more durable benefit than medication once medication is withdrawn.

Overall Strategies for Acute-Phase Treatment of OCD

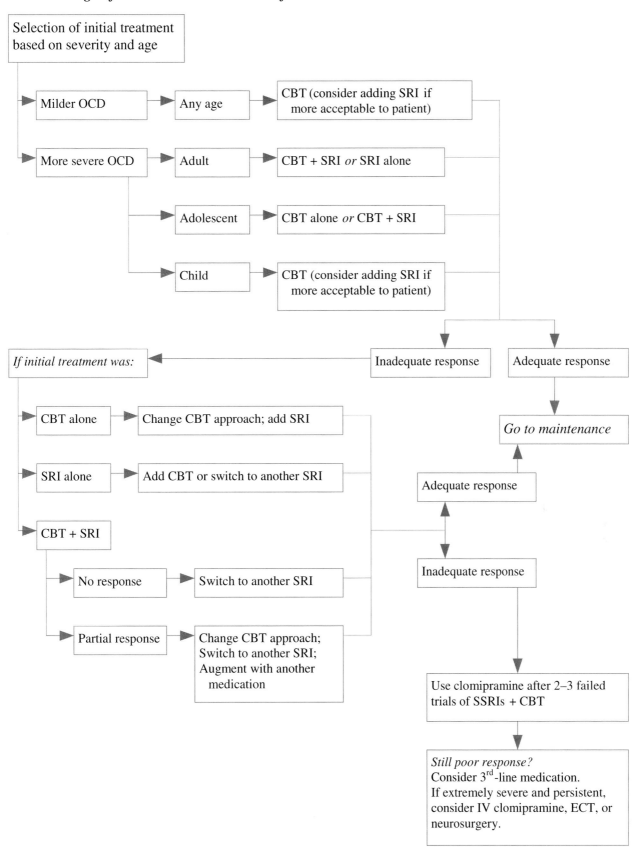

FIGURE 34.1 Expert consensus treatment guidelines for obsessive-compulsive disorder. *(continued)*

Tactics for Duration and Intensity of Treatment During Acute and Maintenance Phases

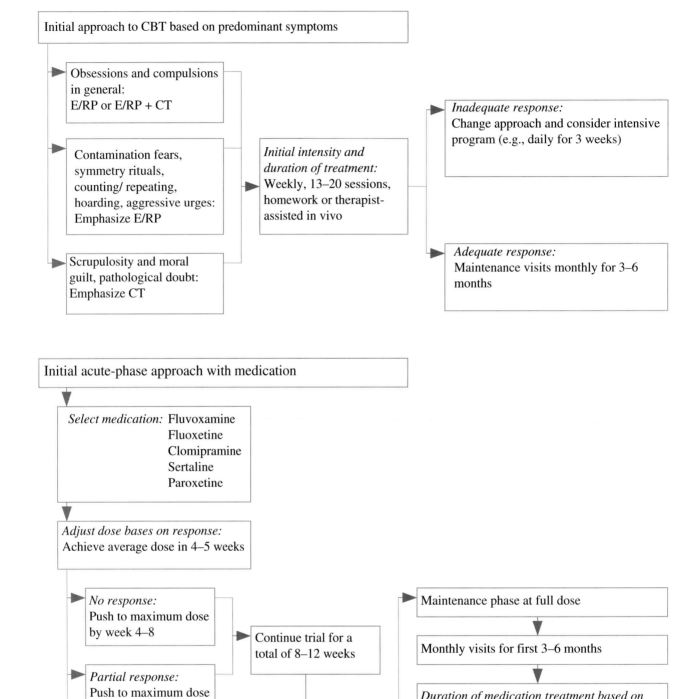

FIGURE 34.1 *(continued)*

440

CONCLUSION

While cynics bemoan our relatively incomplete evidence base, empirically supported unimodal treatments are now available for most disorders seen in clinical practice, including ADHD, OCD, Tourettes syndrome, major depression, schizophrenia, and autism. Despite limitations in the research literature with regard to how best to combine treatments acutely, long-term outcome of combined treatment, effectiveness of drugs and psychosocial interventions across divergent outcome domains and ages, and optimal assessment procedures for selecting whether and how to combine treatments, the empirical literature is also increasingly positive regarding the benefits of short- and longer-term combinations of drug and psychosocial treatments for some, if not all, mentally ill children and adolescents. In addition to the MTA study, which is now examining the long-term impact of early intensive treatment for ADHD, multisite comparative treatment trials, funded by the NIMH, that include a combined treatment arm are underway in pediatric OCD and in adolescent depression. (For more information on the Pediatric OCD Treatment Study (POTS) and on the Treatment of Adolescents with Depression Study (TADS), visit their respective websites: www2.mc.duke.edu/pcaad, and www.nimh.nih.gov). Taken together, these studies and others about to be undertaken in anxiety, eating, and conduct disorders begin to approach the question of which treatment—drug, psychosocial, or combination—is best for which child with a given set of predictive characteristics (March and Curry, 1998; Jensen, 1999). As our understanding of the pathogenesis of mental illness in youth increases, dramatic treatment innovations inevitably will accrue, including knowledge about when and how to combine treatments. Hence, the clinician facing the daunting task of keeping up with the rapid advances in evidence regarding the diagnosis and treatment of mental illness in children and adolescents would be well advised to acquire at least a basic understanding of the tools of evidence-based medicine (Sackett et al., 2000). In the meantime, it is likely that the combination of targeted medication and psychosocial therapies skillfully applied across time affords the most plausible basis for sustained benefit in children, adolescents, and adults suffering from a variety of major mental illnesses.

ACKNOWLEDGMENTS
This work was supported by NIMH Grants 1 K24 MHO1557 to Dr. March and by contributions from the Robert and Sarah Gorrell family.

Portions of this chapter were adapted from: March, J. (in press). Combining medication and psychosocial treatments: an evidence-based medicine approach. *International Review of Psychiatry*.

REFERENCES

Abikoff, H. (1991) Cognitive training in ADHD children: less to it than meets the eye. *J Learn Disab*, 24:205–209.

Ammerman, R., Hersen, M., and Last, C. (1999) *Handbook of Prescriptive Treatments for Children and Adolescents, 2nd ed.* New York: Allyn & Bacon.

Arnold, L.E., Abikoff, H.B., Cantwell, D.P., Conners, C.K., Elliott, G., Greenhill, L.L., Hechtman, L., Hinshaw, S.P., Hoza, B., Jensen, P.S., Kraemer, H.C., March, J.S., Newcorn, J.H., Pelham, W.E., Richters, J.E., Schiller, E., Severe, J.B., Swanson, J.M., Vereen, D., and Wells, K.C. (1997a) National Institute of Mental Health Collaborative Multimodal Treatment Study of Children with ADHD (the MTA). Design challenges and choices. *Arch Gen Psychiatry* 54:865–870.

Arnold, L.E., Abikoff, H.B., Cantwell, D.P., Conners, C.K., Elliott, G., Greenhill, L.L., Hechtman, L., Hinshaw, S.P., Hoza, B., Jensen, P.S., Kraemer, H.C., March, J.S., Newcorn, J.H., Pelham, W.E., Richters, J.E., Schiller, E., Severe, J.B., Swanson, J.M., Vereen, D., and Wells, K.C. (1997b) NIMH Collaborative Multimodal Treatment Study of Children with ADHD (the MTA). Design, methodology and protocol evolution. *J Attention Disord* 2: 141–158.

Barlow, D.H., Gorman, J.M., Shear, M.K., and Woods, S.W. (2000) Cognitive-behavioral therapy, imipramine, or their combination for panic disorder: a randomized controlled trial [see comments]. *JAMA* 283(19):2529–2536.

Barlow, D.H., Levitt, J.T., & Bufka, L.F. (1999) The dissemination of empirically supported treatments: a view to the future. *Behav Res Ther* 37 (Suppl 1):S147–162.

Bergman, D.A. (1999) Evidence-based guidelines and critical pathways for quality improvement. *Pediatrics* 103(1 Suppl E):225–232.

Bernstein, G.A., Borchardt, C.M., and Perwien, A.R. (1996) Anxiety disorders in children and adolescents: a review of the past 10 years. *J Am Acad Child Adolesc Psychiatry* 35:1110–1119.

Bernstein, G.A., Borchardt, C.M., Perwien, A.R., Crosby, R.D., Kushner, M.G., Thuras, P.D., and Last, C.G. (2000) Imipramine plus cognitive-behavioral therapy in the treatment of school refusal. *J Am Acad Child Adolesc Psychiatry* 39:276–283.

Bernstein, G.A., and Shaw, K. (1997) Practice parameters for the assessment and treatment of children and adolescents with anxiety disorders. American Academy of Child and Adolescent Psychiatry. *J Am Acad Child Adolesc Psychiatry* 36(10 Suppl): 69S–84S.

Bernstein, G.A., Warren, S.L., Massie, E.D., and Thuras, P.D. (1999) Family dimensions in anxious-depressed school refusers. *J Anxiety Disord* 13:513–528.

Birmaher, B. (1998) Should we use antidepressant medications for children and adolescents with depressive disorders? *Psychopharmacol Bull* 34:35–39.

Birmaher, B., Brent, D.A., and Benson, R.S. (1998) Summary of the practice parameters for the assessment and treatment of children and adolescents with depressive disorders. American Academy of Child and Adolescent Psychiatry. *J Am Acad Child Adolesc Psychiatry* 37:1234–1238.

Birmaher, B., Yelovich, A.K., and Renaud, J. (1998) Pharmacologic treatment for children and adolescents with anxiety disorders. *Pediatr Clin North Am* 45:1187–1204.

Boyle, M.H., and Jadad, A.R. (1999) Lessons from large trials: the MTA study as a model for evaluating the treatment of childhood psychiatric disorder. *Can J Psychiatry* 44:991–998.

Cohen, J. (1977) *Statistical Power Analyses for the Behavioral Sciences*. New York: Academic Press.

Conners, C. (1995) *Conners' Rating Scales*. Toronto, CA: Multi-Health Systems.

Conners, C., March, J., Wells, K., Frances, A., and Ross, R. (2001) Expert consensus guidelines: treatment of attention-deficit/hyperactivity disorder. *J Attention Disorders* 4 (Suppl 1).

Dunne, J.E. (1997) Introduction: history and development of the practice parameters. *J Am Acad Child Adolesc Psychiatry* 36(10 Suppl):1S-3S.

Frances, A., Kahn, D., Carpenter, D., Frances, C., and Docherty, J. (1998) A new method of developing expert consensus practice guidelines [see comments]. *Am J Manag Care* 4:1023–1029.

Franklin, M.E., Kozak, M.J., Cashman, L.A., Coles, M.E., Rheingold, A.A., and Foa, E.B. (1998) Cognitive-behavioral treatment of pediatric obsessive-compulsive disorder: an open clinical trial. *J Am Acad Child Adolesc Psychiatry* 37:412–414.

Greenhill, L.L., Abikoff, H.B., Arnold, L.E., Cantwell, D.P., Conners, C.K., Elliott, G., Hechtman, L., Hinshaw, S.P., Hoza, B., Jensen, P.S., March, J.S., Newcorn, J., Pelham, W.E., Severe, J.B., Swanson, J.M., Vitiello, B., and Wells, K. (1996) Medication treatment strategies in the MTA Study: relevance to clinicians and researchers. *J Am Acad Child Adolesc Psychiatry* 35:1304–1313.

Greenhill, L.L., Pine, D., March, J., Birmaher, B., and Riddle, M. (1998) Assessment issues in treatment research of pediatric anxiety disorders: what is working, what is not working, what is missing, and what needs improvement. *Psychopharmacol Bull* 34: 155–164.

Greist, J.H., Jefferson, J.W., Kobak, K.A., Katzelnick, D.J., and Serlin, R.C. (1995) Efficacy and tolerability of serotonin transport inhibitors in obsessive-compulsive disorder. A meta-analysis [see comments]. *Arch Gen Psychiatry* 52:53–60.

Guyatt, G.H., and Rennie, D. (1993) Users' guides to the medical literature [editorial]. *JAMA* 270:2096–2097.

Guyatt, G.H., Sackett, D.L., and Cook, D.J. (1993) Users' guides to the medical literature. II. How to use an article about therapy or prevention. A. Are the results of the study valid? Evidence-Based Medicine Working Group. *JAMA* 270:2598–2601.

Guyatt, G.H., Sackett, D.L., and Cook, D.J. (1994) Users' guides to the medical literature. II. How to use an article about therapy or prevention. B. What were the results and will they help me in caring for my patients? Evidence-Based Medicine Working Group. *JAMA* 271:59–63.

Guyatt, G.H., Sinclair, J., Cook, D.J., and Glasziou, P. (1999) Users' guides to the medical literature: XVI. How to use a treatment recommendation. Evidence-Based Medicine Working Group and the Cochrane Applicability Methods Working Group. *JAMA* 281: 1836–1843.

Hersen, M., and Bellack, A.S. (1999) *Handbook of Comparative Interventions for Adult Disorders 2nd ed.* New York, John Wiley & Sons.

Hibbs, E., and Jensen, P. (1996) *Psychosocial Treatments for Child and Adolescent Disorders*. Washington, DC: American Psychological Press.

Hickling, E.J., and Blanchard, E.B. (1997) The private practice psychologist and manual-based treatments: post-traumatic stress disorder secondary to motor vehicle accidents [see comments]. *Behavi Rese Ther* 35:191–203.

Hinshaw, S., March, J., Abikoff, H., Arnold, L., Cantwell, D., Conners, C., Elliott, G., Greenhill, L., Halperin, J., Hechtman, L., Hoza, B., Jensen, P., March, J., Newcorn, J., Pelham, W., Richters, J., Severe, J., Schiller, E., Swanson, J., Veeren, D., Wells, K., and Wigal, T. (1997) Comprehensive asssssment of childhood attention-deficit hyperactivity disorder in the context of a miltisite, multimodal clinical trial. *J Attention Disord* 1: 217–234.

Hyman, S.E. (2000) The millennium of mind, brain, and behavior. *Arch Gen Psychiatry* 57:88–89.

Jensen, P.S., Hinshaw, S.P., Swanson, J.M., Greenhill, L.L., Conners, C.K., Arnold, L.E., Abikoff, H.B., Elliott, G., Hechtman, L., Hoza, B., March, J.S., Newcorn, J.H., Severe, J.B., Vitiello, B., Wells, K., and Wigal, T. (2001) Findings from the NIMH Multimodal Treatment Study of ADHD (MTA): implications and applications for primary care providers. *J Dev Behav Pediatr* 22: 60–73.

Jensen, P.S. (1999) Fact versus fancy concerning the multimodal treatment study for attention-deficit hyperactivity disorder. *Can J Psychiatry* 44:975–980.

Kandel, E., and Squire, L. (2000) Neuroscience: breaking down scientific barriers to the study of brain and mind. *Science* 290:1113–1120.

Kazdin, A.E. (1997) A model for developing effective treatments: progression and interplay of theory, research, and practice. *J Clin Child Psychol* 26:114–129.

Keller, M.B., McCullough, J.P., Klein, D.N., Arnow, B., Dunner, D.L., Gelenberg, A.J., Markowitz, J.C., Nemeroff, C.B., Russell, J.M., Thase, M.E., Trivedi, M.H., and Zajecka, J. (2000) A comparison of nefazodone, the cognitive behavioral–analysis system of psychotherapy, and their combination for the treatment of chronic depression [see comments]. *N Engl J Med* 342:1462–1470.

Kendall, P. (1999) *Child and Adolescent Therapy* 2nd ed. New York: Guilford Press.

King, R.A., Leonard, H., and March, J. (1998) Practice parameters for the assessment and treatment of children and adolescents with obsessive-compulsive disorder. *J Am Acad Child Adolesc Psychiatry* 37(10, Suppl).

Klein, R.G., Abikoff, H., Klass, E., Ganeles, D., Seese, L.M., and Pollack, S. (1997) Clinical efficacy of methylphenidate in conduct disorder with and without attention deficit hyperactivity disorder. *Arch Gen Psychiatry* 54:1073–1080.

Kovacs, M. (1985) The Children's Depression Inventory (CDI). *Psychopharmecol Bull* 21:995–998.

Leonard, H.L., March, J., Rickler, K.C., and Allen, A.J. (1997). Pharmacology of the selective serotonin reuptake inhibitors in children and adolescents. *J Am Acad Child Adoles Psychiatry* 36:725–736.

Levine, M., Walter, S., Lee, H., Haines, T., Holbrook, A., and Moyer, V. (1994) Users' guides to the medical literature. IV. How to use an article about harm. Evidence-Based Medicine Working Group. *JAMA* 271:1615–1619.

Ludwig, A.M., and Othmer, K. (1977) The medical basis of psychiatry. *Am J Psychiatry* 134:1087–1092.

March, J. (1998a) Cognitive behavioral psychotherapy for pediatric OCD. In Jenike, M., Baer, L., and Minichello,?, eds. *Obsessive-Compulsive Disorders 3rd ed.* Philadelphia: Mosby, pp. 400–420.

March, J. (1998b) *Manual for the Multidimensional Anxiety Scale for Children (MASC)*. Toronto: MultiHealth Systems.

March, J. (1999) Current status of pharmacotherapy for pediatric anxiety disorders. In: Beidel, D., ed. *Treating Anxiety Disorders in Youth: Current Problems and Future Solutions (ADAA/NIMH)* Washington, DC: Anxiety Disorders Association of America, pp. 42–62.

March, J. (2000) Child psychiatry: cognitive and behavior therapies.

In: Saddock B. and V., Saddock, eds. *Comprehensive Textbook of Psychiatry/VII* New York: Williams and Wilkins, (pp. 2806–2812).

March, J., Frances, A., Kahn, D., and Carpenter, D. (1997) Expert Consensus guidelines: treatment of obsessive-compulsive disorder. *J Clin Psychiatry* 58(Suppl 4):1–72.

March, J., Mulle, K., and Herbel, B. (1994) Behavioral psychotherapy for children and adolescents with obsessive-compulsive disorder: an open trial of a new protocol driven treatment package. *J Am Acad Child Adoles Psychiatry* 33:333–341.

March, J., Mulle, K., Stallings, P., Erhardt, D., and Conners, C. (1995) Organizing an anxiety disorders clinic. In: March, J., ed. *Anxiety Disorders in Children and Adolesents* New York: Guilford Press, pp. 420–435.

March, J.S., Biederman, J., Wolkow, R., Safferman, A., Mardekian, J., Cook, E.H., Cutler, N.R., Dominguez, R., Ferguson, J., Muller, B., Riesenberg, R., Rosenthal, M., Sallee, F.R., and Wagner, K.D. (1998) Sertraline in children and adolescents with obsessive-compulsive disorder: a multicenter randomized controlled trial [see comments]. *JAMA* 280:1752–1756.

March, J.S., and Curry, J.F. (1998) Predicting the outcome of treatment. *J Abnorm Child Psychol* 26:39–51.

March, J.S., and Leonard, H.L. (1998) OCD in children: research and treatment. In: Swinson, R., Rachman, J., Antony, and Richter, M., eds. *Obsessive-Compulsive Disorder: Theory, research, and Treatment*. New York: Guilford pp. 367–394.

March, J.S., Swanson, J.M., Arnold, L.E., Hoza, B., Conners, C.K., Hinshaw, S.P., Hechtman, L., Kraemer, H.C., Greenhill, L.L., Abikoff, H.B., Elliott, L.G., Jensen, P.S., Newcorn, J.H., Vitiello, B., Severe, J., Wells, K.C., and Pelham, W.E. (2000) Anxiety as a predictor and outcome variable in the multimodal treatment study of children with ADHD (MTA). *J Abnorm Child Psychol* 28:527–541.

McDougle, C.J., Scahill, L., McCracken, J.T., Aman, M.G., Tierney, E., Arnold, L.E., Freeman, B.J., Martin, A., McGough, J.J., Cronin, P., Posey, D.J., Riddle, M.A., Ritz, L., Swiezy, N.B., Vitiello, B., Volkmar, F.R., Votolato, N.A., and Walson, P. (2000). Research Units on Pediatric Psychopharmacology (RUPP) Autism Network. Background and rationale for an initial controlled study of risperidone. *Child Adolesc Psychiatr Clin North Am* 9: 201–224.

MTA Cooperative Group (1999a) A 14-month randomized clinical trial of treatment strategies for attention-deficit/hyperactivity disorder. Multimodal Treatment Study of Children with ADHD. *Arch Gen Psychiatry* 56:1073–1086.

MTA Cooperative Group (1999b) Moderators and mediators of treatment response for children with attention-deficit/hyperactivity disorder: the Multimodal Treatment Study of Children with Attention-Deficit/Hyperactivity Disorder. *Arch Gen Psychiatry* 56:1088–1096.

Norquist, G.S., and Magruder, K.M. (1998) Views from funding agencies. National Institute of Mental Health. *Med Care* 36: 1306–1308.

Pelham, W.E., Jr., Wheeler, T., and Chronis, A. (1998) Empirically supported psychosocial treatments for attention deficit hyperactivity disorder. *J Clin Child Psychol* 27:190–205.

Pliszka, S.R., Greenhill, L.L., Crismon, M.L., Sedillo, A., Carlson, C., Conners, C.K., McCracken, J.T., Swanson, J.M., Hughes, C.W., Llana, M.E., Lopez, M., and Toprac, M.G. (2000a) The

Texas Children's Medication Algorithm Project: Report of the Texas Consensus Conference Panel on Medication Treatment of Childhood Attention-deficit/hyperactivity disorder. Part I. Attention-deficit/hyperactivity disorder. *J Am Acad Child Adolesc Psychiatry* 39:908–919.

Pliszka, S.R., Greenhill, L.L., Crismon, M.L., Sedillo, A., Carlson, C., Conners, C.K., McCracken, J.T., Swanson, J.M., Hughes, C.W., Llana, M.E., Lopez, M., and Toprac, M.G. (2000b) The Texas Children's Medication Algorithm Project: Report of the Texas Consensus Conference Panel on Medication Treatment of Childhood Attention-Deficit/Hyperactivity Disorder. Part II: Tactics. Attention-deficit/hyperactivity disorder. *J Am Acad Child Adolesc Psychiatry* 39:920–927.

Pollack, M.H., Otto, M.W., and Rosenbaum, J.F. (1996) Challenges in Clinical Practice: Pharmacologic and Psychosocial Strategies. New York: Guilford Press, p. 504.

Research Units on Pediatric Psychopharmacology (RUPP). (2001). Fluvoxamine for the treatment of anxiety disorders in children and adolescents. *N Engl J Med* 344:1279–1285.

Richters, J.E., Arnold, L.E., Jensen, P.S., Abikoff, H., Conners, C.K., Greenhill, L.L., Hechtman, L., Hinshaw, S.P., Pelham, W.E., and Swanson, J.M. (1995) NIMH collaborative multisite multimodal treatment study of children with ADHD: I. Background and rationale. *J Am Acad Child Adolesc Psychiatry* 34:987–1000.

Sackett, D., Richardson, W., Rosenberg, W., and Haynes, B. (1997) *Evidence-Based Medicine*. London: Churchill Livingston.

Sackett, D., Richardson, W., Rosenberg, W., and Haynes, B. (2000) *Evidence-Based Medicine, 2nd ed.* London: Churchill Livingston.

Scahill, L., Riddle, M.A., McSwiggin-Hardin, M., Ort, S.I., King, R.A., Goodman, W.K., Cicchetti, D., and Leckman, J.F. (1997) Children's Yale-Brown Obsessive Compulsive Scale: reliability and validity. *J Am Acad Child Adolesc Psychiatry* 36:844–852.

Silverman, W., and Kurtines, W. (1996) *Anxiety and Phobic Disorders: A Pragmatic Approach*. New York: Plenum Press.

Swanson, J. (1993) Effect of stimulant medication on hyperactive children: a review of reviews. *Exceptional Child* 60:154–162.

Van Hasselt, V.B., and Hersen, M. (1993) *Handbook of Behavior Therapy and Pharmacotherapy for Children: A Comparative Analysis*. Boston, MA: Allyn & Bacon.

Weisz, J.R. (2000) Agenda for child and adolescent psychotherapy research: on the need to put science into practice [comment]. *Arch Gen Psychiatry* 57:837–838.

Weisz, J.R., and Hawley, K.M. (1998) Finding, evaluating, refining, and applying empirically supported treatments for children and adolescents [comment] [see comments]. *J Clin Child Psychol* 27: 206–216.

Wells, K. (1995) Family therapy. In: March, J., ed. *Anxiety Disorders in Children and Adolescents* New York: Guilford Press, pp. 401–419.

Wells, K. (in press) Comprehensive vs. matched psychosocial treatment in the MTA study: conceptual and empirical issues. *J Clin Child Psychol*.

Wells, K.C., Pelham, W.E., Jr., Kotkin, R.A., Hoza, B., Abikoff, H.B., Abramowitz, A., Arnold, L.E., Cantwell, D.P., Conners, C.K., Del Carmen, R., Elliott, G., Greenhill, L.L., Hechtman, L., Hibbs, E., Hinshaw, S.P., Jensen, P.S., March, J.S., Swanson, J.M., and Schiller, E. (2000) Psychosocial treatment strategies in the MTA study: rationale, methods, and critical issues in design and implementation. *J Abnorm Child Psychol* 28:483–505.

SPECIFIC DISORDERS AND SYNDROMES

35 | Attention-deficit hyperactivity disorder

THOMAS SPENCER, JOSEPH BIEDERMAN, TIMOTHY WILENS, AND ROSS GREENE

Attention-deficit hyperactivity disorder (ADHD) is the most common juvenile psychiatric disorder presenting to mental health workers, child psychiatrists, and pediatricians. This disorder is one of the major clinical and public health problems because of its associated morbidity and disability in children, adolescents, and adults. Its relevance to society is significant in terms of financial cost, stress to families, and impact on academic and vocational activities, as well as the negative effects on self-esteem.

The *Diagnostic and Statistical Manual of Mental Disorders, 4th ed.* (DSM-IV) recognizes three subtypes of ADHD: a predominantly inattentive subtype, a predominantly hyperactive-impulsive subtype, and a combined subtype (American Psychiatric Association, 1994). These categories acknowledge clinical heterogeneity and reflect a change in emphasis from earlier definitions that stressed motoric symptoms to the current nosology, which emphasizes deficits in the regulation of cognitive function.

Previous discrepancies in geographic prevalence rates of ADHD appear to have been artifacts of differing criteria. Studies using the current accepted definitions of ADHD have documented rates of 2% to 12% in mainland United States, 4% in Germany, 6% in Canada, 7% in New Zealand, and 10% in Puerto Rico (Szatmari, 1992; Bird et al., 1993; Bauermeister et al., 1994). Of note, the co-occurrence of other psychiatric disorders is evident even in these community-based studies (McGee et al., 1985; Anderson et al., 1987; Bird et al., 1988). In a quasi-epidemiologic study of adults, Murphy and Barkley (1996) reported that 4.7% of adults endorsed childhood and current symptoms of ADHD sufficient to meet diagnostic criteria. These self-reported, adult ADHD symptoms were negatively associated with educational attainment and occupational level.

Although its etiology remains unknown, data from family genetic, twin, adoption, and segregation analysis strongly suggest a genetic etiology. Indeed, the genetic contribution appears to be substantial as suggested by the very high heritability coefficients (mean = 0.8) associated with this disorder. While preliminary, molecular genetic studies have implicated several candidate genes, including the dopamine D_2 and D_4 (*DRD4–7*) receptors as well as the dopamine transporter (*DAT-1*) (Faraone et al., 1999). It is of note that both dopamine and norepinephrine neurotransmitters that are thought to mediate the response to ADHD pharmacotherapy, are potent agonists of the D_4 receptor.

Data from follow-up studies indicate that children with ADHD are at risk for maintaining and developing new psychiatric disorders in adolescence and adulthood, including antisocial and substance use disorders (tobacco, alcohol, and drugs). Follow-up data also document that the disorder persists into adulthood in a substantial number of children and that it may be a common adult diagnosis (Spencer et al., 1998d). In recent years, there has been an increasing recognition that ADHD is a highly heterogeneous disorder with high levels of psychiatric comorbidity. Neuroimaging studies have identified subtle anomalies in the frontal cortex and in projecting subcortical structures (Faraone and Biederman, 1999), and dysregulation of catecholamine neurotransmission has been posited to underlie its pathophysiology (Zametkin and Rapoport, 1987).

ASSESSMENT AND EVALUATION

The clinical presentation of ADHD is highly heterogeneous. Recently, the American Academy of Child and Adolescent Psychiatry (AACAP) published practice parameters outlining guidelines for assessment and evaluation of ADHD (Dulcan, 1996). In addition to core symptoms, ADHD affects many areas of function, including academic, social, and behavioral domains. Symptoms diminish in novel or structured environments or in closely supervised settings. Symptoms worsen in other settings, especially those requiring sustained effort and attention to detail. As with all other psychiatric disorders, there is no pathognomonic laboratory test, and clinical interview is the standard for diagnosis. Parents are the primary informers for diagnostic evaluations, providing information about home, school, and peer situations. Children are not considered reliable reporters. Ancillary information from report cards and teachers is often useful. The clinical interview should carefully screen for the presence of other disorders that commonly co-occur with ADHD. Genetic risk factors should be considered and a history of familial ADHD in close relatives should be elicited. Neuropsychological testing is often useful in complicated clinical presentations; however, such testing is to document learning disorders and is not sensitive to ADHD per se.

There are a number of useful standardized scales to monitor severity and treatment outcomes. (reviewed by Conners [1998] and Barkley [1998]) Because of the overlap with other disorders, an ADHD-specific scale is strongly recommended (such as the Conners, SNAP, Dupaul scales) in which symptom items are based on the DSM criteria and do not include items of other disorders (such as anxiety or mood) or nonspecific functional items. Some ADHD scales provide separate ratings of oppositionality or aggression (SNAP, Conners). It may be helpful to monitor symptoms from non-ADHD conditions as well as functional deficits, and thus a broad-spectrum scale may also be employed but should not be used as the primary measure of ADHD severity or anti-ADHD treatment. Normed rating scales provide comparative information on severity based on age and gender; however, such tests are not diagnostic and are not a substitute for the clinical interview.

PHARMACOTHERAPY

A summary of major categories of drugs used in the pharmaco-therapy of ADHD is provided in Table 35.1, and the corresponding treatment algorithm is provided in Table 35.2

Psychostimulants

Commercially available psychostimulants include methylphenidate (Ritalin, Methylin, Metadate, Con-

certa), D-amphetamine (dexedrine, others), D, L-amphetamine (Adderall), and magnesium pemoline (Cylert, others) (see Chapter 20). These sympathomimetic compounds are structurally dissimilar, but share a phenylethylamine backbone with endogenous catecholamines (e.g., dopamine and norepinephrine). The mechanism of action of psychostimulants is thought to be reuptake blockade of catecholamines into presynaptic nerve endings, thereby preventing their degradation by monoamine oxidase. In addition, amphetamine compounds appear to cause retrograde release of catecholamines through the transporter as well as other actions on the vesicular storage of catecholamines (Wilens and Spencer, 1998).

Methylphenidate possesses two asymmetric carbon moieties, giving rise to four optical isomers: d-threo, l-threo, d-erythro, and l-erythro (Patrick et al., 1987). There is stereoselectivity in receptor site binding and its relationship to response. The standard preparation is comprised of the threo racemate as it appears to be the central nervous system (CNS) active form (Patrick et al., 1987; Hubbard et al., 1989). In addition, in rats, the d-methylphenidate isomer shows greater reuptake inhibition of DA and NE than the l-isomer (Patrick et al., 1987). D-Methylphenidate is now available under the brand name Focalin.

Methylphenidate and D-amphetamine are both short-acting compounds, with an onset of action within 30 to 60 minutes and a peak clinical effect seen usually between 1 and 2 hours after administration, lasting 2 to 5 hours. Therefore, multiple daily administrations are required for a consistent daytime response. The amphetamine compound Adderall, the sustained-release preparations of methylphenidate and dextroamphetamine, and pemoline are all intermediate-acting compounds with an onset of action within 60 minutes and a peak clinical effect seen usually between 1 and 3 hours after administration and maintained for up to 8 hours (8 hours with metadate C.D. and Ritalin LA; 12 hours with Concerta), allowing for a single dose for the entire school day. Adderall XR is a 12 hour preparation.

There is a large body of literature documenting the efficacy of stimulants on core features of ADHD (motoric overactivity, impulsivity, and inattentiveness) as well as their substantial effects on cognition, social function, and aggression (Spencer et al., 1996b). Of over 200 controlled studies, most are short-term trials of latency age Caucasian boys. A growing literature suggests, however, that stimulants are very effective through adolescence and into adulthood (Spencer et al., 1995). Recently, a controlled study of stimulants in girls with ADHD documented substantial improvement

TABLE 35.1 *Major Drug Classes Used in the Pharmacotherapy of Attention-Deficit Hyperactivity Disorder*

Drug[a]	Daily Dose[b] (mg/kg)	Daily Dosage Schedule	Main Indications	Common Adverse Effects, Comments
Stimulants				
Dextroamphetamine (Dexedrine)	0.3–1	bid or tid	ADHD MR+ADHD	Insomnia, decreased appetite, weight loss Depression, psychosis (rare, with very high doses) Increase in heart rate and blood pressure (mild) Possible reduction in growth velocity with long-term use Withdrawal effects and rebound phenomena
Mixed salts of L- and D-amphetamine (Adderall) (Adderall XR)	0.5–1.5	Once to bid	Adjunct therapy in refractory depression	D-amphetamine and methylphenidate available in long-acting preparations; effect are less reliable Adderall is long-acting Adderall XR is long-acting
Methylphenidate (Ritalin, Methylin, (Metadate) (Concerta) (Ritalin LA)	1–2 1–2 up to 1.0	bid or tid Once a day		Metadate CD, Ritalin LA, and Concerta are long-acting
d-Methylphenidate (Focalin)	0.25–0.5	bid or tid		
Magnesium pemoline (Cylert)	1–2.5	Once to bid		Pemoline has effect of rare serious hepatotoxicity; requires monitoring of liver function tests
Antidepressants				
Tricyclics (TCAs)				
Tertiary amines Imipramine Amitriptyline Clomipramine	2–5 Dose adjusted according to serum levels (therapeutic window for nortriptyline)	Once or bid	ADHD Enuresis Tic disorder ?Anxiety disorders OCD (Clomipramine)	Mixed mechanism of action (noradrenergic/ serotonergic) Secondary amines are more noradrenergic Clomipramine is primarily serotonergic Narrow therapeutic index Overdoses can be fatal Anticholinergic (dry mouth, constipation, blurred vision) Weight gain
Secondary amines Desipramine Nortriptyline	1–3			Cardiovascular (mild increase) diastolic blood pressure and EKG conduction parameters with daily doses >3.5 mg/kg Treatment requires serum level and EKG monitoring No known long-term side effects Withdrawal effects can occur (severe gastrointestinal symptoms, malaise) Risk of seizures
Monoamine oxidase inhibitors (MAOIs)				
Phenelzine Tranylcypromine	0.5–1 mg/kg	bid	Atypical depression	Difficult medicines to use in juveniles Reserved for refractory cases

(continued)

TABLE 35.1 *Major Drug Classes Used in the Pharmacotherapy of Attention-Deficit Hyperactivity Disorder* (*continued*)

Drug[a]	Daily Dose[b] (mg/kg)	Daily Dosage Schedule	Main Indications	Common Adverse Effects, Comments
Selegiline	0.2–0.4 mg/kg		Treatment-refractory depression	Severe dietary restrictions (high-tyramine foods) Drug–drug interactions Hypertensive crisis with dietetic transgression or with certain drugs Weight gain Drowsiness Changes in blood pressure Insomnia Liver toxicity (remote)

New antidepressants

Selective serotonin reuptake inhibitors (SSRIs)

Fluoxetine, paroxetine, citalopram	0.3–0.9	Once (in the AM)	MD, dysthymia OCD	Mechanism of action is serotonergic (not known to be effective anti-ADHD agents)
Sertraline	1.5–3		Anxiety disorders	
Fluvoxamine	1.5–4.5		Eating disorders ?PTSD	Large margin of safety No cardiovascular effects Irritability Insomnia GI symptoms Headaches Sexual dysfunction Withdrawal symptoms more common in short-acting agents Potential drug–drug interactions (cytochrome P450)
Bupropion (SR)	3–6	bid	ADHD MD Smoking cessation ?Anti-craving effects ?Bipolar depression	Mixed mechanism of action (dopaminergic/ noradrenergic) Irritability Insomnia Drug-induced seizures (in doses >6mg/kg) Contraindicated in bulimics
Venlafaxine (XR)	1–3	Once a day	MD Anxiety disorders ?ADHD ?OCD	Mixed mechanism of action (serotonergic/noradrenergic) Similar to SSRIs Irritability Insomnia GI symptoms Headaches Potential withdrawal symptoms Blood pressure changes
Nefazodone	4–8	Once a day	MD Anxiety disorders ?OCD ?Bipolar depression	Mixed mechanism of action (serotonergic/noradrenergic) Rare liver toxicity Dizziness Nausea Potential interactions with nonsedating antihistamines, cisapride (cytochrome P450) ?Less manicogenic

(continued)

TABLE 35.1 *(continued)*

Drug[a]	*Daily Dose*[b] *(mg/kg)*	*Daily Dosage Schedule*	*Main Indications*	*Common Adverse Effects, Comments*
Mirtazapine	0.2–0.9	Once (in the PM)	MD Anxiety disorders ?Stimulant-induced insomnia ?Bipolar depression	Mixed mechanism of action (serotonergic/noradrenergic) Sedation Weight gain Dizziness ?Less manicogenic
Noradrenergic modulators				
α₂ Agonists				
Clonidine	0.003–0.01	bid or tid	Tourette's syndrome ADHD Aggression/self-abuse Severe agitation Withdrawal syndromes	Sedation (very frequent) Hypotension (rare) Dry mouth Confusion (with high dose) Depression Rebound hypertension Localized irritation with transdermal preparation
Guanfacine	0.015–0.05	Once, bid or tid		Same as clonidine Less sedation, hypotension
Beta-blockers				
Propranolol	1–7	bid	Aggression/self abuse Severe agitation Akathisia	Sedation Depression Risk for bradycardia and hypotension (dose dependent) and rebound hypertension Bronchospasm (contraindicated in asthmatics) Rebound hypertension on abrupt withdrawal

ADHD, attention-deficit hyperactivity disorder; EKG, electrocardiogram; GI, gastrointestinal; MD, major depression; MR, mental retardation; OCD, obsessive-compulsive disorder; PTSD, post-traumatic stress disorder. [a]Trade names are in parentheses. [b]Doses are general guidelines. All doses must be individualized with appropriate monitoring. Weight-corrected doses are less appropriate for obese children.

of ADHD, matching that seen in boys (Sharp et al., 1999). Furthermore, there are a growing number of long-term studies documenting the persistence of stimulant-associated improvements (Hechtman and Abikoff, 1995; Gillberg et al., 1997; Schachar et al., 1997, 1999).

Stimulants have profound affects on social skills and apparent emotional maturity. In several studies, stimulants appeared to "normalize" behaviors of children with ADHD (Whalen, 1989). Investigations of peer relationships in children with ADHD show that those treated with stimulants have increased abilities to perceive peer communications, self-perceptions, and situational cues. These children show improved modulation of the intensity of behavior, improved communication, and greater responsiveness (Whalen et al.,

1990). Additionally, stimulant-associated improvements in social interactions positively influence the social behavior of others in the child's environment (Cunningham et al., 1991; Whalen and Henker, 1992). Parents, teachers, siblings, and peers are more positive toward and less critical of the treated child with ADHD. Thus, when social impairments are associated with ADHD symptoms, pharmacotherapy may be a useful treatment modality.

Consistent with theories on the cognitive underpinnings of ADHD, stimulants have been demonstrated to improve cognitive function as measured by tests of vigilance, impulsivity, reaction time, short term memory, and learning of verbal and nonverbal material in children with ADHD (Barkley, 1977b; Klein, 1987; Rapport et al. 1988). These stimulant-associated improve-

TABLE 35.2 *Pharmacotherapy of Treatment Algorithm for Attention-Deficit Hyperactivity Disorder*

Main characteristics	Pharmacotherapy			
	First Line	Second Line	Third Line	Fourth Line
Inattentiveness, impulsivity, hyperactivity 50% will continue to manifest the disorder into adulthood	Stimulants (70% response; for uncomplicated ADHD; caution in patients with tic disorders)	TCAs (70% response, first line for patients with comorbid MD or anxiety disorders, and for patients with ADHD + tics); requires serum levels and cardiovascular monitoring Bupropion	Clonidine, guanfacine (first line for patients with ADHD + tics)	MAOIs Combined pharmacotherapy for treatment-resistant cases

ments have also been demonstrated in a simulated classroom paradigm (Barkley, 1991; DuPaul et al., 1994). It appears, however, that the primary deficits in ADHD are those of regulation of cognitive function and executive deficits (Reader et al., 1994; Barkley, 1997), cognitive deficits that are not as amenable to measurement by objective tests. In individual children, the more prominent behavioral effects of stimulants have been more useful in clinically monitoring stimulant treatment than cognitive tests per se. Neuropsychological testing may be important to detect additional learning disabilities that would not be responsive to pharmacotherapy (Bergman et al., 1991; Faraone et al., 1993).

While originally it was thought that cognition and behavior were responsive to different doses of stimulants (Sprague and Sleator, 1977), recent studies indicate that both behavior and cognitive performance improve with stimulant treatment in a dose-dependent fashion (Pelham et al., 1985; Klein, 1987; Rapport et al., 1987, 1989a, b; Douglas et al., 1988; Kupietz et al., 1988; Tannock et al., 1989). Also, despite previous concerns, doses that improve behavior rarely constrict attention or cause "overfocusing" (Solanto and Wender, 1989; Douglas et al., 1995).

Common side effects include appetite suppression and sleep disturbances. Usually sleep disturbances can be alleviated by lowering late-afternoon treatment or adding clonidine or other medications (Brown and Gammon, 1992; Prince et al., 1996). Occasionally, mild increases in pulse and blood pressure of unclear clinical significance have been observed (Brown et al., 1984). Stimulant-associated toxic psychosis appears to be rare but resembles a toxic phenomenon (e.g., visual hallucinosis) and not a schizotypal-like exacerbation of psychotic symptoms. Administration of pemoline has been associated with hypersensitivity reactions involving the liver accompanied by elevations in liver function tests (SGOT and SGPT) after several months of treatment (Shevell and Schreriber, 1997). The Food and

Drug Administration (FDA) recommends monitoring liver function every 2 weeks. It is also advisable to educate parents about the warning symptoms of hepatitis. Such symptoms include stomach pain, gastrointestinal (GI) distress, and change of color of urine (darker) or stool (lighter).

There have been long-standing concerns about stimulant-associated growth deficits in children with ADHD; however, no consistent neurohormonal pathophysiology has been identified to explain stimulant-associated height deficits (Spencer et al., 1998b). Preliminary work from our group suggests that ADHD may be associated with temporary deficits (delays) in height, velocity through mid-adolescence that may normalize by late adolescence (Spencer et al., 1996a). Until recently, drug holidays were often advocated to avoid growth problems. Current evidence suggests that drug holidays are not warranted in the absence of documented growth deficits. However, children on stimulants should be monitored for growth progression and evaluated further if growth velocity declines unduly.

While ADHD appears to be a major factor in the impairment attributed to Tourette's Syndrome (Spencer et al., 1998a), it is unclear if the presence of tics has a general impact on the course of ADHD. Our group examined this issue in an ongoing prospective study of ADHD boys (Spencer et al., 1999). We found that boys with ADHD had more tic disorders at baseline and follow-up than controls. However, tic disorders had little impact on the psychosocial functioning of ADHD boys and stimulant treatment was not associated with increased rates, severity, or persistence of tic disorders. Nonetheless, a longitudinal study of children with Tourette's Syndrome and ADHD reported that 30% of study subjects had to discontinue stimulant treatment because of worsening of their tics acutely or over time (Castellanos et al., 1997). Until more is known, it seems prudent to weigh risks and benefits of individual cases, and have appropriate discussions with the patient and family regarding the use of stimulants in individuals with ADHD and tics.

While stimulants are potentially abusable, recent evidence suggests that stimulant treatment substantially reduces the risk for substance abuse generated by ADHD cognitive and behavioral impairments (Biederman et al., 1999b). Moreover, another study has shown that the most commonly abused substance in ADHD adolescents and adults is marijuana and not stimulants (Biederman et al., 1995b). Appropriate education and monitoring are crucial to the safe prescription of psychostimulants in adolescents and adults.

The growing appreciation of the need for treatment throughout the day has led to the development of new long-acting preparations. These compounds employ novel delivery systems to overcome acute tachyphylaxis. Concerta uses an osmotic pump mechanism that creates an ascending profile of methylphenidate in the blood to provide effective extended treatment for 10–12 hours, Concerta is available in 18, 36, and 54 mg to approximate 5, 10 and 15 mg TID dosing of methylphenidate IR. Metadate-CD and Ritalin-LA are both capsules with a mixture of immediate and delayed release beads to provide effective methylphenidate treatment for 8–9 hours. In Metadate-CD, 30% of the beads are immediate release and 70% delayed. Metadate-CD is available in 20 mg capsules to approximate 10 mg BID dosing of Methylphenidate IR. In contrast, with Ritalin-LA, there is a 50:50 ratio of immediate and delayed beads. Ritalin-LA will be available in 20, 30, and 40 mg capsules to approximate 10, 15, and 20 mg BID dosing of methylphenidate IR. Adderall XR is a capsule with a 50:50 ratio of immediate to delayed release beads designed to provide effective amphetamine (Adderall) treatment for 12 hours. Adderall XR is available in 10, 20, and 30 mg capsules to approximate 5, 10, and 15 mg BID dosing (0 and 4 hours) of Adderall. Preparations of beads in capsules (all but Concerta) may be used as sprinkle preparations for children unable to swallow pills.

Methylphenidate as a secondary amine gives rise to four optical isomers: d-threo, l-threo, d-erythro, and l-erythro. There is stereoselectivity in receptor site binding and its relationship to response. The standard preparation is comprised of the threo recemate as it appears to be the CNS active form. Moreover, recent data suggests that the d-methylphenidate isomer is the active form. This has led to the development of a purified d, threo-methylphenidate compound, Focalin. Studies have shown Focalin to be at least as effective as the racemate at half the dosage. Focalin is available in 2.5, 5, and 10 mg to approximate 5, 10, and 20 mg of d,l methylphenidate.

Antidepressants

Tricyclic antidepressants

Tricyclic antidepressants (TCAs) modulate various brain neurotransmitters, especially norepinephrine and serotonin, by blocking reuptake presynaptically. The secondary amines (desipramine, nortriptyline) are more selective for noradrenergic function and have less side effects in sensitive populations. Advantages of this class of drugs include their relative long half life (approximately 12 hours), absence of abuse potential, and putative positive effects on mood and anxiety, sleep, and tics.

There are 33 studies (>1200 subjects) that have evaluated TCAs in children, adolescents, and adults. Most of these studies reported positive effects on ADHD symptoms. Although most TCA studies were relatively brief, lasting a few weeks to several months, nine studies reported enduring effects for up to 2 years. Outcomes in both short and long-term studies were equally positive. While initial reports suggested tolerance to TCAs over time, recent studies have reported sustained improvement for up to a year with desipramine (DMI) (Gastfriend et al., 1985; Biederman et al., 1986) and nortriptyline (Wilens et al., 1993) when a full antidepressant dosage was used. The interindividual relationship between drug dose and serum level is highly variable for DMI and imipramine, as is the relationship between dose and response or side effects. In contrast, nortriptyline appears to have a positive association between dose and serum level (Wilens et al., 1993).

The largest juvenile, controlled trial of a TCA reported favorable results with DMI in 62 clinically referred children with ADHD (Biederman et al., 1989). Many of these children had previously failed to respond to psychostimulant treatment. Sixty-eight percent of DMI-treated patients were considered very much or much improved, compared with only 10% of placebo patients ($p < 0.001$), at an average daily dose of 5 mg/kg. In a further analysis, neither comorbidity with conduct disorder, depression, or anxiety, nor a family history of ADHD yielded differential responses to DMI treatment (Biederman et al., 1993b). In addition, DMI-treated ADHD patients showed a substantial reduction in depressive symptoms compared with placebo-treated patients.

In a prospective placebo-controlled discontinuation trial, we recently demonstrated the efficacy of nortriptyline in doses of up to 2 mg/kg daily in 35 school-aged youth with ADHD (Prince et al., 2000). In that study, 80% of youth responded by week 6 in the open phase. During the discontinuation phase, subjects randomized to placebo lost the anti-ADHD effect. There was a lag in response to medication administration; while the full dosage was achieved by week 2, the full effect evolved slowly over the ensuing 4 weeks. Youth with ADHD receiving nortriptyline also were found to have more modest but statistically significant reductions in oppositionality and anxiety. Nortriptyline was well tolerated, with some weight gain being considered a desirable adverse effect.

Studies of TCAs have uniformly reported a robust rate of response of ADHD symptoms in ADHD subjects with comorbid depression or anxiety (Cox 1982; Biederman et al., 1993b; Wilens et al., 1993, 1995). In addition, studies of TCAs have consistently reported a robust rate of response in ADHD subjects with comorbid tic disorders (Dillon et al., 1985; Hoge and Biederman, 1986; Riddle et al., 1988; Spencer et al., 1993a,b; Singer et al., 1994). For example, in a recent controlled study, Spencer et al. replicated data from a retrospective chart review, indicating that DMI had a robust beneficial effect on ADHD and tic symptoms (Spencer, 1997).

Reports of sudden unexplained death in four ADHD children treated with DMI have engendered concerns about the safety of the use of TCAs in children (Abramowicz, 1990), although the causal link between DMI and these deaths remains uncertain. A rather extensive literature evaluating cardiovascular parameters in TCA-exposed youth consistently identified mostly minor, asymptomatic, but statistically significant, increases in heart rate and electrocardiographic (EKG) measures of cardiac conduction times associated with TCA treatment (Biederman et al., 1993ab). At a National Institutes of Health (NIH) conference, it was noted that the incidence rate of sudden death in children and adolescents of 1–4 100,000 year is unrelated to the presence of a psychiatric disorder or to medication use (D. Atkins, Special Emphasis Panel on Cardiac Arrhythmia's in Children, August 29, 1996). Three-quarters of these deaths are thought to be due to preexisting cardiac conditions such as hypertrophic cardiomyopathy or anomalies of the coronary arteries. Because some of the lesions are small, accurate diagnosis requires meticulous autopsies by cardiac pathologists. A recent report estimated that the magnitude of DMI-associated risk of sudden death in children may not be much larger than the baseline risk of sudden death in this age group (Biederman et al., 1995b). Abnormal EKGs or symptoms pertaining to the cardiovascular system would indicate the need for reassessment of the risks and benefits of treatment with TCAs. Consultation with a pediatric cardiologist may be necessary to establish guidelines for safe use of TCAs in children with an unusual cardiac risk.

Non-tricyclic antidepressants

Bupropion. A part of the structure of bupropion hydrochloride is related to the endogenous amphetamine-like substance phenylethylamine. Accordingly, bupropion appears to possess both indirect dopamine agonist and noradrenergic effects. Bupropion has been shown to be effective in the treatment of ADHD in children in a large, controlled multisite study (N = 72) (Casat et al., 1987; 1989; Conners et al., 1996) and in a comparison with methylphenidate (N = 15) (Barrickman et al., 1995). Similarly, bupropion has been found to be well tolerated and effective in a controlled study of ADHD adults by our group (Wilens et al., 2001) and in a long-term open study of ADHD adults (Wender and Reimherr, 1990). In the adult studies, dosing (300–400 mg) and lag to response (6 to 8 weeks) appeared to be similar to that observed in studies of depression. The slightly increased risk (0.4%) for drug-induced seizures of bupropion has been linked to high doses, to a previous history of seizures, and to eating disorders. Thus, by avoiding these risk factors, and by dividing the daily dose or using the long-acting preparation, the risk of seizures may be comparable to that of other antidepressants. Bupropion is generally well tolerated, and does not have the cardiac conduction difficulties of TCAs or the sexual and GI side effects of the serotonergic antidepressants.

Monoamine oxidase inhibitors. The monoamine oxidase inhibitors (MAOIs) inhibit the intracellular catabolic enzyme monoamine oxidase. There are two types of monoamine oxidase: MAO-A and MAO-B, both of which metabolize tyramine and dopamine. In addition, MAO-A preferentially metabolizes norepinephrine, epinephrine, and serotonin, and MAO-B preferentially metabolizes phenylethylamine (an endogenous amphetamine-like substance) and N-methylhistamine (Ernst, 1996). Some MAOIs are selective for A or B and some are nonselective (mixed). In addition, irreversible MAOIs (e.g., phenelzine, tranylcypromine) are more susceptible to the "cheese effect" than are the reversible agents (e.g., moclobemide).

Preliminary studies suggest that MAOIs are effective in juvenile and adult ADHD. In a controlled trial of clorygline (MAOI-A) and tranylcypromine sulfate (mixed), Zametkin et al. (1985) reported a significant reduction in ADHD symptoms with minimal adverse effects. Feigin et al. (1996) conducted a controlled trial of 10 mg of selegiline (which at low doses is a specific MAOI-B) in children with ADHD and Tourette's syndrome. Selegiline was well tolerated and was associated with a robust ADHD response in the first period of the study.

In open studies of adult ADHD, moderate improvements were reported in studies with pargyline and selegiline (MAOI-Bs) (Wender et al., 1983, 1985). In a controlled study of selegiline in adult ADHD (Ernst 1996), use of active drug failed to produce results different from those with placebo; however, the placebo response was unusually high in that study. In addition, a high dose (60 mg) was more effective than a low dose (20 mg), which suggests that MAOI-A effects may be more helpful in the treatment of ADHD.

A major limitation to the use of MAOIs is the potential for hypertensive crisis (treatable with phentolamine) associated with dietetic transgressions (tyramine-containing foods, i.e., most cheeses) and drug interactions (pressor amines, most cold medicines, amphetamines). A serotonergic syndrome may occur when MAOIs are combined with predominantly serotonergic drugs (e.g., SSRIs). Currently, dietetic restrictions and potential drug–drug interactions limit the use of MAOIs in juveniles. Nonetheless, they may be important to consider in individuals with treatment-refractory ADHD. The ongoing development of reversible and transdermal preparations may lead to MAOIs with a more favorable safety profile.

Selective serotonin reuptake inhibitors. Currently available selective serotonin reuptake inhibitors (SSRIs) include fluoxetine, paroxetine, sertraline, fluvoxamine, and citalopram. At present, expert opinion does not support the usefulness of these serotonergic compounds in the treatment of core ADHD symptoms (National Institute of Mental Health, 1996). Nevertheless, because of the high rates of comorbidity in ADHD, these compounds are frequently combined with effective anti-ADHD agents (see Combined Pharmacotherapy, below). Since many psychotropics are metabolized by the cytochrome P450 system (Nemeroff et al., 1996), which in turn can be inhibited by the SSRIs, caution should be exercised when combining agents, such as the TCAs, with SSRIs.

Venlafaxine. Venlafaxine (Effexor) possesses both SSRI and TCA properties (noradrenergic and serotonergic) and is chemically unrelated to other antidepressants. Several open-label studies of adults with ADHD ($N = 61$) (Adler, et al. 1995; Hornig-Rohan and Amsterdam, 1995; Reimherr et al., 1995; Findling et al., 1996) and one such study of children (Luh et al., 1996) have all shown promising results and support further investigation through controlled trials.

Noradrenergic-Specific Compounds

Other noradrenergic compounds also have been proposed for use in ADHD. One such compound is atomoxetine, which is highly and specifically noradrenergic. Unlike the TCAs, *atomoxetine* has no effects on cardiac conduction or repolarization. Ongoing investigations have documented that atomoxetine is effective for ADHD and is well tolerated. In a controlled trial in adults with ADHD, in addition to subjective symptoms, improvement was noted in inhibitory capacity on the Stroop test, an objective measure of neuropsychological function (Spencer, et al. 1998c). An initial open study of children with ADHD documented robust efficacy as well as excellent tolerability, including a lack of effect on EKG parameters (Spencer et al., 2001). Recently, several large multisite studies have established efficacy and tolerability of atomoxetine in juvenile ADHD (Heiligenstein et al., 2000).

α_{-2}, noradrenergic agonists

Clonidine is an α_{-2}, noradrenergic agonist, and guanfacine is a more selective α_{2a} agonist. Preclinical studies have suggested a possible role for these compounds in enhancing cognitive functioning in the prefrontal cortex (Arnsten et al., 1996). Moreover, a relatively small number of clinical studies (Hunt et al., 1985, 1995; Hunt, 1987; Gunning, 1992; Steingard et al., 1993; Horrigan and Barnhill, 1995) have documented a positive behavioral response with less clear benefit to cognition. A recent placebo-controlled study of guanfacine use in the treatment of ADHD and comorbid tics has shown promising results (Scahill et al, 2001), as further described in Chapter 21 by Newcorn and colleagues in this volume.

Recent reports of death in children who had received clonidine plus other medications have led to heightened concerns about the cardiovascular safety of clonidine. However, due to many mitigating and extenuating circumstances, causality in these cases is uninterpretable (Fenichel, 1995; Popper, 1995; Wilens and Spencer, 1999). For example, one case appeared to be an overdose of other unrelated medication. Moreover, in studies monitoring adverse effects of clonidine, no clinically meaningful EKG changes have been identified. At this time, caution is advised in prescribing this drug.

Buspirone

Buspirone is a nonbenzodiazepine anxiolytic that has recently been tested as an anti-ADHD treatment for children. Buspirone has a high affinity to 5-HT$_{1A}$ receptors, as well as a modest effect on the dopaminergic system and α-adrenergic activity. A recent open study of buspirone (0.5 mg/kg/day) in ADHD children reported less disruptive behavior and improvement in psychosocial function, with only mild side effects (Malhotra and Santosh, 1998). These preliminary findings provide limited support for ongoing controlled trials of buspirone in ADHD treatment.

Cholinergic Drugs

Support for a nicotinic hypothesis of ADHD can be derived from preclinical investigations, associations with cigarette smoking, and recent treatment studies. Nicotine has been shown to enhance dopaminergic neurotransmission (Westfall et al., 1983; Mereu et al., 1987; Dalack et al., 1998). Data suggesting that maternal smoking during pregnancy increases the risk for ADHD in the offspring (Milberger et al., 1996) are consistent with animal data showing that in utero exposure to nicotine increases the risk for an ADHD-like syndrome (Johns et al., 1982; Fung, 1988; Fung and Lau, 1989). ADHD is associated with an increased risk and earlier age of onset of cigarette smoking (Pomerleau et al., 1996; Milberger et al., 1997). In non-ADHD subjects, nicotine has been shown to possess cognitive benefits such as improved temporal memory (Meck and Church, 1987), attention (Peeke and Peeke, 1984; Wesnes and Warburton, 1984; Jones et al., 1992), improved cognitive vigilance (Wesnes and Warburton, 1984; Parrott and Winder, 1989; Jones et al., 1992), and improved executive function (Wesnes and Warburton, 1984).

In adults with ADHD, Levin and colleagues (1996) documented that transdermal nicotine resulted in significant improvement of ADHD symptoms, working memory, and neuropsychological functioning. Similarly, promising results have been reported in a clinical trial of ABT-418, a cholinergic nicotinic activating agent with structural similarities to nicotine. Phase 1 studies of this compound in humans have indicated a low abuse liability, as well as adequate safety and tolerability in elderly adults (Abbott laboratories, unpublished data). In a placebo-controlled trial of a transdermal preparation (75 mg daily), ABT-418 was more effective than placebo (40% vs. 13%; $\chi^2 = 5.3$, $p = 0.021$) in adults with childhood-onset ADHD (Biederman et al., 1999b). Although preliminary, these results suggest that nicotinic and perhaps other cholinergic analogs may be useful anti-ADHD agents.

Antipsychotics

In early ADHD literature, typical antipsychotics for ADHD were found to be mildly efficacious for behav-

ioral symptoms in hyperactive children. However, the lack of cognitive enhancement and the risk of long-term adverse effects (such as tardive dyskinesia) greatly limit their usefulness in the treatment of ADHD.

PSYCHIATRIC COMORBIDITY

Since ADHD is a risk factor for several comorbidies, these conditions can frequently complicate considerations of pharmacotherapy; for example, ADHD is often accompanied by aggressive behavior and conduct disorder. A substantial number of controlled studies have reported improvement in ADHD and aggressive symptoms in ADHD subjects treated with stimulants (Gadow et al., 1990; Kaplan et al., 1990; Pelham et al., 1990; Cunningham et al., 1991; Hinshaw et al., 1992; Livingston et al., 1992; Murphy et al., 1992; Klorman et al., 1994). In these reports, stimulants suppressed physical and nonphysical aggression in children both at home and in school in a dose-dependent fashion. Responsive symptoms included verbal and physical aggression, negative social interactions with peers in group settings, and covert antisocial behavior (stealing, destroying property, but not cheating). There was little effect, however, on social informational processing in these ADHD children. While one report suggests that stimulant treatment ameliorates symptoms of childhood conduct disorder independent of the context of ADHD (Klein et al., 1997), it remains questionable whether premeditated antisocial actions are amenable to stimulant treatment alone.

Stimulants can induce anxiety (Swanson et al., 1978; Gittelman, 1986) or depression (Barkley, 1977a; Gittelman, 1986; Barkley et al., 1990; Wilens and Biederman, 1992) in susceptible patients. In addition, it has been thought that the presence of comorbid mood and anxiety disorders significantly worsen the response of ADHD symptoms to stimulant treatment (Swanson et al., 1978; Voelker et al., 1983; Taylor et al., 1987; Pliszka, 1989; DuPaul et al., 1994; Tannock et al., 1995). Two studies have challenged this view. Diamond and colleagues (1997) reported that despite more physiologic symptoms at baseline, ADHD children with and without anxiety benefited equally from stimulant treatment (Diamond et al., 1999). In the Multimodal Treatment Study of Children with ADHD (MTA), (MTA Cooperative Group, 1999), not only was stimulant treatment equally beneficial in children with and without anxiety but it appeared to improve the anxiety itself. A subsequent analysis by the study authors revealed, however that the construct measured may have been more closely related to an ADHD-related "negative affectivity" than traditional (phobic) anxiety (March et al., 2000).

As may be expected, studies of antidepressants in treatment of ADHD have not shown a differential effect in ADHD children with or without conduct disorder, depression, or anxiety (Biederman et al., 1993b). While DMI-treated ADHD children showed a substantial reduction in depressive symptoms compared with placebo-treated patients (Biederman et al., 1989), DMI appears not to be as powerful an antidepressant in children as the SSRIs. (Bostic et al., 1999). The safety and efficacy of combined SSRI and stimulant pharmacotherapy has been addressed in two open studies and is currently being evaluated in a prospective study conducted by the Resarch Units in Pediatric Psychopharmacology (RUPP) Network (B. *Vitiello*, personal communication).

Despite increasing recognition of the co-occurrence of ADHD and bipolarity (West et al., 1995; Wozniak et al., 1995), little is known about the pharmacotherapy of the combined condition. To evaluate pharmacological approaches for ADHD children who have manic symptoms, we conducted a chart review of 38 children and adolescents over multiple visits (and treatments) to assess correlates of improvement (Biederman et al., 1999a). In this sample we had shown that mood stabilizers (lithium, carbemazepine, valproate) improved manic symptoms but not ADHD (Biederman et al., 1998). A subsequent analysis revealed that mood stabilization was a prerequisite for the successful pharmacologic treatment of ADHD in children. Although TCAs can be helpful in the management of ADHD children with manic-like symptoms, these drugs should be used with caution as they can also have a destabilizing effect on manic symptoms.

COMBINED PHARMACOTHERAPY

Rapport et al. (1993) reported on the safety and efficacy of separate and combined effects of methylphenidate and DMI in 16 hospitalized children. Methylphenidate alone improved vigilance, both methylphenidate and DMI alone produced positive affects on short-term memory and visual problem solving, and their combination produced an effect on the learning of higher-order relationships. The authors speculated that performance on different cognitive measures may be modulated by separate neurotransmitter systems and that the combination produced a useful synergism. The subjects in this study were children with ADHD and comorbid major depression, dysthymia, and anxiety. These investigators (Pataki et al., 1993) also reported that there was no evidence that the combined use of both drugs was associated with unique or serious side effects.

Cohen et al. (1999) reported an absence of a clinically significant pharmacokinetic interaction between DMI and stimulants in children. In their study, 403 serum concentrations from 142 subjects were examined. Pharmacokinetic parameters were similar for both the DMI and DMI + stimulant groups, including the mean weight-corrected dose (mg/kg), weight and dose–normalized DMI serum concentrations [(μg/L)/mg/kg], and DMI clearance (L/kg)/hr.

The safety and efficacy of combined SSRI and stimulant pharmacotherapy have been addressed in two open studies. Gammon and Brown (1993) reported on the successful addition of fluoxetine to stimulants in the treatment of 32 patients with ADHD with comorbid depressive and anxiety disorders (Gammon and Brown 1993). These children with comorbid conditions had failed to respond to methylphenidate alone. Another report detailed the addition of methylphenidate to SSRI treatment (Findling, 1996). Depressed children and adults with comorbid ADHD were treated with either fluoxetine or sertraline. While depressive symptoms remitted, ADHD symptoms persisted. Methylphenidate was added and successfully treated the ADHD symptoms. In both investigations, the combined treatment was well tolerated.

NON PHARMACOLOGIC INTERVENTIONS

Though empirical evidence supporting the effectiveness of psychosocial treatment for ADHD is equivocal, parents and teachers often seek guidance regarding effective nonmedical management of children with ADHD. The development and application of psychosocial treatment procedures for ADHD are grounded in theories related to (a) how human behavior is trained and maintained, and (b) the core deficits underlying ADHD. Such procedures fall roughly into one of two categories. *Operant procedures* (also referred to as *behavior modification* procedures) are based on the notions that (a) human behavior is trained and maintained through its consequences and (b) individuals with ADHD have difficulty considering the consequences of their actions and cause-and-effect relationships, at least at moments when such considerations are most crucial (Pelham and Sams, 1992; Anastopoulos et al. 1998). Operant procedures are aimed at exerting "external control" over behaviors associated with ADHD. By contrast, *cognitive-behavioral procedures* can best be conceived as training "internal control" over behaviors associated with ADHD, and stem from the notions that (a) much of human behavior is governed by cognitive processes and trained through observational learning and modeling, and (*b*) individuals with ADHD have difficulty bringing to bear various internal controls (e.g., sustained attention, impulse control, problem solving) at moments when such controls are most crucial. These procedures have evolved from the early work of Meichenbaum and Goodman (1971), Douglas (1980), and others (see Hinshaw and Earhardt, 1991, for a review).

Briefly, operant programs typically involve application of contingency management procedures at home, or school, or both. Such programs, while varying in form and content (e.g., home-based contingency contracts, home–school daily report cards), involve (*1*) identifying specific target behaviors (e.g., compliance with adult directives, completion of classwork and homework, on-task behavior, etc.), (*2*) developing a menu of specific rewards and punishments (e.g., privilege gain and loss, time-out from reinforcement), and (*3*) establishing a "currency" system (e.g., points, stickers, tokens) to track a child's degree of success in meeting target behaviors and thereby signal the dispensing of rewards or punishments (Pfiffner and O'Leary, 1993; Abramowitz, 1994).

Operant procedures have been shown to be effective at reducing some of the primary and secondary behaviors associated with ADHD, but only while the procedures are actively implemented. In other words, studies have shown that, like medication, the treatment gains achieved by such procedures are not maintained once their active application ends. Treatment gains achieved by operant procedures are typically not as great as those achieved by high doses of stimulant medication. Rarely do ADHD children treated with such procedures progress to within the "normal" range of functioning, and a meaningful percentage fails to show any improvement (Pelham, 1989; Hinshaw et al., 1998). It has been suggested that these limitations are due, at least in part, to the willingness (or lack thereof) of parents and teachers to implement operant programs (Pelham and Murphy, 1986).

The cognitive-behavioral approach has also varied in form and content, and has included the training of skills such as self-instruction, self-evaluation, self-monitoring, self-reinforcement, anger management; and social behavior. Such procedures train children to modify, via self-talk, the cognitions that precede and accompany overt behavior, thereby helping to orient children to the task at hand, organize a behavioral strategy, and regulate performance until it is completed. For example, in problem-solving training (a self-instruction strategy), children are taught to identify the problem at hand, generate alternative solutions, consider the likely outcomes of each solution, monitor and evaluate such outcomes, and self-reward and self-

punish successful or unsuccessful outcomes (Hinshaw and Erhardt, 1991; Hinshaw and Melnick, 1992). These cognitive skills have been trained in individual and group formats, with role-playing and modeling as the primary training tools.

The limited number of studies examining the efficacy of cognitive-behavioral procedures in children with ADHD have produced disappointing findings. In general, cognitive-behavioral interventions have produced minimal, if any, change in the primary and secondary behaviors associated with ADHD (Abikoff, 1985, 1987). However, studies have been limited by the degree to which adults were actively involved in treatment, the mechanisms by which such involvement occurred, the degree to which cognitive-behavioral treatment was individualized, and the duration of treatment.

On the basis of recent theoretical notions of ADHD, Barkley (1997) has provided a rationale for the equivocal findings regarding the effectiveness of cognitive-behavioral treatment of ADHD. Barkley notes that, because of the neurogenetic origin of ADHD, treatments are unlikely to ameliorate the disorder because they cannot correct the underlying neurological substrates or genetic mechanisms contributing to its development. Thus, Barkley has argued that treatment be best understood as management of a chronic developmental condition and should therefore focus on finding the means to cope with, compensate for, and accommodate the developmental deficiencies imposed by the disorder. Further, Barkley has suggested that ADHD be viewed as a disorder of performance (i.e., of doing what one knows) rather than of lacking knowledge (i.e., of knowing what to do). From this perspective, children with ADHD are conceived as unlikely to benefit from interventions aimed at the training of knowledge or skills (as occurs in cognitive-behavioral treatment), because lacking knowledge and skills is not at the core of their difficulties. Thus, it is argued, training more knowledge is not as helpful as altering the motivational parameters associated with the performance of adaptive behaviors at the appropriate points of performance through operant procedures (Barkley, 1997).

More recent studies have examined combinations of medical and nonmedical treatments for ADHD, usually in an effort to determine whether one form of treatment is superior to, or enhances the effectiveness of, another. The largest-scale study examining the relative and combined effectiveness of medical and nonmedical interventions for ADHD is the recently completed MTA study (MTA Cooperative Group, 1999). In this 5-year, six-site project, 579 elementary school–age children with ADHD were randomly assigned to one of four 14-month treatment conditions: behavioral treatment, medication management (usually methylpheni-date), combined behavioral treatment and medication management, and a community comparison group (most of the children in the latter group were receiving medication for ADHD). Key outcome assessment occurred at 9 and 14 months. Children in the behavioral treatment arm received a very intensive combination of predominantly operant treatment ingredients, including school consultation, a classroom aide, an 8-week summer treatment program, and 35 sessions of parent management training. Behavioral treatment was faded prior to the final assessment. By contrast, pharmacotherapy, in both the medication management and combined treatment conditions, was not tapered but rather was ongoing throughout treatment.

Initial reports of findings from the MTA study indicate that, similar to prior findings, medical intervention was significantly more effective than behavioral and community treatments; behavioral treatment only modestly (and nonsignificantly) enhanced the effect of medication alone; and behavioral treatment alone was no more effective than the treatment received by children in the community comparison group (Jensen, 1998). Pelham (1999) has argued that these findings are at least partially attributable to the design of the MTA study–namely, the behavioral treatment was faded over time whereas medical treatment was not. Pelham (1999) has also suggested that the MTA findings actually support the notion that behavioral treatment alone improves the functioning of children with ADHD, as the children who received behavioral treatment alone improved at a level commensurate with that in the community comparison group, most of whom were receiving medical treatment.

Another major concern with the nonmedical treatment component of the MTA study relates to what some might view as a fairly narrow range of treatment ingredients. The behavioral treatment arm (originally referred to as the "psychosocial" treatment arm) included virtually no nonoperant treatment ingredients (the exception was a social skills training program delivered as part of the summer treatment program component). Thus, the MTA study did not apply a full range of available psychosocial treatment options, but rather an extraordinarily intensive and almost exclusively operant treatment package. Attempts to capture the "core" deficit of ADHD—e.g., to characterize all children with ADHD as suffering from a *performance* deficit rather than a *skills* deficit—inevitably belie the heterogeneity of the disorder. While is seems quite the case that many children with ADHD do indeed suffer from a performance deficit, it is just as plausibly the case that others may not have acquired requisite skills because of the developmental lag that typifies the dis-

order. Presumably, children with ADHD who evidence performance deficits might be those who would benefit maximally from a behavioral treatment approach emphasizing motivational strategies. However, those evidencing deficits in cognitive skills might benefit more from an approach emphasizing the training of such skills. Greene and colleagues (Greene, 1995, 1996; Greene and Doyle, 1999) have referred to the "fit" between a child's actual clinical needs and the treatments delivered to address those needs as "child-treatment compatibility."

For example, the social skills deficits of children with ADHD—known to have extremely adverse ramifications for long-term outcomes (Greene et al., 1997, 1999)—may present in diverse ways and with diverse etiologies: some ADHD children may possess fairly intact social skills but, because of the poor impulse control and overactivity associated with the disorder, evidence difficulty exhibiting such skills on a consistent basis in the ongoing stream of behavior. Such children might well benefit from motivational strategies aimed at enhancing the performance of existing skills. However, other children with ADHD might be compromised in a variety of cognitive skills related to social functioning: social problem-solving skills; modulating one's emotions (e.g., anger, frustration); social self-awareness (knowledge and insight about oneself in social settings); and empathy (perspective taking, awareness of others' feelings, and cognizance of the impact of one's behavior on others) (Eslinger, 1996). The training of some of these cognitive skills might be enhanced by medication, but this presumably occurs on a case-by-case basis as well. However, it is difficult to imagine how operant strategies alone would be well suited to the training of such skills. It is also difficult to determine how these complex cognitive skills could be trained and maintained in the types of brief, nonindividualized, nonproximal cognitive-behavioral programs that have typified the literature. These issues were not addressed in the MTA study, and will require further study. It seems nonetheless premature to dismiss the potential role of cognitive-behavioral treatment in children with ADHD, for to do so leaves only a very narrow range of treatment options available to parents and teachers who must interact with and improve the functioning of such children.

CONCLUSIONS

Despite a large body of literature documenting the effectiveness of medication in the treatment of ADHD, there has been public and professional concern regarding the possible inappropriate diagnosis and prescription of ADHD medications. Recently the Council of Scientific Affairs of the American Medical Association addressed these concerns in a scholarly review (Goldman et al., 1998). Several factors were identified that contributed to existing controversies:

1. Like most psychiatric disorders, diagnostic criteria for ADHD are based on history and behavioral assessment. There are no pathognomonic laboratory or radiologic tests to confirm the diagnosis.

2. ADHD is chronic disorder and requires extended treatment.

3. Treatment includes potentially abusable psychotropic medications.

After a review of the voluminous literature, this distinguished panel concluded that ADHD is one of the best researched disorders in medicine; in fact, the overall data on its validity are far more compelling than those for many other medical conditions. They also concluded that there was little evidence of widespread overdiagnosis or misdiagnosis of ADHD or of widespread overprescription of stimulants by physicians.

Consistent with the current emphasis on cognitive dysregulation in ADHD, treatment concerns have expanded from a primarily behavioral focus to include enhancement of executive functions in scholastic as well as other settings. While stimulants have been the most studied compounds, there is a considerable literature indicating an important role for other psychopharmacologic agents. Noradrenergic and dopaminergic modulation appears to be necessary for effective anti-ADHD treatment. In addition, promising evidence of newer cholinergic agents may provide other useful alternatives. As with all psychiatric disorders, comorbid conditions are prominent and may lead to high morbidity and disability if not addressed. As with other areas of medicine, it is sometimes necessary to use multiple agents to treat comorbidity or to achieve an effective response.

REFERENCES

Abikoff, H. (1985) Efficacy of cognitive training intervention in hyperactive children: a critical review. *Clin Psychol Rev* 5: 479–512.

Abikoff, H. (1987) An evaluation of cognitive behavior therapy for hyperactive children. In: Lahey, B. and Kazdin, A., *Advances in Clinical Child Psychology*, Vol. 10. New York: Plenum Press, pp. 171–216.

Abramowicz, M., ed. (1990) Sudden Death in Children Treated with a Tricyclic Antidepressant. *Med Lett Drugs Ther* 32.53.

Abramowitz, A.J. (1994) Classroom interventions for disruptive behavior disorders. *Child Adolesc Psychiatr Clin North Am* 3:343–360.

Adler, L., Resnick, S., Kunz, M. and Devinsky, O. (1995) Open-label trial of venlafaxine in attention deficit disorder. In: *New Clinical Drug Evaluation Unit Program: 34th Annual Meeting Program* Orlando, FL: NIMH.

American Psychiatric Association (1994) *Diagnostic and Statistical Manual of Mental Disorders, 4th ed.*. Washington, DC: American Psychiatric Association Press.

Anastopoulos, A.D., Smith, J.M., and Wier, E.E. (1998) Counseling and training parents. Barkley R.A., eds. *Attention Deficit Hyperactivity Disorder: A handbook for Diagnosis and Treatment*. New York: Guilford Press, pp. 373–393.

Anderson, J.C., Williams, S., McGee, R., and Silva, P.A. (1987) DSM-III disorders in preadolescent children: prevalence in a large sample from the general population. *Arch Gen Psychiatry* 44: 69–76.

Arnsten, A., Steere, J., and Hunt, R. (1996) The contribution of α_2 noradrenergic mechanisms to prefrontal cortical cognitive function: potenial significance to attention deficit hyperactivity disorder. *Arch Gen Psychiatry* 53:448–455.

Barkley, R.A. (1977a) A review of stimulant drug research with hyperactive children. *J Child Psychol Psychiatry* 18:137–165.

Barkley, R. (1997b) Behavioral inhibition, sustained attention, and executive functions: constructing a unifying theory of ADHD. *Psychol Bull* 121:65–94.

Barkley, R.A. (1991) The ecological validity of laboratory and analogue assessment methods of ADHD symptoms. *J Abnorm Child Psychol* 19:149–178.

Barkley, R.A. (1997b) *ADHD and the Nature of Self-Control*. New York: Guilford Press.

Barkley, R.A. (1998) *Attention Deficit Hyperactivity Disorder: A Handbook for Diagnosis and Treatment*. New York: Guilford Press.

Barkley, R.A., McMurray, M.B., Edelbrock, C.S., and Robbins, K. (1990) Side effects of methylphenidate in children with attention deficit hyperactivity disorder: a systemic, placebo-controlled evaluation. *Pediatrics* 86:184–192.

Barrickman, L., Perry, P., Allen, A., Kuperman, S., Arndt, S., Hermann, K., and Schumacher, E. (1995) Bupropion versus methylphenidate in the treatment of attention-deficit hyperactivity disorder. *J Am Acad Child Adolesc Psychiatry* 34:649–657.

Bauermeister, J., Canino, G., and Bird, H. (1994) Epidemiology of disruptive behavior disorders. *Child Adolesc Psychiatr Clini North Am* 3:177–194.

Bergman, A., Winters, L., and Cornblatt, B. (1991). Methylphenidate: effects on sustained attention. In: Greenhill, L. and Osman, B., eds. *Ritalin: Theory and Patient Management*. New York: Mary Ann Liebert, Inc., pp. 223–231.

Biederman, J., Baldessarini, R., Goldblatt, A., Lapey, K., Doyle, A., and Hesslein, P. (1993a) A naturalistic study of 24-hour electrocardiographic recordings and echocardiographic finding in children and adolescents treated with desipramine. *J Am Acad Child Adolesc Psychiatry* 32:805–813.

Biederman, J., Baldessarini, R.J., Wright, V., Keenan, K., and Faraone, S. (1993b), A double-blind placebo controlled study of desipramine in the treatment of attention deficit disorder: III. Lack of impact of comorbidity and family history factors on clinical response. *J Am Acad Child Adolesc Psychiatry* 32:199–204.

Biederman, J., Baldessarini, R.J., Wright, V., Knee, D. and Harmatz, J. (1989) A double-blind placebo controlled study of desipramine in the treatment of attention deficit disorder: I. Efficacy. *J Am Acad Child Adolesc Psychiatry* 28:777–784.

Biederman, J., Gastfriend, D.R., and Jellinek, M.S. (1986) Desipramine in the treatment of children with attention deficit disorder. *J Clin Psychopharmacol* 6:359–363.

Biederman, J., Mick, E., Bostic, J. Prince, J., Daly, J., Wilens, T.,

Spencer, T., Garcia-Jetton, J., Russell, R., Wozniak, J., and Far-aone, S. (1998) The naturalistic course of pharmacologic treatment of children with manic-like symptoms: a systematic chart review. *J Clin Psychiatry* 59:628–637.

Biederman, J., Mick, E., Prince, J., Bostic, J.O., Wilens, T.E., Spencer, T., Wozniak, J., and Faraone, S.V. (1999a) Systematic chart review of the pharmacologic treatment of comorbid attention deficit hyperactivity disorder in youth with bipolar disorder. *J Child Adolesc Psychopharmacol* 9:247–256.

Biederman, J., Thisted, R., Greenhill, L., and Ryan, N. (1995a) Estimation of the association between desipramine and the risk for sudden death in 5- to 14-year-old children. *J Clin Psychiatry* 56: 87–93.

Biederman, J., Wilens, T., Mick, E., Milberger, S., Spencer, T., and Faraone, S., (1995b) Psychoactive substance use disorder in adults with attention deficit hyperactivity disorder: effects of ADHD and psychiatric comorbidity. *Am J Psychiatry* 152:1652–1658.

Biederman, J., Wilens, T., Mick, E., Spencer, T., and Faraone, S.V. (1999b) Pharmacotherapy of attention-deficit/hyperactivity disorder reduces risk for substance use disorder. *Pediatrics* 104:e20.

Bird, H.R., Canino, G., Rubio-Stipec, M., Gould, M.S. and Ribera, J., Sesman, M., Woodbury, M., Huertas-Goldman, S. Pagan, A., Sanchez-Lacay, A., Moscoso, M. (1988) Estimates of the prevalence of childhood maladjustment in a community survey in Puerto Rico: the use of combined measures. *Arch Gen Psychiatry* 45:1120–1126.

Bird, H.R., Gould, M.S., and Staghezza, B.M. (1993) Patterns of psychiatric comorbidity in a community sample of children aged 9 through 16 years. *J Am Acad Child Adolesc Psychiatry* 32:361–368.

Bostic, J., Wilens, T., Spencer, T., and Biederman, J. (1999) Pharmacologic treatment of juvenile depression. *Psychiat Clin North Am* 6:175–191.

Brown, R.T., Wynne, M.E., and Slimmer, L.W. (1984) Attention deficit disorder and the effect of methylphenidate on attention, behavioral, and cardiovascular functioning. *J Clin Psychiatry* 45: 473–476.

Brown, T.E. and Gammon, G.D. (1992) ADHD-associated difficulties falling asleep and awakening: clonidine and methylphenidate treatments. In: Newcorn, J., ed. *Scientific Proceedings of the Annual Meeting: American Academy of Child and Adolescent Psychiatry. Washington, DC*: Washington, DC: American Academy of Child and Adolescent Psychiatry p. 76.

Casat, C.D., Pleasants, D.Z., Schroeder, D.H., and Parler, D.W. (1989) Bupropion in children with attention deficit disorder. *Psychopharmacol Bull* 25:198–201.

Casat, C.D., Pleasants, D.Z., Van Wyck Fleet, J. (1987) A double-blind trial of bupropion in children with attention deficit disorder. *Psychopharmacol Bull* 23:120–122.

Castellanos, F.X., Giedd, J.N., Elia, J., Marsh, W.L., Ritchie, G.F., Hamburger, S.D., and Rapoport, J.L. (1997) Controlled stimulant treatment of ADHD and comorbid Tourette's syndrome: effects of stimulant and dose. *J Am Acad Child Adolesc Psychiatry* 36: 589–96.

Cohen, L.G., Prince, J., and Biederman, J., Wilens, T., Faraone, S.V., Whitt, S., Mick, E., Spencer, T., Meyer, M.C., Polisner, D., Flood, J.G. (1999) Absence of effect of stimulants on the phamacokinetics of desipramine in children. *Pharmacotherapy* 19:746–52.

Conners, C.K. (1998) Rating scales in attention-deficit/hyperactivity disorder: use in assessment and treatment monitoring. *J Clin Psychiatry* 59:24–30.

Conners, K., Casat, C., Gualtieri, T., Weller, E., Reader, M., Reiss,

A., Weller, R., Khayrallah, M. and Ascher, J. (1996) Bupropion hydrochloride in attention deficit disorder with hyperactivity. *J Am Acad Child Adolesc Psychiatry* 35:1314–1321.

Cox, W. (1982) An indication for the use of imipramine in attention deficit disorder. *Am J Psychiatry* 139:1059–1060.

Cunningham, C., Siegel, L., and Offord D. (1991) A dose–response analysis of the effects of methylphenidate on the peer interactions and simulated classroom performance of ADD children with and without conduct problems. *J Child Psychol Psychiatry Allied Disc* 32:439–452.

Dalack, G., Healy, D., and Meador-Woodruff, J. (1998) Nicotine dependence in schizophrenia: clinical phenomena and laboratory findings. *Am J Psychiatry.* 155:1490–1501.

Diamond, I.R., Tannock, R., and Schachar, R.J. (1999) Response to methylphenidate in children with ADHD and comorbid anxiety. *J Am Acad Child Adolesc Psychiatry* 38:402–409.

Dillon, D.C., Salzman, I.J., and Schulsinger, D.A. (1985). The use of imipramine in Tourette's syndrome and attention deficit disorder: case report. *J Clin Psychiatry* 46:348–349.

Douglas, V., Barr, R., Amin, K., O'Neill, M., Britton, B. (1988) Dosage effects and individual responsivity to methylphenidate in attention deficit disorder. *J Child Psychol Psychiatry* 29:453–475.

Douglas, V. Barr. R, Desilets, J. and Sherman, E. (1995) Do high doses of stimulants impair flexible thinking in attention-deficit hyperactivity disorder? *J. Am Acad Child Adolesc Psychiatry* 34: 877–885.

Douglas, V.I. (1980) Treatment and training approaches to hyperactivity: establishing internal or external control. In: Whalen, C. and Henker, B., eds. *Hyperactive children: The Social Ecology of Identification and Treatment.* New York: Academic Press; pp. 283–318.

Dulcan, M. (1997) Practice parameters for the assessment and treatment of children, adolescents, and adults with attention-deficit/hyperactivity disorder. *J Am Acad Child Adolesc Psychiatry* 36: 85S–121S.

DuPaul, G., Barkley, R., and McMurray, M. (1994). Response of children with ADHD to methylphenidate: interaction with internalizing symptoms. *J Am Acad Child Adolesc Psychiatry* 33:894–903.

Ernst, M. (1996) *MAOI treatment of adult ADHD.* Presented at the NIMH Conference on Alternative Pharmacology of ADHD, Washington, DC.

Eslinger, P.J. (1996) Conceptualizing, describing, and measuring components of executive function. In: Lyon G.R. and Krasnegor, N.A., eds. *Attention, Memory, and Executive Function.* Baltimore: Paul H. Brookes Publishing; pp. 367–395.

Faraone, S.V. and Biederman, J. (1999b) The neurobiology of attention deficit hyperactivity disorder. In: Charney, D.S., Nestler, E.J. and Bunney, B.S., eds. *Neurobiology of Mental Illness.* New York: Oxford University Press; pp. 788–801.

Faraone, S.V., Biederman, J. Krifcher Lehman, B., Spencer, T., Norman, D., Seidman, L., Kraus, I., Perrin, J., Chen, W., and Tsuang, M.T. (1993) Intellectual performance and school failure in children with attention deficit hyperactivity disorder and in their siblings. *J Abnorm Pyschol* 102:616–623.

Faraone, S.V. Biederman J. Weiffenbach, B., Keith, T., Chu, M.P., Weaver, A., Spencer, T.J., Wilens, T.E., Frazier, J., Cleves, M., and Sakai J. (1999) Dopamine D4 gene 7-repeat allele and attention deficit hyperactivity disorder. *Am J Psychiatry* 156:768–770.

Feigin, A., Kurlan, R., McDermott, M., Beach, J., Dimitsopulos, Brower, C., Chapieski, L., Trinidad, K., Como, P., and Jankovic, J. (1996) A controlled trial of deprenyl in children with Tourette's syndrome and attention deficit hyperactivity disorder. Neurology 46: 965–968.

Fenichel, R.F. (1995). Combining methylphenidate and clonidine: the role of post-marketing surveillance. *J Child Adolesc Psychopharmacol* 5:155–156.

Findling, R. (1996). Open-label treatment of comorbid depression and attentional disorder with co-administration of SRI's and psychostimulants in children, adolescents, and adults: a case series. *J Child Adolescent Psychopharmacol* 6:165–175.

Findling R., Schwartz, M., Flannery, D., and Manos, M. (1996) Venlafaxine in adults with ADHD: An open trial. J Clin Psychiatry 57:184–189.

Fung, Y.K. (1988). Postnatal behavioural effects of maternal nicotine exposure in rats. *J Pharm Pharmacol* 40:870–872.

Fung, Y.K. and Lau, Y.S. (1989). Effects of prenatal nicotine exposure on rat striatal dopaminergic and nicotinic systems. *Pharmacol Biochem Behav* 33:1–6.

Gadow, K.D., Nolan, E.E., Sverd, J., Sprafkin, J., and Paolicelli, L. (1990) Methylphenidate in aggressive-hyperactive boys: I. Effects on peer aggression in public school settings. *J Am Acad Child Adolesc Psychiatry* 29:710–718.

Gammon, G.D. and Brown, T.E. (1993). Fluoxetine and methylphenidate in combination for treatment of attention deficit disorder and comorbid depressive disorder. *J Child Adolesc Psychopharmacol* 3:1–10.

Gastfriend, D.R., Biederman, J., and Jellinek, M.S. (1985). Desipramine in the treatment of attention deficit disorder in adolescents. *Psychopharmacol Bulle* 21:144–145.

Gillberg, C., Melander, H., Knorring, A., Janols, L., Thernlund, G., Gagglof, B., Wallin, L., Gustafsson, P., and Kopp, S. (1997) Long-term stimulant treatment of children with ADHD symptoms: a randomized, double-blind, placebo controlled trial. *Arch Gen Psychiatry* 54:865–870.

Gittelman, R., ed. (1986) *Anxiety Disorders of Childhood*. New York: Guilford Press.

Goldman, L., Genel, M., Bezman, R., and Slanetz, P. (1998) Diagnosis and treatment of attention-deficit/hyperactivity disorder in children and adolescents. *JAMA* 279:1100–1107.

Greene, R.W. (1995). Students with ADHD in school classrooms: teacher factors related to compatibility, assessment, and intervention. *School Psychol Rev* 24:81–93.

Greene, R.W. (1996) Students with ADHD and their teachers: implications of a goodness-of-fit perspective. In: Ollendick, T.H. and Prinz, R.J., eds. *Advances in Clinical Child Psychology*. New York: Plenum Press, pp. 205–230.

Greene, R.W., Biederman, J., Faraone, S.V., Sienna, M., and Garcia-Jetton, J. (1997), Adolescent outcome of boys with attention-deficit/hyperactivity disorder and social disability: results from a 4-year longitudinal follow-up study. *J Consult Clin Psychol* 65:658–767.

Greene, R.W., Biederman, J., Faraone, S.V., Wilens, T.E., Mick, E., and Blier, H.K. (1999) Further validation of social impairment as a predictor of substance use disorders: findings from a sample of siblings of boys with and without ADHD. *J Clin Child Psychol* 28:349–354.

Greene, R.W. and Doyle, A.E. (1999). Toward a transactional conceptualization of oppositional defiant disorder: implications for treatment and assessment. *Clin Child Fam Psychol Rev* 2:129–148.

Gunning, B. (1992) A controlled trial of clonidine in hyperkinetic children. Thesis, Academic Hospital Rotterdam–Sophia Children's Hospital Rotterdam, The Netherlands.

Hechtman, L. and Abikoff, H. (1995) Multimodal treatment plus

stimulants vs. stimulant treatment in ADHD children: Results from a two-year comparative treatment study. *Scientific Proceedings of the Annual Meeting: American Academy of Child and Adolescent Psychiatry, New Orleans, LA*. Washington, DC: American Academy of Child and Adolescent Psychiatry.

Heiligenstein, J.H., Spencer, T., Faries, D., Biederman, J, and Conners, C.K. (2000), Tomoxetine, a non-stimulant, noradrenergic enhancer for ADHD, doubleblind treatment results. In: Annual Meeting of the American Academy of Child and Adolescent Psychiatry New York: The American Academy of Child and Adolescent Psychiatry.

Hinshaw, S., Heller, T. and McHale, J. (1992). Covert antisocial behavior in boys with attention-deficit hyperactivity disorder: external validation and effects of methylphenidate. *J Consult Clini Psychol* 60:274–281.

Hinshaw, S.P. and Erhardt, D.E. (1991) Attention-deficit hyperactivity disorder. In: Kendall, P.C., ed. *Child and Adolescent Therapy: Cognitive-Behavioral Procedures*. New York: Guilford Press pp. 98–130.

Hinshaw, S.P., Klein, R.G., and Abikoff, H. (1998) Childhood attention-deficit hyperactivity disorder: nonpharmacologic and combination treatments. In: Nathan, P.E. and Gorman, J., ed. *Treatments that Work*. New York, Oxford University Press.

Hinshaw, S.P. and Melnick, S. (1992). Self-management therapies and attention-deficit hyperactivity disorder. Reinforced self-evaluation and anger control interventions. *Behav Modif* 16:253–273.

Hoge, S.K. and Biederman, J. (1986). A case of Tourette's syndrome with symptoms of attention deficit disorder treated with desipramine. *J Clin Psychiatry* 47:478–479.

Hornig-Rohan, M. and Amsterdam, J. (1995) Venlafaxine vs. stimulant therapy in patients with dual diagnoses of ADHD and depression. New Clinical Drug Evaluation Unit Program: 35th Annual Meeting Program. Orlando: FL: pp. Poster # 92.

Horrigan, J.P. and Barnhill, L.J. (1995). Guanfacine for treatment of attention-deficit hyperactivity disorder in boys. *J Child Adolesc Psychophamacol* 5:215–223.

Hubbard, J.W., Srinivas, N.R., Quinn, D., and Midha, K.K. (1989) Enantioselective aspects of the disposition of dl-threo-methylphenidate after the administration of a sustained-release formulation to children with attention deficit disorder. *J Pharm Sci* 78:944–947.

Hunt, R., Arnsten, A., and Asbell, M. (1995). An open trial of guanfacine in the treatment of attention-deficit hyperactivity disorder. *J Am Acad Child Adolesc Psychiatry* 34:50–54.

Hunt, R.D. (1987). Treatment effects of oral and transdermal clonidine in relation to methylphenidate: An open pilot study in ADD-H. *Psychopharmacol Bull* 23:111–114.

Hunt, R.D., Minderaa, R.B., and Cohen, D.J. (1985). Clonidine benefits children with attention deficit disorder and hyperactivity: Report of a double-blind placebo-crossover therapeutic trial. *J Am Acad Child Psychiatry* 24:617–629.

Jensen, P.S. (1998) NIMH multimodal treatment study. *Scientific Proceedings of the Annual Meeting: American Academy of Child and Adolescent Psychiatry, Anaheim, CA*. Washington DC: American Academy of Child and Adolescent Psychiatry.

Johns, J.M., Louis, T.M., Becker, R.F., and Means, I.W. (1982) Behavioral effects of prenatal exposure to nicotine in guinea pigs. *Neurobehav and Toxicol Teratol* 4:365–369.

Jones, G., Sahakian, B., Levy, R., Warburton, D., and Gray, J. (1992) Effects of acute subcutaneous nicotine on attention, information and short-term memory in Alzheimer's disease. *Psychopharmacology* 108:485–494.

Kaplan, S.L., Busner, J., Kupietz, S., Wasserman, E., and Segal, B. (1990) Effects of methylphenidate on adolescents with aggressive conduct disorder and ADDH: a preliminary report. *J Am Acad Child Adolesc Psychiatry* 29:719–723.

Klein, R., Abikoff, H., Klass, E., Gameles, D., Seese, L., and Pollack, S. (1997) Clinical efficacy of methylphenidate in conduct disorder with and without attention deficit hyperactivity disorder. Arch Gen Psychiatry 54:1073–1080.

Klein, R.G. (1987a) Pharmacotherapy of childhood hyperactivity: an update. In: Meltzer, H.Y., *Psychopharmacology: The Third Generation of Progress*. New York: Raven Press, pp. 1215–1225.

Klorman, R., Brumaghim, J., Fitzpatrick, P. Borgstedt, A. and Strauss, J (1994) Clinical and cognitive effects of methylphenidate on children with attention deficit disorder as a function of aggression/oppositionality and age. *J Abnorm Psycho* 103:206–221.

Klorman, R., Brumaghim, J.T., Salzman, L.F., Strauss, J., Borgstedt, A.D., McBride, M.C., and Loeb, S. (1989) Comparative effects of methylphenidate on attention-deficit hyperactivity disorder with and without aggressive/noncompliant features. Psychopharmacol Bull 25:109–113.

Kupietz, S.S., Winsberg, B.G., Richardson, E., Maitinsky, S., and Mendell, N. (1988) Effects of methylphenidate dosage in hyperactive reading-disabled children: I. Behavior and cognitive performance effects. J Am Acad Child Adolesc Psychiatry 27:70–77.

Levin, E., Conners, C., Sparrow, E., Hinton, S., Erhardt, D., Meck, W., Rose, J., and March, J. (1996) Nicotine effects on adults with attention-deficit/hyperactivity disorder. Psychopharmacology 123:55–63.

Livingston, R., Dykman, R., and Ackerman, P. (1992) Psychiatric comorbidity and response to two doses of methylphenidate in children with attention deficit disorder. J Child Adolesc Psychopharamacol 2:115–122.

Luh, J., Pliszka, S., Olvers, R., and Tatum, R. (1996) An open trial of venlafaxine in the treatment of attention deficit hyperactivity disorder: a pilot study. In: New Clinical Drug Evaluation Unit Program: 36th Annual Meeting Program Boca Raton, FL: NIMH.

Malhotra, S. and Santosh, P.J. (1998) An open clinical trial of buspirone in children with attention deficit/hyperactivity disorder. J Am Acad Child Adolesc Psychiatry 37:364–371.

March, J.S., Swanson, J.M., Arnold, L.E., Hoza, B., Conners, C.K., Hinshaw, S.P., Hechtman, L., Kraemer, H.C., Greenhill, L.L., Abikoff, H.B., Elliott, L.G., Jensen, P.S., Newcorn, J.H., Vitiello, B., Severe, J., Wells, K.C., and Pelham, W.E. (2000) Anxiety as a predictor and outcome variable in the multimodal treatment study of children with ADHD (MTA). J Abnorm Child Psychol 28:527–541.

McGee, R., Williams, S., and Silva, P.H. (1985) Factor structure and correlates of ratings of inattention, hyperactivity, and antisocial behavior in a large sample of 9-year old children from the general population. J Consult Clin Psychol 53:480–490.

Meck, W. and Church, R. (1987) Cholinergic modulation of the content of temporal memory. Behav Neuroci 101:457–464.

Meichenbaum, D.H. and Goodman, J. (1971) Training impulsive children to talk to themselves: a means of developing self-control. J Abnorm Psychol 77:115–26.

Mereu, G., Yoon, K., Gessa, G., Naes, L., and Westfall, T. (1987) Preferential stimulation of ventral tegmental area dopaminergic neurons by nicotine. Eur J Pharmacol 141:395–399.

Milberger, S., Biederman, J., Faraone, S., Chen, L., and Jones, J. (1997) ADHD is associated with early imitation of cigarette smoking in children and adolescents. J Am Acad Child Adolesc Psychiatry 36: 37–43.

Milberger, S., Biederman, J., Faraone, S.V., Chen, L., and Jones, J.

(1996) Is maternal smoking during pregnancy a risk factor for attention deficit hyperactivity disorder in children? Am J Psychiatry 153:1138–1142.

Murphy, D., Pelham, W., and Lang, A. (1992) Aggression in boys with attention deficit-hyperactivity disorder: Methylphenidate effects on naturalistically observed aggression, response to provocation, and social information processing. J Abnorm Child Psychol 20:451–466.

Murphy, K. and Barkley, R. (1996) Prevalence of DSM-IV symptoms of ADHD in adult licensed drivers: implications for clinical diagnosis. J Attention Disord 1:147–161.

National Institute of Mental Health (NIMH) (1996). Alternative Pharmacology of ADHD.

Nemeroff, C., DeVane, L., and Pollock, B. (1996) Newer antidepressants and the cytochrome P450 system. Am J Psychiatry 153: 311–320.

Parrott, A.C. and Winder, G. (1989) Nicotine chewing gum (2 mg, 4 mg) and cigarette smoking: comparative effects upon vigilance and heart rate. Psychopharmacology 97:257–261.

Pataki, C., Carlson, G., Kelly, K., Rapport, M., and Biancaniello, T. (1993) Side effects of methylphenidate and desipramine alone and in combination in children. *Am J Psychiatry* 32:1065–1072.

Patrick, K.S., Caldwell, R.W., Ferris, R.M., and Breese, G.R. (1987) Pharmacology of the enantiomers of threo-methylphenidate. *J Pharmacol Exp Ther* 241:152–158.

Peeke, S. and Peeke, H. (1984) Attention, memory, and cigarette smoking. Psychopharmacology 84:205–216.

Pelham, W., Greenslade, K., Vodde-Hamilton, M., Murphy, D., Greenstein, J., Gnagy, E., Guthrie, K., Hoover, M., and Dahl, R. (1990) Relative efficacy of long-acting stimulants on children with attention deficit-hyperactivity disorder: a comparison of standard methylphenidate, sustained-release methylphenidate, sustained-release dextroamphetamine, and pemoline. *Pediatrics* 86: 226–237.

Pelham, W.E. (1989). Behavior therapy, behavioral assessment, and psychostimulant medication in the treatment of attention deficit disorders: an interactive approach. In: Swanson, J. and Bloomingdale, L., eds. *Attention Deficit Disorders (IV): Current Concepts and Emerging Trends in Emotional and Behavioral Disorders of Childhood*. London: Pergamon Press, pp. 169–195.

Pelham, W.E., Jr. (1999) The NIMH multimodal treatment study for attention-deficit hyperactivity disorder: just say yes to drugs alone? Can J Psychiatry 44: 981–990.

Pelham, W.E., Bender, M.E., Caddell, J., Booth, S., and Moorer, S.H., (1985) Methylphenidate and children with attention deficit disorder. Arch Gen Psychiatry 42:948–952.

Pelham, W.E. and Murphy, H.A. (1986) Attention deficit and conduct disorders. In: Hersen, M., ed. *Pharmacological and Behavioral Treatments: An Integrative Approach*. New York: John Wiley and Sons, pp. 108–148.

Pelham, W.E. and Sams, S.E. (1992) Behavior modification. Psychiatr Clin North Am 1:505–518.

Pfiffner, L.J. and O'Leary, S.G. (1993) School-based psychological treatments. In: Matson, J.L., ed. Handbook of Hyperactivity in Children. Boston: Allyn and Bacon.

Pliszka, S.R. (1989) Effect of anxiety on cognition, behavior, and stimulant response in ADHD. J Am Acad Child Adolesc Psychiatry 28:882–887.

Pomerleau, O., Downey, K., Stelson, F., and Pomerleau, C. (1996) Cigarette smoking in adult patients diagnosed with ADHD. J Substance Abuse 7:373–378.

Popper, C.W. (1995) Combining methylphenidate and clonidine:

pharmacologic questions and news reports about sudden death. J Child Adolesc Psychopharmacol 5:157–166.

Prince, J., Wilens, T., Biederman, J., and Wozniak, J. (1996) Clonidine for ADHD related sleep disturbances: a systematic chart review of 62 cases. J Am Acad Child Adolesc Psychiatry 35:599–605.

Prince, J.B., Wilens, T.E., Biederman, J., Spencer, T.J., Millstein, R., Polisner, D.A., and Bostic, J.Q. (2000) A controlled study of nortriptyline in children and adolescents with attention deficit hyperactivity disorder. J Child Adolesc Psychopharmacol 10:193–204.

Rapport, M., Carlson, G., Kelly, K., and Pataki, C. (1993) Methylphenidate and desipramine in hospitalized children: I. Separate and combined effects on cognitive function. J Am Acad Child Adolescent Psychiatry 32:333–342.

Rapport, M.D., DuPaul, G.J., and Kelly, K.L. (1989a) Attention deficit hyperactivity disorder and methylphenidate: the relationship between gross body weight and drug response in children. Psychopharmacol Bull 25:285–290.

Rapport, M.D., Jones, J.T., DuPaul, G.J., Kelly, K.L., Gardner, M.J., Tucker, S.B., and Shea, M.S. (1987) Attention deficit disorder and methylphenidate: group and single-subject analyses of dose effects on attention in clinic and classroom settings. J Clin Child Psychol 16:329–338.

Rapport, M.D., Quinn, S.O., DuPaul, G.J., Quinn, E.P., and Kelly, K.L. (1989b) Attention deficit disorder with hyperactivity and methylphenidate: the effects of dose and mastery level on children's learning performance. J Abnorm Child Psychol 17:669–689.

Rapport, M.D., Stoner, G., DuPaul, G.J., Kelly, K.L., Tucker, S.B., and Shroeler, T. (1988) Attention deficit disorder and methylphenidate: a multilevel analysis of dose–response effects on children's impulsivity across settings. J Am Acad Child Adolesc Psychiatry 27:60–69.

Reader, M.J., Harris, E.L., Schuerholz, L.J., and Denckla, M.B. (1994) Attention deficit hyperactivity disorder and executive dysfunction. Deve Neuropsychol 10:493–512.

Reimherr, F., Hedges, D., Strong, R., and Wender, P. (1995) An open-trial of venlaxine in adult patients with attention deficit hyperactivity disorder. In New Clinical Drug Evaluation Unit Program: 34th Annual Meeting Program. Orlando, FL: NIMH.

Riddle, M.A., Hardin, M.T., Cho, S.C., Woolston, J.L., and Leckman, J.F. (1988) Desipramine treatment of boys with attention-deficit hyperactivity disorder and tics: preliminary clinical experience. J Am Acad Child Adolesc Psychiatry 27:811–814.

Scahill, L., Chappell, P.B., Kim, Y.S., Schultz, R.T., Katsovich, L., Shepherd, E., Arnsten, A.F.T., Cohen, D.J., and Leckman, J.F. (2001) A placebo-controlled study of guanfacine in the treatment of children with tic disorders and attention deficit hyperactivity disorder. Am J Psychiatry 158:1067–1074.

Schachar, R., Tannock, R., Cunninggham, C., and Corkum, P. (1997) Behavioral, situational, and temporal effects of treatment of ADHD with methylphenidate. J Am Acad Child Adolesc Psychiatry 36:754–763.

Sharp, W., Walter, J., Marsh, W., Ritchie, G., Hamburger, S., and Castellanos, X. (1999) ADHD in girls: clinical comparability of a research sample. J Am Acad Child Adolesc Psychiatry 38: 40–47.

Shevell, M. and Schreriber, R. (1997) Peroline-associated hepatic failure: a critical analysis of the literature. Pediatr Neurol: 14–16.

Singer, S., Brown, J., Quaskey, S., Rosenberg, L., Mellits, E., and Denckla, M. (1994) The treatment of attention-deficit hyperactivity disorder in tourette's syndroms: a double-blind placebo-controlled study with clonidine and desipramine. Pediatrics 95: 74–81.

Solanto, M.V. and Wender, E.H. (1989) Does methylphenidate constrict cognitive functioning? J Am Acad Child Adol Psychiatry 28: 897–902.

Spencer, T. (1997) A double-blind, controlled study of desipramine in children with ADHD and tic disorders. In: Scientific Proceedings of the Annual Meeting: American Academy of Child and Adolescent Psychiatry, Toronto. Washington, DC: American Academy of Child and Adolescent Psychiatry.

Spencer, T., Biederman, J., Coffey, B., Geller, D., Wilens, T., and Faraone, S. (1999) The 4-year course of tic disorders in boys with attention-deficit/hyperactivity disorder. Arch Gen Psychiatry 56: 842–847.

Spencer, T., Biederman, J., Harding, M., O'Donnell, D., Faraone, S., and Wilens, T. (1996a) Growth deficits in ADHD children revisited: evidence for disorder-associated growth delays? J Am Acad Child Adolesc Psychiatry 35:1460–1469.

Spencer, T., Biederman, J., Harding, M., O'Donnell, D., Wilens, T., Faraone, S., Coffey, B., and Geller, D. (1998a) Disentangling the overlap between Tourette's disorder and ADHD. J Child Psychol Psychiatry 39: 1037–1044.

Spencer, T., Biederman, J., Heiligenstein, J., Wilens, T., Faries, D., Prince, J., Faraone, S.V., Rea, J., Witcher, J., and Zeras, S. (2001) An open-label, dose-ranging study of atomoxetine in children with attention deficit hyperactivity disorder. J Child Adolesc Psychopharmacol 11:

Spencer, T., Biederman, J., Kerman, K., Steingard, R., and Wilens, T. (1993a) Desipramine in the treatment of children with tic disorder or Tourette's syndrome and attention deficit hyperactivity disorder. J Am Acad Child Adolesc Psychiatry 32:354–360.

Spencer, T., Biederman, J., and Wilens, T. (1998b), Growth deficits in children with attention deficit hyperactivity disorder. Pediatrics 102: 501–506.

Spencer, T. Biederman, J., Wilens, T., Prince, J., Hatch, M., Jones, J., Harding, M., Faraone, S.V., and Seidman, L. (1998c) Effectiveness and tolerability of tomoxetine in adults with attention deficit hyperactivity disorder. Am J Psychiatry 155:693–695.

Spencer, T. Biederman, J., Wilens, T. Steingard, R., Geist, D. (1993b) Nortriptyline in the treatment of children with attention deficit hyperactivity disorder and tic disorder or Tourette's syndrome. Am Acad Child Adolesc Psychiatry 32:205–210.

Spencer, T., Biederman, J., Wilens, T.E. and Faraone, S.V. (1998d) Adults with attention-deficit/hyperactivity disorder: a controversial diagnosis. J Clin Psychiatry 59:59–68.

Spencer, T., Wilens, T., Biederman, J., Faraone, S.V. Ablon, J.S. and Lapey, K. (1995) A double-blind, crossover comparison of methylphenidate and placebo in adults with childhood-onset attention-deficit hyperactivity disorder. Arch Gen Psychiatry 52: 434–443.

Spencer, T.J., Biederman, J., Wilens, T., Harding, M., O'Donnell, D., and Griffin, S. (1996b) Pharmacotherapy of attention deficit hyperactivity disorder across the lifecycle: a literature review. J Acad Child Adolescent Psychiatry 35:409–432.

Sprague, R.L. and Sleator, E.K. (1977). Methylphenidate in hyperkinetic children: differences in dose effects on learning and social behavior. Science 198: 1274–1276.

Steingard, R., Biederman, J., Spencer, T., Wilens, T., and Gonzalez, A. (1993) Comparison of clonidine response in the treatment of attention deficit hyperactivity disorder with and without comorbid tic disorders. J Am Acad Child Adolesc Psychiatry 32:350–353.

Swanson, J., Kinsbourne, M., Roberts, W., and Zucker, K. (1978) Time-response analysis of the effect of stimulant medication on

the learning ability of children referred for hyperactivity. Pediatrics 61:21–24.

Szatmari, P. (1992) The epidemiology of attention-deficit hyperactivity disorders. In: Weiss, G., ed. Attention-Deficit Hyperactivity
Disorder, Vol. 1. Philadelphia: W.B. Saunders, pp. 361–371.

Tannock, R., Ickowicz, A., and Schechar, R. (1995) Differential effects of methylphenidate on working memory in ADHD children
with and without comorbid anxiety. J Am Acad Child Adolesc
Psychiatry 34: 886–896.

Tannock, R., Schachar, R.J., Carr, R.P. and Logan, G.D. (1989)
Dose-response effects of methylphenidate on academic performance and overt behavior in hyperactive children. Pediatrics 84:
648–657.

Taylor, E., Schachar, R., Thorley, G., Wieselberg, H.M. Everitt, B.,
and Rutter, M. (1987) Which boys respond to stimulant medication? A controlled trial of methylphenidate in boys with disruptive behaviour. Psychol Med 17:121–143.

Voelker, S.L., Lachar, D., and Golawski, L.L. (1983). The personality
inventory for children and response to methylphenidate: preliminary evidence for predictive validity. J Pediatr Psychol 8:161–
169.

Wender, P.H. and Reimherr, F.W. (1990) Bupropion treatment of attention-deficit hyperactivity disorder in adults. Am J Psychiatry
147:1018–1020.

Wender, P.H., Wood, D.R., and Reimherr, F.W. (1985) Pharmacological treatment of attention deficit disorder, residual type (ADDRT,
"minimal brain dysfunction", "hyperactivity") in adults. Psychopharmacol Bull 21:222–232.

Wender, P.H., Wood, D.R., Reimherr, F.W., and Ward, M. (1983) An
open trial of pargyline in the treatment of attention deficit disorder, residual type. Psychiatry Res 9:329–336.

Wesnes, K. and Warburton, D. (1984). The effects of cigarettes of
varying yield on rapid information processing performance. Psychopharmacology 82:338–342.

West, S., McElroy, S., Strakowski, S., Keck, P., and McConville, B.
(1995) Attention deficit hyperactivity disorder in adolescent mania. Am J Psychiatry 152:271–274.

Westfall, T., Grant, H., and Perry, H. (1983) Release of dopamine
and 5-hydroxytryptamine from rat striatal slices following activation of nicotinic cholinergic receptors. Gen Pharmacol 14:321–
325.

Whalen, C. (1989). Does stimulant medication improve the peer
status of hyperactive children? J Consult Clin Psychol 57:545–
549.

Whalen, C., Henker, B., and Granger, D. (1990) Social judgement
processes in hyperactive boys: effects of methylpheniddate and
comparisons with normal peers. J Abnorm Child Psychol 18:297–
316.

Whalen, C.K. and Henker, B. (1992) The social profile of attention-
deficit hyperactivity disorder. Child Adolesc Psychiatr Clin North
Am 1:395–410.

Wilens, T. and Biederman, J. (1992) The stimulants. Psychiatr Clin
North Am 15:191–222.

Wilens, T. and Spencer, T. (1998) Amphetamine pharmacology. In :
Tarter, R., Ammerman, R., and Ott, P., eds. Handbook on Substance Abuse: Neurobehavioral Pharmacology. New York: Plenum Press;

Wilens, T.E., Biederman, J., Geist, D.E., Steingard, R., and Spencer,
T. (1993) Nortriptyline in the treatment of attention deficit hy-
peractivity disorder: a chart review of 58 cases, J Am Acad Child
Adolesc Psychiatry 32: 343–349.

Wilens, T.E., Biederman, J., Spencer, T.I. Bostic, J., Prince, J., Monuteaux, M.C. Soriano, J., Fine, C., Abrams, A., Rater, M., and
Polisner, D. (1999a) A pilot controlled clinical trial of ABT-418,
a cholinergic agonist, in the treatment of adults with attention
deficit hyperactivity disorder. Am J Psychiatry 156: 1931–1937.

Wilens, T.E., Biederman, J.B., and Spencer, T. (1995) A systematic
assessment of tricyclic antidepressants in the treatment of adult
attention-deficit hyperactivity disorder. J Nerv Ment Dis 183:48–
50.

Wilens, T.E. and Spencer, T.J. (1999) Combining methylphenidate
and clonidine: a clinically sound medication option. J Am Child
Adolesc Psychiatry 38:614–622.

Wilens, T.E., Spencer, T.J., Biederman J., Girard, K., Doyle, R.,
Prince, J., Polisner, D., Solhkhah, R., Comeau, S., Monuteaux
M.C., and Parekh, A. (2001) A controlled clinical trial of bup-
ropion for attention deficit hyperactivity disorder in adults. Am
J Psychiatry 158:282–288.

Wozniak, J., Biederman, J., Kiely, K., Ablon, S., Faraone, S., Mundy,
E., and Mennin, D. (1995) Mania-like symptoms suggestive of
childhood onset bipolar disorder in clinically referred children. J
Am Acad Child Adolesc Psychiatry 34:867–876.

Zametkin, A., Rapoport, J.L., Murphy, D.L., Linnoila, M., and Ismond, D. (1985) Treatment of hyperactive children with monoamine oxidase inhibitors: I. Clinical efficacy. Arch Gen Psychiatry
42: 962–966.

Zametkin, A.J. and Rapoport, J.L. (1987) Noradrenergic hypothesis
of attention deficit disorder with hyperactivity: a critical review.
In: Meltzer, H.Y., ed. Psychopharmacology: The Third Generation of Progress. New York: Raven Press pp. 837–842.

36 | Depressive disorders

BORIS BIRMAHER AND DAVID BRENT

Major depressive disorder (MDD) is a familial recurrent illness associated with poor psychosocial and academic outcome; an increased risk for other psychiatric disorders, suicide, and suicide attempts; and a high rate of depression and psychological difficulties in adult life (Birmaher et al., 1996b; Goodyer et al., 1997; Lewinsohn et al., 1999; Pine et al., 1998; Rao et al., 1999; Weissman et al., 1999a,b). The prevalence of MDD in children and adolescents is approximately 2% and 6%, respectively (Birmaher et al., 1996b). Thus, early identification and prompt treatment of this disorder at its early stages is critical.

The main aim of this chapter is to review the current pharmacological treatments for children and adolescents with MDD. Although psychotherapy interventions, including cognitive behavior therapy (CBT) and interpersonal psychotherapy (IPT) have also been found efficacious for the acute treatment of adolescents with MDD (e.g., Brent et al., 1997; Mufson et al., 1999), they will not be reviewed here.

DEFINITIONS OF TREATMENT RESPONSE

Before describing the treatment of pediatric MDD, several terms of treatment response and the treatment phases of MDD will be defined (Table 36.1). The definitions depicted have been extensively used in the pediatric and adult literature (e.g., Emslie, et al., 1997a,b; Birmaher et al., 2000a).

ASSESSMENT OF TREATMENT RESPONSE

Treatment response has been traditionally determined by the absence of MDD criteria (e.g., no more than one *Diagnostic and Statistical Manual of Mental Disorder* [DSM] symptom), or more frequently, by a significant reduction (usually >50%) in symptom severity. Using the latter criterion, patients deemed responders may still have considerable residual symptomatology. Therefore, an absolute final score on the Beck Depression Inventory (BDI) ≤9 (Beck, 1967), Hamilton Depression Rating Scale (HDRS) (Hamilton, 1960) ≤7 (17-item HDRS), or Children Depression Rating Scale (CDRS) (Poznanski et al., 1984) ≤28, together with persistent improvement in the patient's functioning for at least 2 weeks or longer, may better reflect a satisfactory response. Overall improvement has also been measured using a score of 1 or 2 (very much or much improved) in the Clinical Global Impression Scale, Improvement (CGI-I) subscale (Guy, 1976).

Functional improvement can be measured using several rating scales, such as a score ≤70 in the Global Assessment of Function (GAF) Scale (GAF) (DSM-IV; American Psychiatric Association, 1994a) or the Children's Global Assessment Scale (C-GAS) (Shaffer et al., 1983).

TREATMENT PHASES

The treatment of MDD has been divided in to three phases (American Academy of Children and Adolescent Psychiatry [AACAP], 1998; American Psychiatric Association [APA], 2000): acute, continuation, and maintenance. The *acute phase* for a youngster with the first episode of depression usually lasts 6–12 weeks and the main goals of treatment are to achieve response and remission of the depressive symptoms. The *continuation phase* usually lasts 4–12 months, during which remission is consolidated to prevent relapses. The *maintenance phase* lasts 1 or more years and the main goal of treatment is the prevention of depression recurrences. Most of the studies in children and adolescents evaluate treatments during the acute phase; there are no controlled trials in continuation or maintenance phases. Therefore, recommendations regarding the continuation and maintenance treatments will be extrapolated from the adult literature, but caution is warranted in doing this because youth may respond differently to continuation and maintenance interventions that have thus far only been tested in adults with MDD (Birmaher et al., 1996a).

TABLE 36.1. *Definitions of Treatment Response*

Term/Phase	Definition
Absence of MDD	≤ 1 symptom of MDD
Subsyndromal depression	2–3 symptoms of MDD
Response	No MDD or a significant reduction in MDD symptoms for at least 2 weeks (see Assessment of Treatment Response)
Remission	A period of at least 2 weeks and less than 2 months with absence of MDD
Recovery	Absence of MDD for ≥2 months
Relapse	An episode of depression during the period of remission
Recurrence	Emergence of symptoms of MDD during the period of recovery (a new episode)

MDD, major depressive disorder.

SYNDROME NOSOLOGY/CLASSIFICATION

Every child and adolescent can be sporadically and appropriately sad. To be diagnosed with MDD, however, children and adolescents need to experience persistent depressed or irritable mood, and markedly diminished interest or pleasure in all or almost all activities needs to be present for at least 2 weeks (APA, 2000). In addition, it is required that at least four of the following symptoms be present: weight loss or gain, insomnia or hypersomnia, psychomotor agitation or retardation, fatigue or loss of energy, feelings of worthlessness or excessive guilt, lack of concentration, and thoughts of death or suicidal ideation or attempts. These symptoms must represent a change from previous functioning and produce psychosocial impairment. These symptoms must not be *solely* attributed to abuse of drugs, use of medications, medical illnesses, bereavement, or other psychiatric disorders such as schizophrenia, schizoaffective disorder, or bipolar disorder.

Overall, the clinical picture of childhood MDD parallels the symptoms of adult MDD (Birmaher et al., 1996b). There are some developmental differences, however. Symptoms of melancholia (e.g., lack of appetite, insomnia, lack of interest in anything), delusions, suicide attempts, especially high-lethality ones, are all less prevalent in young children and increase with age. In contrast, symptoms of anxiety, behavioral problems, and perhaps auditory and visual hallucinations seem to occur more frequently in children (AACAP, 1998; Birmaher et al., 1996a). Also, it appears that the rate of onset of bipolar disorder is higher in early-onset depression (Strober and Carlson, 1982; Geller et al., 1994).

Although the short-term prognosis for depression is good, with up to 90% of affected youths achieving remission in 1–2 years, approximately 70% will experience a second major depressive episode within 2–5 years, and up to 20%–30% will have persistent symptoms of depression (Emslie et al., 1997a,b; Goodyear et al., 1997; Lewinsohn et al., 1999; Rao et al., 1999; Rueter et al., 1999; Weissman et al., 1999a,b; (Birmaher et al., 2000a; Klein et al., 2001). Factors such as age of onset, female sex, severity of the index depressive episode, presence of dysthymia, comorbid attention-deficit hyperactivity disorder (ADHD), conduct and anxiety disorders, and exposure to negative events (e.g., family conflict) have all been associated with poor prognosis (Nolen-Hoeksema et al., 1992; Birmaher et al., 1996b, 2000a,b; Goodyer et al., 1998; Hamilton and Bridge, 1999; Lewinsohn et al., 1999; Rao et al., 1999; Rueter et al., 1999; Weissman et al., 1999a,b; Klein et al., 2001). Approximately 20% of youths with MDD, in particular those with psychotic symptoms, psychomotor retardation, and/or pharmacological induced hypomania, may develop bipolar disorder and require alternative psychopharmacological treatments (Strober and Carlson, 1982; Strober el al., 1993; Geller et al., 1994).

Forty to 70% of children and adolescents with MDD have other coexisting psychiatric problems, including anxiety, and disruptive, substance abuse, and eating disorders (Angold et al., 1999). These comorbid conditions often lead to poorer treatment response of the depression, and to functional impairment and increased use of mental health services (Birmaher et al., 1996b; Brent et al., 1998, 1999b; Emslie et al., 1998). Therefore accurate assessment and treatment of these comorbid conditions are needed. Approximately 70% of children and adolescents with dysthymia will eventually develop MDD, resulting in the presence of both diagnoses, so-called double depression, which usually is associated with a protracted course (Kovacs et al., 1994).

PHARMACOLOGICAL TREATMENT

Psychoeducation and Supportive Therapy

The optimal pharmacological management of child and adolescent MDD may also involve some educative and psychosocial interventions. Education of the patient and family about the disease, nature of treatment, and prognosis is critical to engagement in treatment and enhances compliance (Brent et al., 1993). In addition, there may be family conflicts that interfere with optimal pharamacological outcome that should be addressed (Emslie et al., 1998). Finally, there is evidence that there are psychological *scars* even after the depression remits that may need to be addressed with psychotherapy (e.g., family conflict, poor self-esteem and social skills) (Puig-Antich et al., 1985; Kovacs and Goldston, 1991; Strober et al., 1993); Rao et al., 1995; (Birmaher et al., 2000a; Stein et al., 2000).

The rate of treatment response appears to be equivalent to that of selective serofonin reuptake inhibitors (SSRIs) or either CBT or IPT, and the types of cases not responsive to either type of monotherapy are similar (Brent et al., 1998; Emslie et al., 1998; Mufson et al., 1999).

Because the parents of depressed youth may also be experiencing depression and other psychiatric disorders (Weissman et al., 1987; Klein et al., 2001), parental depression itself may lead to adverse outcomes (Brent et al., 1998). To treat the child successfully, the clinician should assess parents and refer them for their own treatment.

Acute Phase

During the 6–12 weeks of acute pharmacotherapy, the physician usually sees patients weekly or biweekly for monitoring of symptoms, side effects, and dose adjustments, and for support and education. Supportive or more specific forms of psychotherapy such as CBT or IPT should be added to address comorbid conditions or other problems, such as conflicts at home or with peers or academics.

Most child and adolescent studies published thus far have focused on the effects of the tricyclic antidepressants (TCAs) and, more recently, the SSRIs. A few open studies have also shown that monoamine oxidase inhibitors (MAOIs) can be used safely with children and adolescents (Ryan et al., 1988b), but noncompliance with dietary requirements may present a significant problem for minors. Other antidepressants, including the heterocyclics (HTC) (e.g., amoxapine, maprotiline), buproprion, venlafaxine, and nefazodone, have been found to be efficacious for the treatment of depressed adults (APA, 2000), but they have not been well studied for the treatment of MDD in children and adolescents. Therefore, this chapter mainly describes the use of SSRIs and TCAs for youth with MDD.

Selective serotonin reuptake inhibitors

The reports that SSRIs are efficacious for the treatment of adults with MDD (APA, 2000), together with the

findings that SSRIs are efficacious and safe for other childhood psychiatric disorders (e.g., Leonard et al., 1997; RUPP Anxiety Group, 2001), have a relatively safe side effect profile, very low lethality after an overdose, and easy administration, have favored the SSRIs as the first-line medications for the treatment of MDD.

All SSRIs appear to be equally efficacious for the treatment of major depression and, overall, present similar side effect profiles. However, they have some differences, including elimination half-lives, profiles of drug interactions, and the antidepressant activity of their metabolites (e.g., Leonard et al., 1997; Findling et al., 1999; Axelson et al., 2000 a,b).

Open studies with SSRIs for depressed children and adolescents have reported 70% to 90% response rates (e.g., Ambrosini et al., 1999; Strober et al., 1999). A double-blind, placebo-controlled study in a very small sample of adolescents with MDD did not find significant differences between placebo and fluoxetine (Simeon et al., 1990). However, a large 8-week double-blind study for the treatment of children and adolescents with MDD showed that patients on 8 weeks of fluoxetine (20 mg/day) were more likely to show improvement than those on placebo (58% vs 32% on the CGI) (Emslie et al., 1997b). A second study also using fluoxetine (20 mg/day) for 9 weeks replicated the above results, with fluoxetine being superior to placebo (40% vs. 20%, $p = 0.01$), using a CDRS ≤ 28 and a CGI ≤ 2 as the definitions of response (Emslie et al., 2000). In both studies, there were no age or sex-related effects and patients tolerated fluoxetine well. Despite the significant response to fluoxetine, many patients had only partial improvement and a substantial proportion did not remit. The low rate of response suggests that the ideal treatment might require higher doses or greater duration of treatment. In fact, a follow-up of the subjects who participated in the above study noted an improved rate as the duration of treatment increased (Emslie et al., 1998). Also, it is possible that the ideal treatment may involve a combination of pharmacological and psychosocial treatments.

In recent multicenter study comparing the effects of 12 weeks of paroxetine (mean dose at study end: 28 ± 8.5 mg/day), imipramine (mean dose: 205 ± 64 mg/day), and placebo for the treatment of a large sample of outpatient adolescents with MDD ($n = 275$), adolescents taking paroxetine showed significantly better response than those taking placebo (CGI 1 or 2: 65.6% vs 48.3 %, p = 0.02) (Keller et al., 2001). There were no differences in response between the youth taking imipramine and those taking placebo. Approximately 31.5% of the patients taking imipramine were removed from the study for side effects, in contrast to only 9.7%

of those taking paroxetine. Patients with MDD and comorbid ADHD did worse than those without ADHD (Birmaher et al., 2000b).

In adults, the time course of improvement with the SSRIs appears to be similar to that with the TCAs (APA, 2000). Therefore, after 4 to 6 weeks, if a patient has only a partial response, the dosage may be increased.

Side effects. Overall, all SSRIs have similar side effect profiles and patients tend to develop tolerance to some of these side effects over time. While the SSRIs do not show an antidepressant dose–response relationship, the side effects *are* dose-dependent (Leonard et al., 1997; (AACAP, 1998). The most frequent side effects include gastrointestinal symptoms (e.g., nausea, diarrhea), decreased appetite, decreased or more controversial increased weight, headaches, restlessness, jitteriness, tremor, insomnia or hypersomnia, increased diaphoresis, vivid dreams, and sexual dysfunction (painful or delayed ejaculation, anorgasmia). Like other antidepressants, SSRIs may trigger an episode of hypomania or mania in vulnerable patients, but clinicians should be able to differentiate these symptoms from akathisia, jitteriness, and so-called behavioral activation (agitation and disinhibition) (Wilens et al., 1998). Allergic reactions have been reported but, as with any other medications, these need to be differentiated from allergic reactions to the dyes contained in the medications. The SSRIs have been implicated in inducing extrapyramidal symptoms and hyponatremia, and they have been associated with ecchymoses (Leonard et al., 1997; APA, 2000; Lake et al., 2000).

Discontinuation. Especially in SSRIs with shorter half-lives (e.g., paroxetine), sudden or rapid cessation may induce withdrawal symptoms that can mimic a relapse or recurrence of a depressive episode (e.g., tiredness, irritability). Furthermore, there is the clinical impression that rapid discontinuation of antidepressants may induce relapses or recurrences of depression. Therefore, if these medications need to be discontinued, they should be tapered progressively.

Pharmacokinetic studies

In children and adolescents, the half-times for antidepressants such as paroxetine, sertraline, and citalopram are between 14 and 16 hours (Clein and Riddle, 1995; Findling et al., 1999; (Axelson et al., 2000 a,b). This suggests that these medications, particular when prescribed at lower doses, need to be administered twice a day. Otherwise, children and adolescents can experience withdrawal side effects during the evening, and these symptoms can be confused with lack of response or medication side effects. One study suggested that sertraline at doses of 200 mg/day can be administered once a day (Alderman et al., 1998), but further studies are necessary. Pharmacokinetic studies of the other antidepressants are necessary because it appears that youth metabolize these medications faster than the adult populations.

Interactions with other medications

All SSRIs (e.g., Leonard et al., 1997) and in particular fluoxetine, Fluvosamine and paroxetine are metabolized by hepatic cytochrome P450 enzymes. Therefore, it is important to be aware of the possibility that the therapeutic or toxic effects of other medications metabolized by the cytochrome P450 isoenzyme system can be increased. Substantial inhibition of these isoenzymes converts a normal metabolizer into a slow metabolizer with regard to this specific pathway. Inhibition of the hepatic oxidative isoenzymes has been associated with a reduction, to a varying extent, in the clearance of many therapeutic agents, including the TCAs, several neuroleptics, antiarrhythmics, theophylene, terfenadine, benzodiazepines, carbamazepine, and warfarin (for a complete list, see Nemeroff et al., 1996).

The SSRIs also have a high rate of protein binding, which can lead to increased therapeutic or toxic effects of other protein-bound medications. The MAOIs should not be given within 5 weeks after stopping fluoxetine, and at least 2 weeks after other SSRIS, because of the possibility of inducing a serotonergic syndrome.

Tricyclic antidepressants

Outpatient adult studies involving thousands of subjects have shown an approximately 50% to 70% response to TCAs, with drug–placebo differences ranging from 20% to 40% (APA, 2000). In contrast, only 13 double-blind psychopharmacological trials, which include approximately 330 depressed children and adolescents, comparing TCAs (nortriptyline, imipramine, desipramine, amitriptyline) with placebo have been reported. These studies showed a similar response to both the TCAs and placebo (for a review see Birmaher et al., 1996a). These studies need to be considered preliminary because of methodological limitations, in particular the small sample sizes, short-duration trials, and the inclusion of patients with mild depressions, lower levels of neurovegetative symptoms, and comorbid disorders that may have higher response to placebo (Hughes et al., 1990; Birmaher et al., 1996a). However, a recent study comparing imipramine, paroxetine, and placebo (Keller et al., in 2001) in a large sample of adolescents with MDD reported no significant differences in response between those taking imipramine and those taking and placebo, supporting the view that the TCAs are not first-line medications for the treatment of MDD in youth. It is important to emphasize however, that some individual patients may selectively respond to TCAs and not to the newer antidepressants, and the TCAs may be indicated for augmentation of the SSRIs (APA, 2000) and the treatment of comorbid MDD and ADHD (Hughes et al., 1999). A recent report suggested that imipramine, in combination with CBT, may be helpful for short term treatment of adolescents with the combination of MDD and anxiety disorders (Bernstein et al., 2000).

Other antidepressants

Other new antidepressants, including bupropion, venlafaxine, nefazodone, and mirtazapine, have been found to be efficacious in the treatment of depressed adults, but only a few open-label studies have been carried out in children and adolescents (e.g., Daviss et al., 2001). Bupropion and velanfaxine may be useful in treating youth with MDD and ADHD (Plizka, 2000; Daviss et al., 2001). Because of the sedative effects of mirtazapine and trazodone, these medications have been used as adjunctive treatments for patients with severe insomnia.

Acute Treatment—Conclusions and Preliminary Recommendations

Currently, the antidepressants of choice are the SSRIs because they have been shown to be efficacious and safe for the treatment of children and adolescents with MDD, but further research on the other new antidepressants (e.g., bupropion, venlafaxine, nefazodone, mirtazapine) is needed. Patients should be treated with adequate doses for at least 6 weeks before declaring lack of response to treatment (treatment of nonresponders is described below) (AACAP, 1998; Hughes et al., 1999; Fig. 36.1).

It is important to note that specific psychotherapies (CBT or IPT) (Brent et al., 1997; Mufson et al., 1999) are also reasonable initial choices for the acute treatment of a youth with the first *noncomplicated* episode of major depression. Nevertheless, if patients are treated with psychotherapy alone, pharmacotherapy should be added if there is no improvement by 4–6 weeks.

From our clinical experience, we have found that youth with more severe and chronic depressions and those with significant comorbid disorders or who experience parental conflict often fail to respond to either monotherapy alone (Clarke et al., 1992; Brent et al., 1998; Emslie et al., 1998). Therefore, severe and chronic depressions should be treated with both antidepressants and psychotherapy, and other risk factors for poor outcome (e.g., parent depression, ADHD) should be addressed with additional psychosocial and/or pharmacological interventions.

The initial choice of therapy is also dictated by the severity of the depression (e.g., the severity of depressive symptoms impedes an adequate trial of psychotherapy), subtype of depression (e.g., presence of psychosis, seasonal depression, or treatment-resistant depressions) presence of comorbid disorders, prior treatment history, child and parent motivation toward treatment, and the clinician's motivation and expertise in implementing any specific intervention.

Independent of the treatment administered, the patient and family will require education about the nature and treatment of depression, and about support and management of daily problems. Problems at school, academic issues, school refusal, abuse of drugs, exposure to negative events (e.g., abuse, conflict with parents), and peer issues must be addressed. For example, family discord is associated with slower recovery and greater chance of recurrence (Rueter et al., 1999; Birmaher et al., 2000a), and ongoing disappointments have been associated with chronic depression (Goodyer et al., 1998). Therefore, addressing family discord and improving patient coping skills is likely to improve the outcome of either psychosocial or psychopharmacological treatment.

Because of the high degree of comorbidity and the psychosocial and academic consequences of depression, *multimodal pharmacological and psychosocial treatment approaches* are important to consider. (Hughes et al., 1999). For example, a child with MDD and ADHD may not respond to a SSRI alone, and may require either combined treatment with a stimulant and a SSRI, or an alternate approach, such as a TCA, bupropion, or venlafaxine (Plizka, 2000; Daviss et al., 2001). The high incidence of parental mental health problems and the association of family psychopathology and conflicts with poor treatment response (e.g., Rueter et al., 1999; Birmaher et al., 2000a); emphasize the need for evaluation and appropriate referral of parents and siblings of depressed youth.

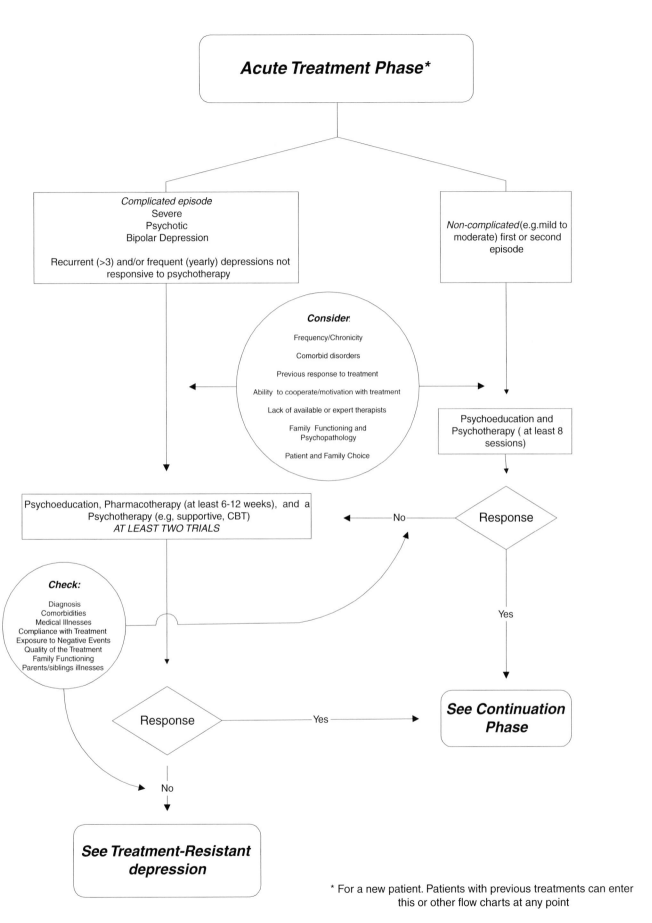

FIGURE 36.1 Major depressive disorder—acute treatment phase.

TREATMENT OF SUBTYPES OF MAJOR DEPRESSIVE DISORDER

Psychotic Depression

Overall, only 20% to 40% of adults with psychotic MDD respond to antidepressant monotherapy, and the range of placebo response is from very low to null (APA, 2000). Although monotherapy with antidepressants may be effective, recovery appears to be greater and more rapid when antidepressants are combined with an antipsychotic. However, the long-term use of the typical neuroleptics in MDD has not been evaluated and carries the risk for tardive dyskinesia (TD). It has therefore been recommended that the antypsychotic be tapered after remission of the depression. The newer antypsychotic medications (e.g., risperidone, olanzapine) may prove to be useful alternatives to the typical neuroleptics and deserve further investigation. Higher blood levels of TCAs appear to be associated with better response (Puig-Antich et al., 1979), and electroconvulsive therapy (ECT) is particularly effective for this subtype of depression in adults (APA, 2000).

Atypical Depression

Patients with atypical depression respond significantly better to the MAOIs and to SSRIs than to TCAs (APA, 2000). This differential response has not been studied in younger patients however.

Seasonal Affective Disorder

Studies in adults, and a few studies in children and adolescents have suggested that bright-light therapy is efficacious for the treatment of seasonal affective disorder (SAD) (see review by Swedo et al., 1997). The most widely used protocol consists of using a light box with 10,000 lux at a 1-foot distance from the face of the patient for 30 minutes every morning, starting in the late fall to early winter. Treatment can be extended to 1 hour in cases of partial response. Studies of use of light visors and other head-mounted devices have been inconclusive. It is unclear at which time of the day light exposure is more efficacious; some patients may respond better during the morning hours. At the same time, morning hours may be difficult during the school year or for adolescents who refuse to wake up early. Bright-light therapy has been associated with some side effects, such as headaches and eye strain. Some authors have recommended an ophthalmological evaluation before initiating light therapy, but others have questioned the usefulness of this practice unless patients have had previous eye illnesses. Treatment with light may induce episodes of hypomania or mania in vulnerable patients.

Bipolar Depression

Many of the children and adolescents seen for treatment of depression are experiencing their first depressive episode. Because the symptoms of unipolar and bipolar depression are similar, it is difficult to decide whether a patient needs only an antidepressant or concomitant use of mood stabilizers. As noted above, symptoms and signs such as psychosis, psychomotor retardation, or family history of bipolar disorder may warn the clinician about the risk of the child developing a manic episode.

There are no studies in youth with bipolar depression, and there are few controlled pharmacological studies in adults (Compton and Nemeroff, 2000). Given the possibility that antidepressants may induce mania or rapid cycling, it has been recommended that the patient be started first on a mood stabilizer (lithium carbonate, valproate, carbamazepine) (APA, 1994b) and then, if necessary, an antidepressant can be added. However, in one controlled study, a large sample of depressed bipolar-II patients were successfully treated with fluoxetine alone, without a significant increase in manic switches (Amsterdam et al., 1998). Therefore, patients with bipolar-II depression, in particular those with sporadic periods of hypomania, may respond to a SSRI or bupropion, without mood stabilizers. Clinicians should nonetheless be aware that antidepressants might induce rapid cycling in vulnerable patients.

In adults, mood stabilizers reduce the risk of cycling and have modest antidepressant effects (APA, 1994b). For patients with bipolar depression who do not respond to mood stabilizers alone, an antidepressant should be added to the treatment. It appears that bipolar depressed patients may be less likely to respond to TCAs than patients with unipolar depressions, who may show a more favorable response to bupropion, SSRI, or MAOIs. Furthermore, some studies, but not all, have also suggested that bupropion and the MAOIs are less likely to produce mania and less rapid cycling (APA, 1994b; Compton and Nemeroff, 2000).

Although there are continuation and maintenance guidelines for the use of antidepressants for unipolar depression, it is not clear how long a patient with bipolar depression should be treated with these medications. Rates of recurrence of bipolar depression of approximately 60% have been observed in patients taking adequate doses of lithium, alone or in combination with imipramine (APA, 1994b). As the TCAs have not been shown to be efficacious for youth with

MDD (Birmaher et al., 1996b; Keller et al., 2001), and in adults they appear to be poor antidepressants for patients with bipolar depression or may induce rapid cycling (APA, 1994b, 2000), it remains to be seen whether the combination of mood stabilizers and other antidepressants such as bupropion and SSRIs will yield more complete prophylaxis.

Treatment—Resistant Depression

Similar to reports in the adult literature (APA, 2000), approximately 20%-30% of youth with MDD have a partial (moderate response on the CGI improvement scale, presence of significant symptoms of MDD but not the full syndrome) or no response to treatment (e.g., Birmaher et al., 2000a). Patients with partial response have a significantly higher rate of relapse during the first 6 months following therapy and have significantly more psychosocial, occupational, and medical problems (APA, 2000). Moreover, chronic depressions usually do not remit spontaneously and are not responsive to placebo (APA, 2000), indicating the need for aggressive treatment of patients with these conditions (Fig. 36.2)

The first step in the management of patients with treatment-resistant depression is to establish nonresponse. Several definitions of nonresponse have been used, including the presence of a significant number of depressive symptoms, less than 50% improvement as measured by rating scales (e.g., the CDRS), and no change or worsening in the CGI. Once it has been established that the patient has not responded, it is crucial to try to find the underlying cause. The most common reasons for treatment failure are inappropriate diagnosis, inadequate drug dosage or length of drug trial, lack of compliance with treatment, comorbidity with other psychiatric disorders (e.g., dysthymia, anxiety, ADHD, covered substance abuse, personality disorders) or comorbid medical illnesses (e.g., hypothyroidism), existence of bipolar depression, and exposure to chronic or severe life events (e.g., abuse, chronic conflicts) that require different modalities of therapy (Brent et al., 1998; Emslie et al, 1998; APA, 2000).

There are very few pharmacological studies of children and adolescents with treatment—refractory depression. After noncompliance with treatment has been ruled out, on the basis of adult literature, the following strategies have been recommended: (1) optimizing the initial treatment, (2) switching to either a different agent from the same group (e.g., one SSRI to another SSRI) or an agent from a different group (e.g., a SSRI to venlafaxine); (3) augmentation or combination, (4) ECT, and (5) use of other treatments (e.g., IV clomi-

pramine, transcraneal magnetic stimulation [TMS]) (for reviews see Thase and Rush, 1997; AACAP, 1998; APA 2000; Martis and Janicak, 2000). All of these strategies require implementation *in a systematic fashion.*

Psychoeducation of the patient and family is required to avoid the development of hopelessness in both the patient and family, and the clinician. Comparing these strategies with other treatments of medical disorders can be useful to help patients and their families understand the medication plan and to improve compliance with and tolerance of treatment. In this instance the example of hypertension is appropriate: diuretics may be used alone, or combined with other antihypertensives in different trials, according to response.

Optimizing initial treatments

Although few studies have evaluated the efficacy of this strategy, the initial treatment should be maximized when possible by increasing the length of the trial and/or the dosage.

Extending the initial medication trial. For patients with at least a *partial response* after receiving a therapeutic dosage of antidepressant for 6 weeks, the first and simplest strategy will be, if the patient's clinical and functional status allows, to extend the treatment for another 2 to 4 weeks (Thase and Rush, 1997; APA, 2000).

Increasing the dosage. This strategy can be used for partial responders, but in occasional cases of patients with no response, increasing the dosage for another 2–3 weeks may help (APA, 2000).

Switching strategies

For patients who do not respond to a specific antidepressant medication or who do not tolerate its side effects, other antidepressants *of the same class or different classes* (e.g., venlafaxine for a patient treated with a SSRI) can be tried. The few adult studies published thus far suggest that it is more efficacious to switch antidepressant classes than to stay within the same class, because of the probable heterogeneity in underlying depression mechanisms. Also, it has been suggested that severe depressions appear to respond better to antidepressants with both serotonergic and adrenergic properties (e.g., venlafaxine) (Poirier and Boyer, 1999).

Studies in adult depressed populations have shown a

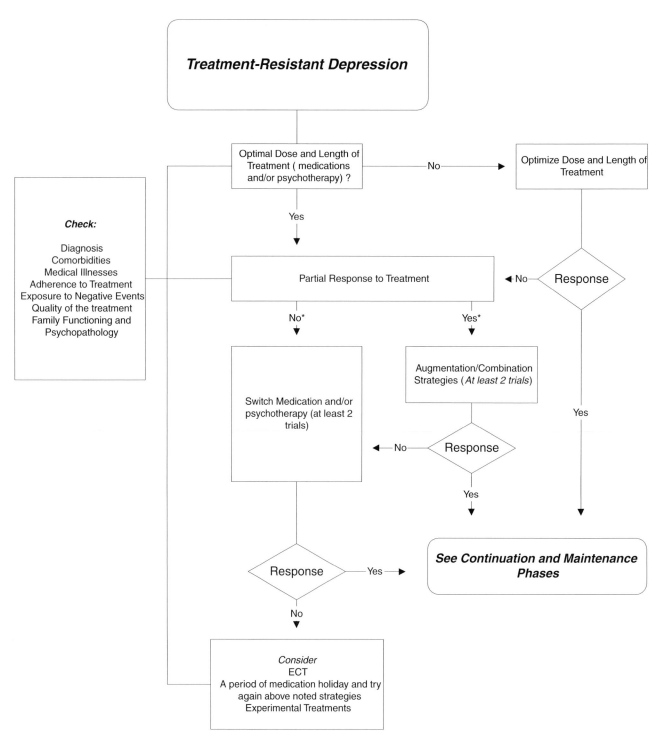

FIGURE 36.2 Management of treatment resistant depression.

10% to 30% response when a TCA is replaced with another TCA, a 20%–50% response rate when a TCA is switched to a heterocyclic antidepressant (e.g., amoxapine, nomifensine), a 30% to 70% rate when a TCA or a heterocyclic antidepressant is switched to a SSRI, and an approximately 60% rate when a SSRI is switched to a TCA (Thase and Rush, 1997). Clinical experience suggests that a patient who has not responded to a particular SSRI has about a 50% chance of responding to a different SSRI (Joffe et al., 1996), but this strategy needs further investigation.

The MAOIs have been found to be beneficial for patients who have not responded to other medications (Thase and Rush, 1997; APA, 2000). An open study suggested that adolescents with depression who did not respond to TCAs responded to MAOIs (Ryan et al., 1988b). However, it is possible that these adolescents did not respond to TCAs because this group of medications is not efficacious for the treatment of pediatric MDD (Birmaher et al., 1996a).

Augmentation or combination strategies

The most common augmentation or combination strategies include adding lithium carbonate at therapeutic levels for a period of 4 weeks, adding 1-triiodothyronine (T_3) (25–50 μ/day), using stimulants, and combining a SSRI with a TCA (APA, 2000; Bauer et al., 2000). In adults, the combination of lithium and antidepressants has yielded a response rate of 50% to 65% in studies in which lithium was administered at therapeutic levels for at least 4 weeks (e.g., Thase and Rush, 1997; APA, 2000). The interval before response to augmentation with lithium has been reported to be from several days to 3 weeks (APA, 2000). After this period, the chances of observing improvement with lithium decrease.

In adolescents with MDD, an open study showed significant improvement of refractory depressive symptoms after augmentation of TCA treatment with lithium (Ryan et al., 1988a). Another open-label study did not replicate this finding (Strober et al., 1992).

Case reports have suggested that adding stimulant medications or combining a SSRI and a TCA or bupropion may also be effective (APA, 2000), but these combinations need to be done with caution, given the possibility of drug interactions (e.g., SSRIs' cytochrome inhibition leading to toxic TCA levels). Additionally, in adults, the combination of antidepressants and psychotherapy (CBT, IPT) for patients with severe or treatment-resistant depression has been found useful (APA, 2000; Keller et al., 2000).

Electroconvulsive therapy

Electroconvulsive therapy is one of the most efficacious treatments for adults with nonresistant (70% response) and resistant MDD (50% response) (APA, 2000). Because of the invasiveness of this treatment, however, it remains the treatment of choice only for the most severe, incapacitating forms of resistant depression. No studies have been carried out among adolescents, but anecdotal reports have suggested that adolescents with refractory depression may respond to ECT without significant side effects (Rey and Walter, 1997). Approximately 60% of adult patients treated successfully with ECT tend to relapse after 6 months (APA, 2000). Therefore, they must also receive maintenance treatment with antidepressants and sometimes maintenance ECT. There are no reports of use of maintenance ECT in adolescents.

Other treatments

Other innovative treatments such as intravenous clomipramine (CMI) and TMS have been used for the treatment of depressed adults who have not responded to standard treatment. In adolescents, intravenous clomipramine has been shown to be efficacious for patients who have failed to respond to other antidepressant treatments (Sallee et al., 1997).

Some randomized control trials have shown that TMS is efficacious and safe for the treatment of adults with MDD (with and without treatment-resistant depressions) (e.g., Grunhaus et al., 2000; Martis and Janicak, 2000). However, the use of TMS has not been standardized and there is controversy regarding the methodology used in some studies.

TREATMENT OF COMORBID CONDITIONS AND SUICIDALITY

Comorbid disorders may influence the onset, maintenance, and recurrence of depression (Birmaher et al., 1996a,b). Therefore, in addition to the treatment of depressive symptoms, it is of prime importance to treat the comorbid conditions that frequently accompany the depressive disorder.

For example, depressed adolescents with comorbid ADHD respond less well to treatment (Emslie et al., 1998; Hamilton and Bridge, 1999; Birmaher et al., 2000b). For these patients, it has been suggested that the ADHD be initially treated and if depressive symptoms persist after stabilization of the ADHD, a SSRI

(Hughes et al., 1999; Plizka, 2000). This strategy has not been validated, however. Recently an open study using bupropion suggested that this medication can be efficacious to treat both MDD and ADHD (Daviss et al., 2001), although its effect on ADHD is not as impressive as that obtained with stimulants (Conners et al., 1996).

Comorbid anxiety has been associated with differential treatment response. This association predicts at times a better response to CBT and TCAs (Hughes et al., 1990; Brent et al., 1998). Treatment of comorbid anxiety, which most often precedes depression, is essential because the treatment contributes to improvement and may prevent future depressive episodes (Kovacs et al., 1989; Hayward et al., 2000). Fortunately, pharmacotherapy and psychotherapy treatments found useful for the treatment of MDD have also been found to be beneficial for treatment of youths with anxiety disorders (Kendall, 1994; RUPP Anxiety Group, 2001).

Suicidal ideation and behavior are common symptoms accompanying major depression and are more likely to occur in the face of comorbid disruptive disorders and/or substance abuse (e.g., Gould et al., 1996). Assessment of suicidality, securing any lethal agents (e.g., medications, firearms), and development of no-suicide contracts with the patient and family are essential components of management of the suicidal, depressed patient. Patients who cannot agree to a no-suicide contract require inpatient hospitalization. Treatment of the underlying depression may be necessary but not sufficient to prevent recurrent attempts, insofar as placebo-controlled medication trials in adults show greater improvement in depression associated with medication, but equal rates of attempts and completions in medication plus placebo conditions (Khan et al., 2000). Other contributors to suicidality, such as sexual abuse, use of drugs and alcohol, ADHD, conduct problems, impulsivity and aggression, homosexuality personality disorders, and family discord, must be assessed and targeted (Brent et al., 1999b).

Other comorbid conditions, such as obsessive-compulsive, conduct, eating, and post-traumatic stress disorders, have also been found to affect the treatment response and need to be addressed for the successful treatment of depressed youths (Birmaher et al., 1996b; Goodyer et al., 1997; Brent et al., 1998).

CONTINUATION THERAPY

To consolidate the response and to prevent relapse of symptoms, *all patients* should be offered continuation treatment for at least 6 months after complete remission of symptoms. (Fig. 36.3). Those who have shown difficulty achieving remission (≥ 3 months), those who have factors associated with persistent depression, such as subsyndromal symptoms of depression, early onset, family history of recurrent depressions, dysthymia, comorbid disorders, or suicidality, and those who are exposed to stressors (e.g., family discord) or have a history of recurrent depressions (Birmaher et al., 1996b; AACAP, 1998) should be treated for at least 1 year. During this phase, patients are seen biweekly or monthly, depending on the patient's clinical status, functioning, support systems, environmental stressors, and motivation for treatment, and the existence of other psychiatric and/or medical disorders. The patient and family should be taught to recognize early signs of relapse.

PHARMACOTHERAPY STUDIES

Although not studied in children and adolescents, on the basis of studies with adults, antidepressants must be continued during the continuation phase, at the same dosage used to attain remission of acute symptoms, provided that there are no significant side effects or dose-related negative effects on the patient's compliance (APA, 2000). In adults, continuation pharmacotherapy treatment during this phase reduces the risk of relapse—from 40%–60% to 10%–20%—with TCAs, SSRIs, and lithium carbonate, all of which have been found to be significantly more effective than placebo in preventing relapses (APA, 2000). Overall, over 50% of adult patients (APA, 2000) and adolescents (Wood et al., 1996) randomized to placebo relapsed during continuation trials, most within 3 months of having their medication discontinued.

If at the end of the continuation phase it is decided that the antidepressants should be discontinued, this should be done gradually (e.g., over 6 weeks) to avoid withdrawal effects such as sleep disturbance, irritability, or gastrointestinal symptoms, which may lead the clinician to misinterpret the need for continued medication treatment. Clinical practice has suggested that rapid discontinuation of antidepressants may precipitate a relapse or recurrence of depression. In children and adolescents, it is recommended that treatment be discontinued while they are on extended vacations, rather than during the school year.

Follow-up of depressed youth and adults has shown that, despite successful acute psychotherapy or pharmacological treatment, the rate of relapse or recurrence at 6 to 12 months is about 40% to 60%, particularly in those who discontinue treatment (Vostanis et al.,

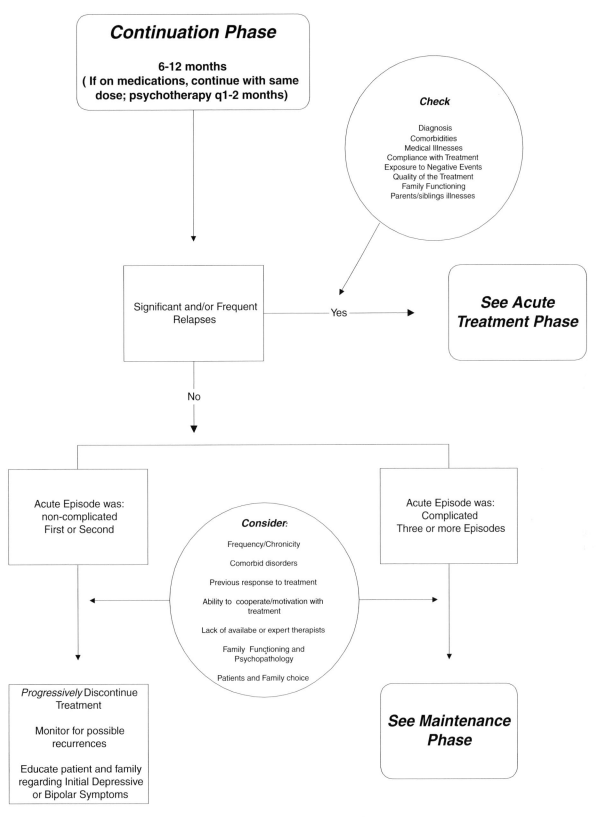

FIGURE 36.3 Major depressive disorder—continuation treatment phase.

477

1996; Wood et al., 1996; Emslie et al., 1998; Birmaher et al., 2000a). Naturalistic studies of children and adolescents and controlled trials in adults show that continuation medication and/or psychotherapy can reduce relapses (Fava et al., 1996; Kroll et al., 1996; Mufson and Fairbanks, 1996; Emslie et al., 1998). Patients treated with psychotherapy alone or in combination with medications should continue psychotherapy biweekly to monthly, depending on the presence of factors that increase the risk of relapse. The patient and family should be taught to recognize early signs of relapse.

If relapse does occur, it should first be determined whether the patient was compliant with treatment. If the patient was not compliant, antidepressant medication should resume. If the patient was compliant and had been previously responding to the medication (without significant side effects), the existence of ongoing stressors (e.g., conflict, abuse) or comorbid medical or psychiatric disorders should be considered (anxiety disorder, ADHD, substance abuse, dysthymia, bipolar disorder, eating disorder).

In this case, and depending on the specific circumstances, an increase in the medication dosage, a change to another medication, augmentation strategies, or psychotherapy may be indicated. For patients receiving only psychotherapy, adding medications and/or utilizing new psychotherapeutic strategies may be considered.

MAINTENANCE THERAPY

After the patient has been asymptomatic for a period of approximately 6–12 months (continuation phase), the clinician has to decide *who* should receive maintenance therapy, *which* therapy to use, and for *how long*. The main goal of the maintenance phase is to prevent recurrences. This phase may last from 1 year to much longer, and is typically conducted at a visit frequency of every 1 to 3 months, depending on the patient's clinical status, functioning, support systems, environmental stressors, and motivation for treatment, and the existence of other psychiatric or medical disorders (Fig. 36.4).

Who Should Receive Maintenance Therapy?

The recommendation for maintenance therapy depends on several factors, such as severity of the present depressive episode (e.g., suicidality, psychosis, functional impairment), number and severity of prior depressive episodes, chronicity, comorbid disorders, family psy-

chopathology, presence of support, patient and family willingness to adhere to the treatment program, and contraindications to treatment.

Factors associated with increased risk for recurrence in naturalistic studies of depressed children and adolescents may serve as guidance to the clinician to decide who needs maintenance treatment. These factors include history of prior depressive episodes, female sex, late onset, suicidality, double depression, subsyndromal symptoms, poor functioning, personality disorders, exposure to negative events (e.g., abuse, conflicts), and family history of recurrent MDD (≤2 episodes) (Birmaher et al., 1996 a,b; Goodyer et al., 1998; Lewinsohn et al., 1999; Rao et al., 1999; Rueter et al., 1999; Weissman et al., 1999a, b; Klein et al., 2001).

In depressed *adults* (APA, 2000), patients who have only a single, uncomplicated episode of depression, or those with mild episodes or with lengthy intervals between episodes (e.g., 5 years) should probably not start maintenance treatment. There is also consensus that adult patients with three or more episodes (especially if they occur in a short period of time or have deleterious consequences) and those with chronic depression should receive maintenance treatment.

It is still debated whether patients with two previous episodes should receive maintenance treatment. Overall, maintenance treatment has been recommended for adult depressed patients with two episodes who have one or more of the following criteria (Depression Guideline Panel, 1993): (*1*) a family history of bipolar disorder or recurrent depression, (*2*) early onset of the first depressive episode (before age 20), and (*3*) both episodes were severe or life threatening and occurred during the past 3 years. Given that depression in youth has similar clinical presentation, sequelae, and natural course as in adults, these guidelines should probably be applied for youth with two previous major depressive episodes.

Which Treatment?

Practically, unless there is any contraindication (e.g., medication side effects), the treatment that was efficacious in inducting remission of the acute episode should be used for maintenance therapy. Patients who are maintained only on medication should be offered psychotherapy to help them cope with the psychosocial scars induced by the depression. Further, many depressed youths live in environments charged with stressful situations and their parents usually have psychiatric disorders. In these instances multimodal treatments are particularly needed.

In adults, pharmacological and psychosocial thera-

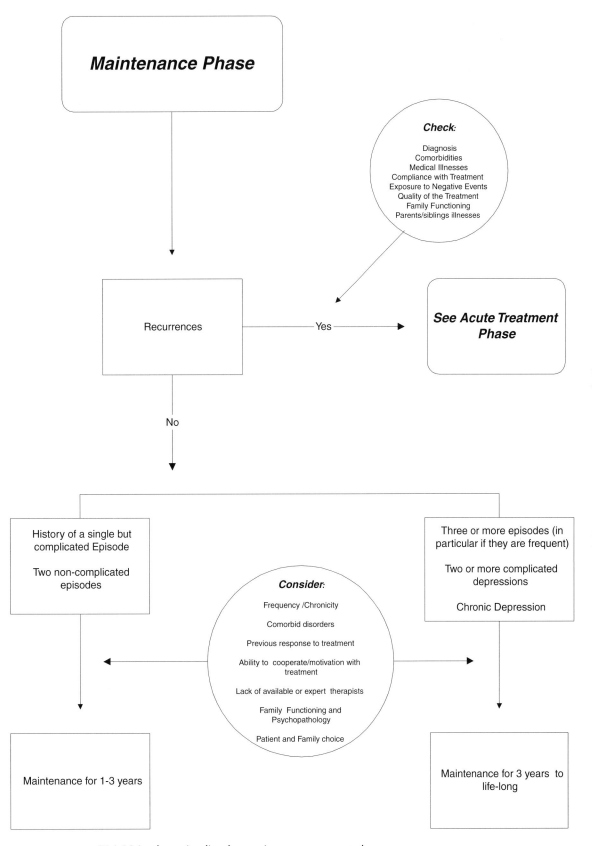

FIGURE 36.4 Major depressive disorder—maintenance treatment phase.

pies have been found to be efficacious in the prevention of depressive recurrences (APA, 2000). There are no controlled psychopharmacological or psychotherapy maintenance studies of children and adolescents. One open investigation with a small sample of depressed adolescents showed that acute treatment with IPT was associated with a low risk of depressive recurrences after 1 year of finishing the therapy (Mufson et al., 1996). Also, CBT seems to be helpful in preventing progression from subsyndromal to full-blown depression (Clarke et al., 1995). Because it is important to develop preliminary treatment maintenance guidelines in children and adolescents with depressive disorders, psychotherapy and pharmacological adult maintenance studies are briefly reviewed below.

In selecting the medication for maintenance therapy, clinicians should consider the profile of side effects and the way these may affect a patient's compliance. For example, dry mouth, weight gain, increased sweating, sexual dysfunction, and polyuria (if patients are taking lithium) may be troublesome and induce discontinuation of treatment. In addition, in children and adolescents, the potential long-term consequences of using antidepressant medications (e.g, chronic inhibition of serotonin, tachycardia induced by TCAs) are not known. Other factors, such as patients' embarrassment with friends, the idea of having their minds "controlled" by a medication the perception that taking medications is a sign of weakness, and uncertainty about the risk of relapse in spite of doing well on medication, should be addressed with both patients and their parents.

How Long Should the Maintenance Phase Last?

It is recommended that adult patients with second episodes of depression and who fulfill the criteria for maintenance therapy noted above be maintained for several years (up to 5 years in adult studies), using the same dosage of the antidepressant used to achieve clinical remission during the acute-treatment phase. Maintenance therapy for patients with three or more episodes of MDD, patients with second episodes associated with psychosis, severe impairment, and severe suicidality, and those who proved very difficult to treat should be considered for longer periods of time, even for the life of the patient (AACAP, 1998).

In summary, during the maintenance treatment phase, both psychosocial and pharmacological treatments have been found to be beneficial in preventing recurrences. However, as yet, in adults the evidence is stronger for pharmacotherapy. Also, it is not clear whether psychosocial treatments are efficacious in pre-

venting recurrences for severe depressions. Psychotic, bipolar, and chronic depressions all require the use of medications.

The TCAs, SSRIs, and lithium have been found to be efficacious for the prevention of depressive recurrences in adults (APA, 2000). However, given the noted advantages of the SSRIs and their efficacy in the acute treatment of MDD and dysthymia, this group is considered the first-choice medication for Intervention.

For most children and adolescents, multimodal therapies are recommended. However, if antidepressant medications are used alone, psychosocial maintenance strategies should be implemented to help the patient manage inner and interpersonal conflicts, improve coping and social skills, deal with the psychosocial and personal scars left by the depression, and improve academic and social functioning. The reduction of family stress, promotion of a supportive environment, and the effective treatment of parents and siblings with psychiatric disorders may also help diminish the risk for recurrence.

REFERENCES

Alderman, J., Wolkow, R., Chung, M., and Johnston, H.F. (1998) Sertraline treatment of children and adolescents with obsessive-compulsive disorder or depression: pharmacokinetics, tolerability, and efficacy. *J Am Acad Child Adolesc Psychiatry*, 37:386–394.

Ambrosini, P.J., Wagner, K.D., Biederman, J., Glick, I., Tan, C., Elia, J., Hebeler, J., Rabinovich, H., Lock, J., and Geller, D. (1999) Multicenter open-label sertraline study in adolescent outpatients with major depression. *J Am Acad Child Adolesc Psychiatry* 38: 566–572.

American Academy of Child and Adolescent Psychiatry (AACAP) (1998) Practice parameters for the assessment and treatment of children and adolescents with depressive disorder. *J Am Acad Child Adolesc Psychiatry* 37(10 Suppl):63S–83S.

American Psychiatric Association (APA) (1994a) *Diagnostic and Statistical Manual of Mental Disorders (DSM-IV)*, (4th ed.) Washington, DC.

American Psychiatric Association (APA) (1994b) Practice guideline for the treatment of patients with bipolar disorder. *Am J Psychiatry* 41:1–35.

American Psychiatric Association (APA) (2000) Practice for the treatment of patients with major depressive disorder [revision] *Am J Psychiatry* 157:(Suppl): 1–45.

Amsterdam, J.D., Garcia-Espana, F., Fawcett, J., Quitkin, F.M., Reimherr, F.W., Rosenbaum, J.F., Schweizer, E., and Beasley, C. (1998) Efficacy and safety of fluoxetine in treating bipolar II major depressive episode. *J Clin Psychopharmacol* 18:435–440.

Angold, A., Costello, E.J., and Erkanli, A. (1999) Comorbidity. *J Child Psychol Psychiatry* 40:57–87.

Axelson, D., Perel, J., Rudolph, G., Birmaher, B., and Brent, D. (2000a) Sertraline pediatric/adolescent PK-PD parameters: dose/plasma level ranging for depression [abstract]. *Clin Pharmacol Ther* 67:169.

Axelson, D., Perel, J., Rudolph, G., Birmaher, B., Nuss, S., and Brent, D. (2000b) Significant differences in pharmacokinetics/dynamics of ± citalopram between adolescents and adults: Implications for clinical dosing [abstract]. *Proceedings of the 39th Annual Meeting of the American College of Neuropsychopharmacology.* San Juan, Puerto Rico, p. 122.

Bauer, M., Bschor, T., Kunz, D., Berghoefer, A., Strohle, A., and Muller-Oerlinghausen, B. (2000) Double-blind, placebo-controlled trial of the use of lithium to augment antidepressant medication in continuation treatment of unipolar major depression. *Am J Psychiatry* 157:1429–1435.

Beck, A.T. (1967) *Depression: Clinical, Experimental and Theoretical Aspects.* New York: Harper & Row.

Bernstein, G.A., Borchardt, C.M., Perwien, A.R., Crosby, R.D., Kushner, M.G., Thuras, P.D., and Last, C.G. (2000) Imipramine plus cognitive-behavioral therapy in the treatment of school refusal. *J Am Acad Child Adolesc Psychiatry* 39:276–283.

Birmaher, B., Brent, D.A., Kolko, D., Baugher, M., Bridge, J., Holder, D., Iyengar S., and Ulloa, R.E (2000a) Clinical outcome after short-term psychotherapy for adolescents with major depressive disorder. *Arch Gen Psychiatry* 57:29–36.

Birmaher, B., McCafferty, J.P., Bellow, K.M., and Beebe, K.L. (2000b) Comorbid ADHD and disruptive behavior disorders as predictors of response in adolescents treated for major depression. Presented at the *American Psychiatric Association Annual Meeting*, Chicago, IL.

Birmaher, B., Ryan, N.D., Williamson, D.E., Brent, D.A., and Kaufman, J. (1996a) Childhood and adolescent depression: A review of the past 10 years—Part II. *J Am Acad Child Adolesc Psychiatry* 35:1575–1583.

Birmaher, B., Ryan, N.D., Williamson, D., Brent, D., Kaufman, J., Dahl, R., Perel, J., and Nelson, B. (1996b) Childhood and adolescent depression: a review of the past 10 years—Part I. *J Am Acad Child Adolesc Psychiatry* 35:1427–1439.

Brent, D.A., Baugher, M., Bridge, J., Chen, J., and Beery, L. (1999a) Age and sex-related risk factors for adolescent suicide. *J Am Acad Child Adolesc Psychiatry* 38:1497–1505.

Brent, D.A., Holder, D., Birmaher, B., Baugher, M., Roth, C., Iyengar, S., and Johnson, B. (1997) A clinical psychotherapy trial for adolescent depression comparing cognitive, family, and supportive therapy. *Arch Gen Psychiatry* 54:877–885.

Brent, D.A., Kolko, D., Birmaher, B., Baugher, M., and Bridge, J. (1999b) A clinical trial for adolescent depression: predictors of additional treatment in the acute and follow-up phases of the trial. *J Am Acad Child Adolesc Psychiatry* 38:263–270.

Brent, D.A., Kolko, D., Birmaher, B., Baugher, M., Bridge, J., Roth C., and Holder, D. (1998) Predictors of treatment efficacy in a clinical trial of three psychosocial treatments for adolescent depression. *J Am Acad Child Adolesc Psychiatry* 37:906–914.

Brent, D.A., Poling, K., McCain, B., and Baugher, M. (1993) A psycho educational program for families of affectively ill children and adolescents. *J Am Acad Child Adolesc Psychiatry* 32:770–774.

Clarke, G.N., Hawkins, W., Murphy, M., Sheerer, L.B., Lewiston, P.M., and Seeley, J.R. (1995) Targeted prevention of unipolar depressive disorder in an at-risk sample of high school adolescents: a randomized trial of a group cognitive intervention. *J Am Acad Child Adolesc Psychiatry* 34:312–321.

Clarke, G.N., Hops, H., Lewinsohn, P.M., Andrews, J.A., Seeley, J.R., and Williams, J. (1992) Cognitive behavioral group treatment of adolescent depression: prediction of outcome. *Behav Ther* 23:341–354.

Clein, P.D. and Riddle, M.A. (1995) Pharmacokinetics in children and adolescents. *Child Adolesc Psychiatr Clin North Am* 4:59–75.

Comton, M.T. and Nemeroff, C.B. (2000) The treatment of bipolar depression. *J Clin Psychiatry* 61:57–67.

Connors, C.K., Cast, C.D., Guiltieri, C.T., Welder, E., Mark, R., Reissue, A., Khayrallah, M., and Ascher, J. (1996) Bupropion hydrochloride in attention deficit hyperactivity disorder. *J Am Acad Child Adolesc Psychiatry* 35:1314–1321.

Daviss, W.B., Bentivoglio, P., Racusin, R., Brown, K., Bostic, J., and Wiley, L. (2001) Bupropion sustained release in adolescents with comorbid attention deficit hyperactivity. *J Am Acad Child Adolesc Psychiatry* 40:307–314.

Depression Guideline Panel (1993) *Depression in Primary Care: Vol I. Treatment of Major Depression. Clinical Practice Guidelines.* Rockville, MD: U.S. Department of Health and Human Services, Public Health Services, Agency for Health Care Policy and Research.

Emslie, G.J., Heiligenstein, J.H., Hoog, S.L., Judge, R., Brown E.B., and Nilsson, M. (2000) Fluoxetine for acute treatment of depression in children and adolescents: a placebo controlled randomized clinical trial. Presented at the 39th Annual Meeting of the American College of Neuropsychopharmacology, San Juan, Puerto Rico.

Emslie, G.J., Rush, A.J., Weinberg, W.A., Gullion, C.M., Rintelmann, J., and Hughes, C.W. (1997a) Recurrence of major depressive disorder in hospitalized children and adolescents. *J Am Acad Child Adolesc Psychiatry* 36:785–792.

Emslie, G.J., Rush, A.J., Weinberg, W.A., Kowatch, R.A., Carmody, T., and Mayes, T.L. (1998) Fluoxetine in child and adolescent depression: acute and maintenance treatment. *Depress Anxiety* 7:32–39.

Emslie, G., Rush, A.J., Weinberg, A.W., Kowatch, R.A., Hughes, C.W., Carmody, T., and Rintelmann J. (1997b) A double-blind, randomized placebo-controlled trial of fluoxetine in depressed children and adolescents. *Arch Gen Psychiatry* 54:1031–1037.

Fava, G.A., Grandi, S., Zielezny, M., Rafanelli, C., and Caneatrari, R. (1996) Four-year outcome for cognitive behavioral treatment of residual symptoms in major depression. *Am J Psychiatry* 153:945–947.

Findling, R.L., Reed, M.D., Myers, C., Riordan, M.A., Fiala, S., Branicky, L., Waldorf, B., and Blumer, J.L. (1999) Paroxetine pharmacokinetics in depressed children and adolescents. *J Am Acad Child Adolesc Psychiatry* 38:952–959.

Geller, B., Fox, L.W., and Clark, K.A. (1994) Rate and predictors of prepubertal bipolarity during follow-up of 6- to 12 year-old depressed children. *J Am Acad Child Adolesc Psychiatry* 33:461–468.

Goodyer, I.M., Herbert, J., and Altham, P.M. (1998) Adrenal, steroid secretion and major depression in 8-to 16-year-olds, III. Influence of cortisol/DHEA ratio at presentation on subsequent rates of disappointing life events and persistent major depression. *Psychol Med* 28:265–73.

Goodyer, I.M., Herbert, J., Secher, S.M., and Pearson, J. (1997) Short-term outcome of major depression: I. Comorbidity and severity at presentation as predictors of persistent disorder. *J Am Acad Child Adolesc Psychiatry* 36:179–187.

Gould, M.S., Fisher, P., Parides, M., Flory, M., and Shaffer, D. (1996) Psychosocial risk factors of child and adolescent completed suicide. *Arch Gen Psychiatry* 53:1155–1162.

Grunhaus, L., Dannon, P.N., and Schreiber, S. (2000) Repetitive transcraneal magnetic stimulation is as effective as electroconvulsive therapy in the treatment of nondelusional major depressive disorder: an open study. *Biol Psychiatry* 47:314–324.

Guy, W. (1976) Clinical Global Improvement Scale. In: *Assessment*

Manual of Psychopharmacology. Rockville, MD: National Institute of Mental Health, p. 76.

Hamilton, J.D. and Bridge, J. (1999) Outcome at 6 months of 50 adolescents with major depression treated in a health maintenance organization. *J Am Acad Child Adolesc Psychiatry* 38: 1340–1346.

Hamilton, M. (1960) A rating scale for depression. *J Neurol Neurosurg Psychol* 23:56–61.

Hayward, C., Killen, J.D., Kraemer, H.C., and Barr Taylor, C. (2000) Predictors of panic attacks in adolescents. *J Am Acad Child Adolesc Psychiatry* 39:207–214.

Hughes, C., Preskorn, S., Weller, E., Weller, R., Hassanein, R., and Tucker, S. (1990) The effect of concomitant disorders in childhood depression on predicting treatment response. *Psychopharmacol Bull* 26:235–238.

Hughes, C.W., Emslie, G.J., Crismon, M.L., Wagner, K.D., Birmaher, B., Geller, B., Pliszka, S., Ryan, N., Strober, M., Trivedi, M.H., Toprac, M.G., Sedillo, A., Llana, M.E., Lopez, M., Rush, A.J., and Texas Consensus Conference Panel on Medication Treatment of Childhood Major Depressive Disorder (1999). The Texas childhood medication algorithm project: report of the Texas Consensus Conference Panel on Medication Treatment of Childhood Major Depressive Disorder. *J Am Acad Child Adolesc Psychiatry* 38:1442–1454.

Joffe, R.T., Levitt, A.J., Sokolov, S.T.H., and Toung, L.T. (1996) Response to an open trial of a second SSRI in major depression. *J Clin Psychiatry* 57:114–115.

Keller, M.B., McCullough, J.P., Klein, D.N., Asrnow, B., Dunner, D.L., Gelenberg, A.J., Markowitz, J.C., Nemeroff, C.B., Russell, J.M., Thase, M.E., Trivedi, M.H., and Zajecka, J. (2000) A comparison of nefazodone, the cognitive behavioral-analysis system of psychotherapy, and their combination for the treatment of chronic depression. Multicenter study. Randomized controlled trial. *N Engl J Med* 342:1462–1470.

Keller, M.B., Ryan, N.D, Strober, M., Klein, R.G., Kutcher, S.P., Birmaher, B., Hagino, O.R., Koplewicz, H., Carlson, G.A., Clarke, G.N., Emslie, G.J., Feinberg, D., Geller, B., Kusumakar, V., Papatheodorou, G. Sack, W.H., Sweeney, M., Wagner, K.D., Weller, E.B., Winters, N.C., Oakes, R. and McCafferty, J.P. (2001) Efficacy of paroxetine in the treatment of adolescent major depression: a randomized, controlled trial. *J Am Acad Child Adolesc Psychiatry* 40:762–772.

Kendall, P.C. (1994) Treating anxiety disorders in children: results of a randomized clinical trial. *J Consult Clin Psychol* 62:100–110.

Khan, A., Warner, H.A., and Brown, W.A. (2000) Symptom reduction and suicide risk in patients treated with placebo in antidepressant clinical trials: an analysis of the Food and Drug Administration database. *Arch Gen Psychiatry* 57:311–317.

Klein, D.N., Lewinsohn, P.M., Seeley, J.R., and Rohde, P. (2001) A family study of major depressive disorder in a community sample of adolescents. *Arch Gen Psychiatry* 58:13–20.

Kovacs, M,. Akiskal, S., Gatsonis, C., and Parrone, P.L. (1994) Childhood-onset dysthymic disorder. *Arch Gen Psychiatry* 51: 365–374.

Kovacs, M., Gatsonis, C., Paulauskas, S.L., and Richards C. (1989) Depressive disorders in childhood. IV. A longitudinal study of comorbidity with and risk for anxiety disorders. *Arch Gen Psychiatry* 46:776–782.

Kovacs, M. and Goldston, D. (1991) Cognitive and social cognitive development of depressed children and adolescents. *J Am Acad Child Adolesc Psychiatry* 30:388–392.

Kroll, L., Harrington, R., Jayson, D., Fraser, J., and Gowers, S. (1996) Pilot study of continuation cognitive-behavioral therapy

for major depression in adolescent psychiatric patients. *J Am Acad Child Adolesc Psychiatry* 35:1156–1161.

Lake, M.B., Birmaher B., Wassick S., Mathos, K., and Yelovich, A.K. (2000) Bleeding and selective serotonin reuptake inhibitors in childhood and adolescence. *J Child Adolesc Psychopharmacol* 10: 35–38.

Leonard, H.L., March, J., Rickler, K.C., and Allen, A.J. (1997) Review of the pharmacology of the selective serotonin reuptake inhibitors in children and adolescents. *J Am Acad Child Adolesc Psychiatry* 36:725–736.

Lewinsohn, P.M., Allen, N.B., Seeley, J.R., and Gotlib, I.H. (1999) First onset versus recurrence of depression: differential processes of psychosocial risk. *J Abnorm Psychol* 108:483–489.

Martis, B. and Janicak, P.G. (2000) Transcranial magnetic stimulation for major depression: therapeutic possibilities. *Int Drug Ther Newsletter*, July 1–10.

Mufson, L. and Fairbanks, J. (1996) Interpersonal psychotherapy for depressed adolescents: a one-year naturalistic follow-up study. *J Am Acad Child Adolesc Psychiatry* 35:1145–1155.

Mufson, L., Weissman, M.M., Moreau, D., and Garfinkel R. (1999) Efficacy of interpersonal psychotherapy for depressed adolescents. *Arch Gen Psychiatry* 56:573–579.

Nemeroff, C.B., DeVane, C.L., and Pollock, B.G. (1996) Newer antidepressants and the cytochrome P450 system. *Am J Psychiatry* 153:311–320.

Nolen-Hoeksema, S., Girgus, J.S., and Seligman, M.E.P. (1992) Predictors and consequences of childhood depressive symptoms: a 5-year longitudinal study. *J Abnorm Psychiatry* 101:405–422.

Pine, D.S., Cohen. P., Gurley. D., Brook. J., and Ma, Y. (1998) The risk for early-adulthood anxiety and depressive disorders in adolescents with anxiety and depressive disorders. *Arch Gen Psychiatry* 55:56–64.

Pliszka, S. (2000) Patterns of psychiatric comorbidity with attention-deficit hyperactivity disorder. *Child Adolesc Clin North Am* 9: 1056–4993.

Poirier, M.F. and Boyer, P. (1999) Venlafaxine and paroxetine in treatment-resistant depression: double-blind, randomized comparison. *Br J Psychiatry* 175:12–16.

Poznanski, E.O., Freeman, L.N., and Mokros, H.B. (1984) Children's Depression Rating Scale–Revised. *Psychopharmacol Bull* 21:979–989.

Puig-Antich, J., Lukens, E., Davies, M., Goetz, D., Brennan-Quattrock, J., and Todak, G. (1985) Psychosocial functioning in prepubertal depressive disorders. II. Interpersonal relationships after sustained recovery from the affective episode. *Arch Gen Psychiatry* 42:511–517.

Puig-Antich, J., Perel, J., Lupatkinm, W., Chambers, W.J., Shea, C., Tabrizi, M.A., and Stiller, R.L. (1979) Plasma levels of imipramine (IMI) and desmethylimipramine (DMI) and clinical response in prepubertal major depressive disorder. A preliminary report. *J Amer Acad Child Psychiatry* 18:616–627.

Rao, U., Dahl, R.E., Ryan, N.D., Birmaher, B., Williamson, D.E., Giles, D.E., Kaufman, J., Rao, R., and Nelson, B. (1995) Unipolar depression in adolescents: Clinical outcome in adulthood. *J Am Acad Child Adolesc Psychiatry* 34:566–578.

Rao, U., Hammen, C., and Daley, S.E. (1999) Continuity of depression during the transition to adulthood: a 5-year longitudinal study of young women. *J Am Acad Child Adolesc Psychiatry* 38: 908–915.

Research Units of Pediatric Psychopharmacology (RUPP) Anxiety Group (2001) Flovoxamine for anxiety in children. *N Engl J Med* 344:1279–1285.

Rey, J.M. and Walter, G. (1997) Half a century of ECT use in young people. *Am J Psychiatry* 154:595–602.

Rueter, M.A., Scaramella, L., Wallace, L.E., and Conger, R.D. (1999) First onset of depressive or anxiety disorders predicted by the longitudinal course of internalizing symptoms and parent–adolescent disagreements. *Arch Gen Psychiatry* 56:726–732.

Ryan, N., Meyer, V., Dachille, S., Mazzie, D., and Puig-Antich, J. (1988a) Lithium antidepressant augmentation in TCA-refractory depression in adolescents. *J Am Acad Child Adolesc Psychiatry* 27:371–376.

Ryan, N., Puig-Antich, J., Rabinovich, H., Fied, J., Ambrosini, P., Meyer, V., Torres, D., Dachille, S., and Mazzie, D. (1988b) MAOIs in adolescent major depression unresponsive to tricyclic antidepressant. *J Am Acad Child Adolesc Psychiatry* 27:755–758.

Sallee, F.R., Vrindavanam, N.S., Deas-Nesmith, D., Carson, S.W., and Sethuraman, G. (1997) Pulse intravenous clomipramine for depressed adolescents: a double-blind, controlled trial. *Am J Psychiatry* 154:668–673.

Shaffer, D., Gould, M.S., Brasic, J., Ambrosini, P., Fisher, P., Bird, H., and Aluwahlia, S. (1983) A Children's Global Assessment Scale (CGAS). *Arch Gen Psychiatry* 40:1228–1231.

Simeon, J., Dinicola, V., Ferguson, H., and Copping, W. (1990) Adolescent depression: a placebo-controlled fluoxetine treatment study and follow-up. *Prog Neuropsychopharmacol Biol Psychiatry* 14:791–795.

Stein, D., Williamson, D.E., Birmaher, B., Brent, D.A., Kaufman, J., Dahl, R.E., and Ryan, N.D. (2000) Parent–child bonding and family functioning in depressed children and children at high-risk and low risk for future depression. *J Am Acad Child Adolesc Psychiatry* 39:1220–1226.

Strober, M. and Carlson, G. (1982) Bipolar illness in adolescents with major depression: clinical, genetic, and psychopharmacologic predictors in a three-to four-year prospective follow-up investigation. *Arch Gen Psychiatry* 39:549–555.

Strober, M., DeAntonio, M., Schmidt-Lackner, S., Pataki, C., Freeman, R., Rigali, J., and Rao, U. (1999) The pharmacotherapy of depressive illness in adolescents: an open-label comparison of fluoxetine with imipramine-treated historical controls. *J Clin Psychiatry* 60:164–169.

Strober, M., Freeman, R., Rigali, J., Schmidt, S., and Diamond, R. (1992) The pharmacotherapy of depressive illness in adolescence: II. Effects of lithium augmentation in nonresponders to imipramine. *J Am Acad Child Adolesc Psychiatry* 31:16–20.

Strober, M., Lampert, C., Schmidt, S., and Morrell, W. (1993) The course of major depressive disorder in adolescents: I. Recovery and risk of manic switching in a follow-up of psychotic and nonpsychotic subtypes. *J Am Acad Child Adolesc Psychiatry* 32:34–42.

Swedo, S., Allen, A.J., Glod, C.A., Clark, C.H., Teicher, M.H., Richter, D., Hoffman, C., Hamburger, S.D., Dow, S., Brown, C., and Rosenthal, N.E. (1997) A controlled trial of light therapy for the treatment of pediatric seasonal affective disorder. *J Am Acad Child Adolesc Psychiatry* 36:816–821.

Thase, M.E. and Rush, A.J. (1997) When at first you don't succeed: sequential strategies for antidepressant nonresponders. *J Clin Psychiatry* 58:23–29.

Vostanis, P., Feehan, C., Grattan, E., and Bickerton, W.A. (1996) A randomized controlled outpatient trial of cognitive-behavioral treatment for children and adolescents with depression: 9-month follow-up. *J Affect Disord* 40:105–116.

Weissman, M.M., Gammon, G.D., John, K., Merikangas, K.R., Prusoff, B.A., and Sholomskas, D. (1987) Children of depressed parents: increased psychopathology and early onset of major depression. *Arch Gen Psychiatry* 44:847–853.

Weissman, M.M., Wolk, S., Goldstein, R.B., Moreau, D., Adams, P., Greenwald, S., Klier, C.M., Ryan, N.D., Dahl, R.E., and Wickramaratne, P.J. (1999a) Depressed adolescents grownup. *JAMA* 281:1707–1713.

Weissman, M.M., Wolk, S., Wockramaratne, P.J., Goldstein, R., Adams, P., Greenwald, S., Ryan, N.D., Dahl, R.E., and Steinberg, D. (1999b) Children with prepubertal-onset major depressive disorder and anxiety grown up. *Arch Gen Psychiatry* 56:794–801.

Wilens, T.E., Wyatt, D., and Spencer, T.J. (1998) Disentangling disinhibition. *J Am Acad Child Adolesc Psychiatry* 37:1225–1227.

Wood, A., Harrington, R., and Moore, A. (1996) Controlled trial of a brief cognitive-behavioral intervention in adolescent patients with depressive disorders. *J Child Psychol Psychiatry* 37:737–746.

37 | Bipolar disorder

GABRIELLE A. CARLSON

The association of periods of excited, volatile behavior and withdrawn, depressed behavior has long been recognized. There is current consensus that uncomplicated, classical manic depression (including episodes of euphoric mania, depression, and normal mood state) occurs in adolescents, but it is relatively uncommon in prepubertal children. However, chronic manic symptoms superimposed on a wide variety of other types of psychopathology appear to be much more common and may be a subtype of mania. The extent to which mood dysregulation in young people is part of a larger bipolar spectrum (Akiskal et al., 2000) is uncertain and under investigation. Increasingly, mood-incongruent psychotic symptoms, briefer hypomania (which people may not identify as abnormal), and dimensions of temperament are considered part of a spectrum of *bipolarity*. Whether bipolar spectrum is valid in children is unclear and remains controversial: outside the United States, for example, early-onset bipolar disorder is rarely reported. When it is diagnosed, it generally lacks externalizing disorder comorbidity (Thomsen et al., 1992; Reddy et al., 1997; Rasenen et al., 1998; Srinath et al., 1998). One suspects that these countries are restricting their definition of bipolar disorder to that of the classical variety.

The primary focus of this chapter is the assessment and treatment of the child or adolescent with *manic* symptoms. Considerations regarding bipolar depression are dealt with in Chapter 36.

PHENOMENOLOGY AND DIFFERENTIAL DIAGNOSIS

Although the terms are used interchangeably, there is a difference between bipolar disorder and manic episode. *Bipolar disorder* characterizes the type of disorder afflicting patients during their lifetime. They may be experiencing no problems, current mania, hypomania, depression, or minor symptoms. If one is doing a family study, it may not matter what types of symptoms (if any) are *currently* occurring. In a treatment study, it matters considerably if one is treating mania,

hypomania, or depression. Table 37.1 reviews *the Diagnostic and Statistical Manual of Mental Disorders, 4th ed.* (DSM IV) criteria for bipolar disorder and for an acute manic episode.

Patients whose first episodes of mania or bipolar depression occur between ages 30 to 60 years appear to have clearer episodes of mood disorder, have mania characterized by euphoria and irritability (rather than irritability alone), and be less likely to develop substance addiction (though they may engage in substance abuse as part of their acute episodes). Although psychosis occurs frequently and can be severe, in such late-onset cases confusion with other disorders is usually not a problem. Finally, this more classical presentation is generally responsive to lithium (Carlson, 2000).

Adolescent- and young adult–onset of bipolar disorder may also be classical. Severe psychosis, which used to be misdiagnosed as schizophrenia, substance-induced psychosis, borderline personality disorder, or severe "adolescent turmoil" are alternative diagnoses given to youths who have, or will ultimately develop, bipolar disorder. Adhering to diagnostic criteria and obtaining information on prior functioning, acuity of onset, type of mood, and psychotic symptoms significantly cut down on diagnostic error (Carlson et al., 1994). Moreover, in teen-onset bipolar patients, unequivocal episodes of mania and depression occur in patients with prior childhood psychopathology, and these young people appear to have a stormier course of illness than those with uncomplicated bipolar disorder (Strober et al., 1998; Carlson et al., 2000a).

Younger children with manic symptoms tend to have severe functional impairment and comorbid psychopathology such as anxiety dysregulation, disruptive behaviors, and developmental delays that further complicate their clinical picture. In addition, these children may have mood symptoms that merge with other disorders, making manic episodes difficult to define. Irritability is part of the clinical picture of depression, anxiety, attention-deficit hyperactivity disorder (ADHD), and oppositional defiant disorder (ODD). Poor concen-

TABLE 37.1 *DSM-IV Criteria for the Diagnosis of Bipolar I Disorder*

Diagnostic criteria for 296.4 bipolar I disorder, most recent episode manic

A. Currently (or most recently) in a manic episode (see below)

B. There has previously been at least one major depressive episode, manic episode, or mixed episode (see below).

C. The mood episodes in criteria A and B are not better accounted for by schizoaffective disorder and are not superimposed on schizophrenia, schizophreniform disorder, delusional disorder, or psychotic disorder not otherwise specified.

Specify (for current or most recent episode):

Severity/psychotic/remission speficifers
With catatonic features
With postpartum onset

Specify:

Longitudinal course specifiers (with and without interepisode recovery)
With seasonal pattern (applies only to the pattern of major depressive episodes)
With rapid cycling

Criteria for manic episode

A. Distinct period of abnormally and persistently elevated, expansive, or irritable mood, lasting at least 1 week (or any duration if hospitalization is necessary)

B. During the period of mood disturbance, three (or more) of the following symptoms have persisted (four if the mood is only irritable) and have been present to a significant degree:

Inflated self-esteem or grandiosity
Decreased need for sleep (e.g., feels rested after only 3 hours of sleep)
More talkative than usual or pressure to keep talking
Flight of ideas or subjective experience that thoughts are racing
Distractibility (i.e., attention too easily drawn to unimportant or irrelevant external stimuli)
Increase in goal-directed activity (either socially, at work or school, or sexually) or psychomotor agitation
Excessive involvement in pleasurable activities that have a high potential for painful consequences (e.g., engaging in unrestrained buying sprees, sexual indiscretions, or foolish business investments)

C. The symptoms do not meet criteria for a mixed episode.

D. The mood disturbance is sufficiently severe to cause marked impairment in occupational functioning or in usual social activities or relationships with others, or to necessitate hospitalization to prevent harm to self or others, or there are psychotic features.

E. The symptoms are not due to the direct physiological effects of a substance (e.g., a drug of abuse, a medication, or other treatment) or a general medical condition (e.g., hyperthyroidism).

tration and distractibility are also part of the clinical picture of depression, ADHD, and anxiety. Sleep disorders occur in anxiety and depression. Children with ADHD often put up struggles at bedtime and rise earlier than their parents. It is the reduced *need* for sleep that represents a change in previous functioning that characterizes mania. Because children may have mania *and* another disorder, the question of mania *or* another diagnosis becomes particularly complicated. Treatment decisions may be quite different depending on diagnostic conclusions. A child with pure mania might well have the hyperactivity and inattention mitigated with mood stabilizers, while a child with comorbid ADHD may not (Carlson et al., 1992b). A child whose panic attacks are mistaken for manic episodes may not be given a potentially beneficial selective serotonia reuptake inhibitor (SSRI). Mania appearing like anxiety, by contrast, needs to be identified, as such a course of treatment could worsen their manic symptoms. There is limited information concerning the impact of mood stabilizers on these comorbid disorders, so clinicians have little in the way of objective data to guide their practice.

Differential diagnosis is also increasingly complicated by secondary agitation that occurs when a child is on multiple medications (Wilens et al., 1998). It is sometimes necessary to hospitalize a child and discontinue all medications to really separate baseline disorder from secondary, medication-related reactions.

To summarize, comorbidities on which a manic syndrome can be superimposed include ADHD, ODD, conduct or pervasive developmental disorders, Tourette's syndrome, or medical conditions such as brain tumors, multiple sclerosis, temporal lobe seizures, human immune-deficiency syndrome (HIV), and endocrinopathies such as hyperthyroidism and Cushing's syndrome (James and Javaloyes, 2001). *Organic affective syndrome*, a condition given separate designation in DSM I–IIIR, is now subsumed under *mood disorder due to a general medical condition* in DSM IV. Substance induced mood disorder has a similar "due to . . ." designation.

Family Studies

Offspring of parents with bipolar disorder have an almost three fold increased risk for developing a mental disorder, and a fourfold risk for an affective disorder, as compared to the offspring of parents with no mental disorder (LaPalme et al., 1997). Families of patients with early-onset bipolar disorder have higher than expected rates of substance abuse, unipolar depression, antisocial personality, and comorbid bipolar disorder with ADHD. Biederman et al. (2000) have concluded that this comorbid bipolar plus ADHD condition is familial, as evidenced by the fact that the two conditions seemed to co-segregate in certain families. This observation and findings from Duffy et al. (1998) showing that offspring of lithium-responsive parents have less psychopathology and a more benign course of mood disorder lend further support to the notion that classic and comorbid or complicated bipolar disorder may be different entities.

DIAGNOSTIC ASSESSMENT AND CLINICAL EVALUATION

The National Institute of Mental Health (NIMH) Roundtable on prepubertal bipolar disorder (Nottelman et al., 2001) recommended two basic definitions for bipolar disorder: a narrow phenotype that adheres strictly to bipolar I (BP-I) and bipolar II (BP-II) criteria (with mania, hypomania, and depression clearly delineated) and a broader phenotype that "encompasses more heterogeneity, basically bipolar NOS (not otherwise specified), and that includes children who do not quite meet criteria, but still are impaired by symptoms of mood instability." However, even "strictly adhering" has areas of controversy. Much of the difficulty hinges on the definition of *episode* and the fact that children's growth and development present a moving target. In other words, there may not be a stable baseline of personality and function with which to compare a change from the way the person usually functions. Also, most conditions fluctuate—even ADHD. Distinguishing between symptomatic fluctuations, exacerbations during periods of stress or less structure, and superimposed mania is not always easy. Finally, symptoms of "euphoric mood, recognized as excessive" and "grandiosity" (uncritical self-confidence [reaching] delusional proportions) are characteristic of mania and not part of the symptomatology of other disorders. However, there really are no developmental norms for key symptoms. Certainly hyperactivity and inattention have to be assessed within the context of developmental level. Additionally, Caplan et al. (2000) have discussed the evolution of logical thinking during school-age years. The ability to distinguish grandiose thinking from inflated self-esteem from immature thinking is relevant in this, and one would expect that emotion regulation in terms of euphoria and irritability would also change with development.

Screening

It is often helpful to have parents provide information addressing the child's birth and developmental, medical, and previous treatment history (including medications) prior to being evaluated (see Chapter 31 in this volume). Comprehensive rating scales that address symptoms of attention deficit disorder, ODD, conduct disorder, depression, anxiety, and pervasive developmental disorders should also be completed as clinically indicated (see Hart and Lahey, 1999 and Chapter 32 in this volume for a review). Child Behavior Checklist (Achenbach, 1991) factors that are typically elevated in mania are anxiety/depression, attention problems, and aggressive behavior (Biederman et al., 1995), but social problems and thought problems are often clinically significant as well (Carlson and Kelly, 1998). The Child Symptom Inventory (CSI, Gadow and Sprafkin, 1994), a DSM-IV–based parent report, is a useful instrument for a range of psychiatric diagnoses. As always, these rating instruments only guide the subsequent interview, rather than replacing it. Although the use of pencil-and-paper instruments is not as rigorous as a structured diagnostic interview, it is more practical in a clinical setting.

Structured Interviews

In a research setting, structured interviews need to be done in conjunction with a comprehensive psychiatric evaluation and mental status examination, given the following:

1. Most structured interviews do not ascertain information about conditions that used to be on axis II or axis III: pervasive developmental disorders, learning and language disorders, or medical or neurological disorders.

2. If one strictly follows the structured interview, some children may have some symptoms of many disorders but not meet criteria for any of them.

3. A child may not really understand what is meant by certain terms. Concrete thinking is typical of children, and although more abstract thinking should be possible as the child approaches adolescence, learning-disabled and language-disordered children (and their parents) may endorse symptoms that are absent or deny symptoms that are present. If the interview consists only of having the child or parent answer yes/no questions (without having to provide examples), it may be impossible to know whether there are communication problems.

Although designers of structured interviews have tried hard to operationalize and detail symptom questions (see Angold and Fisher, 1999, for a review), interviews for mood disorders are only as good as the interviewers. Interviews vary in their approach; most have screening questions, which typically include elated mood, decreased need for sleep and racing thoughts. The Diagnostic Interview for Children and Adolescents (DICA; Reich, 2000) and the Diagnostic Interview Schedule for Children (DISC; Shaffer et al., 2000), which are more respondent based, use the following format: "Have you ever had a time when. . . ." followed by a description of the symptom in question; for example, for elated mood: "Has there been a time in your life when you felt really super-happy? Not just because something good was happening, but so happy and excited that you couldn't believe how good you felt?" The interviewer then asks whether this episode was "a lot different from the way you usually are?", followed by whether others noticed or were worried. At the end, the interviewer ascertains if these symptoms occurred together, caused impairment, required treatment, or were drug or alcohol induced. All versions of the Kiddie Schedule for Affective Disorders and Schizophrenia (K-SADS) are interviewer based and allow for more flexibility in asking questions. However, there are examples of questions. The interviewer needs to understand the disorder well enough to listen for examples the patient gives and to determine whether these examples are applicable to the disorder in question. The Washington University (ST. Louis, MO) K-SADS provides precise anchors (Geller et al., 2001). The K-SADS–Present and Lifetime Version (K-SADS-PL; Kaufman et al., 1997) provides advice on when to rate and when not to rate the symptom.

Irritability is a particularly vexing symptom to ascertain and, interestingly, one generally asked in the depression section of structured interviews. In the DICA, irritability is asked in the context of being in a "crabby or bad mood." In the K-SADS, irritability is more general: "Was there ever a time you got annoyed, irritated or cranky at little things?"

Aggressive, agitated, explosive behavior is a frequent complaint of parents seeking treatment for their child, and both parents and children often place this behavior within the context of irritability or mood swings. The most common reasons given for such explosions are being denied something the child wants, being frustrated when something does not work out, provocation by peers, being surprised by a change in plans, and during transitions from one activity to another. These precipitants are not synonymous and may have diagnostic implications. For example, children with pervasive developmental disorders may become explosive with change. A low frustration tolerance is associated with ADHD. Fatigue is an important precipitant of irritability. Medical conditions should also be considered. One of the most "manic" children on our inpatient service was a boy who had sleep apnea. His mania attenuated after a tonsillectomy. Children who develop insomnia on stimulants may become irritable because of inadequate sleep. Some children explode quickly but calm down readily. By contrast, others may not explode often, but are upset for hours. During pretreatment assessment one needs to make these distinctions to monitor treatment response. It is not clear whether there is a specific kind of irritability unique to mania.

Rating Scales

Rating scales can be used to track mania (including mood lability), depression, anxiety, ADHD, aggression, and psychosis. However, mania scales are limited (Altman, 1998) and have not been examined in pediatric populations. The Young-Mania Rating Scale (YMRS; Young et al., 1978) has been used increasingly in drug studies of children (e.g., Kowatch et al., 2000). To date, however, the YMRS has not demonstrated treatment sensitivity in children, and published reliability and validity data are currently limited to one study of 21 children with bipolar disorder (Fristad et al., 1992; 1995). The YMRS was developed as a severity measure to be completed after spending time with a hospitalized manic adult. However, insofar as the instrument is used to get information from parents about the child, it is being used as a history-gathering as well as a severity measure. Some items (e.g., insight) are simply not designed for children. Axelson et al. (1999) have recently examined mania items from the K-SADS and have developed a rating scale that is a much more promising and ecologically valid approach to assessing children and adolescents. In addition, the Neuropsychiatric Rating Schedule (Max et al., 1998), which was developed to assess organic mood syndrome, has a good measure of mood lability.

Aggression is an important component of mood disorders. Thus, a measure that captures the frequency and severity of the child's outbursts, such as the Overt Aggression Scale (OAS; Yudofsky et al., 1986), may be useful. This rating was evaluated in one inpatient study, and appears to be reliable and valid (Kafantaris et al., 1996). Behavior disorder rating scales that measure ADHD and ODD are also likely to be useful. As noted above, our clinic uses a combined Child and Adolescent Symptom Inventory both at baseline and to follow treatment response, as it provides a comprehensive rating of symptoms (Grayson and Carlson, 1991; Gadow et al., 1999).

Child Mental Status

A child mental status examination is obviously imperative and will not be reviewed in its entirety here. However, there are a few important issues specific to bipolar disorder worthy of mention. It is necessary to spend time with the child to assess the presence or absence of pervasive developmental disorder, language or thought disorder, anxiety, depression, and suicidal behavior, as well as illicit substance use. Although younger children may not be able to describe symptoms such as racing thoughts and flight of ideas reliably, it is necessary to inquire and observe the child during the interview to decide if these are present. For example, a child may deny distractibility and nevertheless appear quite distractible with frequent topic shifts in conversation. Conversely, a child may say he has "racing thoughts," but appear perfectly calm and nonimpaired. Although multiple informants have been the mainstay and frustration of child psychiatry, direct observation of the child during the clinical interviews is essential in the assessment of mania.

Communication disorders (receptive and/or expressive language disorder) interfere with obtaining accurate information and may mimic thought disorder. Although it is not possible to diagnose a communication disorder without standardized testing, it is useful to have a consistent language task to obtain a language sample from the child. Tasks include having the child tell a well-known fairy tale, or to read a picture story like *A Boy, A Dog and A Frog*, by Mercer Mayer (1967) and relate the story back. Such a framework may help to distinguish a thought disorder from a language disorder. Communication disorders can complicate a child's academic and social ability and are not likely to be sensitive to current pharmacological interventions. As an extreme example of this point, a recently evaluated 12-year-old child with "rule out bipolar disorder" had a language ability of a 7-year-old, could not read, and had been receiving mood stabilizers for 6 years with everyone "waiting for the drug to kick in." Failure to identify these specific developmental disorders deprived him of much needed special educational services.

Parents and children may differ in their responses to the presence or absence of certain symptoms. When there are such differences, the clinician needs to meet with both parties simultaneously and to come to a consensus about the symptom and about the source of the disagreement.

TREATMENT OF BIPOLAR DISORDER

General Considerations

The relative absence of systematic studies of bipolar patients under age 18 forces clinicians to extrapolate data from adult studies. There are four major types of studies that provide information on subjects with bipolar disorder: double-blind, placebo-controlled studies of patients with acute mania; prospective open-label studies of patients with bipolar disorder (which includes mania, hypomania, manic symptoms, or bipolar NOS, people at risk for mania because of their family history, and those with a history of mania who are not currently manic); case series; and anecdotal reports.

Summary of Data from Controlled Treatment Studies of Acute Mania in Adults

A thorough discussion of this topic is beyond the scope of this chapter. However, a recent review of controlled studies of mood stabilizers (Keck et al, 2000) provides a reasonable summary. Pooling response data from five studies (from 1954 to 1994) and 124 acute manic patients revealed that 70% of the patients had at least partial improvement with lithium treatment. Response took 2–3 weeks, was superior to antipsychotics in ameliorating affective symptoms, produced an improvement in psychosis, but was less effective in treating psychomotor agitation. DSM-III and earlier criteria were used to diagnose the patients in these trials, so these samples may not be comparable to patients in more modern studies. Table 37.2 summarizes a compilation of clinical

TABLE 37.2 *Predictors of Lithium Response*

Good Response	Poor Response
Euphoric mania	Dysphoric, mixed mania
Mania, depression, interval sequence	Rapid cycling
Rapid-onset of retarded depression	Slow-onset/chronic depression
Mood congruent psychotic features	Mood incongruent features
Absence of neurotic personality traits	Personality disorders
Good intermorbid function	Comorbid psychopathology (e.g., anxiety)
No substance abuse	Substance abuse
Primary mood disorder	Secondary mood disorder
Good family/social support network	Severe family dysfunction
<11 lifetime episodes	>11 manic episodes; >4 depressive episodes

features traditionally associated with good and poor response to lithium treatment (Abou-Saleh, 1993). Most of the poor-response criteria are in fact compatible with mixed bipolar disorder or BP-II disorder in which comorbidity, poor intermorbid function, and severe and chronic lifetime disruption are the rule.

Divalproex sodium (DVP) provided a significant reduction in manic symptoms in 54% of patients from three controlled studies. Especially when an oral loading dose of 20 mg/kg/day is used, rapid antimanic effects may be observed between 3 and 5 days. Mixed episodes and the presence of depressive symptoms are associated with better response to DVP than to lithium.

Carbamazepine (CBZ) has been compared to placebo once, to lithium in two controlled trials, and to chlorpromazine in one trial. Pooling these data revealed a 50% response to CBZ, 56% for lithium, and 68% for chlorpromazine. Onset of response to CBZ was 7–14 days.

Controlled trials of combinations of mood stabilizers with single mood stabilizer, or of the newer anticonvulsants (e.g., lamotrigine and topiramate) are in process. Open trials have included add-on medications and heterogeneous samples.

Prior to the availability of atypical antipsychotics, typical antipsychotics were used to diminish the acute agitation of mania. Onset of action is typically observed within 3 to 7 days. In a meta-analysis of chlorpromazine trials, efficacy was 54%, which was substantially less than that of lithium, but comparable to that of other mood stabilizers (range, 12%–70%). Risk of extrapyramidal effects and tardive dyskinesia limits the use of these medications beyond the acute phase.

Of the atypical antipsychotics, clozapine, olanzapine, and risperidone have been studied the most. Clozapine was used to treat 10 treatment refractory acutely manic patients and 15 schizomanic patients. Using reduction in the YMRS score as the outcome measure, 72% improved (non–rapid cycling, bipolar patients). Comparison of olanzapine (5–20 mg) with placebo showed significant reduction of the YMRS in 49% vs. 24% of subjects by 3 weeks, with significant change evident by the first week. In a trial comparing risperidone at 6 mg with haloperidol at 10 mg and low-dose lithium (800–1200 mg/day) efficacy was similar over the 28 days of the trial.

Systematic studies of combinations of mood stabilizers and atypical antipsychotics, or of benzodiazepines and mood stabilizers, were not included in Keck et al. (2000) review.

The other major class of medications examined systematically is the calcium channel blockers. The more methodologically sound studies suggested that verapamil may be better than placebo, but not as good as lithium in reducing manic symptoms. Nimodipine was superior to placebo in nine rapid cycling patients, in a crossover design study.

Inpatient Treatment Studies of Acute Mania in Patients Age 18 and Under

There are no randomized, double-blind, controlled studies of hospitalized children and adolescents with acute mania. Two systematic, albeit open, studies of lithium in hospitalized, acutely manic adolescents had response rates of 67%–80% in classic manic adolescents, and 33%–40% in manic adolescents with prior ADHD (Strober et al., 1988; 1998). In a discontinuation study in which manic adolescents stabilized on lithium were subsequently assigned double-blind to placebo or continuation treatment, the response rate was 53.5%, and the presence of prior ADHD made no difference in outcome (Kafantaris et al., 1998). However, the presence of psychosis decreased the likelihood of lithium response and antipsychotic medication was necessary for stabilization. Naturalistic discontinuation of lithium (because of noncompliance) after stabilization resulted in relapse rates of 90% vs. 37.5% for those remaining on lithium (Strober et al., 1990). A NIMH multisite study is currently examining this issue more systematically.

More common are case series and open trials of mood stabilizers for acute mania (see Davanzo and McCracken, 2000 for review). These studies, some of which were done in the 1970s and 1980s with classical adolescent manic patients, showed promise for the use of lithium in the treatment of mania. In some early studies, response to lithium was a requirement for diagnosis, a circular criterion that would undoubtedly have increased the response rate.

There are two studies of hospitalized children with mania or manic symptoms. The first, a controlled trial of lithium in 11 children (7 of whom were treated under double-blind, placebo-controlled conditions), found that 6 showed improvement over an 8-week period of hospitalization, but only 3 were well enough to be discharged on lithium. Long-standing concurrent ADHD complicated assessment of response (Carlson et al., 1992a), and the addition of methylphenidate was necessary to achieve an improvement in attention span and hyperactivity (Carlson et al., 1992b). An open trial of lithium in 10 acutely manic/psychotic prepubertal children showed positive response in all (Varanka et al., 1988).

There are also two open studies of adolescents hospitalized for acute mania and treated with DVP (West et al., 1994, 1995; Papatheodorou et al., 1995). Papatheordorou's study included 15 well-diagnosed manic adolescents, of whom 13 completed a 7-week trial. Eight showed marked improvement and four showed at least a 50% reduction in symptoms (for an overall response rate of 75%). West et al. (1994, 1995) reviewed 11 hospitalized, acutely manic adolescents who had failed lithium and/or antipsychotic treatment alone. The addition of DVP to these regimens (serum concentrations of 38 to 94, and mean of 74 μg/mL) led to improvements in 9 out of 11 subjects, according to chart information. Five hospitalized teens with mixed mania given a loading dose of valproate (20 mg/kg) tolerated the dose well. Two of five showed at least a 50% reduction in mania scores by the time of discharge. Finally, a naturalistic study of hospitalized adolescents ($n = 36$) treated with DVP for various disorders showed promising results in 20 bipolar patients. In this study, 16 patients were diagnosed with mixed mania and 4 had classic mania. Improvements in manic, aggressive, or mood lability symptoms were observed in 70%–80% of the bipolar patients (Deltito et al., 1998).

There are three reports (Hsu and Starzinsi, 1986; Woolston, 1999; Craven and Murphy, 2000) on a total of six bipolar adolescents treated with CBZ—three with acute mania, two of whom responded (Hsu and Starzinski, 1986). As in studies of adults, antipsychotic and/or antianxiety medications were frequently used adjunctively in subjects of these reports. Gabapentin, topiramate, and lamotrigine have been minimally studied for the treatment of acute mania in youth. Davanzo and McCracken review these limited data in Chapter 25 in this volume.

Electroconvulsive therapy (ECT) has been described in the treatment of refractory mania in two prepubertal children (Hill et al., 1997). Rey and Walter (1997) have also summarized the literature on juvenile ECT, including its use in mania in adolescents (also see Chapter 30 in this volume).

Outpatient Studies of Bipolar Children and Adolescents

There are several controlled trials of young outpatients with bipolar and bipolar spectrum conditions. Geller et al. (1998) studied 25 adolescents in a 6-week, double-blind, placebo-controlled study. Twelve received lithium, of whom 4 had BP-I (presumably acute mania), 4 had BP-II (presumably hypomania), and 4 had major depression with bipolar predictors. All had concurrent substance abuse. There were no significant differences in outcome between active and placebo groups, except in

substance abuse recurrences, which declined only in the lithium group. A randomized, but open, trial over 8 weeks examined use of lithium, DVP, and CBZ in 42 outpatient children and adolescents. Twenty were diagnosed with BP-I (mean YMRS score of 24.6, and 22 with BP-II (mean YMRS score of 19.7). Overall, 46% responded to DVP, 42% responded to lithium, and 34%, to CBZ (Kowatch et al., 2000). The sample sizes in these studies were too small to comment on response by diagnostic subtype, and may have contributed to the seemingly large effect sizes reported (1.63, 1.06, and 1.00 for DVP, lithium, and CBZ, respectively).

An industry-sponsored discontinuation trial of DVP involving 40 children and adolescents with bipolar illness show improvement in 22 patients after 8–10 weeks of treatment. However, rescue medication was necessary in enough subjects that the discontinuation design could not be carried out (Wagner, personal communication, January 2002). In a review of one clinician's series of 196 patients treated with lithium over the course of 10 years, Delong and Aldershof (1987) broke down their clinical sample of children and adolescents by diagnostic group. Subgroups had either clear mood disorder or other disorders with manic-like symptoms. The authors determined response by whether or not patients were continued on lithium over a 10-month period. They additionally commented on whether relapse occurred upon discontinuation. Because their experience reflects how mood stabilizers appear to be used in clinical practice, some detail is enlightening:

Response for Mood disorder
• 66% (39 of 59) patients with manic depression showed a positive response, and of these, 11 discontinued without relapse.
• 17% (5 of 29) with unipolar depression, were classified as responders; 2 discontinued after 13 and 24 months, respectively.

Response for manic-like behavior
• 38% (3 of 8) of ADHD patients with affective symptoms showed a positive response; all discontinued ultimately without further problems.
• 56% (5 of 9) with explosive/aggressive behavior showed a positive response; 2 discontinued and did not need further treatment. The absence of recurrence in these patients makes the diagnosis of bipolar disorder suspect.
• 71% (4 of 7) were offspring of lithium-responding parents, 1 successfully stopped after 3 years and was doing well at 52 months.

In a somewhat similar vein, Biederman et al. (1998) used survival analysis to determine the effect of mood stabilizers and other medications on the course of manic-like symptoms in children and adolescents who attended the Massachusetts General Hospital Child Psychopharmacology Clinic. The occurrence of manic symptoms significantly predicted the subsequent prescription of mood stabilizers and use of mood stabilizers predicted decreases in manic symptoms (rate ratio = 4.9, 95% CI = 1.2–20.8). However, improvement was gauged over a 2-year period and associated with a substantial risk for relapse. In this regard, mood stabilzers were not associated with acute response, and the condition was not acute mania.

Chart reviews and open trials of outpatients with bipolar disorder and bipolar spectrum disorder have been published for 28 risperidone- and 23 olanzapine-treated treated children and adolescents (Frazier et al., 1999; 2001). Significant decreases in mania, depression, and aggression ratings occurred over the course of treatment; however, other medications were also used simultaneously. Additional anecdotal information exists for olanzapine (Soutullo et al., 1999; Chang and Ketter, 2000), quetiapine (Schaller and Behar, 1999), and clozapine (Fuchs, 1994).

Case reports have also been published on the utility of gabapentin (Soutullo et al., 1998), verapamil (Kastner and Friedman, 1992), nimodipine (Davanzo et al., 1999), lecithin (Schreier, 1982), and melatonin (Robertson and Tanguay, 1997). Taken together, these uncontrolled and small sample studies do not provide much in the way of useful information, but they do indicate what clinicians are doing to manage children and adolescents with bipolar symptoms.

Summary

These data suggest that there is more available information for use of lithium than for other mood stabilizers, and that adolescents hospitalized with adolescent-onset, acute mania have rates of response between 50% and 80%. Supplementation with sedating medication appears to be common but not systematically evaluated. Children hospitalized with mania also respond to lithium, but their comorbid disorders often need separate attention. Open trials with DVP in hospitalized adolescents are also supported. There is much less information on CBZ and there are no data on newer anticonvulsants such as lamotrigine, topiramate, or gabapentin. These data are largely consistent with data from studies of hospitalized adults with classic mania.

In outpatient samples with an assortment of bipolar and bipolar spectrum disorders, the frequency and magnitude of response are lower for all mood stabilizers (40%–50%) than in adult studies. This lower response may be related to greater heterogeneity in the samples due to problems of diagnostic uncertainty. Case series for atypical antipsychotics are encouraging, but more systematic data are needed.

AN APPROACH TO THE TREATMENT OF ACUTE MANIA IN YOUNG PEOPLE

The first step in the treatment of a patient with bipolar illness at any age is establishing the diagnosis and deciding if one is treating acute mania (classical, mixed, psychotic, rapid cycling), hypomania, or bipolar spectrum/bipolar NOS. The latter may be characterized by chronic manic symptoms complicating other comorbidities or by severe mood swings that do not meet full criteria for mania. Although the medications used and the sequence in which they are introduced are similar for various types of mania, the probability and completeness of recovery (i.e., prognostic implications) may depend on the type of mania being treated.

The treatment of a hospitalized child or adolescent who truly meets criteria for acute, psychotic mania or is having an episode of clear, mixed mania can follow similar algorithms used for adults. Figure 37.1 combines data from the Expert Consensus Guidelines (Sachs et al., 2000) with specifics based on data from child and adolescent studies. Euphoric mania, or a pattern of mania followed by depression and euphoria, may be treated with lithium or DVP. However, mixed manic and rapid cycling episodes respond better to DVP, with CBZ as the second-line alternative. There are more data on atypical antipsychotics as adjunctive medications to substantiate their use than on benzodiazepines, although these medications (lorazepam and clonazepam) are helpful in treating severely agitated children and adolescents and may mitigate the need for restraints. Rapid stabilization strategies have been used for DVP (West et al., 1995) and lithium (Weller and Weller, 1986), but are reserved for hospitalized children. Medication response of a bipolar parent is also something to consider in selecting a first medication. Parent medication response may select a more homogeneous group of bipolar subjects and influence the likelihood of positive response (Duffy et al., 1998).

In children or adolescents managed as outpatients, where compliance is less enforcible, medications are ideally introduced gradually and one at a time. This approach permits gradual achievement of therapeutic levels while minimizing side effects and enhances treat-

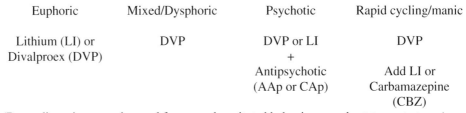

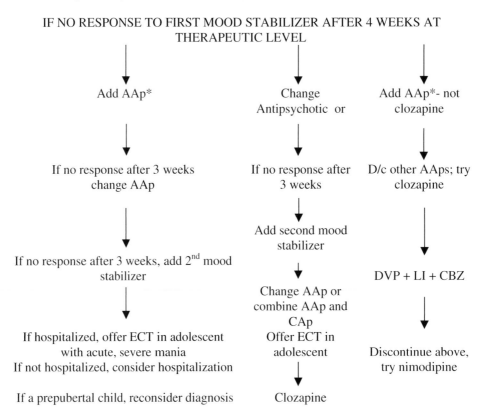

FIGURE 37.1 Suggested medication algorithm for juvenile mania. Reasons for failure of mania treatment have included the following: continued treatment with medications inducing manic episodes (e.g., concurrent SSRIs or other antidepressants), seizure disorder, other CNS disorders, Tourette's disorder, sleep apnea, mistaking panic attacks for manic episodes, mistaking explosive outbursts for manic episodes, and not recognizing concurrent substance abuse. *If there is no evidence that a particular strategy has produced a change, don't continue it. At each medication change, check rating scales for which symptoms are ongoing. Keep in mind that the condition being treated may not be true bipolar disorder. AAp, atypical antipsychotic; CAp, conventional antipsychiotic, ECT, electroconvulsive therapy.

ment compliance. If there is only partial response, in the absence of systematic data, the addition of either a second mood stabilizer or an atypical antipsychotic is equally supportable. Finally, emerging data suggest that the atypical neuroleptics are likely to be helpful as an additional strategy, but this needs to be more systematically studied.

Bipolar Disorder Not Otherwise Specified

Children with chronic manic symptoms (i.e., lacking episodes) are most accurately diagnosed as bipolar NOS (Nottelman et al., 2001). The chief symptoms in children with manic symptoms/bipolar NOS appear to be mood lability and explosive behavior. The explosive episodes are often, but not always, superimposed on long-standing ADHD. Once other reasons for aggressive behavior have been ruled out, one should follow the algorithm for acute mania, keeping in mind that the same treatments that ameliorate mood instability are also medications used for aggression (see Chapter 50 in this volume).

Diagnostic Hospitalization

Hospitalizing nonresponsive manic patients and discontinuing medications can be a helpful diagnostic intervention (Carlson and Fahim, 1998). There comes a point when it is difficult to differentiate the primary disorder from the secondary effects of multiple therapies. There may be environmental situations driving the behavioral dysregulation that can only be clarified in a hospital setting. Alternatively, adverse effects of one medication in a cocktail of multiple medications are difficult to identify without discontinuation. Because there is a possibility that the clinical picture may worsen with discontinuation of pharmacotherapy, this procedure may need to be carried out on an inpatient service. This kind of hospitalization may need to be argued for vigorously with managed-care companies because answers are usually not forthcoming in a few days.

Psychopharmacologic Treatment of Comorbid Disorders

There is no evidence that treating manic symptoms with mood stabilizers diminishes the symptoms of ADHD (Carlson et al., 1992b; Frazier et al., 2001). Lithium has been combined with methylphenidate in children with comorbid ADHD and manic symptoms with some suggestion of a synergistic effect (Carlson et al., 1992b). Children with ADHD and stimulant-induced rebound, depressive symptoms, or increased irritability do not appear to be at greater risk to develop bipolar disorder than those without such adverse events (Carlson et al., 2000b). Nevertheless, it is clear that some bipolar children destabilize on stimulants (Koehler-Troy et al., 1986), making their attentional problems very difficult to treat. In those instances, second- and third-line medications for ADHD (such as the α agonists or bupropion) may be useful. The concurrent use of antidepressants and mood stabilizers raises particular concerns, as discussed in more detail in Chapter 36 in this volume.

Comorbid substance abuse may also complicate the course and treatment of bipolar disorder and its treatment (Carlson et al., 1999). Short-term lithium (Geller et al., 1998) and DVP (Donovan and Nunes, 1998) appear to be somewhat helpful in bipolar spectrum conditions accompanied by substance abuse. Management of substance abuse is also important. For example, in a 2-year follow-up of hospitalized manic youth, the substance-abusing bipolar patients who continued to use drugs had more manic episodes and generally poorer functioning than their early-onset, non–substance-abusing bipolar peers. Cessation of substance abuse was associated with fewer episodes and greater functional improvement at the 4-year follow-up point (Carlson et al., 1999).

Maintenance Treatment

An awesome question facing young persons with bipolar disorders is whether they will require lifelong treatment with medication. With adults who have experienced several episodes, one can use their life experience to help decide the relative merits of long-term continuation. For young people taking mood stabilizers after only one or at most two episodes, the issue is far more complex. Data from adult studies for both recurrence of major depression in non-bipolar patients, as well as those with bipolar disorder, suggest that continuation of pharmacotherapy for up to 2 years reduces the risk of recurrence (e.g., Bowden et al., 2000) In the absence of guidance from longitudinal studies, we encourage adolescents to continue medication until completion of high school college or trade school, or past an anticipated major life stressor (starting a new job, getting married, etc). If discontinuation, is insisted upon, it should come when the impact on life is likely to be minimal, and when there is ongoing monitoring to avert a manic episode early on should one occur. Discontinuation should be undertaken very gradually, as there is evidence for an increased likelihood of mania upon rapid discontinuation of lithium (Suppes et al., 1991).

Although adolescents who discontinue maintenance treatment have a high (92%) rate of relapse compared to those who maintain lithium treatment (37%) (Strober et al., 1990), reliable continuation of medication is a serious problem in bipolar adolescents, particularly those with comorbid behavior disorders (Carlson et al., 2000a).

The most effective acute and maintenance treatment occur when patient, family members, and treating staff collaborate. This requires a comprehensive approach, and can include this following actions:

1. Educate family members and the patient about the characteristics of the disorder(s) being treated, e.g., euphoric mania, mixed mania, psychotic mania, severe

depression with a history of hypomania, rapid cycles, episodes of rage and/or aggression, that fit a bipolar NOS framework.

2. Help the child and family focus on aspects of disorder over which they have some control (e.g., maintaining adequate sleep, sensible nutrition, and regular schedules is important in people with bipolar disorder). Because children with bipolar spectrum disorders are at high risk for ADHD and perhaps learning disability, they will need appropriate educational planning. Adolescents need to understand the increased risk of mania induction with continued substance abuse (Carlson et al., 1999). If there are other family members with mood or other psychiatric disorders, treatment should be recommended for them. Parent education may also include the importance of consistent limit-setting and anger reduction strategies to limit the impact of explosive behavior on their family (e.g., Greene, 1998).

3. Discuss advantages, limitations, and risks of medication use, as well as the following consequences of lack of such use:

a. Inform parents and patients about the importance of following the exact prescription, of keeping medications secure, and of participating in safety monitoring.

b. Maintain standard safety monitoring with baseline bloodwork: complete blood cell count (CBC), platelets, fasting blood sugar, tests of liver and renal functioning, cholesterol levels, and thyroid tests. Although serious blood, liver, thyroid, and kidney effects are rare in children, it is prudent to establish a normal baseline in these laboratory values and to monitor levels during treatment. Serum drug levels, height, weight, and menstrual patters should also be monitored.

c. Have separate baselines for the major symptom areas being addressed to track time and response. In the case of acute mania without other psychopathology, a mania rating scale suffices. When mania is comorbid with ADHD or aggressive outbursts, those symptoms should be monitored. In the case of bipolar depression, the depression needs to be followed.

d. Set up a priority and order of drugs for trial, and prepare staff, patient, and family for a stepwise approach. In outpatient settings, go from least complicated to most complicated interventions. Consider the more complicated drugs that need closer observation or where risks are higher for inpatient settings.

e. Give each drug and dosage adequate time to work.

SUMMARY

Bipolar spectrum disorders are a serious group of conditions. Their onset in childhood or adolescence has the potential to exert a reactive impact on development, as well as on life in general. Accurate assessment of the bipolar symptoms and concomitant conditions is imperative to provide comprehensive treatment. Unfortunately, support for effective treatment in young people is limited, and to some extent, clinicians must proceed with treatment without the benefit of empirical support.

REFERENCES

Abou-Saleh, M.T. (1993) Who responds to prophylactic lithium therapy? *Br J Psychiatry Suppl* 21:20–26.

Achenbach, T.M. (1991) *Manual for the Child Behavior Checklist 4–18 and 1991 Profile.* University of Vermont, Department of Psychiatry, Burlington, VT.

Akiskal, H.S., Bourgeois, M.L., Angst, J., Post, R., Moeller, H.-J., and Hirschfelt, R. (2000) Re-evaluating the prevalence of and diagnostic composition within the broad clinical spectrum of bipolar disorders. *J Affect Disord* 59:S5–S30.

Altman, E., (1998) Rating scales for mania: is self-rating reliable? *J Affect Disord* 50:283–286. Angold, A., and Fisher, P.W. (1999) Interviewer-based interviews. In: Shaffer, D., Lucas, C.P., and Richters, J.E., eds. *Diagnostic Assessment in Child and Adolescent Psychopathology.* New York: Guilford Press, pp. 34–61.

Axelson, D.A., Birmaher, B., Brent, D.A., and Ryan, N. (1999) The KSADS-Mania Rating Scale for Pediatric Bipolar Disorder. Presented at the 46th Annual Meeting of the American Academy of Child and Adolescent Psychiatry, New York, NY.

Biederman, J., Faraone, S.V., Wozniak, J., and Monuteaux, M.C. (2000) Parsing the associations between bipolar, conduct, and substance use disorders: a familial risk analysis. *Biol Psychiatry* 48:1037–1044.

Biederman, J., Mick, E., Bostic, J.Q., Prince, J., Daly, J., Wilens, T.E., Spencer, T., Garcia-Jetton, J., Russell, R., Wozniak, J., and Faraone, S.V. (1998) The naturalistic course of pharmacologic treatment of children with maniclike symptoms: a systematic chart review. *J Clin Psychiatry* 59:628–637.

Biederman, J., Wozniak, J., Kiely, K., Ablon, S., Faraone, S., Mick, E., Mundy, E., and Kraus, I. (1995) CBCL Clinical Scales discriminate prepubertal children with structured-interview-derived diagnosis of mania from those with ADHD. *J Am Acad Child Adolesc Psychiatry* 34:133–140.

Bowden, C.L., Lecrubier, Y., Mauer, M., Goodwin, G., Greil, W.I., Sachs, G., and von Knorring, L. (2000) Maintnance therapies for clasic and other forms of bipolar disorder. *J Affect Disord* 59: S57–S67.

Caplan, R., Guthrie, D., Tang, B., Komo, S., and Asarnow, R.F. (2000) Thought disorder in childhood schizophrenia: replication and update of concept. *J Am Acad Child Adolesc Psychiatry* 39: 771–778.

Carlson, G.A. (2000) Very early onset bipolar disorder, Does it Exist in Childhood: In: Rapoport, J, ed. *Onset of Adult Psychopathology—Clinical and Research Advances.* APPI Press, pp. 303–332.

Carlson, G.A., Bromet, E.J., and Lavelle, J. (1999) Medication treatment in adolescents vs adults with psychotic mania. *J Child Adolesc Psychopharmacol* 9:221–231.

Carlson, G.A., Bromet, E.J., and Sievers, S.B. (2000a) Phenomenology and outcome of youth and adult onset subjects with psychotic mania. *Am J Psychiatry* 157:213–219.

Carlson, G.A. and Fahim, F. (1998) "George." *J Affect Disord* 51: 195–198.

Carlson, G.A., Fennig, S., and Bromet, E.J. (1994) The confusion between bipolar disorder and schizphrenia in youth. Where does it stand in the 1990s. *J Am Acad Child Adolesc Psychiatry* 33: 453–460.

Carlson, G.A., and Kelly, K.L. (1998) Manic symptoms in psychiatrically hospitalized children—what do they mean? *J Affect Disord* 51:123–135.

Carlson, G.A., Loney, J., Salisbury, H., Kramer, J.R., and Arthur, C. (2000b) Stimulant treatment in young boys with symptoms suggesting childhood mania: a report from a longitudinal study. *J Child Adolesc Psychopharmacol* 10:175–184.

Carlson, G.A., Rapport, M.D., Pataki, C., and Kelly, K.K. (1992a) Lithium in hospitalized children at 4 and 8 weeks: affective, behavioral and cognitive effects. *J Child Psychol Psychiatry* 33:411–425.

Carlson, G.A., Rapport, M.D., Pataki, C., and Kelly, K.K. (1992b) The effects of methylphenidate and lithium on attention and activity level. *Am Acad Child Adolesc Psychiatry* 31:262–270.

Chang, K.D., and Ketter, T.A. (2000) Mood stabilizer augmentation with olanzapine in acutely manic children. *J Child Adolesc Psychopharmacol* 10: 45–49.

Craven, C., and Murphy, M. (2000) Carbamazepine treatment of bipolar disorder in an adolescent with cerebral palsy. *J Am Acad Child Adolesc Psychiatry* 39:680–681.

Davanzo, P.A., Krah, N., Kleiner, J., and McCracken, J. (1999) Nimodipine treatment of an adolescent with ultradian cycling bipolar affective illness. *J Child Adolesc Psychopharmacol* 9:51–61.

Davanzo, P.A., and McCracken, J.T. (2000) Mood stabilizers in the treatment of juvenile bipolar disorder. *Child Adolesc Psychiatr Clin North Am* 9:159–182.

Delong, G.R., and Aldershof, A.L. (1987) Long-term experience with lithium treatment in childhood; correlation with clinical diagnosis. *Am Acad Child Adolesc Psychiatry* 26:389–394.

Deltito, A.J., Levitan, J., Damore, J., Hajal, F., and Zambenedetti, M. (1998) Naturalistic experience with the use of divalproex sodium on an in-patient unit for adolescent psychiatric patients. *Acta Psychiatri Scand* 97:236–240.

Donovan, S.J., and Nunes, E.V. (1998) Treatment of comorbid affective and substance use disorders. Therapeutic potential of anticonvulsants. *Am J Addictions* 7:210–220.

Duffy, A., Alda, M., Kutcher, S., Fusee, C., and Grof, P. (1998) Psychiatric symptoms and syndromes among adolescent children of parents with lithium-responsive or lithium-nonresponsive bipolar disorder. *Am J Psychiatry* 155:431–433.

Frazier, J.A., Biederman, J., Tohen, M., Feldman, P.D., Jacobs, T.G., Toma, V., Rater, M.A., Tarazi, R.A., Kim, G.S., Garfield, S.B., Sohma, M., González-Heydrich, J., Risser, R.C., and Nowlin, ZM (2001) A prospective open-label trial of olanzapine monotherapy in children and adolescents with bipolar disorder. *J Child Adolesc Psychopharmacol* 11:239–250.

Frazier, J.A., Meyer, M.C., Biederman, J., Wozniak, J., Wilens, T.E., Spencer, T.J., Kim, G.S., and Shapiro, S. (1999) Risperidone treatment for juvenile bipolar disorder: a retrospective chart review. *J Am Acad Child Adolesc Psychiatry* 38:960–965.

Fristad, M.A., Weller, E.B., and Weller, R.A. (1992) The Mania Rating Scale: can it be used in children? A preliminary report. *J Am Acad Child Adolesc Psychiatry* 31:252–257.

Fristad, M.A., Weller, R.A., and Weller, E.B. (1995) The Mania Rating Scale (MRS): further reliability and validity studies with children. *Ann Clin Psychiatry* 7:127–132.

Fuchs, D.C. (1994) Clozapine treatment of bipolar disorder in a young adolescent. *J Am Acad Child Adolesc Psychiatry* 33:1299–1302.

Gadow, K.D., and Sprafkin, J. (1994) Child Symptom Inventories Manual. Stony Brook, NY: Checkmate Plus, Ltd.

Gadow, K.D., Sverd, J., Sprafkin, J., Nolan, E.E., and Grossman, S. (1999) Long-term methylphenidate therapy in children with comorbid attention-deficit hyperactivity disorder and chronic multiple tic disorder. *Arch Gen Psychiatry* 56:330–336.

Geller, B., Cooper, T.B., Sun, K., Zimerman, B., Frazier, J., Williams, M., and Heath, J. (1998) Double-blind and placebo-controlled study of lithium for adolescent bipolar disorders with secondary substance dependency. *J Am Acad Child Adolesc Psychiatry* 37: 171–178.

Geller, B., Zimerman, B., Williams, M., Bolhofner, K., Craney, J.L., DelBello, M.P., and Soutullo, C. (2001) Reliability of the Washington University in St. Louis Kiddie Schedule for Affective Disorders and Schizophrenia (WASH-U-KSADS) mania and rapid cycling sections. *J Am Acad Child Adolesc Psychiatry* 40:450–455.

Grayson, P. and Carlson, G.A. (1991) The utility of a DSM-III-R-based checklist in screening child psychiatric patients. *J Am Acad Child Adolesc Psychiatry* 30:669–672.

Greene, R.W. (1998) *The Explosive Child*. New York: Harper-Collins.

Hart, E.L. and Lahey, B.B. (1999) General behavior rating scales. In: Shaffer, D., Lucas, C.P., Richters, J.E., eds. *Diagnostic Assessment in Child and Adolescent Psychopathology*. New York: Guilford Press, pp. 65–90.

Hill, M.A., Courvoisie, H., Dawkins, K., Nofal, P., and Thomas, B. (1997) ECT for the treatment of intractable mania in two prepubertal male children. *Convul Thera* 13:74–82.

Hsu, L.K.G. and Starzynski, J.M. (1986) Mania in adolescence. *J Clin Psychiatry* 47:596–599.

James, A.C.D. and Javaloyes A.M. (2001) Practioner review: the treatment of bipolar disorder in children and adolescents. *J Child Psychol Psychiatry* 42:439–451.

Kafantaris, V., Coletti, D.J., Dicker, R., Padula, G., and Pollack, S. (1998) Are childhood psychiatric histories of bipolar adolescents associated with family history, psychosis, and response to lithium treatment? *J Affect Disord* 51:153–164.

Kafantaris, V., Lee, D.O., Magee, H., Winny, G., Samuel, R., Pollack, S., and Campbell, M. (1996) Assessment of children with the overt aggression scale. *J Neuropsychiatry Clin Neurosci* 8:186–193.

Kastner, T. and Friedman, D.L. (1992) Verapamil and valproic acid treatment of prolonged mania. *J Am Acad Child Adolesc Psychiatry* 31:271–275.

Kaufman, J., Birmaher, B., and Brent D. (1997) Schedule for Affective Disorders and Schizophrenia for School-Age Children–Present and Lifetime Version (K-SADS-PL). *J Am Acad Child Adolesc Psychiatry* 36: 980–988.

Keck, P.E., Jr., Mendlwicz, J., Calabrese, J.R., Fawcett, J., Suppes, T., Vestergaard, P.A., and Carbonell, C. (2000) A review of randomized, controlled clinical trials in acute mania. *J Affect Disord* 59:S31–S39.

Koehler-Troy, C., Strober, M., and Malenbaum, R. (1986) Methylphenidate-induced mania in a prepubertal child. *J Clin Psychiatry* 47:566–567.

Kowatch, R.A., Suppes, T., Carmody, T.J., Bucci, J.P., Hume, J.H.,

Kromelis, M., Emslie, G.J., Weinberg, W.A., and Rush, A.J. (2000) Effect size of lithium, divalproex sodium, and carbamazepine in children and adolescents with bipolar disorder. *J Am Acad Child Adolesc Psychiatry* 39:713–720.

Lapalme, M., Hodgins, S., and LaRoche, C. (1997) Children of parents with bipolar disorder: a metaanalysis of risk for mental disorders. *Can J Psychiatry* 42:623–631.

Lee, D.O., Steingard, R.J., Cesena, M., Helmers, S.L., Riviello, J.J., and Mikati, M.A. (1996) Behavioural side effects of gabapentin in children. *Epilepsia* 37:87–90.

Licamele, W.L., and Goldberg, R.L. (1989) The concurrent use of lithium and methylphenidate in a child. *J Am Acad Child Adolesc Psychiatry* 28:785–787.

Max, J.E., Castillo, C.S., Lindren, S.D., and Arndt, S. (1998) The Neuropsychiatric Rating Schedule: reliability and validity. *J Am Acad Child Adolesc Psychiatry* 37:297–304.

Mayer, M. (1967) *A Boy, A Dog and A Frog.* New York: The Dial Press.

National Institute of Mental Health (2001) National Institute of Mental Health Research Round table on Prepubertal Bipolar Disorder. *J Am Acad Child Adolesc Psychiatry* 40:871–878.

Nurnberger, J. and Berrettini, W. (1998) *Psychiatric Genetics.* London: Chapman Hall.

Papatheodorou, G., Kutcher, S.P., Katic, M., and Szalai, J.P. (1995) The efficacy and safety of divalproex sodium in the treatment of acute mania in adolescents and young adults: an open clinical trial. *J Clin Psychopharmacol* 15:110–116.

Rasanen, P., Tiihonen, J., and Hakko, H. (1998) The incidence and onset-age of hospitalized bipolar affective disorder in Finland. *J Affect Disord* 48:63–68.

Reddy, Y.C., Girimaji, S., and Srinath, S. (1997) Clinical profile of mania in children and adolescents from the Indian subcontinent. *Can J Psychiatry* 42:841–846.

Reich, W. (2000) Diagnostic Interview for Children and Adolescents (DICA). *J Am Acad Child Adolesc Psychiatry* 39:59–66.

Rey, J.M., and Walter, G. (1997) Half a century of ECT use in young people. *Am J Psychiatry* 154:595–602.

Robertson, J.M., and Tanguay, P.E. (1997) Case study: the use of melatonin in a boy with refractory bipolar disorder. *J Am Acad Child Adolesc Psychiatry* 36:822–825.

Sachs, G.S. and Thase, M.E. (2000) Bipolar disorder therapeutics: maintenance treatment. *Biol Psychiatry* 48:573–581.

Schaller, J.L., and Behar, D. (1999) Quetiapine for refractory mania in a child. *J Am Acad Child Adolesc Psychiatry* 38:498–499.

Schreier, H.A. (1982) Mania responsive to lecithin in a 13-year-old girl. *Am J Psychiatry* 139:108–110.

Shaffer, D., Fisher, P., Lucas, C.P., Dulcan, M.K., and Schwab-Stone, M.E. (2000) NIMH Diagnostic Interview Schedule for Children Version IV. Description, differences from previous versions and reliability of some comon diagnoses. *J Am Acad Child Adolesc Psychiatry* 39:28–38.

Soutullo, C.A., Casuto, L.S., and Keck, P.E., Jr. (1998) Gabapentin in the treatment of adolescent mania: a case report. *J Child Adolesc Psychopharmacol* 8:81–85.

Soutullo, C.A., Sorter, M.T., Foster, K.D., McElroy, S.L., and Keck, P.E. (1999) Olanzapine in the treatment of adolescent acute mania: a report of seven cases. *J Affect Disord* 53:279–283.

Srinath, S., Janardhan Reddy, Y.C., Girimaji, S.R., Seshadri, S.P., and Subbakrishna, D.K. (1998) A prospective study of bipolar disorder in children and adolescents from India. *Acta Psychiatr Scand* 98:437–442.

Strober, M., DeAntonio, M., Schmidt-Lackner, S., Freeman, R., Lampert, C., and Diamond, J. (1998) Early childhood attention deficit hyperactivity disorder predicts poorer response to acute lithium therapy in adolescent mania. *J Affect Disord* 51:145–151.

Strober, M., Morrell, W., Burroughs, J., Lampert, C., Danforth, H., and Freeman, R. (1988) A family study of bipolar I disorder in adolescence. *J Affect Disord* 15:255–268.

Strober, M., Morrell, W., Lampert, C., and Burroughs, J. (1990) Relapse following discontinuation of lithium maintenance therapy in adolescents with bipolar I illness: a naturalistic study. *Am J Psychiatry* 147:457–461.

Suppes, T., Baldessarini, R.J., and Faedda, G.L. (1991) Risk of recurrence following discontinuation of lithium in bipolar disorder. *Arch Gen Psychiatry* 48:1082–1088.

Thomsen, P.H., Møller, L.L., Dehlholm, B., and Brask B.H. (1992) Manic-depressive psychosis in children younger than 15 years: a register-based investigation of 39 cases in Denmark. *Acta Psychiatr Scand* 85:401–406.

Varanka, T.M., Weller, R.A., and Weller, E.B. (1988) Lithium treatment of manic episodes with psychotic features in prepubertal children. *Am J Psychiatry* 145:1557–1559.

Weller, E.B., Weller, R.A., and Fristad, M.A. (1986) Lithium dosage guide for prepubertal children: a preliminary report. *J Am Acad Child Psychiatry* 25:92–95.

West, S.A., Keck P.E., Jr., and McElroy, S.L. (1995) Oral loading doses in the valproate treatment of adolescents with mixed bipolar disorder. *J Child Adolesc Psychopharmacol* 5:225–231.

West, S.A., Keck P.E., Jr., McElroy, S.L., Strakowski, S.M., Minnery, K.L., McConville, B.J., and Sorter, M.T. (1994) Open trial of valproate in the treatment of adolescent mania. *J Child Adolesc Psychopharmacol* 4:263–267.

Wilens, T.E., Wyatt, D., and Spencer, T.J. (1998) Disentangling disinhibition. *J Am Acad Child Adolesc Psychiatry* 37:1225–1227.

Woolston, J.L. (1999) Case study: carbamazepine treatment of juvenile-onset bipolar disorder. *J Am Acad Child Adolesc Psychiatry* 38:335–338.

Young, R.C., Biggs, J.T., Ziegler, V.E., and Meyer, D.A. (1978) A rating scale for mania: reliability, validity and sensitivity. *Br J Psychiatry* 133:429–435.

Yudofsky, S.C., Silver, J.M., Jackson, W., Endicott, J., and Williams, D. (1986) The Overt Aggression Scale for the objective rating of verbal and physical aggression. *Am J Psychiatry* 143:35–39.

38 | Anxiety disorders

MICHAEL J. LABELLARTE AND GOLDA S. GINSBURG

Research on pediatric anxiety disorders, the most prevalent psychiatric disorders in children and adolescents, has burgeoned in the last 20 years. The rise in research on pediatric anxiety coincided with the establishment of the broad diagnostic category "Anxiety Disorders of Childhood and Adolescence" in the *Diagnostic and Statistical Manual of Mental Disorders, 3rd ed.* (DSM-III; American Psychiatric Association [APA], 1980). New knowledge on the validity of pediatric anxiety diagnoses spurred changes in the classification and criteria of pediatric anxiety disorders in the Diagnostic and Statistical Manual *of Mental Disorders, 4th ed.* (DSM-IV; American Psychiatric Association, 1994). Among the most significant changes were the elimination of the broad diagnostic category "Anxiety Disorders of Childhood and Adolescence," and the elimination of the diagnostic categories "Avoidant Disorder" and "Overanxious Disorder," which were subsumed under the "adult" disorders social phobia (SoP) and generalized anxiety disorder (GAD), respectively.

Anxiety disorders unique to childhood, such as separation anxiety disorder (SAD), are now categorized as "Disorders Usually First Diagnosed During Infancy, Childhood or Adolescence" in the (DSM-IV (APA, 1994) and the *Diagnostic and Statistical Manual for Mental Disorders, 4th ed., Text Revision* (DSM-IV-TR; APA, 2000). The remaining anxiety disorders, i.e., panic disorder (PD), agoraphobia (AG), specific phobia (SpP), SoP, obsessive-compulsive disorder (OCD), posttraumatic stress disorder (PTSD), acute stress disorder (ASD), and GAD, can be diagnosed in children or adults. However, the diagnostic criteria for these anxiety disorders in children differ slightly from those for adults.

The validity of anxiety disorder diagnoses in children and adolescents is tied to reliable and valid pediatric anxiety assessment tools. This chapter focuses on up-to-date clinical assessment methods, as well as treatment modalities for the most common anxiety disorders in children and adolescents. The Assessment section includes an overview of anxiety screens, semistructured diagnostic interviews, anxiety rating scales, observational assessment methods, and physiological assessment methods. The Treatment section includes a review of psychopharmacotherapy and cognitive-behavior therapy (CBT) for pediatric anxiety disorders. Strategies for pediatric dosing and monitoring of selected anxiolytics are presented along with strategies for combining psychosocial and pharmacological treatment.

ASSESSMENT

Choosing the best pediatric anxiety assessment method is complicated by the vast number and variable quality of extant instruments. The first step in choosing an anxiety assessment tool is to identify the specific goal of the assessment, as different methods are better suited to attain certain goals or outcomes than others (Ronan, 1996; Silverman and Kurtines, 1996). For instance, pediatricians in a large health maintenance organization (HMO) may want an instrument to help screen for anxiety problems (to make an appropriate referral), while a child psychiatrist might want an instrument to assist in making a differential diagnosis. Table 38.1 identifies common goals and corresponding anxiety assessment instruments to guide practitioners. Whenever possible, multiple informants should be used (e.g., child, parent, teacher, and clinician ratings) in assessing pediatric anxiety.

Diagnostic Interviews

The use of structured and semistructured interview schedules for diagnosing anxiety disorders (and other psychiatric disorders) has increased because of problems with reliability and validity of psychiatric diagnoses derived from unstructured clinical interviews (Edelbrock and Costello, 1984). Structured and semistructured interviews are most useful for diagnosis (including differential diagnosis) and treatment planning. These instruments also facilitate the gathering of de-

TABLE 38.1 *Questions and Measures used to Assess Childhood Anxiety and Identify Assessment Goals*

Question	Measure
A. Is anxiety excessive for this child?	Multidimensional Anxiety Scale for Children (MASC) Screen for Child Anxiety-Related Emotional Disorders (SCARED)
B. Does this child have an anxiety disorder?	Anxiety Disorders Interview Schedule for Children (ADIS-C/P) Kiddie Schizophrenia and Affective Disorders Schedule (K-SADS)
C. Does the child have a comorbid psychiatric disorder?	ADIS-C/P, K-SADS, Youth Self-Report (YSR), Child Behavior Checklist (CBCL)
D. How severe or impairing is the anxiety disorder?	Clinical Global Impressions-Severity (CGI-S) Global Assessment of Function (GAF)
E. What are contributing contextual factors?	a. Situational: behavioral observation, daily diary b. Family: parent–child interaction, parental psychopathology c. Social: social skills and competence, friendships and peer network d. School: Teacher Report Form (TRF), academic performance and skills
F. What is the treatment plan?	B, C, and D as well as cognitive measures and coping skills measures
G. Is the treatment working?	Pediatric Anxiety Rating Scale (PARS) CGI-S and CGI-Improvement; also A–F to create a comprehensive battery to compare mid-and post-treatment

tailed information on severity of symptoms, impairment, duration of illness, and lifetime occurrences of illness.

Although several interview schedules are now available for assessing children, only the Anxiety Disorders Interview Schedule for Children (ADIS-C/P; Silverman & Albano, 1999a) was specifically designed to assess pediatric anxiety disorders. Consequently, the ADIS-C/P, a semistructured clinician-rated interview, provides the most detailed coverage of pediatric anxiety symptoms and disorders. This instrument also has psychometric support, including reliability and validity, and is often considered the gold standard of diagnostic interviews for assessing pediatric anxiety disorders (Silverman and Nelles, 1988; Silverman and Eisen, 1992; Rapee, et al., 1994; Silverman and Rabian, 1995). Although the ADIS-C/P is routinely used for diagnosing anxiety disorders in psychosocial treatment research, psychopharmacological treatment studies of pediatric anxiety disorders tend to rely on a version of the Kiddie Schedule for Affective Disorders and Schizophrenia (K-SADS; Kaufman et al., 1996). In fact, only one of

the controlled psychopharmacological studies described below used the ADIS-C/P. Fortunately, recently designed treatment studies have included the ADIS-C/P, facilitating comparisons of modalities across treatment studies.

While structured diagnostic interviews have generally improved the reliability of diagnoses, reliability and validity for specific anxiety disorders vary considerably among interview schedules and much work remains to be done in this area. Another limitation of structured diagnostic interviews is the time needed for administering (approximately 2–3 hours) them and the requirement for considerable clinician training. An additional problem with existing diagnostic interviews is that they fail to assess the overall severity of anxiety symptoms across disorders; they link severity to one specific disorder, based on the current (or past) version of the DSM. Changes in the DSM criteria for childhood anxiety disorders overlap of symptoms among anxiety disorders, and high rates of comorbidity among anxiety disorders in youth highlight the limitation of this method for assessing the overall severity of anxiety symptoms. This issue is particularly relevant when assessing global changes in anxiety severity in the context of treatment outcome studies. To address this issue, clinical researchers have turned to clinician-rated scales to assess anxiety severity.

Clinician-Rated Measures

Few clinician-rated instruments have been developed for assessing symptom severity of pediatric anxiety disorders. Among the extant instruments are the Hamilton Anxiety Rating Scale (HAM-A; Clark and Donovan, 1994), the Children's Yale-Brown Obsessive Compulsive Scale (CY-BOCS; Scahill et al., 1997a), and the recently developed Pediatric Anxiety Rating Scale (PARS; Research Units for Pediatric Pharmacology [RUPP] Anxiety Study Group, 2000). The HAM-A focuses predominantly on physiological or somatic symptoms of anxiety, and the psychometric properties of this measure have only been examined in adolescents; no data are available for children. The CY-BOCS, a widely used measure, assesses symptomatology specific to OCD. The psychometric properties have been well established in both child and adolescent populations and this instrument is often considered the gold standard for assessing severity of OCD symptoms in youth.

The PARS, developed to fill a gap in clinician-rated assessments of pediatric anxiety, was modeled after the CY-BOCS and Yale Global Tic Severity Scale (YGTSS; Leckman et al., 1989). The PARS consists of a 50-item symptom checklist, scored by the interviewing clinician as present or absent (yes/no) during a specific rating period (e.g., past week). Symptoms are then rated by the clinician along seven severity/interference dimensions, using a 6-point scale (0, least severe to 5, most severe). Preliminary psychometric properties have been encouraging; the coefficient for test–retest over a 1- to 3-week period was 0.55, and interrater reliability was 0.97 (Walkup, 1999).

Self-Report Rating Scales

A frequently used method for assessing pediatric anxiety is self-report rating scales. Self-report (and parent-report) measures are most useful for screening and assessing the degree to which a child's anxiety is "normative" in the context of developmental, gender, and cultural factors. In addition, self-report measures are useful to monitor changes in anxiety symptomatology over time or in relation to treatment. They are quick and inexpensive, and require little training to administer.

Among the many self-report instruments that exist, some, such as the Multidimensional Anxiety Scale for Children (MASC; March et al., 1997) and the Screen for Anxiety-Related Emotional Disorders (SCARED; Birmaher et al., 1997; 1999), assess a broad range of anxiety symptoms, while others assess one specific disorder or domain of anxiety (e.g., obsessive and compulsive behaviors, social anxiety, worry, fears, etc.).

Despite their advantages, self-report scales cannot be used for diagnosis, are dependent on the child's cognitive abilities (i.e., to read and comprehend items), and are vulnerable to response bias because they rely solely on the child's perspective to interpret items. Moreover, earlier self-report anxiety rating scales lacked discriminant and construct validity. For instance, scores on these scales could not differentiate children with anxiety disorders from children with other internalizing or externalizing disorders (e.g., Hodges et al., 1982; Perrin and Last, 1992). Many of these scales assessed a diffuse global state of "negative affectivity" rather than anxiety per se (Finch, et al., 1989; King et al., 1991). The newer rating scales, such as the MASC (March et al., 1997) and SCARED (Birmaher et al., 1997), have begun to address these issues by demonstrating both discriminant and construct validity.

Observational Methods

Observational methods of assessing anxiety in real life or analogue situations are a useful adjunct to the mental status examination in a clinical setting. These methods generally involve the child or others (e.g., trained raters, parents, teachers, clinicians) monitoring anxiety-related behaviors. This approach helps document the frequency and severity of anxiety symptoms as well as their antecedents and consequences. Observational methods may be unstructured or structured.

When children are the "observers," these procedures are referred to as *self-monitoring*. A commonly used unstructured self-monitoring approach involves a child systematically recording several factors into a daily diary, including *(1)* the situations in which they feel fear or anxiety, *(2)* the actions they took in that situation (i.e., whether they confronted or avoided the situation), *(3)* accompanying cognitions, and *(4)* a rating of fear (e.g., ranging from 0, not at all afraid or anxious, to 10, very very afraid or anxious). An example of a more structured approach involves a child-completed checklist for certain events that occurred during the week and whether anxious feelings or thoughts occurred during the events (Beidel et al., 1991). Few data exist supporting the psychometric properties of these self-monitoring instruments, but they are useful clinical tools and are commonly used during psychosocial treatments.

A behavioral observation coding system is generally used when other informants, such as trained clinicians or researchers, are observers of anxious behavior. Several observational systems have been developed to assess anxiety (for a review see Barrios and Hartman, 1997). These observational systems can be used in both naturalistic and analogue situations and many have been designed for assessing anxiety during stressful medical procedures. Psychometric properties of these coding systems have been strong, with high coefficients for interrater reliability and concurrent validity. Examples of these methods include the Preschool Observation Scale of Anxiety (Glennon and Weisz, 1978) and the Observer Rating Scale of Anxiety (Melamud and Siegel, 1975).

Most clinicians are likely to find the use of an analogue observational procedure more feasible than a naturalistic observational procedure, and most do not rely on behavioral coding systems. One example of such a procedure is called the Behavioral Approach Task (BAT; Lang and Lazovik, 1963). These procedures are generally individualized and involve asking a child to confront or approach a feared object or situation. Examples of tasks might include asking children to talk about themselves for 5 minutes in front of a small audience (for SoP), to approach a dog (for SpP), to leave the clinic with the examiner without the parent (for SAD), etc. Coding schemes vary with respect to which behaviors get observed but generally include whether the child can engage in the task, for how long, and if relevant, the distance approach. Because these procedures are not used in a standardized manner (e.g., differing instructions, individualized situations, etc.), the reliability and validity of BAT procedures vary.

Physiological Methods

Data on the physiological assessment of pediatric anxiety are limited. The most common physiological assessments include measuring a child's heart or pulse rate, electrodermal activity (e.g., finger or palm sweat), and cortisol levels (see King, 1994, for a review). Although some data on the psychometric properties of physiological measures exist (e.g., Beidel, 1991), reliability and validity data are sparse and/or unremarkable because of the complexities of this type of assessment, individual differences in arousal patterns, and the instruments' sensitivity to nonanxiety influences. More recent studies suggest indices of respiration may be a potential marker for presence of an anxiety disorder in children (Pine et al., 2000).

PSYCHOPHARMACOLOGICAL TREATMENT

The psychopharmacology of anxiety disorders is anchored by neurotransmitter hypotheses involving γ-aminobutyric acid (GABA), serotonin (5-HT), and norepinephrine (NE). Currently, a number of psychotropic medications have a Food and Drug Administration (FDA) indication for treatment of adult anxiety disorders, including anxiolytics such as benzodiazepines (BZs) and buspirone; antidepressants such as selective serotonin reuptake inhibitors (SSRIs), tricyclic antidepressants (TCAs), venlafaxine, and phenelzine; and a miscellaneous group of agents, including an antihistamine (hydroxyzine), and older sedatives such as mephobarbital and meprobamate. In contrast, only doxepin ($\geq$ 12 years of age) and meprobamate ($\geq$ 6 years of age) have FDA indications for non-OCD anxiety disorders that include pediatric age groups; however, neither indication is based on adequate controlled treatment data (Riddle et al., 1998). Many of the medications in Table 38.2 have never been studied for treatment of pediatric anxiety using adequate methodology, and are not likely to be studied further because of questionable promise (e.g. antihistamines) and/or safety concerns (e.g., monoamine oxydase inhibitors [MAOIs] and meprobamate). Many of the pharmacotherapy studies discussed below are limited by small sample size and lack of reliable and valid anxiety rating scales.

Selective Serotonin Reuptake Inhibitors

The SSRIs have supplanted the TCAs as clinical treatment options because of their anxiolytic potential, ease

TABLE 38.2 *Pediatric Dosage for Anxiety Disorders*

| Medication | Dose/Day | |
	Children	Adolescents
Fluvoxamine[a]	50–150 mg	100–300 mg
Imipramine[a]	2–5 mg/kg/day	2–5 mg/kg/day
Clonazepam[b]	0.125–0.5 mg	0.5–2 mg
Buspirone	10–20 mg	15–60 mg
Venlafaxine	1–4.5 mg/kg/day	1–4.5 mg/kg/day
Nefazodone	50–100 mg	100–200 mg
Alternatives		
Sertraline[a]	25–100 mg	50–150 mg
Paroxetine[a]	5–20 mg	10–40 mg
Fluoxetine[a]	5–20 mg	10–40 mg
Citalopram[a]	5–20 mg	10–40 mg
Nortriptyline[a]	1–3 mg/kg/day	1–3 mg/kg/day
Lorazapam[b]	0.5–2 mg	2–4 mg

[a]Alternatives within drug class.
[b]Adjunctive alternatives.

of use, and safety and tolerability profiles. Five medications have been investigated in large controlled studies of pediatric OCD: *(1)* clomipramine (Flament et al., 1985; Leonard et al., 1989; DeVeaugh-Geiss, et al., 1992); *(2)* fluvoxamine (Riddle et al., 2001); *(3)* sertraline (March et al., 1998); *(4)* paroxetine (Emslie et al., 2000); and *(5)* fluoxetine (Geller et al., 2001). Clomipramine, fluvoxamine, and sertraline have FDA indications for children and adolescents with OCD. Experience with SSRIs in controlled pediatric OCD studies has led researchers and clinicians to consider SSRIs as treatment options for non-OCD anxiety disorders.

The recently published landmark, double-blind study of 128 children and adolescents (ages 6–16 years) with GAD, SoP, and/or SAD compared fluvoxamine (50–250 mg/day) plus supportive (non-CBT) therapy to placebo plus supportive therapy (RUPP Anxiety Study Group, 2001). The inclusion of subjects with separate but overlapping anxiety disorders is similar to the methodology used in numerous controlled CBT treatment studies of pediatric anxiety disorders discussed in the next section. Based on ratings of the Clinical Global Impression-Improvement scale (CGI-I; Rapaport et al., 1985), 76% of the fluvoxamine-treatment group responded, compared to 29% of the placebo group. About one-third of responders had statistically significant CGI-I ratings by week 2 of treatment. More than 50% of subjects treated with fluvoxamine had a >50 % improvement in PARS ratings. The effect size of the fluvoxamine–anxiety study was large (1.1). In contrast, the effect size of the largest published SSRI–pediatric OCD studies ranged from 0.4 (March et al., 1998; Riddle et al., 2001) to 0.5 (Geller et al., 2001). Furthermore, the effect size of imipramine (IMI) on school avoidance has ranged from 0.29 (Bernstein et al., 2000) to 0.73 (Gittleman-Klein and Klein, 1971). The most commonly reported adverse effects in the RUPP anxiety study included hyperactivity and gastrointestin (GI) distress. Long-term (12-month) safety and efficacy data involving fluvoxamine treatment of pediatric anxiety disorders are being analyzed.

A recently published study compared sertraline (a logical SSRI selection due to its FDA indication for OCD) to placebo in a nine-week treatment study of 22 children and adolescents (ages 5–17 years) with GAD as a primary diagnosis (Rynn et al., 2001). Comorbidity exclusion criteria were strict, and only six subjects had symptoms of another anxiety disorder, e.g. subsyndromal separation anxiety disorder. Sertraline (up to 50 mg/day) was superior to placebo on all primary outcome measures (e.g., HAM-A total, psychic, and somatic factor scores; CGI-I and CGI-S) beginning at week four of treatment. Based on the CGI-I, 90% (10/11) of the sertraline treatment group responded, compared to 10% (1/10) of the placebo group. Restlessness, dry-mouth, and leg spasms occurred twice as often in subjects treated with sertraline compared to placebo; gastrointestinal complaints were much less common in the sertraline group.

Prior to the fluvoxamine–anxiety disorders study, only one placebo-controlled study of a SSRI for pediatric anxiety had been published. Fluoxetine (12–27 mg/day) was superior to placebo in a study of 15 children (ages 6–11 years) with elective mutism, a subset of social phobia now called *selective mutism* (Black and Uhde, 1994). Fluoxetine treatment was superior to placebo on 28 of 29 rating items, however, only parent ratings of Mutism CGI and Global Change CGI showed a statistically significant difference between treatment groups. No clinician-rated outcome measure showed a statistically significant difference between treatment groups. The small number of subjects further limits the generalizability of the study, and the focus on selective mutism, limits the applicability of the results to children and adolescents with more common anxiety disorders.

Tricyclic Antidepressants

The most often cited publication of psychopharmacological treatment for pediatric anxiety is a study of IMI for 35 subjects (ages 6–14 years) with school phobia who received concomitant behavior treatment (Gittle-man-Klein and Klein, 1971). This study introduced the formulation that separation anxiety likely accounted for school phobia in many children. Eighty-one percent of subjects returned to school after 6 weeks of IMI treatment (100–200 mg/day), compared to 47% of subjects treated with placebo. Imipramine was also superior to placebo, based on global improvement ratings by child, parent, and psychiatrist. Interestingly, all children treated with IMI rated themselves as much improved or better, compared to 21% of the placebo treatment group. No outcome measure showed significant improvement after the first 3 weeks of treatment, when the initial treatment dose of 75 mg/day was being titrated (mean dose at week 3 was 107 mg/day vs. 152 mg/day at week 6). Imipramine was well tolerated in the study.

In a similar study of children (ages 6–15 years) with SAD, the same investigator group (Klein et al., 1992) was not able to replicate the treatment effect of IMI, based on ratings of global improvement and the Children's Manifest Anxiety Scale (CMAS). Fewer subjects ($n = 21$) were included in the 6 week medication treatment phase than in the previous study because more than 20 enrolled subjects responded to 4 weeks of behavioral treatment and therefore were not randomized to IMI treatment. Compared to the earlier study, there was a much larger placebo-response rate, potentially due to less severe anxiety symptoms (subjects in this study did not have school refusal). Accounting for both study outcomes, the authors suggested that IMI "need not be precluded" from treatment of pediatric anxiety disorders, but the effect of IMI suggested in the prior study cannot be regularly expected.

Several controlled studies of IMI involved less homogeneous samples of anxious children. Neither IMI nor alprazolam (a BZ) was superior to placebo in an 8-week study of 24 children (ages 7–18 years) with school refusal, which included subjects with anxiety and depression (Bernstein et al., 1990). A more recent placebo-controlled study of IMI + CBT for 47 adolescents (ages 12–18 years) with school refusal, anxiety, and/or depression was "designed to address the limitations" of previous studies of TCA treatment for pediatric anxiety disorders (Bernstein et al., 2000). Accordingly, sample size was based on proposed power analysis; IMI dose and serum level were monitored to ensure adequate exposure (mean IMI dose 180 mg/day; mean serum IMI 180 µg/L; and mean IMI + DMI 250 µg/L at week 3 and week 8); and CBT was manual based and closely monitored. Fifty-four percent of subjects treated with IMI + CBT met remission criteria (defined as ≥ 75% school attendance at the end of the study), compared to 17% of subjects treated with placebo + CBT. No between-group differences were noted on measures of anxiety (Anxiety Rating for Children-Revised, [ARC-R]; and depression (Children's Depression Rating Scale-Revised [CDRS-R]; Poznanski and Mokros, 1995); significant numbers of both treatment groups improved. A naturalistic follow-up study of 41 subjects who returned at one year showed that most of the subjects remained in school, however, the subgroup that attended follow-up study also had better attendance at the end of the controlled treatment study, compared to the subgroup that did not attend follow-up study (Bernstein et al., 2001). Sixty-four percent of the subjects still met criteria for an anxiety disorder at 1 year follow-up.

The final controlled TCA study to be discussed here involved a different TCA, clomipramine. This agent showed no significant treatment benefits in 51 subjects (ages 9–14 years) with school refusal (Berney, et al., 1981). The dose range of clomipramine in the school refusal study (40–75 mg/day) was much lower than the clomipramine dose ranges (75–250 mg/day) in the definitive pediatric OCD studies cited above (Flament et al., 1985; Leonard et al., 1989; Deveaugh-Geiss et al., 1992). However, clomipramine's potent anticholingeric profile and the potential cardiotoxicity of all TCAs likely preclude its use in future controlled studies of non-OCD anxiety disorders in children and adolescents.

Buspirone

The extent of buspirone experience in children and adolescents is limited to open studies and case reports. There are no published double-blind placebo-controlled studies of buspirone for pediatric anxiety disorders or any other psychiatric disorder. Results of a recently completed large ($n = 350$; ages 6–17 years), industry-sponsored, multisite study of buspirone for children (15–30 mg/day) and adolescents (45–60 mg/day) with GAD have not been published or presented at open academic conferences. Until such data are made available, the use of buspirone for treatment of pediatric anxiety disorders remains speculative.

Benzodiazepines

Despite the history of robust BZ anxiolytic impact in adults, controlled studies, open studies, and case reports of BZs for pediatric anxiety have not been impressive. Concerns about BZ-related adverse events, such as behavioral disihnhibition, have since slowed interest in controlled studies of BZs for treatment of pediatric anxiety disorders. Three small placebo-controlled studies of BZs for pediatric anxiety disorders have been published and none demonstrated

efficacy. The earliest controlled study was a comparison of alprazolam (0.75–4 mg/day), IMI (50–175 mg/day), and placebo for 24 children with school refusal (Bernstein, et al., 1990). Next was a study of alprazolam (0.5–3.5 mg/day) for 30 children (ages 8–16 years) with overanxious disorder and/or avoidant disorder (Simeon et al., 1992). The authors cited the small number of subjects, short duration of treatment (4 weeks), and relatively low-treatment dose of alprazolam (0.04 mg/kg/day) as factors influencing the study results. The final study involved 4 weeks of clonazepam (0.5–2 mg/day) for 15 children (ages 7–13 years) with one or more anxiety disorders; most subjects had a diagnosis of SAD (Graee et al., 1994).

Other Psychopharmacological Treatments

Potential treatment role for pediatric anxiety disorders

Venlafaxine is FDA indicated for GAD in adults. A controlled study of venlafaxine for pediatric GAD is underway, however, no controlled pediatric study of venlafaxine treatment for any psychiatric disorder has been published.

A large study demonstrated efficacy of nefazodone for social phobia in adults (Van Amerigen et al., 1999), but no controlled pediatric study of nefazodone treatment for anxiety disorders or any psychiatric disorder has been published. *The package insert for nefazopone (2002) now includes a black-box warning about potential hepatotoxicity, so liver function tests need to be closely monitored.*

Doubtful treatment role for pediatric anxiety disorders

Although no controlled psychopharmacological study has demonstrated efficacy, antihistamines have been commonly used to treat pediatric anxiety symptoms, based on extrapolation from adult data and anecdotal experience. Diphenhydramine (200–800 mg/day) was sedating but not convincingly anxiolytic in treatment of 'neurotic disorder' in a study discussed below (Korein et al., 1971). Other anticholinergic adverse effects, including irritability and potential for confusion, further discourage use of antihistamine as a potential anxiolytic. In adults, clonidine may have acute antianxiety effects that fade due to tolerance (Uhde et al., 1989), so clonidine has no consistent role in treating anxiety disorders. Despite the lack of evidence supporting its use, clonidine has been used anecdotally for treatment of pediatric anxiety, based on models of NE blockade. The availability of more compelling treatment efficacy data for pediatric anxiety, as well as adverse effect profile including sedation, irritability, hypotension, and potential for bradycardia all make clonidine a poor choice for the treatment of pediatric anxiety disorders.

There are no controlled studies and little open data to inform use of beta-blockers in treatment of pediatric anxiety disorders.

Neuroleptics, sedatives, MAOIs, and antihistamines have been used for treatment of anxiety disorders (referred to as "neurosis") in early studies of pediatric psychopharmacology. The earliest pediatric psychopharmacology treatment studies of anxiety included medication treatment for a neurotic subgroup of children with meprobamate (a propanediol, a minor tranquilizer), prochlorperazine (a neuroleptic), and perphenazine (a neuroleptic) (Cytryn et al., 1960; Eisenberg et al., 1961), as well as chlorpromazine (a neuroleptic) and diphenhydramine (Korean et al., 1971). Another treatment strategy involving subjects with imprecise diagnoses demonstrated that phenelzine (a MAOI) plus chlordiazepoxide was superior to phenobarbitol (a sedative) plus placebo in a double-blind crossover study of 32 depressed children, including a "phobic" subgroup ($n = 15$) (Frommer, 1967). Global improvement in the phobic subgroup was not significantly different from improvement in the "mood disorder" subgroup of depressed children.

MEDICATION DOSING

Are Pharmacokinetic Data Useful for Dosing?

Available pharmacokinetic (PK) studies of medications with potential to treat pediatric anxiety disorders have been open studies that examine PK parameters and monitor adverse effects in children and adolescents. None of the pediatric PK studies described below were designed as dose finding studies, and none of the studies were able to describe a clear association between dose or exposure and specific adverse effect. However, pediatric PK data can be useful to guide dosing and adverse effect monitoring to the extent that the weight-adjusted PK parameters inform extrapolation based on comparable studies of adult PK. The following summary of PK studies is based on multiple-dose PK studies.

Children (especially females) have higher exposure to fluvoxamine than adolescents and adults (Labellarte et al., in press), and children and adolescents have higher exposure to nefazodone than adults (Findling et al., 2000). Children and adolescents demonstrate linear kinetics and exposure to sertraline similar to those of adults (Alderman, et al., 1998); children also seem to

generate similar plasma concentrations of fluoxetine (Wilens et al., 2000). Children and adolescents have lower exposure to venlafaxone than adults (Derivan et al., 1995), and children and adolescents clear low doses of paroxetine faster than adults (Findling et al., 1999). Children metabolize and eliminate diazepam faster than adults, and children achieve peak concentration sooner and eliminate TCAs faster than adults (Coffey, 1993).

Recommended Dosing

Table 38.2 demonstrates recommended medication dosing for pediatric anxiety disorders. Two types of dosing strategies are recommended. A typical daily dose range is recommended for medications with no specific dose-related adverse effects, and a mg/kg/day dose range is recommended for medications with dose-related adverse effects. The IMI dose of 3–5 mg/kg/day or the equivalent (i.e., NTP 1–3 mg/kg/day) appears to be a safe dose for treatment of children and adolescents (Popper, 2000). A rational dose range for venlafaxine (regular-release and extended-release preparations) in children and adolescents is 1–4.5 mg/kg/day. Venlafaxine extended-release (Effexor XR) is administered once daily (instead of bid or tid with regular-release venlafaxine) and is available in capsules ranging from 37.5 to 150 mg. Blood pressure should be monitored in children taking venlafaxine, and blood pressure, pulse, electrocardiogram (EKG), and serum level should be monitored in children taking a TCA.

Other SSRIs may be selected as an alternative to fluvoxamine in the event that fluvoxamine cannot be used. Sertraline is the first option because of efficacy for pediatric GAD (Rynn et al., 2001); paroxetine is an option because of controlled treatment data for adolescent depression (Keller et al., 2000) and OCD (see Chapter 39); and fluoxetine is an option because of controlled treatment data for pediatric depression (Emslie et al., 1997). Lorazepam is included as a short acting alternative to clonazepam. Nortriptyline, which is less anticholinergic and thus may be better tolerated, is included as an alternative to IMI.

PSYCHOSOCIAL TREATMENT

A recent review of studies published in the past decade (ADAA/NIMH, 1999) identified a total of 9 controlled and 15 uncontrolled psychosocial treatment outcome studies. In the last 2 years, at least four additional controlled treatment outcome studies for pediatric anxiety (excluding PTSD and OCD) have been published, and several large trials are underway. Although various psychosocial treatment approaches have been used to treat pediatric anxiety (e.g., psychodynamic, family systems, cognitive, behavioral, play therapy, etc.), only cognitive-behavioral interventions are well represented by randomized controlled studies.

Cognitive-behavioral treatments emerged from a combination of learning-theory principles (Francis and Beidel, 1995) and are generally short term (ranging between 10 and 16 weeks). Four CBT strategies dominate the treatment literature for pediatric anxiety. These include: *(1) exposure* (based on classical conditioning), which generally involves gradual imagined, and in vivo confrontation to fear- and /anxiety-provoking stimuli, and systematic desensitization (gradual exposure paired with relaxation techniques); *(2) contingency management* (based on operant conditioning), which includes modification of external factors influencing anxiety through positive reinforcement, shaping, and extinction; *(3) cognitive strategies* (based on cognitive theory), which includes identification and modification of internal factors (i.e., thoughts) influencing anxiety through self-instruction training, problem solving, and improving self-talk: and *(4) modeling* (based on social learning theory), which includes demonstration of appropriate behavior in anxiety-provoking situations. A fifth strategy, *exposure and response prevention* (E/RP) has been found to be useful for pediatric OCD (March, 1998; March et al., 1994; DeHann et al., 1998; Franklin et al., 1998).

Taken together, CBT treatment studies have several methodological strengths, including the use of structured diagnostic interviews, random assignment, manualized treatment protocols and checks for treatment fidelity, long term follow-up, independent/blind evaluators, and multi-informant, multimethod assessments. Extant studies also vary along numerous dimensions (e.g., diagnostic target group, treatment modality, age of participants, outcome measures, involvement of parents, length of treatment follow-up, type of comparison group, etc.), making comparisons across studies more difficult. In addition, the findings are based on those participants who completed treatment, rather than on intent-to-treat analyses. Thus, response rates may be inflated. Additional methodological problems include unclear severity rating of anxiety symptoms, an over-reliance on self-report rating scales, overly stringent inclusion and exclusion criteria, and treatments that combine various ingredients, which make determining the relative impact of specific cognitive and behavioral strategies difficult.

Despite these limitations, CBT treatments have proven to be efficacious for a majority of child and adolescent subjects with anxiety disorders. Indeed, across studies, between 50% and 80% of treated children no longer meet diagnostic criteria for their anxiety disorder after CBT. In light of the previous success of CBT, current efforts by pediatric anxiety researchers are focused on improving the efficacy of existing individual CBT treatments. These efforts include examining (1) the relative benefit of individual CBT to more stringent comparison conditions to control for nonspecific therapeutic factors, (2) the impact of administering CBT in group formats, and (3) the advantages of including parents more centrally in the treatment (i.e., family-based approaches). Finally, initial efforts toward prevention have also begun. A summary of this literature is presented next.

Individual Cognitive Behavior Therapy

Kendall and colleagues were the first to demonstrate the efficacy of individual CBT in children and adolescents using the 16-week Coping Cat program (Kendall, 1994; Kendall et al., 1997). The program involves cognitive (i.e., recognizing and modifying distorted cognitions and attributions, devising coping plans, evaluating performance, and administering self-reinforcement) and behavioral (i.e., imagined and in vivo exposures, relaxation training) components. The children (ages 9–13 years) were randomly assigned to either a CBT ($n = 27$) or a wait-list control (WLC) condition ($n = 20$). A multimethod approach to assessing treatment outcome was used, including diagnosis (via the ADIS-C/P), several self-, parent-, and teacher-rating scales, and behavioral observations. Overall, the treatment group displayed significantly greater improvement than that of the WLC group on most measures at post-treatment. Specifically, 64% of those treated, compared to 5% of the WLC group, no longer met criteria for an anxiety disorder. Furthermore, 1- and 3-year follow-up assessments revealed that improvements were maintained (Kendall and Southam-Gerow, 1996). Kendall's program (or key ingredients) has been replicated and adapted and tested by other researchers and continues to show efficacy compared to WLC conditions (e.g., Barrett et al., 1996; Kendall et al., 1997; Mendolowitz et al., 1999; Silverman et al., 1999b).

In contrast to the studies above, studies comparing individual CBT to other active treatments (a more stringent control condition than WLC) have been less convincing. For instance, two studies have compared individual CBT to an education support (ES) condition. In the ES treatment, educational presentations about anxiety and supportive psychotherapy were used with no specific instructions or encouragement to engage in exposure. In the first study, anxious youth with school refusal (*n* = 56, ages 6–17 years) were randomly assigned to either CBT or ES. Both conditions were equally effective in reducing school absenteeism, anxiety, and depression (Last et al., 1998).

In one of the few dismantling studies, Silverman and colleagues (1999c) compared ES to both an exposure-based behavioral and cognitive intervention for childhood phobias (including SpP, SoP, and AG) in a sample of 81 children (ages 6–16 years). At post-treatment, children in all three groups showed equal improvements on most measures of anxiety. The only outcome measure that showed differences was diagnostic status: fewer children receiving cognitive treatment continued to meet their primary diagnosis, compared to those in the behavioral or ES conditions, whose results were not different from each other's.

One explanation for the unexpected success of ES in these studies is that ES may contain similar treatment elements integral to CBT, such as psychoeducation and information about cognitive and behavioral principles. Participants in the ES condition may have been able to extrapolate key CBT elements and apply the approaches to anxiety situations without therapist direction. Taken together, these results suggest that further delineation of the unique characteristics of each modality of treatment is needed to identify the essential ingredients of effective treatments.

Group Cognitive Behavior Therapy

Group treatments attempt to harness the benefits of using peers in treatment and are believed to increase social support, provide modeling opportunities and credible corrective instruction and feedback, and reduce feelings of stigma and isolation. For children with social anxiety, group treatments incorporate "natural" weekly exposures (a key treatment ingredient of CBT). Group treatments may also be more cost-effective than individual approaches. Several studies have examined the efficacy of group CBT for anxious youth relative to either a WLC, individual CBT, or another treatment. Overall, findings are promising for group CBT, with response rates being similar to those of individual CBT (e.g., Albano et al., 1995; Barrett, 1998; Silverman et al., 1999b); Hayward et al., 2000).

In a recent study, Flannery-Schroeder and Kendall (2000) compared group and individual CBT to a WLC in 37 children (ages 8–14 years) with GAD, SAD, and/or SoP. Treatment outcome was evaluated using diagnostic interviews and child, parent, and teacher reports of anxiety and other measures of psychosocial functioning at post-treatment and 3-month follow-up. At post-treatment, significantly more children in the indi-

vidual (73%) and group (50%) CBT conditions did not meet diagnostic criteria for their primary anxiety disorder, compared to those in the WLC (8%). Children in both active treatments were also significantly less anxious according to the self-, parent-, and teacher-rating scales than those in the WLC. Few differences were found between the two treatment groups, including on measures of social functioning. Treatment gains in both groups were maintained at 3-month follow-up.

Finally, Beidel and colleagues (2000) evaluated the relative effectiveness of Social Effectiveness Training for Children (SET-C), a group behavioral treatment, and "Testbusters" (TB), a nonspecific treatment control involving study skills and test-taking strategies, for SoP in children. In their study, children (*n* = 67, ages 8–12 years) were randomly assigned to SET-C or TB. Findings revealed that children in SET-C showed greater improvements than those in the TB conditions across multiple measures of anxiety. For instance, at post-treatment, 67% of children receiving SET-C treatment no longer met diagnostic criteria for SoP, compared to 5% of those receiving TB. The number of children treated with SET-C who were diagnosis-free at 6-month follow-up increased to 85%; this results suggests continued gains even after treatment was completed. In summary, group CBT is as effective as individual treatments, and for some disorders (such as social phobia) may be the preferred modality.

Family-Based Cognitive Behavior Therapy

As noted above, recent efforts have focused on enhancing the efficacy of individual CBT for pediatric anxiety disorders. One approach has been to incorporate parents more centrally in the therapeutic process. Conceptually, this approach has been driven by research indicating that anxiety disorders run in families (because of both environmental/learning and biological factors) and by the identification of specific parenting behaviors associated with increased anxiety in children (Ginsburg et al., 1995). Several recent controlled trials of CBT (using either individual or group formats) have involved parents more centrally in the treatment process. Overall, findings are encouraging for this format of CBT (e.g., Barrett et al., 1996; Cobham et al., 1998; Mendlowitz et al., 1999; Silverman et al., 1999b; Spence et al., 2000).

Silverman and colleagues (1999b) compared the efficacy of a 12-week CBT program for youth (*n* = 56, ages 6–16 years) with SoP, avoidant disorder, and GAD. The treatment was based on the transfer-of-control treatment model. Briefly, this model is based on the assumption that effective long-term child change involves a gradual transfer of control of knowledge and skills for anxiety reduction, where the sequence is generally from therapist to parent to child (see Ginsburg et al., 1995; Silverman and Kurtines, 1996, for a detailed description of this model). The treatment involved weekly parent, child, and conjoint group sessions in which children and their parents were taught CBT strategies. Parents were specifically taught contingency management (e.g., rewarding approach behavior and using extinction for anxious avoidant behavior) in addition to other strategies to help reduce and manage their child's anxiety. Findings supported the efficacy of the CBT treatment over the WLC on diagnostic status (64% vs. 13%) as well as self- and parent-report measures of anxiety.

In an effort to clarify the benefits of parental involvement over individual treatment, Barrett and colleagues (1996), treated 79 children (ages 7–14 years) with a modified version of the Coping Cat program. They compared (1) individual CBT, (2) CBT plus family anxiety management (FAM), and (3) a WLC. Family anxiety management included discipline training, anxiety management of parental distress, and communication and problem-solving skills for parents. Results indicated that while youth in both active treatments improved, the combination of CBT + FAM was superior to CBT alone, based on the outcome measure of diagnosis-free status at post-treatment assessment (84% vs. 57%) and at 12-month follow-up (96% vs. 70%). Children in both active treatments were similar on self- and parent-report measures. Both CBT treatments were superior to WLC, replicating earlier studies by Kendall and colleagues (1994; 1997).

In a unique study, Cobham and colleagues (1998) examined the role of both parental involvement and parental anxiety in the treatment of child anxiety. Using a randomized controlled design, the authors compared individual CBT only and individual CBT plus parent anxiety management (PAM) in 67 children (ages 7–14 years). Both of these treatments were compared in families in which the child alone or child and parent presented with excessive anxiety. Among families with anxious children only, CBT plus PAM was as effective as CBT alone (80% and 82% diagnosis-free status at post-treatment). However, in families where both the child and parent were anxious, the CBT + PAM treatment was more efficacious (77% were diagnosis-free at post-treatment compared to 39% in the CBT-only group). Treatment gains were maintained at 6- and 12-month follow-up.

In summary, although the mechanisms by which parental involvement impacts the treatment of pediatric anxiety remains unclear, these initial findings suggest that involving parents in the treatment of pediatric anxiety, particularly when parental anxiety is present, is associated with a positive treatment response.

COMBINING COGNITIVE BEHAVIOR THERAPY AND ANXIOLYTICS

An editorial that accompanied the RUPP Anxiety Study Group Publication on Fluoxamine (2001) echoed the ongoing debate over CBT, pharmacotherapy, or both to treat pediatric anxiety disorders (Coyle 2001). No controlled comparison of CBT and psychopharmacotherapy exists for pediatric anxiety disorders, and there are no controlled data to inform sequencing or combination effects of CBT used with medication treatment. A number of controlled pharmacological studies of pediatric anxiety listed above provided concomitant psychotherapy in addition to medication as part of the dedication to routine clinical management. However, many of the psychosocial approaches in those "combination studies" were nonspecific, and the specific modalities (i.e., behavioral therapy) were not manualized. Because they were not designed as controlled comparison studies, the unintentional combined pharmacotherapy–psychosocial treatment studies in pediatric anxiety disorders rarely produced noteworthy data regarding timing of treatment modality or relative impact of psychosocial versus pharmacological treatment.

One exception is the behavioral therapy used in the controlled study of IMI for SAD discussed above (Klein et al., 1992). About half of the 45 subjects enrolled in the study responded to behavioral therapy in the initial 4-week treatment phase prior to medication treatment. The authors noted about half of the subjects who responded to behavioral treatment and did not meet randomization criteria still "continued to have clinically significant separation anxiety requiring treatment." Given the results prior to medication randomization, Klein and colleagues (1992) further suggested that behavioral therapy be considered a potential first treatment for SAD before medication treatment.

The other example is the manualized CBT used in the IMI study of school refusal, anxiety, and depression (Bernstein et al., 2000). Although few children receiving CBT and placebo went back to school, a majority of subjects treated with CBT improved significantly on measures of anxiety, regardless of IMI or placebo treatment. The results are consistent with the results of controlled CBT studies described above.

The lack of definitive psychopharmacological treatment data and pharmacotherapy vs. CBT comparison data makes any approach to a medication–CBT algorithm preliminary. Table 38.3 is a list of treatment op-

TABLE 38.3 *Treatment Options for Pediatric Anxiety Disorders*

Anxiety Characteristics	Treatment Options
Mild–Moderate Severity	CBT[a] or fluvoxamine
Severe	
Psychological duress Prominent avoidance Physiological symptoms Impairment in 3 or more areas	CBT ± fluvoxamine
Partial Response to Treatment	Maintain CBT + fluvoxamine Adjunct: addition of clonazepam[b] Augment: addition of other serotonergic agent[c]

[a]CBT, cognitive behavior therapy.
[b]Adjunctive alternatives: lorazepam.
[c]Augmenting strategies: add lithium, buspirone, etc.

tions for target symptoms of pediatric anxiety, based on the logic of two previously published treatment algorithms for pediatric anxiety disorders (Labellarte et al., 1999). Psychopharmacotherapy can be combined with other important approaches to anxiety treatment, e.g., psychoeducation, parent management training, and CBT, regardless of which medication treatment is utilized.

For mild to moderate anxiety, we recommend the conservative approach of beginning with CBT and including medication if CBT is ineffective or only partially effective. However, severe anxiety that involves duress, prominent avoidance behavior, physiological symptoms, or marked impairment, requires a combination of CBT and medication as an initial intervention. Furthermore, children and families with low motivation (i.e., those unlikely to participate in CBT assignments) or having a poor subjective sense of anxiety may require medication treatment as one of the initial interventions.

SUMMARY

Pediatric anxiety disorders are among the most common psychiatric conditions. Additional research into family studies, genetic studies, pathophysiology, and course of illness are needed to inform current nosological systems and clinical interventions. Currently, several assessment methods are available for detecting and diagnosing these disorders. The selection of methods will rely on the specific goal of the assessment. The large treatment effect of fluvoxamine for treatment of

pediatric anxiety disorders is groundbreaking and has opened the door to a generation of research for newer serotonergic agents for pediatric anxiety disorders. However, numerous efficacy studies support CBT for pediatric anxiety disorders; several studies support psychopharmacotherapy. Comparison of CBT, psychopharmacotherapy, and the combination of the two is being planned as a large multimodal treatment study. A study of medication combination treatment is underway for pediatric anxiety disorders and comorbid ADHD. Large, multisite controlled studies of serotonergic agents for pediatric anxiety disorders (OCD, SoP, GAD, SAD) are currently in the data collection phase. Controlled psychopharmacological studies of pediatric PTSD are likely.

REFERENCES

Albano, A.M., Marten, P.A., Holt, C.S., Heimberg, R.G., and Barlow, D.H. (1995) Cognitive-behavioral group treatment for social phobia in adolescents: a preliminary study. *J Nerv Ment Dis 183*: 649–656.

ADAA/NIMH (1999). *Conference on Treating Anxiety Disorders in Youth: Current Problems and Future Solutions.* Anxiety Disorders Association of America.

Alderman, J., Wolkow, R., Chung, M., and Johnston, H.F. (1998). Sertraline treatment of children and adolescents with obsessive-compulsive disorder or depression: pharmacokinetics, tolerability, and efficacy. *J Am Acad Child Adolesc Psychiatry* 37:386–394.

American Psychiatric Association (1980) *Diagnostic and Statistical Manual of Mental Disorders, 3rd ed.* Washington, DC: American Psychiatric Association Press.

American Psychiatric Association (1994) *Diagnostic and Statistical Manual of Mental Disorders, 4th ed.* Washington, DC: American Psychiatric Association Press.

American Psychiatric Association (2000) *Diagnostic and Statistical Manual of Mental Disorders, 4th ed., Text Revision.* Washington, DC: American Psychiatric Association Press.

Barrett, P.M. (1998) Evaluation of cognitive-behavioral group treatments for childhood anxiety disorders. *J Clin Child Psychol* 27: 459–468.

Barrett, P.M., Dadds, M.M., Rapee, R.M., and Ryan, S.M. (1996) Family intervention for childhood anxiety. *J Consult Clin Psychol* 64:333–342.

Barrios, B.A. and Hartman, D.P. (1997) Fears and anxieties. In Mash, E.J. and Terdal, eds. *Assessment of Childhood Disorders, 3rd ed.* New York: Guilford Press, pp. 230–327.

Beidel, D.C. (1991) Determining the reliability psychophysiological assessment in childhood anxiety. *J Anxiety Disord* 5:139–150.

Beidel, D.C., Neal, A.M., and Lederer, A.S. (1991) The feasibility and validity of a daily diary for the assessment of anxiety in children. *Behav Ther* 22:505–517.

Beidel, DC, Turner, S.M., and Morris, T.L. (2000) Behavioral Treatment of Childhood Social Phobia. *J Consult Clin Psychology* 68: 1072–1080.

Berney, T., Kolvin, I., Bhate, R.F., Garsioe, R.F., Jeans, J. Kay, B. and Scarth, L. (1981) School phobia: a therapeutic trial with clomipramine and short—term outcome. *Br J Psychiatry* 138:110–118.

Bernstein, G.A., Borchardt, C.M., Perwein, A.R., et al. (2000) Imipramine plus cognitive-behavioral therapy in in the treatment of school refusal. *J Am Acad Child Adolesc Psychiatry* 39:276–283.

Bernstein, G.A., Crosby, R.D. Perwein, A.R., and Borchardt, C.M.

(1996) Anxiety Rating for Children—Revised: Reliability and Validity. *J Anxiety Disord* 10:97–114.

Bernstein, G.A., Hektner, J.M., Borchardt, C.M., and McMillan, M.H. (2001) Treatment of school refusal: one-year follow-up. *J Am Acad Child Adolesc Psychiatry* 40:206–213.

Bernstein, G.A., Garfinkel, B.D., and Borchardt, C.M. (1990) Comparative studies of pharmacotherapy for school refusal. *J Am Acad Child Adolesc Psychiatry* 29:773–781.

Birmaher, B., Brent, D.A., Chiappetta, L., Bridge, J., Monga, S., and Baugher, M. (1999) Psychometric properties of the Screen for Child Anxiety–Related Emotional Disorders (SCARED): a replication study. *J Am Acad Child Adolesc Psychiatry* 38:1230–1236.

Birmaher, B., Khetarpal, S., Brent, D., Cully, M., Balach, L., Kaufman, J., and McKenzie-Neer, S. (1997) The Screen for Child Anxiety–Related Emotional Disorders (SCARED): scale construction and psychometric characteristics. *J Am Acad Child Adolesc Psychiatry* 36:545–553.

Black, B., and Uhde, T.W. (1994) Treatment of elective mutism with fluoxetine: a double-blind, placebo-controlled study. *J Am Acad Child Adolesc Psychiatry* 33:1000–1006.

Clark, D.B. and Donovan, J.E. (1994) Reliability and Validity of the Hamilton Anxiety Rating scale in an Adolescent Sample. *J am Acad Child Adolesc Psychiatry* 33:354–360.

Cobham, V.E., Dadds, M.R., and Spence, S.H. (1998) The role of parental anxiety in the treatment of childhood anxiety. *J Consult Clin Psychol* 66:893–905.

Coffey, B. (1993) Review and update: benzodiazapines in childhood and adolescence. *Psychiatr Ann* 23:332–339.

Coyle, J.T. (2001) Drug treatment of anxiety disorders in children. *N Engl J Med* 344:1326–1327.

Cytryn, L., Gilbert, A., and Eisenberg (1960) The effectiveness of tranquilizing drugs plus supportive psychotherapy in treating behavior disorders of children: a double-blind study of eighty outpatients. *Am J Orthopsychiatry* 30:113–128.

DeHann, E., Hoogduin, K.A.L., Buitelaar, J.K., and Keijsers, G.P.J. (1998) Behavior therapy versus clomipramine for the treatment of OCD in children and adolescents. *J Am Acad Child Adolesc Psychiatry* 37:1022–1029.

Derivan, A., Aguiar, L., Upton, G.V., Martin, P., D'Amico, D., Troy, S., Ferguson, J., and Preskorn, S. (1995) Poster presented at the 42nd Annual Meeting of the American Academy of Child and Adolescent Pychiatry, New Orleans, LA, October 17–22. Scientific Proceedings.

DeVeaugh-Geiss, J., Moroz, B., and Biederman, J. (1992) Clomipramine hydrochloride in childhood and adolescent obsessive-compulsive disorder—a multicenter trial. *J Am Acad Child Adolesc Psychiatry* 31:45–49.

Edelbrock, C. and Costello, A. (1984) Structured psychiatric interviews for children and adolescents. In: Goldstein, G. and Hersen, M., eds. *Handbook of Psychological Assessment*. New York: Pergamon Press pp. 276–290.

Eisenberg, L., Gilbert, A., Cytryn, L., and Molling, P.A. (1961) The effectiveness of psychotherapy alone and in conjunction with perphenazine or placebo in the treatment of neurotic and hyperkinetic children. *Am J Psychiatry* 117:1088–1093.

Emslie, G.J., Rush, A.J., Weinberg, W.A., Gullion, C.M. Rintelmann, J., and Hughes, C.W. (1997) A double-blind, placebo controlled trial of fluoxetine in children and adolescents with depression. *Arch Gen Psychiatry* 54:1031–1037.

Emslie, G.J., Wagner, K., Riddle, M., Birmaher, B., Geller, B., Rosenberg, D., Gallagher, D., and Carpenter, D. (2000) Efficacy and safety of paroxetine in juvenile OCD. Poster presented at the 47th Annual Meeting of the American Academy of Child and Adoles-cent Pychiatry in New York, NY, October 24–29. Scientific proceedings.

Finch, A.J., Lipovsky, J.A., and Casat, C.D. (1989) Anxiety and depression in children and adolescents: negative affectivity or separate constructs? In: Kendall, P.C. and Watson, D. eds. *Anxiety and Depression: Distinctive and Overlapping Features*. San Diego: Academic Press, pp. 171–196.

Findling, R.L., Preskorn, S.H., Marcus, R.N., Magnus, R.D., D'Amico, F., Marathe P. and Reed, M.D., (2000) Nefazodone pharmacokinetics in depressed children and adolescents. *J Am Acad Child Adolesc Psychiatry* 39:1008–1016.

Findling, R.L., Reed, M.D., Myers, C., O'Riordan, M.A. Fiala, S., Branicky L., Waldorf, B., and Blumer, J.L. (1999) Paroxetine pharmacokinetics in depressed children and adolescents. *J Am Acad Child Adolesc Psychiatry* 38:952–959.

Flament, M., Rapoport, J.L., Berg, C., Sceery W., Kilts, C., Mellstrom, B. and Lawolka, M. (1985). Clomipramine treatment of childhood obsessive-compulsive disorder. *Arch Gen Psychiatry* 42:977–988.

Flannery-Schroeder, and Kendall, P.C. (2000) Group and Individual Cognitive Behavioral Treatment for Youth with Anxiety Disorders: A Randomized Trial. *Cognitive Ther Research* 24:251–278.

Francis, G. and Beidel, D. (1995) Cognitive Behavioral Psychotherapy in: March, J.S. *Anxiety Disorders in Children and Adolescents* New York: Guilford Press, pp. 321–340.

Franklin, M.E., Kozak, M.J., Cashman, L.A., Coles, M.E., Rheingold, A.A., and Foa, E.B. (1998) Cognitive-behavioral treatment of pediatric obsessive-compulsive disorder: an open clinical trial. *J Am Acad Child Adolesc Psychiatry* 37:412–419.

Frommer & A (1967) Treatment of Childhood Depression with Antidepressant Drugs and *Br M & D J* 1:729–732.

Geller, D.A., Hoog, S.L., Heiligenstein, J.H. (2001) Fluoxetine treatment for obsessive-compulsive disorder in children and adolescents: a placebo-controlled clinical trial. *J Am Acad Child Adolesc Psychiatry* 40:773–779.

Ginsburg, G.S., Silverman, W.K., and Kurtines, W.M. (1995) Family involvement in treating children with phobic and anxiety disorders: a look ahead. *Clin Psychol Rev* 15:457–473.

Gittleman-Klein, R. and Klein, D. (1971) Controlled imipramine treatment of school phobia. *Arch Gen Psychiatry* 25:204–207.

Gittleman-Klein, R. and Klein, D. (1973) School phobia: diagnostic considerations in light of imipramine effects. *J Nerv Ment Dis* 156:199–215.

Glennon, B., and Weisz, J.R. (1978) An observational approach to the assessment of anxiety in young children. *J Consult Clin Psychol* 46:1246–1257.

Graae, F., Milner, J., Rizzotto, L., and Klein, R.G. (1994) Clonazepam in childhood anxiety disorders. *J Am Acad Child Adolesc Psychiatry* 33:372–376.

Hayward, C., Varady, S., Albano, A.M., et al. (2000) Cognitive-behavioral group therapy for social phobia in female adolescents: results of a pilot study. *J Am Acad Child Adolesc Psychiatry* 39: 721–726.

Hodges, K., McKnew, D., Cytryn, L. Stern, L., and Kline, J. (1982) The Child Assessment Schedule (CAS) diagnostic interview: a report on reliability and validity. *J Am Acad Child Psychiatry*. 21: 468–473.

Kaufman, J., Birmaher, B., Brent, D., et al. (1996) Schedule for Affective Disorders and Schizophrenia for School-aged Children—Present and Lifetime Version (K-SADS-PL): initial reliability and validity data. *J Am Acad Child Adolesc Psychiatry* 36: 980–988.

Keller, M.B., Ryan, N.D., Strober, M., Klein, R.G., Kutcher, S.P.,

Birmaher, B., Hagino, O.R., Koplewicz, H., Carlson, G.A., Clarke, G.N., Emslie, G.J., Feinberg, D., Geller, B., Kusumakar, V., Papatheodorou, G., Sack, W.H., Sweeney, M., Wagner, K.D., Weller, E.B., Winters, N.C., Oakes, R., and McCafferty, J.P. (2001) Efficacy of paroxetine in the treatment of adolescent major depression: a randomized, controlled trial. *J Am Acad Child Adolesc Psychiatry* 40:762–772.

Kendall, P.C. (1994) Treating anxiety disorders in children: Results of a randomized clinical trial. *J Consult Clin Psychol* 62:200–210.

Kendall, P.C., Flannery-Schroeder, E., Panichelli-Mindel, S.M., Southam-Gerow, M., Henin, A., and Warman, A. (1997) Therapy for youths with anxiety disorders: a second randomized clinical trial. *J Consult Clin Psychol* 65:366–380.

Kendall, P.C. and Southam-Gerow, M.A. (1996) Long-term follow-up of a cognitive-behavioral therapy for anxiety-disordered youths. *J Consult Clin Psychol* 64:724–730.

King, N.J. (1994) Physiological Assessment. In: Ollendick, T.H., King, N.J., and Yule, W. (eds.) International Handbook of Phobic and Anxiety Disorder in Children and Adolescents. Plenum.

King, N.J., Ollendick, T.H., and Gullone, E. (1991) Negative affectivity in children and adolescents: relations between anxiety and depression. *Clin Psychol Rev* 11:441–459.

Klein, R.G., Kopelwicz, H.S., and Kanner, A. (1992) Imipramine treatment in children with separation anxiety disorder. *J Am Acad Child Adolesc Psychiatry* 31:21–28.

Korein, J., Fish, B., Shapiro, T., Gerner E.W., and Levidow, T. (1971) WWG and behavioral affects of drug therapy in children. Chlorpromazine and diphenhydramine. *Arch Gen Psychiatry* 24:552–563.

Labellarte, M.J., Ginsburg, G.S., and Riddle, M.A. (1999) The treatment of anxiety disorders in children and adolescents. *Biol Psychiatry* 46:1567–1578.

Labellarte, M., Zumbrunnen, T., Brennan, J., Biederman, J., Connor, J., Emslie, J., Ferguson, J., Khan, A., Ruckle, J., Sallee, R., and Riddle, M. (in press) Multiple-dose pharmacokinetics of fluvoxamine in children and adolescents. *J Am Acad Child Adolesc Psychiatry*.

Lang, N.J. and Lazovik, A. (1963) Experimental Desensitization of Phobia. *J Abnormal Soc Psychology* 66:519–525.

Last, C.G., Hansen, C., and Franco, N. (1998). Cognitive-Behavioral Treatment of School Phobia; *J Am Acad Child Adolesc Psychiatry* 37:404–411.

Leckman, J.F., Riddle, M.A., Hardin, M.T., Ort, S.I., Swartz, K.L., Stevenson, J., and Cohen, D.J. (1989) The Yale Global Tic Severity Scale (YGTSS): initial testing of a clinical-rated scale of tic severity. *J Am Acad Child Adolesc Psychiatry* 28:566–573.

Leonard, H.L., March, J., and Rickler, K.C. (1997) Pharmacology of selective serotonin reuptake inhibitors in children and adoescents. *J Am Acad Child Adolesc Psychiatry* 36:725–736.

Leonard, H.L., Swedo, S.E., Rapaport, J.L., et al. (1989) Treatment of obsessive-compulsive disorder with clomipramine and desipramine in children and adolescents: a double-blind crossover comparison. *Arch Gen Psychiatry* 46:1088–1092.

March, J.S., Biederman, J., Wolkow, R., Safferman, A., Mardekian, J., Cook, E.H., et al. (1998) Sertraline in children and adolescents with obsessive-compulsive disorder: a multicenter randomized controlled trial. *JAMA* 280:1752–1756.

March, J.S., Mulle, K., and Herbel, B. (1994) Behavioral therapy for children and adolescents with obsessive-compulsive disorder: an open trial with a protocol driven package. *J Am Acad Child Adolesc Psychiatry* 33:333–341.

March, J. and Mulle, K. (1998). **OCD** in children and adolescents: a cognitive-behavioral treatment manual. Guilford Press.

March, J.S., Parker, J., Sullivan, K., Stallings, P., and Conners, C.K. (1997) The Multidimensional Anxiety Scale for Children (MASC): factor structure, reliability, and validity. *J Am Acad Child Adolesc Psychiatry* 36:554–565.

Melamud, B.G. and Seigel, L.J. (1975) Reductions of anxiety in children facing hospitalization and surgery by use of filmed modeling. *J Consult Clin Psychol* 43:511–521.

Mendlowitz, S.L., Manassis, K., Bradley, S., Scapillato, D., Miezitis, S., and Shaw, B. (1999) Cognitive-behavioral group treatments in childhood anxiety disorders: the role of parental involvement. *J Am Acad Child Adolesc Psychiatry* 38:1223–1229.

Perrin, S. and Last, C.G. (1992) Do childhood anxiety measures measure anxiety? *J Abnorm Child Psychol* 20:567–578.

Pine, D., Klein, R.G., Coplan, J.D., et al. Pappla, Hoven, C.W., Martinez, J., Kovalenko, P., Mandell, D.J., Moreau, D., Klein, D.F., and Gorman, J.M. et al. (2001) Differential carbon-dioxide sensitivity in childhood anxiety disorders and normal comparison group. *Arch Gen Psychiatry* 57:960–967

Popper, C.W. (2000). Pharmacologic alternatives to psychostimulants for the treatment of attention-deficit/hyperactivity disorder. *Child Adolesc Psychaiatr Clin N Amer* 9:605–646.

Poznanski, E.O. and Mokros, H.B. (1995) Children's Depression Rating Scale, Revised (CDRS-R). Los Angeles: Western Psychological Services.

Rapee, R.M., Barret, P.M., Dadds, M.R., and Evans, L. (1994) Reliability of the DSM-III-R childhood anxiety disorders using structured interview: interrater and parent–child agreement. *J Am Acad Child Adolesc Psychiatry* 33:984–992.

Rapoport, J., Conners, C.K., and Reatig, N. eds. (1985) Clinical Global Impression (CGI) Scale. *Psychopharmacol Bull* 21:839–843.

Research Units for Pediatric Psychopharmacology (RUPP) Anxiety Study Group (2001) Fluvoxamine for the treatment of anxiety disorders in children and adolescents. *N Engl J Med* 344:1279–1285.

Riddle, M.R., Reeve, E.A., Yaryura-Tobias, J.A., et al. (2001) Fluvoxamine for children and adolescents with obsessive-compulsive disorder: a randomized, controlled, multicenter trial. *J Am Acad Child Adolesc Psychiatry* 40:222–229.

Riddle, M.R., Subramanium, G., and Walkup, J.T. (1998) Efficacy of psychiatric medications in children and adolescents: a review of controlled studies. *Psychiatr Clin North Am* 5:269–285.

Ronan, K. (1996) Building a reasonable bridge in childhood anxiety assessment: a practitioners resource guide. *Cognit Behav Pract* 3:63–90.

Rynn, M.A., Siqueland, L., and Rickels, K. (2001) Placebo-controlled trial of sertraline in the treatment of children with generalized anxiety disorder. *Am J Psychiatry* 158:2008–2014.

Scahill, L., Riddle, M.A., King, R.A., Hardin, M.T., Rasmusson, A., Makuch R.W., and Leckman, J.F. (1997b) Fluoxetine has no marked effect on tic symptoms in patients with Tourette's syndrome: a double-blind placebo controlled study. *J Child Adolesc Psychopharmacol* 7:75–85.

Scahill, L., Riddle, M.A., McSwiggin-Hardin, M., ORT, S.T. King, R.A., Goodman, W.K., Cicahet D., and Leckman, J.F. Children's Yale-Brown Obsessive Compulsive Scale: reliability and validity. J Am Acad Child Adolesc Psychiatry 36:844–852.

Silverman, W.K., Albano, A., & Barlow, D. (1999). The anxiety disorder interview schedule for children for DSM-IV (ADIS-C/P-IV). New York: Psychological Corporation.

Silverman, W.K. and Eisen, A.R. (1992) Age differences in the reliability of parent and child reports of child anxious symptomatology using a structured interview. *J Am Acad Child Adolesc Psychiatry* 31:117–124.

Silverman, W.K. and Kurtines, W.K. (1996) *Childhood Anxiety and Phobic Disorders: a Pragmatic Perspective.* New York: Plenum Press.

Silverman, W.K., Kurtines, W.M., Ginsburg, G.S., Weems, C.F., Lumpkin, P.W., and Carmichael, D.H. (1999b) Treating anxiety disorders in children with group cognitive behavior therapy: a randomized clinical trial. *J Consult Clin Psychol* 67:995–1003.

Silverman, W.K., Kurtines, W.M., Ginsburg, G.S., Weems, C.F., Rabian, B. and Serafini, L.T. (1999c) Contingency management, self-control, and education support in the treatment of childhood phobic disorders: a randomized clinical trial. *J Consult Clin Psychol* 67:675–687.

Silverman, W.K., and Nelles, W.B. (1988) The Anxiety Disorders Interview Schedule for Children. *J Am Acad Child Adolesc Psychiatry* 27:772–778.

Silverman, W.K., and Rabian, B. (1995) Test–retest reliability of the DSM-III-R anxiety childhood disorders symptoms using the Anxiety Disorders Interview Schedule for Children. *J Anxiety Dis* 9: 1–12.

Simeon, J.G., Ferguson, H.B., Knott, V., Roberts, N., Gauthier, B., Dubois, C., and Wiggins, D. (1992) Clinical, cognitive, and neurophysiological effects of alprazolam in children andadolescents with overanxious and avoidant disorders. *J Am Acad Child Adolesc Psychiatry* 31:29–33.

Simeon, J.G., Knott, V.J., Dubois, C., Wiggins, D., Geraets, I., Thatte, S., and Miller, W. (1994) Buspirone therapy of mixed anxiety disorders in childhood and adolescence: a pilot study. *J Child Adolesc Psychopharmacol* 4:159–170.

Spence, S.H., Donovan, C., and Brechman-Toussaint, M. (2000) The treatment of childhood social phobia: the effectiveness of a social skills training-based, cognitive-behavioral intervention, with and without parental involvement. *J Child Psychol Psychiatry* 41: 713–726.

Spencer, T., Biederman, J., and Wilens, T. (2000) Pharmacotherapy of attention deficit hyperactivity disorder. *Child Adolesc Psychiatr Clin North Am* 9:77–97.

Uhde, T.W., Stein, M.B., Vittone, B.J., Siever, L.J., Boulenger, J.P., Klein, E., and Mellman, T.A. Behavioral and physiological effects of short-term and long-term administration of clonidine in panic disorder. *Arch Gen Psychiatry* 46:353.

Van Amerigen, M.V., Mancini, C., and Oakman, J.M. (1999) Nefazodone in social phobia. *J Clin Psychiatry* 60:96–100.

Walkup, J. (1999) The Pediatric Anxiety Rating Scale (PARS): a reliability study. Poster presented at the 46th Annual Meeting of the American Academy of Child and Adolescent Psychiatry, New York, NY, October 19–24. 1999. Scientific proceedings.

Wilens T, Cohen LG, Beiderman J, Abrams A, neft D, Melnick K, Kurtz D, and Sinha V (2000, poster). Pharmacokinetics of fluoxetine in pediatric patients. Scientific Proceedings of the 47th Annual Meeting of The American Academy of Child And Adolescent Psychiatry. October 24–29, 2000). New York, NY.

39 | Obsessive-compulsive disorder

DANIEL A. GELLER AND THOMAS SPENCER

Once thought rare, obsessive-compulsive disorder (OCD) is now recognized as a relatively common disorder affecting children and adolescents, and mental health professionals are almost certain to encounter such affected youth. Epidemiological studies in the United States and elsewhere report prevalence rates of around 2% in the adolescent population. In one epidemiological study (Flament et al., 1988), several adolescents identified with clinical OCD had been neither diagnosed nor treated, suggesting that, at that time, the disorder was underrecognized. While the secretive nature of obsessional symptoms might delay diagnosis, extensive research over the last decade into the clinical phenomenology, etiology, pathogenesis, and treatment of pediatric OCD has greatly increased awareness of this disorder.

Early intramural research from the National Institute of Mental Health (NIMH) regarding the efficacy of clomipramine for pediatric OCD was followed by a number of industry-sponsored multisite trials of antiobsessional drugs. There is now a body of data that, while more meager than in adult OCD, provides a rational basis for pediatric psychopharmacologists to treat the child or adolescent with OCD. Indeed, because the phenotype of OCD is relatively unambiguous and since the introduction of the serotonin reuptake inhibitor antidepressants (starting with fluoxetine in 1987), more empirical data regarding the pharmacotherapy of juvenile OCD have been obtained in the last 10 years than for almost any other psychiatric disorder of youth.

DEFINITION AND NOSOLOGY

Obsessions are defined as intrusive, repetitive thoughts, ideas, images, or impulses that are anxiety provoking and unwanted ("worries"). They are typically recognized as being unwanted and excessive (ego dystonic), even in very young children, and the anxiety they cause leads to the performance of compulsive behaviors that serve to reduce anxiety ("rituals"), thus setting up a reinforced cycle of obsessions and compulsions. To meet criteria for the full *Diagnostic and Statistical Manual of Mental Disorders, 4th ed.* (DSM IV) clinical syndrome, obsessions and compulsions must be time consuming (usually taken as at least 1 hour per day), cause subjective distress (suffering), and cause functional impairment in one or more domains of life. That the phenotype of OCD is remarkably similar at all ages is reflected in the DSM IV nosology, which makes no specific allowances for age at onset or variable developmental expression of the disorder. The only exception is the specifier "with poor insight" that might be said to apply particularly to younger subjects. Although DSM IV uses a categorical approach to diagnosis (a reasonable one, since a decision to use medication often follows), obsessions are extremely common if not ubiquitous in the population—up to 20% in one report (Apter et al., 1996).

CLINICAL FEATURES

Phenotypic Presentation

Despite overall similarities (Table 39.1), there may be some differences in the phenotypic expression of OCD across the life cycle. In a recent examination of this subject (Geller et al., 2001a), several differences between children, adolescents, and adults were noted in the frequency of particular obsessions and compulsions. Children and adolescents had much higher rates of aggressive obsessions (including fears of catastrophic events, such as death or illness in self or loved ones) than adults (63% vs. 69% vs. 31%, $p < 0.001$). These were the most common obsessions in the pediatric age group and may be understood in the context of expected developmental stages of attachment and independence that could affect the clinical picture of OCD in younger children.

Religious obsessions, by contrast, were overrepresented in adolescents (36%), compared with children (15%) and adults (10%) ($p < 0.001$), and sexual obsessions were underrepresented in children (11%),

511

TABLE 39.1 *Symptoms of Obsessions and Compulsions in Children, Adolescents, and Adults with Obsessive-Compulsive Disorder*

	Children (n=46)		Adolescents (n=55)		Adults (n=560)		
	n	(%)	n	(%)	n	(%)	p-*value*
Obsessions							
Aggressive/ catastrophic	29	(63)	38	(69)	174	(31)	<0.001[b,c]
Religious	7	(15)	20	(36)	56	(10)	<0.001[a,c]
Sexual	5	(11)	20	(36)	134	(24)	0.011[a,b,c]
Contamination	24	(52)	35	(64)	280	(50)	0.15
Somatic	15	(33)	20	(36)	185	(33)	0.88
Compulsions							
Hoarding	14	(30)	20	(36)	101	(18)	0.001[b,c]
Counting	20	(44)	23	(42)	202	(36)	0.40
Confessing/asking	15	(33)	11	(20)	190	(34)	0.11
Checking	29	(63)	36	(65)	342	(61)	0.80
Ordering/arranging	17	(37)	18	(33)	157	(28)	0.36
Washing	22	(48)	31	(56)	280	(50)	0.63

[a]Significance between children and adolescents, $p < 0.05$.
[b]Significance between children and adults, $p < 0.05$.
[c]Significance between adolescents and adults, $p < 0.05$.

compared with adolescents (36%) and adults (24%) ($p = 0.011$). Since adolescents had selectively higher rates of sexual and religious obsessions and preoccupation with these subjects are prominent in adolescents, these findings also suggest that OCD symptoms follow themes and conflicts appropriate to developmental stages. For compulsions, only hoarding was seen more often in children and adolescents than in adults (30% and 36% vs. 18%, respectively, $p = 0.001$). The great majority of subjects in all groups had both multiple obsessions and compulsions. Poor insight was noted more often in child OCD cases (18%) than in adolescent (6%) and adult (6%) OCD subjects($p = 0.01$). Insight is developmentally sensitive; children may have a limited ability to cognitively process their obsessional ideation, self-evaluate their compulsive behavior, or adequately articulate their OCD symptoms.

Clear environmental precipitating factors were identified in some children, ranging from 15% to 54%, compared with 29% of adult subjects in one report (Rasmussen and Eisen, 1998). Examples include maternal hemorrhage and sudden hospitalization, death of a grandparent, reading the book *Outbreak* (about a lethal virus), and watching a TV program about AIDS. Although symptoms tend to wax and wane over time, they are usually persistent to some degree and may vary over time so that the presenting constellation may

change (Rettew et al., 1992). In a number of studies, parents were noted to be intimately involved in their children's rituals, especially in reassurance seeking, a form of verbal checking.

Age at Onset and Gender

Onset is usually insidious or subacute in most pediatric OCD subjects, with the notable exception of *p*ediatric *a*utoimmune *n*europsychiatric *d*isorders *a*ssociated with *s*treptococcal infections (PANDAS)–related OCD, which, by definition, has a dramatic or acute onset (see Chapter 14 in this volume). In a recent review of 11 reported clinical series comprising 419 juvenile OCD patients, age at onset ranged from 7.5 to 12.5 years (mean 10.3 years) while mean age at assessment was 13 years, indicating a long lag between onset and referral. By contrast, the mean age at OCD onset in adult studies was 21 years, suggesting a bimodal distribution of incidence for this disorder. This review also found male predominance in most pediatric studies, with an average 3:2 male:female ratio. In contrast, both the Epidemiologic Catchment Area study (Karno et al., 1988) and Black's (1974) review of 11 adult studies of both OCD inpatient and outpatients encompassing 1336 subjects found a female preponderance (51.4%) in adult OCD subjects.

Comorbidity

One of the most relevant issues in the treatment of OCD in children and adolescents is that it only infrequently occurs as a single disorder (Fig. 39.1). All clinical reports and even epidemiological (non-referred) samples report lifetime comorbidity rates of well over 50% (Geller et al., 2000). Although tic disorders are the only ones shown to be consistently part of the phenotype (and perhaps genotype) of childhood-onset OCD, they are not the most commonly observed comorbid disorders. Mood disorders, including major depression and bipolar disorder, disruptive behavior disorders, and other, frequently multiple, anxiety disorders, are even more common and influence the pharmacological and behavioral management of the child with OCD.

Both comorbid tic disorders and disruptive behavior disorders aggregate predominantly in preadolescent males, while comorbid mood disorders increase significantly after puberty (Geller et al., 2001a). Other anxiety disorders are prevalent at all ages, although developmentally sensitive diagnoses, such as separation anxiety disorders, are seen more frequently in children than adolescents. Subjects referred to both specialized and nonspecialized clinical settings have a similar spectrum and frequency of comorbid psychopathology and the evaluation of such children is not complete without adequately delineating the full spectrum of psychiatric comorbidity.

In summary, OCD occurring in children and adolescents is a highly prevalent disorder with some no-table developmental differences from OCD in adults. They include a preadolescent peak of onset, male predominance, and a developmentally sensitive phenotype. It is highly comorbid with mood and anxiety disorders as well as tic and disruptive behavior disorders. While a discussion of the neurobiology and pathophysiology of pediatric OCD is beyond the scope of this chapter, it seems likely that OCD is a heterogeneous disorder with multiple etiologies and a final common phenotypic pathway (for more discussion see Chapters 12 and 14).

ASSESSMENT AND EVALUATION

Although the DSM-IV criteria for OCD are straightforward, clinicians may be frustrated in their attempt to accurately diagnose OCD in some cases. Reasons for this include an insidious or subclinical onset, waxing and waning course, varying symptom constellation, sometimes secretive obsessional ideation (which is experienced as embarrassing), and poor insight in some subjects. Tell-tale clinical signs may include red, chapped, or bleeding hands, blocked toilets, lengthy showers, or other bathroom rituals, and avoidance behaviors.

The children's version of the Yale-Brown Obsessive Compulsive Scale (CY-BOCS) is a 10-item anchored ordinal scale (0–4) that rates the clinical severity of the disorder by scoring the time occupied, degree of life interference, subjective distress, internal resistance, and

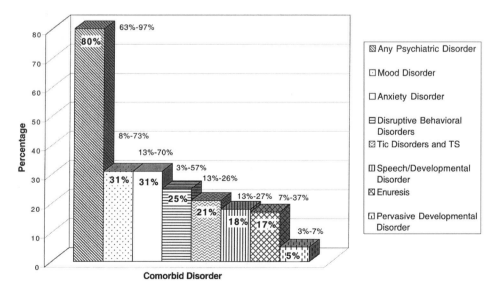

FIGURE 39.1 Comorbidity: mean range. TS, Tourette's Syndrome.

degree of control for both obsessions and compulsions. It has been validated for use with pediatric subjects (Scahill et al., 1997a) and has been shown to be sensitive to change with treatment. It also includes a symptom checklist of over 60 symptoms of obsessions and compulsions categorized by the predominant theme involved such as contamination, hoarding, washing, checking, etc.

In a recent report, the mean CY-BOCS score at initial assessment (23 ± 6.5) did not differ between child and adolescent OCD subjects. It should be noted that although the CY-BOCS is an anchored ordinal scale, it is not linear and lacks sensitivity to change when symptoms are severely impairing. For example, "time occupied" is scored as 4 when more than 8 hours/day are spent in either obsessions or compulsions, while 4 hours/day would rate a score of 3—i.e., a 50% decrease in time lowers this item score by one point (out of 5 ordinal scores). It is for this reason that a decrease in CY-BOCS score of more than 25% is considered clinically significant improvement and a number of controlled studies have used a 25% reduction to define a positive response. The CY-BOCS remains the gold standard for both baseline evaluation as well as for monitoring effects of treatment.

It should be apparent from the above discussion that careful attention to the presence of comorbid disorders is mandatory at baseline and over the course of treatment, since new disorders such as major depressive disorder may emerge after some years. Interviews of the child or adolescent as well as the parents are essential if the full spectrum of obsessional, compulsive, and other symptoms is to be elucidated. Using a best-estimate method to synthesize information from all sources will result in the most comprehensive assessment of the pediatric subject. Structured diagnostic assessments that provide lifetime anamnesis of psychopathology will avoid the common errors of omission of comorbidity but such assessments are not always possible. Functional assessment using global measures such as Global Assessment of Function (GAF) scores or Clinical Global Impression (CGI) scales as well as educational indices are easier and provide useful information. While teacher and school information is desirable, it is a notable fact that some youth can have clinically impairing OCD that is not apparent to school personnel. However, our data show that there is a considerable educational and psychosocial burden from OCD and its associated comorbid psychopathology in children.

The differential diagnoses include several disorders with overlapping behaviors that have either a compulsive quality or impulse control deficits. The stereotypies and perseverative behavior of the pervasive develop-

mental disorders are undertaken as preferred activities, and not in response to anxiety or ego dystonic ideation. Habit or impulse control disorders such as trichotillomania, compulsive nail biting, or skin picking also lack specific cognitions that precede the behavior, though sensory premonitions or a sense of tension may occur prior to them.

In adults with OCD there appears to be an overlap with eating disorders (Pigott et al., 1994), but this is much less common in pediatric samples. On occasion, youth may meet criteria for both OCD and another OCD-related diagnosis.

TREATMENT—GENERAL PRINCIPALS

Behavioral Therapy

While this chapter focuses on pharmacological therapies, the reader should be aware of the important role of cognitive behavior therapy (CBT) and family involvement in the management of the child and adolescent patient with OCD. Therapist-assisted, hierarchy-based exposure and response prevention (E/RP) has been shown to be a durable treatment for OCD and a well-constructed technical manual is available (March and Mulle, 1998). While the extant literature regarding CBT in young OCD patients does not achieve the scientific rigor of drug trials because of methodological difficulties and small numbers, there is little doubt that CBT is an effective treatment for some children. This is reflected in the Expert Consensus Guidelines for treatment of OCD (March et al., 1997) and the American Academy of Child and Adolescent Psychiatry Practice Parameters for OCD (King et al., 1998) that recommend CBT, with or without medication, as a first-line intervention in youth.

Unfortunately, research is lacking as to how to predict which subjects will benefit most from CBT. Experience indicates that absence of comorbid disorders and good insight will increase the chances for successful CBT, the latter permitting a subject to tolerate anxiety-provoking stimuli without ritualizing based on intact reality testing. However, in very young children, insight may not be necessary for a good outcome since parents control so many of the contingencies of the CBT. In contrast, the presence of a concurrent major depressive disorder, other (multiple) anxiety disorders, or disruptive behavior disorders could severely limit the response to CBT in some children.

Severe functional impairment, CY-BOCS scores in the severe range (26), poor insight, and lack of family resources or skilled therapists for adequate CBT should influence a clinician toward earlier introduction of medication. If CBT alone is used first, then 13 to 20 outpatient sessions are usually adequate, with refresher sessions as needed. Failure to respond to a well-delivered trial of CBT in a compliant patient after about 4 weeks is an indication for SSRI medication. For an excellent discussion of this decision-making process, the reader is referred to Chapter 34 in this volume. The combination of CBT and medication might be more effective than either one alone. CBT may reduce relapse rates in those withdrawn from medication.

The take-home message for clinicians is that a decision to treat with medication without prior discussion of CBT with parent or guardian is probably not true "informed consent."

TREATMENT—REVIEW OF PUBLISHED STUDIES

At this time at least 19 studies, including over 1100 pediatric subjects, reporting on medication experience in OCD have been published (Table 39.2). All showed that serotonergic medications are effective in the short- and medium-term treatment of OCD. Most studies were acute trials lasting 10 to 13 weeks but five reported that efficacy could be maintained over at least 1 year of treatment (Leonard et al., 1991; DeVeaugh-Geiss et al., 1992; Geller et al., 1995; Cook et al., 2001). Eleven studies ($n = 913$) used prospectively designed controlled trials with either placebo (Flament et al., 1985; DeVeaugh-Geiss et al., 1992; Riddle et al., 1992, 2001; Scahill et al., 1997b; March et al., 1998; Geller et al., 2001b; 2001c; Geller et al., 2002) or desipramine (Leonard et al., 1989; 1991). The latter studies indicated that antiobsessional specificity of the serotonergic agents was distinct from antidepressant activity.

Some authors (Flament et al., 1987) found that response to treatment with clomipramine was correlated with a marked decrease in platelet serotonin concentration and monoamine oxidase (MAO) activity. Changes in cerebrospinal fluid (CSF) neuropeptides and monoamine metabolites have also been described with chronic clomipramine administration (Swedo et al., 1992; Altemus et al., 1994). Despite these observations, the exact mechanism of action of serotonergic drugs (and the "serotonin hypothesis") remains unproven, although it is thought they mediate their effects via down-regulation of the presynaptic 5-HT1D autoreceptor (Rauch et al., 1994).

Assessing Response

In most double-blind, placebo-controlled studies, responder analysis rates, defined as at least a 25% re-duction in CY-BOCS scores at end point, were quite modest, ranging from 42% for fluvoxamine to 49% for fluoxetine and 53% for sertraline. Clinician- and subject-rated global improvement ratings indicated a somewhat higher proportion of those deemed much or very much improved (e.g., 60% for clomipramine). Although an initial double-blind study using clomipramine suggested a low placebo response rate in children with OCD (8%), subsequent studies have found substantial placebo responder rates (defined as above), ranging from 37% for sertraline, 26% for fluvoxamine, to 25% for fluoxetine. Translated into quantitative measures, analyses of the above double-blind, placebo-controlled studies using an intent-to-treat model typically showed an absolute decrease in CY-BOCS scores, ranging from 6 to 9.5, a 30%–38% decrement from baseline CY-BOCS scores. This apparently limited effect size may actually reflect a dramatic clinical response due to the nonlinear properties of the CY-BOCS scale, and is similar to that observed in treatment studies of adults with OCD. Though incomplete, the significant response to the SRI's over placebo in children with OCD provides a clear indication for their use. However, as measured by the CY-BOCS, studies indicate that, even in the presence of a positive response, residual OCD symptoms frequently remain, since post-treatment scores of 15 to 20 indicate mild to moderate OCD. Thus, for many children and adolescents with OCD, even when treated, persistent low-grade symptoms and impairment are the norm.

Although systematic dose–response data are not available for pediatric subjects, robust doses have been used in published studies. For example, clomipramine doses were up to 3 mg/kg or 200 mg/day, while the doses for sertraline (mean = 178 mg/day), fluvoxamine (mean = 165 mg/day), paroxetine (mean = 32 mg/day), and fluoxetine (up to 60 mg/day) all indicate the need for relatively high dosing in this condition. Low initial doses and slow titration schedules are recommended, however, to avoid adverse events and age and weight should be taken into consideration (Table 39.3). Molecular and secondary synaptic changes are rate-limited biological processes that cannot be altered by administrative dictates, and patience is often required in titration of the SRIs, especially clomipramine. Most experts agree that an adequate trial of a SRI consists of at least 10–12 weeks of treatment at maximal tolerated dose, despite the observation that mosts SRIs show statistically significant improvement over placebo after just 3 weeks of treatment (5 weeks in the placebo-controlled fluoxetine trial, where the titration schedule was more gradual). In addition, further gradual symptomatic improvement may accrue beyond the first 12 weeks of treatment.

TABLE 39.2 *Pharmacological Treatment Studies in Pediatric Obsessive-Compulsive Disorder*

Reference	Medication and Dose	Design of Study (n), Age	Results	Adverse Events	Comments
Flament et al., 1985	Clomipramine Mean dose 141 (±30) mg/day	10-week randomized, double-blind, placebo-controlled cross-over (19) Mean age 14.5 (±2.3) years (range 10–18)	75% showed marked to moderate improvement Response independent of depressive symptoms	Tremor, dry mouth, dizziness, constipation, sweating One subject had grand mal seizure One subject developed psychotic symptoms	Response not predicted by baseline measures Outcome not correlated with age, mode or age at onset, severity or duration
Leonard et al., 1989	Clomipramine Mean dose 150 (±53) mg/day or 3 (±0.7) mg/k/day	10-week randomized, double-blind, controlled, cross-over with desipramine (48) Mean age 13.9 (±2.9) years (range 6–18)	Clomipramine significantly superior to desipramine 64% relapsed when switched from clomipramine to desipramine Little placebo response	Dry mouth, tremor, tiredness, constipation, dizziness, sweating	Depressive symptoms were higher in the desipramine group
Liebowitz et al., 1990	Fluoxetine Dose 60–80 mg/day	8-week open label (8) Adolescent (range 12–17 years)	≥ 50% improved clinically	Nausea, jitteriness, headache, agitation	—
Riddle et al., 1990	Fluoxetine Modal dose 20 mg/day (10–40/day)	20-week open label (10) Age range 8–15 years	50% response rate using clinician rating scale	Behavioral agitation, nausea	—
Como and Kurlan, 1991	Fluoxetine Dose 20–40mg/day	Open label in subjects with Tourette's disorder over 3–8 months (13) Mean age 12 (±3.2) years	54% response rate 35% mean reduction in Leyton Obsessional Inventory-Child Version scores	Dyspepsia, nausea	—
Leonard et al., 1991	Clomipramine Mean dose 135 (±58) mg/day	8-month double-blind desipramine substitution during clomipramine maintenance treatment over 17 (±8.3) months. (26) Mean age 14.7 (±3.3) years (range 8–19)	89% relapsed on desipramine, compared to 18% on clomipramine Younger age predicted increased risk for relapse	Dry mouth, tiredness, constipation, dizziness, sleep disturbance	OCD symptoms varied in severity over time Residual symptoms noted in maintenance clomipramine treatment Of subjects with relapse off clomipramine 38% in first month and 62% in second month
DeVeaugh-Geiss, 1992	Clomipramine Dose 3mg/k/day up to 200 mg/day	Multicenter 8-week randomized, double-blind, placebo-controlled trial, with 1-year open-label extension phase (60) Age range 10–17 years	CY-BOCS score decreased 37% in treated group, compared to 8% in placebo group 60% were rated very much improved Response was maintained over 1-year extension	Dry mouth, somnolence, dizziness, fatigue, tremor, constipation, decreased appetite	Low placebo response
Riddle et al., 1992	Fluoxetine Dose 20 mg/day	20-week randomized, double-blind, placebo-controlled, cross-over (14) Mean age 11.8 (±2.3) years (range 8–15)	CY-BOCS score decreased 44% in fluoxetine group vs. 27% in placebo (p = 0.17) CGI-improvement fluoxetine > placebo (p<.05). 3 of 6 subjects relapsed when switched from flx to placebo	Insomnia, fatigue, nausea, motor activation, increased tics, suicidal ideation	Plasma fluoxetine level correlated with change in OCD scores

Study	Medication/Dose	Study design	Outcome	Adverse effects	Comments
Kurlan et al 1993	Fluoxetine Dose 20–40 mg/day	4-month pilot double-blind, placebo-controlled, randomized trial in Tourette's syndrome and comorbid OCD (11) Mean age 13 (±2.6) years (range 10–18)	No significant change in measures of OCD symptoms Trend toward improvement in tic severity, attention and social functioning	Mild irritability, fatigue, agitation seen in both groups	All boys Haloperidol and clonidine allowed as concomitant treatment for tics
Apter et al., 1994	Fluvoxamine Dose 200 mg/day (range 100–300/day)	8-week open-label variable-dose (14) Age range 13–18 years	CY-BOCS score decreased 29% from baseline in Fluvoxamine group	Dermatitis, insomnia, hyperactivity, excitement, anxiety, tremor, nausea	Significant efficacy not noted until sixth week of treatment Inpatient group with severe comorbid disorders, including anorexia and schizophrenia
Geller et al., 1995	Fluoxetine Mean dose 50 mg/day or approx 1 mg/k/day	Retrospective clinical review of fluoxetine treatment in an outpatient clinic (38) Mean age 12.3 (±0.5) years	74% moderate/marked improvement using CGI-I scale 47% reduction in symptoms using GGI-S scale	Behavioral activation, insomnia, somnolence, weight and appetite change	Response equal in child & adolescent subjects Response maintained over average period of 19 months
Scahill et al 1997b	Fluoxetine Dose fixed at 20 mg/day	20-week fixed-dose double-blind placebo-controlled, crossover trial (14 with Tourette's including 5 with comorbid OCD) Age range 8–33 years	Y-BOCS decreased 37.5% (p=0.04) in flx subjects. OCD subjects withdrawn to placebo showed a 55% increase in OC symptoms. No effect on tics shown	Motor restlessness, insomnia, decreased appetite, fatigue, increased motor tics	Motor restlessness observed more often in younger subjects
Thompson, 1997	Citalopram Dose 40 mg/day in 21/23 subjects	10-week open label trial inpatient and outpatient (23) Mean age 13 (±2.5) years (range 9–18)	Significant 31% reduction in CY-BOCS score 18/23 subjects showed marked to moderate improvement	Sedation, tremor, dry mouth, insomnia, agitation, hyperactivity, erectile dysfunction AE's mostly transient	Inpatients and outpatients did equally well Concurrent behavioral therapy
March et al., 1998	Sertraline Mean dose 167 mg/day, 57% of children and 82% adolescents at 200 mg/day at endpoint	Multisite 12-week randomized, double blind placebo-controlled, flexible dose (187 [107 children and 80 adolescents]) Mean age 12.6 years (range 6–17)	Significant CY-BOCS decrease ≥ 25% in 53% of sertraline group vs. 37% of placebo (p = 0.03). 42% rated as much or very much improved vs. 26% in placebo group using NIMH CGI-I scale (p = 0.02)	Insomnia, nausea, agitation and tremor	No predictors of outcome found
Rosenberg et al., 1999	Paroxetine Mean dose 41 mg/day (10–60/day)	12-week open label trial (20) Age range 8–17 years	Significant 29% mean reduction in CY-BOCS score over baseline 55% subjects had ≥30% decrease CY-BOCS	Hyperactivity/behavioral activation, headache, insomnia, gastrointestinal distress, anxiety, drowsiness, dry mouth, increased tics	Significant improvement seen in 4th week Behavioral activation improved with dose reduction

(continued)

TABLE 39.2 *Pharmacological Treatment Studies in Pediatric Obsessive-Compulsive Disorder (continued)*

Reference	Medication and Dose	Design of Study (n), Age	Results	Adverse Events	Comments
Riddle et al., 2001	Fluvoxamine Mean dose 165 mg/day (50–200)	Multi-site, 10-week, randomized, double-blind, placebo-controlled trial, flexible dose with 1-year open-label extension phase (120) Mean age 13 years (range 8–17)	Significant 25% mean reduction of CY-BOCS cf. 14% in placebo at week 10 Significant improvement in CGI scores over placebo Significant improvement noted as early as week 1, maximum at week 3 Responder analysis ≥25% decrease on CY-BOCS 42% fluvoxamine vs. 26% placebo ($p = 0.07$)	Well tolerated overall. AEs were mostly transient Insomnia, asthenia (fatigue loss of energy, tiredness, weakness), agitation, hyperkinesias, somnolence	Children 8–12 years had higher proportion of responders
Geller et al., 2001c	Fluoxetine Mean dose 25 mg/day (20–60mg/day); well tolerated	Multisite 13-week, randomized double-blind, placebo-controlled study, flexible dose (103) Mean age 11.4 (± 3) years (range 7–17)	Responders (defined as ≥40% reduction on CY-BOCS): 49% fluoxetine vs. 25% placebo ($p = 0.03$). Mean decrease in CY-BOCS scores 9.5 fluoxetine vs. 5.2 placebo ($p = 0.03$) Significant difference between groups after week 5 All secondary outcome OCD measures significant improvement for fluoxetine 55% rated as much or very much improved	Well tolerated overall Diarrhea, hyperkinesia more common (NS) in fluoxetine group Slight weight loss (0.2 kg) in fluoxetine group ($p = 0.002$).	2:1 randomization to fluoxetine or placebo Slow titration schedule; max dosing at week 7
Geller et al, 2001b	Paroxetine Mean dose 33 mg/day (10–60 mg/day)	32-week, randomized, two phase, double-blind, placebo-controlled withdrawal from open label treatment (335 phase I, 193 phase II) Mean age 12 years (range 8–17)	Response rates in patients with comorbid ADHD, tic disorder, or oppositional defiant disorder (56%, 53%, and 39%, respectively) were significantly less than in patients with OCD only (75%, ITT LOCF; $p < 0.05$). Psychiatric comorbidity was associated with a greater overall relapse rate (56% for ≥2, 46% for 1 comorbid disorder vs. 32% for no comorbidity; $p = 0.04$).	Headache, asthenia, insomnia most commonly reported AEs. Impaired concentration. Behavioral AEs (agitation, hostility, hyperkinesia) more likely in younger subjects (< 12 years)	Comorbid disorders *not* excluded; the largest systematic controlled study of naturalistically ascertained pediatric OCD subjects
Geller et al., 2002	Paroxetine Mean dose 30mg/day(10–50 mg/day)	10-week, randomized, double-blind, placebo-controlled, flexible-dose study (203) Age range 7–17 years	Baseline CY-BOCS = 25 Mean decrease in CY-BOCS scores was 9 points for patients receiving paroxetine vs. 5 points for patients receiving placebo ($p = 0.03$) Significant difference in response rates (defined by >25% decrease in CY-BOCS scores) in favor of paroxetine	Hyperkinesia, agitation, decreased appetite, gastrointestinal upset, and fatigue	Efficacy demonstrated No unexpected safety or adverse event findings

AE, adverse effect; CGI-I, Clinical Global Impression—Improvement; CGI-S, Clinical Global Impression—Severity; CY-BOCS, Children's Yale-Brown Obsessive-Compulsive Scale; ITT LOCF, Intent-to-Treat, Last Observation Carried Forward; OCD, obsessive-compulsive disorder.

TABLE 39.3 *Dose Range for Serotonin Reuptake Inhibitors in Preadolescents and Adolescents with Obsessive-Compulsive Disorder*

| Drug | Starting Dose (mg) | | Typical Dose Range (mg) (Typical Mean Dose)[a] |
	Preadolescent	Adolescent	
Clomipramine[b]	12.5–25	25	50–200
Fluoxetine[c]	5–10	10–20	10–80 (25)
Sertraline[c]	12.5–25	25–50	50–200 (178)
Fluvoxamine[b]	12.5–25	25–50	50–300 (165)
Paroxetine[d]	5–10	10	10–60 (32)
Citalopram[c]	5–10	10–20	10–60

[a]Mean daily doses were used in controlled trials.

[b]Doses <25 mg/day may be administered by compounding 25 mg into 5 mL suspension.

[c]Oral concentrate is commercially available.

[d]Oral suspension is available.

Predictors of Response

Factors that predict a positive response to drug therapy have not been well established. Early studies suggested that age of onset, gender, severity, and duration of illness, or type of symptoms did not predict initial response (Leonard and Rapoport, 1989; DeVeaugh-Geiss et al., 1992).

A potential limitation of most of the controlled studies discussed above relates to the numerous exclusion criteria used for patient selection. For example, in order to find homogenous samples, major depression, bipolar disorder, Tourette's disorder, psychosis (clomipramine, fluvoxamine and fluoxetine trials), primary psychiatric disorder other than OCD (clomipramine and sertraline trials), and attention deficit/hyperactivity disorder (ADHD), autism, or other developmental disorders (clomipramine and fluoxetine trials) were excluded. Thus it remains unknown how well these controlled studies will generalize to more naturalistic clinical populations that are highly comorbid and where exclusion criteria are not applied.

Preliminary evidence that this issue is an important one for clinicians derives from post hoc analyses of the double-blind, placebo-controlled paroxetine withdrawal study (Geller et al., 2001b), in which no strict exclusionary criteria were applied. In that study, 193/335 (58%) patients had at least one psychiatric disorder in addition to OCD and 102/335 (30%) had multiple (≥2) other disorders. The response rates in patients with comorbid ADHD, tic disorder, or oppositional defiant disorder (56%, 53%, and 39%, respectively) were significantly less than in patients with OCD only (75%, [ITT LOCF]; $p < 0.05$). Psychiatric comorbidity was also associated with a greater overall relapse rate (32% for no comorbid disorder vs. 46% for ≥1 comorbid disorder, $p = 0.04$, and 56% for 2 comorbid disorders). However, a subsequent double-blind, placebo-controlled, randomized study where any predominant axis I disorder other than OCD was excluded, paroxetine showed significant superiority over placebo.

TREATMENT GUIDELINES AND OUTCOME

Selecting an Initial Agent

Although the SSRIs differ in potency and selectivity, it is not known which SSRI will be most effective for which type of patient. Furthermore, since no direct comparisons or meta-analyses are available in the pediatric literature, there is no evidence that one compound is superior to another. Thus the choice of an initial agent should take into account the pharmacokinetics, adverse event profiles, and potential for drug–drug interactions of the various SSRIs. Several important pharmacokinetic variables include the half-life of the compound, presence of active metabolites, the linear or nonlinear nature of its clearance, and its capacity to inhibit various cytochrome P450 (CYP) enzymatic pathways in the liver (for a complete discussion, see Chapter 22). Paroxetine and fluvoxamine have nonlinear kinetics and interfere with (autoinhibit) their own metabolism. Thus, the half-life of a single dose of paroxetine (10 hours) becomes twice as long with multiple dosing (Lane and Baldwin, 1997). This quality may be more important when decreasing rather than increasing medication, since rapidly falling levels are more common with nonlinear kinetics and may predispose to the SSRI discontinuation syndrome that is seen most commonly with clomipramine (31%), paroxetine (20%), and fluvoxamine (14%) (Coupland et al., 1996). Fluoxetine has an active metabolite, norfluoxetine, with a very long half-life (4–7 days), which delays the achievement of steady-state plasma levels.

Perhaps the most important characteristic of the antiobsessional medications is their degradation by and inhibition of the CYP subsystems. Clinically significant drug–drug interactions are possible in a number of common situations in which combined pharmacotherapy is employed. For example, the combination of a SSRI that potently inhibits CYP 2D6 (fluoxetine and paroxetine) system may cause markedly elevated, even dangerous, serum levels of clomipramine that utilizes this same metabolic pathway. Fluvoxamine as an inhibitor of CYP1A2 and CYP2C19 may also increase clomipramine levels. Many other medications are removed by the CYP2D6 (tricyclics, haloperidol, codeine, beta-blockers, risperidone, thioridazine, perphenazine, nefazodone), CYP1A2 (chlorpromazine, clozapine, tricyclics, cisapride, verapamil), and CYP3A4 (carbamazepine, alprazolam, steroids, nifedipine, erythromycin) enzymes, creating other potential interactions.

Because of the potential arrythmogenic properties of clomipramine, it is usually not employed as a first-line agent in uncomplicated OCD. Its use mandates an evaluation of the pediatric patient's medical condition and cardiac status in particular. Baseline evaluation should include a systems review and inquiry regarding a personal or family history of heart disease. A history of nonfebrile seizures should also be noted but is not an absolute contraindication to clomipramine. If in doubt, a general pediatric examination to include auscultation of the heart and measurement of pulse and blood pressure is indicated. A baseline (pretreatment) electrocardiogram (EKG) should be requested. While changes in conduction intervals and heart rate may occur, these are rarely of clinical significance. The prudent practitioner will evaluate and document EKG parameters.

Guidelines regarding *un*acceptable EKG indices for the use (or increase) of clomipramine have been recommended by the Federal Drug Administration (FDA) as follows: (*1*) PR interval > 200 ms; (*2*) QRS interval > 30% increased over baseline or > 120 msec; (*3*) blood pressure > 140 systolic or 90 diastolic; and (*4*) heart rate > 130 bpm at rest (Puig-Antich et al., 1979, 1987; Biederman, 1991). Finally, a prolonged QTc (corrected QT interval = 450 msec) is associated with an increased risk of ventricular tachyarrythmias and is a contraindication for clomipramine use (or further increase). Despite these concerns, clomipramine remains an important and perhaps unique drug in the armamentarium of antiobsessional medications.

Treating the Comorbid Patient

Treatment of the comorbid patient presents a number of challenges (Fig. 39.2). The phenotype of OCD and Tourette's disorder (TD) is encountered frequently as there is a bidirectional overlap between the two conditions. In a review of 11 clinical studies, TD was found in an average of 21% of juvenile OCD subjects (Geller et al., 1998). These subjects are more often male with an earlier age at onset and positive family history of OCD and tics. Kurlan et al. (1993) suggested that obsessional symptoms might respond less well to the SSRIs in these subjects.

There are anecdotal reports that the SSRIs, especially at higher doses, may exacerbate or even induce tics in some OCD patients (Riddle et al., 1992; Fennig et al., 1994). However, because tics often diminish when anxiety is reduced, SSRIs alone may be sufficient for both disorders. Several SSRIs have dopaminergic (sertraline) or noradrenergic (fluoxetine) activity that could theoretically affect the expression of tics in a patient with comorbid OCD and TD. Furthermore, since tics themselves are usually not clinically impairing (Spencer et al., 1999), they often do not require specific pharmacotherapy even when present. If tics are severe, then traditional treatments, including the neuroleptics and the α agonist agents clonidine or guanfacine, may be indicated in addition to SSRIs, with attention to potential cardiovascular and other drug–drug interactions. Although not typically a first-line drug for the young OCD patient, clomipramine may have a unique role in those subjects with both tic and disruptive behavior disorders, since it is metabolized to desmethylclomipramine, a secondary amine tricyclic antidepressant that is identical to desipramine with a chloride atom substitution. These agents have noradrenergic properties and been reported to be useful in the treatment of both ADHD (Biederman et al., 1989) and tic disorders (Spencer et al., 1993), so clomipramine may offer the potential advantage of targeting more than one set of symptoms. Unfortunately, systematic data on this interesting possibility are lacking.

When major depression is present as a comorbid disorder in OCD youth, the primary medication strategy remains unchanged and straightforward, although severe depression may require hospitalization of the affected patient or addition of mood stabilizers. However, the clinical picture becomes rapidly more complex when symptoms of hypomania emerge, as they may in the presence of the SSRIs. Whether the behavioral activation seen frequently in SSRI-treated children and adolescents represents organic driving of a true mood disorder and an underlying bipolar diathesis is unknown. Nonetheless, it presents a pressing clinical concern in those subjects whose OCD symptoms require aggressive SSRI dosing but who invariably develop impairing mood instability with such treatment. Mood stabilizers and/or atypical neuroleptics are sometimes needed in these circumstances to permit treatment of the OCD symptoms.

Managing disruptive behavior disorders in juvenile OCD also presents challenges, because, as with tics and OCD, the pharmacological approaches to ADHD and OCD diverge. These children with OCD are more globally impaired than non-comorbid children and carry the full psychoeducational burden of both dis-

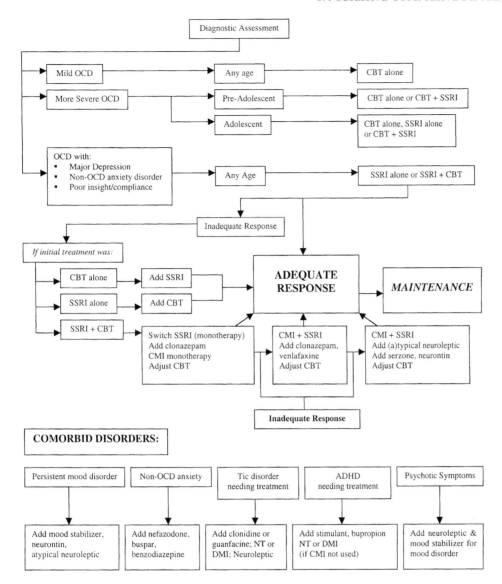

FIGURE 39.2 Treatment algorithm for pediatric obsessive-compulsive disorder (OCD). In adjusting cognitive behavior therapy (CBT), increase frequency or intensity, or alter the setting or format, e.g., have it be home based or day treatment. CMI, clomipramine; DMI, desipramine; NT, nortriptyline; SSRI, selective serotonin reuptake inhibitor (fluoxetine, fluvoxamine, paroxetine, sertraline, citalopram).

orders (Geller et al., 2001a). Despite theoretical concerns and anecdotal reports that stimulants may exacerbate obsessions, there are nonetheless some patients who will respond positively to the stimulants once their OCD is controlled. Other agents, including bupropion and Clonidine, may also be helpful.

Psychotic symptoms must be distinguished from obsessions with poor or variable insight and overvalued ideation. Other positive or negative symptoms of a psychotic disorder may be present and the nature of the obsessions is often atypical and associated with a de-

teriorating course. A concomitant mood disorder may be the source of an affective psychosis and should be treated aggressively. The addition of typical or atypical neuroleptics should be considered.

Obsessional symptoms found in children with pervasive developmental disorder present diagnostic and nosological dilemmas. There are a very few children who seem genuinely to meet criteria for both diagnoses, for example, with rather typical contamination concerns and cleaning behaviors. Since the SSRIs are effective in symptomatic management of both these disorders (Cook et al., 1992; Gordon et al., 1993; Mc-Dougle et al., 1996), drug treatment is similar, though low doses are advised, and behavioral activation may be more likely in this population.

Duration of Treatment

Optimal duration of treatment for children with OCD is unknown. Most authors (March et al., 1997; Grados et al., 1999) recommend 9 to 18 months of treatment after symptom resolution or stabilization, followed by a very gradual taper (25% per 1–2 months). Relapse upon discontinuation is common (Flament et al., 1990; Leonard et al., 1993). Long term maintenance after 3–4 mild or 2–3 severe relapses is recommended.

Adverse Events

Adverse events are relatively common with clomipramine (dry mouth 63%, sedation 46%, dizziness 41%, tremor 33% as well as constipation, flushing, sweating, and memory impairment) (DeVeaugh-Geiss et al., 1992). Adverse events, though less frequent, are also quite common with the SSRIs and involve mainly the central nervous system (insomnia, agitation, hyperkinesia, loss of energy, fatigue, somnolence, tremor) and gastrointestinal system (nausea, dyspepsia, diarrhea). One should also remember to discuss sexual dysfunction as a potential side effect of the SSRIs in teenagers. Behavioral activation (behavioral side effects, disinhibition) deserves special mention, because it is relatively frequent (Riddle et al., 1991) and may limit the usefulness of these medications. It may have a delayed onset that parallels the reduction in anxiety and may follow a honeymoon period of rapid improvement. Like other adverse events, it appears to be dose dependent and in our experience, it is more frequent in preadolescent patients. All the SSRIs have the potential to produce this reaction and it is unclear whether it is more common with any particular agent. If dose reduction is not possible, addition of a mood stabilizer may be required to permit antiobsessional treatment (see Treating the Comorbid Patient, above). Significant weight gain may occasionally occur with SSRI treatment.

AUGMENTATION STRATEGIES FOR TREATMENT RESISTANCE

Failure to respond to an initial medication trial does not predict failure to respond to another drug. If no or little clinical response is noted after 8–10 weeks using maximal therapy or adverse events are unacceptable, a switch to another SSRI or to clomipramine is indicated (Fig. 39.2). For patients with only partial therapeutic response after several successive SSRI trials, augmentation strategies may be useful. In adults, a personal or family history of chronic tic disorder was associated with a positive response to haloperidol augmentation to fluvoxamine (McDougle et al., 1994). Case reports also support this approach in children (Hawkridge et al., 1996). Clonazepam was also shown to be helpful in adults (Hewlett, 1993) and children (Leonard et al., 1994) with OCD but sedation as well as behavioral disinhibition in children in particular may limit the use of clonazepam.

Several reports also suggest that adjunctive risperidone (Giakas, 1995; Jacobsen, 1995; Lombroso et al., 1995; McDougle et al., 1995; Ravizza et al., 1996; Stein et al., 1997)or olanzapine (Peris and Szerman, 2000) may be helpful in treatment-resistant OCD. Systematic data in pediatric samples are needed, however, before such an approach can be recommended, and there are anecdotal reports of increased obsessions and anxiety with the atypical neuroleptics (Alzaid and Jones, 1997; Andrade, 1998; Mottard and de la Sablonniere, 1999).

A more common approach in difficult to treat cases would be the combination of clomipramine with a SSRI; several reports lend support to this practice (Simeon and Thatte, 1990; Figueroa et al., 1998). In this situation, careful attention to the potential pharmacokinetic interactions discussed above are recommended. Sertraline and citalopram are least likely to elevate tricyclic levels due to less potential CYP interactions. By expert consensus, second- (venlafaxine) and third-line (nefazadone and gabapentin) agents may be used when clinical response is inadequate despite a lack of controlled data. Venlafaxine may be substituted for a more typical SSRI while nefazadone or gabapentin may be added to either clomipramine or a SSRI. The combination of venlafaxine with other SSRIs is not generally recommended as it may increase the risk of a serotonin syndrome. The addition of nefazadone to SSRIs presents a lesser risk.

Outcome Studies

In one review of eight outcome studies with a mean length of follow-up of 7 years (range 2–22 years), an average of 50% of subjects still met the diagnosis of OCD at follow-up (range 23%–70%) (Geller et al., 1998). This finding is similar to that reported in a recent 40-year follow-up of adult OCD patients (Skoog and Skoog, 1999). Onset severity appears not to be related to outcome. Drug improvement could generally be maintained over time but a poor psychosocial outcome, with failure to achieve social developmental milestones, were noted in four studies. Comorbidity continued to be common in the studies reviewed but it is unknown whether comorbid conditions affect the long-term outcome in children and adolescents with OCD. Leonard et al. (1993), in a follow-up study found a family history of axis I psychopathology, poor initial response after 5 weeks of treatment, and a lifetime history of tics to be predictors of poorer outcome. One prospective study (Ravizza et al., 1995) suggested that an earlier age at onset was associated with a worse clinical outcome in adult subjects. Childhood-onset OCD has been reported by many authors to be a more highly familial form of the disorder (Pauls et al., 1995; Nestadt et al., 2000).

Novel Treatments

Immune-mediated neuropsychiatric disorders of childhood are discussed in Chapter 14. Immune modulation therapies are still investigational, but a few points will be helpful to the practicing psychopharmacologist in this area. A throat culture, antistreptolysin O (ASO), and anti DNAase B titer should be obtained in any child with OCD, tics, or choreiform movements who has an acute onset of symptoms, an acute exacerbation of symptoms, loss of a previous medication response, or a dramatic change in behavior. Furthermore, inter-episode antibody levels are recommended to demonstrate a later rise associated with an intercurrent streptococcal infection and subsequent increase of OCD or tic symptoms. A single titer during symptom exacerbation is of limited use, since a rise in antibody levels cannot be demonstrated at that time. In the absence of documented group A beta-hemolytic streptococcal infection, antibiotics are not indicated for the treatment of the OCD child. However, in those with PANDAS-related symptoms, standard antiobsessional drugs may not be as effective until the underlying infection is treated. A low index of suspicion is the best course. Intravenous clomipramine has been shown to be useful in small controlled studies in adults, but the cardiovascular risks have thus far precluded any trials in the pediatric age group.

The treatment algorithm depicted in Figure 39.2 is derived from the Texas Childhood Major Depression Medication Algorithm (Hughes and Preskorn, 1994), the Expert Consensus Guidelines for the Treatment of OCD (March et al., 1997) and the American Academy of Child and Adolescent Psychiatry (AACAP) practice parameters for the treatment of child and adolescent OCD (King et al., 1998). Data are weighted hierarchically from controlled clinical trials, open-label and retrospective analyses and expert consensus opinion. Such algorithms are not "one size fits all" and are not intended to define a standard of care or include all methods of care.

FUTURE RESEARCH

Specific treatments guided by clinical, etiological (e.g., PANDAS), or genetic subtypes are the focus of ongoing efforts. Systematic augmentation trials using the atypical neuroleptics or the beta-blocker pindolol are needed. Family-based behavioral interventions are also under study.

ACKNOWLEDGMENTS

This work was supported by the Tourette Syndrome Association Foundation, the Obsessive Compulsive Foundation, and NIMH K08 MH01481.

REFERENCES

Altemus, M., Swedo, S., Leonard, H., Richter, D., Rubinow, D., Potter, W., and Rapoport, J. (1994) Changes in cerebrospinal fluid neurochemistry during treatment of obsessive-compulsive disorder with clomipramine. *Arch Gen Psychiatry* 51:794–803.

Alzaid, K. and Jones, B.D. (1997) A case report of risperidone-induced obsessive compulsive symptoms. *J Clin Psychopharmacol* 17:58–59.

Andrade, C. (1998) Risperidone may worsen fluoxetine-treated OCD. *J Clin Psychiatry* 59:255–256.

Apter, A., Fallon, T.J., Jr., King, R.A., Ratzoni, G., Zohar, A.H., Binder, M., Weizman, A., Leckman, J.F., Pauls, D.L., Kron, S., and Cohen, D.J. (1996) Obsessive-compulsive characteristics: from symptoms to syndrome. *J Am Acad Child Adolesc Psychiatry* 35:907–912.

Apter, A., Ratzoni, G., King, R., Weizman, A., Iancu, I., Binder, M., and Riddle, M. (1994) Fluvoxamine open-label treatment of adolescent inpatients with obsessive-compulsive disorder or depression. *J Am Acad Child Adolesc Psychiatry* 33:342–348.

Biederman, J. (1991) Sudden death in children treated with a tricyclic antidepressant: a commentary. *J Am Acad Child Adolesc Psychiatry* 30:495–497.

Biederman, J., Baldessarini, R., Wright, V., Knee, D., and Harmatz, J. (1989) A double-blind placebo controlled study of desipramine in the treatment of attention deficit disorder: I. Efficacy. *J Am Acad Child Adolesc Psychiatry* 28:777–784.

Black, A. (1974) The natural history of obsessional neurosis. In: Beech, H., ed. *Obsessional States*. London: Methuen, pp. 1–23.

Como, P.G. and Kurlan, R. (1991) An open-label trial of fluoxetine for obsessive-compulsive disorder in Gilles de la Tourette's Syndrome. *Neurology* 41:872–874.

Cook, E., Rowlett, R., Jaselskis, C., and Leventhal, B. (1992) Fluoxetine treatment of children and adults with autistic disorder and mental retardation. *J Am Acad Child Adolesc Psychiatry* 31:739–745.

Cook, E.H., Wagner, K., March, J.S., Biederman, J., Landau, P., Wolkow, R., and Messig, M. (2001) Long-term sertraline treatment of children and adolescents with obsessive-compulsive disorder. *J Am Acad Child Adolesc Psychiatry* 40:1175–1181.

Coupland, N.J., Bell, C.J., and Potokar, J.P. (1996) Serotonin reuptake inhibitor withdrawal. *J Clin Psychopharmacol* 16:356–362.

DeVeaugh-Geiss, J., Moroz, G., Biederman, J., Cantwell, D., Fontaine, R., Greist, J., Reichler, R., Katz, R., and Landau, P. (1992) Clomipramine hydrochloride in childhood and adolescent obsessive-compulsive disorder: a multicenter trial. *J Am Acad Child Adolesc Psychiatry* 31:45–49.

Fennig, S., Fennig, S., Pato, M., and Weitzman, A. (1994) Emergence of symptoms of Tourette's syndrome during fluvoxamine treatment of obsessive-compulsive disorder. *Br J Psychiatry* 164:839–841.

Figueroa, Y., Rosenberg, D., Birmaher, B., and Keshavan, M. (1998) Combination treatment with clomipramine and selective serotonin reuptake inhibitors for obsessive-compulsive disorder in children and adolescents. *J Child Adolesc Psychopharmacol* 8:61–67.

Flament, M., Koby, E., Rapoport, J., Berg, C., Zahn, T., Cox, C., Denckla, M., and Lenane, M. (1990) Childhood obsessive-compulsive disorder: a prospective follow-up study. *J Child Psychol Psychiatry* 31:363–380.

Flament, M., Whitaker, A., Rapoport, J., Davies, M., Berg, C., Kalikow, K., Sceery, W., and Shaffer, D. (1988) Obsessive compulsive disorder in adolescence: an epidemiological study. *J Am Acad Child Adolesc Psychiatry* 27:764–771.

Flament, M.F., Rapoport, J.L., Berg, C.J., Sceery, W., Kilts, C., Mellstrom, B., and Linnoila, M. (1985) Clomipramine treatment of childhood obsessive-compulsive disorder: a double-blind controlled study. *Arch Gen Psychiatry* 42:977–983.

Flament, M.F., Rapoport, J.L., Murphy, D.L., Berg, C.J., and Lake, C.R. (1987) Biochemical changes during clomipramine treatment of childhood obsessive-compulsive disorder. *Arch Gen Psychiatry* 44:219–225.

Geller, D., Biederman, J., Agranat, A., Kim, G.S., Hagermoser, and L.M. (2001a) Developmental aspects of obsessive compulsive disorder: findings in children, adolescents and adults. *J Nerv Ment Dis* 189(7):471–477.

Geller, D., Biederman, J., Emslie, G., and Carpenter, D. (2001b) Comorbid psychiatric illness and response to treatment in pediatric OCD. Presented at Scientific *Proceedings of the American Psychiatric Association, New Orleans, LA.*

Geller, D., Biederman, J., Faraone, S.V., Frazier, J., Coffey, B.J., Kim, G., and Bellordre, C.A. (2000) Clinical correlates of obsessive compulsive disorder in children and adolescents referred to specialized and non-specialized clinical settings. *Depress Anxiety* 11:163–168.

Geller, D.A., Biederman, J., Jones, J., Park, K., Schwartz, S., and Coffey, B. (1998) Is juvenile obsessive-compulsive disorder a developmental subtype of the disorder? A review of the pediatric literature. *J Am Acad Child Adolesc Psychiatry* 37:420–427.

Geller, D., Biederman, J., Reed, E., Spencer, T., and Wilens, T. (1995) Similarities in response to fluoxetine in the treatment of children and adolescents with obsessive-compulsive disorder. *J Am Acad Child Adolesc Psychiatry* 34:36–44.

Geller, D.A., Hoog, S.L., Heiligenstein, J.H., Ricardi, R.K., Tamura, R., Kluszynski, S., Jacobsen, J.G., and Team TFPOS (2001c) Fluoxetine treatment for obsessive-compulsive disorder in children and adolescents: a placebo-controlled clinical trial. *J Am Acad Child Adolesc Psychiatry* 40:773–779.

Geller, D.A., Wagner, K., Emslie, G., Murphy, T., Gallagher, D., Gardner, C., and Carpenter, D. (2002) Efficacy of Paroxetine in Pediatric OCD: Results of a Multicenter Study. Scientific Proceedings of the American Psychiatric Association. Philadelphia: 2002.

Giakas, W.J. (1995) Risperidone treatment for a Tourette's disorder patient with comorbid obsessive-compulsive disorder. *Am J Psychiatry* 152:1097–1098.

Gordon, C., State, R., Nelson, J., Hamburger, S., and Rapoport, J. (1993) A double-blind comparison of clomipramine, desipramine, and placebo in the treatment of autistic disorder. *Arch Gen Psychiatry* 50:441–447.

Grados, M., Scahill, L., and Riddle, M.A. (1999) Pharmacotherapy in children and adolescents with obsessive-compulsive disorder. *Child Adolesc Psychiatr Clin North Am* 8:617–634.

Hawkridge, S., Stein, D.J., and Bouwer, C. (1996) Combined pharmacotherapy for TS and OCD. *J Am Acad Child Adolesc Psychiatry* 35:703–704.

Hewlett, W.A. (1993) The use of benzodiazepines in obsessive compulsive disorder and Tourette's syndrome. *Psychiatr Ann* 23:309–316.

Hughes, C. and Preskorn, S. (1994) Pharmacokinetics in child/adolescent psychiatric disorders. *Psychiatr Ann* 24:76–82.

Jacobsen, F.M. (1995) Risperidone in the treatment of affective illness and obsessive-compulsive disorder. *J Clin Psychiatry* 56:423–428.

Karno, M., Golding, J., Sorenson, S., and Burnam, A. (1988) The epidemiology of obsessive-compulsive disorder in five U.S. communities. *Arch Gen Psychiatry* 45:1094–1099.

King, R., Leonard, H., and March, J. (1998) Practice parameters for the assessment and treatment of children and adolescents with obsessive compulsive disorder. *J Am Acad Child Adolesc Psychiatry* 37:275–455.

Kurlan, R., Deeley, C., McDermott, M., and McDermott, M. (1993) A pilot controlled study of fluoxetine for obsessive-compulsive symptoms in children with Tourette's syndrome. *Clin Neuropharmacol* 16:167–172.

Lane, R., and Baldwin, D. (1997) Selective serotonin reuptake inhibitor-induced serotonin syndrome: review. *J Clin Psychopharmacol* 17:208–221.

Leonard, H.L., and Rapoport, J.L. (1989) Pharmacotherapy of childhood obsessive-compulsive disorder. *Psychiatr Clin North Am* 12:963–970.

Leonard, H.L., Swedo, S.E., Lenane, M.C., Rettew, D.C., Cheslow, D.L., Hamburger, S.D., and Rapoport, J.L. (1991) A double-blind desipramine substitution during long-term clomipramine treatment in children and adolescents with obsessive-compulsive disorder. *Arch Gen Psychiatry* 48:922–927.

Leonard, H., Swedo, S., Lenane, M., Rettew, D., Hamburger, S., Bartko, J., and Rapoport, J. (1993) A 2- to 7-year follow-up study of 54 obsessive-compulsive children and adolescents. *Arch Gen Psychiatry* 50:429–439.

Leonard, H., Swedo, S., Rapoport, J., Koby, E., Lenane, M., Cheslow, D., and Hamburger, S. (1989) Treatment of obsessive-compulsive disorder with clomipramine and desipramine in children and adolescents. *Arch Gen Psychiatry* 46:1088–1092.

Leonard, H.L., Topol, D., Bukstein, O., Hindmarsh, D., Allen, A.J., and Swedo, S.E. (1994) Clonazepam as an augmenting agent in the treatment of childhood-onset obsessive-compulsive disorder. *J Am Acad Child Adolesc Psychiatry* 33:792–794.

Liebowitz, M., Hollander, E., Fairbanks, J., and Campeas, R. (1990) Fluoxetine for adolescents with obsessive-compulsive disorder. *Am J Psychiatry* 147:370–371.

Lombroso, P.J., Scahill, L., King, R.A., and Lynch, K.A. (1995) Risperidone treatment of children and adolescents with chronic tic disorders: a preliminary report. *J Am Acad Child Adolesc Psychiatry* 34:1147–1152.

March, J.S., Biederman, J., Wolkow, R., Safferman, A., Mardekian, J., Cook, E.H., Cutler, N.R., Dominguez, R., Ferguson, J., Muller,

B., Riesenberg, R., Rosenthal, M., Sallee, F.R., and Wagner, K.D. (1998) Sertraline in children and adolescents with obsessive-compulsive disorder: a multicenter randomized control trial. *JAMA* 280:1752–1756.

March, J.S., Frances, A., Carpenter, D., and Kahn, D.A. (1997) The Expert Consensus Guideline Series: treatment of obsessive-compulsive disorder. *J Clin Psychiatry* 58:5–72.

March, J.S., and Mulle, K. (1998) *OCD in Children and Adolescents: A Cognitive-Behavioral Treatment Manual.* New York: Guilford Press.

McDougle, C., Goodman, W., Leckman, J., Lee, N., Heninger, G., and Price, L. (1994) Haloperidol addition in fluvoxamine-refractory obsessive compulsive disorder: a double-blind, placebo-controlled study in patients with and without tics. *Arch Gen Psychiatry* 51:302–308.

McDougle, C.J., Kresch, L.E., Goodman, W.K., Naylor, S.T., Volkmar, F.R., Cohen, D.J., and Price, L.H. (1995) A case-controlled study of repetitive thoughts and behavior in adults with autistic disorder and obsessive-compulsive disorder. *Am J Psychiatry* 152: 772–777.

McDougle, C.J., Naylor, S.T., Cohen, D.J., Volkmar, F.R., Heninger, G.R., and Price, L.H. (1996) A double-blind, placebo-controlled study of fluvoxamine in adults with autistic disorder. *Arch Gen Psychiatry* 53:1001–1008.

Mottard, J.P., and de la Sablonniere, J.F. (1999) Olanzapine-induced obsessive-compulsive disorder. *Am J Psychiatry* 156:799–800.

Nestadt, G., Samuels, J., Bienvenu, J.O., Grados, M., Hoehn-Saric, R., Liang, K., LaBuda, M., Riddle, M., and Walkup, J. (2000) A family study of obsessive compulsive disorder. *Arch Gen Psychiatry* 57:358–363.

Pauls, D., Alsobrook, J., II, Goodman, W., Rasmussen, S., and Leckman, J. (1995) A family study of obsessive-compulsive disorder. *Am J Psychiatry* 152:76–84.

Peris, M.D., and Szerman, N. (2000) Efficacy of serotonin reuptake inhibitors and olanzapine in obsessive compulsive disorder. In: 4th International Obsessive Compulsive Disorder Conference, St. Thomas, USA.

Pigott, T.A., L'Heureux, F., Dubbert, B., Bernstein, S., and Murphy, D.L. (1994) Obsessive-compulsive disorder: comorbid conditions. *J Clin Psychiatry* 55:15–27.

Puig-Antich, J., Perel, J.M., Lupatkin, W., Chambers, W.J., Shea, C., Tabrizi, M., and Stiller, R.L. (1979) Plasma levels of imipramine (IMI) and desmethylimipramine (DMI) and clinical response in prepubertal major depressive disorder. *J Am Acad Child Psychiatry* 18:616–627.

Puig-Antich, J., Perel, J.M., Lupatkin, W., Chambers, W.J., Tabrizi, M.A., King, J., Goetz, R., Davies, M., and Stiller, R.L. (1987) Imipramine in prepubertal major depressive disorders. *Arch Gen Psychiatry* 44:81–89.

Rasmussen, S.A., and Eisen, J.L. (1998) Epidemiology and clinical features of obsessive compulsive disorders. In: Jenike, M.A., Baer, L., and Minichiello, W.E. eds. *Obsessive Compulsive Disorders—Practical Management, 3rd ed.* Boston: Mosby, pp. 12–43.

Rauch, S.L., Jenike, M.A., Alpert, N.M., Baer, L., Breiter, H.C.R., Savage, C.R., and Fischman, A.J. (1994) Regional cerebral blood flow measured during symptom provocation in obsessive-compulsive disorder using oxygen 15–labeled carbon dioxide and positron emission tomography. *Arch Gen Psychiatry* 51:62–70.

Ravizza, L., Barzega, G., Bellino, S., Bogetto, F., and Maina, G. (1995) Predictors of drug treatment response in obsessive-compulsive disorder. *J Clin Psychiatry* 56:368–373.

Ravizza, L., Barzega, G., Bellino, S., Bogetto, F., and Maina, G. (1996) Therapeutic effect and safety of adjunctive risperidone in

refractory obsessive-compulsive disorder (OCD). *Psychopharmacol Bull* 32:677–682.

Rettew, D.C., Swedo, S.E., Leonard, H.L., Lenane, M.C., and Rapoport, J.L. (1992) Obsessions and compulsions across time in 79 children and adolescents with obsessive-compulsive disorder. *J Am Acad Child Adolesc Psychiatry* 31: 1050–1056.

Riddle, M.A., Hardin, M.T., King, R., Scahill, L., and Woolston, J.L. (1990) Fluoxetine treatment of children and adolescents with Tourette's and obsessive compulsive disorders: preliminary clinical experience. *J Am Acad Child Adolescent Psychiatry* 29:45–48.

Riddle, M., King, R., Hardin, M., Scahill, L., Ort, S., Chappell, P., Rasmusson, A., and Leckman, J. (1991) Behavioral side effects of fluoxetine in children and adolescents. *J Child Adolesc Psychopharmacol* 1:193–198.

Riddle, M.A., Reeve, E.A., Yaryura-Tobias, J.A., Yang, H.M., Claghorn, J.L., Gaffney, G., Greist, J.H., Holland, D., McConville, B.J., Pigott, T., and Walkup, J.T. (2001) Fluvoxamine for children and adolescents with obsessive compulsive disorder: a randomized, controlled, multicenter trial. *J Am Acad Child Adolesc Psychiatry* 40:222–229.

Riddle, M., Scahill, L., King, R., Hardin, M., Anderson, G., Ort, S., Smith, J., Leckman, J., and Cohen, D. (1992) Double-blind, crossover trial of fluoxetine and placebo in children and adolescents with obsessive-compulsive disorder. *J Am Acad Child Adolesc Psychiatry* 31:1062–1069.

Rosenberg, D.R., Stewart, C.M., Fitzgerald, K.D., Tawile, V., and Carroll, E. (1999) Paroxetine open-label treatment of pediatric outpatients with obsessive-compulsive disorder. *J Am Acad Child Adolesc Psychiatry* 38:1180–1185.

Scahill, L., Riddle, M.A., King, R.A., Hardin, M.T., Rasmusson, A., Makuch, R.W., and Leckman, J.F. (1997b) Fluoxetine has no marked effect on tic symptoms in patients with Tourette's syndrome: a double-blind placebo-controlled study. *J Child Adolesc Psychopharmacol* 7:75–85.

Scahill, L., Riddle, M., McSwiggin-Hardin, M., Ort, S.I., King, R.A., Goodman, W.K., Cicchetti, D., and Leckman, J.F. (1997a) Children's Yale-Brown Obsessive Compulsive Scale: reliability and validity. *J Am Acad Child Adolesc Psychiatry* 36:844–852.

Simeon, J. and Thatte, S. (1990) Treatment of adolescent obsessive-compulsive disorder with clomipramine-fluoxetine combination. *Psychopharmacol Bull* 26:285–290.

Skoog, G., and Skoog, I. (1999) A 40-year follow-up of patients with obsessive-compulsive disorder. *Arch Gen Psychiatry* 56:121–127.

Spencer, T., Biederman, J., Harding, M., O'Donnell, D., Wilens, T., Faraone, S., Coffey, B., and Geller, D. (1999) Disentangling the overlap between Tourette's disorder and ADHD. *J Child Psychol Psychiatry* 39:1037–1044.

Spencer, T., Biederman, J., Kerman, K., Steingard, R., and Wilens, T. (1993) Desipramine treatment of children with attention deficit hyperactivity disorder and tic disorder or tourette's syndrome. *J Am Acad Child Adolesc Psychiatry* 32:354–360.

Stein, D.J., Bouwer, C., Hawkridge, S., and Emsley, M.B. (1997) Risperidone augmentation of serotonin reuptake inhibitors in obsessive-compulsive and related disorders. *J Clin Pscyhiatry* 58:119–122.

Swedo, S.E., Leonard, H.L., Kruesi, M.J., Rettew, D.C., Listwak, S.J., Berrenttini, W., Stipetic, M., Hamburger, S., Gold, P.W., Potter, W.Z., and Rapoport, J.L. (1992) Cerebrospinal fluid neurochemistry in children and adolescents with obsessive-compulsive disorder. *Arch Gen Psychiatry* 49:29–36.

Thompson, P.H. (1997) Child and adolescent obsessive-compulsive disorder treated with citalopram: findings from an open trial of 23 cases. *J Child Adolesc Psychopharmacol* 7:157–166.

40 | Tourette's syndrome and other tic disorders

ROBERT A. KING, LAWRENCE SCAHILL, PAUL J. LOMBROSO, AND JAMES LECKMAN

The fluctuating chronic motor and phonic tics that characterize Tourette's syndrome (TS) are often a substantial source of distress or impairment and hence the target of therapeutic intervention. In addition to these pathognomonic symptoms, however, many individuals with TS also suffer from various other psychological difficulties, including obsessions, compulsions, impulsivity, attentional difficulties, depression or mood lability, various anxiety symptoms, and a range of neuropsychological deficits (King et al., 1999a). For many individuals, these comorbid difficulties may be a greater source of impairment or distress than the tics per se.

The breadth, prevalence, and nature of this penumbra of tic-associated symptoms have been the subject of controversy (Comings and Comings, 1987; King et al., 1999a). There seems general agreement that around half of individuals with TS also have substantial obsessive-compulsive symptoms and that this association likely reflects a shared underlying genetic diathesis. Attention-deficit hyperactivity disorder (ADHD) is also quite common in clinical samples of youngsters with TS (on the order of 60%–70%) (Spencer et al., 2001), but this increased risk is not found in some community samples of individuals with TS (Apter et al., 1993), raising the question to what extent the association between TS and ADHD seen in clinical samples may be influenced by referral bias. Further longitudinal community-based epidemiological studies, such as that of Peterson et al. (2001), are needed to clarify this issue. Although some comorbid difficulties, such as depression, may reflect the cumulative psychosocial burden of tics and associated obsessive-compulsive symptoms, neurobiological findings demonstrating increased autonomic lability in individuals with TS suggest that many of the psychological vulnerabilities of individuals with TS are not simply secondary to the social stigma

or psychological burden of tics alone (Chappell et al., 1994).

One of the clinician's most important tasks is thus to identify the principal sources of distress and impairment and to prioritize the targets for pharmacological intervention. Although tic reduction may be the first priority in some cases, in other cases it may be a child's ADHD, depression, or compulsions that may have the first claim on the clinician's interventional efforts. Even when the tics are not themselves the initial target of treatment, the TS-related nature of the child's depression, ADHD, or obsessive-compulsive disorder (OCD) may have important implications for the choice of agents, therapeutic response, or possible side effects.

We begin with a consideration of each of the major TS-associated symptom realms, and the medications commonly used in their treatment, before returning to the overall coordination of care for individuals with TS.

INDICATIONS FOR TREATMENT

The mere presence of tics does not by itself mandate a trial of anti-tic medication. Tics warrant treatment only if they are a source of substantial interference in the patient's everyday life. This interference may take the form of disrupting concentration, causing pain or injury, disturbing classmates, provoking teasing or other forms of stigma, or disturbing the child's self-esteem. There is no evidence that giving or withholding anti-tic medication influences the long-term natural history of tic severity for better or for worse.

It is important for both the clinician and parents to understand the usual natural history of tics. The characteristic temporal pattern of tics is one of short-term bouts or bursts and longer-term waxing and waning. Statistical studies of the temporal dynamics of tics suggest that periods of relative quiescence are likely to be followed by bursts of tic activity and that periods of bursting are likely to be followed by relative quiescence. This pattern appears to hold over both short periods of time (e.g., minutes to days) and long periods of time, with the transition between bursting and quiescence going rather abruptly from one extreme to the other (Peterson and Leckman, 1998). Although some exacerbations are clearly related to stressful or exciting life events (Surwillo et al., 1978; Silva et al., 1995), it may not be possible to discern a precipitant for a given exacerbation. In the majority of childhood cases, there is a natural improvement or remission of tics (but not necessarily associated difficulties) as youngsters move into later adolescence and young adulthood (Leckman et al., 1998).

This natural fluctuation of tics complicates clinical decision making about initiating medication and dose adjustment, as well as conducting drug efficacy studies. The clinician is often consulted when the child has a tic exacerbation and the child's and parents' distress is at its peak. There is an understandable impulse to begin or increase medication at such times, yet either with or without a change in medication, it may well be that tic severity will regress toward its previous mean over the next few weeks. Hence, while supporting and remaining in active contact with the patient and family, it is usually wise (save in the case of seriously disruptive or physically injurious tics) to refrain from medication changes unless the exacerbation has persisted for more than a week or two. This helps to prevent the pitfall of increasing medication to relatively large doses over time, with resulting adverse effects and greater difficulty reducing the dosage without causing rebound exacerbations.

The natural fluctuations of tics and the occasional improvement of tics on placebo mandate caution in interpreting open-label trials and anecdotal reports of alternative treatments. For example, a 12-week double-blind, placebo-controlled study of clonidine found that in the placebo group (who also received the usual supportive care and regular contact with the treating clinicians), tic severity, as rated independently by parents, patient, and clinicians, improved 11%–13%. Other placebo-controlled studies report placebo response rates on the order of 6%–11% (Gilbert et al., 2000); (Sallee et al., 2000b; Scahill et al., submitted).

Many parents of children with TS are frightened of drug treatment and some are categorically opposed. As with most areas of pediatric psychopharmacology, the decision to initiate medication or not is best approached as a collaborative decision, involving the parents, clinician, and (if old enough) the child, rather than an area for dogmatic pronouncement. It is appropriate to explicate the following risks and benefits of giving or withholding a trial of medication:

• *Risks of treatment*: The known and unknown possible side effects, which vary by class.
• *Benefits of treatment*: The real and present likelihood of reduction of burdensome symptoms (relative benefit depends on severity of tics and associated distress). Discus the level of improvement that can be expected as well as the time to onset of therapeutic effect.
• *Risks of withholding treatment*: The real and present likelihood of continued immediate and long-term distress and impairment due to symptoms in light of known natural history and impact of given symptom (tic, ADHD, and/or OCD).
• *Benefit of withholding treatment*: Avoiding potential side effects. The possibility of spontaneous decrease in symptoms is more likely with tics, depending on severity history; this is unlikely with ADHD or OCD symptoms.

Placing the decision regarding medication in this nondogmatic context often helps to address a priori objections to medication, especially if coupled with the assurance that dose adjustment will be a collaborative enterprise between clinician and family, with the goal of minimizing potential side effects. Similarly, this careful weighing of the risks and benefits can serve to temper unreasonably high expectations about the level of improvement that the medication can achieve.

TYPICAL NEUROLEPTICS

As competitive inhibitors of postsynaptic D_2 receptors, neuroleptics decrease dopaminergic input from the substantia nigra and ventral tegmental area into the basal ganglia.

The typical neuroleptics have been the best studied and most potent agents for the treatment of tics (Table 40.1). Of these, haloperidol and pimozide have been the most extensively studied in controlled or head-to-head trials. Applying these studies to clinical practice is complicated by the fact that older studies (such as Shapiro et al., 1989) used higher dose ranges of these two drugs (e.g., 2–20 mg/day for haloperidol, 2–48 mg/day for pimozide) than are currently the practice. Historically, haloperidol has been considered more potent than pimozide. Thus, most drug-to-drug comparison studies used pimozide doses approximately twice those of haloperidol. A recent crossover study of 22 youngsters using numerically comparable doses of pimozide and haloperidol (mean daily doses 3.4 and

TABLE 40.1 *Controlled Studies with Antipsychotic Agents for Tic Reduction*

Medication	Reference	Patients (n)	Design	Dose Range	Improvement (%)
Haloperidol	Shapiro et al., 1989	57	Crossover	1–10 mg/day	66[a]
Pimozide	Shapiro et al., 1989	57	Crossover	2–20 mg/day	52[a]
Pimozide	Shapiro and Shapiro, 1984	20	Crossover	4–9 mg/day	44[b]
Risperidone	Scahill et al., submitted	34	Parallel	1–2.5 mg	36[a]
Tiapride	Eggers et al., 1988	16	Crossover	6 mg/kg	44[b]
Ziprasidone	Sallee et al., 2000b	28	Parallel	5–40 mg/day	35[a]

[a]Based on clinician measure.
[b]Based on tic counts.

3.5 mg, respectively) found a 40% improvement over baseline for pimozide, compared to 27% for haloperidol (Sallee et al., 1997). At this moderately high dose level, haloperidol was associated with three times the frequency of dose-limiting side effects, such as extrapyramidal symptoms, depression, anxiety, or sedation, as that of pimozide (9/22 subjects for haloperidol, 3/22 for pimozide). Follow-up studies suggest that over the long term (1–15 years), patients are significantly more likely to remain on pimozide than haloperidol (Sandor et al., 1990).

Fluphenazine, a typical neuroleptic of the phenothiazine class, has been less widely used for treatment of tics than haloperidol or pimozide. A controlled trial of haloperidol, fluphenazine, and trifluoperazine found comparable tic-reducing efficacy, but greater sedation and extrapyramidal side effects for haloperidol; fluphenazine was the best tolerated (Borison et al., 1982). In an open-label trial with 21 subjects who had an unsatisfactory response to haloperidol, fluphenazine had a superior side effect profile to that of haloperidol in the dose range employed (mean dose of fluphenazine, 7 mg/day, range 2–15 mg/day) (Goetz et al., 1984). In this group selected for an unsatisfactory response to haloperidol, 11 of the 21 subjects (52%) had a better response to fluphenazine than haloperidol, 6 subjects had a comparable response, and 2 subjects preferred haloperidol.

Side Effects of Typical Neuroleptics

The side effects of typical neuroleptics are extensively discussed in Chapters 26 and 41 in this volume. Given its potent calcium channel blocking properties, additional considerations apply to the use of pimozide. The use of pimozide requires caution regarding the possibility of QT prolongation, and we typically obtain an electrocardiogram (EKG) to measure the QTc interval at baseline, and obtain a repeat EKG during the dose adjustment period, after reaching a maintenance level, and annually thereafter. Because pimozide is metabolized by the cytochrome P450 (CYP) 3A4 isoenzyme, inhibition of the enzyme can dramatically increase serum pimozide levels to toxic, even fatal levels (Desta et al., 1999, Flockhart et al., 2000). Thus, concomitant use of drugs that inhibit the CYP 3A4 isoenzyme, such as erythromycin and clarithromycin, should be avoided. Rare cases of toxicity due to impaired drug metabolism caused by genetic polymorphisms of CYP loci have been reported (Sallee et al., 2000a).

Dosing of Typical Neuroleptics

General considerations in dose adjustment

The frequency of sedation on neuroleptics, the latency of response, the natural fluctuation of tics, and the occurrence of rebound exacerbations following discontinuation or abrupt decreases in dose of neuroleptics support the wisdom of starting with low doses and making upward or downward adjustments of dosage slowly. Large or rapid increases in dosage in response to every increase in tics can lead to patients' ratcheting up over time to ever higher and higher doses, with each attempt at decreasing the dosage being met by a rebound exacerbation. As noted earlier, the overall goal is to find the lowest dosage necessary to reduce tics to tolerable levels; in our experience, exceeding the levels suggested below usually provide little additional benefit and increase the risk of troublesome side effects.

Haloperidol

Haloperidol is usually started with an evening dose of 0.25 or 0.5 mg; if this is tolerated well over 4–7 days, another 0.25 or 0.5 mg can be added in the morning, if needed. The total daily dose can be raised, as tolerated and as needed, by 0.25–0.5 mg increments every

5 to 7 days, alternating between the morning and evening dose, to a total daily dose of 0.75 to 2.5 mg. Therapeutic and adverse effects should be closely monitored in the dose adjustment phase.

Pimozide

The typical starting dose of pimozide is 0.5 mg in young children or 1 mg day in larger children. The dosage may be increased in 0.5 to 1 mg increments every 5 to 7 days over a 3 to 4-week period. The total dose in children typically ranges from 2–4 mg/day given in divided doses.

ATYPICAL NEUROLEPTICS

Many families are reluctant to consider the use of typical neuroleptics for children with tics because of the perceived, albeit low, risk of tardive dyskinesia (TD). The development of the atypical neuroleptics, which are combined serotonergic (5-HT$_2$) and dopaminergic (D$_2$) antagonists with an apparently lower risk of TD, has provided effective and, to many patients, more acceptable, treatment alternatives to the typical neuroleptics. Among this group of antipsychotics, there is preliminary evidence for the tic-suppressing efficacy of risperidone (Bruun and Budman, 1996; Bruggeman et al., 2001; van der Linden et al., 1994; Lombroso et al., 1995; Scahill et al., submitted) and ziprasidone (Sallee et al., 2000b) in reducing tics. Although these two agents are potent blockers at the 5-HT$_2$ site, they also have D$_2$ blocking properties (Sallee et al., 2000b). In contrast, clozapine, a weak D$_2$-blocker, but potent 5-HT$_2$-blocker, is not effective in reducing tics (Caine et al., 1979). Taken together, these positive findings with risperidone and ziprasidone, compared to negative results with clozapine, suggest that D$_2$ blockade is important for tic suppression (Chappell et al., 1997). Other atypical antipsychotics include olanzapine, which has modest D$_2$ affinity, and quetiapine, which has only a weak affinity for D$_2$ receptors. To date, only open label studies (Stamenkovic et al., 2000; Budman et al., 2001; Bhadrinath, 1998) and one small double-blind cross over comparison with pimozide (Onofrj et al., 2000) have been published regarding the use of olanzapine for tics. Only a single case report on two subjects has been published on the use of quetiapine in the treatment of tics (Parraga et al., 2001).

In open-label trials in children and adults, risperidone was helpful in reducing tics (dose range in children 1–3 mg in two divided doses), with minimal side effects in the short term. A recently completed 8-week, randomized, double-blind, placebo-controlled trial examined the efficacy of risperidone in reducing tic severity in 34 medication-free subjects (30 males, 4 females) with TS who ranged in age from 8 to 62 years (mean = 19.7 ± 17.01 years) (Scahill et al., submitted). Of these, 26 subjects were less than 18 years of age (mean age 11.1 ± 2.20). After 8 weeks of treatment, the 16 subjects in the risperidone group showed a 32% reduction in tic symptoms from baseline, significantly greater than the 7% reduction seen in the placebo group (N = 18). When evaluated separately, the 12 pediatric subjects randomized to risperidone showed a comparable reduction in tic symptoms. No extrapyramidal symptoms were observed. Two pediatric subjects on risperidone showed increased social anxiety, which resolved with dose reduction in one subject, but resulted in discontinuation in the other. There was a statistically significant mean increase of 6.6 lbs in the risperidone group compared to no change in the placebo group. In a 12-week double-blind parallel group study of 50 patients (age 10–65 years old) comparing risperidone (mean daily dose, 3.8 mg/day) and pimozide (mean dose, 2.9 mg), risperidone appeared to have the advantage of fewer spontaneously reported acute extrapyramidal symptoms and less insomnia (Bruggeman et al., 2001). However, patients under 18 year old gained significantly more weight on risperidone than on pimozide (4.5 kg vs. 2.7 kg).

Olanzapine has shown encouraging results, in doses ranging from 2.5 to 20 mg/day, in two open trials involving a total of 30 adults with TS (Budman et al., 2001; Stamenkovic et al., 2000). A 52-week double-blind crossover study of olanzapine (5 or 10 mg) versus pimozide (2 or 4 mg) in four adult patients with TS conducted by Onofrj et al. (2000) found olanzapine superior to pimozide in terms of tic reduction, sedation, and patient preference. The small sample size limits the clinical import of these findings.

Ziprasidone is a new atypical neuroleptic that, in addition to 5-HT$_2$ and D$_2$ blocking properties, also has 5-HT$_{1A}$ agonist and norepinepherine- and serotonin-reuptake blocking effects that may contribute to its anxiolytic and antidepressant effects. Ziprasidone was evaluated in an 8-week multisite double-blind study in 28 children (ages 7–17) with tic disorder (Sallee et al., 2000b). Children randomized to ziprasidone (increased weekly in 5 mg increments to a mean dose of 28.2 ± 9.6 mg/day in two divided doses) showed an average 35% decrease in tics, significantly better that the 7% improvement in the placebo group. Side effects of ziprasidone included transient sedation, insomnia, and akathisia; there were no significant changes in cardiac conduction and weight gain was comparable to that in the placebo group. Studies of normal volunteers find that ziprasidone increases QTc by 9–14 msec, which is greater than that observed with risperidone, olanzapine, quetiapine, or haloperidol (package insert summary, 2001). Beyond the need for periodic EKG monitoring similar to that recommended above for pimozide, the clinical implications of this finding are unclear.

Marked weight gain is a common problem with both typical and atypical antipsychotics. In a recent review, Taylor and McAskill (2000) rank ordered the available atypical antipsychotics with respect to risk for weight gain as follows: clozapine, olanzapine, risperidone, and ziprasidone. Close monitoring is required in light of the magnitude of the weight gain associated with the atypical agents.

Clarifying the relative merits of the different atypical neuroleptics will require further comparative studies. Ziprasidone appears to have a lesser propensity to induce weight gain, but may have greater propensity to prolong QTc (United States Food and Drug Administration website: http://www.fda.gov/cder/foi/label/2001/20825lbl.pdf). Although there are future plans for a liquid preparation, currently the smallest available capsule size of ziprasidone is 20 mg, making dose adjustment difficult in children.

Dosing

The same general principles apply to adjusting the dosages of the typical and atypical neuroleptics (see above).

Risperidone is typically started at 0.5 mg with similar increments every 5–7 days while monitoring therapeutic response and adverse effects. The typical dose range is 1–3mg in divided doses. There are no data on the appropriate dose range of olanzapine for children and adolescents with TS; beginning with a starting daily dose of 2.5 mg, increasing gradually as needed to up to 10 mg/day seems reasonable in light of the dose range used in childhood-onset schizophrenia (Grothe et al., 2000)

OTHER DOPAMINERGIC MODULATING DRUGS

A variety of other antidopaminergic agents have also been studied in small samples for the control of tics.

Tetrabenazine

Tetrabenazine is a non-neuroleptic that is a weak postsynaptic antagonist of dopamine and depletes presynaptic dopamine vesicles by interfering with reuptake and storage. In the United States, tetrabenazine is currently available only as an investigational drug. It has been studied for the treatment of choreiform movements, Huntington's disease, and, in a small open-label trial, Tourette's syndrome. Of 17 patients with TS treated with the drug, 11 (65%) had a modest decrease in tics, using a crude measure of tic severity (Jankovic and Orman, 1988).

Tiapride and Sulpiride

Tiapride and sulpiride are neuroleptics of the substituted benzamide class. These selective D_2 blockers have weak antipsychotic properties and are not available in the United States, although they are commonly used in Europe for the treatment of tics. In a pair of 6-week controlled trials involving 27 children with TS, at doses ranging from 4 to 6 mg/kg/day, tiapride was superior to placebo and produced a 30%–44% decrease in videotaped tic counts (Eggers et al., 1988).

In an uncontrolled retrospective study of 63 patients with TS, ages 10–68 years, many of whom were on other medications, sulpiride produced a positive response in 60% of subjects (Robertson et al., 1990). The modal daily dose of responders was 400 mg (dose range 200–1000 mg/day). Drowsiness, depression, akathisia, and weight gain were common side effects.

Pergolide

Pergolide is a mixed D_2–D_1 agonist used to increase dopaminergic activity in Parkinson's disease. In lower doses, it is believed to have greater effect on presynaptic D_2 autoreceptors than on postsynaptic receptors, which, ultimately, reduces dopaminergic transmission. In a 6-week open-label trial of pergolide in 32 patients (ages 7–19 years) with TS, three-quarters of subjects reported an improvement of at least 50% in tic severity, at a mean dose of 177 ± 61μg in three divided doses.

Gilbert et al. (2000) studied pergolide in 24 children (ages 7–17 years old) with TS using a 6-week placebo-controlled crossover design. On pergolide (mean dose 200μg, range 150–300μg), children had a significantly greater mean decrease in the total tic severity score on the Yale Global Tic Severity Scale (YGTSS) (38% for pergolide vs. 11% for placebo). There were no differences in side effects between placebo and pergolide. The crossover design makes it difficult to interpret the findings of this study. For example, during the first arm of the study, the mean decrease in tic severity was the same across the two treatment groups.

THE α₂ AGONISTS: CLONIDINE AND GUANFACINE

From the observation that tics were exacerbated by stress, and because cerebrospinal fluid findings suggested possible alterations in central nervous system catecholamine metabolism, Cohen and colleagues (1979) used clonidine in the treatment of TS in what was among the first theory-based treatments for the disorder.

Initially developed as centrally acting antihypertensive agents, clonidine, guanfacine, and related drugs stimulate specific α_2-adrenergic receptors in the brain. At low doses they stimulate presynaptic α_2 adrenergic receptors. Molecular cloning techniques demonstrate at least three subtypes of α_2 receptors, each with distinctive anatomical distribution and functions that may account for the distinctive effects of the various drugs in this class (see Chapter 21.)

By activating presynaptic autoreceptors in brain stem locus ceruleus neurons (where most noradrenergic fibers have their origin), clonidine reduces norepinepherine release and turnover. This inhibitory effect on noradrenergic locus ceruleus neurons, as well as direct effects on thalamic α_{2B} receptors, are most likely responsible for the sedative effects of clonidine (Berridge and Foote, 1991; Buzsaki et al., 1991).

In contrast, guanfacine has only one-tenth the potency of clonidine in inhibiting locus ceruleus–mediated norepinepherine release (Engberg and Eriksson, 1991). As animal studies (Li et al., 1999) suggest, guanfacine appears to have its beneficial effects through direct action on postsynaptic α_{2A} receptors in the prefrontal cortex, with consequent beneficial effects on impulsivity, attention, and working memory (Avery et al., 2000 Arnsten and van Dyck, 1997; Scahill et al., 2001). This selectivity of action appears to account for guanfacine's cognitive enhancing effects while minimizing the sedative and hypotensive effects that are more characteristic of clonidine (Ernsberger et al., 1990; Mao et al., 1999).

Other clinically significant differences between clonidine and guanfacine include guanfacine's longer half-life (12–23 hours, vs. clonidine's 12–16 hours) and the absence of rebound increases in blood pressure, which have been observed following abrupt withdrawal of clonidine (Wilson et al., 1986).

Clonidine

In school-age children, clonidine is usually started at 0.05 mg (half of a 0.01mg tablet) in the morning. If tolerated without difficulty for a few days, an afternoon and then early evening dose can be added. The dosage can be increased in one-quarter to half tablet increments every 3 to 4 days to a total dose of 0.15–0.3 mg day in three or four divided doses. Smaller children may have to start with a quarter tablet. Plasma levels of clonidine peak about 3–5 hours after an oral dose. The acute clinical effect of an oral dose also begins to diminish after about 3–5 hours. The most common side effect is sedation, which is typically most evident 30 to 60 minutes after each dose. Clonidine can also cause depressed mood and/or irritability. Mid-sleep awakening is common. Whether this is due to the drug's sedative effects wearing off or more subtle effects on sleep architecture is not clear.

Although most children do not experience significant changes in pulse or blood pressure on clonidine (Leckman et al., 1991), isolated cases of potentially clonidine-related hyper- or hypotension have been reported (Cantwell et al., 1997). The child's history regarding preexisting heart disease, arrhythmia, or hypotension should be taken before initiating medication. It is prudent to monitor blood pressure and pulse at baseline and during dose adjustment. Acute-onset dizziness or syncope, especially if exercise related, requires closer monitoring or medical consultation. Most studies do not find significant EKG changes in children on clonidine (Leckman et al., 1991; Kofoed et al, 1999), but idiosyncratic changes in EKG have been reported in children on clonidine (Cantwell et al., 1997); most of these affected children were receiving clonidine in combination with methylphenidate and/or other agents. Baseline and follow-up EKG have been recommended in some practice guidelines (American Academy of Child and Adolescent Psychiatry [AACAP]-ADHD guidelines; Cantwell et al., 1997), but not others (Gutgesell et al., 1999). Although blood pressure is generally not a problem with clonidine, patients and families should be educated about the potential for rebound increases in blood pressure, heart rate, tics, and anxiety with abrupt discontinuation or missed doses (Leckman et al., 1986; Cantwell et al., 1997).

Because the smallest tablet size for clonidine is currently 0.1 mg, it may be difficult to adjust the dosage for younger children. In such cases, it is possible to compound an oral liquid preparation that permits more accurate adjustment of pediatric doses (Levinson and Johnson, 1992)

Clonidine is also available as a transdermal patch (Catapres-TTS [transdermal therapeutic system]) that has the advantages of avoiding the need for repeated doses during the day and of reportedly lower rates of dry mouth and drowsiness (Burris, 1993). Steady-state plasma levels are reached within 2–3 days after applying the patch and clonidine concentrations reportedly diminish gradually over 2–3 days following patch removal, without rebound hypertension in adult hypertensives treated with the patch. The patch is available in three sizes, formulated to deliver 0.1, 0.2, or 0.3 mg of clonidine per day. Although the patch can be divided to reduce correspondingly the amount delivered, the manufacturer recommends against cutting the patches, "as careless manipulation may damage the rate-controlling membrane" (P. A. Bowers, Boehringer Ingelheim Pharmaceuticals, personal communication, 1991). Local skin irritation, probably due to the occlusive effects of the patch, occurs in about one-half of patients; a more serious allergic contact dermatitis, with local erythema, induration, and vesiculation, occurs in about 15% of patients on the patch. Such reactions are worrisome, as it appears that the reaction appears to be clonidine-specific and rarely occurs with placebo TTS patches (Bowers, ibid).

Guanfacine

Given its longer-half life, guanfacine usually requires fewer daily doses than clonidine. Treatment is usually begun with 0.5 mg in the morning (0.25 mg in smaller children) and, if tolerated, after 3 or 4 days, adding a second 0.5 mg dose mid-afternoon. Subsequent increases might be made every 3 or 4 days in 0.5 mg increments as tolerated, up to a total daily dose of between 1.5 and 4 mg/day given in three divided doses. Side effects of guanfacine other than initial sedation are typically mild. In the double-blind study by Scahill et al. (2001), these included mild decrease in blood pressure early in treatment, mid-sleep awakening, and constipation. Horrigan and Barnhill (1998) observed hypomanic-like agitation and excitation in 5 out of 95 children receiving guanfacine; the symptoms appeared abruptly within the first week of administration and all 5 of the children were reported to have a personal or family risk factor for bipolar disorder. Increased plasma valproate concentrations, when coadministered with guanfacine, have been reported in two children (Ambrosini and Sheikh, 1998).

Other Tic-Suppressant Agents

Nicotine/mecamylamine

Nicotine chewing gum was reported to be effective in decreasing tics in 8 of 10 children with TS when given in conjunction with ongoing haloperidol treatment (Sanberg et al., 1989). McConville and colleagues (1992) evaluated the effect on tics of 30 minutes of chewing gum containing 2 mg of nicotine. Five patients with TS received the gum alone and 10 patients received the gum in combination with ongoing treatment

with haloperidol. The nicotine gum alone had only a modest effect compared to the combined treatment, but under both conditions improvement was transitory. Furthermore, the bitter taste of the gum and accompanying gastrointestinal symptoms were unpleasant. In two open clinical trials in patients with TS whose tics were inadequately controlled by neuroleptic treatment, Silver and colleagues (Silver et al., 1995, 1996) found that application of a transdermal nicotine patch (7 or 14 mg) for 24 hours produced a substantial decrease in tics that was sustained for 2–3 weeks or longer. Seventy patients whose tics persisted despite an optimal dose of haloperidol were randomly assigned by Silver et al. (2001a) to treatment by addition of either a daily nicotine (7 mg/24 hours) or placebo transdermal patch for 19 days. On the 6th day, haloperidol dosage was reduced by half. Compared to those receiving placebo, those who completed all 19 days of the nicotine patch showed significant improvement on a global scale that included various associated symptoms in addition to tics. However, on the clinician-rated tic severity scales of the YGTSS, significant improvement was largely confined to improvement in motor tics as rated at day 5 while still on an optimal dose of haloperidol. By day 19, the apparent beneficial effects of the nicotine patch on motor and phonic tic severity was no longer evident. These findings suggest that, as with a recent study with baclofen (Kurlan, 2001), patients' reported subjective impression of improvement may have been due to nonspecific psychophysiological effects of the nicotine, rather than to treatment-related changes in tic severity per se. In the nicotine group, the side effects of nausea (71%) and vomiting (40%) were common and several patients had to discontinue the patch after a couple of hours, because of nausea. In an open study, Dursan and Reveley (1997) applied two 10 mg transdermal nicotine patches for 2 consecutive days to five patients with TS, four of whose symptoms were not controlled by haloperidol alone and one who had never been medicated. Tic severity ratings decreased by 50% for up to 4 weeks without side effects, but the decrease was not sustained at 16 weeks.

In two retrospective case studies of 24 child and adult patients, Sanberg et al. (1998) and Silver et al. (2000) reported that mecamylamine (a nicotine antagonist used as an antihypertensive) in doses up to 5 mg daily significantly reduced tic severity in 22 of 24 patients, with many patients also reporting improved mood and irritability, but details of concomitant medication and duration of treatment were unclear. However, an 8 week double-blind, placebo-controlled study of 61 subjects with TS using mecamylamine at up to 7.5 mg/day as a monotherapy found no significant differences between mecamylamine and placebo in tic severity (Silver et al. 2001).

It is speculated that both nicotine and mecamylamine may act via prolonged inactivation of acetylcholinergic nicotinic-receptor subtypes (Young et al., 2001). In the absence of larger series or controlled double-blind studies, however, the effectiveness of nicotinergic agents in augmenting neuroleptic treatment of tics remains unclear.

Androgen modification

The higher prevalence of tics in males and the exacerbating effects of anabolic steroids suggested the possibility that manipulation of steroid hormones might be helpful in the treatment of TS. Despite some promising case studies (Peterson et al., 1994), however, a double-blind, placebo-controlled, crossover study of the androgen receptor blocker flutamide, in 13 adults with TS, failed to find significant benefits (Peterson et al., 1998).

Botulinum

Given the successful use of botulinum in the treatment of dystonia, injections of dilute botulinum toxin have been studied in several open trials (reviewed by Kwak et al., 2000) and in one randomized double blind study with TS patients (Marras et al., 2001). Jankovic and colleagues treated 45 patients (age range 8 to 69 years) with TS in two open-label studies (Jankovic, 1994; Kwak, et al., 2000). Thirty-nine of the 45 patients reported at least moderate improvement; the duration of maximum benefit was 12.3 ± 10.7 weeks, with a mean number of 3.3 ± 3.6 visits. Of the subgroup of 30 patients who described the presence of premonitory urges, 26 reported marked improvement in their tics and the associated premonitory urge. In most cases, the benefit was limited to the anatomical area of the injection. The most common side effects were neck weakness, ptosis, and mild transient dysphagia. Injection appeared to be most effective for eyelid and vocal tics. Direct injection of the vocal cords was reported to be effective in three cases reports of severe vocal tics, but was also accompanied by the side effect of hypophonia (see Kwak et al., 2000).

In an open trial, Awaad (1999) treated 186 children (133 boys, 53 girls) with intramuscular botulinum toxin. Injections were administered every 6–9 months, except in 23 patients who received injections after 13–19 months of sustained improvement. As rated on the YGTSS and by blinded tic counts from videotape samples, 35 (18.8%) of subjects "experienced complete

control of their motor tics, but less significant improvement in their vocal tics" (p. 318). The report did not distinguish between tics involving the muscle groups injected and other motor tics. Four patients whose vocal cords were injected experienced a 30% reduction in tics. The most common side effects were soreness, transient neck weakness, and ptosis.

A randomized, double-blind, placebo-controlled crossover trial of botulinum toxin for the treatment of simple motor tics was conducted in 20 patients, ages 15–55, 18 of whom completed the study (Marras et al., 2001); (Table 40.2). As rated blindly on a 12-minute videotape sample, the proportional change in treated tics per minute was −39% during the botulinum toxin phase in contrast to an increase of +5.8% during the placebo phase. Half of the patients noted weakness of the injected muscles that was not functionally disabling, Two patients reported inner restlessness, accompanied by an increased urge to perform the treated tic. Two others felt that the decrease in the treated tic prompted a new "replacement" tic. Despite improvement in the treated tic, there was no significant evidence of overall improvement.

Taken together, these studies suggest that botulinum toxin injection may be useful for ameliorating specific severe or impairing tics, but does not produce overall improvement of tics at untreated sites.

Baclofen

Baclofen, a muscle relaxant that influences GABA neurotransmission, has been studied in one large open trial (Awaad, 1999) and one small double-blind placebo-controlled trial in 10 children with TS (Singer et al., 2001). In the open-label trial, Awaad (1999) treated 264 children with TS (198 boys, 66 girls) with 10 mg/day of baclofen, increased by weekly increments of 10 mg/day until improvement was noted or side effects appeared. At a mean dose of 30 mg/day (range 10–80 mg/day), 250 subjects (95%) had significant decrease in motor and vocal tics as measured by the YGTSS "within 1–2 weeks." However, the report did not provide baseline or follow-up scores on the YGTSS, making it impossible to compare these results with other studies. The most common side effect was sedation.

Singer et al. (2001) treated 10 children, ages 8–14 years, with baclofen (20 mg, tid) in a randomized-sequence double-blind, placebo-controlled, crossover study. The mean improvement in tic severity as measured by the YGTSS total tic score was 14% for baclofen, compared with 7% worsening for placebo. This difference was not significant. When the authors evaluated the Impairment scale of the YGTSS, however,

TABLE 40.2 *Controlled Studies with Non-antipsychotic Agents for Tic Reduction*

Medication	Reference	Patients (n)	Design	Dose Range	Improvement (%)
Baclofen	Singer et al., 2001	9	Crossover	60 mg	15.1%[a]
Botulinum toxin	Marras et al, 2001	20	Crossover	N/A	39%[b]
Clonidine	Leckman et al., 1991	40	Parallel	0.03–.06 mg/kg	35[c]
Pergolide	Gilbert et al., 2000	24	Crossover	150–300 mg	35[c]

[a]Based on clinician measure, change in tic severity subscale was not significant.
[b]Based on tic counts
[c]Based on clinician measure

there was a significant difference between groups, with baclofen being superior to placebo. Because this scale measures the impact of tics on the person's life, rather than tic severity per se, it is difficult to interpret over the course of a brief clinical trial (Scahill et al., 1999; Kurlan, 2001). In this trial, it is simply unclear what aspect of the subjects' functioning actually improved on baclofen.

Other agents

Small open-label pilot studies or challenge studies have been reported for the treatment of tics with various agents such as topiramate (Abuzzahab and Brown, 2001), levodopa (Black and Mink, 2000), low-dose naloxone (van Wattum et al., 2000), donepezil (Hoopes, 1999), cyproterone (Izmir and Dursun, 1999), and ondansetron (Toren et al., 1999). The safety and effectiveness of the chronic use of these agents, especially in children, requires more systematic studies.

General Treatment Approach to Tic Symptoms

In children for whom the primary focus of treatment is mild tics, and in whom a decision has been made to proceed with medication treatment, our general approach is to begin with guanfacine or clonidine (in that order), especially if there is concurrent ADHD symptomatology. Although these agents are less potent than the neuroleptics, they have fewer known worrisome side effects. In children whose tics are not adequately controlled by an α-adrenergic agent, our next choice would be to begin a low dose of a neuroleptic, with the choice between the available agents determined by the degree of concern regarding potential side effects (e.g., potential QTc prolongation with pimozide and ziprasidone; excess weight gain on risperidone or olanzapine; neurological side effects with haloperidol). On balance, we probably would start with risperidone in

most cases. It is sometimes necessary to try two or three neuroleptics before finding an agent that is effective for tics at a tolerable level of side effects. As discussed above, both upward and downward adjustments should be made gradually, bearing in mind the natural fluctuation of tics and the problem of rebound tic exacerbations. If no neuroleptic provides sufficient relief from tics at a tolerable level of side effects, there are several options: brief application of a nicotine patch, pergolide, or in the case of specific troublesome focal tics, botulinum injection. (In the United States, tiapride, sulpiride, and tetrabenazine are not available.) The efficacy and indications for baclofen and mecamylamine remain unclear because of the small number of subjects studied systematically to date.

In light of the potential serious side effects of long-term neuroleptic treatment, how long children should remain on such agents for treatment of tics is an important unanswered question. Rapid fluctuations in dosage risk enhancing receptor sensitivity and rebound exacerbations. Only one controlled study has attempted to evaluate the long-term effectiveness of chronic neuroleptic therapy in children with TS (Tourette Syndrome Study Group, 1999). Ten children who had been on pimozide for at least 3 months were randomly assigned to placebo substitution or maintenance therapy with pimozide. The medication taper was carried out over a 2-week period, a relatively rapid discontinuation. Tic symptoms recurred within 1 month after randomization (mean = 37 days), with three of the four subjects randomized to placebo experiencing symptom relapse. Children in the long-term pimozide group maintained tic control for an average of 231 days, with only 1 of 6 subjects dropping out prior to the 2-month mark. The relatively rapid pace of discontinuation may have increased the likelihood of relapse. Thus, in the absence of guidance from large-scale controlled studies concerning the duration of neuroleptic treatment in TS, it is appropriate on an annual basis to consider dose reduction if tics are stable. If a small dose reduction does not produce a recrudescence of tic symptoms after a few weeks, it may be worth considering further reduction.

In addition to pharmacological interventions for severe tics, individual and family psychotherapeutic interventions and school consultation are essential to address the various stresses the child may be experiencing, as these can be major exacerbants of tics. Habit reversal techniques may also be use for specific troublesome tics (King et al., 1999b).

Although stereotaxic neurosurgery has been used in some adults with intractably severe tic disorder (Babel et al., 2001), it is hard to justify its consideration in children, given the usual trend toward improvement of tics in later adolescence (Peterson and Leckman, 1998).

PHARMACOLOGICAL TREATMENT OF ATTENTION-DEFICIT HYPERACTIVITY DISORDER IN INDIVIDUALS WITH TOURETTE'S SYNDROME

The ADHD symptoms accompanying TS are often a greater source of impairment for children than tic symptoms per se (Stokes et al., 1991). Given the high rates of comorbid ADHD in children with tic disorder, the treatment of ADHD symptoms in the context of tics represents a common therapeutic challenge.

Stimulants and Tic Disorder

The use of stimulant drugs in children with personal or family histories of tics has been a topic of considerable controversy. The de novo onset or worsening of tics following stimulants has been noted in several case reports and retrospective case series (Lowe et al., 1982; Erenberg et al. 1985; Lipkin et al., 1994; Varley et al., 2001) and in prospective or placebo-controlled studies that excluded children with tics at baseline (Borcherding et al., 1990, Barkley et al., 1992).

Gadow et al. (1995), however, found no increase in tics in a placebo-controlled trial of methylphenidate in children with ADHD and a tic disorder. Other trials of stimulants in such children have found little or no *average* increase in tic severity scores, but clinically significant increases of tics in a handful of subjects severe enough to prompt discontinuation of the stimulant (Castellanos et al., 1997; Law and Schachar, 1999) or to require addition of a medication to control their tic symptoms (Gadow et al., 1999). A multicenter, double-blind, placebo-controlled, parallel group study of methylphenidate and clonidine, used alone or in combination in 136 children with ADHD and a comorbid chronic tic disorder, reported that clonidine and methylphenidate were superior to placebo for ADHD symptoms. Moreover, the combined use of methylphenidate and clonidine produced the greatest level of improvement in ADHD symptoms. There were no serious side effects associated with the combination. The proportion of subjects who reported an increase of tics was no greater among those receiving methylphenidate (20%) than among those on clonidine alone (26%) or placebo (22%); the worsening of tics however, limited upward adjustment in the dose of methylphenidate in a third of these subjects (Tourette's Syndrome Study Group, 2002). On balance, then, although many children can tolerate stimulant medication without exacerbation of preexisting tics, a subgroup of children do exhibit an unacceptable tic exacerbation or de novo tics in response to stimulant treatment.

Nonstimulant Alternatives for Treatment of Combined attention-deficit hyperactivity disorder and tic disorder

α-Adrenergic Agents: Clonidine and Guanfacine

The α-adrenergic agents clonidine or guanfacine may be useful alternatives or adjuncts to stimulants in children with combined ADHD and tics. Clonidine can be helpful in diminishing hyperactivity and impulsivity in children with TS, although clonidine-induced sedation can itself be an iatrogenic cause of irritability. In a double-blind, placebo-controlled withdrawal trial in 10 children with tic disorders and ADHD, a 37% increase in core ADHD symptoms was observed following withdrawal from clonidine (Hunt et al., 1985). In a 3-month randomly assigned open-label trial in 24 subjects with ADHD plus aggressive oppositional defiant or conduct disorder, equal numbers of subjects were assigned to either clonidine alone, clonidine plus methylphenidate, or methylphenidate alone (Connor et al., 2000). All groups showed improvement in ADHD symptoms. In a placebo-controlled trial in children with tic disorder, clonidine produced a significant 39% reduction in the Conners impulsivity/hyperactivity factor score (compared to none in the placebo group, Leckman et al., 1991).

A recent 8-week placebo-controlled study of guanfacine in 34 children (ages 7–14 years) with a mild to moderate tic disorder and ADHD found guanfacine significantly superior to placebo in reducing the core symptoms of ADHD, as evidenced by a 36% decrease in scores on teacher rating scales, compared to an 8% decrease for the placebo group. This difference was evident both for the inattentive and hyperactive/impulsive subscales as well as the total score. In addition, guanfacine was associated with decreased continuous performance test errors and improved Clinical Global Improvement Scale ratings (Scahill et al., 2001). No EKG changes and only transient changes in blood pressure and pulse were noted in a few children on guanfacine; one subject withdrew because of sedation. The medication was started at 0.5 mg at bedtime, with increases in 0.5 mg increments every 4 days to a maximum of 3.0 mg/day in three divided doses. In this sample of children with mild tics, there was a 30% decrease in the total tic score of the YGTSS, compared to no change on placebo.

On the basis of relatively limited empirical data, stimulants are now widely prescribed to children with ADHD (with or without tics) in combination with guanfacine, clonidine, or other agents. Reports of the death of four children who had been prescribed clonidine and methylphenidate raised questions about the safety of this combination (Popper, 1995). Although careful review suggested that neither drug alone nor the combination was responsible, it is clear that further studies of the safety and efficacy of such combinations are needed (Swanson et al., 1999; Wilens and Spencer, 1999a, b). It is troubling that despite the absence of such studies (other than the recent Tourette's Syndrome Study Group study, 2002), such combinations are being prescribed to very large numbers of children (Jensen et al., 1999).

Other nonstimulant alternatives

Other alternatives to the stimulants that have been studied for treatment of ADHD in children and adults include the tricyclic antidepressants desipramine and nortriptyline; the newer antidepressants bupropion, venlafaxine, and atomoxetine; the beta-blocker pindolol; and the selective monoamine oxidase inhibitor, deprenyl. Across these agents, the number of controlled studies varies from none (nortriptyline) to four (bupropion). Only deprenyl and desipramine have been studied in children with ADHD and tic disorders.

Desipramine. Singer et al., (1995) compared clonidine (0.05–0.2 mg/day) and desipramine (25–100 mg/day) in a double-blind, placebo-controlled crossover study in 37 children (ages 7–13 years old) with combined ADHD and TS. Desipramine produced a significant improvement in ADHD outcome measures and was superior to placebo. Clonidine was not different

from placebo. Desipramine did not increase tic severity and clonidine did not diminish it.

Biederman et al. (1989a,b) also found desipramine (at the relatively high mean dose of 4.6 mg/kg/day) to be safe and effective for treatment of ADD. Despite these positive results, however, concerns about prolonged cardiac conduction times and the reports of several sudden deaths of children on desipramine have left many clinicians and parents reluctant to use the drug (Riddle, et al., 1993). Another less well–studied tricyclic, nortriptyline, which some believe to have less potential cardiotoxicity, has shown promise in a retrospective study in children with ADHD plus tic disorder (Spencer et al., 1993b).

Buproprion. Buproprion has been studied in four controlled studies. In one study, buproprion, in doses ranging from 50 to 200 mg/day in divided doses, was generally well tolerated and produced an improvement of 30%–50% on teacher and parent ADHD rating scales, comparable in effect to methylphenidate (Barrickman et al., 1995) and superior to placebo (Conners et al., 1996). However, buproprion, especially in high doses, has been associated with seizures in children, and Conners et al. (1996) noted drug-related electroencephalographic (EEG) changes in a few children. Case reports have also suggested that bupropion may accentuate tic symptoms (Spencer et al. 1993a).

Pindolol. The antihypertensive beta-blocker pindolol was studied in 32 subjects in a crossover study comparing pindolol (20 mg, twice daily), methylphenidate, and placebo (Buitelaar et al., 1996). Pindolol significantly reduced ADHD symptoms, but two subjects developed nightmares and hallucinations on the medication. Because lower doses were not examined in this study, it is possible that lower doses may be effective and better tolerated.

Deprenyl. Deprenyl, a selective monoamine oxidase B inhibitor that enhances dopaminergic function, is used in the treatment of Parkinson's disease. An open-label study (Jankovic et al., 1994) suggested that deprenyl could be effective for the treatment of ADHD in children with TS. A placebo-controlled crossover study (Feigin et al., 1996) of 24 subjects with ADHD and a tic disorder found that deprenyl was safe and effective at doses ranging from 5 to 10 mg/day. Only one subject showed an increase in tics. Interpretation of these results, however, is hampered by the clear evidence of an order effect. Subjects who received active drug first showed a 37% improvement in ADHD symptoms, but those who received deprenyl in the second arm of the study showed no improvement. At low doses (5–10 mg/day), deprenyl does not require dietary restrictions. However, data on drug interaction in non-Parkinson populations are limited.

The mechanism of deprenyl's action is unclear. In addition to enhancing dopaminergic activity in the brain by inhibiting dopamine degradation, deprenyl is metabolized into various stimulant metabolites. In spontaneously hyperactive rats used in an animal model of ADHD, chronic deprenyl administration improved impulsivity (but not hyperactivity or attention) along with altering levels of noradrenaline, dopamine, and serotonin and their metabolites (Boix et al., 1998).

General Approach to Pharmacotherapy of Attention-Deficit Hyperactivity Disorder Symptoms in Children with Tourette's Syndrome

The approach to treatment planning for ADHD in a child with a tic disorder entails a careful discussion of the alternatives with the family. Although recent data show that stimulants can be well tolerated and effective in many children with tics, there is a risk that tics may flare up following exposure to a stimulant. The available evidence clearly indicates nonetheless that stimulants are the most effective medications for ADHD. Presented with these pros and cons, many families are able to express a clear preference, often based on which symptoms have been most problematic for the child. We usually select from stimulants or the α-2 agonists, with guanfacine being our preference over clonidine for ADHD. The more difficult clinical situation is the child with prominent ADHD and a history of positive response to a stimulant followed by an exacerbation of tics. In these cases, we discuss with parents the possibility of combined treatment. For example, we might start with guanfacine and evaluate the response in the domains of ADHD and tics. We might then add low doses of methylphenidate in an effort to boost the effect of guanfacine while remaining at stimulant dose levels that may be less likely to induce an increase in tics. It is of course essential to remind parents that this clinically derived strategy has not been formally evaluated.

PHARMACOLOGICAL TREATMENT OF OBSESSIVE-COMPULSIVE DISORDER IN INDIVIDUALS WITH CHRONIC TIC DISORDER

For a general consideration of the pharmacotherapy of childhood OCD, see the related chapter by Daniel Geller (Chapter 39), as well as King et al. (1998) and Grados et al. (1999).

Tic-related forms of OCD differ from cases of OCD without personal or family history of tics in terms of phenomenology, genetic and neurobiological features, and treatment response (Miguel et al., 2001). Compared to non-tic related OCD, tic-related OCD appears to have a male preponderance, earlier onset, and a predominance of obsessions and compulsions concerning (1) aggression, sex, and religion; and (2) need for symmetry or exactness and compulsions involving repeating, counting, and ordering or arranging (King et al., 1999a); in addition, tic-related compulsions are more likely to be associated with "just-right" phenomena and urges, rather than anxiety.

Studies of the use of the specific serotonin-uptake inhibitors (SSRIs) to treat OCD suggest that, compared to non–tic-related OCD, tic-related OCD is less responsive to SSRI monotherapy (McDougle et al., 1993, 1994). Addition of a neuroleptic, such as haloperidol (McDougle et al., 1994), risperidone (McDougle et al., 2000), or olanzapine (Bogetto et al., 2000), appears to be useful in improving treatment-resistant individuals' response to a SSRI. It is unclear whether this pattern of treatment response is specifically associated with a comorbid tic disorder; the pattern of obsessive compulsive symptoms characteristic of TS; or yet some other predictors.

Although there are a variety of case reports regarding the use of the SSRIs in children with combined tic disorder and OCD (e.g., Wehr and Namerow, 2001), comorbid TS has been an exclusionary criteria for many of the double-blind controlled studies of SSRIs in childhood OCD. Only a few systematic studies have looked at the use of these agents in children with TS (Riddle et al., 1988, 1990; Kurlan et al., 1993; Scahill et al., 1997). In general, the SSRIs are well tolerated in children with TS, with the most common troublesome side effect, as with other children, being behavioral activation (Riddle et al., 1991). Although tic exacerbations or de novo tics have been reported in association with SSRI administration (Delgado et al., 1990; Fennig et al, 1994), this is relatively uncommon; in a double-blind, placebo-controlled study of fluoxetine in children with TS, overall tic severity was not affected (Scahill et al., 1997), although one subject experienced a dramatic increase in tics at 20 mg daily. More systematic studies are needed to clarify the treatment responsivity to the various SSRIs of the different obsessive-compulsive symptom factors in children with TS-related OCD and the indications, efficacy, and safety of neuroleptic augmentation.

CONCLUSION

The treatment of chronic tic disorder remains a clinical challenge that requires thoughtful prioritizing of the symptoms to be addressed, vigilance in watching for potential side effects, a clinical feel for the natural history of the disorder, and patience and caution in the choice and adjustment of medication. Because of the prevelance of comorbid psychopathology, polypharmacy is common. With all the attendant hazards of side effects and unpredictable interactions, careful periodic review of the number and dosages of agents used is essential. Attention to the quality of the child's functioning in school, at home, and with peers is also necessary to have an accurate picture of the sources of impairment (e.g., the tics per se, compulsion, impulsivity, inattention, sedation or agitation secondary to medication, learning disabilities) and to minimize stressors that may exacerbate tics and other symptoms. Given the changing pattern, severity, and impact of symptoms over the childhood years, optimal treatment requires an ongoing relationship with the child and family that can address the neurological and psychosocial vicissitudes of the disorder over the course of development (Leckman et al., 1999).

REFERENCES

Abuzzahab, F.S. and Brown VL. (2001) Control of Tourette's syndrome with topiramate. *Am J Psychiatry* 158:968.

Ambrosini, P.J. and Sheikh, R.M. (1998) Increased plasma valproate concentrations when coadministered with guanfacine. *J Child Adolesc Psychopharmacol* 8:143–147.

Apter, A., Pauls, D.L., Bleich, A., Zohar, A.H., Kron, S., Ratzoni, G., Dycian, A., Kotler, M., Weizman, A., Gadot, N., and Cohen, D.J. (1993) An epidemiological study of Gilles de la Tourette's syndrome in Israel. *Arch Gen Psychiatry* 50:734–738.

Arnsten, A.F.T. and van Dyck, C.H. (1997) Monoamine and acetylcholine influences on higher cognitive functions in nonhuman primates: relevance to the treatment of Alzheimer's disease. In: Brioni, J.D. and Decker, M.W., eds. *Pharmacological Treatment of Alzheimer's Disease*: Molecular and Neurobiological Foundations. New York: John Wiley & Sons, pp. 63–86.

Avery, R., Franowicz, J.C.S., Studholme C., van Dyck C.H., and Arnsten, A.F.T. (2000) The alpha-2A adrenoceptor agonist, guanfacine, increases regional cerebral blood flow in dorsolateral prefrontal cortex and improves accuracy in monkeys performing a spatial working memory task. *Neuropsychopharmacology* 23:240–249.

Awaad Y. (1999) Tics in Tourette syndrome: new treatment options. *J Child Neurol.* 14:316–319.

Babel, T.B., Warnke, P.C. and Ostertag, C.B. (2001) Immediate and long-term outcome after infrathalamic and thalamic lesioning for intractable Tourette's syndrome. *J Neurol Neurosurg Psychiatry* 70:666–671.

Barkley, R.A., McMurray, M.B., Edelbrock, C.S., and Robbins, K. (1992) Side effects of methylphenidate in children with attention deficit hyperactivity disorder: a systemic, placebo-controlled evaluation. *Pediatrics* 86:184–192.

Barrickman, L., Perry, P., Allen, A., Kuperman, S., Arndt, S., Herrmann, K., and Schumacher, E. (1995) Buproprion versus methylphenidate in the treatment of attention-deficit hyperactivity disorder. *J Am Acad Child Adolesc Psychiatry* 34: 649–657.

Berridge, C.W., and Foote, S.L. (1991) Effects of locus coeruleus activation on electroencephalographic activity in neocortex and hippocampus. *J Neurosci* 11:3135–3145.

Bhadrinath, B.R. (1998) Olanzapine in Tourette syndrome [letter]. *Br J Psychiatry* 172:366.

Biederman, J., Baldessarini, R.J., Wright, V., Knee, D., and Harmatz, J.S. (1989a) A double-blind placebo controlled study of desipramine in the treatment of ADD: I. Efficacy. *J Am Acad Child Adolesc Psychiatry* 28:777–784.

Biederman, J., Baldessarini, R.J., Wright, V., Knee, D., Harmatz, J.S., and Goldblatt, A. (1989b) A double-blind placebo controlled study of desipramine in the treatment of ADD: II. Serum drug levels and cardiovascular findings. *J Am Acad Child Adolesc Psychiatry* 28:903–911.

Black, K.J. and Mink, J.W. (2000) Response to levodopa challenge in Tourette syndrome. *Mov Disord* 15:1194–1198.

Bogetto, F., Bellino, S., Vaschetto, P., and Ziero, S. (2000) Olanzapine augmentation of fluvoxamine-refractory obsessive-compulsive disorder (OCD): a 12-week open trial. *Psychiatry Res* 96:91–98.

Boix, F. Qiao, S.W., Kolpus, T., and Sagvolden, T., (1998) Chronic L-deprenyl treatment alters brain monoamine levels and reduces impulsiveness in an animal model of attention-deficit/hyperactivity disorder. *Behav Brain Res* 94:153–62.

Borcherding, B.G., Keysor, C.S., Rapoport, J.L., Elia, J., and Amass, J. (1990) Motor/vocal tics and compulsive behaviors on stimulant drugs: is there a common vulnerability? *Psychiatry Res* 33:83–94.

Borison, R.L., Ang, L., Chang, S., Dysken, M., Comaty, J.E. and Davis, J.M. (1982) New pharmacological approaches in the treatment of Tourette syndrome. *Adv Neurol* 35:377–382.

Bruggeman, R., van der Linden, C., Buitelaar, J.K., Gericke, G.S., Hawkridge, S.M., and Temlett, J.A. (2001) Risperidone versus pimozide in Tourette's disorder: a comparative double-blind parallel-group study. *J Clin Psychiatry* 62:50–56.

Bruun, R.D. (1998) Subtle and underrecognized side effects of neuroleptic treatment in children with Tourette's disorder. *Am J Psychiatry* 145:621–624.

Bruun, R.D., and Budman, C.L. (1996) Risperidone as a treatment for Tourette's syndrome. *J Clin Psychiatry* 57:29–31.

Budman, C.L., Gayer, A., Lesser, M., Shi, Q., and Bruun, R.D. (2001) An open-label study of the treatment efficacy of olanzapine for Tourette's disorder. *J Clin Psychiatry* 62:290–294.

Buitelaar, J.K., Van der Gaag, R.J., Swaab-Barneveld, H., and Kuiper, M. (1996) Pindolol and methylphenidate in children with attention-deficit hyperactivity disorder. Clinical efficacy and side-effects. *J Child Psychol Psychiatry* 37:587–595.

Burris, J.F., (1993) The USA experience with the clonidine transdermal therapeutic system. *Clin Auton Res* 3:391–396.

Buzsaki, G., Kennedy, B., Solt, V.B., and Ziegler, M. (1991) Noradrenergic control of thalamic oscillation: the role of α-2 receptors. *Eur J Neurol* 3:222–229.

Caine, E.D., Polinsky, R.J., Kartzinel, R., and Ebert, M.H. (1979) The trial use of clozapine for abnormal involuntary disorders. *Am J Psychiatry* 136:317–320.

Cantwell, D.P., Swanson, J., and Connor, D.F. (1997) Case study: adverse response to clonidine. *J Am Acad Child Adolesc Psychiatry* 36:539–544.

Castellanos, F.X., Giedd, J.N., Elia, J., Marsh, W.L., Ritchie, G.F., Hamburger, S.D., and Rapoport, J.L. (1997) Controlled stimulant treatment of ADHD and comorbid Tourette's syndrome: effects of stimulants and dose. *J Am Acad Child Adolesc Psychiatry* 36: 589–596.

Chappell, P., Riddle, M., Anderson, G., Scahill, L., Hardin, M., Walker, D., Cohen, D., and Leckman, J. (1994) Enhanced stress responsivity of Tourette syndrome patients undergoing lumbar puncture. *Biol Psychiatry* 36:35–43.

Chappell, P.B., Scahill, L.D., and Leckman, J.F. (1997) Future therapies of Tourette syndrome. *Neurol Clin* 15:429–50.

Cohen, D.J., Young, J.G., Nathanson, J.A., and Shaywitz, B.A. (1979) Clonidine in Tourette's syndrome. *Lancet* 2:551–553.

Comings, D.E. and Comings, B.G. (1987) A controlled study of Tourette's syndrome. *Am J Hum Genet* 41:407–866.

Conners, C.K., Casat, C.D., Gualtieri, C.T., Weller, E., Reader, M., Reiss, A., Weller R.A., Khayrallah, M., and Ascher, J. (1996) Bupropion hydrochloride in attention deficit disorder with hyperactivity. *J Am Acad Child Adolesc Psychiatry* 34:1314–1321.

Connor, D.F., Barkely, R.A., and Davis, H.T. (2000) A pilot study of methylphenidate, clonidine, or the combination in ADHD comorbid with aggressive oppositional defiant or conduct disorder. *Clin Pediatr* 39:15–25.

Delgado, P.L., Goodman, W.K., Price, L.H., Heninger, G.R., and Charney, D.S. (1990) Fluvoxamine/pimozide treatment of concurrent Tourette's and obsessive-compulsive disorder. *Br J Psychiatry* 157:762–765.

Desta, Z., Kerbusch, T., and Flockhart, D.A. (1999) Effect of clarithromycin on the pharmacokinetics and pharmacodynamics of pimozide in healthy poor and extensive metabolizers of cytochrome P450 2D6 (CYP2D6). *Clin Pharmacol Ther* 65:10–20.

Dursun, S.M., and Reveley, M.A. (1997) Differential effects of transdermal nicotine on microstructural analyses of tics in Tourette's syndrome: an open study. *Psycholo Med* 27:483–487.

Eggers, C.H., Rothenberger, A., and Berghaus, U. (1988) Clinical and neurobiological findings in children suffering from tic disease following treatment with tiapride. *Eur Arch Psychiatry Neurol Sci* 237:223–229.

Engberg, G., and Eriksson, E. (1991) Effects of a-2-adrenoceptor agonists on locus coeruleus firing rate and brain noradrenaline turnover in EEDQ-treated rats. *Naunyn Schmiedebergs Arch Pharmacol* 343:472–477.

Erenberg, G., Cruse, R.P., and Rothner, A.D. (1985) Gilles de la Tourette's syndrome: effects of stimulant drugs. *Neurology* 35: 1346–1348.

Ernsberger, P., Giuliano, R., Willette, R.N., Reis, D.J. (1990) Role of imidazole receptors in the vasodepressor response to clonidine analogs in the rostral ventrolateral medulla. *J Pharmacol Exp Ther* 253:408–418.

Feigin, A., Kurlan, R., McDermott, M.P., Beach, J., Dimitsapulos, T., Brower, C.A., Chapieski, L., Trinidad, K., Como, P., and Jankovic, J. (1996) A controlled trial of deprenyl in children with Tourette's syndrome and attention deficit hyperactivity disorder. *Neurology* 46:965–968.

Fennig, S., Naisberg, Fennig, S., Pato, M., and Weitzman, A. (1994) Emergence of symptoms of Tourette's syndrome during fluvoxamine treatment of obsessive-compulsive disorder. *Br J Psychiatry* 164:839–841.

Flockhart, D.A., Drici, M.D., Kerbusch, T., Soukhova, N., Richard, E., Pearle, P.L., Mahal, S.K., and Babb, V.J. (2000) Studies on the mechanism of a fatal clarithromycin-pimozide interaction in a patient with Tourette syndrome. *J Clin Psychopharmacol* 20:317–24.

Gadow, K.D., Sverd, J., Sprafkin, J., Nolan, E.E., and Ezor, S.N. (1995) Efficacy of methylphenidate for attention-deficit hyperactivity disorder in children with tic disorder. *Arch Gen Psychiatry* 52:444–455.

Gadow, K.D., Sverd, J., Sprafkin, J., Nolan, E.E., and Grossman, S. (1999) Long-term methylphenidate therapy in children with comorbid attention-deficit hyperactivity disorder and chronic multiple tic disorder. *Arch Gen Psychiatry* 56:330–336.

Gilbert, D.L., Sethuraman, G., Sine, L., Peters, S., and Sallee, F.R. (2000) Tourette's syndrome improvement with pergolide in a randomized, double-blind, crossover trial. *Neurology* 54:1310–1315.

Goetz, C.G., Tanner, C.M., and Klawans, H.L. (1984) Fluphenazine and multifocal tic disorders. *Arch Neurol* 41:271–272.

Golden, G.S. (1985) Tardive dyskinesia in Tourette syndrome. *Pediatr Neurol* 1:192–194.

Grados, M., Scahill, L., and Riddle, M.A. (1999) Pharmacotherapy in children and adolescents with obsessive-compulsive disorder. *Child Adolesc Psychiatry Clin North Am* 8:617–634.

Grothe, D.R., Calis, K.A., Jacobsen, L., Kumra, S., DeVane, C.L., Rapoport, J.L., Bergstrom, R.F., and Kurtz, D.L. (2000) Olanzapine pharmacokinetics in pediatric and adolescent inpatients with childhood-onset schizophrenia. *J Clin Psychopharmacol.* 20: 220–225.

Gutgesell, H., Atkins, D., Barst, R., Buck, M., Franklin, W., Humes, R., Ringel, R., Shaddy, R., and Taubert, K. (1999) Cardiovascular monitoring of children and adolescents receiving psychotropic drugs. *Circulation* 99:979–982.

Hoopes, S.P. (1999) Donepezil for Tourette's disorder and ADHD. *J Clin Psychopharmacol* 19:381–382.

Horrigan, J.P. and Barnhill, J. (1998) Does guanfacine trigger mania in children? *J Child Adolesc Psychopharmacol* 8:149–150.

Hunt, R.D., Minderaa, R.B., and Cohen, D.J. (1985) Clonidine benefits children with attention-deficit disorder and hyperactivity: report of a double-blind placebo-crossover therapeutic trial. *J Am Acad Child Adolesc Psychiatry* 24:617–629.

Izmir, M. and Dursun, S.M. (1999) Cyproterone acetate treatment of Tourette's syndrome. *Can J Psychiatry* 44:710–711.

Jankovic, J. (1994) Botulinum toxin in the treatment of dystonic tics. *Mov Disord* 9:347–349.

Jankovic, J. (1993) Deprenyl in attention deficit associated with Tourette's syndrome. *Arch Neurology* 50:286–288.

Jankovic, J. and Orman, J. (1988) Tetrabenazine therapy of dystonia, chorea, tics, and other dyskinesias. *Neurology* 38:391–394.

Jensen, P.S., Bhatara, V.S., Vitiello, B., Hoagwood, K., Feil, M., and Burke, L.B. (1999) Psychoactive medication prescribing practices for U.S. children: gaps between research and clinical practice. *J Am Acad Child Adolesc Psychiatry* 38:557–565.

Kelly, D.L., Conley, R.C., Love, R.C., Horn D.S., and Ushchak, C.M. (1998) Weight gain in adolescents treated with risperidone and conventional antipsychotics over sixth months. *J Child Adolesc Psychopharmacol* 8:151–159.

King, R.A., Leckman, J., and Scahill, L. (1999a) Associated forms of psychopathology: obsessive-compulsive disorder, anxiety, and depression. In: Leckman, J.F. and Cohen, D.J., eds. *Tourette's Syndrome—Tics, Obsessions, Compulsions: Developmental Psychopathology and Clinical Care.* New York: John Wiley and Sons, pp. 43–62.

King, R.A., Leonard, H., and March, J. (1998) Practice parameters on the assessment and treatment of children with obsessive compulsive disorder. *J Am Acad Child Adolesc Psychiatry* 37(Suppl): 27S–45S.

King, R.A., Scahill, L., and Findley D. (1999b) Psychosocial and behavioral treatments in Tourette's syndrome. In: Leckman, J.F. and

Cohen, D.J., eds. *Tourette's Syndrome—Tics, Obsessions, Compulsions: Developmental Psychopathology and Clinical Care.* New York: John Wiley and Sons, pp. 338–359.

Kofoed, L., Tadepalli, G., Oesterheld, J.R., Awadallah, S., and Shapiro, R. (1999) Case series: clonidine has no systematic effects on PR or QTc intervals in children. *J Am Acad Child Adolesc Psychiatry* 38:1193–1196.

Kurlan, R. (2001) New treatments for tics? *Neurology* 56:580–581.

Kurlan, R., Como, P.G., Deeley, C., McDermott, M., and McDermott, M.P. (1993) A pilot-controlled study of fluoxetine for obsessive-compulsive symptoms in children with Tourette's syndrome. *Clin Neuropharmacol* 16:167–172.

Kwak, C.H., Hanna, P.A., and Jankovic, J. (2000) Botulinum toxin in the treatment of tics. *Arch Neurol* 57:1190–1193.

Law, S.F. and Schachar, R.J. (1999) Do typical clinical doses of methylphenidate cause tics in children treated for attention-deficit hyperactivity disorder? *J Am Acad Child Adolesc Psychiatry* 38: 944–951.

Leckman, J.F., Hardin, M.T., Riddle, M.A., Stevenson, J., Ort, S.I., and Cohen, D.J. (1991) Clonidine treatment of Gilles de la Tourette's syndrome. *Arch Gen Psychiatry* 48:324–328.

Leckman, J.F., King, R.A., Scahill, L., Findley, D., Ort, S.I., and Cohen, D.J. (1999) Yale approach to assessment and treatment. In: Leckman, J.F. and Cohen D.J., eds. *Tourette's Syndrome—Tics Obsessions, Compulsions: Developmental Psychopathology and Clinical Care.* New York: John Wiley and Sons, pp. 285–309.

Leckman, J.F., Ort, S., Caruso, K.A., Anderson, G.M., Riddle, M.A., and Cohen, D.J. (1986) Rebound phenomena in Tourette's syndrome after abrupt withdrawal of clonidine. *Arch Gen Psychiatry* 43:1168–1176.

Leckman, J.F., Zhang, H., Vitale, A., Lahnin, F., Lynch, K., Bondi, C., Kim, Y.S., and Peterson, B.S. (1998) Course of tic severity in Tourette syndrome: the first two decades. *Pediatrics* 102:14–19.

Levinson, M.L. and Johnson, C.E. (1992) Stability of an extemporaneously compounded clonidine hydrochloride oral liquid. *Am J Hosp Pharm* 49:122–125.

Li, B.M., Mao, Z.M., Wang, M., and Mei, Z.T. (1999) Alpha-2 adrenergic modulation of prefrontal cortical neuronal activity related to spatial working memory in monkeys. *Neuropsychopharmacology* 21:601–610.

Lipkin, P.H., Goldstein, I.J., and Adesman, A.R. (1994) Tics and dyskinesias associated with stimulant treatment in attention-deficit hyperactivity disorder. *Arch Pediatr Adolesc Med* 1994; 148:859–861.

Lombroso, P.J., Scahill, L., King, R.A., Lynch, K.A., Chappel, P.B., Peterson, B.S., McDougle, C.J., and Leckman, J.F. (1995) Risperidone treatment of children and adolescents with chronic tic disorders: a preliminary report. *J Am Acad Child Adolesc Psychiatry* 34:1147–1152.

Lowe, T.L., Cohen, D.J., Detlor, J., Kremenitzer, M.W., and Shaywitz, B.A. (1982) Stimulant medications precipitate Tourette's syndrome. *JAMA* 26:1729–1731.

Marras, C., Andrews, D., Sime, E., and Lang, A.E. (2001) Botulinum toxin for simple motor tics: a randomized, double-blind, controlled clinical trial. *Neurology* 56:605–610.

Mao, Z.M., Arnsten, A.F.T., Li, B.M. (1999) Local infusion of alpha-1 adrenergic agonist into the prefrontal cortex impairs spatial working memory performance in monkeys. *Biol Psychiatry* 46: 1259–1265.

McConville, B.J., Sanberg, P.R., Fogelson, M.H., King, J., Cirna, R., Parker, K.W., and Norman, A.B. (1992) The effects of nicotine plus haloperidol compared to nicotine only and placebo nicotine

only in reducing tic severity and frequency in Tourette's disorder. *Biolo Psychiatry* 15:832–840.

McDougle, C.J., Epperson, C.N., Pelton, G.H., Wasylink, S., and Price, L.H. (2000) A double-blind, placebo-controlled study of risperidone addition in serotonin reuptake inhibitor-refractory obsessive-compulsive disorder. *Arch Gen Psychiatry* 57:794–801.

McDougle, C.J., Goodman, W.K., Leckman, J.F., Barr, L.C., Heninger, G.R., and Price, L.H. (1993) The efficacy of fluvoxamine in obsessive compulsive disorder: effects of comorbid chronic tic disorder. *J Clin Psychopharmacol* 13:354–358.

McDougle, C.J., Goodman, W.K., Leckman, J.F., Lee, N.C., Heninger, G.R., and Price, L.H. (1994) Haloperidol addition in fluvoxamine-refractory obsessive compulsive disorder: a double-blind placebo-controlled study in patients with and without tics. *Arch Gen Psychiatry* 51:302–308.

Miguel, E.C., do Rosario-Campos, M.C., Shavitt, R.G., Hounie, A.G., and Mercandante, M.T., (2001) The tic-related obsessive-compulsive disorder: phenotype and treatment implications. In: Cohen, D.J., Jankovic, J., Goetz, C., eds. *Tourette Syndrome and Associated Disorders* (*Adv Neurol* Vol 85). Philadelphia: Lippincott-Williams & Wilkins, pp. 43–56.

Onofrj, M., Paci, C., D'Andreamatteo, G., and Toma, L., (2000) Olanzapine in severe Gilles de la Tourette syndrome: a 52-week double-blind cross-over study vs. low-dose pimozide. *J Neurol.* 247:443–446.

Parraga, H.C., Parraga, M.I., Woodward, R.L., and Fenning, P.A. (2001) Quetiapine treatment of children with Tourette's syndrome: report of two cases. *J Child Adolesc Psychopharmacol* 11:187–191.

Peterson, B.S., and Leckman, J.F. (1998) The temporal dynamics of tics in Gilles de la Tourette syndrome. *Biol Psychiatry* 44:1337–1348.

Peterson, B.S., Leckman, J.F., Scahill L., Naftolin, F., Keefe, D., Charest, N.J., King, R.A., Hardin, M.T., and Cohen, D.J., (1994), Steroid hormones and Tourette's syndrome: early experience with antiandrogen therapy. *J Clin Psychopharmacol* 14:131–135.

Peterson, B.S., Pine, D.S., Cohen, P., and Brook, J.S., (2001) Prospective, longitudinal study of tic, obsessive-compulsive, and attention-deficit/hyperactivity disorders in an epidemiological sample. *J Am Acad Child Adolesc Psychiatry* 40:685–695.

Peterson, B.S., Zhang, H., Anderson, G.M., and Leckman, J.F. (1998) A double-blind, placebo-controlled, crossover trial of an antiandrogen in the treatment of Tourette's syndrome. *J Clin Psychopharmacol.* 18:324–331.

Popper, C.W., (1995) Combining methylphenidate and clonidine: pharmacologic questions and new reports about sudden death. *J Child Adolesc Psychopharmacol* 5:157–166.

Riddle, M.A., Geller, B., and Ryan, N. (1993) Another sudden death in a child treated with desipramine. *J Am Acad Child Adolesc Psychiatry* 32:792–797.

Riddle, M.A., Hardin, M.T., King, R., Scahill, L., and Woolston, J.L. (1990) Fluoxetine treatment of children and adolescents with Tourette's and obsessive compulsive disorders: preliminary clinical experience. *J Am Acad Child Adolesc Psychiatry* 29:45–48.

Riddle, M.A., King, R.A., Hardin, M.T., Scahill, L., Ort, S.I., and Leckman, J.F. (1991) Behavioral side effects of fluoxetine in children and adolescents. *J Child Adolesc Psychopharmacol* 3:193–198.

Riddle, M.A., Leckman, J.F., Hardin, M.T., Anderson, G.M., and Cohen, D.J. (1988) Fluoxetine treatment of obsessions and compulsions in patients with Tourette's syndrome. *Am J Psychiatry* 145:1173–1174.

Robertson, M.M., Schnieden, V., and Lees, A.J., (1990) Management of Gilles de la Tourette syndrome using sulpiride. *Clin Neuropharmacol* 13:229–235.

Sallee, F.R., DeVane, C.L., and Ferrell, R.E., (2000a) Fluoxetine-related death in a child with cytochrome P-450 2D6 genetic deficiency. *J Child Adolesc Psychopharmacol.* 10:27–34.

Sallee, F.R., Kurlan, R., Goetz, C.G., Singer, H., Scahill, L., Law, G., Dittman, V.M., and Chappell, P.B. (2000b) Ziprasidone treatment of children and adolescents with Tourette's syndrome: a pilot study. *J Am Acad Child Adolesc Psychiatry* 39:292–299.

Sallee, F.R., Nesbitt, L., Jackson, C., Sine, L., and Sethuraman, G. (1997) Relative efficacy of haloperidol and pimozide in children and adolescents with Tourette's disorder. *Am J Psychiatry* 154: 1057–1062.

Sanberg, P.R., McConville, B.J., Fogelson, H.M., Manderscheid, P.Z., Parker, K.W., Blythe, M.M., Klykylo, W.M., and Norman, A.B. (1989) Nicotine potentiates the effects of haloperidol in animals and in patients with Tourette syndrome. Biomedi Pharmacother. 43:19–23.

Sanberg, P.R., Shytle, R.D., and Silver, A.A., (1998) Treatment of Tourette's syndrome with mecamylamine. *Lancet* 352: 705–6.

Sandor, P., Musisi, S., Moldofsky, H., and Lang, A. (1990) Tourette syndrome: a follow-up study. *J Clin Psychopharmacol.* 10:197–199.

Scahill, L., Chappell, P.B., Kim, Y.S., Schultz, R.T., Katsovich, L., Shepherd, E., Arnsten, A.F., Cohen, D.J., and Leckman, J.F. (2001) A placebo-controlled study of guanfacine in the treatment of children with tic disorders and attention deficit hyperactivity disorder. *Am J Psychiatry* 158:1067–1074.

Scahill, L., King, R.A., Schultz, R.T., and Leckman, J.F. (1999) Selection and use of diagnostic and clinical rating instruments. In: Leckman, J.F., and Cohen, D.J., eds. *Tourette's Syndrome—Tics, Obsessions, Compulsions: Developmental Psychopathology and Clinical Care.* New York: John Wiley and Sons, pp. 310–324.

Scahill, L., Leckman, J.F., Schultz, R.T., Katsovich, L., and Peterson, B.S. (submitted) A placebo-controlled trial of risperidone in Tourette syndrome.

Scahill, L. Riddle, M.A., King, R.A., Hardin, M.T., Rasmusson, A., Makuch, R.W., and Leckman, J.F. (1997) Fluoxetine has no marked effect on tic symptoms in patients with Tourette's syndrome: a double-blind placebo-controlled study. *J Child Adolesc Psychopharmacol* 7:75–85.

Shapiro, A.K., and Shapiro, E. (1984) Controlled study of pimozide vs. placebo in Tourette's syndrome. *J Am Acad Child Adolesc Psychiatry* 23:161–173.

Shapiro, E., Shapiro, A.K., Fulop, G., Hubbard, M., Mandell, J., Nordlie, J., and Phillips, R.A. (1989) Controlled study of haloperidol, pimozide, and placebo for the treatment of Gilles de la Tourette's syndrome. *Arch Gen Psychiatry* 46:722–730.

Silver, A.A., Shytle, R.D., and Sanberg, P.R. (2000) Mecamylamine in Tourette's syndrome: a two-year case study. *J Child Adolesc Psychopharmacol* 10:59–68.

Silva, R.R., Munoz, D.M., Barickman, J., and Friedhoff, A.J. (1995) Environmental factors and related fluctuation of symptoms in children and adolescents with Tourette's disorder. *J Child Psychol Psychiatry* 36:305–312.

Silver, A.A., Shytle, R.D., Philipp, M.K., and Sanberg, P.R. (1996) Case study: long-term potentiation of neuroleptics with transdermal nicotine in Tourette's syndrome. *J Am Acad Child Adolesc Psychiatry* 35:1631–1636.

Silver, A.A., Shytle, R.D., Philip, M.K., Sanberg, P.R. Transdermal nicotine in Tourette's syndrome. In: Clarke, P.B.S., Quik, M., and Thurau, K., eds. *The Effects of Nicotine on Biological Systems. Advances in Pharmacological Sciences.* Birkhauser Publishers.

Silver, A.A., Shytle, R.D., and Sanberg, P.R. (2000) Mecamylamine in Tourette's syndrome: a two-year retrospective case study. *J Child Adolesc Psychopharmacol* 10:59–68.

Silver, A.A., Shytle, R.D., Philipp, M.K., Wilkinson, B.J., McConville, B., and Sanberg, P.R. (2001a) Transdermal nicotine and haloperidol in Tourette's disorder: a double-blind placebo-controlled study. *J Clin Psychiatry* 62:707–714.

Silver, A.A., Shytle, R.D., Sheehan, K.H., Sheehan, D.V., Ramos, A., and Sanberg, P.R. (2001b) Multicenter, double-blind, placebo-controlled study of mecamylamine monotherapy for Tourette's disorder. *J Am Acad Child Adolesc Psychiatry* 40:1103–1110.

Singer, H., Brown, J., Quaskey, S., Rosenberg, L.A., Mellits, E.D., and Denckla, M.B. (1995) The treatment of attention-deficit hyperactivity disorder in Tourette's syndrome: a double-blind placebo-controlled study with clonidine and desipramine. *Pediatrics* 95:74–81.

Singer, H.S., Wendlandt, J., Krieger, M., and Giuliano, J. (2001) Baclofen treatment in Tourette syndrome: a double-blind, placebo-controlled, crossover trial. *Neurology* 56:599–604.

Spencer, T., Biederman, J., Coffey, B.J., Geller, D., Faraone, S., and Willens, T. (2001) Tourette disorder and ADHD. In: Cohen, D.J., Jankovic, J., and Goetz, C., eds. *Tourette Syndrome and Associated Disorders (Adv Neurol* Vol. 85). Philadelphia: Lippincott-Williams & Wilkins, pp. 57–77.

Spencer, T., Biederman, J., Steingard, R., and Wilens, T. (1993a) Bupropion exacerbates tics in children with attention-deficit hyperactivity disorder and Tourette's syndrome. *J Am Acad Child Adolesc Psychiatry* 32:211–214.

Spencer, T., Biederman, J., Wilens, T., Steingard, R., and Geist, D. (1993b) Nortriptyline treatment of children with attention-deficit hyperactivity disorder and tic disorder or Tourette's syndrome. *J Am Acad Child Adolesc Psychiatry* 32:205–210.

Stamenkovic, M., Schindler, S.D., Aschauser, H.N., DeZwaan, M., Willinger, U., Resinger, E., and Kasper, S. (2000) Effective open-label treatment of Tourette's disorder with olanzapine. *Int Clin Psychopharmacol* 15:23–28.

Stokes, A., Bawden, H.N., Camfield, P.R., Backman, J.E., and Dooley, M.B. (1991) Peer problems in Tourette's disorder. *Pediatrics* 87: 936–942.

Surwillo, W.W., Shafii, M., and Barrett, C.L. (1978) Gilles de la Tourette syndrome: a 20-month study of the effects of stressful life events and haloperidol on symptom frequency. *J Nerv Ment Dis* 166: 812–816.

Swanson, J.M., Connor, D.F., and Cantwell, D. (1999) Combining methylphenidate and clonidine: Ill-advised. *J Am Acad Child Adolesc Psychiatry* 38:617–619.

The Tourette's Syndrome Study Group. (2002) Treatment of ADHD in children with Tourette's Syndrome; a randomized controlled trial. *Neurology* 58:527–536.

Taylor, D.M., and McAskill, R. (2000) Atypical antipsychotics and weight gain—a systematic review. *Acta Psychiatr Scand* 101:416–432.

Toren, P., Laor, N., Cohen, D.J., Wolmer, L., and Weizman, A. (1999) Ondansetron treatment in patients with Tourette's syndrome. *Int Clin Psychopharmacol* 14:373–376.

Tourette Syndrome Study Group (1999) Short-term versus longer term pimozide therapy in Tourette's syndrome: a preliminary study. *Neurology* 56:874–877.

The Tourette's Syndrome Study Group. (2002) Treatment of ADHD in children with Tourette's Syndrome; a randomized controlled trial. *Neurology* 58:527–536.

van der Linden, C., Bruggeman, R., and Van Woerkom, T. (1994)

Serotonin–dopamine antagonist and Gilles de la Tourette's syndrome: an open pilot dose-titration study with risperidone. *Mov Disord* 9:687–688.

van Wattum, P.J., Chappell, P.B., Zelterman, D., Scahill, L.D., Leckman, J.F. (2000) Patterns of response to acute naloxone infusion in Tourette's syndrome. *J* 15:1252–1254.

Varley, C.K., Vincent, J., Varley, P., and Calderon, R. (2001) Emergence of tics in children with attention deficit hyperactivity disorder treated with stimulant medications. *Compr Psychiatry* 42: 228–233.

Wehr, A.M., and Namerow, L.B. (2001) Citalopram for OCD and Tourette's syndrome. *J Am Acad Child Adolesc Psychiatry* 40: 740–741.

Wilens, T.E. and Spencer, T.J. (1999a) Combining methylphenidate and clonidine: a clinically sound medication option. *J Am Acad Child Adolesc Psychiatry* 38:614–616.

Wilens, T.E. and Spencer, T.J. (1999b) "Combining methylphenidate and clonidine": affirmative rebuttal. *J Am Acad Child Adolesc Psychiatry* 38: 619–622.

Wilson, M.F., Haring, O., Lewin, A., Bedsole, G., Stepansky, W., Fillingim, J., Hall, D., Roginsky, M., McMahon, F.G., and Jagger, P. (1986) Comparison of guanfacine versus clonidine for efficacy, safety and occurrence of withdrawal syndrome in step-2 treatment of mild to moderate essential hypertension. *Am J Cardiol* 57:43E–49E.

Young, J.M., Shytle, R.D., Sanberg, P.R., and George, T.P. (2001) Mecamylamine: New therapeutic uses and toxicity/risk profile. *Clin Ther* 23:532–565.

41 | Early-onset schizophrenia

HELMUT REMSCHMIDT AND JOHANNES HEBEBRAND

Schizophrenic psychoses in childhood are important but rare disorders within the spectrum of the psychoses. Since the descriptions of Homburger (1926) and Lutz (1937/38), there is no doubt about the existence of schizophrenic psychoses in childhood. According to Bleuler (1911) and Lutz (1937/38) about 4% of schizophrenic psychoses begin before the 15th year of life, and 0.5% to 1%, before the 10th year. There is a remarkable increase in frequency during adolescence, and with increasing age the symptomatology becomes quite similar to that of adult patients. Accordingly, the classification is much easier during adolescence than during childhood. It is not clear if the criteria of the current classification systems (*International Classification of Disease, 10th ed.* [ICD-10] and the *Diagnostic and Statistical Manual of Mental Disease, 4th ed.* [DSM-IV]) are appropriate for schizophrenic disorders in younger children, e.g., below the age of 10 or 12 years. Many of these children suffer from other early developmental, cognitive, and/or emotional disorders, thus complicating an adequate classification within a system that was primarily constructed for the adult type of schizophrenia. It may be that there are two types of childhood and adolescent schizophrenia: one type that can clearly be diagnosed using the prototype of adult symptomatology without remarkable developmental precursors, and another one complicated by an additional and complex developmental disorder that may modify the expression of symptoms in an age- and stage-appropriate way. For practical purposes, the current classification systems can be used, but we should always be aware that they reflect our current knowledge and do not describe clear-cut nosological entities.

CLASSIFICATION, EPIDEMIOLOGY, AND ASSESSMENT

Classification

According to Werry (1992), we can distinguish between early-onset schizophrenia (EOS) beginning in childhood or adolescence (before the ages of 16 or 17) and very early-onset schizophrenia (VEOS, onset before age 13). Werry separates the latter group because that definition is more precise than the term *prepubertal*. He further states that a review of the studies of childhood schizophrenia is complicated by the fact that before ICD-9 and DSM-III, all psychotic disorders of childhood were aggregated into the single category of childhood schizophrenia.

Psychoses manifested during adolescence may not have precursor symptoms in childhood (Rutter, 1967; Remschmidt, 1975a, 1975b). The subdivision according to premorbid personality and psychosocial adaptation also seems to be important in positive and negative schizophrenia in adolescence, because there is a relationship between poor premorbid adjustment and negative schizophrenia in adulthood (Andreasen and Olsen, 1982).

About 50% of children and adolescents with schizophrenia show characteristic symptomatology in their premorbid personality (Stutte, 1969): they have been described as withdrawn, shy, introverted, sensitive, and anxious. It is not clear whether these personality characteristics directly predispose them to schizophrenia, or whether they enhance the constitutional vulnerability of those children. Again, there is a large body of evidence for neurobiological and neurodevelopmental deficits in schizophrenic children and adolescents prior to the full manifestation of their disorder (Remschmidt 1993; 2002).

Epidemiology

Until the publication of Kolvin (1971), the disorders now subsumed under the label of autism spectrum disorders (Wing, 1996) or developmental pervasive disorders (American Psychiatric Association [APA], 1994) were referred to as "childhood schizophrenia" (Bender, 1969). Kolvin demonstrated different age-of-onset patterns between autism and EOS, which was the beginning of the notion that these disorders are separate nosological entities. Early-onset schizophrenia can be

543

subdivided into VEOS (onset before age 13) and EOS proper (onset before age 16 or 17) (for review see Gillberg, 2001).

Very early–onset schizophrenia (13 years or under)

The prevalence of very early–onset psychoses is very rare, and seems to be below 2 in one million children in the general population (Gillberg, 1984; Steffenburg & Gillberg 1986; Burd et al., 1987; Gillberg and Steffenburg; 1987, Gillberg et al., 1991). The male/female ratio in these young cases is about 2:1 or even higher (Werry, 1992). The youngest ages of onset reported in the literature are 3 years in one case (Russell et al., 1989) and 5 years in some other cases (Caplan et al., 1989; Green et al., 1992).

As far as symptomatology is concerned, there is considerable age-dependent variation (Asarnow, 1994), with well-formulated delusions being extremely rare. However, hallucinations and disorganized thinking do occur (Garralda, 1984; Watkins et al., 1988; Caplan et al., 1990). There is some evidence that VEOS is probably associated with a lower IQ than that in the general population (Gillberg, 2001): about 10%–20% score about 70 or below in standardized intelligence testing (Green et al., 1992; Werry, 1992), and mental retardation as well as language delay, language abnormalities, and delays in motor development are all considered premorbid features. The same applies to attention deficits and hyperactivity (Asarnow et al., 1991; Asarnow, 1994).

Early-onset schizophrenia (13–19 years of age)

According to a review by Gillberg (2001), there is some evidence that the incidence of schizophrenia occurs about 50 times less often before the age of 15 years than after (Beitchman, 1985). In a study in Sweden, 0.23% of all 20-year-old individuals living in Göteborg in the early 1980s who had been hospitalized for schizophrenia ranged in age from 13 to 19. In inpatient child and adolescent psychiatric settings, up to 5% of 13- to 19-year-olds are typically diagnosed with schizophrenia.

The male/female ratio varies to some extent and is characterized in the younger patients by a preponderance of males (ratio from 1.4:1 to 2.4:2), with an equal ratio observed in older individuals (Werry, 1992). Several studies found a significant increase in the frequency of the diagnosis of schizophrenia between the ages of 13 and 18 years (Gillberg et al., 1986; Remschmidt, 2001), and onset during adolescence seems to be more acute than in VEOS (Werry, 1992). There seems to be a weak to moderate association of schizophrenia with low IQ during adolescence as well (Gillberg, 2001). With increasing age, the symptomatology becomes more similar to that of schizophrenia in adults. The diagnosis of EOS has a high stability over time, and follow-up studies show that outcome and prognosis are poor (Gillberg et al., 1993).

Assessment

Diagnostic criteria (ICD-10 and DSM-IV)

The publication of DSM-IV in 1994 (American Psychiatric Association 1994), ICD-10 (clinical guidelines) in 1992 (World Health Organization, 1992) and ICD-10 (research criteria) in 1993 (World Health Organization, 1993) led to a greater convergence between the DSM and ICD classification systems (for details see Hollis, 2001; Remschmidt, 2001).

Table 41.1 gives an overview of the classification of

TABLE 41.1 *Comparison of ICD-10 and DSM-IV Classifications of Schizophrenia and Related Disorders*

Schizophrenia, Schizotypal, and Delusional Disorders (ICD-10)	Schizophrenia and Other Psychotic Disorders (DSM-IV)
Schizophrenia	**Schizophrenia**
Paranoid schizophrenia	Paranoid type
Hebephrenic schizophrenia	Disorganized type
Catatonic schizophrenia	Catatonic type
Undifferentiated schizophrenia	Undifferentiated type
Post-schizophrenic depression	
Residual schizophrenia	Residual type
Simple schizophrenia	
Classification of course possible	Classification of course possible
Schizotypal disorder	Schizophreniform disorder
Persistent delusional disorder	Delusional disorder
Acute and transient psychotic disorder	Brief psychotic disorder
Induced delusional disorder	Shared psychotic disorder (folie à deux)
Schizoaffective disorder with subtype: manic, depressive, and mixed	Schizoaffective disorder with bipolar subtype, depressive subtype
	Psychotic disorder due to a general medical condition
	Substance-induced psychotic disorder

schizophrenia and other psychotic disorders according to ICD-10 and DSM-IV. Many categories correspond. One major difference between ICD-10 and DSM-IV concerns the minimally required period of presence of schizophrenic symptoms for the diagnosis of schizophrenia (ICD-10: 1 month; DSM-IV: 6 months). The schizophrenic subtypes in the two systems are broadly comparable and share the same labels except the DSM-IV "disorganized type" (295.1), which is equivalent to ICD-10 "hebephrenic schizophrenia" (F20.1). An important difference is the inclusion of the category of "simple schizophrenia" (F20.6) in ICD-10, which is characterized by insidious onset of social withdrawal, oddities of conduct, and deteriorating social performance over a period of at least 1 year without active psychotic symptoms. There is no equivalent category in DSM-IV. The ICD-10 places "schizotypal disorder" (F21) in the broad group of "schizophrenia and other psychotic disorders," while in DSM-IV, "schizotypal personality disorder" (301.22) is placed in the section of personality disorders.

"Schizophreniform "disorder" in DSM-IV is somewhat different from "schizotypal" disorder" in ICD-10. The diagnosis of schizophreniform disorder requires the identical criteria of schizophrenia (criterion A), except for two differences: the total duration of the illness is at least 1 month, but less than 6 months (criterion B), and impaired social or occupational functioning during some part of the illness is not required. The delusional disorder in DSM-IV corresponds more or less to the category "persistent delusional disorder" of ICD-10, and "brief psychotic disorder" (DSM-IV) is similar to the ICD-10 category "acute and transient psychotic disorder," whereas the "shared psychotic disorder" of DSM-IV corresponds to "induced delusional disorder" of ICD-10.

Clinical Presentation

The clinical presentation of EOS comprises cognitive symptoms, emotional symptoms, and changes in social functioning, disturbances of speech and language, and motor disturbances.

Cognitive symptoms include distortions of thinking, delusions, and hallucinations. Thought distortions comprise thought insertion, breaks and interpolations in the train of thought, thought echo, or incoherent and vague thinking that sometimes cannot verbally be expressed in a comprehensible way.

Delusions may include ideas of references, beliefs of being persecuted, bodily changes, delusions of control, and a variety of other types of delusions. As far as delusions are concerned, systematized delusions are very rare in childhood (below the age of 12) and become more frequent during adolescence.

Hallucinations manifest themselves mainly as threatening voices giving comments or commands to the patient, or as auditory hallucinations without a verbal structure, such as laughing, humming, or whistling. Auditory hallucinations are the most frequent, while visual hallucinations or those involving smell or taste or other bodily sensations are rare. Visual hallucinations are, if occurring at all, more frequently found in younger children (below the age of 13) and raise differential diagnostic questions, as they also can occur in intoxications.

Emotional symptoms and changes in social functioning include blunted affect, mood disturbances such as irritability, fearfulness, and suspicion, negative symptoms such as marked apathy, paucity of speech, or incongruity of emotional responses resulting in social withdrawal and lowering of social performance.

Disturbances of speech and language are characterized by paucity of speech or logorrhea, perseverations, or speech stereotypies, sometimes also by echolalia and phonographism. Neologisms can also occur. With regard to these symptoms, the differential diagnosis regarding autism is important, especially in children below the age of 8.

Motor disturbances are manifold and can extend from clumsiness and motor dysharmony to strange postures, stupor, and symptoms of catatonia. Bizarre movements and motor stereotypies such as finger stereotypies are frequent. Initially, and also during the course of the disorder, compulsive acts or rituals resulting in strange and unexpected movements can also be observed.

Assessment Instruments

Many instruments exist for use in children and adolescents with suspected psychotic disorders (see Table 41.2) (for details see Hollis, 2001). The instruments can be divided into two categories: diagnostic interviews and symptom rating scales. Whereas the diagnostic interviews have been constructed with the aim of arriving at categorial diagnoses according to the DSM- or ICD-10 systems, the symptom rating scales have a broader focus and are constructed with the aim of assessing psychopathological symptoms on a continuous scale (e.g., positive symptoms, negative symptoms, thought disorders, functional impairment). In contrast to the diagnostic interviews, they produce scores on certain dimensions, thus following the di-

TABLE 41.2 *Assessment Instruments for Evaluating Schizophrenic Symptoms in Children*

Instrument	Description	Informant	Age range (years)
Clinical interviews			
Schedule for Affective Disorders and Schizophrenia for School-Age Children, Epidemiologic version (K-SADS-E) (Orvaschel and Puig-Antich, 1987)	Semistructured diagnostic interview designed to assess past and current DSM-III and DSM-III-R disorders	Parent Child	6–17
Interview for Childhood Disorders and Schizoprenia (ICDS) (Russel et al., 1989)	Semistructured interview	Parent Child	6–18
Child and Adolescent Psychiatric Assessment (CAPA) (Angold et al., 1995)	Semistructured interview Focus on past 3 months; includes severity ratings	Parent Child	8–18
Diagnostic Interview for Children and Adolecents (DICA) (Herjanic and Reich, 1982)	Highly structured interview designed to assess DMS-III and III-R diagnoses Available in computerized version	Parent Child	6–17
The NIMH Diagnostic Interview Schedule for Children (NIMH DISC) (National Institute of Mental Health [NIMH], 1992)	Highly structured interview designed to give DSM-III and III-R diagnoses Available in computerized version	Parent Child	9–17
Rating scales			
Positive and Negative Syndrome Scale for Children and Adolescents (K-PANSS) (Fields et al., 1994)	Rating scale for positive and negative symptoms and other symptoms	Interviewer rating Parent/Child	6–16
Children's Psychiatric Rating Scale (CPRS) (Fish, 1985)	Symptoms ratings based on severity/degree of abnormality Good coverage of schizophrenic symptoms	Interviewer rating Child	Up to 15
Children's Global Assessment Scale (C-GAS) (Shaffer et al., 1983)	Rating of severity of fuctional impairment on a 0–100 scale	Rating based on review of all available sources	4–16
Thought disorder scales			
Kiddie-Formal Thought Disorder Story Game and Kiddie Formal Thought Disorder Scale (K-FTDS) (Caplan et al., 1989)	Procedures for eliciting and scoring speech samples	Child	5–13
Thought Disorder Index (TDI) (Arboleda and Holzmann, 1985)	Codes thought disorder from speech samples	Child	5–16

Instruments organized according to Hollis (2001); adapted from Asarnow (1994).

mensional approach to schizophrenia. For the diagnosis of child and adolescent schizophrenia, it is important to collect all information available, not only from and about the child but also from other sources. Usually, a battery is used that includes rating scale data from parents, children, and teachers, whenever possible. Moreover, we feel that the most valid diagnoses integrate data from all available sources by using either the "best estimate" (Leckman et al., 1982) or PLASTIC (Prospective, Longitudinal, All Source, Treatment, Impairment, and Clinical presentation) procedures (Young et al., 1987). This information is included in the schedules described in Table 41.2. This approach is different from the use of schedules in adult psychiatry, which usually rely only on the information gathered only or primarily from the patient.

Diagnostic interview schedules

The most commonly used instruments are listed in table 41.2 and can be subdivided into two groups: first, semi-structured interviews such as the Kiddie Schedule for Affective Disorders, and Schizophrenia, Epidemiologic version (K-SADS-E), the Interview for Childhood Disorders and Schizophrenia (ICDS) and the Children and Adolescent Psychiatric Assessment (CAPA). These interviews are investigator based and require a high level of training, and the interviewer has to decide whether an item is satisfactorily fulfilled or whether further questions are required to get the relevant information. The second group comprises highly structured interviews such as the Diagnostic Interview for Children and Adolescents (DICA) and the National Institute of Mental Health Diagnostic Interview Schedule for Children (NIMH-DISC). These instruments are respondent based, which implies that the responsibility is placed on the person who is investigated rather than on the interviewer.

Rating scales

Rating scales provide a continuous measure of psychotic symptoms or global functioning. They can significantly contribute to a categorial diagnosis, by providing measures of symptom variability or symptom change over time. In addition, they are very useful for checking the social functioning of the patient. According to Hollis (2001), three main types of rating scales are available *(1)* general psychotic symptom rating scales such as the Kiddie Positive and Negative Syndrome Scale (K-PANSS) and the Children's Psychiatric Rating Scale (CPRS), which cover a broad range of positive and negative psychotic symptoms, *(2)* global rating scales such as the Children's Global Assessment Scale (C-GAS), which provide an overall measure of severity of the disturbance, and *(3)* thought disorder scales, including the Kiddie Formal Thought Disorder Story Game (K-FTDS) and the Thought Disorder Index (TDI). By means of these scales, it is possible to measure specifically thought disorders in children.

Rating scales are rarely used for diagnostic purposes of arriving at an ICD or DSM diagnosis. However, they have great advantages for the quantitative assessment of several areas of psychopathology and can be used to construct Receiver/Response Operating Characteristic (ROC) curves (Verhulst and Koot, 1992). Using ROC curves offers the possibility of devising multiple cutoffs on a rating scale, either for the distinguishing of cases from non-cases, or for the measurement of the severity of true cases, thus following a dimensional rather than a categorial approach.

Differential Diagnosis

A list of major differential diagnoses for psychotic symptoms in children and adolescents, including their clinical characteristics and differentiating features, is presented in Table 41.3 (for details see Hollis, 2001).

TREATMENT AND REHABILITATION

The treatment of EOS requires a coordinated team approach and is based upon several components that have to be individually tailored to meet the needs of the patient and family. The treatment components comprise pharmacotherapy, individual psychotherapy, family oriented measures as well as specific measures of rehabilitation, described in several recent reviews (AACAP 2000; 2001; Remschmidt et al., 1996; 2001; Lambert, 2001)

Pharmacological Treatment

Classification of antipsychotics

Antipsychotics can be classified according to three main principles: chemical structure, receptor binding profile, and clinical profile. The clinical profile covers several effects such as antipsychotic efficacy, sedation, and side effects (see Table 41.4). Together with the receptor binding profile, this has led to the classification of antipsychotics into two main groups: typical and atypical. The receptor binding profile is essential for the pharmacological action and the clinical efficacy of all antipsychotics agents, subdivided into the three groups: typical high-potency antipsychotics, typical moderate and low-potency antipsychotics, and atypical antipsychotics (for review see Remschmidt et al., 2001, and Chapter 34 in this volume).

Typical or classical antipsychotics, especially typical high-potency antipsychotics, have been found to be effective mainly in the positive symptoms of schizophrenia and cause extrapyramidal side effects (EPS). Both effects have been attributed to their high dopamine receptor antagonism (especially D_2). Typical low-potency antipsychotics lead to sedation. Atypical antipsychotics have a different receptor affinity pattern, targeting mainly serotoninergic receptors (especially $5\text{-}HT_{2A}$). Therefore they are probably especially effective in positive as well as negative symptoms, and cause weight gain. Up to 60 % of nonresponders to typical antipsychotics improve under the atypical antipsychotic clozapine. An important strategy in the pharmacological treatment of acute psychotic states is the differentiation of positive and negative symptoms. Table 41.4

TABLE 41.3 *Differential Diagnosis of Early-Onset Psychoses*

Differential Diagnosis	Symptoms
Drug-induced psychoses	High incidence Best known substances include hallucinogens, cocaine, and amphetamines Psychotic symptoms may also occur with the withdrawal of alcohol, sedatives, hypnotics, and anxiolytics The following symptoms may occur: persecutory delusions, perceptual distortions, and vivid hallucinations in any modality, most classically visual and tactile hallucination of insects crawling under the skin (formication) Substance abuse history may be elicited from the history and confirmed by finding urinary metabolites Confirmation of schizophrenia can only be made if the psychotic symptoms persist for at least a month following drug withdrawal
Conduct and emotional disorders	Hallucinations are usually transient and fragmentary Negative symptoms are unusual Misdiagnosis arises when undue emphasis is placed on symptoms such as ideas of reference
Affective psychoses (psychotic depression and bipolar disorder)	Positive symptoms may occur and the onset is often rapid with relatively good premorbid functioning Distinctions such as mood congruency can be difficult to apply Negative symptoms may occur in depression
Asperger's syndrome and autistic spectrum disorders	Positive symptoms may develop (DSM-IV does not exclude a diagnosis of schizophrenia in cases of PDD/autism as long as prominent delusions or hallucinations are present for a month) Social and cognitive impairments are more long-standing Progressive deterioration of functioning prior to onset is less marked
Neurodegenerative disorders	Very rare disorders include juvenile metachromatic leukodystrophy, adrenoleucodystrophy, Wilson's disease These conditions are associated with movement disorders, particularly gait disturbance. It is important to attempt to distinguish between primary and secondary (antipsychotic related) movement disorders These conditions are characterized by a progressive loss of cognitive skills (in contrast to the more relative decline seen in schizophrenia and other developmental disorders, where a loss of previously learned skill is unusual)
Temporal lobe epilepsy	Association between epilepsy and psychosis has been described Consciousness is always impaired and patients seem retarded and absent minded and tend to perseverate Automatisms may be seen, such as lip smacking or picking at clothes Hallucinations are usually visual and may be vivid in content; however, memory of the episodes may be incomplete or fragmentary. Differentiation of this group of seizures from schizophrenia is based on presence of clouding of consciousness and their brief and episodic nature, with partial amnesia for the episodes
Multiple complex developmental disorder (MCDD)	Impaired regulation of affective state and anxiety Impaired social behavior and sensitivity Impaired cognitive processing No diagnosis of autism Duration of symptoms longer than 6 months Occurrence before age 6 years Increased risk for becoming schizophrenic in adolescence or later

Adopted from Towbin et al. (1993) and Hollis (2001).

demonstrates the effects of typical and atypical antipsychotics with regard to their efficacy on both positive and negative symptoms, sedation, EPS, and anticholinergic reactions.

Indications and contraindications

Typical (classical) antipsychotics have been proposed for a wide range of disorders. In the context of EOS the following indications exist: acute treatment, maintenance treatment, and relapse prevention of schizophrenic disorders acute treatment and maintenance treatment of schizoaffective disorders treatment of organic mental disorders with psychotic features and treatment of mental and behavioral disorders due to psychoactive and other substance use.

Contraindications for the use of antipsychotics are acute intoxications with sedative agents, and patients with leukopenia should not be medicated with tricyclic neuroleptics (mainly clozapine). If drugs with high anticholinergic properties are used, patients with pylorus stenosis, glaucoma, and prostatatic hypertrophy must be excluded. Further restrictions are Parkinson's syndrome, seizures, allergic reactions, diseases of the hematological system, hypotension or cardiovascular diseases, liver and kidney diseases, prolactin-dependent tumors, asthma or bronchospasm, and pheochromocytoma.

TABLE 41.4 *Effects and Side Effects of Antipsychotics*

Generic Name	Brand Names (Where Available)	Effects on Positive Symptoms	Effects on Negative Symptoms	Sedation	Extrapyramidal Symptoms	Anticholinergic Reactions	Neuroleptic Potency	Usual Oral Dosage (Usual Depot Dose IM)
Typical high potency antipsychotics								
Benperidol	Glianimon (D) Anquil (UK) Frenactil (F, Be)	++	++	+	++(+)	+	100	1–6mg/day
Flupenthixol (-decanoate)	Fluanxol (D, US, CAN, F, Ch) Depixol (UK)	++	++	+	++(+)	+	50	2–10mg/day (20–100mg/2–4 weeks)
Fluphenazine (-decanoate)	Lyogen (D) Dapotum (D) Prolixin (CAN, US) Permitil (CAN, US) Modecate (CAN, UK)	+++	++	+(+)	+++	+	30	5–20mg/day (12.5–100mg/2–4 weeks)
Fluspirilene	Imap (D) Redeptin (UK)	+++	++	+	+++	+	300	(2–10mg/week)[a]
Haloperidol (-decanoate)	Haldol (D, UK, US, CAN, F, Ch, NL, Be, It, Is, Port) Haldol-Decanoat(e) (D, UK, US, F, It, Ch)	+++	++	+	+++	+	60	2–20mg/day (50–300mg/2–4 weeks)
Perphenazine (-enanthate)	Decentan (D, It) Trilafon (CAN, US, Be, NL, Ch) Fentazin (UK) Etrafon (CAN, US) Trilafan (F)	+++	++	++	+++	+(+)	8	12–64mg/day (50–200 mg/2 weeks)
Pimozide	Orap (D, UK, US, CAN, F) Opiran (F)	+++	++	+	+++	+	50	4–20 mg/day
Typical moderate and low potency antipsychotics								
Chlorpromazine	Megaphen (D) Thorazine (CAN, US) Largactil (UK, F)	+++	++	+++	++	+++	1	150–600mg/day
Chlorprothixene	Truxal (D) Taractan (D, US, F)	++	++	+++	+(+)	+++	0.8	150–600mg/day
Levomepromazine	Neurocil (D) Nozinan (UK, CAN, US, F, Be, It, Ch, NL) Levoprome (US)	++	++	+++	+(+)	+++	0.8	75–600mg/day
Perazine	Taxilan (D)	++	++	++	+	++(+)	0.5	75–600mg/day

(continued)

TABLE 41.4 *Effects and Side Effects of Antipsychotics (continued)*

Generic Name	Brand Names (Where Available)	Effects on Positive Symptoms	Effects on Negative Symptoms	Sedation	Extrapyramidal Symptoms	Anticholinergic Reactions	Neuroleptic Potency	Usual Oral Dosage (Usual Depot Dose IM)
Pipamperone	Dipiperon (D, F, Ch, NL, Be) Atosil (D)			++	+	+	0.2	120–360mg/day
Promethazine	Phenergan (US, UK, Be, Ch, NL)			+++	+	++		50–400mg/day
Sulpiride	Dogmatil (D, F, Be, NL, E, Jpn) Dolmatil (UK) Sulpitil (UK)	++	+++	+	+(+)	+(+)	0.5	100–800mg/day
Thioridazine	Mellaril (D, UK, US, F, Be, NL, Ch, It) Mellaril (CAN, US)	++	++	+++	+(+)	+++	0.7	200–700mg/day
Tiapride	Tiapridex (D) Equilium (F) Tiapridal (F, Be)			+	+	+		300–600mg/day
Atypical antipsychotics								
Amisulpride	Solian (D, CAN, F, Be)	+++	+++	+	+	+		250–800mg/day
Clozapine	Leponex (D, F, Be) Clozaril (UK, US, CAN)	+++	+++	+++	+	+++	0.5–2	25–600mg/day
Olanzapine	Zyprexa (D,UK,US,CAN)	+++	+++	++	+(+)	++	8–20	5–20mg/day
Quetiapine	Seroquel (D, UK, US, CAN)	+++	+++	+	+	+(+)		150–750mg/day
Risperidone	Risperdal (D, UK, US, CAN, F)	+++	+++	+	+(+)	+	50	1–12mg/day
Zotepine	Nipolept (D) Lodpin (Jpn)	+++	+++	++	+(+)	++	2	75–300mg/day

Be, Belgium; CAN, Canada; Ch, China; D, Germany; E, Spain (Espagna); F, France; Is, Israel; It, Italy; Jpn, Japan; NL, The Netherlands; Port; Portugal; UK, United Kingdom; US, United States.
+, none or low; ++, moderate; +++, high; ᵃAvailable only as depot.
Adapted from Remschmidt et al. (2001).

Special considerations for atypical antipsychotics

The main indications for atypical antipsychotics are the acute and maintenance treatment of schizophrenic disorders, with an emphasis on the treatment of refractory and chronic disorders. However, because of the lower risk of EPS and in particular of tardive dyskinesia, there is a tendency toward a wider range of indications for some of the atypical neuroleptics. Favorable effects in drug-induced psychoses have been demonstrated for olanzapine. Clozapine seems effective in the treatment and relapse prevention of manic episodes and bipolar disorders, and risperidone has been shown to have good efficacy in conduct disorders and in the pervasive developmental disorders.

Treatment of Acute States

In general, schizophrenic psychoses have to be treated by a multimodal approach including medication, psychotherapeutic interventions, and in chronic cases, rehabilitation. During the acute state of the psychosis, inpatient treatment and antipsychotic medication are required as the most important components. Drug treatment is the most important component during the first inpatient phase.

Until recently, only typical high-potency antipsychotics were used for acute psychotic states, which have been found to be effective against positive symptoms such as delusions and hallucinations, and also have quite a good effect on agitation, aggression, tension, and formal thought disorders. Haloperidol was the most frequently used agent. Currently, the atypical antipsychotics, mainly clozapine, olanzapine and risperidone, have replaced the typical antipsychotics for treatment during the acute phase, but also for maintenance treatment. In addition, amisulpride, quetiapine, and zotepine have also been used, but experience with these compounds in EOS is very limited.

Table 41.5 summarizes existing studies on the use of atypical antipsychotics in EOS. As the table demonstrates, most studies have been carried out with clozapine, only three with olanzapine and two with risperidone each, and only one study has assessed use of amisulpride and one quetiapine.

Table 41.5 also contains the dosages used, the outcome measures, and the main results. In addition to the informations of Table 41.5, the clinical experiences with the use of atypical antipsychotics can be described as follows (Remschmidt et al., 2000).

Clozapine

In some countries, the treatment guidelines for clozapine require that patients have failed to respond to or have not tolerated other atypical or standard antipsychotic medications. Because of the risk of agranulocytosis, the absence of any hematological anomaly (number of white blood cells than 3500/mm³, normal differentiatial blood count) is required. Before initiating treatment, patients must have a baseline white blood cell and differential count. During treatment, white blood cell count has to be monitored (frequency and duration depends on country—e.g., United States: weekly during the first 6 months of treatment, bimonthly thereafter, and 4 weeks after discontinuation; United Kingdom: weekly during the first 18 weeks and at least every 2-weeks for the first year, then at least every 4 weeks and 4 weeks after discontinuation; Germany: weekly for the first 18 months and subsequently every 4 weeks). In addition, total and differential blood counts must be administered if any symptoms or hints of agranulocytosis occur. The dosages applied to adolescent patients typically range from 100 to 600 mg/day.

Efficacy in short-term treatment. From studies in adult schizophrenia, it is evident that clozapine treatment has at least the same or superior antipsychotic effect, compared to typical antipsychotics. In some studies, clozapine was superior with regard to symptom reduction in severe and acute schizophrenic patients. As the guidelines do not allow the use of clozapine as a first-choice drug, most patients have been treated before with at least two atypical or typical antipsychotics. Only one controlled trial has assessed the efficacy of clozapine in child and adolescent psychiatry. In this study (Kumra et al., 1996), clozapine was found to be superior to haloperidol in all measures of psychosis, and showed a striking superiority for both positive and negative symptoms.

Efficacy in maintenance treatment. Studies in adult schizophrenia concerning maintenance treatment have been especially interesting, because the majority of the patients were nonresponders to conventional antipsychotics. These studies demonstrate the superior efficacy of clozapine as maintenance treatment in therapy-refractory psychoses treated by classical antipsychotics. Beyond that, it could be demonstrated that clozapine was effective in reducing recurrence rates and duration of hospitalization. The superior efficacy of clozapine, although not its effects on recurrence or hospital stay, have also been demonstrated in adolescents suffering from chronic schizophrenia (Schulz et al., 1996, 1997).

Olanzapine

For olanzapine, the literature for adolescent schizophrenia is sparse; adult patients are generally treated

TABLE 41.5 *Reports on Use of Atypical Antipsychotics in Children and Adolescents with Schizophrenia*

No. of subjects (Trial Type)	Diagnosis and Comorbidity	Mean age [Years (Range)]	Treatment Duration	Mean Dose mg/day (Range)[a]	Outcome Measures	Results	Reference
Clozapine							
21 (open)	Schizophrenia	18.1 (57%<18)	133 days	352 (150–800)	Symptom checklist	80% improved	Siefen and Remschmidt, 1986
57 (open)	Schizophrenia (n = 53), mood disorders (n = 2), PDD (n = 2)	16.8 (10–21)	311 days (1–75 months)	285 (75–800)	NA	88% improved, 7% no change, 5% worse	Schmidt et al., 1989; Blanz and Schmidt, 1993
11 (open)	Schizophrenia	(12–18)	6 week	370 (125–900)	BPRS, CGAS, BHS, SAPS, SANS, AIMS	>50% improved	Frazier et al., 1994; Gordon et al., 1994
36 (open)	Schizophrenia	(14–22)	154 days	330 (50–800)	SANS, SAPS	75% improved, 8% no change, 17% worse	Remschmidt et al., 1994
13 (open)	Schizophrenia	16.6 (14–17)	NA	240	BPRS	77% improved	Levkovitch et al., 1994
6 (open)	Psychosis with TD or PTSD	NA	NA	300	NA	% improved	Mandoki, 1994
11[b] (open)	Schizophrenia	14.1 (6–18)	6 weeks	350	BPRS, BHS	Improved[c]	Piscitelli et al., 1994
31 (open)	Schizophrenia	NA	NA	NA	NA	Improved	Abczynska et al., 1995
20 (open)	Schizophrenia	(14–22)	30 weeks	307 (75–600)	BPRS, SAPS, SANS	Improved[d]	Schulz et al., 1996
21 (controlled)	Schizophrenia	14.0 ± 2.3	6 weeks	176 ± 149	BPRS, CGI, BHS, SAPS, SAS, AIMS	Positive + negative symptoms improved, clozapine > haloperidol (p = 0.04–0.002)	Kumra et al., 1996
11 (open)	Schizophrenia	11.3 (9–13)	16 weeks	230 (200–300)	PANSS, BPRS, CGI	4/11 improved	Turetz et al., 1997
Olanzapine							
8 (retrospective study)	Schizophrenia	NA	NA	(5–20)	CGI	8/8 as effective as clozapine	Mandoki, 1997
8 (open)	Schizophrenia	15.3 (6–18)	8 weeks	17.5 (12.5–20); 0.27/kg (0.15–0.41/kg)	BPRS, SAPS, SANS, CGI	2/8 drug responders, 1/8 partial responder	Kumra et al., 1998

n (design)	Diagnosis	Age	Duration	Dose[a]	Scales	Results	Reference
15 (open)	Schizophrenia	9.4 ± 1.99 (6–13)	11.3 days	5	0–3 Likert scale rating of psychotic improvement	13/15 improved, 5/15 showed significant improvement	Sholevar et al., 2000
Risperidone							
5 (open)	Schizophrenia	(12–17)	NA	(4–5)	CGI	3/4 improved in CGI	Quintana and Keshavan, 1995
10 (open)	Schizophrenia	15.1 (11–18)	6 weeks	6.6 (4–10)	PANSS, BPRS, CGI	9 improved, 1 no change; p < .01	Armenteros et al., 1997
Amisulpride							
27[e] (controlled)	Schizophrenia (n = 21), schizotypal (n = 6)	20 ± 4	6 weeks	50 (n = 14), placebo (n = 13)	SANS, SAPS, BPRS, MADRS	21/27 improved in negative symptoms; 6/27 worse/dropped	Paillere-Martinot et al., 1995
Quetiapine							
10 (open)	Psychosis	(12.3–15.9)	23 days	200 and 800	BPRS, CGI, SANS, SAS	Positive and negative symptoms improved	McConville et al., 2000

Abbreviations: AIMS, Abnormal Involuntary Movement Scale; BHS, Bunney-Hamburg Scale; BPRS, Brief Psychiatric Rating Scale; CGAS, Children's Global Assessment Scale; CGI, Clinical Global Impression Scale; MADRS, Montgomery-Asberg, Depression Rating Scale; NA, not available; PANSS, Positive and Negative Syndrome Scale; PDD, pervasive develpomental disorder; PTSD, post-traumatic stress disorder; SANS, Scale for the Assessment of Negative Symptoms; SAPS, Scale for the Assessment of Positive Symptoms; SAS, Simpson-Angus Scale for EPS; TD, Tourette's disorder.

[a] mg/kg are cited when available.
[b] 8 patients in open trials, 3 in blind trials.
[c] Clinical improvement exhibited a consistent linear relationship with plasma clozapine concentrations but not with clozapine treatment.
[d] No specific data are available about patients improvement with clozapine treatment.
[e] Study includes young adults as well.
Modified according to Quintana and Keshavan (1995); Toren et al. (1998), and McConville et al. (2000).

with dosages between 5 and 20 mg/day. As Table 41.5 demonstrates, there are three open trials. In the study by Kumra et al. (1998), 8 patients with EOS were treated with olanzapine. The mean age was 15.3 years, and the mean duration of the illness 4.6 years. The patients were markedly ill, as demonstrated by the mean score on the Brief Psychiatric Rating Scale (BPRS) of 53.2 − 15.3 at baseline. The results of this trial demonstrate significant improvement in symptomatology, indicated by a 17% improvement on the BPRS, a 27% improvement on the Scale for the Assessment of Negative Symptoms (SANS) and a 1% improvement on the Scale for the Assessment of Positive Symptoms (SAPS). In terms of the Clinical Global Impression (CGI) scale, three patients were rated as much improved and two as minimally improved. In a follow-up investigation (follow-up intervals 3–14 months), half of the subjects continued olanzapine, and the other half discontinued treatment because of inadequate response or adverse side effects. Weight gain after a 6-week period of treatment was quite striking, and was a particular problem for adolescents.

Risperidone

Several investigations in adult patients with schizophrenia have demonstrated the significant improvement of positive and negative symptoms, comparable to the efficacy of haloperidol. Until now, there are no controlled studies on the use of risperidone in EOS. There are only two open trials that demonstrated an improvement of schizophrenic symptomatology at mean dosages between 4 and 6.6 mg/day (see Table 41.5). In the study by Armenteros et al. (1997), risperidone produced clinically and statistically significant improvement in 10 schizophrenics on the PANSS for schizophrenia, the BPRS, and the CGI scale, at a mean daily dosage of 6.6 mg. The reported side effects in this study included mild somnolence during dose finding (8 of 10 subjects), acute dystonic reactions (2/10), parkinsonism (3/10), mild orofacial dyskinesia (1/10), blurred vision (1/10), impaired concentration (1/10), and weight gain (8/10; mean weight gain: 4.85 kg). The side effect profile suggests that risperidone may be more closely related to the typical antipsychotics, especially at higher doses. For example, at a dosage of 6 mg/day and more, risperidone can cause EPS at a rate comparable to that of the typical antipsychotics.

Several case reports suggest good efficacy of risperidone in child and adolescent schizophrenia (for review see Toren et al., 1998).

Amisulpride

Several clinical trials with adults have demonstrated that amisulpride is effective in improving positive and negative symptoms of schizophrenia (Möller, 2000). There is one clinical trial including adolescent and young adulthood schizophrenia (Paillere-Martinot, 1995). Amisulpride was generally well tolerated and improved both positive and negative symptoms.

Quetiapine

There is only one study in (open trial) examining the efficacy of quetiapine in the treatment of EOS (McConville et al., 2000). Patientes were treated with 100 or 400 mg/day. Quetiapine was well tolerated and improved both positive and negative symptoms as determined by the BPRS, the CGI Scale, and the Modified SANS. Quetiapine pharmacokinetics were dose proportional in adolescents and resembled those reported in adult patients. The most common side effects in the study were postural tachycardia and insomnia. The EPS occurred and improved during the course of treatment. There were no serious adverse events or clinically important changes in hematology or clinical chemistry.

Figure 41.1 shows a decision tree for treatment with antipsychotics in EOS. Treatment is usually initiated with an atypical antipsychotic medication. Depending on the individual reaction (efficacy and side effects), the current medication can be switched or maintained. Only after two different compounds are not effective or not tolerated should treatment with clozapine be initiated.

Although EOS is mainly treated today with atypical antipsychotics, sometimes conventional antipsychotics must still be used. This applies in cases where atypical antipsychotics are not effective or are not tolerated. In some of these cases, haloperidol can still be used as well as other typical antipsychotics, such as fluphenazine or perphenazine. They should also be initiated at a low dosage. Dosages should be increased until improvement of the symptoms or the maximally recommended dosage is reached. When sufficient improvement has been achieved, readjustment of dosage is recommended, because lower dosages are often sufficient for maintenance treatment. If the acute psychotic state is complicated by aggression, tension, and/or psychomotor agitation, typical high-potency antipsychotics (e.g., haloperidol) can be combined with typical moderate—or low-potency antipsychotics such as chlorpromazine, or alternatively for a limited time with a benzodiazepine. However, benzodiazepines should be only used for a limited time span.

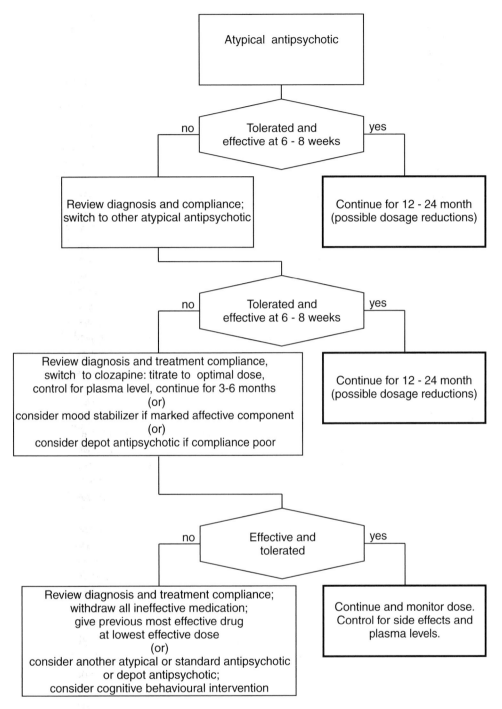

FIGURE 41.1 A decision tree for antipsychotic treatment selection in childhood and adolescence (adapted and modified from Clark and Lewis 1998).

Prevention of Relapses

A high risk of relapse is inherent to schizophrenic psychoses. A relapse is often triggered by emotional stress. It is very important to prevent a relapse by either maintaining low-dose oral medication or by switching to a depot antipsychotic. In some cases, this cannot be avoided. Especially when compliance is a problem, a depot medication may help to keep the patient free of psychotic symptoms. Frequently used depot antipsychotics are haloperidol-decanoate, fluphenazine-decanoate, and fluspirilene, which are given in relatively low dosages (see Table 41.4). In EOS, relapse prevention is more important than in adulthood, as the majority of patients have not yet finished school or started a professional career.

Conclusions

The following guidelines are suggested with regard to the use of antipsychotic medication:

1. Atypical and typical antipsychotics are to some extent comparable with regard to their clinical efficiency. They differ remarkably, however, with regard to their side effect profiles. Therefore, atypical antipsychotics are currently preferred in the initial treatment of EOS.

2. All antipsychotics should be administered in adequate dosages, using the lowest dosage that is effective.

3. It is imperative that children and adolescents who are being treated with antipsychotics and their parents be informed about the disorder and the effects and side effects of the medication. All of this information must be documented in the patient's chart. Furthermore, effects and side effects must be monitored during long-term treatment.

4. Antipsychotic medication must always start at low dosages and be increased slowly to reach steady-state levels. Treatment should not be interrupted suddenly, except in cases of emergency or pronounced adverse effects.

5. It is important to differentiate between nonresponse and noncompliance in the group of patients who do not respond to treatment.

6. First-episode patients seem to be more sensitive to side effects and may require lower doses than chronic patients. At the same time, they usually respond better to treatment, but many of them will relapse.

7. It is recommended that first-episode patients remain on antipsychotic treatment for a period of 1 to 2 years as a measure to prevent relapses.

8. In case of acute dystonia or parkinsonism, antiparkinsonian agents are the therapy of choice. If akathisia occurs, the drug should be given at a reduced dosage or discontinued. Benzodiazepines or propanolol can also be helpful for the treatment of akathisia. In case of acute dystonia or parkinsonism, antiparkinsonian agents are the therapy of choice. If akathisia occurs, the drug should be given at a reduced dose or discontinued. Benzodiazepines or propanolol can also be helpful for the treatment of akathisia. One of the major adverse effects of atypical antipsychotics is weight gain, for which no appropriate treatment is available (Bromel et al., 1998; Kraus et al., 1999).

Psychotherapeutic Measures

Cognitive and other behavioral approaches

Behavioral interventions based on basic learning principles started in the 1970s and were introduced under the term of *token economy programs*. They were administered individually, as well as in groups, and were mainly focused on the training of everyday activities such as self-sufficiency. Later on, the focus of behavioral therapy shifted towards more complex programs, such as social skills training, which is based on an analysis of each patient's interpersonal strengths and weaknesses and forms the basis of a more individualized therapeutic approach. Social skills training for schizophrenic patients includes several techniques, such as modeling prosocial behaviors, problem-centerd group discussions, model learning (e.g., by video demonstrations or role-play enhanced with video feedback), and in vivo exercises. Examples of potential skills to be trained include maintaining eye contact, reacting more quickly to interpersonal communication, varying voice intonation, and reinforcing prosocial responses from others.

Social competence training is often carried out in a group therapy setting and focuses on the management of everyday situations and the training of situation-appropriate behavior. Participants learn to express their own wishes and desires, to accept at the same time the needs and wishes of the other patients, to accept proposals as well as criticism, and to behave appropriately in a given situation. Group members are encouraged to express their emotions and to interact in a respectful rather than an egocentric way. Especially during adolescence, other common problems are addressed, such as social roles, identity and independence, contact with the opposite sex, and overall behavior at school, at work, or in peer groups. A number of controlled studies, all in adults, have demonstrated good results of social skills training, with improvements of up to 70% in social functioning and a shortened hospital stay. Several groups have emphasized the high correlation between poor results obtained for social competence training and cognitive deficits. They have therefore tried to integrate cognitive variables into the treatment procedure (Hoggarty et al., 1986; Jackson et al., 1998).

These experiences have led to highly structured manualized therapy techniques involving video- and audiolearning materials, as well as written instructions to optimize the learning situation (Lieberman and Eckman, 1989). One of these integrated approaches has been evaluated in young schizophrenic patients. This Integrative Psychological Therapy Program for Schizophrenic Patients (IPT) program (Brenner et al., 1993) consists of five standardized therapeutic components: cognitive differentiation, social perception, verbal communication, social skills, and interpersonal problem solving. The program originated from the classical social skills training technique extended to the area of communication. Most of the tasks, assigned to the different therapeutic components, are realistic and focused on everyday situations. Patients are encouraged to discuss and describe the respective situations with the aim of achieving a more realistic assessment, learning in the process from one another. This program has now been modified for adolescents with schizophrenia (Kienzle et al., 1997) and seems to offer a promising approach that still needs to be evaluated systematically.

Cognitive psychotherapeutic techniques have further been developed since their introduction by Beck et al. (1979), who demonstrated their effectiveness in the treatment of depression. Several studies have extended Beck's cognitive therapy to adulthood schizophrenia with encouraging clinical results. The efficacy of cognitive-behavioral approaches could be demonstrated in several key areas in schizophrenia, especially therapy-resistant hallucinations and delusions. Several approaches have also addressed therapeutic efforts in the treatment of associated symptoms such as anxiety and depression. In addition, cognitive-behavioral techniques have been shown to be effective in treatment of chronic schizophrenia, resulting in reduction of distress and disruption due to hallucinations and delusions. In some studies anxiety and depression associated with schizophrenia could also be reduced to some extent. The value of these techniques in children and adolescents has yet to be demonstrated.

Emotional management therapy

Therapeutic methods addressing the patient's emotional state are rare. The emotional state of schizo-

phrenic patients is very important: approximately 20% of all schizophrenic psychoses in adolescents start with a depressive episode (Remschmidt et al., 1973), but depressive symptoms are also extremely important over the course of the disorder. Depression in a patient entering a rehabilitation treatment program has been found to be a predictor of poor outcome at 1-year follow-up (Remschmidt et al., 1988). Schizophrenic patients have been found to be slower and less accurate at the recognition of emotional stimuli than normal controls and depressive patients (Gaebel and Wölwer, 1992; Heimberg et al., 1992), especially in situations characterized by stress and tension (Bellack, 1996). Emotional management therapy (EMT) has been designed to help people develop and refine specific strategies for coping with the impact of distress, anxiety, and dysfunction in information processing (Hodel and Brenner, 1996). According to its authors, EMT consists of two subprograms (Hodel et al., 1998). The first is devoted to the patients' ability to describe their physiological and cognitive reaction patterns when confronted by stress, fear, or excitement, and to the learning of relaxation techniques. The second subprogram addresses the description of subjective experiences in various emotional states and the development of coping strategies in relation to any consequent emotional distress. This therapy has been administered to young schizophrenic patients and in the early stages of their psychotic disorder (Kienzle and Martinius, 1995). In one study schizophrenic patients were randomly assigned either to the EMT group or to a comparison group (Hodel et al., 1998). All patients were additionally on neuroleptic medication. After 4 weeks of the EMT program, there were some significant improvements in the EMT group. These improvements were mainly in the areas of cognitive functioning. There were no significant differences between the groups in emotional well-being or social functioning. The trial undertaken involved a short therapy phase (4 weeks), and the therapy sessions might not have been intensive enough. In conclusion, EMT has not yet been demonstrated to be an effective treatment method for young patients with schizophrenia in the subacute stage of the first episode. However, as there is no doubt that the emotional sphere is of great importance in the course of the disorder, this approach should receive further investigation.

Group programs

Group programs have been thought to be helpful in the treatment of young schizophrenic patients, as they might reduce feelings of alienation and demonstrate to patients that others suffer from similar problems, thus giving support to participants in group activities. Group therapies were originally developed to enhance self-esteem and to modify attitudes and behavior through the corrective experience of supportive group processes. Initial adaptations with focus on special symptoms were developed in the 1970s, originating from social-cognitive theories (Bandura, 1977; 1986). Many of the above-mentioned psychotherapeutic and educational techniques for the treatment of schizophrenic patients have been performed in group programs. The main aspects of group program treatment can be subdivided into focused approaches, devoted to a special area of intervention, and integrative approaches that try to cover a wider range of problem areas with the aim of general improvement in different areas, expressed by better integration of the patients. Focused group programs have been established for improvement of skills (e.g., social skills training, problem solving, communication) and education (e.g., information about illness and treatment, management of medication and relapses). Integrative approaches include different areas of functioning that are typically impaired in schizophrenic patients.

Since schizophrenic patients have impairments in focusing attention and are often highly sensitive to social overstimulation, group programs have to be well structured and supportive. Mainly insight-oriented and conflict-enhancing group therapies are not appropriate (Schooler and Spohn, 1982; Leszcz et al., 1985). Especially in acute psychotic states, the use of group therapies has been questioned and even considered harmful (Kanas et al. 1980; Ciompi, 1982). A recent study used an integrated group approach and included a group of patients with a first schizophrenic episode, ages 16 to 30 years. This group was compared to other patients who received conventional treatment. There were no significant differences on any outcome measure between the two groups (Albiston et al., 1998).

Family-oriented measures

The families of children and adolescents with schizophrenic psychoses have to be included in the planning and design of therapy. Empirical research has shown, however, that ambitious family therapy designs have not reaped the benefits hoped for. Studies using the concept of expressed emotion have shown that emotional factors within the family play an important role in relapses of the disorder. Therefore, in every child and adolescent with schizophrenia, one must decide on the extent to which the family should be integrated into the therapeutic process. This depends on the patient, the disorder, and the structure and stability of the family.

Family interventions in childhood or adolescent onset schizophrenia comprise a combination of psychoeducational and behavioral approaches that support the patient and the family and that are used to attempt to reduce high levels of expressed emotion by family members, especially criticism and hostility. From adult psychiatry settings there is evidence that reducing the amount of expressed emotion is associated with a reduction of subsequent relapse rates and with better social functioning (Penn and Mueser, 1996; Dixon and Lehmann, 1995). Attempts to replicate findings from adult psychiatry have not so far been successful, and studies have failed to replicate the concept of expressed emotion in children (Asarnow et al., 1994). Recently, one study in schizophrenic adolescents demonstrate that standard plus family intervention was able to reduce the institutional length of stay, as compared to standard treatment alone (Lenior et al., 2001). In about 30% to 40% of children and adolescents with schizophrenia, there is no ready possibility for reintegration into their families after inpatient treatment (Remschmidt et al., 2001). For this group, a special rehabilitation program is necessary.

Specific measures of rehabilitation

Residential rehabilitation for adolescents with schizophrenia may be indicated because of either the nature or the course of the illness. In particular, it may be advisable if there are marked negative symptoms after treatment of the acute episode, or when reintegration into the family is impossible. Residential rehabilitation is also advisable when there are specific educational issues. The rehabilitation of adolescents with psychotic illnesses involves the coordination of a number of interrelated measures that should be included in a comprehensive rehabilitation program. A prototypical rehabiliation program has been developed in connection with the Department of Child and Adolescent Psychiatry of the Philipps-University of Marburg at the Leppermuehle Rehabilitation Centre near Marburg (Martin and Remschmidt, 1983; Martin, 1991). This rehabilitation program is of about two years duration and includes the following components (Martin, 1991; Remschmidt et al., 2001): medical treatment, individual supportive psychotherapy, occupational therapy, opportunities for basic academic and professional qualifications, and a wide range of living options, from a staffed therapeutic community setting to smaller, supervised units integrated within the local community.

As a result of the high staffing levels of such a unit,

it is often possible to deal with mild relapses in the unit itself. It must be emphasized, however, that without the support of and close contact with the clinic and, in particular, the ability to admit a patient immediately when required, the work at the Leppermuehle Center would be untenable. Short or relatively short hospital admissions do not break the routine of the rehabilitation process.

An attempt was made to predict the success of the program after 1 year by variables present at the beginning of rehabilitation. The results are summarized here (Remschmidt et al., 1991):

1. Schizophrenic adolescents who are characterized by deficits in cognitive functioning, subjective complaints, and psychopathological symptoms do profit from a structured 1-year rehabilitation program. Most of these deficiencies improved considerably.

2. However, this improvement does not occur in all patients. It applies to a subgroup of schizophrenic patients characterized by higher cognitive abilities and less somatic and psychiatric symptoms. Interestingly, this differentiation is independent on the classical subtypes of schizophrenia (hebephrenic, paranoid, or schizoaffective).

3. The status at the end of the 1-year rehabilitation program could best be predicted by the depression score at the beginning of rehabilitation, which is in line with a result of an earlier study using an independent sample (Remschmidt et al., 1988).

CONCLUSIONS

There is no doubt about the existence of EOS (before the age of 16) and VEOS (manifestation before the age of 13). There is a continuity between these disorders and adult schizophrenia, (see Chapter 15 in this volume), but the prognosis of EOS and VEOS is much poorer. Therefore, early diagnosis and early intervention is most important. Although the diagnostic criteria (in ICD-10 and DSM-IV) are the same for adults and children with schizophrenia, the diagnosis in young patients is much more difficult because of the interference with developmental processes and the sometimes not fully expressed symptomatology. This can make the differential diagnosis quite difficult. Treatment is always based upon a multidimensional approach, including antipsychotic medication, psychotherapeutic and family-oriented measures, as well as clear information about the disorder, the components of treatment, and rehabilitation measures. As far as pharmacological treatment is concerned, atypical antipsychotics are now the first-line medication in treatment. They are effective on positive and negative symptoms and produce less adverse effects than typical antipsychotics, especially with regard to EPS. However, they produce other side effects, among which weight gain is a great concern, especially for young people. Therefore, initiatives have been undertaken to develop new antipsychotic medications with minimal or no effect on weight, but having the same efficacy as that of the currently available atypical antipsychotics. Ziprazodone and aripiprazole have been identified as such medications, which hopefully will improve the pharmacological treatment component. Programs in the field of cognitive behavioral approaches and emotional management therapy are also promising and are currently being studied. Finally, more institutions for rehabilitation are necessary, because, despite the array of modern treatment components, a chronic course in about 30% of EOS cannot be avoided, and long-lasting and intensive measures of rehabilitation have been demonstrated to be effective.

ACKNOWLEDGMENT

The authors thank Dr. Philip Heiser for his help with tables and with the literature search, and Ms. Le Guillarme for her editorial assistance.

REFERENCES

Abczynska, M., Kazmirek, Z., Syguda, J., and Terminska, K. (1995) Own experience (1989–1994) in the treatment of adolescent schizophrenic paranoid syndromes with Leponex produced by Sandoz Company. *Psychiatr Pol* 29:79–85.

Albiston, D.J., Francey, S.M., and Harrigan, S.M. (1998) Group programmes for recovery from early psychoses. *Br J Psychiatry* 172 (Suppl. 33):117–121.

American Academy of Child and Adolescent Psychiatry (2000) Summary of the practice parameters for the assessment and treatment of children and adolescents with schizophrenia. *J Am Acad Child Adolesc Psychiatry* 39:1580–1582.

American Academy of Child and Adolescent Psychiatry (2001) Practice parameters for the assessment and treatment of children and adolescents with schizophrenia. *J Am Acad Child Adolesc Psychiatry* 40:45–23 S (supplement).

American Psychiatric Association (1994) *Diagnostic and Statistical Manual of Mental Disorders*, 4th ed. Washington, DC: American Psychiatric Association.

Andreasen, N.C. and Olsen, S. (1982) Negative and positive schizophrenia: definition and validation. *Arch Gen Psychiatry* 39:789–794.

Angold, A., Prendergast, M., Cox, A., Harrington, R., Simonoff, E., and Rutter, M. (1995) The Child and Adolescent Psychiatric Assessment (CAPA). *Psychol Med* 25:739–753.

Arboleda, C. and Holzman, P. (1985) Thought disorder in children at risk for psychosis. *Arch Gen Psychiatry* 42:1004–1013.

Armenteros, J.L., Whitaker, A.H., Welikson, M., Stedge, D.J., and

Gorman, J. (1997) Risperidone in adolescents with schizophrenia: an open pilot study. *J Am Acad Child Adolesc Psychiatry* 36:694–700.

Asarnow, J.R. (1994) Annotation: childhood-onset schizophrenia. *J Child Psychol Psychiatry* 35:1345–1371.

Asarnow, J.R., Asarnow, R.F., Hornstein, N., and Russell, A.T. (1991) Childhood-onset schizophrenia: developmental perspectives on schizophrenic disorders. In: Walker, E.F., ed. *Schizophrenia: A Life Course Developmental Perspective*. New York: Academic Press, pp. 92–122.

Asarnow, J.R., Thompson, M.C., and Goldstein, M.J. (1994) Childhood-onset schizophrenia: a follow-up study. *Schizophr Bull* 20: 599–617.

Bandura A. (1977) *Social Learning Theory*. Englewood Cliffs, NJ: Prentice-Hall.

Bandura, A. (1986) *Social Foundations of Thought and Action*. Englewood Cliffs, NJ: Prentice-Hall.

Beck, A.T., Rush, A.J., Shaw, B.F., and Emery, G. (1979) *Cognitive Therapy of Depression*. New York: Guilford Press.

Beitchman, J.H. (1985) Childhood schizophrenia. A review and comparison with adult-onset schizophrenia. *Psychiatr Clin North Am* 8:793–814.

Bellack, A.S. (1996) Defizitäres Sozialverhalten und Training sozialer Fertigkeiten: Neue Entwicklungen und Trends. In: Böker, W. and Brenner, H.D. eds. *Integrative Therapie der Schizophrenie*. Bern: Huber, pp. 191–202.

Bender, L. (1969) A longitudinal study of schizophrenic children with autism. *Hosp Community Psychiatry* 20:230–237.

Blanz, B., and Schmidt, M.H. (1993) Clozapine for schizophrenia [letter; comment]. *J Am Acad Child Adolesc Psychiatry* 32:223–224.

Bleuler, E. (1911) Dementia praecox oder die Gruppe der Schizophrenien. In: Aschaffenburg, G. ed. *Handbuch der Psychiatrie, special part, section 4*. Leipzig: Deuticke, pp. 1–420.

Brenner, H.D., Roder, V., and Merlo, M.C.G. (1993) Verhaltenstherapeutische Verfahren bei schizophrenen Erkrankungen. In: Möller, H.J., ed. *Therapie Psychiatrischer Erkrankungen*. Stuttgart: Enke, pp. 222–230.

Bromel, T., Blum, W.F., Ziegler, A., Schulz, E., Bender, M., Fleischhaker, C., Remschmidt, H., Krieg, J.C., and Hebebrand, J. (1998) Serum leptin levels increase rapidly after initiation of clozapine therapy. *Mol Psychiatry* 3:76–80.

Burd, L., Fisher, W., and Kerbeshian, J. (1987) A prevalence study of pervasive developmental disorders in North Dakota. *J Am Acad Child Adolesc Psychiatry* 26:704–710.

Caplan, R., Guthrie, D., Tanguay, P., Fish, B., and David-Lando, G. (1989) The Kiddie Formal Thought Disorder Scale (K-FTDS): clinical assessment, reliability and validity. *J Am Acad Child Adolesc Psychiatry* 28:408–416.

Caplan, R., Perdue, S., Tanguay, P., and Fish, B. (1990) Formal thought disorder in childhood onset schizophrenia and schizotypal personality disorder. *J Child Psychol Psychiatry* 31:1103–1114.

Ciompi, L. (1982) How to improve the treatment of schizophrenia: a multicausal concept and its theoretical components. In: Stierlin, H., Wynne, L., and Wirschung, M., eds. *Psychosocial Intervention in Schizophrenia: An Interactional View*. New York: Springer-Verlag, pp. 53–66.

Clark, A.F. and Lewis, S.W. (1998) Treatment of schizophrenia in childhood and adolescence. *J Child Psychol Psychiatry* 39:1071–1081.

Dixon, L.B. and Lehmann, A.F. (1995) Family interventions for schizophrenia. *Schizophr Bull* 21:631–643.

Fields, J., Grochowski, S., Linenmayer, J., Kay, S., Grosz, D., Hyman,

R., and Alexander, G. (1994) Assessing positive and negative symptoms in children and adolescents. *Am J Psychiatry* 151:249–253.

Fish, B. (1985) Children's Psychiatric Rating Scale. *Psychopharmacol Bull* 21:753–765.

Frazier, J.A., Gordon, C.T., McKenna, K., Lenane, M.C., Jih, D., and Rapoport, J.L. (1994) An open trial of clozapine in 11 adolescents with childhood-onset schizophrenia. *J Am Acad Child Adolesc Psychiatry* 33:658–663.

Gaebel, W. and Wölwer, W. (1992) Facial expression and emotional face recognition in schizophrenia and depression. *Eur Arch Psychiatry Clin Neurosci* 242:36–52.

Garralda, M.E. (1984) Hallucinations in children with conduct and emotional disorders; I. The clinical phenomena. *Psychol Med* 14: 589–596.

Gillberg, C. (1984) Infantile autism and other childhood psychoses in a Swedish urban region. Epidemiological aspects. *J Child Psychol Psychiatry* 25:35–43.

Gillberg, C. (2001) Epidemiology of early onset schizophrenia. In: Remschmidt, H., ed. *Schizophrenia in Children and Adolescents*. Cambridge; UK: Cambridge University Press, pp. 43–59.

Gillberg, C. and Steffenburg, S. (1987) Outcome and prognostic factors in infantile autism and similar conditions: a population-based study of 46 cases followed through puberty. *J Autism Dev Dis* 17:273–287.

Gillberg, C., Steffenburg, S., and Schaumann, H. (1991) Is autism more common now than 10 years ago? *Br J Psychiatry* 158:403–409.

Gillberg, C., Wahlström, J., Forsman, A., Hellgren, L., and Gillberg, I.C. (1986) Teenage psychoses—epidemiology, classification and reduced optimality in the pre-, peri- and neonatal periods. *J Child Psychol Psychiatry* 27:87–98.

Gillberg, I.C., Hellgren, L., and Gillberg, C. (1993) Psychotic disorders diagnosed in adolescence. Outcome at age 30 years. *J Child Psychol Psychiatry* 34:1173–1185.

Gordon, C.T., Frazier, J.A., McKenna, K., Giedd, J., Zametkin, A., Zahn, T., Hommer, D., Hong, W., Kaysen, D., Albus, K.E., et al. (1994) Childhood-onset schizophrenia: an NIMH study in progress. *Schizophr Bull* 20:697–712.

Green, W., Padron-Gayol, M., Hardesty, A.S., and Bassiri, M. (1992) Schizophrenia with childhood onset: a phenomenological study of 38 cases. *J Am Acad Child Adolesc Psychiatry* 35:968–976.

Heimberg, C., Gur, R., and Erwin, R.J. (1992) Facial emotion discrimination: III. Behavioural findings in schizophrenia. *Psychiatry Res* 42:253–265.

Herjanic, B. and Reich, W. (1982) Development of a structured psychiatric interview for children: agreement between child and parent on individual symptoms *J Abnorm Child Psychol* 10:307–324.

Hodel, B. and Brenner, H.D. (1996) Ein Trainingsprogramm zur Bewältigung von maladaptiven Emotionen bei schizophrenen Erkrankungen. Erste Ergebnisse und Erfahrungen. *Nervenarzt* 67: 564–571.

Hodel, B., Brenner, H.D., Merlo, M.C.G., and Teuber, J.F. (1998) Emotional management therapy in early psychosis. *Br J Psychiatry* 172(Suppl 33):128–133.

Hoggarty, G.E., Anderson, C.M., Reiss, D.J., Kornblith, S.J., Greenwald, D.P., Javna, C.D., and Madonia, M.J. (1986) Family psychoeducation, social skills training and maintenance chemotherapy in the aftercare treatment of schizophrenia. I. One-year effects of a controlled study on relapse and expressed emotions. *Arch Gen Psychiatry* 43:633–642.

Hollis, C. (2001) Diagnosis and differential diagnosis. In: Remschmidt, H., ed. *Schizophrenia in Children and Adolescents.* Cambridge; UK: Cambridge University Press, pp. 82–118.

Homburger, A. (1926) *Vorlesungen über Psychopathologie des Kindesalters.* Berlin: Springer.

Jackson, H., McGorry, P., Edwards, J., Ulbert, C., Henry, L., Frency, S., Maude, D., Cocks, J., Power, P., Harrigan, S., and Dudgeon, P. (1998) Cognitively oriented psychotherapy for early psychoses (COPE). *Br J Psychiatry* 172(Suppl 33):93–100.

Kanas, N., Rogers, M., Kreth, E., Patterson, L., and Campbell, R. (1980) The effectiveness of group psychotherapy during the first three weeks of hospitalization: a controlled study. *J Nerv Ment Dis* 168:487–492.

Kienzle, N., Braun-Scharm, H., and Hemme, M. (1997) Kognitive, psychoedukative und familientherapeutische Therapiebausteine in der stationären jugendpsychiatrischen Versorgung. In: Dittmar, V., Klein, H.E., and Schön D., eds. *Die Behandlung schizophrener Menschen. Integrative Therapiemodelle und ihre Wirksamkeit.* Regensburg: Roderer, pp. 39–152.

Kienzle, N. and Martinius, J. (1995). Modifikationen und Adaptationen des IPT für die Anwendung bei schizophrenen Jugendlichen. In: Roder, V., Brenner, H.D., Kienzle, N., and Hodel, B. eds. *Integriertes psychologisches Therapieprogramm für schizophrene Patienten (IPT).* Weinheim: Psychologie-Verlagsunion, pp. 171–182.

Kolvin, I. (1971) Studies in the childhood psychoses. *Br J Psychiatry* 118:381–419.

Kraus, T., Haack, M., Schuld, A., Hinze-Selch, D., Kuhn, M., Uhr, M., and Pollmacher, T. (1999) Body weight and leptin plasma levels during treatment with antipsychotic drugs. *Am J Psychiatry* 156:312–314.

Kumra, S., Frazier, J.A., Jacobsen, L.K., McKenna, K., Gordon, C.T., Lenane, M.C., Hamburger, S.D., Smith, A.K., Albus, K.E., Alaghband-Rad, J., and Rapoport, J.L. (1996) Childhood-onset schizophrenia. A double-blind clozapine-haloperidol comparison. *Arch Gen Psychiatry* 53:1090–1097.

Kumra, S., Jacobsen, L.K., Lenane, M.C., Karp, B.I., Frazier, J.A., Smith, A.K., Bedwell, J., Lee, P., Malanga, C.J., Hamburger, S.D., and Rapoport, J.L. (1998) Childhood-onset schizophrenia: an open-label study of olanzapine in adolescents. *J Am Acad Child Adolesc Psychiatry* 37:377–385

Kutcher, S. (1998) The identification of akathisia. *Child Adolesc Psychopharmacol News* 3:11–12.

Lambert, L.T. (2001) Identification and management of schizophrenia in childhood. *J Child Adolesc Psychiat Nursing* 14:73–80.

Leckman, J.F., Sholomskas, D., Thompson, W.D., Belanger, A., and Weissman, M.M. (1982) Best estimate of lifetime psychiatric diagnoses. A methodological study. *Arch Gen Psychiatry* 39:879–883.

Lenior, M.E., Dingemans, P.M.A.J., Linseen, D.H., Haan, L. de, and Schene, A.H. (2001) Social functioning and the course of early onset schizophrenic. *Brit J Psychiatry* 179:53–58.

Leszcz, M., Yalom, I.D., and Norden, M. (1985) The value of inpatient group psychotherapy: patients' perceptions. *Int J Group Psychother* 35:411–433.

Levkovitch, Y., Kaysar, N., Kronnenberg, Y., Hagai, H., and Gaoni, B. (1994) Clozapine for schizophrenia [letter]. *J Am Acad Child Adolesc Psychiatry* 33:431.

Lieberman, R.P. and Eckman, T.A. (1989) Zur Vermittlung von Trainingsprogrammen für soziale Fertigkeiten an psychiatrischen Einrichtungen: Möglichkeiten der praktischen Umsetzung eines neuen Rehabilitationsansatzes. In: Böker, W. and Brenner, H.D.; eds. *Schizophrenie als systemische Störung. Die Bedeutung intermediärer Prozesse für Theorie und Therapie.* Bern: Huber, pp. 256–267.

Lutz, J. (1937/38) Über die Schizophrenie im Kindesalter. Part 1. *Schweiz Arch Neurol, Neurochirurg Psychiatrie* 39:335–332.

Mandoki, M. (1994) Anti-aggressive effects of clozapine in children and adolescents [abstract]. Proceedings of the Annual Meeting, Society for Biological Psychiatry, Philadelphia. *Biol Psychiatry* 35 (Suppl):469.

Mandoki, M. (1997) Olanzapine in the treatment of early onset schizophrenia in children and adolescents. *Biol Psychiatry* 35(Suppl 7S):S22.

Martin, M. (1991) *Der Verlauf der Schizophrenie im Jugendalter unter Rehabilitationsbedingungen.* Stuttgart: Enke.

Martin, M. and Remschmidt, H. (1983) Ein Nachsorge- und Rehabilitationsprojekt für jugendliche Schizophrene. *Z Kinder Jugendpsychiatrie* 11:234–242.

McConville, B.J., Arventis, L.A., Thyrum, P.T., Yeh, C., Wilkinson, L.A., Chaney, R.O., Foster, K.D., Sorter, M.T., Friedman, L.M., Brown, K.L., and Heubi, J.E. (2000) Pharmacokinetics, tolerability, and clinical effectivness of quetiapine fumarate: an open-label trial in adolescents with psychotic disoreders. *J Clin Psychiatry* 61:252–260.

Möller, H.J. (2000) Neue bzw. atypische Neuroleptika bei schizophrener Negativsymptomatik. *Nervenarzt* 71:345–353.

National Institute of Mental Health (NIMH) (1992) The NIMH Diagnostic Interview Schedule for Children. Rockville, MD: National Institute of Mental Health.

Orvaschel, H. and Puig-Antich, J. (1987) Schedule for Affective Disorders and Schizophrenia for School-age Children: Epidemiological Version. Unpublished manuscript. Medical College of Pennsylvania, Eastern Pennsylvania Psychiatric Institute.

Pailere-Martinot, M.L., Lecrubier, Y., Martin, J.L., and Aubin, F. (1995) Improvement of some schizophrenic deficit symptoms with low dose of amisulpride. *Am J Psychiatry* 152:130–133.

Parmar, R. (1993) Attitudes of child psychiatrists to electroconvulsive therapy. *Psychiatry Bull* 17:12–13.

Penn, D.L. and Mueser, K.T. (1996) Research update on the psychosocial treatment of schizophrenia. *Am J Psychiatry* 153:607–617.

Piscitelli, S.C., Frazier, J.A., McKenna, K., Albus, K.E., Grothe, D.R., Gordon, C.T., and Rapoport, J.L. (1994) Plasma clozapine and haloperidol concentrations in adolescents with childhood-onset schizophrenia: association with response. *J Clin Psychiatry* 55(9, Suppl B): 94–97.

Quintana H. and Keshavan, M. (1995) Case study: risperidone in children and adolescents with schizophrenia. *J Am Acad Child Adolesc Psychiatry.* 34:1292–1296.

Remington, G. (1997) Selecting a neuroleptic and the role of side effects. *Child Adolesc Psychopharmacol News* 2:1–5.

Remschmidt, H. (1975a). Neuere Ergebnisse zur Psychologie und Psychiatrie der Adoleszenz. *Z. Kinder Jugendpsychiatrie* 3:67–101.

Remschmidt, H. (1975b) Psychologie und Psychopathologie der Adoleszenz. *Monatsschr Kinderheilkd* 123:316–323.

Remschmidt, H. (1993) Schizophrenic psychoses in children and adolescents. *Triangle* 32:15–24.

Remschmidt, H. (2001) Definition and classification. In: Remschmidt, H., ed. *Schizophrenia in Children and Adolescents.* Cambridge; UK: Cambridge University Press, pp. 24–42.

Remschmidt, H. (2002) Early-onset schizophrenia as a progressive deteriorating disorder: evidence from child psychiatry *J Neural Transm* 109:101–117.

Remschmidt, H., Brechtel, B., and Mewe, F. (1973) Zum Krankheitsverlauf und zur Persönlichkeitsstruktur von Kindern und Jugendlichen mit endogen-phasischen Psychosen und reaktive Depressionen. *Acta Paedopsychiatr* 40:2–17.

Remschmidt, H., Hennighausen, K., Clement, H.-W., Heiser, P., and Schulz, E. (2000): Atypical neuroleptics in child and adolescent psychiatry. *Eur Child Adolesc Psychiatry* 9 (Suppl 1): 9–19.

Remschmidt, H., Martin, M., Albrecht, G., Gerlach, G., and Rühl, D. (1988) Der Voraussagewert des Initialbefundes für den mittelfristigen Rehabilitationsverlauf bei jugendlichen Schizophrenen. *Nervenarzt* 59:471–476.

Remschmidt, H., Martin, M., Hennighausen, K., and Schulz, E. (2001) Treatment and rehabilitation. In: Remschmidt, H., ed. *Schizophrenia in Children and Adolescents*. Cambridge, UK: Cambridge University Press, pp. 192–267.

Remschmidt, H., Martin, M., Schulz, E., Gutenbrunner, C., and Fleischhaker, C. (1991) The concept of positive and negative schizophrenia in child and adolescent psychiatry. In: Marneros, A., Andreasen, N.C., and Tsuang, M.T., eds. *Negative and Positive Schizophrenia*. Bern-Heidelberg: Springer, pp. 219–242.

Remschmidt, H., Schulz, E., and Herpertz-Dahlmann, B. (1996) Schizophrenic psychoses in childhood and adolescence. A guide to diagnosis and drug choice. *CNS Drugs* 6:100–112.

Remschmidt, H., Schulz, E., and Martin, M. (1994) An open trial of clozapine in thirty-six adolescents with schizophrenia. *J Child Adolesc Psychopharmacol* 4:31–41.

Russell, A.T., Bott, L., and Sammons, C. (1989) The phenomenology of schizophrenia occurring in childhood. *J Am Acad Child Adolesc Psychiatry* 28:399–407.

Rutter, M. (1967) Psychotic disorders in early childhood. In: Coppen, A.J. and Walk, A., eds. *Recent Developments in Schizophrenia*. Ashford: Headly Brothers, pp. 133–158.

Schooler, C. and Spohn, H.E. (1982) Social dysfunction and treatment failure in schizophrenia. *Schizophr Bull* 8:85–98.

Schmidt, M.H., Trott, G.E., Blanz, B., et al. (1989) Clozapine medication in adolescents. In: Stefanis, C.N., Rabavilas, A.D., and Soldatos, C.R., eds. *Psychiatry: A World Perspective, Vol 1. Proceedings of the 8th World Congress of Psychiatry, Athens, Greece, October 12–19*. Amsterdam: Excerpta Medica; pp. 1100–1104.

Schulz, E., Fleischhaker, C., Clement, H.-W., and Remschmidt, H. (1997) Blood biogenic amines during clozapine treatment of early-onset schizophrenia. *J Neural Transm* 104:1077–1089.

Schulz, E., Fleischhaker, C., and Remschmidt, H. (1996) Correlated changes in symptoms and neurotransmitter indices during maintenance treatment with clozapine or conventional neuroleptics in adolescence and young adulthood schizophrenia. *J Child Adolesc Psychopharmacol* 6:119–131.

Shaffer, D., Gould, M.S., Brasic, J., Ambrosini, P., Fisher, P., Bird, H., and Aluwahlia, S. (1983) A children's global assessment scale (CGAS). *Arch Gen Psychiatry* 40:1228–1231.

Sholevar EH. Baron DA, Hardie TL. Treatment of childhood-onset schizophrenia with olanzapine. *J Child Adolesc Psychoparmacol*. 2000 Summer; 10(2):69–78.

Siefen, G. and Remschmidt, H. (1986) Results of treatment with clozapine in schizophrenic adolescents. *Z Kinder Jugendpsychiatrie* 14:245–247.

Steffenburg, S. and Gillberg, C. (1986) Autism and autistic-like conditions in Swedish rural and urban areas: a population study. *Br J Psychiatry* 149:81–87.

Stutte, H. (1969) Psychosen des Kindesalters. In: Schmidt, F. and Asperger, H., eds. *Neurologie-Psychologie-Psychiatrie (Handbuch der Kinderheilkunde)*, Vol VIII/1. Berlin: Springer, pp. 908–938.

Tobwin, K.E., Dykens, E.M., Pearson, G.S., and Cohen, D.J. (1993) Conceptualizing borderline syndrome of childhood and childhood schizophrenia as a developmental disorder. *J Am Acad Child Adolesc Psychiatry* 32:775–782.

Toren, P., Laor, N., and Weizman, A. (1998) Use of atypical neuroleptics in child and adolescent psychiatry. *J Clini Psychiatry* 59: 644–656.

Turetz, M., Mozes, T., Toren, P., Chernauzan, N., Yoran-Hegesh, R., Mester, R., Wittenberg, N., Tyano, S., and Weizman, A. (1997) An open trial of clozapine in neuroleptic-resistant childhood-onset schizophrenia. *Br J Psychiatry* 170:507–510.

Verhulst, F. and Koot, H. (1992). *Child Psychiatric Epidemiology: Concepts, Methods and Findings. Assessment and Diagnosis*. London: Sage, pp. 42–96.

Watkins, J.M., Asarnow, R.F., and Tanguay, P.E. (1988) Symptom development in childhood onset schizophrenia. *J Child Psychol Psychiatry* 29:865–878.

Werry, J.S. (1992) Child and adolescent (early onset) schizophrenia: a review in light of DSM-III-R. *J Autism Dev Dis* 22:601–624.

Wing, L. (1996) Autism spectrum disorder. *BMJ*. 312:327–328.

World Health Organization (1992) *The ICD-10 Classification of Mental and Behavioral Disorders. Clinical Descriptions and Diagnostic Guidelines*. Geneva: World Health Organization.

World Health Organization (1993) *The ICD-10 Classification of Mental and Behavioral Disorders. Diagnostic Criteria for Research*. Geneva: World Health Organization.

Young, J.G., O'Brien, J.D., Gutterman, E.M., and Cohen, D. (1987) Research on the clinical interview. *J Am Acad Child Adolesc Psychiatry* 26:613–620.

42 | Autistic and other pervasive developmental disorders

CHRISTOPHER J. MCDOUGLE AND DAVID J. POSEY

The assessment and treatment of autistic disorder and other pervasive developmental disorders (PDDs) requires a multidisciplinary team approach. Initial interventions are largely based on educational programming and behavior management principles, particularly for preschool- and school-aged children and adolescents. Speech therapy is usually essential and physical and occupational therapy are often needed as well. Despite these extensive therapeutic efforts, many children, adolescents, and adults with PDDs remain significantly impaired. Under these conditions, drug treatment is often necessary and appropriate.

Adequate drug treatment studies focused on subjects with a specific subtype of PDD, other than autistic disorder, have not been completed. Many trials have included mixed samples of subjects with autistic disorder, Asperger's disorder, and PDD not otherwise specified (NOS). Because of the extreme rarity of Rett's disorder and childhood disintegrative disorder, almost no systematic drug treatment studies have been done in subjects with these subtypes of PDD. More recently, researchers have been conducting drug studies of adults with PDDs, in addition to those of children and adolescents. The results from these investigations allow for some evaluation of the effects of developmental factors on drug efficacy and tolerability.

Drugs that have primary effects on the core social impairment of autistic disorder and other PDDs have not yet been developed. Currently, the pharmacotherapy of this group of disorders involves the identification and treatment of associated symptoms, including motor hyperactivity, inattention, irritability, aggression toward self, others, or the environment, and interfering repetitive thoughts and behavior. Improvement in some aspects of social behavior can occur as a result of a reduction in these associated target symptoms.

This chapter will first define the five subtypes of PDD included in the *Diagnostic and Statistical Manual of Mental Disorders, 4th ed.* (DSM-IV) (American Psychiatric Association, 1994) and discuss the differential diagnosis of PDDs. Aspects of clinical practice, including assessment and evaluation, and measurement of symptom severity and change will follow. The chapter will review results from drug treatment studies with a focus on more recent controlled trials. Novel treatment strategies are discussed. A suggested treatment algorithm is provided.

DSM-IV SUBTYPES OF PERVASIVE DEVELOPMENTAL DISORDERS

The PDDs are characterized by severe and pervasive impairment in several areas of development, including reciprocal social interaction, communication, or the presence of stereotyped behavior, interests, and activities. These abnormalities occur relative to the individual's level of development or mental age. These disorders are usually evident in the first 1 to 3 years of life and are often associated with some degree of mental retardation. The PDDs are sometimes observed among a diverse group of identifiable biological abnormalities (e.g., chromosomal abnormalities, congenital infections, structural abnormalities of the brain). In the majority of cases, however, the etiology remains unknown. Previously, terms like "psychosis" and "childhood schizophrenia" were used to refer to individuals with these disorders. There is now considerable evidence, however, to demonstrate that PDDs are distinct from schizophrenia. There are five subtypes of PDD in the DSM-IV. They include autistic disorder, Rett's disorder, childhood disintegrative disorder, Asperger's disorder, and PDD NOS.

Autistic Disorder

Autistic disorder is characterized by a severe impairment in the development of social interaction and communication skills and a markedly restricted repertoire of activity and interests. The clinical presentation varies significantly depending on the level of development and age of the individual.

The clinical features must include delays or abnormalities in social interaction, language, or imaginative play before the age of 3 years. One or 2 years of relatively normal development can occur, although there is usually no period of clearly normal development. In some cases, regression in language, usually manifest as complete loss of speech after a child has acquired from 5 to 10 words, occurs. If there is a period of normal development, it cannot extend past the age of 3 years.

In nearly 75% of cases, there is a comorbid diagnosis of mental retardation, usually in the moderate range (intelligence quotient [IQ] 35–50). Motor hyperactivity, inattention, irritability, aggression toward self, others or property, and interfering repetitive thoughts and behavior are often present. The disorder is sometimes observed in association with an identifiable medical condition (e.g., encephalitis, phenylketonuria, tuberous sclerosis, fragile X syndrome, anoxia at birth, maternal rubella). Seizures may develop, often in adolescence, in up to 25% to 33% of cases. The disorder is four to five times more common in males than in females, although females often have a more severe degree of cognitive impairment. Earlier epidemiological studies identified rates of autistic disorder of 2 to 5 cases per 10,000, although more recent estimates of prevalence are higher (Chakrabarti and Fombonne, 2001). Language skills and IQ are the strongest predictors of eventual outcome.

Rett's Disorder

Rett's disorder differs from autistic disorder in its characteristic sex ratio and distinctive pattern of abnormal development. The disorder is much less common than autistic disorder and has been diagnosed almost exclusively in females. Following apparently normal prenatal and perinatal development through the first 5 months of life, there is a characteristic pattern of head growth deceleration, loss of previously acquired purposeful hand skills, intermittent hyperventilation, and the appearance of ataxic gait or trunk movements. Difficulties in social interaction, particularly during the preschool years, may occur but these tend to be time limited. Severe or profound mental retardation, seizures, and significant expressive and receptive language impairment are typical. A mutation in the gene (*MECP2*) encoding X-linked methyl-CpG-binding protein 2 (MeCP2) has been identified as the cause of some cases of Rett's disorder (Amir et al., 1999).

Childhood Disintegrative Disorder

Childhood disintegrative disorder differs from autistic disorder in that there is a distinctive pattern of regression after at least 2 years of normal development. In autistic disorder, some abnormalities in development are usually noted within the first year of life. After the first 2 years, but before the age of 10, the child with childhood disintegrative disorder has a significant loss of previously acquired skills in at least two of the following areas: expressive or receptive language, social skills or adaptive behavior, bowel or bladder control, play, or motor skills. The onset may be insidious or abrupt, and in most cases occurs between the ages of 3 and 4 years. The disorder has been reported in association with metachromatic leukodystrophy and Schilder's disease, although the etiology remains unknown in most cases. Childhood disintegrative disorder is usually associated with severe mental retardation, appears to be very rare, and is more common among males. Previously, the disorder was termed Heller's syndrome, dementia infantilis, or disintegrative psychosis.

Asperger's Disorder

Asperger's disorder can be distinguished from autistic disorder by the lack of delay in language and cognitive development, in addition to no significant abnormality in the development of age-appropriate self-help skills, adaptive behavior (other than in social interaction), and curiosity about the environment in childhood. Motor milestones may be delayed, and motor clumsiness is often observed. The disorder appears to be more common in males. Asperger's disorder is usually recognized somewhat later than autistic disorder, frequently in the context of school. All-encompassing preoccupations or circumscribed interests are typically present and can be quite interfering.

Pervasive Developmental Disorder Not Otherwise Specified

Pervasive developmental disorder NOS is diagnosed when there is a severe and pervasive impairment in the development of reciprocal social interaction. Impairment in verbal and nonverbal communication skills and stereotyped behavior, interests, and activities may be present, but the criteria are not met for a specific PDD, schizophrenia, schizotypal personality disorder, or avoidant personality disorder. This category includes presentations associated with late age at onset, atypical or subthreshold symptomatology, or all of these.

DIFFERENTIAL DIAGNOSIS OF PERVASIVE DEVELOPMENTAL DISORDERS

Periods of developmental regression may occur in normal development, but these are neither as severe or as prolonged as in the PDDs. Childhood-onset schizophrenia usually develops after years of normal, or near-normal, development. A comorbid diagnosis of schizophrenia can be made if an individual with a PDD develops the features of the disorder with active-phase symptoms of delusions or hallucinations that last for at least 1 month. In contrast to the PDDs, in selective mutism, the individual typically shows appropriate communication in certain settings and does not have the severe impairment in social interaction and the restricted repertoire of behaviors. Similarly, in expressive language disorder and mixed receptive-expressive language disorder, there is a language impairment, but it is not associated with a qualitative abnormality in social relatedness and stereotyped patterns of behavior. In individuals with severe or profound mental retardation, it can be difficult to determine if a comorbid diagnosis of a PDD should be made. An additional diagnosis of a PDD can be made when there are qualitative deficits in social interaction and communication and the specific features of a PDD are present. Although motor stereotypies are common among the PDDs, a comorbid diagnosis of stereotypic movement disorder is not made when these occur as part of the presentation of the PDD. Childhood disintegrative disorder must be differentiated from a dementia with onset during infancy or childhood. Childhood disintegrative disorder usually occurs in the absence of an identifiable general medical condition, whereas dementia will typically result from the direct physiological effects of a known etiological agent. Asperger's disorder must be differentiated from obsessive-compulsive disorder (OCD) and schizoid personality disorder. In contrast to OCD, Asperger's disorder is characterized by a significant impairment in social relatedness and a more restricted pattern of interests and activities. Compared with schizoid personality disorder, Asperger's disorder is characterized by stereotyped behaviors and interests and by more severely impaired social interaction. Symptoms of motor hyperactivity and inattention occur frequently in individuals with PDDs, particularly in younger-aged individuals. A comorbid diagnosis of attention-deficit/hyperactivity disorder

(ADHD) is not made if these symptoms occur exclusively during the course of the PDD.

CLINICAL PRACTICE

Assessment and Evaluation

Review of diagnostic instruments

Arnold et al. (2000) recently reviewed the challenges in assessment in multisite randomized clinical trials of subjects with autistic disorder. The Autism Diagnostic Interview–Revised (ADI-R) (Lord et al., 1994), currently regarded by many as the gold standard among diagnostic instruments for autistic disorder, was reviewed and discussed. The ADI-R is a clinician-administered, semistructured instrument designed to aid in the diagnosis of children, adolescents, and adults for whom the diagnosis of autistic disorder or another PDD is being considered. The ADI-R incorporates the DSM-IV and *International Classification of Diseases, 10th ed.* (ICD-10) (World Health Organization, 1993) diagnostic criteria. The ADI-R consists of 111 items and usually takes 2 to 4 hours to complete, using a parent or other primary caregiver as the principal informant. Because of the lengthy time of administration, the ADI-R is primarily used for research purposes. A shorter version is available, although it lacks published reliability and validity data at this time.

The ADI-R follows a series of questions that are organized developmentally. Results obtained for each of the ADI-R individual items are scored on a 4-point scale, usually rating behavior from absent to constantly present. The onset of target behaviors is coded to the nearest month. Based on these results, a 41-item algorithm is completed. The algorithm is divided into three subscales corresponding to the three primary areas of impairment of PDDs: reciprocal social interaction, communication, and repetitive behaviors. Interrater reliability on individual and overall scores on the ADI-R has been excellent (Lord et al., 1997). Cutoff values for the diagnosis of autistic disorder have been established for each subscale and overall score, although not for the diagnosis of the other subtypes of PDD. The ADI-R is an excellent instrument for confirming the clinical diagnosis of autistic disorder. It is not designed to reflect change and thus is not useful as an outcome measure.

Medical Work-up

All subjects should receive a complete physical examination, including a neurological exam. If focal signs are found on neurological exam, magnetic resonance imaging of the brain should be considered. If there is clinical evidence for seizure activity, a sleep-deprived electroencephalogram should be pursued. All children should have adequate hearing and vision screening. We recommend having blood and urine obtained for ruling out fragile X syndrome and abnormalities in amino/organic acid metabolism, respectively. A blood lead level should also be considered in the presence of any learning or cognitive delay. Prior to initiating treatment with drugs with significant potential for negative effects on hepatic or cardiac function, baseline liver function tests and an electrocardiogram should be obtained. Baseline measures of vital signs, height, and weight should also be made and monitored. For drugs associated with the potential development of acute and chronic extrapyramidal symptoms, the Abnormal Involuntary Movement Scale (AIMS) (Rapoport et al., 1985) and Simpson-Angus Scale (Simpson and Angus, 1970) should be administered at baseline and periodically throughout the treatment course.

Psychological Work-up

Although the determination of IQ may not be essential prior to the use of psychotropic agents in individuals with PDDs, preliminary data suggest that particular classes of drugs might be more efficacious and/or better tolerated in individuals with different cognitive abilities. In the study described above by Arnold et al. (2000), IQ assessment was also addressed. In the first study by the National Institute of Mental Health (NIMH)–sponsored Research Units on Pediatric Psychopharmacology (RUPP) Autism Network (McDougle et al., 2000b), the Wechsler-III Intelligence Scale for Children (WISC-III) (Wechsler, 1991) was used preferentially when possible. Children for whom the WISC-III was not feasible were given the Leiter International Test of Intelligence–Revised (Roid and Miller, 1997). If the Leiter test did not prove feasible, the Mullen Scale of Early Development (Mullen, 1995) was given. Because these tests have different standard deviations, identical scores are not strictly comparable. Moreover, not all of these tests provide a mental age. Furthermore, there is a discontinuity across tests of constructs as to what constitutes intelligence. The WISC-III, for example, assesses verbal IQ, performance IQ, and full-scale IQ, whereas the Leiter-R emphasizes performance IQ.

Other intelligence tests were considered for use in the RUPP Autism Network studies, but were not chosen for various reasons (Arnold et al., 2000). The Kaufman Assessment Battery for Children (K-ABC) General Cognitive Index is not strictly comparable to an IQ,

the Differential Ability Scale does not provide a well-recognized measure for deriving an IQ, and the current Stanford-Binet Intelligence Scale tends to be verbally loaded. In summary, additional intelligence test development is needed to improve studies of drug treatment in subjects with PDDs.

Symptom Severity and Measurement of Change

Review of rating scales

A number of rating scales used to measure change in various symptom clusters affecting individuals with PDDs were reviewed and described in the publication by Arnold et al. (2000) referred to above. A number of interfering symptoms that affect individuals with PDDs are potential targets of pharmacotherapy. These include motor hyperactivity and inattention, aggression towards self, others, and property, irritability and agitation, and ritualistic and repetitive behavior. Not all individuals present with this entire range of maladaptive behaviors. As discussed earlier, no pharmacological agent has been developed that directly targets and improves the social and communication abnormalities that are core features of PDDs.

Due to the heterogeneity in clinical presentation among individuals with PDDs, it is important to identify at baseline the predominant symptoms that are targets of treatment. A number of rating scales have been developed for measuring symptom change in other diagnostic groups that have some applicability to individuals with PDDs. Some of these scales were chosen for the RUPP Autism Network's initial study of risperidone (Arnold et al., 2000). The Aberrant Behavior Checklist (ABC) (Aman et al., 1985) irritability subscale encompasses such targets of treatment as tantrums, aggression, and self-injury. It was selected as one of the primary outcome measures for the initial study of risperidone in children and adolescents with autistic disorder. The second primary outcome measure chosen was the Clinical Global Impression (CGI) global improvement item score (Guy, 1976), which is based on careful examination of all areas of possible improvement. In order to measure change in repetitive behavior, the compulsion subscale from the Children's Yale-Brown Obsessive Compulsive Scale (CY-BOCS) (Scahill et al., 1997) was chosen.

To date, no comprehensive scale has been developed for assessing change in the entire range of maladaptive behaviors associated with PDDs for use in drug treatment studies. The development of such an instrument will be a significant challenge. The measurement of subtle changes in social behavior is difficult and consideration will need to be given to the differences in target symptom manifestation that occur throughout development in individuals with PDDs. Until a more comprehensive scale is developed, clinicians and researchers will continue to utilize rating scales that measure change in particular symptom clusters of target behaviors that were likely developed for use in different diagnostic groups.

Strengths and weaknesses of currently available rating scales

As mentioned above, scales have not been developed specifically for measuring change in the various maladaptive behaviors associated with PDDs for drug treatment studies. As a result, existing scales have had to be adapted for use in studies involving subjects with PDDs. An example is the use of the CY-BOCS to measure change in the core symptom of repetitive behavior in such individuals. Repetitive behaviors and preoccupations are frequent and prominent in individuals with autistic disorder and other PDDs. In some ways, these symptoms are similar to the obsessions and compulsions of individuals with OCD. Unlike the obsessive-compulsive symptoms of adolescents and adults with OCD, in which symptoms are ego-dystonic, however, the rituals and preoccupations often do not seem to bother the individual with PDD. Nonetheless, these symptoms can be severely impairing through time consumption and irritable reactions to interruption. This is one of the core autistic features that may be drug-responsive.

To evaluate repetitive behavior as a secondary outcome measure in the RUPP Autism Network's study of risperidone, the compulsion subscale of the CY-BOCS was altered (Scahill et al., 1997). The adaptation expanded the symptom checklist to include repetitive behaviors associated with autistic disorder, such as spinning objects, staring, twirling, and repetition of words and phrases. The probes for resistance and control were adapted to the parent as the informant. This is an example of the need to modify or adapt existing rating scales to meet the special needs and challenges of conducting drug treatment studies in PDDs.

REVIEW OF PUBLISHED STUDIES

Early Drug Treatment Studies

Beginning in the 1960s, a number of agents, including lysergic acid diethylamide, methysergide, levodopa, triiodothyronine, imipramine, and 5-hydroxytryptophan were studied in autistic disorder. Many of these trials were limited by the lack of diagnostic standard-

ization and inadequate study design. In general, none of these drugs resulted in consistent target symptom reduction.

Fenfluramine

The identification of elevated whole blood serotonin (5-HT) in a large minority of autistic children is one of the most consistent findings in biological psychiatry (Schain and Freedman, 1961). Following reports that the indirect 5-HT agonist fenfluramine decreased blood and brain 5-HT in animals, this drug underwent extensive investigation. Early enthusiasm generated by small open-label reports was not sustained as most controlled studies found no consistent beneficial effects for fenfluramine as a drug treatment for autistic disorder (Campbell et al., 1988). Furthermore, increasing evidence of possible neurotoxic effects of the drug on 5-HT neurons in animals and the association of fenfluramine with primary pulmonary hypertension and (in combination with phentermine) valvular heart disease have eliminated its use as a safe agent.

Typical antipsychotics

Most of the available typical antipsychotic drugs have been studied in heterogeneous diagnostic groups of children that included autistic subjects. Many of these early trials lacked adequate methodology and employed nonstandardized outcome measures. Most of these investigations were direct comparisons of two drugs, usually low-potency antipsychotics, and did not include a placebo control. While some of these drugs were effective for motor hyperactivity, agitation, and stereotypies, significant sedation and adverse cognitive effects were common. As a result, studies of higher-potency conventional antipsychotics were next pursued.

Campbell and co-workers conducted several controlled studies of haloperidol in autistic children (Campbell et al., 1978; Cohen et al., 1980; Anderson et al., 1984, 1989). Haloperidol, in doses of 1 to 2 mg/day, was found to be more effective than placebo for withdrawal, stereotypy, hyperactivity, affective lability, anger, and temper outbursts. Acute dystonic reactions and withdrawal and tardive dyskinesias were not infrequent, however.

Naltrexone

The opioid antagonist naltrexone was subsequently investigated as a treatment for the associated target symptoms of autistic disorder, in addition to the core social impairment. Results from open-label trials and small controlled investigations were encouraging. Larger controlled studies involving children, adolescents, and adults with autistic disorder, however, failed to identify improvement in the majority of maladaptive behaviors, including impaired social relatedness (Willemsen-Swinkels et al., 1995, 1996). Naltrexone was well tolerated and effective for reducing motor hyperactivity.

β adrenergic agents, buspirone, and mood stabilizers

Numerous other drugs have been studied in PDDs, although most of the studies were either uncontrolled or contained a small number of subjects (Posey and McDougle, 2000; McDougle, 2002). For example, β-adrenergic blockers have been reported to reduce aggression and self-injury in some small open-label trials in autistic adults. Hypotension and bradycardia were common dose-related adverse effects. Small open-label trials have found mixed results with the 5-HT$_{1A}$ partial agonist buspirone. Controlled studies of putative mood stabilizers, including lithium, valproic acid, carbamazepine, gabapentin, and topiramate have not been reported in well-defined groups of subjects with PDDs.

More Recent Drug Treatment Studies

Atypical antipsychotics

Considerable interest has been generated with the development of the atypical antipsychotics (Potenza and McDougle, 1998). Reports have now appeared in which clozapine, risperidone, olanzapine, or quetiapine were used in the treatment of autistic disorder and other PDDs. The reader is referred to other recent publications that provide a more comprehensive review of atypical antipsychotics in autistic disorder and other PDDs (McDougle et al., 2000b; Posey and McDougle, in press).

Clozapine. There has been only one published report to date describing the use of clozapine in autistic disorder (Zuddas et al., 1996). Three children with marked hyperactivity, fidgetiness, or aggression were given clozapine. Improvement was noted in the three subjects after 3 months' treatment at dosages up to 200 mg/day. The scarcity of reports describing the use of clozapine in autistic disorder might reflect concern regarding the risk of agranulocytosis or seizures in children or adolescents that is associated with the drug. Because autistic individuals typically have an impaired ability to communicate effectively and often a high

pain threshold, infections secondary to a decreased white blood cell count may not be identified in a timely manner. Additionally, as described earlier, many individuals with autistic disorder have comorbid seizure disorders. Furthermore, the necessary frequent blood draws would not be ideal for children in general, nor for those with autistic disorder, in particular.

Risperidone. A number of open-label reports describing improvement in aggression, self-injury, ritualistic behavior, irritability, impulsivity, hyperactivity, and social relatedness in children, adolescents, and adults with autistic disorder and other PDDs with risperidone have been published (McDougle et al., 2000b). Only one controlled study of risperidone, or any atypical antipsychotic for that matter, has been published in individuals with autistic disorder and other PDDs (McDougle et al., 1998b). In that study, 31 adults with autistic disorder ($n = 17$) or PDD NOS ($n = 14$) entered the 12-week trial. For study completers, 8 (57%) of 14 treated with risperidone (mean ± SD dose, 2.9 ± 1.4 mg daily; range 1–6 mg/day) were categorized as responders compared with none of 16 in the placebo group. Risperidone was particularly effective for reducing interfering repetitive behavior, along with aggression toward self, others, and property. In general, risperidone was well tolerated. Thirteen (87%) of 15 subjects randomized to risperidone had at least one adverse effect, although this included only mild, transient sedation in nine subjects. Five (31%) of 16 subjects given placebo demonstrated an adverse effect (agitation in all five cases). Interestingly, the weight gain that has been observed with risperidone in the treatment of many children and adolescents with PDDs did not occur to the same degree in this study of adults.

On the basis of these results and other clinical, preclinical and safety data, the RUPP Autism Network chose risperidone as the first drug to study in children and adolescents with autistic disorder (McDougle et al., 2000b). When completed, this investigation will be the largest drug study conducted to date in autistic disorder, with an anticipated sample size of 101 children and adolescents.

Olanzapine. To date, case reports and an open-label case series have described positive responses to the atypical antipsychotic olanzapine in subjects with PDDs. In the case series, six of seven children, adolescents, and adults with autistic disorder and other PDDs (mean age, 20.9 +/− 11.7 years; range 5–42 years) who completed the 12-week open-label trial were responders (Potenza et al., 1999). Significant improvement in overall symptoms of autistic disorder, motor restlessness or hyperactivity, social relatedness, affectual reactions, sensory responses, language usage, self-injurious behavior, aggression, irritability or anger, anxiety, and depression was observed. Significant changes in repetitive behavior did not occur for the group. The mean dose of olanzapine was 7.8 +/− 4.7 mg daily (range 5–20 mg/day). The drug was well tolerated, with the most significant adverse effects being increased appetite and weight gain in six subjects and sedation in three.

Quetiapine. Only one report of quetiapine in the treatment of autistic disorder has been published (Martin et al., 1999). Six males with autistic disorder, 6.2 to 15.3 years of age (mean age, 10.9 +/− 3.3 years), entered a 16-week open-label trial of quetiapine. The mean daily dose of quetiapine was 225 +/− 108 mg (range 100–350 mg/day). Overall, there was no statistically significant improvement between baseline and end point for the group as a whole on various rating scales. Two subjects completed the entire 16-week trial; both were considered responders, based on CGI scores. However, only one of these two subjects continued to benefit from longer-term treatment with quetiapine. The other four subjects dropped out because of lack of response and sedation (three subjects) and a possible seizure during the fourth week of treatment (one subject). Other significant side effects included behavioral activation, increased appetite, and weight gain (range 0.9–8.2 kg).

Ziprasidone. To date, no publications have appeared on the use of ziprasidone in autistic disorder and other PDDS. The drug was recently released in the United States and is reported to be associated with less weight gain than the other available atypical antipsychotics.

Serotonin reuptake inhibitors

In Kanner's 1943 landmark description of 11 autistic children, the repetitive nature of behavior, speech, and modes of social interaction were designated as core clinical elements of the syndrome (Kanner, 1943). Verbal and motor rituals, obsessive questioning, a rigid adherence to routine, a preoccupation with details, and an anxiously obsessive desire for the maintenance of sameness and completeness were all noted. These phenomena remain as core elements in the diagnostic criteria for autistic disorder in DSM-IV.

Abnormalities in 5-HT function have been identified in subjects with autistic disorder and other PDDs

(McDougle et al., in press). Taken with the efficacy of serotonin reuptake inhibitors (SRIs) in the treatment of OCD (McDougle, 1999) and the high prevalence of interfering repetitive thoughts and behavior in subjects with PDD (McDougle et al., 1995, 2000a), researchers have been studying the clinical response and side effect profile of SRIs in children, adolescents, and adults with PDDs.

Clomipramine. In the first controlled investigation of clomipramine in autistic disorder, the drug was found to be more efficacious than desipramine and placebo on standardized ratings of autistic disorder and anger, as well as ratings of repetitive and compulsive behaviors (Gordon et al., 1992). Seven subjects with autistic disorder, ages 6 to 18 years (means age, 9.6 years), completed the 10-week double-blind, crossover trial of clomipramine (mean dose, 129 mg daily) and desipramine (mean dose, 111 mg daily) following a 2-week single-blind, placebo phase. In general, the side effects were relatively minor and did not differ between the two drugs. Mild sleep disturbance, dry mouth, and constipation were observed, and one patient developed a minor tremor on clomipramine. Two subjects taking desipramine developed uncharacteristic and severe irritability and temper outbursts. The parents of all seven subjects chose to have their children continue on clomipramine after completion of the study.

As a follow-up to this pilot study, a larger double-blind comparison of clomipramine, desipramine, and placebo was conducted in children and adolescents with autistic disorder (Gordon et al., 1993). Following a 2-week single-blind, placebo phase, 12 subjects completed a 10-week double-blind, crossover comparison of clomipramine and placebo, and 12 different subjects completed a similar comparison of clomipramine and desipramine. The latter study included data from the seven subjects who participated in the original pilot study described above. Clomipramine (mean dose, 152 mg daily) was superior to both placebo and desipramine (mean dose, 127 mg daily) on ratings of autistic symptoms, including stereotypies, anger, and ritualized behaviors, with no difference between desipramine and placebo. Clomipramine was equal to desipramine and both drugs were superior to placebo for reducing motor hyperactivity. One child developed prolongation of the corrected QT interval (0.45 seconds) and another developed severe tachycardia (resting heart rate, 160–170 beats/minute) during clomipramine treatment. A third child experienced a grand mal seizure.

Subsequent open-label studies of clomipramine have been published with mixed results and increased recognition of adverse effects. Clomipramine treatment of five young adults (ages 13 to 33 years) with autistic disorder led to ratings of "much improved" on the CGI in four patients, with improvement seen in social relatedness, obsessive-compulsive symptoms, aggression, and self-injurious behavior (McDougle et al., 1992). In another study, 11 consecutively referred children and adolescents with developmental disabililties and chronic stereotypies or self-injurious behavior were treated with clomipramine (Garber et al., 1992). Four of the subjects (ages 13 to 20 years) had been diagnosed with autistic disorder and of them, three had a significant reduction in stereotypic, self-injurious behavior with clomipramine at doses of 50 to 125 mg daily. Adverse effects included constipation, aggression, rash, and enuresis. In another open-label study, clomipramine at 200 mg daily was associated with decreased abnormal motor movements and compulsions in five autistic boys ages 6 to 12 years (Brasic et al., 1994).

A large prospective, open-label study reported on clomipramine (mean dose, 139 mg daily) treatment of 35 adults diagnosed with different subtypes of PDD (Brodkin et al., 1997). Of the 33 subjects who completed the 12-week study, 18 (55%) were categorized as responders, based on the CGI with improvement seen in aggression, self-injurious behavior, interfering repetitive thoughts and behavior, and social relatedness. Thirteen of the 33 subjects had significant adverse effects such as seizures (in three patients, including two who had preexisting seizure disorders stabilized on anticonvulsants), weight gain, constipation, sedation, agitation, and anorgasmia.

A number of published reports have suggested that younger children may tolerate clomipramine less well and show a decreased response compared to adolescents and adults with PDDs. In one study, eight children (ages 3.5 to 8.7 years) were treated with clomipramine (mean dose, 103 mg daily) for 5 weeks in a prospective, open-label fashion (Sanchez et al., 1996). Of the seven children who completed the study, only one child was judged moderately improved on a clinical global consensus rating. Adverse effects were frequent and included urinary retention requiring catheterization, constipation, drowsiness, and increased aggression and irritability. In a follow-up publication to a study described above, in which five autistic children had an initial positive response to clomipramine (Brasic et al., 1994), it was reported that the drug was eventually discontinued in all cases because of adverse effects or continued unmanageable behavior (Brasic et al., 1998). Adverse effects included the serotonin syndrome, increased seizure frequency, and exacerbation of agitation and aggressiveness requiring hospitalization.

Because of their better side effect profile compared with clomipramine, including their lower propensity to decrease the seizure threshold, selective SRIs (SSRIs) have been receiving increasing attention as a treatment for the interfering symptoms associated with autistic disorder and other PDDs.

Fluvoxamine. To date, only one double-blind, placebo-controlled study of a SSRI in subjects with autistic disorder has been published (McDougle et al., 1996). Fluvoxamine (mean dose, 276.7 mg daily) or placebo was given to 30 autistic adults for 12 weeks. Eight (53%) of 15 subjects who received fluvoxamine and none who received placebo were categorized as "much improved" or "very much improved" on the CGI. Fluvoxamine was significantly more effective than placebo for reducing repetitive thoughts and behavior, maladaptive behavior, and aggression. In addition, fluvoxamine reduced inappropriate repetitive language usage. Adverse effects included nausea and sedation, which were transient and of minor severity.

In contrast to the encouraging results from this study of fluvoxamine in autistic adults, a 12-week double-blind, placebo-controlled study in children and adolescents with autistic disorder and other PDDs found the drug to be poorly tolerated, with limited efficacy at best (C.J. McDougle and co-workers, unpublished data). Thirty-four patients (5 female, 29 male; age range 5–18 years, mean age, 9.5 years), 12 of whom met criteria for autistic disorder, 8 for Asperger's disorder, and 14 for PDD NOS, participated. Of the 16 subjects randomized to placebo, none demonstrated any significant change in target symptoms. Adverse events that occurred in the placebo-treated subjects included increased motor hyperactivity (2), insomnia (2), dizziness and/or vertigo (1), agitation (1), diarrhea (1), decreased concentration (1), and increased self-stimulation (1). Eighteen of the subjects were randomized to fluvoxamine (dosage range 25–250 mg daily; mean dose, 106.9 mg/day). The drug was begun at 25 mg every other day and increased by 25 mg every 3 to 7 days, as tolerated. Only one of the fluvoxamine-treated children demonstrated a significant improvement with the drug. Fourteen of the children randomized to fluvoxamine demonstrated adverse effects (insomnia [9], motor hyperactivity [5], agitation [5], aggression [5], increased rituals [2], anxiety [3], anorexia [3], increased appetite [1], irritability [1], decreased concentration [1], and increased impulsivity [1]).

The marked difference in efficacy and tolerability of fluvoxamine in children and adolescents with autistic disorder and other PDDs in this study, compared with that of autistic adults, underscores the importance of developmental factors in the pharmacotherapy of these subjects. This differential drug response is consistent with the hypothesis that ongoing brain development has a significant impact on the subjects' ability to tolerate and respond to a drug, at least with respect to fluvoxamine and possibly other SSRIs. Developmental changes in brain 5-HT function may contribute to these widely varying clinical responses between subjects with autistic disorder and other PDDs of different age groups.

Fluoxetine. Several case reports and case series have been published describing fluoxetine treatment of autistic subjects. To date, no controlled studies of fluoxetine in autistic disorder have appeared.

In a large case series, Cook and associates (1992) found fluoxetine (10 to 80 mg daily), given in an open-label manner, effective in 15 of 23 subjects (ages 7 to 28 years) with autistic disorder as determined by the CGI. Intolerable side effects, including restlessness, hyperactivity, agitation, elated affect, decreased appetite, and insomnia, occurred in 6 of 23 subjects.

In a retrospective case analysis, fluoxetine (20 to 80 mg daily) and paroxetine (20 to 40 mg daily) were found to be effective in approximately one-quarter of adults (mean age, 39 years) with "intellectual disability" and autistic traits (Branford et al., 1998). The sample consisted of all intellectually disabled subjects who had been treated with a SSRI over a 5-year period within a health-care service in Great Britain. The mean duration of treatment was 13 months. Target symptoms were perseverative behaviors, aggression, and self-injurious behavior. Six of 25 subjects treated with fluoxetine and 3 of 12 subjects given paroxetine were rated as "much improved" or "very much improved" on the CGI.

In another study, 37 children (ages 2.25 to 7.75 years) with autistic disorder were given fluoxetine in an open-label fashion at doses ranging from 0.2 to 1.4 mg/kg daily (DeLong et al., 1998). Eleven of the children had an "excellent" clinical response and 11 others had a "good" response. Improvement was seen in behavioral, cognitive, affective, and social areas. Interestingly, language acquistion seemed to improve with fluoxetine treatment. Drug-induced hyperactivity, agitation, and aggression were frequent causes of discontinuation of fluoxetine.

Sertraline. To our knowledge, no controlled studies of sertraline in subjects with autistic disorder or other PDDs have been published, although a number of open-label reports have appeared. In a 28-day trial of sertraline (at doses of 25 to 150 mg daily) in nine adults with mental retardation (five of whom had autistic disorder), significant decreases in aggression and self-injurious behavior occurred in eight subjects as rated on the CGI severity scale (Hellings et al., 1996). In a case series of nine autistic children (ages 6 to 12 years) treated with sertraline (25 to 50 mg daily), eight showed significant improvement in anxiety, irritability, and "transition-induced behavioral deterioration" or "need for sameness" (Steingard et al., 1997). Three of the responders demonstrated a return of symptoms after 3 to 7 months. Two children experienced agitation when the dose was raised to 75 mg daily.

A large prospective, open-label study of 42 adults with PDDs (including patients with autistic disorder, Asperger's disorder, and PDD NOS) found sertraline (mean dose, 122 mg/day) effective for improving aggression and interfering repetitive behavior, but not impaired social relatedness as assessed by a number of measures over the course of the 12-week study (McDougle et al., 1998a). As determined by a CGI global improvement item score of "much improved" or "very much improved," 15 of 22 subjects with autistic disorder, none of 6 with Asperger's disorder, and 9 of 14 with PDD NOS were categorized as responders. Those subjects with autistic disorder and PDD NOS showed significantly more improvement with sertraline than those with Asperger's disorder; the authors hypothesized that this might have been because those diagnosed with Asperger's disorder were less impaired at baseline. Three of the 42 subjects dropped out of the study because of intolerable agitation and anxiety.

Paroxetine. Only a few reports, none of them controlled, have appeared on the use of paroxetine in autistic disorder. Paroxetine at 20 mg/day decreased self-injurious behavior in a 15-year-old boy with "high-functioning" autistic disorder (Snead et al., 1994). In another report, paroxetine's effectiveness for a broader range of symptoms, including irritability, temper tantrums, and interfering preoccupations, was reported in a 7-year-old boy with autistic disorder (Posey et al., 1999). The optimal dose of paroxetine was 10 mg daily; an increase of paroxetine to 15 mg/day was associated with agitation and insomnia. As described earlier, a retrospective case analysis found paroxetine to be effective in approximately 25% of adults with PDD NOS (Branford et al., 1998).

In a 4-month open-label study of 15 adults with severe and profound mental retardation (seven with PDD), paroxetine at doses of 20 to 50 mg daily was significantly effective for symptoms of aggression at 1-month, but not at 4-month follow-up (Davanzo et al., 1998). The investigators hypothesized that adaptive changes may have occurred in 5-HT receptor density, availability of 5-HT, or in 5-HT transporter sensitivity.

Citalopram. To date, there have been no published reports on the effects of citalopram, a SSRI which has been recently introduced in the United States, in patients with autistic disorder or other PDDs.

Psychostimulants and α_2-adrenergic agonists

The pharmacological management of motor hyperactivity and impaired attentional mechanisms in individuals with PDDs has proven particularly challenging for clinicians and researchers. These symptoms are most prominent in younger autistic children. Thus, these symptoms are largely present during a time when educational programming and interventions are most critical.

The psychostimulants, such as methylphenidate and dextroamphetamine, are effective treatments for these symptoms in individuals with ADHD. Early controlled studies of these agents in autistic children, however, produced mixed results at best (Campbell et al., 1972, 1976). In a double-blind, crossover study of methylphenidate and placebo, 10 autistic children, ages 7 to 11 years, received doses of 10 or 20 mg twice daily for 2 weeks (Quintana et al., 1995). Statistically significant improvement was seen on the Conners Teacher Questionnaire (Conners, 1989) and on the hyperactivity factor, irritability factor, and total score of the ABC. Adverse effects were minimal. The authors' impression was that the effects of methylphenidate were modest. Following completion of the study, it was necessary to add haloperidol to the treatment regimen of 2 of the 10 children because of continued symptoms of aggression. Most recently, Handen and colleagues (2000) treated 13 children (ages 5.6 to 11.2 years) with autistic disorder in a double-blind, placebo-controlled crossover study of methylphenidate (0.3–0.6 mg/kg/dose). Eight subjects responded to methylphenidate, based on a 50% decrease on the Teachers Conners Hyperactivity Index, compared to placebo. Adverse effects included social withdrawal, dullness, sadness, and irritability, especially at the 0.6 mg/kg dose. Anecdotal reports from physicians in clinical practice and in academic centers commonly describe the onset or exacerbation of irritability, insomnia, and aggression in individuals with PDDs with psychostimulant treatment.

The α_2-adrenergic agonist clonidine has been shown to be an effective treatment for some individuals with autistic disorder and other PDDs. In a small double-blind, placebo-controlled study of clonidine (4–10 μg/kg daily) in eight children with autistic disorder, statistically significant improvement was recorded in hyperactivity and irritability on some teacher and parent ratings (Jaselskis et al., 1992). No significant drug–placebo

differences were identified on clinician ratings of videotaped observations, however. Adverse effects included hypotension, sedation, and irritability. In contrast, transdermal clonidine (5 μ/kg daily) was reported to be effective in a double-blind, placebo-controlled crossover study (4 weeks in each treatment phase) involving nine males (ages 5–33 years) with autistic disorder (Fankhauser et al., 1992). Significant improvement was seen on the CGI, and hyperactivity and anxiety were also reduced. The most common adverse effects were sedation and fatigue.

Guanfacine is an α_2-adrenergic agonist with a longer half-life than clonidine, which may be less sedating and cause less pronounced hypotension (Arnsten et al., 1988). To date, only one report of guanfacine treatment in PDDs has been published (Posey et al., 2001). In that study, which was retrospective in nature, 19 (23.8%) of 80 subjects (10 female, 70 male; mean age, 7.7 +/− 3.5 years, age range 3 to 18 years) were rated as responders on the CGI after a mean duration of treatment of 10 months. The greatest response rates were seen in the symptoms of tics, insomnia, hyperactivity, and inattention. Subjects with PDD NOS and Asperger's disorder showed a greater rate of global response than those with autistic disorder. Guanfacine (0.25 to 9 mg daily in divided doses, mean daily dose, 2.6 +/− 1.7 mg) was well tolerated, with the most common adverse effect being transient sedation.

To more rigorously address the pharmacotherapy of symptoms of hyperactivity and inattention in PDD, the NIMH-sponsored RUPP Autism Network is conducting a controlled investigation of methylphenidate versus placebo in children and adolescents with PDDs. Nonresponders to methylphenidate will have the opportunity to enter a prospective, open-label trial of guanfacine.

Novel Treatment Strategies

Secretin

Recent interest has surrounded the polypeptide hormone secretin, which is secreted primarily by the endocrine cells in the upper gastrointestinal (GI) tract. This interest was generated by a report by Horvath and colleagues (1998) that described significant improvement in social relatedness and language usage in three children with PDDs who were administered secretin during a diagnostic work-up for GI disturbance. Subsequently, four double-blind, placebo-controlled studies have been completed with all four finding no significant difference on primary outcome measures between intravenous secretin and placebo (Owley et

TABLE 42.1 *Recent Controlled Trials of Drug Treatment for Autistic Disorder*

Reference	Design	Patients (Age)	Drug (Dose)	Results Comments	Adverse Effects Comments
Gordon et al., 1993	2-week, single-blind, placebo washout 10-week, double-blind, crossover	4 females 8 males (7–15 years)	Clomipramine for 5 weeks (152 ± 56 mg/day) Placebo for 5 weeks	Clomipramine > placebo for autistic symptoms, anger/uncooperativeness, hyperactivity, and obsessive-compulsive symptoms	One subject developed prolongation of corrected QT interval (0.45 seconds) on clomipramine. Another subject developed severe tachycardia (resting heart rate, 160 to 170 beats/minute) on clomipramine
Gordon et al., 1993	2-week, single-blind, placebo washout 10-week, double-blind, crossover	5 females 7 males (6–18 years)	Clomipramine for 5 weeks (152 ± 56 mg/day) Desipramine for 5 weeks (127 ± 52 mg/day)	Clomipramine > desipramine for autistic symptoms, anger/uncooperativeness, and obsessive-compulsive symptoms Clomipramine = desipramine for hyperactivity	One subject had a grand mal seizure on clomipramine. Eight of 12 subjects developed increased irritability, temper outbursts, and aggression on desipramine
Quintana et al., 1995	2-week, drug-free period 1-week, double-blind, crossover	4 females 6 males (7–11 years)	Methylphenidate (10 mg twice daily) for 1 week (20 mg twice daily) for 1 week Placebo for 1 week	Methylphenidate > placebo for hyperactivity and irritability (teacher-rated) Methylphenidate = placebo for hyperactivity (parent-rated)	Irritability 4% Headache 1% Stomache ache 3% Lack of appetite 20% Insomnia 5% Not different from placebo
Willemsen-Swinkels et al., 1995	2-week, single-blind, placebo period 4-week, double-blind, crossover with 4-week washout period	5 females 27 males 7 with autistic disorder 16 with autistic disorder and SIB 9 with SIB (18–46 years)	Naltrexone for 4 weeks (50 mg [n = 18]) or (150 mg [n = 14]) Placebo for 4 weeks	Placebo > naltrexone (50 mg) for autistic symptoms and SIB Placebo = naltrexone (150 mg) for autistic symptoms and SIB Naltrexone associated with increased stereotypic behavior	One subject developed acute and severe increase in SIB and acting-out behavior. Another subject complained of nausea and tiredness. Three subjects developed sedation. Liver function tests were normal
Willemsen-Swinkels et al., 1996	2-week, baseline period Double-blind, crossover with 4-week washout period	4 females 16 males (2.8–7.4 years)	Naltrexone for 4 weeks (20 mg/day) Placebo for 4 weeks	Naltrexone = placebo (parent-rated) Naltrexone > placebo for hyperactivity and irritability (teacher-rated)	None
McDougle et al., 1996	12-week, double-blind, placebo-controlled, parallel groups	3 females 27 males (18–53 years)	Fluvoxamine for 12 weeks (276.7 ± 41.7 mg/day) Placebo for 12 weeks	Fluvoxamine, 8 of 15 responders Placebo, 0 of 15 responders Fluvoxamine > placebo for repetitive phenomena, maladaptive behavior, aggression, and autistic symptoms	Three subjects reported nausea and two experienced sedation on fluvoxamine
McDougle et al., 1998b	12-week, double-blind, placebo-controlled, parallel groups	9 females 21 males (18–43 years)	Risperidone for 12 weeks (2.9 ± 1.4 mg/day) Placebo for 12 weeks	Risperidone, 8 of 14 responders Placebo, 0 of 16 responders Risperidone > placebo for repetitive phenomena, aggression, anxiety, depression, irritability, and autistic symptoms	Transient sedation 9 Dry mouth 1 Agitation 2 Weight gain 2 Enuresis 2 Dyspepsia 1 Diarrhea 1 Constipation 1 Abnormal gait 1 Sialorrhea 1 All of above experienced while on risperdone.

(continued)

TABLE 42.1 *Recent Controlled Trials of Drug Treatment for Autistic Disorder (continued)*

Reference	Design	Patients (Age)	Drug (Dose)	Results Comments	Adverse Effects Comments
Handen et al., 2000	3-week, double-blind, placebo-controlled, crossover	3 females 10 males (5.6–11.2 years)	Methylphenidate (0.3 mg/kg/dose) for 1 week Methylphenidate (0.6 mg/kg/dose) for 1 week Placebo for 1 week	Methylphenidate, 8 of 13 responders Placebo, 2 of 13 responders Methylphenidate > placebo for hyperactivity and inappropriate speech	Adverse effects included crying, tantrums, aggression, skin picking, irritability, and social withdrawal while on methylphenidate.
King et al., 2001	1-week, single-blind, placebo run-in 4-week, double-blind, placebo-controlled, parallel groups	5 females 34 males (5–15 years)	Amantadine hydrochloride (2.5 mg/kg/day) for 1 week (5 mg/kg/day) for 3 weeks Placebo for 4 weeks	Amantadine hydrochloride, 9 of 19 responders (parent-rated) Placebo, 7 of 19 responders (parent-rated) Amantadine hydrochloride, 10 of 19 responders (clinician-rated) Placebo, 5 of 20 responders (clinician-rated) Amantadine hydrochloride > placebo for hyperactivity and inappropriate speech (clinician-rated)	Four subjects experienced insomnia and two subjects, somnolence while on amantadine hydrochloride

SIB, self-injurious behavior.

al., 1999; Sandler et al., 1999; Chez et al., 2000, Dunn-Geier et al., 2000). Based upon the results of these systematic studies, secretin cannot be recommended as a treatment for PDDs.

Mirtazapine

Mirtazapine is an antidepressant with a novel mechanism of action affecting both 5-HT and noradrenergic function. A recent systematic, open-label study found that 9 (34.6%) of 26 subjects (5 females, 21 males; mean age, 10.1 +/− 4.8 years, age range 3.8–23.5 years) with autistic disorder and other PDDs were "much improved" or "very much improved" on the CGI after a mean duration of treatment of 5 months (Posey et al., 2001). The dosage range for mirtazapine was 7.5 to 45 mg/day with a mean daily dose of 30.29 mg +/− 12.64 mg. Target symptoms of aggression, self-injury, irritability, hyperactivity, anxiety, depression, and insomnia showed improvement. Adverse effects were transient and minimal and included increased appetite, irritability, and sedation. Based upon these preliminary data, a double-blind, placebo-controlled trial appears warranted.

Glutamatergic Compounds

Potential drug treatments affecting glutamatergic function have been identified for a number of neuropsy-

chiatric disorders (Krystal et al., 1999). A hypothesis regarding a dysregulation in glutamatergic function in autistic disorder has been proposed (Carlsson, 1998).

Lamotrigine is an anticonvulsant drug that attenuates some forms of cortical glutamate release via inhibition of sodium, calcium, and potassium channels. An open-label case series (Uvebrant and Bauziene, 1994) and a case report (Davanzo and King, 1996) described improvement in "autistic symptoms" and self-injurious behavior, irritability, disturbed sleep, and social impairment in autistic children and an 18-year-old female with profound mental retardation, respectively, who were treated for epilepsy.

Amantadine hydrochloride is a noncompetitive antagonist at the N-methyl-D-aspartate (NMDA) subclass of glutamate receptor. King et al. (2001) recently published results from a double-blind, placebo-controlled trial involving 39 subjects (age range, 5 to 19 years) with autistic disorder. After a 1-week single-blind, placebo run-in, subjects received a single daily dose of amantadine (2.5 mg/kg/day) or placebo for the next week, and then twice-daily dosing (5.0 mg/kg/day) for the subsequent 3 weeks. There was no statistically significant difference in parent-rated measures of irritability and hyperactivity between amantadine and placebo. In the amantadine group, there were statistically significant improvements in absolute changes in clinician-rated measures of hyperactivity and inappropriate speech. The drug

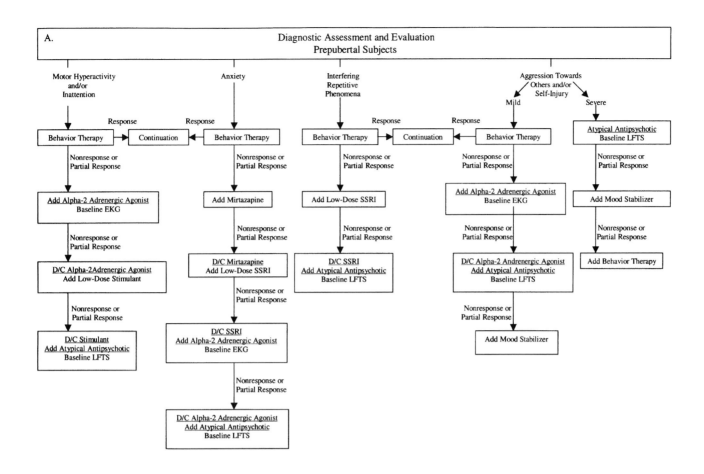

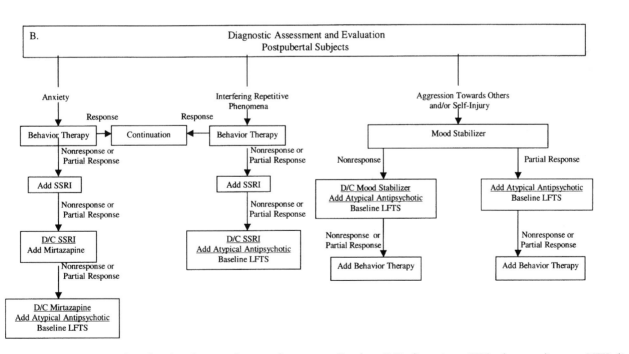

FIGURE 42.1 Treatment algorithm for pharmacotherapy of target symptoms associated with autistic and other pervasive developmental disorders. D/C, discontinue; EKG, electrocardiogram; LFTS, liver function tests; SSRI, selective serotonin reuptake inhibitor.

was well tolerated and the investigators suggested that additional study of glutamatergic dysfunction in autistic disorder will be important.

Neuroimmune therapies

An extensive body of literature regarding immune abnormalities in autistic disorder has been published (van Gent et al., 1997). Viral and autoimmune mechanisms, among others, have been proposed. To date, a limited number of treatment studies have been conducted in this area. In one study, DelGiudice-Asch et al. (1999) reported that open-label, intravenous immunoglobulin was of only limited benefit in a minority of subjects, if at all. In another study, 10 children with "regressive"-onset autistic disorder completed an 8-week open-label trial of the antibiotic vancomycin (Sandler et al., 2000). Entry criteria included antecedent broad-spectrum antimicrobial exposure followed by chronic persistent diarrhea, deterioration of previously acquired skills, and then autistic features. Eight of the 10 children were noted to show improvement in communication and behavior during the study. Upon drug discontinuation, the children's symptoms returned to baseline levels. The investigators concluded that a possible gut flora-brain connection warrants further investigation. To date, controlled studies of drugs that have direct effects on immune function have not been conducted in autistic disorder.

CONCLUSIONS

Significant advances have been made in the pharmacological treatment of autistic disorder and other PDDs since biological research began in this area in the late 1950s. Despite this progress, only a limited number of double-blind, placebo-controlled studies have been published (results from selected controlled studies since 1990 [$n > 10$] are summarized in Table 42.1). Recent action by the NIMH to fund the RUPP Autism Network has resulted in completion of the largest controlled drug treatment study in autistic disorder to date. Ongoing efforts by the federal government and other funding sources will be necessary to support continued research for this understudied and underserved population. Future research should include additional controlled trials of atypical antipsychotics in individuals with autistic disorder and other subtypes of PDD. In particular, assessment of longitudinal efficacy and safety is needed with these agents. Larger controlled studies of SSRIs in pre- versus postpubertal individuals with autistic disorder will be important. In these trials, the optimal dos-

age for age and developmental level and the duration of an adequate treatment trial should be determined. Novel treatment approaches, including those affecting glutamatergic and immune function, should also be pursued. A suggested treatment algorithm for the pharmacotherapy of target symptoms associated with autistic disorder and other PDDs is presented in Figure 42.1.

ACKNOWLEDGMENTS
The authors wish to thank Ms. Robbie Smith for preparing the manuscript. This work was supported in part by a Daniel X. Freedman Psychiatric Research Fellowship Award (Dr. Posey), a National Alliance for Research in Schizophrenia and Depression (NARSAD) Young Investigator Award (Dr. Posey), a Research Unit on Pediatric Psychopharmacology Contract (N01MH70001) from the National Institute of Mental Health to Indiana University (Drs. McDougle and Posey), a National Institutes of Health Clinical Research Center Grant (M01-RR00750) to Indiana University, and the State of Indiana Division of Mental Health.

REFERENCES

Aman, M.G., Singh, N.N., Stewart, A.W., and Field, C.J. (1985) The Aberrant Behavior Checklist: a behavior rating scale for the assessment of treatment effects. *Am J Ment Defic* 89:485–491.

American Psychiatric Association (1994) *Diagnostic and Statistical Manual of Mental Disorders, 4th ed.* Washington, DC: American Psychiatric Association.

Amir, R.E., Van den Veyver, I.B., Wan, M., Tran, C.Q., Francke, U., and Zoghbi, H.Y. (1999) Rett syndrome is caused by mutations in X-linked *MECP2*, encoding methyl-CpG-binding protein 2. *Nat Genet* 23:185–88.

Anderson, L.T., Campbell, M., Adams, P., Small, A.M., Perry, R., and Shell, J. (1989) The effects of haloperidol on discrimination learning and behavioral symptoms in autistic children. *J Autism Dev Disord* 19:227–239.

Anderson, L.T., Campbell, M., Grega, D.M., Perry, R., Small, A.M., and Green, W.H. (1984) Haloperidol in the treatment of infantile autism: effects on learning and behavioral symptoms. *Am J Psychiatry* 141:1195–1202.

Arnold, L.E., Aman, M.G., Martin, A., Collier-Crespin, A., Vitiello, B., Tierney, E., Asarnow, R., Bell-Bradshaw, F., Freeman, B.J., Gates-Ulanet, P., Klin, A., McCracken, J.T., McDougle, C.J., McGough, J.J., Posey, D.J., Scahill, L., Swiezy, N.B., Ritz, L., and Volkmar, F. (2000) Assessment in multisite randomized clinical trials of patients with autistic disorder: the autism RUPP network. *J Autism Dev Disord* 30:99–111.

Arnsten, A.F.T., Cai, J.X., and Goldman-Rakic, P.S. (1988) The alpha-2 adrenergic agonist guanfacine improves memory in aged monkeys without sedative or hypotensive side effects: evidence for alpha-2 receptor subtypes. *J Neurosci* 8: 4287–4298.

Branford, D., Bhaumik, S., and Naik, B. (1998) Selective serotonin reuptake inhibitors for the treatment of perseverative and maladaptive behaviours of people with intellectual disability. *J Intellect Disabil Res* 42:301–306.

Brasic, J.R., Barnett, J.Y., Kaplan, D., Sheitman, B.B., Aisemberg, P., Lafargue, R.T., Kowalik, S., and Clark, A. (1994) Clomipramine ameliorates adventitious movements and compulsions in prepubertal boys with autistic disorder and severe mental retardation. *Neurology* 44:1309–1312.

Brasic, J.R., Barnett, J.Y., Sheitman, B.B., Lafargue, R.T., Kowalik, S., Kaplan, D., Tsaltas, M.O., Ahmad, R., Nadrich, R.H., and Mendonca, M.F. (1998) Behavioral effects of clomipramine on prepubertal boys with autistic disorder and severe mental retardation. *CNS Spectrums* 3:39–46.

Brodkin, E.S., McDougle, C.J., Naylor, S.T., Cohen, D.J., and Price, L.H. (1997) Clomipramine in adults with pervasive developmental disorders: a prospective open-label investigation *J Child Adolesc Psychopharmacol* 7:109–21.

Campbell, M., Adams, P., Small, A.M., Curren, E.L., Overall, J.E., Anderson, L.T., Lynch, N., and Perry, R. (1988) Efficacy and safety of fenfluramine in autistic children. *J Am Acad Child Adolesc Psychiatry* 27:434–439.

Campbell, M., Anderson, L.T., Meier, M., Cohen, I.L., Small, A.M., Samit, C., and Sachar, E.J. (1978) A comparison of haloperidol and behavior therapy and their interaction in autistic children. *J Am Acad Child Psychiatry* 17:640–655.

Campbell, M., Fish, B., David, R., Shapiro, T., Collins, P., and Koh, C. (1972) Response to triiodothyronine and dextroamphetamine: a study of preschool schizophrenic children. J Autism Child Schizophr 2:343–358.

Campbell, M., Small, A.M., Collins, P.J., Friedman, E., David, R., and Genieser, N. (1976) Levodopa and levoamphetamine: a crossover study in young schizophrenic children. *Curr Therap Res* 19: 70–86.

Carlsson, M.L. (1998) Hypothesis: is infantile autism a hypoglutamatergic disorder? Relevance of glutamate-serotonin interactions for pharmacotherapy. *J Neural Transm* 105:525–535.

Chakrabarti, S. and Fombonne, E. (2001) Pervasive developmental disorders in preschool children. *JAMA* 285:3093–3099.

Chez, M.G., Buchanan, C.P., Bagan, B.T., Hammer, M.S., McCarthy, K.S., Ovrutskaya, I., Nowinski, C.V., and Cohen, Z.S. (2000) Secretin and autism: a two-part clinical investigation. *J Autism Dev Disord* 30:87–94.

Cohen, I.L., Campbell, M., Posner, D., Small, A.D., Triebel, D., and Anderson, L.T. (1980) Behavioral effects of haloperidol in young autistic children: an objective analysis using a within-subjects reversal design. *J Am Acad Child Adolesc Psychiatry* 19: 665–677.

Conners, C.K. *Conners Rating Scales manual.* North Tonowanda, New York: Multi-Health Systems, 1989.

Cook, E.H., Rowlett, R., Jaselskis, C., and Leventhal, B.L. (1992) Fluoxetine treatment of children and adults with autistic disorder and mental retardation. *J Am Acad Child Adolesc Psychiatry* 31: 739–745.

Davanzo, P.A., Belin, T.R., Widawski, M.H., and King, B.H. (1998) Paroxetine treatment of aggression and self-injury in persons with mental retardation. *Am J Ment Retard* 102:427–437.

Davanzo, P.A. and King, B.H. (1996) Open trial of lamotrigine in the treatment of self-injurious behavior in an adolescent with profound mental retardation. *J Child Adolesc Psychopharmacol* 6: 273–279.

DelGiudice-Asch, G., Simon, L., Schmeidler, J., Cunningham-Rundles, C., and Hollander, E. (1999) Brief report: a pilot open clinical trial of intravenous immunoglobulin in childhood autism. *J Autism Dev Disord* 29:157–160.

DeLong, G.R., Teague, L.A., and Kamran, M.M. (1998) Effects of fluoxetine treatment in young children with idiopathic autism. *Dev Med Child Neurol* 40:551–562.

Dunn-Geier, J., Ho, H.H., Auersperg, E., Doyle, D., Eaves, L., Matsuba, C., Orrbine, E., Pham, B., and Whiting, S. (2000) Effect of

secretin on children with autism: a randomized controlled trial. *Dev Med Child Neurol* 42:796–802.

Fankhauser, M.P., Karumanchi, V.C., German, M.L., Yates, A., and Karumanchi, S.D. (1992) A double-blind, placebo-controlled study of the efficacy of transdermal clonidine in autism. *J Clin Psychiatry* 53:77–82.

Garber, H.J., McGonigle, J.J., Slomka, G.T., and Monteverde, E. (1992) Clomipramine treatment of stereotypic behaviors and self-injury in patients with developmental disabilities. *J Am Acad Child Adolesc Psychiatry* 31:1157–1160.

Gordon, C.T., Rapoport, J.L., Hamburger, S.D., State, R.C., and Mannheim, G.B. (1992) Differential response of seven subjects with autistic disorder to clomipramine and desipramine. *Am J Psychiatry* 149:363–366.

Gordon, C.T., State, R.C., Nelson, J.E., Hamburger, S.D., and Rapoport, J.L. (1993) A double-blind comparison of clomipramine, desipramine, and placebo in the treatment of autistic disorder. *Arch Gen Psychiatry* 50:441–447.

Guy, W. (1976) *ECDEU Assessment Manual for Psychopharmacology (NIMH Publication No. 76–338).* Washington, DC: U.S. Department of Health, Education, and Welfare, National Institute of Mental Health.

Handen, B.L., Johnson, C.R., and Lubetsky, M. (2000) Efficacy of methylphenidate among children with autism and symptoms of attention-deficit hyperactivity disorder. *J Autism Dev Disord* 30: 245–255.

Hellings, J.A., Kelley, L.A., Gabrielli, W.F., Kilgore, E., and Shah, P. (1996) Sertraline response in adults with mental retardation and autistic disorder. *J Clin Psychiatry* 57:333–336.

Horvath, K., Stefanatos, G., Sokolski, K.N., Wachtel, R., Nabors, L., and Tildon, J.T. (1998) Improved social and language skills after secretin administration in patients with autistic spectrum disorders. *J Assoc Acad Minor Phys* 9:9–15.

Jaselskis, C.A., Cook, E.H. Jr., Fletcher, K.E., and Leventhal, B.L. (1992) Clonidine treatment of hyperactive and impulsive children with autistic disorder. *J Clin Psychopharmacol* 12:322–327.

Kanner, L. (1943) Autistic disturbances of affective contact. *Nerv Child* 2:217–250.

King, B.H., Wright, D.M., Handen, B.L., Sikich, L., Zimmerman, A.W., McMahon, W., Cantwell, E., Davanzo, P.A., Dourish, C.T., Dykens, E.M., Hooper, S.R., Jaselskis, C.A., Leventhal, B.L., Levitt, J., Lord, C., Lubetsky, M.J., Myers, S.M., Ozonoff, S., Shah, B.G., Snape, M., Shernoff, E.W., Williamson, K., and Cook, E.H. (2001) Double-blind, placebo-controlled study of amantadine hydrochloride in the treatment of children with autistic disorder. *J Am Acad Child Adolesc Psychiatry* 40:658–665.

Krystal, J.H., D'Souza, D.C., Petrakis, I.L., Belger, A., Berman, R.M., Charney, D.S., Abi-Saab, W., and Madonick, S. (1999) NMDA agonists and antagonists as probes of glutamatergic dysfunction and pharmacotherapies in neuropsychiatric disorders. *Harv Rev Psychiatry* 7:125–143.

Lord, C., Pickles, A., McLennan, J., Rutter, M., Bregman, J., Folstein, S., Fombonne, E., Leboyer, M., and Minshew, N. (1997) Diagnosing autism: analyses of data from the Autism Diagnostic Interview. *J Autism Dev Disord* 24:501–517.

Lord, C., Rutter, M., and Le Couteur, A. (1994) Autism Diagnostic Interview-Revised: a revised version of a diagnostic interview for caregivers of individuals with possible pervasive developmental disorders. *J Autism Dev Disord* 24:659–685.

Martin, A., Koenig, K., Scahill, L., and Bregman, J. (1999) Open-label quetiapine in the treatment of children and adolescents with autistic disorder. *J Child Adolesc Psychopharmacol* 9:99–107.

McDougle, C.J. (1999) The neurobiology and treatment of obsessive-compulsive disorder. In Charney, D.S., Nestler, E.J., and Bunney, B.S., eds. *The Neurobiology of Mental Illness*. New York: Oxford University Press, pp. 518–533.

McDougle, C.J. (2002) Current and emerging therapeutics of autistic disorder and related pervasive developmental disorders. In Davis, K.L., Charney, D., Coyle, J.T., and Nemeroff, C., eds. *Neuropsychopharmacology—The Fifth Generation of Progress*. Philadelphia: Lippincott—Williams & Wilkens, pp. 565–576.

McDougle, C.J., Brodkin, E.S., Naylor, S.T., Carlson, D.C., Cohen, D.J., and Price, L.H. (1998a) Sertraline in adults with pervasive developmental disorders: a prospective open-label investigation. *J Clin Psychopharmacol* 18:62–66.

McDougle, C.J., Holmes, J.P., Carlson, D.C., Pelton, G.H., Cohen, D.J., and Price, L.H., (1998b) A double-blind placebo-controlled study of risperidone in adults with autistic disorder and other pervasive developmental disorders. *Arch Gen Psychiatry* 55:633–641.

McDougle, C.J., Kresch, L.E., Goodman, W.K., Naylor, S.J., Volkmar, F.R., Cohen, C.J., and Price, L.H. (1995) A case-controlled study of repetitive thoughts and behavior in adults with autistic disorder and obsessive-compulsive disorder. *Am J Psychiatry* 152:772–777.

McDougle, C.J., Kresch, L.E., and Posey, D.J. (2000a) Repetitive thoughts and behavior in pervasive developmental disorders: treatment with serotonin reuptake inhibitors. *J Autism Dev Disord* 30:425–433.

McDougle, C.J., Naylor, S.T., Cohen, D.J., Volkmar, F.R., Heninger, G.R., and Price, L.H. (1996) A double-blind, placebo-controlled study of fluvoxamine in adults with autistic disorder. *Arch Gen Psychiatry* 53:1001–1008.

McDougle, C.J., Posey, D.J., and Potenza, M.N. (in press) Neurobiology of serotonin function in autism. In: Hollander, E. and Delaney, K., eds. *Diagnosis and Treatment of Autism*. New York: Marcel Dekker.

McDougle, C.J., Price, L.H., Volkmar, F.R., Goodman, W.K., Ward-O'Brien, D., Nielsen, J., Bregman, J., and Cohen, D.J. (1992) Clomipramine in autism: preliminary evidence of efficacy. *J Am Acad Child Adolesc Psychiatry* 31:746–750.

McDougle, C.J., Scahill, L., McCracken, J.T., Aman, M.G., Tierney, E., Arnold, L.E., Freeman, B.J., Martin, A., McGough, J.J., Cronin, P., Posey, D.J., Riddle, M.A., Ritz, L., Swiezy, N.B., Vitiello, B., Volkmar, F.R., Votolato, N.A., and Walson, P. (2000b) Research Units on Pediatric Psychopharmacology (RUPP) Autism Network: background and rationale for an initial controlled study of risperidone. *Child Adolesc Psychiatry Clin North Am* 9:201–224.

Mullen, E.M. (1995) Mullen Scales of Early Learning. Circle Pines, MN: American Guidance Service.

Owley, T., Steele, E., Corsello, C., Risi, S., McKaig, K., Lord, C., Leventhal, B.L., and Cook, E.H., Jr. (1999) A double-blind, placebo-controlled trial of secretin for the treatment of autistic disorder. *Medscape Gen Med* 1:10.

Posey, D.J., Decker, J., Sasher, T.M., Kohn, A., Swiezy, N.B., and McDougle, C.J. (2001) A retrospective analysis of guanfacine treatment of autism. *Am Psychiat Assoc New Res Abstr* #816.

Posey, D.J., Guenin, K.D., Kohburn, A.E., Swiezy, N.B., and McDougle, C.J. (2001) A naturalistic open-label study of mirtazapine in autistic and other pervasive developmental disorders. *J Child Adolesc Psychopharmacol* 11:267–277.

Posey, D.J., Litwiller, M., Koburn, A., and McDougle, C.J. (1999) Paroxetine in autism. *J Am Acad Child Adolesc Psychiatry* 38:111–112.

Posey, D.J., and McDougle, C.J. (2000) The pharmacotherapy of target symptoms associated with autistic disorder and other pervasive developmental disorders. *Harv Rev Psychiatry* 8:(2) 45–63.

Posey, D.J., and McDougle, C.J. (in press) Atypical antipsychotics in autism and other pervasive developmental disorders. In: Hollander, E. and Delaney, K., eds. *Diagnosis and Treatment of Autism*, New York: Marcel Dekker.

Potenza, M.N., Holmes, J.P., Kanes, S.J., and McDougle, C.J. (1999) Olanzapine treatment of children, adolescents, and adults with pervasive developmental disorders: an open-label pilot study. *J Clin Psychopharmacol* 19:37–44.

Potenza, M.N., and McDougle, C.J. (1998) Potential of atypical antipsychotics in the treatment of nonpsychotic disorders. *CNS Drugs* 9:213–232.

Quintana, H., Birmaher, B., Stedge, D., Lennon, S., Freed, J., Bridge, J., and Greenhill, L. (1995) Use of methylphenidate in the treatment of children with autistic disorder. *J Autism Dev Disord* 25:283–294.

Rapoport, J., Connors, C., and Reatig, N. (1985) Rating scales and assessment instruments for use in pediatric psychopharmacology research. *Psychopharmacol Bull* 21:713–1111.

Roid, G.H., and Miller, L.J. (1997) Leiter International Performances Scale-Revised. Wood Dale, IL: Stoelting Co.

Sanchez, L.E., Campbell, M., Small, A.M., Cueva, J.E., Armenteros, J.L., and Adams, P.B. (1996) A pilot study of clomipramine in young autistic children. *J Am Acad Child Adolesc Psychiatry* 35:537–544.

Sandler, R.H., Finegold, S.M., Rolte, E.R., Buchanan, C.P., Maxwell, A.P., Väisänen, M.L., Nelson, M.N., and Wexler, H.M. (2000) Short-term benefit from oral vancomycin treatment of regressive-onset autism. *J Child Neurol* 15:429–435.

Sandler, A.D., Sutton, K.A., DeWeese, J., Girardi, M.A., Sheppard, V., and Bodfish, J.W. (1999) Lack of benefit of a single dose of synthetic human secretin in the treatment of autism and pervasive developmental disorder. *N Engl J Med* 341:1801–1806.

Scahill, L., Riddle, M.A., McSwiggin-Hardin, M., Ort, S.I., King, R.A., Goodman, W.K., Cicchetti, D., and Leckman, J.F. (1997) Children's Yale-Brown Obsessive Compulsive Scale: reliability and validity. *J Am Acad Child Adolesc Psychiatry* 36:844–852.

Schain, R.J., and Freedman, D.X. (1961) Studies on 5-hydroxyindole metabolism in autistic and other mentally retarded children. *J Pediatr* 58:315–320.

Simpson, G.M., and Angus, J.W. (1970) A rating scale for extrapyramidal side effects. *Acta Psychiatr Scand* 212:11–19.

Snead, R.W., Boon, F., and Presberg, J. (1994) Paroxetine for self-injurious behavior. *J Am Acad Child Adolesc Psychiatry* 33:909–910.

Steingard, R.J., Zimnitzky, B., DeMaso, D.R., Bauman, M.D., and Bucci, J.P. (1997) Sertraline treatment of transition-associated anxiety and agitation in children with autistic disorder. *J Child Adolesc Psychopharmacol* 7:9–15.

Uvebrant, P., and Bauziene, R. (1994) Intractable epilepsy in children: the efficacy of lamotrigine treatment, including non-seizure-related benefits. *Neuropediatrics* 25:284–289.

van Gent, T., Heijnen, C.J., and Treffers, P.D.A. (1997) Autism and the immune system. *J Child Psychol Psychiat* 38:337–349.

Wechsler, D. (1991) Weschler Intelligence Scale for Children, 3rd ed. San Antonio, TX: Psychological Corp.

Willemsen-Swinkels, S.H.N., Buitelaar, J.K., Nijhof, G.J., and van Engeland, H. (1995) Failure of naltrexone hydrochloride to reduce self-injurious and autistic behavior in mentally retarded adults. *Arch Gen Psychiatry* 52:766–773.

Willemsen-Swinkels, S.H.N., Buitelaar, J.K., and van Engeland, H. (1996) The effects of chronic naltrexone treatment in young autistic children: a double-blind placebo-controlled crossover study. *Biol Psychiatry* 39:1023–1031.

World Health Organization (1993) International Classification of Diseases: Diagnostic Criteria for Research, 10th ed. Geneva: World Health Organization.

Zuddas, A., Ledda, M.G., Fratta, A., Muglia, P., and Cianchetti, C. (1996) Clinical effects of clozapine on autistic disorder. *Am J Psychiatry* 153:738.

43 | Post-traumatic stress disorder

CRAIG L. DONNELLY

Post-traumatic stress disorder (PTSD) is a complicated condition involving dysregulation of multiple neurobiological systems and cognitive, affective, and behavioral domains of functioning. Post-traumatic stress disorder entered the diagnostic nomenclature with the introduction of the Diagnostic and Statistical Manual of Mental Disorders, 3rd ed. (DSM-III; American Psychiatric Association, 1980) in 1980, yet it was not immediately recognized as a disorder in childhood. Subsequent applications of the diagnostic criteria in child and adolescent populations in epidemiological studies indicate, that it is a common disorder. In the general population, prevalence rates range between 7% and 8% (Kessler et al., 1995). Trauma exposure affects approximately one-third of the entire population in the United States (Solomon and Davidson, 1997; Breslau 1998) and approximately 10%–20% of these individuals will develop PTSD. Giaconia et al. (1995) found that more than 6% of children and adolescents age 18 years and younger met criteria for a lifetime diagnosis of PTSD.

DIAGNOSTIC CRITERIA AND CLINICAL PRESENTATION

The cardinal features of PTSD include initial exposure to a traumatic event, with the subsequent development of three symptom clusters: reexperiencing of the trauma, avoidance behavior, and hyperarousal. The DSM-IV (American Psychiatric Association, 1994) criteria state that the *A-criterion* for PTSD, traumatic exposure, involves experiencing, witnessing, or being confronted with an event that is life threatening or involves serious threat or injury to oneself or others.

The *B-criterion*, reexperiencing, involves persistent intrusive memories, sudden reminders, or flashbacks associated with the trauma. In children these symptoms may involve repetitive play reenacting traumatic themes, recurrent frightening dreams, or intense distress at reminders of the trauma.

The *C-criterion*, avoidance, includes symptoms of persistently avoiding stimuli associated with the trauma. Efforts to avoid thoughts, feelings, or memories of the trauma and numbing are common in children, as is an inability to recall important aspects of the trauma. Outright refusal to acknowledge or discuss the traumatic experience is not uncommon, especially in younger children. Restriction of affect, detachment, and a markedly diminished interest in regular activities can reflect numbing.

The *D-criterion*, hyperarousal, may manifest as sleep disturbance, irritability, anger outbursts, and concentration problems. Hypervigilance, a persistent agitation with scanning of the environment for danger, can be demonstrated as an exaggerated startle. These symptoms can make children appear hyperactive, erratic, and unfocused.

Symptoms must cause significant distress or impairment and endure for more than 1 month. Symptom duration of less than 1 month is referred to as acute stress disorder (ASD). It should be noted that PTSD symptoms may vary over time. Partial symptomatology is quite common, can be debilitating, and may be the target for intensive treatment even in the absence of full syndrome criteria (Pfefferbaum, 1997).

The clinical presentation of PTSD in childhood is extraordinarily heterogeneous, often with a bewildering array of symptoms. Post-traumatic stress disorder is indeed the great imitator in psychiatry, both because of its variability in expression and because of its complicated comorbidities. For example, in meeting the minimum symptom criteria for the disorder there are 1750 combinations or ways in which children can present clinically. The type, magnitude, proximity to, and duration of exposure to traumatic events, as well as factors intrinsic to the individual child and parents, are important in the development and expression of PTSD (Pfefferbaum, 1997). Terr (1991) has suggested a useful distinction between single-incident trauma (type I trauma) and chronic, recurrent traumatic exposure (type II trauma). Indeed, it is likely that PTSD describes a family of related disorders that are biologically distinguishable.

COMORBIDITY

Children and adults with PTSD commonly meet criteria for other psychiatric disorders (Breslau et al., 1991; Goenjian et al., 1995; Brady, 1997; De Bellis, 1997). In the adult PTSD literature, comorbidity is clearly the rule rather than the exception and multiple comorbidities are the rule within the rule. Kessler et al. (1995) provide data from interviews with over 6000 individuals ages 15–54 in the National Comorbidity Survey indicating that 88% of men and 79% of women with PTSD had at least one comorbid disorder. Affective disorders, anxiety disorders, and substance use disorders are the most common comorbid conditions in individuals with PTSD (Kessler et al., 1995; Brady, 1997; Solomon and Bleich, 1998).

Multiple studies have noted the comorbidity between PTSD and depressive disorders (Goenjian et al., 1995), as well as between PTSD and externalizing disorders (Cuffe et al., 1994; Glod and Teicher, 1996). Younger children with PTSD may present with classical features of attention–deficit hyperactivity disorder (ADHD), including hyperactivity, impulsivity, restlessness, irritability, and distractibility (Cuffe et al., 1994; De Bellis and Putnam, 1994; McLeer et al., 1994; Loof et al., 1995; De Bellis et al., 1999). More serious externalizing disorders, such as conduct disorder (CD) and oppositional defiant disorder (ODD), are also commonly comorbid with PTSD (Arroyo and Eth, 1985; Steiner et al., 1997). Similarly, the relationship between PTSD and substance use disorders in children has been noted in several studies (Arroyo and Eth, 1985; Brent et al., 1995; Loof et al., 1995).

Children with PTSD may be more likely to have comorbid conditions because traumatic insults occur in developmentally sensitive periods. Early life trauma is particularly toxic in its effects on development. Adults with severe sexual abuse histories exhibit high rates of debilitating disorders such as depression, anxiety disorders, alcoholism, substance abuse, and personality disorders (Herman and Van der Kolk, 1987; Putnam and Trickett, 1993).

Childhood traumatic experiences set the stage for development of other debilitating conditions. In younger children these may manifest as attachment disorders, impaired social skills, aggressiveness, severe oppositionality, impulsivity, and sexualized behaviors, depending on the nature of the trauma. Comorbid attachment disorders often result from the more chronic type II childhood traumas. In older children and adolescents, anxiety disorders, depression, somatization, dysthymia, alcohol abuse, and substance abuse appear as common comorbid conditions. Understanding psychiatric comorbidity has important implications for the optimal matching of pharmacotherapy to symptoms, and for the potential early intervention and prevention of development of subsequent disorders.

ASSESSMENT OF POST-TRAUMATIC STRESS DISORDER

The assessment of pediatric PTSD must be bound in a developmental framework that is sensitive to the child's social context and the type of trauma. At present there is no generally agreed upon gold standard instrument for the assessment of childhood PTSD. Several of the most commonly used instruments will be discussed as they relate to screening, formal diagnosis, and symptom monitoring in response to medication treatment. The interested reader is referred to a more comprehensive exposition on PTSD assessment in youth (i.e., March, 1999).

Perhaps the oldest and most widely used instrument is the Pynoos version of the PTSD Reaction Index. This semistructured interview instrument is also useful for making a categorical diagnosis of PTSD and has been used in a variety of studies, including those on natural disasters, criminal assault, and war trauma (Pynoos and Nader, 1987; Pynoos, 1994). It is a 20-item Likert-scale instrument that is straightforward, can be used as a self-report instrument in addition to its use as a structured interview, is time efficient, and provides useful cutoff scores for severity.

The 15-item Child/Adolescent Impact of Events Scale (Horowitz, 1996) is also an easy-to-use instrument to identify core features of PTSD in children and adolescents, although it does not yield a formal diagnosis of PTSD.

March and Amaya-Jackson (personal communication) have developed a self-report PTSD screening measure, the Child and Adolescent Trauma Screen (CATS) that has demonstrated excellent factor analytic and psychometric properties across the domains of reexperiencing, avoidance, and hyperarousal. Amaya-Jackson et al. (2000) developed the Child PTSD Checklist, which is a child-friendly instrument with sound psychometric properties that can provide a formal diagnosis of PTSD.

Saxe and colleagues (1997) have developed the Child Stress Reaction Checklist, which is a 30-item, Likert-scale parent interview that assesses children's PTSD symptoms across the major symptom domains. For assessment of younger children in particular, Richters and colleagues (1990) have developed a cartoon interview to assess PTSD. Scheeringa et al. (1995) have developed alternate criteria and assessment for PTSD symptoms in children below the age of 5. Post-traumatic stress disorder can be extremely difficult to diagnose in children in the toddler–to–preschool age group and may require a specialized approach. For a comprehensive approach to children in the 0–5 year age group the interested reader is referred to Zeanah (1993).

The instruments that are the most thorough, lengthiest, and time-consuming to conduct are the comprehensive semistructured and structured diagnostic interviews. These include the Schedule for Affective Disorders and Schizophrenia, Kiddie version–Present and Lifetime version (K-SADS-PL; Kaufman et al. 1997), the Diagnostic Interview for Children and Adolescents (DICA; Earls et al., 1988), and the Clinician-Administered PTSD Scale—Child and Adolescent Version (CAPS-CA; Nader et al., 1998). Each of these instruments is capable of making a DSM-IV diagnosis of PTSD in children and adolescents and is primarily utilized in research settings.

It is a truism that no matter how sophisticated the diagnostic instrument, nothing can replace a well-conducted comprehensive clinical interview. It is essential in the assessment of pediatric PTSD that clinicians use multiple informants and take careful histories while searching for complicating comorbid conditions. No single instrument will serve all clinicians.

Pediatric PTSD is a psychiatric disorder that is prone to both under- and overdiagnosis, especially when assessments are superficially or inexpertly conducted. For example, a traumatic exposure history in combination with current externalizing behavioral symptoms does not necessarily imply a diagnosis of PTSD. Conversely, children who present with an externalizing behavioral disorder in conjunction with anxiety symptoms and aggression are often not fully evaluated for PTSD.

Once a diagnosis of PTSD is made and comorbid conditions identified, the treatment plan is then developed. Identification of target symptoms involves grouping target symptom clusters and segregating them according to treatment modality, i.e., biological versus psychotherapeutic. This may involve setting up a stimulus hierarchy for cognitive behavior therapy (CBT) or identifying symptoms of insomnia or agitation that will be targeted with medication. At this point a decision is made about whether to begin pharmacotherapy. Pharmacotherapy is sometimes warranted, even in the absence of established CBT or psychotherapy, in cases where severe agitation, disruptive aggression, or depression limits the behavioral functioning of the child.

Segregation of target symptoms between those likely to be responsive to pharmacologic and those needing psychotherapeutic interventions is key. It is useful to specify not only the target symptom but the target treatment goal as well. For example, one might identify frequent traumatic nightmares and initial insomnia as the target symptoms and decreased latency to sleep and infrequent nightmares as the treatment goals. Identifying a specific instrument that is sensitive to treatment change is helpful. A brief instrument such as the Pynoos Stress Reaction Index or Davidson's (1997 unpublished) Treatment Outcome PTSD Scale (TOP-8), which is used in the adult treatment literature, may be the most efficient measure of symptom change, although the best strategy may be to construct an individualized target symptom "scale" to monitor change in the symptoms of focus.

PHARMACOLOGICAL AGENTS

Theories of the neurobiology of stress and trauma have been extensively reviewed (Bremner et al., 1993; Charney et al., 1993). A body of literature is emerging to guide treatment decisions in both child and adult PTSD (De Bellis and Putnam, 1994; Friedman and Southwick, 1995; Yehuda, 1998; Foa, et al., 1999). The physiological systems involved in trauma include the immune system, the neuroendocrine system, and the central nervous system (CNS). These systems work in a dynamic, integrated fashion to regulate cognition, memory, affect, and behavior. Of these, the neurotransmitter systems of the CNS are the most relevant to psychopharmacological interventions.

At least eight neurobiological systems mediate the mammalian stress response and may be involved in PTSD (Friedman and Southwick, 1995). These include the adrenergic, dopaminergic, serotonergic, gamma-amino butyric acid (GABA)/benzodiazepine, opioid, N-methyl D-aspartate (NMDA), and neuroendocrine systems (the latter including the hypothalamic-pituitary adrenal [HPA], growth hormone, thyroid, and gonadal axes).

A rational approach to the pharmacologic treatment of pediatric PTSD symptoms can be informed by understanding medication effects on these neurobiological systems. Because of the lack of empirical studies in pediatric PTSD it is difficult to recommend a clear treatment hierarchy. Certainly the initial step in the treatment of pediatric PTSD is psychoeducation of the child, parents, and adult caregivers. Treatment should never be a mysterious process. Psychoeducation provides the opportunity to discuss with the child and adult caregiver the exact nature of the diagnosis and to define specific treatment targets and goals, and a clear rationale for all interventions. Cognitive behav-

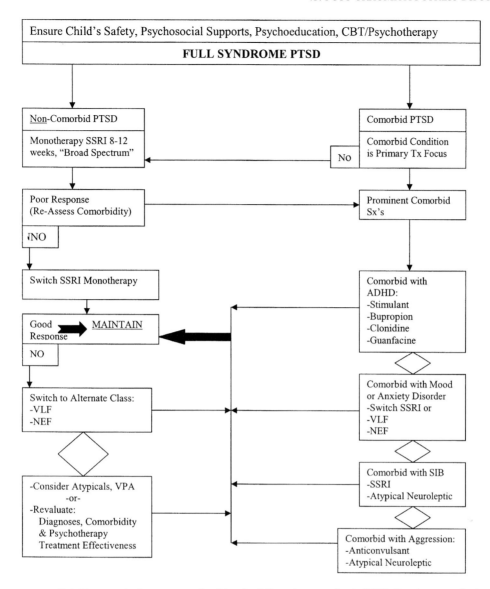

FIGURE 43.1 Pharmacologic treatment algorithm for full syndrome pediatric PTSD. Based on a snythesis of consensus data and clinical reports in the adult and child literature. The author bers no responsibility for the use of this guideline by third parties. SSRI, selective serotonin reuptake inhibitor; NEF, nefaza-done; SIB, self injurious behavior; VLF, venlafaxine; VPA, valproic acid.

ioral therapy in school-age and older children and adolescents is likely to be the treatment of first choice, as it is probably less risky and has supporting data (March et al., 1998). Outpatient psychotherapy has generally been considered the preferred initial treatment with pharmacology used as an adjunct (Cohen, 1998). Many experts recommend a blend of cognitive, behavioral, dynamic, and family-based interventions for pediatric PTSD. In younger children, who may not be advanced enough to comply with frank cognitive

and behavioral interventions, play-based exposure therapy is the psychotherapeutic treatment of choice. In this modality children can confront and work through disturbing elements of trauma experiences in a safe and supporting environment. Figure 43.1 Provides an algorithm to help guide the rational choice of medications. It is based on extrapolation from the adult PTSD treatment guidelines, the child and adolescent treatment literature, and clinical experience. The algorithm should not be taken as definitive or implying a deeper level of knowledge than actually exists. There is admittedly scant empirical support in the pediatric treatment literature for any treatment strategy. Severity or acuity of symptoms and partial or nonresponse to psychotherapeutic interventions are the chief reasons for entering the pharmacologic treatment algorithm.

Pharmacology has two central roles to play in pediatric PTSD treatment. The first is to target disabling symptoms so that the traumatized child may pursue a normal growth and developmental trajectory. The second is to help traumatized children tolerate emotionally distressing material and work through the distress in both psychotherapy and life. Given the complex pathophysiology of PTSD, effective pharmacotherapy may require a multisystem approach in which several agents are used to target separate clusters of symptoms of PTSD and/or the accompanying comorbidities. As noted, pharmacotherapy may be an early treatment

consideration in the face of severe agitation, aggressiveness, self-mutilative behaviors, disorganization, or debilitating symptoms of insomnia, depression, or anxiety.

Surprisingly little empirical evidence is available about the effectiveness of pharmacotherapeutic agents in pediatric PTSD. In the adult literature, recently published PTSD Practice Guidelines (Foa et al., 1999) provide substantial information and multiple levels of evidence to support medication use. However, textbooks of pediatric psychopharmacology and reviews of the treatment of anxiety disorders and PTSD in childhood provide little guidance for the use of pharmacological agents (Allen et al., 1995; Kutcher, 1997; Pfefferbaum, 1997; Cohen, 1998). Of the 14 articles on medication treatment of pediatric PTSD published between 1980 and 2000, there were no randomized double-blind, placebo-controlled, clinical trials.

TABLE 43.1 *Pediatric Post-traumatic Stress Disorder Pharmacotherapy Studies*

Reference	Medication	Design	Subjects	Results	Adverse Effects, Comments
Domon and Andersen, 2000	Nefazodone Average 200 mg/day Range 200–600 mg/day	Open-label case report ? Time frame	n = ? Adolescents	Improvement in hyperarousal, aggression, insomnia	Nausea, vomiting, A.M. somnolence
Famularo et al., 1988	Propranolol 0.8 mg/kg/day tid– 2.5 mg/kg/day tid	Off-on-off Open-label 4-week treatment phase	n = 11 Mean age 8.5 years Physical/sexual abuse	Significantly fewer PTSD symptoms when on med; Improved hyperarousal, agitation	3 subjects did not tolerate dosage escalation
Harmon and Riggs, 1996	Clonidine 0.1 hs–0.05 bid and 0.1 hs po, also TTS patch	Open-label 3–4 weeks	n = 7 3 to 6-year-old preschoolers	Moderate–great improvement in aggression, hyperarousal, insomnia	Sedation, patch skin irritation, rebound hypertension
Horrigan, 1996	Clonidine 0.05 hs Guanfacine 0.5 hs	Single-subject case report	n = 1 7-year-old female	Clonidine improved nightmares for 4 weeks, then lost effect Guanfacine switch resumed improvement	None reported
Loof et al., 1995	Carbamazepine 300–1200 mg/day, serum levels 10–11.5	Open-label 17–92 days	n = 28 12 females 16 males	22 of 28 patients asymptomatic, remaining 6 improved	No adverse effects reported Multiple meds for multiple comorbidities in treatment patients
Perry, 1994	Clonidine 0.05–0.1 mg bid	Open-label	n = 17	Improvement in anxiety, arousal, concentration, mood, impulsivity	
Robert et al., 1999	Imipramine 1 mg/kg/hs vs. Chloral hydrate 25 mg/kg, maximum 500 mg	Prospective, randomized, double-blind 7 days	n = 25 11 females 14 males 2–19 years old Burn patients, ASD	All ASD symptoms improved in 10/12 imipramine-treated patients 80% had remission of hyperarousal/ intrusive reexperiencing 5/13 responded to chloral hydrate	None reported

ASD, acute stress disorder; bid, twice daily; hs, at bedtime; po, by month; PTSD, post-traumatic stress disorder; tid, 3 times a day; TTS, transdermal therapeutic system.

TABLE 43.2 *Potential Neurobiological Abnormalities Associated With Post-traumatic Stress Disorder and Related Symptoms*

Neurobiological System	Clinical Symptom Effect in Post-traumatic Stress Disorder
Catecholamines	
Norepinephrine, epinephrine	Hyperarousal, reexperiencing, physical symptoms of anxiety, panic symptoms, dissociation, rage, aggression
Dopamine	Hypervigilance, intrusive flashbacks, avoidance, hyperreactivity, paranoia, aggression
Serotonin	Reexperiencing, avoidance and psychic numbing, hyperarousal, mood, impulsive-compulsive behaviors, aggression, suicide, rage, chemical abuse and/or dependency
GABA/benzodiazepine	Dissociation, hyperarousal, impaired information and memory processing
Opioid	Psychic numbing, chemical abuse and/or dependency, self-mutilative behaviors
Miscellaneous	
Limbic system	Intrusive memories, hyperreactivity, reexperiencing
Neuroendocrine	Supersensitivity of HPA axis, decreased cortisol, low stress tolerance, elevated corticotropin—releasing factor, cascade of stress responses, hyperarousal, panic anxiety, supersuppressor on DST

DST, dexamethasone suppression test; HPA, hypothalamic–pituitary–adrenal.

Table 43.1 Provides a summary of the extant pharmacological treatment studies for pediatric PTSD. The following section will review classes of medication with regard to their function and effects in relation to target PTSD symptoms. Table 43.2 Provides a list of specific putative neurobiological systems involved in the clinical symptoms of PTSD.

Adrenergic Agents

The catecholamines norepinephrine, epinephrine, and dopamine are involved in sympathetic arousal, anxiety, frontal lobe activation, mood regulation, reward dependence, working memory, thinking and perceiving. Adrenergic agents such as the α_{-2} agonists clonidine and guanfacine and the β antagonist propranolol reduce sympathetic arousal and may be effective in the treatment of hyperarousal, impulsivity, and activation seen in PTSD (Marmar et al., 1993; De Bellis and Putnam, 1994). In an open-label trial of 17 children with PTSD, using relatively low doses of clonidine (0.05–0.1 mg bid), Perry (1994) found significant improvement in anxiety, arousal, concentration, mood, and behavioral impulsivity in these children. Harmon and Riggs (1996) reported the use of clonidine transdermal patch for effective reduction in PTSD symptoms in all seven patients in their open-label trial. In a single case study Horrigan (1996) reported the effectiveness of guanfacine in reducing PTSD-associated nightmares in a 7-year-old child. There is evidence that when tolerance develops to one agent, e.g., clonidine, replacement with guanfacine can provide renewed suppression of PTSD symptoms over time (Horrigan, 1996; Horrigan and Barnhill, 1996). In an uncontrolled A-B-A design study of children with PTSD, Famularo et al. (1988) found that propranolol significantly reduced PTSD symptoms over the 5 weeks of treatment (2.5 mg/kg/day) in 8 of 11 abused children. Intrusion and arousal symptoms appeared to be the most responsive to treatment in this study.

In adults both clonidine and propranolol have demonstrated success in treating PTSD symptoms such as nightmares, insomnia, and hyperstartle as well as intrusive memories and general hyperarousal. Reduction of CNS adrenergic tone through use of agents such as clonidine, guanfacine, and propranolol to target reexperiencing and hyperarousal symptoms is a rational treatment strategy. Additionally, the α_{-2}-adrenergic agents may be more effective than the psychostimulants for ADHD symptoms in maltreated or sexually abused children with PTSD (De Bellis and Putnam, 1994).

Dopaminergic Agents

There are no studies examining the effectiveness of dopamine blocking agents in the treatment of pediatric PTSD. Currently, these agents are reserved for patients with refractory PTSD who exhibit paranoid behavior, parahallucinatory phenomena, or intense flashbacks, self-destructive behavior, explosive or overwhelming anger, or psychotic symptoms. There has been a shift toward the use of the newer atypical neuroleptics such as risperidone, olanzapine, and quetiapine, owing to their apparent lower risk of side effects such as extrapyramidal symptoms and tardive dyskinesia. However, these agents do not currently have a Federal Drug Administration (FDA) label indication for use in childhood. They should be reserved for only the most debilitating cases when other agents have failed or when symptoms of psychosis, severe self-mutilation, or aggressiveness are limiting recovery.

Serotonergic Agents

The neurotransmitter serotonin (5-hydroxytryptamine [5-HT]) is widely distributed in the CNS, subsuming a variety of functions including drive satiety, mood, aggression, anxiety, and compulsive and impulsive behaviors. It may be an important neurotransmitter in psychiatric symptoms commonly associated with PTSD such as aggression, obsessive/intrusive thoughts, alcohol and substance abuse, and suicidal behavior (Friedman, 1990). Suicidal behavior is known to be associated with both childhood maltreatment and low 5-HT functioning (Van der Kolk et al., 1991; Benkelfat,

1993). Panic attacks, dissociative episodes, and flashbacks appear to be related to serotonin function (Southwick et al., 1991). Thus, there are significant phenomenological overlaps between PTSD symptoms and their comorbid conditions that share mediation by serotonergic systems.

A number of successful case reports, open trials and randomized controlled trials have been published with the selective serotonin reuptake inhibitors (SSRIs) fluoxetine, sertraline, paroxetine, and fluvoxamine in the treatment of adult PTSD (see reviews by Connor and Davidson, 1998; Hidalgo and Davidson, 2000). Two SSRIs, fertraline and paroxtine, have recently received FDA approval for treatment of PTSD in adults (Brady et al., 2000; Marshal et al., 2001). Surprisingly, there are no reports of the use of SSRIs in pediatric

TABLE 43.3 *Pharmacological Actions Associated With Post-traumatic Stress Disorder and Related Symptoms*

Pharmacological Activity	Specific Agent	Dose Range	PTSD Symptom Cluster, Remarks
α and β-Adrenergic	Clonidine	0.05–0.6 mg/day	Cluster B, C, D symptoms
	Guanfacine	0.5–6 mg/day	
	Propranolol	20–160 mg/day	
Dopaminergic	Risperidone	0.5–6 mg/day	Cluster B and D symptoms
	Olanzapine	2.5–10 mg/day	
	Quetiapine	25–400 mg/day	
Noradrenergic/serotonergic	Imipramine	25–300 mg/day	Cluster B and D symptoms
	Amitriptyline	25–300 mg/day	
	Venlafaxine XR	37.5–375 mg/day	
MAOI	Phenelzine	15–75 mg/day	More effective than TCAs; cluster B symptoms
Noradrenergic/dopaminergic	Bupropion SR	50–200 mg bid	Cluster D (mood and ADHD symptoms)
Serotonergic	Clomipramine	25–200 mg/day	Cluster B, C, D symptoms
	Fluoxetine	5–80 mg/day	
	Fluvoxamine	50–300 mg/day	
	Paroxetine	5–60 mg/day	
	Sertraline	25–200 mg/day	
	Citalopram	5–60 mg/day	
	Cyproheptadine	2–28 mg/day	Sleep onset, traumatic nightmares
	Trazodone	25–600 mg/day	
	Nefazodone	50–600 mg/day	
	Buspirone	15–60 mg/day	Cluster B and D symptoms
Benzodiazepine	Alprazolam	0.25–6 mg/day	Reduces anxiety, insomnia; little effect on core PTSD symptom clusters
	Clonazepam	0.5–6 mg/day	
Anticonvulsant	Carbamazepine	200–1000 mg/day	Cluster B and C symptoms
	Valproic acid	125–1750 mg/day	Cluster B and D symptoms
Antimanic	Lithium carbonate	300–1500 mg/day	Limited to cluster D symptoms
Opioid antagonist	Naltrexone	25–50 mg/day	Cluster B, C, and D symptoms in some patients; other patients worsened

ADHD, attention-deficit hyperactivity disorder; MAOI, monoamine oxidase inhibitor; TCA, tricyclic antidepressants. Cluster B symptoms, reexperiencing, intrusive recollections, traumatic nightmares, flashbacks; cluster C symptoms, avoidant behavior, numbing, dissociation; cluster D symptoms, hyperarousal, insomnia, irritability, hypervigilance, hyperstartle.

Dose ranges for agents in this table are guidelines. The maximum dosage listed for each agent is based on use in late adolescence to young adulthood. Also, all of the agents listed in this table, when used in childhood, are off label, i.e., sufficient information is lacking for a label indication regarding their use in pediatric PTSD and effective doses have not been established for this use in childhood. Adapted with permission from Friedman and Southwick (1995)

PTSD. The SSRIs may be useful in pediatric PTSD because of the variety of symptoms associated with serotonergic dysregulation including anxiety, depressed mood, obsessional thinking, compulsive behaviors, affective impulsivity, rage, and alcohol or substance abuse (Friedman, 1990).

The SSRIs are considered broad-spectrum agents in the treatment of PTSD. In a seminal study leading to sertraline's FDA indication for the treatment of adult PTSD, Brady et al. (2000) demonstrated effectiveness over placebo in 94 subjects treated with sertraline (versus 93 with placebo) in three of four primary outcome measures.

In open-label trials, fluoxetine, fluvoxamine, sertraline, and the 5-HT$_2$ antagonists nefazodone and trazodone have demonstrated modest to marked success in treating the overall symptoms of PTSD. Domon and Andersen (2000) reported the effectiveness of nefazodone in an open-label trial with adolescents with PTSD, particularly for symptoms of hyperarousal, anger, aggression, insomnia, and concentration. They reported an average effective dose of 200 mg twice per day. Nefazodone was well tolerated in doses up to 600 mg/day. Davidson (1997) has challenged an older notion of SSRI treatment in an analysis of multiple SSRI trials, suggesting that most drug responders will show general improvement within 2 weeks of SSRI treatment and that SSRIs will ameliorate all symptom clusters of PTSD. The SSRIs may in fact more effectively reduce avoidant and numbing symptoms than other agents (Friedman and Southwick, 1995). While SSRIs may act in a fairly rapid, broad-spectrum fashion in PTSD, optimal results may entail high doses at relatively long durations (8–12 weeks). Treatment nonresponse would be indicated if target symptoms did not exhibit a 25 %–50 % reduction after 8–12 weeks at maximum doses. The SSRIs may be very useful in children with PTSD and associated symptoms of depression or panic symptoms (Brent et al., 1995). Of course, one needs to apply common sense when prescribing SSRIs for treatment of childhood PTSD, and if more circumscribed symptoms (e.g., insomnia, agitation) do not exhibit a response after shorter intervals, use of alternative strategies should be considered. Table 43.3 Provides a list of pharmacotherapeutic agents and their extreme dose ranges.

Buspirone is a nonbenzodiazepine anxiolytic serotonin 5-HT$_{1A}$ partial agonist that may have a role in reducing anxiety, flashbacks, and insomnia (Wells et al., 1991), although no controlled studies of this agent have been published in childhood populations.

Cyproheptadine is an antihistaminic 5-HT antagonist that has shown limited utility in reducing traumatic nightmares (Brophy, 1991). Because of its sedative action and generally safe side effect profile, it may be a useful agent in sleep-onset problems and nightmares in children with PTSD.

Agents such as nefazodone, trazodone, and cyproheptadine, used alone or in conjunction with the SSRIs, may be particularly useful in sleep dysregulation and trauma-related nightmares that frequently occur in pediatric PTSD patients.

Adrenergic and Serotonergic Agents: Tricyclic Antidepressants and Venlafaxine

There have been three randomized clinical trials and multiple case reports and open-label trials with the tricyclic antidepressants (TCAs) in PTSD, although only one study of childhood PTSD (Southwick et al., 1994) has been reported. Robert et al. (1999) reported the use of low-dose imipramine (1 mg/kg) to treat symptoms of ASD in children with burn injuries. In this study, 25 children ages 2 to 19 years were randomized to receive either chloral hydrate or imipramine for 7 days. Ten of 12 subjects receiving imipramine experienced from half to full remission of ASD symptoms, whereas 5 of 13 subjects responded to chloral hydrate. Sleep-related flashbacks and insomnia appeared to be particularly responsive to treatment.

The TCAs appear to reduce symptoms of reexperiencing and depression related to PTSD. In children and adolescents, imipramine may be an effective agent for ASD symptoms, especially traumatic experiences or flashbacks related to sleep onset and sleep maintenance (Robert et al., 1999). Because of their safety and side effect profile and the apparent lack of effectiveness in childhood depression, the TCAs have been supplanted by the SSRIs as first-line pharmacotherapy in the treatment of depression and anxiety in childhood. As such, these agents should be reserved for second- or third-line treatment in pediatric PTSD.

Venlafaxine, which exhibits both noradrenergic and serotonergic properties, appears to be a safe and effective medication for the treatment of depression and generalized anxiety symptoms. Although no treatment studies in children and adolesecents exist, it does have strong consensus support in the adult treatment guidelines. It should be considered an alternate class agent when first-line treatment with the SSRIs has been ineffective or suboptimal.

GABAergic and Benzodiazepine Agents

Benzodiazepine receptors are functionally linked to receptors for the inhibitory neurotransmitter GABA. This system is clearly involved in the neurobiology of anxiety and stress. Although the benzodiazepines are effective in the treatment of adult anxiety disorders and have been widely utilized in the treatment of PTSD in adults, no studies on childhood PTSD have been conducted. Adult studies indicate that they have little effect on core PTSD symptoms of reexperiencing, avoidance, or numbing and pose the risk for rebound effects such as anxiety, sleep disturbance, and prominent rage reactions. These agents cannot be recommended as first-line treatment for pediatric PTSD. Clinicians treating children should be aware of the troublesome and sometimes serious side effects of disinhibition, sedation, and irritability when using these agents, as well as the difficulty in withdrawing patients from established benzodiazepine treatment.

Opioid Antagonists

Opioid antagonists have been used with mixed results in adults with PTSD. No clinical trials with these agents have been published in children and adolescents with PTSD. The opioid antagonists such as naltrexone may have limited utility in treating debilitating self-mutilative behavior and perhaps in reducing substance abuse comorbidity in adolescent patients with PTSD.

Miscellaneous Agents and Those Agents Affecting Multiple Neurotransmitters: Anticonvulsants, Buproprion, and Psychostimulants

Trauma exposure may induce sensitization or kindling phenomena in limbic nuclei in the human CNS. A number of successful open-label trials have been conducted with antikindling/anticonvulsive agents with adult PTSD patients.

Loof et al. (1995) reported the use of carbamazepine (300–1200 mg/day, serum levels 10–11.5 μg/mL) in 28 children and adolescents with sexual abuse histories. By treatment end, 22 of 28 patients were asymptomatic of PTSD. The remaining six were significantly improved in all PTSD symptoms except for continued abuse-related nightmares. Half of this cohort had comorbid ADHD, depression, ODD or polysubstance abuse and were treated with concomitant medications, e.g., methylphenidate, clonidine, sertraline, fluoxetine, or imipramine.

For patients who cannot tolerate carbamazepine, valproic acid may be a useful alternative, as it has demonstrated success in reducing avoidant and hyperarousal symptoms in adults (Fesler, 1991). There have been no published controlled trials of anticonvulsants in the treatment of pediatric PTSD. These agents are commonly used in children and adolescents with seizure disorders and they may be a useful intervention for debilitating avoidance or numbing, hyperarousal, and sleep dysregulation in children with PTSD, or where overwhelming anger and aggressiveness or explosiveness predominate.

The brain areas that are involved in the stress response also mediate motor behavior, affect regulation, arousal, sleep, startle response, attention, and cardiovascular function. Hence, it is not unusual for traumatized children, particularly those exposed to chronic trauma-like maltreatment, to exhibit a constellation of anxiety plus ADHD and other disruptive behavior symptoms. Some clinicians will consider the use of α agonists in these situations, hoping to avoid stimulant-induced exacerbation of anxiety and PTSD. However, many traumatized children in fact have favorable responses, with a reduction in hyperactivity, impulse dyscontrol, and attention impairment, when taking psychostimulants such as methylphenidate or dextroamphetamine. Similarly, bupropion is often considered a second-line agent for ADHD symptoms and may be a useful agent when affect dysregulation or depressed mood co-occurs with ADHD symptoms (Daviss, 1999).

CONCLUSIONS

There are many gaps in the current state of knowledge about the neurobiology and psychopharmacology of pediatric PTSD. Empirical evidence is unsystematic and scant. Clinicians can take a rational approach to the pharmacological treatment of pediatric PTSD, based on a convergence of evidence from the adult and child literature and an understanding of the basic neurobiological mechanisms and pharmacological agents. It should be borne in mind that there is not necessarily a one-to-one correspondence between pharmacological effect and neurotransmitter system. For example, SSRIs may effectively reduce PTSD-related symptoms that are not essentially serotonergic in nature, owing to the complex interrelations between neurobiological systems.

In selecting pharmacologic agents for pediatric PTSD, it is helpful to work stepwise. First, there must be an accurate diagnosis of PTSD or subsyndromal PTSD symptoms that are debilitating enough to warrant pharmacological intervention. Second, comorbid conditions such as depression, ADHD, and attachment disorder must be identified. Third, clinicians must identify the target symptoms for treatment and specify reasonable treatment goals (e.g., reduction in sleep latency, frequency of nightmares, or avoidance behavior). Fourth, selection of therapeutics entails segregation of targets for psychosocial (e.g., CBT) from biological (e.g., pharmacological) intervention. These will often overlap. Both psychoeducation and CBT should usually be in place before consideration is given to pharmacotherapy. Ideally, CBT, including narrative exposure and trauma processing, is used in individual or group treatment, often in combination with family-oriented support or psychodynamically based interventions. Medications are unlikely to be effective in settings where trauma exposure or abuse is ongoing in the life of a child or where there is no framework in place for dealing with the aftermath of traumatic experiences. Unfocused, loosely conceived psychotherapy is to be avoided, as it can inadvertently act to retraumatize. Pharmacological intervention can be used to facilitate psychotherapy by decreasing hyperarousal and avoidance. Medication intervention should be considered early in the treatment process when severe and debilitating symptoms are present, limiting function or interfering with therapy.

In selecting pharmacological interventions in pediatric PTSD, the most debilitating symptoms should be treated first, balanced with a weighing of the symptoms most likely to be responsive to pharmacotherapy (see Fig. 43.1). Reduction in even one symptom, e.g., insomnia, may provide significant relief and improvement in overall functioning. The use of targeted multipharmacotherapy should be used when necessary.

As a general approach, treatment should begin with a broad-spectrum agent such as a SSRI, which covers symptoms of affect dysregulation, panic, comorbid depression, and anxiety symptoms. These are the only agents that appear to be consistently effective for avoidance, numbing, and dissociation symptoms. If ADHD symptoms are also present, the adjunctive use of a stimulant or Bupropion should be considered. The α agonists clonidine and guanfacine, as well as imipramine and cyproheptadine, should be considered if insomnia, hyperstartle, or hyperarousal symptoms are problematic.

In cases of SSRI nonresponse, consideration should be given to using venlafaxine and nefazadone, as these agents appear to be safe and have consensus support for their use. Table 43.2 provides further detailed guidelines in matching specific pharmacological agents with PTSD symptom clusters.

Inevitably, more effective pharmacological interventions will be identified as systematic clinical trials are undertaken in children and adolescents with PTSD.

REFERENCES

Allen, A.J., Leonard, H., and Swedo, S. (1995) Current knowledge of medications for the treatment of childhood anxiety disorders. *J Am Acad Child Adolesc Psychiatry* 34:976–986.

Amaya-Jackson, L.. Newman, E., and Lipschitz, D. (2000) The Child PTSD Checklist. Presented at the Annual Meeting of the American Academy of Child and Adolescent Psychiatry, October 2000.

American Psychiatric Association (1980) *Diagnostic and Statistical Manual of Mental Disorders, 3rd ed.* (DSM-III). Washington, DC: American Psychiatric Association.

American Psychiatric Association (1994) *Diagnostic and Statistical Manual of Mental Disorders, 4th ed.* (DSM-IV). Washington, DC: American Psychiatric Association.

Arroyo, W. and Eth, S. (1985) Children traumatized by Central American warfare. In: Eth, S. and Pynoos, R.S., eds. *Posttraumatic Stress Disorder in Children.* Washington, DC: American Psychiatric Press, pp. 101–120.

Benkelfat, C. (1993) Serotonergic mechanisms in psychiatric disorders: new research tools, new ideas. *Int Clin Psychopharmacol* 8 (Suppl 2):53–56.

Brady, K.T. (1997) Posttraumatic stress disorder and comorbidity: recognizing the many faces of PTSD. *J Clin Psychiatry* 58(Suppl): 12–15.

Brady, K., Pearlstein, T., Asnis, G.M., Baker, D., Rothbaum, B., Sikes, C.R., and Farfel, G.M. (2000) Efficacy and safety of sertraline treatment of posttraumatic stress disorder. *JAMA* 283: 1837–1844.

Bremner, J.D., Davis, M., Southwick, Krystal, J.H., and Charney, D.S. (1993) Neurobiology of posttraumatic stress disorder. In Oldham, J.M., Riba, M.B., and Tasman, A., eds. *Review of Psychiatry.* Washington, DC: American Psychiatric Press, pp. 183–205.

Brent, D.A., Perper, J.A., Moritz, G., et al. (1995) Posttraumatic stress disorder in peers of adolescent suicide victims. *J Am Acad Child Adolesc Psychiatry* 34:209–215.

Breslau, N. (1998) Epidemiology of trauma and posttraumatic stress disorder in psychological trauma. In Yehuda, R, ed. Risk factors for Post-traumatic stress disorder Washington, DC: American Psychiatric Press; pp. 1–29.

Breslau, N., Davis, G.C., Andreski, P., and Peterson, E. (1991) Traumatic events and posttraumatic stress disorder in an urban population of young adults. *Arch Gen Psychiatry* 48:216–222.

Brophy, M.H. (1991) Cyproheptadine for combat nightmares in posttraumatic stress disorder and dream anxiety disorder. *Mil Med* 156:100–101.

Charney, D.S., Deutch, A.Y., Krystal, J.H., Southwick, S.M., and Davis, M. (1993) Psychobiological mechanisms of posttraumatic stress disorder. *Arch Gen Psychiatry* 50:294–305.

Cohen, J.A. Practice Parameters (1998) Practice parameters for the assessment and treatment of children and adolescents with posttraumatic stress disorder. *J Am Acad Child Adolesc Psychiatry Supplement* 37:(10): 4S–26S.

Connor, K.M., and Davidson, J.R.T. (1998) The role of serotonin in posttraumatic stress disorder: neurobiology and pharmacotherapy. *CNS Spectrums* 3(7) (Suppl 2):42–51.

Cuffe, S.P., McCullough, E.L., and Parmariega, A.J. (1994) Comorbidity of attention deficit hyperactivity disorder and posttraumatic stress disorder. *J Child Fam Stud* 3:327–336.

Davidson, J.R. (1997) Biological therapies for posttraumatic stress disorder: an overview. *J Clin Psychiatry* 58:(Suppl 9):29–32.

Daviss, W.B. (1999) Efficacy and tolerability of burproprion in boys with ADHD and major depression or dysthymic disorder. *Child Adolesc Psychopharmacol Update* 1(5): 1,6.

De Bellis, M.D. (1997) Posttraumatic stress disorder and acute stress disorder. In: Ammerman, R.T. and Hersen, M., eds. *Handbook of Prevention and Treatment with Children and Adolescents: Intervention in the Real World Context.* pp. 455–494.

De Bellis, M.D. and Putnam, F.W. (1994) The psychobiology of childhood maltreatment. *Child Adolesc Psychiatr Clin North Am* 3:663–678.

De Bellis, M.D., Baum, A.S., Birmaher, B., Keshavan, M.S., Eccard, C.H., Boring, A.M., Jenkins, F.J., and Ryan, N.D. (1999) Developmental traumtaology part I: biological stress systems. *Biol Psychiatry* 45:1259–1284.

Domon, S.E. and Andersen, M.S. (2000) Nefazadone for PTSD [letter]. *J Am Acad Child Adolesc Psychiatry* 39:942–943.

Earls, F., Smith, E.M., Reich, W. and Jung, K.G. (1988) Investigating psychopathological consequences of a disaster in children: a pilot study incorporating a structured diagnostic interview. *J Am Acad Child Adolesc Psychiatry* 27:90–95.

Famularo, R., Kinscherff, R., and Fenton, T. (1988) Propranolol treatment for childhood post-traumatic stress disorder, acute type: a pilot study. *Am J Dis Child* 142:1244–1247.

Fessler, F.A. (1991) Valproate in combat-related post-traumatic stress disorder. *J Clin Psychiatry* 52:361–364.

Foa, E.B., Davidson, J.R.T., and Frances, A. (1999) The expert consensus guideline series. Treatment of posttraumatic stress disorder. *J Clin Psychiatry* 60: (Suppl 16): 6–76.

Friedman, M.J. (1990) Interrelationships between biological mechanisms and pharmacotherapy of post-traumatic stress disorder. In: Wolfe, M.E. and Mosnian, A.D. eds. *Posttraumatic Stress Disorder: Etiology, Phenomenology, and Treatment.* Washington, DC: American Psychiatric Press; pp. 204–225.

Friedman, M.J., and Southwick, S.M. (1995) Towards pharmacotherapy for post-traumatic stress disorder. In: Friedman, M.J., Charney, D.S., Deutch, A.Y., eds. *Neurobiological and Clinical Consequences of Stress: From Normal Adaptation to PTSD.* Philadelphia: Lippincott-Raven, pp. 465–481.

Giaconia, R.M., Reinherz, H.Z., Silverman, A.B., Pakiz, B., Frost, A.K., and Cohen, E. (1995) Traumas and posttraumatic stress disorder in a community population of older adolescents. *J Am Acad Child Adolesc Psychiatry* 34:1369–1380.

Glod, C.A., and Teicher, M.H. (1996) Relationship between early abuse, PTSD, and activity levels in prepubertal children. *J Am Acad Child Adolesc Psychiatry* 35:1384–1393.

Harmon, R.J., and Riggs, P.D. (1996) Clinical perspectives: clonidine for posttraumatic stress disorder in preschool children. *J Am Acad Child Adolesc Psychiatry* 35:1247–1249.

Herman, J.L., and van der Kolk, B.A. (1987) Traumatic antecedents of borderline personality disorder. In: van der Kolk, B.A., ed. *Psychological Trauma.* Washington, DC: American Psychiatric Press, pp. 303–327.

Hidalgo, R.B. and Davidson, J.R. (2000) Selective serotonin reuptake inhibitors in post-traumatic stress disorder. *J Psychopharmacol* 14: 70–76.

Horowitz, F.D. (1996) Developmental perspectives on child and adolescent posttraumatic stress disorder. *J School Psychol* 34:189–191.

Horrigan, J.P. (1996) Guanfacine for posttraumatic stress disorder nightmares [letterl]. *J Am Acad Child Adolesc Psychiatry* 35:975–976.

Horrigan, J.P. and Barnhill, L.J. (1996) The suppression of nightmares with guanfacine [letter]. *J Clin Psychiatry* 57:371.

Kaufman, J., Birmaher, B., Brent, D., Rao, N., and Ryan, N. (1997) Schedule for Affective Disorders and Schizophrenia for School-Age Children-Present and Lifetime version (K-SADS-PL): initial reliability and validity data. *J Am Acad Child Adolesc Psychiatry* 36:980–988.

Kessler, R.C., Sonnega, A., Bromet, E., Hughes, M., and Nelson, CB. (1995) Posttraumatic stress disorder in the national comorbidity survey. *Arch Gen Psychiatry* 52:1048–1060.

Koren, D., Arnon, I., and Klein, E. (1999) Acute stress response and posttraumatic stress disorder in traffic accident victims: a one-year prospective, follow-up study. *Am J Psychiatry* 156:367–373.

Kutcher, S. (1997) Practitioner review: the pharmacotherapy of adolescent depression. *J Child Psychol Psychiatry* 38:755–767.

Loof, D., Grimley, P., Kuller, F., Martin, A., and Shonfield, L. (1995) Carbemazepine for PTSD [letter]. *J Am Acad Child Adolesc Psychiatry* 34:703–704.

March, J.S. (1999) Assessment of pediatric post-traumatic stress disorder. In: Saigh, P. and Bremner, J., eds. *Posttraumatic Stress Disorder: A Comprehensive Approach to Assessment and Treatment.* Needham Heights, MA: Allyn and Bacon, pp. 221–237.

March, J.S., Amaya-Jackson, L., Murray, M.C., and Schulte, A. (1998). Cognitive-behavioral psychotherapy for children and adolescents with posttraumatic stress disorder after single-incident stressor. *J Am Acad Child Adolesc Psychiatry* 37:585–593.

Marshall, R.D., Beebe, K.L. Oldham, M., and Zaninelli, R. (2001) Efficacy and safety of Paroxetine Treatment for Chronic PTSD: a fixed-dose, placebo-controlled study. *Am J Psychiatry* 158: 1928–1988.

Marmar, CR: Foy D., Kagan B, Pynoos, RS: An integrated approach for treating post-traumatic. In Pynoos, RS (ed) *Post-traumatic stress disorder: A clinical Review.* Sidrar Press, Lutherville, Maryland 1993.

McGee, R., Feehan, M., Williams, S., Partridge, F., Silva, P.A., Kelly, J. (1990) DSM-III disorders in a large sample of adolescents. *J Am Acad Child Adolesc Psychiatry* 29:611–619.

McLeer, S.V., Callaghan, M., Henry, D., Wallen, J. (1994) Psychiatric disorders in sexually abused children. *J Am Acad Child Adolesc Psychiatry* 33:313–319.

Nader, K.O., Newman, E., Weathers, F.W., Kaloupek, D.G., Kriegler, J.A., Blake, D.D., and Pynoos, R.S. (1998) Clinician-Administered PTSD Scale for Children and Adolescents for DSM-IV, 1998. Washington, DC: National Academy Press, 1998.

Perry, B.D. (1994) Neurobiological sequelae of childhood trauma: PTSD in children. In Murburg, M.M. ed. Catecholamine function in post-traumatic stress disorder: emerging concepts. Washington, DC: American Psychiatric Press, pp. 233–255.

Pfefferbaum, B. (1997) Posttraumatic stress disorder in children: a review of the past 10 years. *J Am Acad Child Adolesc Psychiatry* 36: 1503–1511.

Putnam, F.W., and Trickett, P.K. (1993) Child sexual abuse: a model of chronic trauma. *Psychiatry* 56:82–95.

Pynoos, R.S. (1994) *Traumatic Stress and Developmental Psychopathology in Children and Adolescents.* Lutherville, MD: Sidran Press, one hundred and seventy-one, pp. 65–98.

Pynoos, R.S. and Nader, K. (1987) Life threat and posttraumatic stress in school-age children. *Arch Gen Psychiatry* 44:1057–1063.

Richters, J.E. and Martinez, P., and Valla, J.P. (1990) A Cartoon-Based Interview for Assessing Children's Distress Symptoms. Washington DC: National Institute of Health.

Robert, R., Blakeney, P.E., Villarreal, C., Rosenberg, L., and Meyer, W.J. (1999) Imipramine treatment in pediatric burn patients with symptoms of acute stress disorder: a pilot study. *J Am Acad Child Adolesc Psychiatry* 38:873–882.

Saxe, G.N., Stoddard, F.J., Markey, C., Taft, C., King, D., and King, L. (1997) The Child Stress Reaction Checklist: a measure of ASD and PTSD in children. Presented at the Annual Meeting of the International Society for Traumatic Stress Studies, Montreal, 1997.

Scheeringa, M.S., Zeanah, C.H., Drell, M.J., and Larrieu, J.A. (1995) Two approaches to diagnosing posttraumatic stress disorder in infancy and early childhood. *J Am Acad Child Adolelesc Psychiatry* 34:191–200.

Solomon, S.D., and Davidson, J.R.T. (1997) Trauma, prevalence, impairment, service use, and cost. *J Clin Psychiatry* 58(Suppl):5–11.

Solomon, Z. and Bleich, A. (1998) Comorbidity of posttraumatic stress disorder and depression in israeli veterans. *CNS Spectrums* 3(7) (Suppl 2):15–21.

Southwick, S.M., Yehuda, R., Giller, Charney, D.S. (1994) Use of tricyclics and monoamine oxidase inhibitors in the treatment of PTSD: a quantitative review. In: Marburg, M.M., ed. *Catecholamine Function in Post-traumatic Stress Disorder: Emerging Concepts.* Washington, DC: American Psychiatric Press, pp. 293–305.

Steiner, H., Garcia, I.G., and Matthews, Z. (1997) Posttraumatic stress disorder in incarcerated juvenile delinquents. *J Am Acad Child Adolesc Psychiatry* 36:357–365.

Terr, L. (1991) Childhood traumas: an outline and overview. *Am J Psychiatry* 148:10–20.

Van der Kolk, B.A., Perry, J.C., and Herman, J.L. (1991) Childhood origins of self-destructive behavior. *Am J Psychiatry* 148:1655–1671.

Wells, G.B., Chu, C., and Johnson, R. (1991) Buspirone in the treatment of post-traumatic stress disorder. *J Clin Psychiatry* 55:517–522.

Yehuda, R. (1998) Recent developments in the neuroendocrinology of posttraumatic stress disorder. *CNS Spectrums* 3(7) (Suppl 2): 22–29.

Zeanah, C.H. ed. (1993) *Handbook of Infant Mental Health.* New York: Guilford Press.

44 | Eating disorders

KATHERINE A. HALMI

Eating disorders are best conceptualized as syndromes, which are classified on the basis of the clusters of symptoms they present. The two major and best-documented eating disorders, anorexia nervosa (AN) and bulimia nervosa (BN), are best understood with a multidimensional model. In this model these disorders begin with dieting, and behaviors and influences antecedent to the dieting experience propel the symptoms into a full-blown eating disorder. The antecedent conditions consist of biological vulnerability, psychological predisposition, and social influences. As the dieting continues, starvation effects, weight loss, nutritional effects, and psychological changes occur. Both psychological and physiological reinforcements of the maladaptive eating behavior continue a cycle of the core dysfunctional eating behaviors. The numerous treatment approaches for AN and BN reflect studies representing the various categories of this multidimensional model for eating disorders. (Halmi, 1994)

Anorexia nervosa is characterized by weight loss, an intense fear of gaining weight, a distorted body image, and amenorrhea. *Bulimia nervosa* is mainly distinguished by its central feature of binge eating. In this disorder individuals engage in some sort of compensatory behavior to counteract the potential weight gain from calories ingested during bingeing. They are also overly concerned about their physical appearance.

Both AN and BN can be chronic, the consequences of AN being much more severe, both physically and mentally. A third newly defined eating disorder termed *binge eating disorder* is still being studied to determine if it is indeed a separate entity. Those with binge eating disorder do not have the concern with weight and shape present in AN and BN.

There are variants of the well-defined eating disorders mentioned above that often cause considerable distress and impairment. These are currently referred to as *eating disorders not otherwise specified* and are usually treated with strategies targeted towards their specific symptoms.

Eating disorders have been described since the earliest times in Western civilization. The most prominent examples of irreversible self-starvation are the fasting female saints of the Middle Ages (Bell, 1985). It is likely that the psychobiological vulnerability factors that induce the development of irreversible starvation in medieval saints are similar to those that spurred the emergence of AN in twentieth century women. Although binge eating and purging behavior are certainly described in Roman civilization, the disorder BN as we define it today has not been so well documented.

DIAGNOSTIC CRITERIA

The specific criteria for AN and BN according to the *Diagnostic and Statistical Manual of Mental Disorders, 4th ed.* (DSM-IV) are given in Tables 44.1 and 44.2 (American Psychiatric Association, 1994).

CLINICAL DESCRIPTION

Anorexia Nervosa

Anorectic patients constantly think about food and how fat they are. Although they may deny this, one can assume they are preoccupied with the slenderness of their bodies by observing their frequent mirror gazing and by listening to their incessant concerns about feeling fat and flabby. They often collect recipes and prepare elaborate meals for others, another indication they are preoccupied with food. Anorectic persons lose weight by different methods. The restricting subtypes lose weight by drastically reducing their total food intake and disproportionately decreasing the intake of high-carbohydrate and fatty foods. Some of these individuals will develop rigorous exercising programs and others will simply be as active as possible at all times. Individuals of the binge eating/purging type also rigorously diet but lose control and regularly engage in binge eating followed by purging behavior. The latter consists of self-induced vomiting, and/or misuse of laxatives, diuretics, or enemas. Some of these individuals

TABLE 44.1 *Anorexia Nervosa (307.1 AN)*

A. Refusal to maintain body weight at or above a minimally normal weight for age and height (e.g., weight loss leading to maintenance of body weight less than 85% of that expected; or failure to make expected weight gain during period of growth, leading to body weight less than 85% of the expected)

B. Intense fear of gaining weight or becoming fat, even though underweight

C. Disturbance in the way in which one's body weight or shape is experienced, undue influence of body weight or shape on self-evaluation, or denial of the seriousness of the current low body weight

D. In postmenarcheal females, amenorrhea, i.e., the absence of at least three consecutive menstrual cycles (A woman is considered to have amenorrhea if her periods occur only following hormone, e.g., estrogen, administration.)

Specify type

Restricting type: during the current episode of AN, the person has not regularly engaged in binge-eating or purging behavior (i.e., self-induced vomiting or the misuse of laxatives, diuretics, or enemas)

Binge-eating/purging type: during the current episode of AN, the person has regularly engaged in binge-eating or purging behavior (i.e., self-induced vomiting or the misuse of laxatives, diuretics, or enemas)

Source: *Diagnostic and Statistical Manual of Mental Disorders*, Fourth Edition, (1994). Washington DC: American Psychiatric Association.

do not binge eat but routinely purge after eating small amounts of food. There is a frequent association in those patients who binge and purge with other impulsive behaviors such as suicide attempts, self-mutilation, stealing, and substance abuse. Adolescents usually refuse to eat with their families or in public places. Many of their weight-reducing behaviors make it very difficult for a physician to realize that the weight reduction is actually secondary to a willful, self-induced weight loss regimen.

Anorectic adolescents have a peculiar way of handling food. They will hide carbohydrate-rich foods, such as candies and cookies in secretive places. They hoard large quantities of candies and carry them in their pockets and purses. If forced to eat in public, they will often try to dispose of their food surreptitiously to avoid eating. They will spend a great deal of time cutting food into small pieces and rearranging the food on their plate. If confronted about their peculiar behavior, they will flatly deny it or refuse to discuss it.

In the AN patients who engage in self-induced vomiting or abuse laxatives and diuretics, hypokalemic alkalosis may develop. These patients often have elevated serum bicarbonate, hypochloremia, and hypokalemia.

Patients with electrolyte disturbances have physical symptoms of weakness, lethargy, and, at times, cardiac arrhythmias. The latter condition may result in sudden cardiac arrest, a cause of death in patients who purge. Elevation of serum enzymes reflects fatty degeneration of the liver and is present in both the emaciated anorectic phase and during refeeding. Elevated serum cholesterol levels tend to occur more frequently in younger patients and return to normal with weight gain. Carotenemia is often observed in the malnourished anorectic patients.

Anorectic patients are usually brought to professional attention by family members after the patients have lost a large amount of weight. If they seek help on their own it is usually because of their subjective distress over the somatic and psychological consequences of starvation. These include weakness, fatigue, difficulty concentrating, sleep disturbances, and depression. Because individuals with AN have considerable denial of the seriousness of their problem, they are often unreliable historians. Thus it is necessary to ob-

TABLE 44.2 *Bulimia Nervosa (307.51 BN)*

A. Recurrent episodes of binge eating. An episode of binge eating is characterized by both of the following:

1. Eating, in a discrete period of time (e.g., within any 2-hour period), an amount of food that is definitely larger than most people would eat during a similar period of time and under similar circumstances
2. A sense of lack of control over eating during the episode (e.g., a feeling that one cannot stop eating or control what or how much one is eating)

B. Recurrent inappropriate compensatory behaviors in order to prevent weight gain, such as self-induced vomiting; misuse of laxatives, diuretics, enemas, or other medications; fasting; or excessive exercise

C. The binge eating and inappropriate compensatory behaviors both occur, on average, at least twice a week for 3 months

D. Self-evaluation is unduly influenced by body shape and weight.

E. The disturbance does not occur exclusively during episodes of AN.

Specify type

Purging type: during the current episode of BN, the person has regularly engaged in self-induced vomiting or the misuse of laxatives, diuretics, or enemas

Nonpurging type: during the current episode of BN, the person has used other inappropriate compensatory behaviors, such as fasting or excessive exercise, but has not regularly engaged in self-induced vomiting or the misuse of laxatives, diuretics, or enemas

Source: *Diagnostic and Statistics Manual of Mental Disorders*, Fourth Edition (1994). Washington DC: American Psychiatric Association.

tain information from parents and other sources to have sufficient information for an adequate assessment of the patient.

Bulimia Nervosa

Binge eating is the predominant symptom of BN. It is simply defined as eating more food than most people eat in similar circumstances and in a similar period of time. The sense of losing control is a significant subjective aspect that occurs in binge eating. Abdominal pain or discomfort, self-induced vomiting, sleep, or social interruption usually terminates the bulimic episode, which is followed by feelings of guilt, depression, or self-disgust. Bulimic patients often use cathartics for weight control and have an eating pattern of alternate binges and fasts. The food consumed during a binge usually has a high dense calorie content and a texture that facilitates rapid eating. Bulimic patients have a fear of not being able to stop eating voluntarily. Frequent weight fluctuations occur, but without the severity of weight loss present in AN. Most bulimic patients do not eat regular meals and have difficulty feeling satiety at the end of a normal meal. They usually prefer to eat alone and at their homes. About one-fourth to one-third of BN patients have a previous history of AN.

Most bulimic patients (60%–80%) have a lifetime history of depression (Braun et al., 1994). They have problems with interpersonal relationships, self-concept, and impulsive behavior and show high levels of anxiety and compulsivity. Chemical dependency is not unusual in this disorder, alcohol abuse being the most common. Bulimics will abuse amphetamines to reduce their appetite and lose weight (Braun et al., 1994).

Bulimic patients who purge differ from binge eaters who do not purge in that the latter tend to have less body image disturbance and less anxiety concerning eating. Bulimic persons who do not purge tend to be obese. The physical and medical complications of bulimic patients are described in the Assessment section below.

Long-term follow-up research has shown that about one-fourth of AN patients will recover and the rest will have either partial or no improvement. Mortality rates at 10 years are 6.6% and at 30 years are 18%–20% after presentation for treatment (Theander, 1985; Eckert et al., 1995). Most follow-up studies of AN show patients with an earlier age onset (under age 18) to have a better chance of recovery. Purging behavior, self-induced vomiting, and laxative abuse are usually predictive of a worse outcome (Eckert et al., 1995).

Follow-up studies between 5 and 10 years after onset of illness show that about one-half of BN patients fully recover while one-fifth continue to meet full criteria for that disorder. Relapse is a serious problem for bulimics, as about one-third of recovered bulimics relapse within 4 years after treatment. About 20% of bulimics seem to sustain an unremitting bulimic disorder (Keel and Mitchell, 1997).

ASSESSMENT

Interview Information for Diagnosis

The interview information necessary for the diagnosis of AN and BN and for diagnosis of their common comorbid psychiatric diagnoses is listed in Tables 44.3 and 44.4. It is important to remember that most AN patients deny their symptoms and are not motivated for

TABLE 44.3 *Interview Information for Diagnosis of Anorexia Nervosa and Bulimia Nervosa*

A. Weight history
1. Greatest weight patient has achieved, age at that time
2. Least weight (after weight loss) the patient has achieved, age at that time
3. Present weight

B. Eating behavior
1. Changes in eating pattern with family (e.g., eating alone)
2. Dieting behavior—what does patient eat and when?
3. Bingeing episode? Describe

C. Purging behavior
1. Self-induced vomiting
2. Laxative abuse
3. Diuretic abuse
4. Enemas

D. Preoccupations and rituals concerning food and weight
1. Frequency of patient weighing self
2. Mirror gazing, comments about being fat
3. Collecting recipes, increased interest in cooking and baking
4. Constant calorie counting and concern of fat content of foods
5. Fear of being unable to stop eating
6. Peculiar eating rituals

E. Activity
1. Jogging—how far and for how long
2. Bike riding—how far and for how long
3. Exercising—what type and how long
4. General overactivity at home (paces, never sits)

F. Menstrual history
1. Age onset of menses
2. Date of last menstrual period
3. Regularity of cycles

TABLE 44.4 *Interview Information on Common Comorbid Behavior and Psychiatric Diagnoses*

A. Depression
1. Sleep disturbance
2. Irritability and difficulty concentrating
3. Crying spells
4. Suicidal thoughts

B. Impulsive behavior
1. Drug abuse
2. Alcohol abuse
3. Suicide attempts
4. Self-mutilation, cutting on body

C. Anxiety symptoms
1. Obsessive, compulsive behaviors
2. Social phobia
3. Generalized anxiety and fearfulness
4. Panic attacks

D. Personality disorders
1. Pattern of instability in interpersonal relationships, self-image, affect
2. Pattern of social inhibition, feelings of inadequacy, hypersensitivity to negative evaluation
3. Pattern of dependent, submissive behavior with difficulty separating from parents
4. Preoccupation with orderliness, perfectionism, and control

treatment. Because of this, it is usually necessary to interview family members or close friends to obtain an idea of their actual behavior. Many adolescent anorectics have delayed psychosocial and sexual development and adults often have a markedly decreased interest in sex with the onset of AN. In contrast, bulimic patients often have promiscuous problems with sex.

In obtaining a weight history it is important to know if the patient has had previous episodes of being underweight or has been previously obese. In either case the patient will have a more difficult time in responding to treatment. To obtain food intake information, patients should be asked what they have had to eat from the time they arise in the morning until they go to bed at night. It is especially important to find out about purging behavior, since that can be associated with medical problems (see below). Behaviors listed under D. in Table 44.3 specifically reflect the frantic concern with food and weight. Obtaining an activity history is helpful in assessing the severity of the patient's commitment to losing weight. Table 44.4 lists the interview information necessary to obtain the comorbid psychiatric diagnoses commonly found in eating disorders. Depression is the most frequent comorbid disorder in both AN and BN. For example, in a 10-year follow-up study of AN, Halmi et al. (1991) found 68% of the patients had a lifetime history of major depressive disorder, and Brewerton et al. (1995) found that 63% of BN patients had major depressive disorder.

The obsessions and rituals of patients with an eating disorder have been compared with the compulsions of patients with obsessive-compulsive disorder (OCD) (Thiel et al., 1995). The actual prevalence of OCD in AN was found to be only 21% in the Halmi et al. (1991) study and 18% in Braun et al.'s (1994) study. In a review of 51 studies, Holderness et al. (1994) concluded that the relationship between substance abuse and BN (and bulimic behaviors) is far stronger than that with AN. Bulimic anorectics reported more substance use and abuse than restricting anorectics but less than patients with BN. A variety of drugs made up the substances of abuse; most commonly they were cannabis, cocaine, stimulants, and over-the-counter pills such as diet pills. The comorbidity between eating disorders and personality disorders has also been extensively studied. Herzog et al. (1992) examined the rates of comorbid axis II diagnoses among 210 women seeking treatment for AN, BN, or AN binge/purge subtype. They found that of the 210 subjects, 27% had at least one personality disorder. Overall, the AN binge/purge subtypes showed the highest prevalence of personality disorders, at 39%. Consistent with previous reports, the highest rates of borderline personality disorder were found in the bulimic and anorectic–bulimic groups, while avoidant personality disorder was most prevalent among the anorectic and anorectic–bulimic groups. In the Braun et al. (1994) study, 68.6% of 72 eating disorder patients had at least one personality disorder. It is important to obtain information for comorbid psychiatric diagnoses so that an effective treatment strategy can be devised for the eating disorder patient.

Self-rating and semistructured interview scales

Three self-rating scales and two semistructured interview scales useful in the clinical assessment of eating disorders are summarized in Table 44.5 (Wilson and Smily, 1989).

Physical examination abnormalities

These abnormalities are presented in Table 44.6. The findings on physical examination are due to emaciation or purging behavior. Dry, cracking skin, lanugo hair, bradycardia, and hypotension are found in patients who are underweight. Nutritional rehabilitation and

TABLE 44.5 *Eating Disorder Assessment Scales*

Instrument	Size	Description	Rater	Reference
Eating Disorder Inventory 2 (EDI-2)	91 items	11 subscales	Self-report	Garner, 1991
Body Shape Questionnaire (BSQ)	34 items	single score	Self-report	Cooper et al., 1987
Three Factor Eating Questionnaire (TFEQ)	51 items	3 subscales	Self-report	Stunkard and Messick, 1995
Eating Disorder Examination (EDE)	DSM-IV, ED diagnoses	4 subscales	Semistructured interview	Fairburn and Cooper, 1993
Yale-Brown-Cornell Eating Disorder Scale (YBC-EDS)	8 items	2 subscales	Semistructured interview	Mazure et al., 1994

weight gain will change these findings. Calluses on the dorsum hand are from placing the hand in the throat to self-induce vomiting. Perioral dermatitis, enlarged parotid glands, teeth enamel erosion, and periodontitis are all secondary to self-induced vomiting. Arrhythmias are usually due to hypokalemia, which is caused by the purging behavior.

Laboratory tests

The laboratory abnormalities in eating disorders are listed in Table 44.7 The common laboratory findings secondary to emaciation are leukopenia with a relative lymphocytosis and reduced bone density. The former is restored with nutritional rehabilitation but the reduced bone density is seldom corrected. Nutritional rehabilitation can prevent further reduction of bone density (Newman and Halmi, 1989).

Electrolyte abnormalities are associated with poor

fluid intake, vomiting, laxative abuse, and diuretic abuse in both AN and BN patients. A metabolic alkalosis may occur in those who engaged in purging behavior. This results in low serum chloride and low serum potassium levels (hypokalemia) and elevated serum bicarbonate levels. This condition produces physical symptoms of weakness, lethargy, and, at times, cardiac arrhythmias. Hypomagnesemia may be present and interfere with the correction of hypokalemia. Hypophosphatemia may occur in anorectics as a result of poor dietary intake. It can also be a dangerous complication of refeeding. Inorganic phosphate moves intracellularly as it is required for protein synthesis, in

TABLE 44.7 *Laboratory Abnormalities in Eating Disorders*

Laboratory Findings	Cause
Complete blood count	
Leukopenia with a relative lymphocytosis	Starvation
Anemia	Starvation
Serum and plasma	
Hypokalemia	Purging, diuretic abuse
Hypochloremic metabolic alkalosis	Purging
Hyperamylasemia	Purging
Hypercholesterolemia	Starvation
Hypercarotinemia	Ingestion of high-carotene foods
Electrocardiogram	
Q-T and T-wave changes	Hypokalemia, cardiomyopathy from ipecac
Photon absorptiometry	
Reduced bone density	Starvation

TABLE 44.6 *Physical Examination Abnormalities in Eating Disorders*

Physical Symptoms	Cause
Dry, cracking skin	Dehydration, loss of subcutaneous fat
Lanugo hair	Starvation
Calluses on dorsum of hand	Self-induced vomiting with hand
	Friction against teeth
Perioral dermatitis	Vomiting
Enlarged parotid glands (chipmunk face)	Vomiting
Teeth enamel erosion and caries	Vomiting
Periodontitis	Vomiting
Bradycardia	Starvation
Hypotension	Starvation and fluid depletion
Arrhythmias	Hypokalemia from purging

glucose phosphorylation. This may result in a sudden drop in serum phosphatase levels, which can aggravate mild cardiac dysfunction.

Electrocardiograph (EKG) changes are common and usually reflect electrolyte disturbances. The EKG changes include low voltage, sinus bradycardia, and ST segment depression. At times cardiac arrhythmias occur with hypokalemia. In the latter, myocardial repolarization may be delayed, resulting in a prolonged QT interval. The QT interval reflects electrical signals from the start of ventricular depolarization to repolarization, the stage that prepares the ventricles for the next beat. The repolarization–depolarization process needs to happen more rapidly as the heart rate increases. The QTc, the corrected QT interval adjusts for this. Patients with hypokalemia are vulnerable to having prolonged QTc, which may be associated with ventricular tachycardia, Torsade de Pointes, and sudden death. Adverse affects can occur when the $CYP_{450}3A_4$ enzyme system is inhibited by certain medications, leading to elevated levels of medication that prolong the QT interval. Patients who use ipecac to induce vomiting may develop a cardiomyopathy from ipecac intoxication. This may cause an irreversible condition of cardiac failure that usually results in death. Symptoms of pericardial pain, dyspnea, and generalized muscle weakness associated with hypotension, tachycardia, and EKG abnormalities should alert one to possible ipecac cardiac intoxication (Halmi, 1985).

Delayed gastric emptying has been inconsistently observed in patients with both AN and BN. Emaciated anorectic patients frequently have feelings of fullness and bloating but these may or may not be associated with delayed gastric emptying (Robinson and McHugh, 1995). Persistent laxative abuse may decrease the motility of the colon and increase complication of constipation. Patients who binge and purge are at risk for acute dilatation of the stomach or esophageal tears, which are usually accompanied by shock. Impaired temperature regulation has been observed in emaciated AN patients with an abnormal autonomic response to cold.

TREATMENT

Psychopharmacological Treatment

Anorexia nervosa

Medication should be considered an adjunct treatment for AN. Although many medications have been used in the treatment of AN, there are few large-scale, controlled studies demonstrating the efficacy of pharma-cotherapy in the treatment of AN. One of the first systematic open studies reported on the treatment of AN with chlorpromazine was by Crisp (1965). Those who were treated with chlorpromazine gained weight faster and were discharged sooner than patients on the same unit who did not receive the medication. None of these were randomly assigned controlled studies. Clinical experience has shown this medication to be particularly helpful in the severely ill patient who is overwhelmed with constant thoughts of losing weight and has uncontrollable behavioral rituals. It is best to start chlorpromazine at low doses of 10 mg tid and increase the dosage gradually, monitoring blood pressure and side effects. It should be noted that these studies were conducted in hospitalized patients and the major outcome measure was weight gain.

Two other randomly assigned placebo-controlled studies with the antipsychotics, pimozide (Vandereycken and Pierloot, 1982) and sulpiride (Vandereycken, 1984) failed to demonstrate any benefit for overall weight gain compared to placebo.

Cyproheptadine, an antihistaminic and antiserotonergic drug used especially in children with allergy based asthma, was investigated in three studies for a weight gain effect in AN patients. All were placebo-controlled studies of hospitalized patients. Two studies showed no effect on weight gain (Vigirsky and Loriaux, 1997; Goldberg el al., 1979). A third study in which 72 anorectic patients were randomly assigned to amitriptyline, cyproheptadine, and placebo showed that both cyproheptadine and amitriptyline had a marginal effect in decreasing the number of days necessary to achieve a normal weight. Cyproheptadine, in high doses such as 24 to 28 mg/day, had an unexpected antidepressant effect, demonstrated by a significant decrease on the Hamilton Depression Rating Scale (Halmi et al., 1986). With the bulimic subgroups of anorectic patients, cyproheptidine had a negative effect, compared with both placebo and amitriptyline (Halmi et al., 1986). Cyproheptadine has the advantage of not having the tricyclic antidepressant (TCA) side effects of reducing blood pressure and increasing heart rate. This characteristic makes the drug especially attractive for use in emaciated anorectic patients.

In another study examining amitriptyline a smaller dosage, 75 mg, was used. Several different clinical settings were involved and there was a total smaller number of patients than in earlier studies. This study showed no effect of the drug over placebo in weight gain (Biederman et al., 1985). Clomipramine, studied in a placebo-controlled randomly assigned design showed no advantage of the active drug over placebo in the rate of weight gain. In this study the medication was given at a dose of 50 mg; thus, the low dosage might have contributed to the lack of a significant finding (Lorey and Crisp, 1980).

Two open, uncontrolled studies suggested some efficacy for fluoxetine in weight gain and improvement of anorectic symptoms in AN patients (Freeman and Thompson, 1987, Solyan et al 1989). A recent report compared low-weight anorectic hospitalized patients who were receiving a serotonin reuptake inhibitor (SSRI) with those who were not. Baseline weight and other psychopathological measures did not differ between the groups. The SSRI treatment in these low-weight individuals had little impact on weight or other clinically meaningful variables (Ferguson et al., 1999). These findings supported clinical observations that SSRIs have little effect in low-weight individuals.

Two studies, both with methodological limitations, have examined fluoxetine in the prevention of relapse in AN patients who had some weight rehabilitation. In one study (Kayl, 1996); a double-blind, placebo-controlled study of fluoxetine, patients with some weight restoration and who were receiving a variety of other therapies were randomized to fluoxetine (n = 16) or placebo (n = 19) for 1 year. Relapse rates were dramatically higher in the placebo group then in the active treatment group (84% vs. 37%). Depression, anxiety, and obsessive-compulsive symptoms also improved in those patients receiving fluoxetine. In another study, Strober et al. (1997) examined a 2-year course of fluoxetine following hospitalization for AN. These patients also had some weight restoration. The 33 patients receiving fluoxetine were compared with historical matched controls discharged from the same program with no fluoxetine treatment. In this study, fluoxetine showed no benefit over the 24-month follow-up.

At the present time there is no strong support for psychopharmacological agents as the sole means of treating AN. It will be beneficial to have results from trials examining fluoxetine for relapse prevention and in conjunction with psychotherapeutic treatments for AN. Medication seems to be more effective after some weight restoration has occurred. For severely obsessive-compulsive anxious and agitated anorectic patients, chlorpromazine or a newer atypical antipsychotic drug such as olanzapine, which has fewer side effects than the phenothiazines, may be useful. In the restricting type of AN patient who is emaciated, cyproheptadine in high doses may be helpful as an adjunct treatment in a structured setting for facilitating weight gain and decreasing depressive symptomatology.

Bulimia nervosa

Studies of antidepressant medication in the treatment of bulimia have been based on the observation that mood disturbance is frequently present in this disorder. Over a dozen double-blind, placebo-controlled trials of antidepressants, such as desipramine, imipramine, amitriptyline, nortriptyline, phenelzine, and fluoxetine, have been conducted in normal-weight outpatients with BN. The variety of medications have included TCAS, monoamine oxidase inhibitors (MAOI) and heterocyclic compounds. The dosage of antidepressant medications used was similar to that for the treatment of depression. In almost all trials the antidepressants were significantly more effective than placebo in reducing binge eating. These medications also improved mood and reduced eating disorder symptoms such as preoccupations with shape and weight. The effect on reducing binge eating occurred irrespective of the presence of depression. Overall, the complete abstinence rate from bingeing and purging was only 20%–25%. Most of the above studies were of short duration, varying between 8 and 12 weeks. For a review of these studies see Walsh et al. (1991).

The SSRIs are best tolerated by bulimic patients, which makes them a logical first choice. However, the only controlled studies showing efficacy in bulimia patients have used fluoxetine (Fluoxetine Bulimia Nervosa Collaborative Study Group, 1992). The tricyclics have more side effects and are generally less well tolerated. In particular, weight gain associated with them reduces compliance in bulimic patients. Monoamine oxidase inhibitors such as phenelzine are contraindicated because of the required dietary restrictions that bulimic patients are not likely to follow, especially during binge episodes.

It is important to note that 60 mg of fluoxetine showed a therapeutic effect, while 20 mg showed no difference compared to placebo (Fluoxetine Bulimia Nervosa Collaborative Study Group, 1992). There are no data at present to provide guidelines for the length of time that bulimic patients should stay on the antidepressant medication.

Of the various mood-stabilizing agents being used in treating bulimic patients, only lithium was studied in a placebo-controlled, randomized trial, which was negative. Lithium is risky to use because of the dehydration experienced in bulim patients, which may result from purging behavior and thus rapidly increase lithium blood levels to a toxic level.

The serotonergic agonist drug fenfluramine was

shown to be ineffective in a controlled trial with BN (Russell et al., 1988).

Relapse prevention with medication has been studied in BN as well as AN. In 1991 Walsh et al. placed bulimics who had a 50% or more reduction in binge eating on desipramine in maintenance treatment. About half of the patients relapsed below the 50% reduction within 4 months, despite continued use of the medication. In a second multicenter collaborative study examining the efficacy of fluoxetine maintenance in bulimic patients who had responded to the drug with a 50% reduction of symptoms, the patients who were maintained on the active drug were significantly less likely to relapse than those who were switched to placebo at the end of the acute treatment phase (Romano, 1999).

Several studies have compared medication therapy with cognitive behavior therapy (CBT) and with a combination of drug and CBT in the treatment of BN. In a study by Mitchell et al. (1990), the CBT program was superior to drug treatment and placebo in terms of improvement in eating symptoms. In terms of eating disorder variables, there was no additional benefit from adding the drug to psychotherapy, but there was some benefit with this combination for mood and anxiety variables.

In another study with desipramine, Agras et al. (1992) studied the effect of the drug, of individual CBT, and of the combination of the two and again found CBT to be superior to drug therapy alone, with no added benefit from using the combination to effect eating disorder symptoms. There was some evidence that the combination was superior for dietary restraint thinking.

In a five-cell design study, Walsh et al. (1997) compared CBT, supportive therapy (a time and contact control), each combined with medication (involving desipramine followed by fluoxetine in those who did not achieve abstinence on desipramine, or placebo), and medication management alone. The CBT was superior to supportive therapy and active drug was superior to placebo. The best results were achieved with a combination of CBT plus active drug. Results from CBT plus placebo were roughly equivalent to those with medication management alone.

Antidepressant medications have been shown to have a significant impact in the treatment of BN. Fluoxetine is the only drug that is Federal Drug Administration (FDA) approved for BN and it is has been studied with the largest number of patients. Studies contrasting drug therapy with CBT suggest that, if drug therapy is used, it should be used in conjunction with CBT.

Cognitive Behavior Therapy

Anorexia nervosa

Initial behavior therapy interventions were focused on principles of operant conditioning and were designed to restore weight during inpatient treatment (Agras et al., 1974). These interventions were highly effective, but patients lost weight and relapsed when they were discharged from the hospital program.

Bemis (1978) devised a cognitive therapy for AN, which involved a modification of negative thinking and dysfunctional assumptions about eating and body shape and weight. Controlled CBT treatment studies for AN are rare. Another study (Channon et al., 1989) compared individual outpatient CBT with strictly behavioral treatment and a supportive control treatment. Six- and 12-month follow-up showed that all three groups gained weight and had improved psychosocial functioning. The methodological limitations, including small sample size, make it difficult to generalize the data from this study. In another study, (Serfaty et al., 1999.) AN patients were assigned to either 20 sessions of individual CBT or dietary counseling. All 10 patients in the dietary counseling dropped out before the 6-month outcome evaluation, in contrast to a 92% retention rate for those who had CBT. At 6 months, 70% of the patients who had received CBT no longer met criteria for AN.

Bulimia nervosa

Most CBT for BN is based on a model that emphasizes both cognitive and behavioral factors in the maintenance of the disorder (Fairburn et al., 1997). A manual published in 1993 (Fairburn and Cooper, 1993) is the standard for CBT in bulimia. The model emphasizes that societal cultural pressures on women to be thin lead to an overvaluing of the importance of body weight and shape. This in turn produces restriction of food intake, which causes women to become both physiologically and psychologically susceptible to periodic loss of control over eating, thus they binge eat. Purging and other extreme forms of weight control are attempts to compensate for the effect of binge eating. Purging reduces the patient's anxiety about potential weight gain and disrupts learned satiety that regulates food intake. Bingeing and purging cause distress and lower self-esteem and thus lead to more dietary restriction and subsequent binge eating. Binge eating becomes a means for regulating negative affect by serving to blunt or distract from sources of personal distress. Binge eating can become a negative reinforcement and a potent factor in the maintenance of the disorder. The CBT treatment involves developing a regular pattern of eating, expanding foods to previously avoided foods, developing more constructive skills for coping with high-risk situations for bingeing and purging, modifying abnormal attitudes, and preventing relapse at the conclusion of the acute treatment. Treatment is time limited, directive, and problem oriented.

For BN, CBT is the most effective treatment proven in 35 controlled studies. About 40%–50% of patients are abstinent from both bingeing and purging at the end of treatment (16–20 weeks). Improvement by reducing bingeing and purging occurs in a 70% to 90% of patients. Another 30% who do not show improvement immediately post-treatment show improvement to full recovery 1 year after treatment. In BN patients, CBT interrupts the self-maintaining cycle of bingeing and purging and alters the individual's dysfunctional cognitions and beliefs about food, weight, body image, and overall self-concept.

Cognitive behavior therapy has shown to be consistently superior to waiting-list groups, which show no improvement across the range of measures. In addition to beneficial effects on bingeing and purging, CBT reduces dietary restraint and the intensity of concerns about shape and weight. Therapeutic changes are maintained at 1 year post-treatment (Agras et al., 1999).

Individual and group CBT have been compared in only one study. In this study, with five to six patients in a group using a modification of the Fairburn manual, individual treatment was more effective at reducing binge eating and vomiting than the group adaptation (Jelch et al., 1990).

GUIDELINES FOR LEVEL OF TREATMENT AND MEDICAL MANAGEMENT

Inpatient Treatment

Hospitalization for eating disorder depends on the weight status of the patient, the presence of medical complications, and the presence of related psychiatric comorbidities, such as depression, suicidal behavior, and OCD. Hospitalization for AN may be brief or extended. Inpatient brief hospitalization (7–14 days) is for patients who have (1) relapsed from previous treatment or have been ill for less than 6 months; (2) a weight loss of 10%–15% from normal weight if they have relapsed, or 16%–20% if this is their first episode; (3) hypokalemic alkalosis with serum potassium < 2.5 mEq/L; and (4) cardiac arrhythmias. To promote rapid weight gain, patients can be placed on a liquid formula

for 5 to 7 days and then given regular meals on trays, which can be monitored for calories ingested for an additional 3 to 5 days. This allows the patient to eat food for a few days before leaving the structured program. Patients should be monitored for access to the bathroom. During hospitalization they can participate in multiple group therapy sessions, which should include groups for body image and specific eating disorder problems; self-esteem, self-confidence, and self-expression groups; female issue groups; and a movement—control exercise group. Younger patients should participate in intensive family counseling. Discharge planning should include consideration of a transition to partial hospitalization program.

An extended hospital treatment program for the AN patient is 14 to 60 days and is for patients who have a weight loss > 20% of normal, a history of repeated hospitalizations for more than 6 months, a psychotic depression or serious suicide attempt, incapacitating obsessions and compulsions related or not to the eating disorder, and serious comorbid medical conditions such as edema, hypoproteinemia, and severe anemia. Treatment should begin with a liquid formula and appropriate medical treatment along with highly monitored 24-hour surveillance to prevent purging, exercising, and other self-defeating behaviors. In addition to multiple group sessions as described above, individual therapy, family counseling (for those younger than 18), and a cognitive-behavioral ward milieu to prevent bingeing and purging and to ensure normal ingestive behavior would be ideal.

Hospitalized patients respond best in a specialized inpatient eating disorder setting that can provide a team of individuals who are highly skilled in multidisciplinary management of AN patients. Medical management consists of weight restoration, nutrition rehabilitation, rehydration, and correction of serum electrolytes. Daily monitoring of weight, food and calorie intake, and urine is necessary.

Most patients with BN can be effectively treated as outpatients. Medical hospitalizations result from consequences of purging activities, such as frequent vomiting and abuse of laxatives and diuretics, which can create electrolyte imbalances and dehydration. These patients are at risk for developing cardiac arrhythmias due to hypokalemia. If the patient's serum potassium falls below 2.5 mEq/L, the patient should be hospitalized. Other medical emergencies are gastric dilatation and esophageal tears (both are rare). Cardiac failure caused by cardiomyopathy from ipecac intoxication is a medical emergency.

Hospitalization is necessary for bulimics who have severe depression or a suicide plan, or have engaged in repeated current self-injury such as cutting. Hospitalization may also be required for severe functional impairment and inability to function from persistent bingeing and purging.

Hospitalized treatment is usually 5 to 14 days. The first aim of inpatient treatment for a bulimic patient should be to stop the bingeing and purging behavior. This not only helps to correct electrolyte imbalances and dehydration but is also the first step for reestablishing normal eating behavior. The bulimic patient should receive sufficient calories to maintain weight within a normal range. Access to bathrooms should be restricted and supervised to prevent surreptitious vomiting.

Partial Hospitalization or Day Program

Partial hospitalization programs for both AN and BN patients, can provide a transition from inpatient treatment for patients with a history of repeated hospitalizations and severe chronic illness or with severe comorbid personality disorder or substance abuse problems. It is also suitable for patients who have had a recent relapse of weight loss and a return of poor anorectic behavior causing a severe impairment of function. Bulimics who are nonfunctioning from bingeing and purging may require a day program.

This type of program should offer cognitive-behavioral group therapy and individual therapy. It should be able to provide medication if necessary, structured meals, and nutritional counseling and meal planning. Group therapies, e.g., social skills training, are also useful.

Outpatient Treatment

Outpatient treatment for AN should be considered if the patient is in her first episode with no previous treatment and/or relapse after resuming a normal weight. Outpatient treatment can also occur following partial hospitalization or inpatient treatment programs.

For the anorectic patient, outpatient treatment should be considered if the weight loss has been gradual, such as over 3 months or longer, and the weight is within 75% to 80% of a normal weight for age, height, and bone structure, and if the patient has normal serum electrolytes. For the bulimic patient, outpatient treatment should be considered for the first episode with no previous treatment or for a relapse after abstinence from bingeing and purging.

Essential elements of outpatient treatment for anorexia include a cognitive-behavioral format in which monitoring occurs with daily food records and weekly weighing. A cognitive view of the maintenance of an-

orexia needs to be presented to the patient and should include psychological and physical effects of starvation and a cost–benefit analysis. Cognitive restructuring and problem-solving techniques should be taught to the patient to deal with interpersonal problems and eating behavior. Family counseling is essential for all patients under age 18 and is advised for patients over 18 living with their parents. For the AN patient, it may be necessary to attend sessions several times a week at the beginning of treatment with the frequency of sessions gradually decreasing to weekly and then bimonthly over a period of a year.

Because of the decreased length of stay imposed by managed care companies, patients are being transferred prematurely to outpatient settings. Unlike many other patients with psychiatric disorders, those with disordered eating are usually resistant to treatment and become noncompliant in outpatient settings where they are not closely monitored by staff. A deteriorating condition leads to rehospitalization, which ultimately is not an overall cost-effective treatment strategy.

For the BN patient a brief, structured, and highly controlled inpatient milieu may effectively break the binge–purge cycle. The patient can then be maintained in an outpatient setting. Short-term hospitalization is not as effective for patients with AN, as shown by the higher rates of readmission as length of stay decreases (Weiseman et al, 2001). Specific sets of hospital discharge criteria need to be tested with appropriate research methodology.

REFERENCES

Agras, W., Rossiter, E.M., Arnow, and Schneider, J.A. (1992) Pharmacologic and cognitive-behavioral treatment for bulimia nervosa: a controlled comparison. *Am J Psychiatry* 149:82–87.

Agras, W., Walsh, B.T., Fairburn, C., Wilson, G.T., Kraemer, H. (1999) A multicenter comparison of cognitive-behavioral therapy an interpersonal psychotherapy for bulimia nervosa.

Agras, W.S., Barlow, D., Chapin, H., Abel, G., and Leitenberg H. (1973) Behavior modification of anorexia nervosa. *Arch Gen Psychiatry* 30:274–286.

American Psychiatric Association (1994) *Diagnostic and Statistical Manual of Mental Disorders, 4th ed.* Washington, DC: American Psychiatric Association Press.

Bell, R. (1985) *Holy Anorexia.* Chicago: University of Chicago Press.

Bemis, K.N. (1978) Current approaches to the etiology and treatment of anorexia nervosa. *Psychol Bull* 85:593–617.

Biederman, J., Herzog, D.B., and Rivinus, T.M. (1985) amitriplyline in the treatment of anorexia nervosa. *J Clin Psychophormocol* 5: 10–25.

Braun, D., Sunday, S., and Halmi, K.A. (1994) Psychiatric comorbidity in patients with eating disorders. *Psychol Med* 24:859–967.

Brewerton, T.D., Lydiard, R.B., Herzog, D.B., and Brotman A.W. (1995) Comorbidty of axis I psychiatric diagnoses in bulimia nervosa. *J Clin Psychiatry* 56:77–80.

Channon, S., de Silva, P., and Hemsley (1989) A controlled trial of cognitive behavioral and behavioral treatment of anorexia nervosa. *Behav Res J her.* 27:529–535.

Cooper, P., Taylor, M., Cooper, Z., and Fairburn, C. (1987) The development and validation of the body shape questionnaire. *Int J Eat Disord.* 6:485–494.

Crisp, A. (1965) A treatment regime for AN. *Br J Psychiatry* 112: 505–512.

Eckert, E.D., Halmi, K.A., Marchi, P., and Cohey, J. (1995) Ten-year follow-up of anorexia nervosa: clinical course and outcome. *Psychol Med* 25:143–156.

Fairburn, C.G. and Cooper, Z. (1993) The Eating Disorder Examination, 12th ed. In: Fairburn, C.B. and Wilson, G.T., eds. *Binge Eating: Nature, Assessment, and Treatment.* New York: Guilford Press, pp. 317–360.

Fairburn, C., Jones, R., Peveler, R., and Hope R. (1993) Psychotherapy and bulimia nervosa: longer-term effects of interpersonal therapy, behavior therapy and cognitive behavioral therapy. *Arch Gen Psychiatry* 50:419–428.

Fairburn, C.G., Welch, Doll, H., and Davies, B. (1997) Risk factors for bulimia nervosa. *Arch Gen Psychiatry* 54:509–517.

Ferguson, C., Lavia, M., Crossan, P., and Kaye, W. (1999) Are serotonin selective reuptake inhibitors effective in underweight anorexia nervosa? *Int J Eat Disord* 25:11–17.

Fluoxetine Bulimia Nervosa Collaborative Study Group (1992) Fluoxetine in the treatment of bulimia nervosa: a multicenter, placebo-controlled, double-blind trial. *Arch Gen Psychiatry* 49:139–147.

Freemon, C.P., Hampson, M. (1987) Fluoxetine as a treatment for bulimis nervosa. *Int J Obesity* 2: 171–173.

Garner, D.M. (1991) Eating Disorder Inventory–2 Professional Manual. Obessa, FL: Psychological Assessment Resources.

Goldberg, S.C., Halmi, K.A., Eckert, E.D., Casper, R.C., and Davis, J.M. (1979) Cyproheptadine in anorexia nervosa. *Bri J Psychiatry* 134:71–78.

Halmi, K.A. (1994) A multi-modal model for understanding and treating eating disorders. *J Women Health* 3:487–493.

Halmi, K.A. (1985) Medical aberrations in bulimia nervosa. In: Kaye, W. and Gwirtzman, H., eds. *Normal Weight Bulimia: Physiology and Treatment.* pp. 37–46.

Halmi, K.A., Eckert, E.D., Ladu, T., and Cohen, J. (1986) anorexia nervosa: treatment efficacy of cyproheptadine and amitriptyline. *Arch Gen Psychiatry* 43:177–181.

Halmi, K.A., Eckert, E., Marchi, P., and Cohen, J. (1991) Comorbidity of psychiatric diagnosis in anorexia nervosa. *Arch Gen Psychiatry* 48:712–718.

Halmi, K.A. and Falk, J.R. (1981) Common physiological changes in anorexia nervosa. *Int J Eat Disord* 1:16–27.

Herzog, D.B., Keller, M., and Lavori, P., (1992) The prevalence of personality disorders in 210 women with eating disorders. *J Clin Psychiatry* 53:147–152.

Holderness, C.C., Brooks-Gunn, J., and Warren M.P. (1994) Comorbidity of eating disorders and substance abuse review of the literature. *Int J Eat Disord* 16:1–34.

Kaye, W. (1996) The use of fluoxetine to prevent relapse in anorexia nervosa. Presented at the Annual Meeting of the Eating Disorder Research Society, Pittsburgh, PA, November, 1996.

Keel, P.K. and Mitchell, J.E. (1997) Outcome in bulimia nervosa. *Am J Psychiatry* 154:313–321.

Lacey, H. and Crisp, A.H. (1980) The impact of clomipramine on refeeding anorexia nervosa. *Postgrad Med J* 1:79–83.

Mazure, C.M., Halmi, K.A., Sunday, S.R., and Romana, S. (1994) Yale-Brown-Cornell Eating Disorder Scale: development, use, reliability and validity. *J Psychaitr Res* 28:425–445.

Mitchell, J.E. (1989) A placebo-controlled, double-blind crossover study of naltrexone in patients with normal weight bulimia. *J Clin Psychopharm* 9:94–97.

Mitchell, J.E., Pyle R., and Eckert, E.D. (1990) A comparison study of antidepressants and structured intensive group psychotherapy in the treatment of bulimia nervosa. *Arch Gen Psychiatry* 47: 149–157.

Newman, M. and Halmi, K.A. (1989) The relationship of bone density to estradiol and cortisol in AN and bulimia nervosa. *Psychiatry Res* 29:105–112.

Robinson, P. and McHugh, T. (1995) A physiology of starvation that sustains eating disorders. In: Szmukler, J., Dare, C., Treasure, J., eds. *Handbook of Eating Disorders.* New York: John Wiley & Sons, pp. 109–123.

Romano, S. (1999) A relapse prevention trial of bulimia nervosa using fluoxetine. Presented at the 152nd Annual Meeting of the American Psychiatric Association. Washington, DC, May 15–20, 1999.

Russell, G.F.M., Checkley, S.A., and Feldman, F. (1988) A control trial of D-fenfluramine in bulimia nervosa. *Clin Neuropharmacol* 11:146–159.

Solyom, L., Solyon, C., Ledwidge, B. (1989) Fluoxetine treatment of low weight chronic anorexia nervosa. *J Clin Psychopharmacol* 10:421–425.

Serfaty, M., Jurhington, D., Heap, M., Ledsham, L., and Jolley, E., (1999) Cognitive therapy vs. dietary counselling in the outpatient treatment of anorexia nervosa. *Europ. Eating Dis. Rev.* 7:334–350.

Strober, M., Freeman, R., and DeAntonio M., (1997) Does adjunctive fluoxetine influence the post-hospital course of anorexia nervosa? *Psychopharmacol Bull* 33:425–431.

Stunkard, A. and Messick, S. (1985) The Three-Factor Eating Questionnaire to measure dietary restraints, disinhibition and hunger. *J Psychosom Res* 29:71–83.

Telch, C.F., Agras, W., Rossiter, E.N., and Wilfley, D. (1990) Group cognitive-behavioral treatment for the nonpurging bulimic: an initial evaluation. *J Consult Clin Psychol* 58:629–635.

Theander, S. (1985) Outcome and prognosis in anorexia nervosa and bulimia: results of previous investigations compared with those of a Swedish long-term study. *J Psychiatr Res* 19:493–508.

Thiel, A., Brooks, A., Ohlmeier, M., Jacoby, G. (1995) Obessive-compulsive disorder in anorexia and bulimia nervosa. *Am J Psychiat* 152:72–75.

Vandereycken, W. (1984) Neuroleptics in the short term treatment of anorexia nervosa: a double-blind placebo-control study with sulpiride. *Br J Psychiatry* 144:288–292.

Vandereycken, W. and Nierloo, T.R. (1982) Pimozide combined with behavior therapy in the short term treatment of anorexia nervosa. *Acta Psychiatr Scand* 66:445–450.

Vigersky, R.A. and Loriaux D.L. (1977) The Effect of Cyproheptadine in anorexia nervosa: a Double-Blind Trial. In: Vigersky, R.A., ed. *Anorexia Nervosa* NY: Roven Press.

Walsh, B., Hadigan, C, Devlin, M., and Gladis, M. (1991) Long-term outcome of antidepressants treatment for bulimia nervosa. *Am Psychiatry* 148:1206–1212.

Walsh, B.T., Wilson, G.T., Loeb, K.L., and Devlin, M. (1997) Medication and psychotherapy in the treatment of bulimia nervosa. *Am J Psychiatry* 154:523–531.

Weisman, C., Sunday, S., Klapper, F., Harris, W., Halmi K.A. (2001) Changing patterns of hospitalization in eating disorder patients. *Int J Eat Disord* 30: 69–74.

Wilson, G.T. and Smith D. (1989) Assessment of bulimia nervosa: an evaluation of the eating disorders examination. *Int J Eat Disord* 8:173–179.

PART

III-C SPECIAL CLINICAL POPULATIONS

45 | Substance-abusing youths

JAMES G. WAXMONSKY AND TIMOTHY WILENS

Substance abuse continues to be one of the most common and serious mental health disorders, with a 27% lifetime prevalence in American society (Kessler et al., 1997). Substance use disorders (SUD) are increasingly conceptualized as having their developmental roots in childhood, as 30% to 50% of SUD begin in childhood or adolescence (Kandel, 1992; Kessler et al., 1997). According to the most recent epidemiological data presented in the 1999 Monitoring the Future Study, over half (55%) of all 12th graders have used at least one illicit substance in their lifetime, an 11% increase in just the last 8 years. Moreover, the data indicate an earlier onset of first use. For example, use in eighth graders has more than doubled in the past 8 years (Johnston et al., 2000).

Early onset of use is particularly concerning as studies have shown that onset of drinking by age 14 is correlated with significantly higher rates of alcohol abuse and dependence than drinking that begins in late adolescence or adulthood (Dewit et al., 2000). Early onset of SUD is associated with higher rates of psychiatric comorbidity (Kandel et al., 1999) and delinquent behavior (Cloninger et al., 1981). In addition, biochemical differences have been observed in subjects whose SUD developed early in life, as compared to those with later-onset SUD, including increased rates of abnormal serotonergic functioning in the brain and variable responses to pharmacological challenges (Johnson et al., 2000). Pediatric substance use has also been correlated with increased rates of suicide, risky sexual behaviors, school dropout (Crum et al., 1992), and motor vehicle accidents (Weinberg et al., 1998; Kaminer, 1999). In addition, recent research suggests that the adolescent brain may be particularly vulnerable to alcohol-induced brain damage (De Bellis et al., 2000).

Current data suggest that the treatment of pediatric SUD requires a multi-integrated strategy. The recent American Academy of Child and Adolescent Psychiatry (AACAP) Practice Parameters recommend that each treatment plan be tailored to the individual patient and take into consideration the patient's current developmental status (Bukstein, 1997). Psychosocial interventions are an integral part of the treatment plan. A variety of psychosocial interventions have been implemented successfully in youth with SUD, including family therapy (Ozechowski, et al., 2000) cognitive behavior therapy (Kaminer and Burleson, 1999), and multisystemic therapy (Henggeler, 1999). In all of the various therapies, the social environment, particularly the immediate family, plays an influential role in the successful treatment of pediatric SUD, even more so than with adults (Bergmann et al., 1995). Pharmacotherapy, an emerging treatment modality, appears to be an effective component of the SUD treatment plan.

The pharmacotherapy of SUD across the life span is an intense area of research, but few studies are being done with pediatric populations, as evidenced by the AACAP Practice Parameters' description of the existing research on the pharmacotherapy of adolescent SUD as "limited" (Bukstein, 1997). As a paucity of pediatric literature exists, clinicians have relied on findings in adults to develop pediatric treatment protocols. However, the generalizability of the diagnostic criteria and treatment data for adult SUD to pediatric populations remains unclear (Bukstein et al., 1989; Bukstein et al., 1992).

One complicating factor in the treatment of SUD in youth is the extensive overlap with psychiatric disorders, as psychiatric comorbidity appears to be the rule, more than the exception, for youth with SUD. Psychiatric disorders have been observed in up to 75% to 85% of such youth (Stowell and Estroff, 1992; Hovens et al., 1994; Kandel et al., 1999), and youth with SUD are three times more likely to have a current psychiatric illness than those without SUD (Kandel et al., 1999). In addition, there is evidence to suggest that among all patients with SUD, those ages 15 to 24 have the highest rate of psychiatric comorbidity (Kandel et al., 1999). More specifically, conduct disorder (CD) occurs in 50% to 75 % of youth with SUD (Bukstein et al., 1992; Hovens et al., 1994; Wilens et al., 1997a; Weinberg et al., 1998), attention-deficit hyperactivity disorder (ADHD) occurs in 30% to 60%, (Wilens et al., 1996, 1997a; Riggs, 1998), and mood disorders occur

TABLE 45.1 *Classification of Pharmacological Agents for Treatment of Substance Use Disorders in Youth*

Class	Modality of Action	Examples
Aversion	Production of an aversive reaction when an illicit substance is used	Disulfiram for alcohol use disorders
Substitution	Replacement of illicit substance with controlled use of prescribed agent that works at same receptors as illicit agent	Methadone, buprenorphine for opiate use disorders
Craving reduction	Reduction of psychological craving for specific substances	Naltrexone for alcohol and buproprion for nicotine use disorders
Treatment of comorbid psychiatric illness	Improvement in comorbid psychopathology that leads to decreased drive to use substances and/or increases probability that SUD treatment will be successful	Antidepressants and mood stabilizers in subjects with affective disorders and SUD
Prevention	Primary prevention of SUD in at-risk populations through treatment of existing psychiatric illness	Pharmacotherapy of ADHD reduces the risk for future development of SUD

ADHD, attention deficit hyperactivity disorder; SUD, substance use disorder.

in 30% to 75% (DeMilio, 1989; Bukstein et al., 1992; Stowell and Estroff, 1992; Wilens et al., 1997a; Kandel et al., 1999). Comorbidity is a major clinical concern, as patients with psychiatric disorders and SUD have more complicated treatment courses and higher rates of relapse (Bukstein et al., 1989; Wilens et al., 1998; Wise et al., 2001; Rohde et al., 2001). To help conceptualize the role of pharmacotherapy in pediatric SUD, Kaminer (1995) has proposed categorizing the existing agents by their mechanism of action: aversion, craving reduction, substitution, and treatment of comorbid psychiatric disorders. In addition, we have added a fifth category, the use of pharmacotherapy as preventive treatment for at-risk populations (see Table 45.1).

SUMMARY OF EXISTING PEDIATRIC LITERATURE

In this chapter, we will provide a systematic review of the available literature on the pharmacotherapy of pediatric addictions, and representative studies will be summarized for each of the aforementioned classes (see Table 45.2). Treatment of nicotine addictions will not be addressed in this chapter. Overall, there is a paucity of published studies on the pharmacological treatment of youth with SUD (*n* 12). Many are case reports with limited details and of short duration (*n* 5). There are six open studies that primarily address comorbid disorders with the assumption that treatment of the SUD will be more effective once the psychiatric symptoms have improved. The literature search revealed only one placebo-controlled study of a pharmacological intervention for pediatric SUD (Geller et al., 1998).

Aversive Agents

The aversive agents diminish substance use by producing an aversive reaction when a specific illicit substance is consumed. For example, disulfiram (Antabuse) prevents the breakdown of acetaldehyde, a toxic metabolite of alcohol, producing a noxious reaction when alcohol is consumed. While aversive agents have been in existence for decades, studies of their effectiveness in adults have produced mixed results (Kaminer, 1994b; Garbutt et al., 1999). Likewise, there is only one published case report on the use of aversive therapy for pediatric SUD. Myers and associates (1994) reported on the use of disulfiram (Antabuse) for two teens with alcohol dependence. Both patients were briefly abstinent, but then became noncompliant and quickly relapsed.

Agents of Substitution

Agents of substitution diminish substance use by binding to the same receptors as the illicit substance, allowing the patient to shift from the illicit substance to controlled use of the prescribed substituting agent. Methadone, which decreases craving and withdrawal symptoms of heroin and other opiates by blocking the μ-opiate receptor, is the most frequently used agent in this class.

While there are extensive data on the use of methadone substitution therapy in adult opiate-dependent patients, there are only two published studies on opiate substitution therapy in adolescents and most of these subjects were 18 years of age or older (Hopfer et al., 2000). This lack of research is particularly concerning, given the recent increase in heroin use among adolescents (Hopfer et al., 2000). Two newer substitution agents, L-oc acetylmethadol (LAAM) and buprenorphine, offer alternatives to methadone, but remain untested in youth with SUD (Kranzler et al., 1999).

Dopamine agonists, including the stimulants, have been used as substitution agents in cocaine-dependent adults, but with little success (Kranzler et al., 1999). For example, one controlled study has found that stimulant medications neither increased nor decreased craving for cocaine (Grabowski et al., 1997). No studies of substituting agents have been done in youth with cocaine abuse or dependence.

Anticraving Agents

This class of medications diminishes substance use by reducing psychological craving for specific illicit substances. The most studied agent in this class is naltrexone (ReVia), an opiate antagonist that has gained Federal Drug Administration (FDA) approval for the treatment of alcohol addiction in adults. Other anticraving agents awaiting approval for alcohol addiction include nalmefene and acamprosate (Garbutt et al., 1999). Recent research found that ondansetron (Zofran), a serotonin antagonist, significantly reduced alcohol consumption in adults whose SUD began prior to age 25. Ondansetron (Zofran) was significantly less effective in adult subjects whose SUD began after age 25, highlighting its potential, but yet untested, use in adolescents with SUD (Johnson et al., 2000).

Since some aspects of craving for substances appear to have an obsessional quality, the craving-reducing capacity of antiobsessional medications have been evaluated. These studies have generally shown that the antidepressants and antimanic agents are not effective for craving reduction in patients without comorbid psychiatric disorders (Donovan and Nunes, 1998; Garbutt et al., 1999). There are mixed data on the efficacy of desipramine for cocaine dependence in adults (O'Brien, 1996; Kranzler et al., 1999). Buproprion (Wellbutrin) has been approved for smoking cessation and its potential as an anticraving agent for other substances is actively being explored.

There are several published case reports on the use of anticraving agents in adolescents. Kaminer (1992, 1994b) has reported on the use of desipramine for cocaine dependence in three adolescents, observing short-term success in one patient. Lifrak et al. (1997) reported on use of naltrexone (ReVia) in three adolescents with alcohol dependence, observing a positive response in all three cases with no significant adverse events after 6 months of use. However, Hopfer and colleagues (2000) report significant compliance difficulties when using naltrexone (ReVia) in youth with SUD. Presently, there are no controlled trials of anticraving agents in youth with SUD.

Agents that Treat Comorbid Psychopathology

Research has shown that patients with psychiatric disorders and SUD have a more complicated treatment course and higher rates of substance relapse, suggesting that the SUD outcome may be directly related to the underlying psychiatric disorder (Bukstein et al., 1989 Rohde, et al., 2001 Wilens et al., 1998; Wise et al., 2001). Therefore, pharmacotherapy of comorbid psychiatric symptoms may lead to improvement in the SUD. In adults, treatment with lithium, anticonvulsants, and the antidepressants have reduced substance use in patients with comorbid affective disorders (Garbutt et al., 1999; Donovan and Nunes, 1998). Additionally, buproprion (Wellbutrin) was found to be effective in reducing SUD as well as ADHD symptoms in one small open study of adults (Levin et al., 1998).

The majority of pharmacotherapy studies done in youth with SUD have been completed in groups with psychiatric comorbidity. In the one controlled study of youth with SUD and comorbid psychiatric illness, Geller et al. (1998) completed a randomized, placebo-controlled study evaluating the use of lithium in a group of adolescents with affective dysregulation and substance dependence. All patients were in outpatient treatment for the duration of the study but did not receive any other psychotropic medications besides lithium ($n = 13$) or placebo ($n = 12$). After 6 weeks, only the lithium group (average blood level = 0.9 mEq/L) had a statistically significant decrease in the number of positive urine tests ($p = 0.042$). However, there was no difference in severity of the affective symptoms between the two groups (measured via the Kiddie Schedule for Affective Disorders and Schizophrenia [K-SADS]). No subjects discontinued the lithium because of adverse events, although subjects receiving lithium did report higher rates of polyuria and polydipsia.

Donovan et al. (1996, 1997) completed an open study evaluating the use of valproic acid (Depakote) in adolescent outpatients with marijuana abuse or dependence and "explosive mood disorder" (mood symptoms were not classified using the DSM IV Diagnostic System). Eight subjects were prescribed 1000 mg of valproic acid (Depakote) for 5 weeks, in addition to regular therapy sessions, but did not receive any other psychotropic medications. All subjects showed a significant improvement in their marijuana use ($p < 0.007$) and their affective symptoms ($p < 0.001$), although both outcomes were measured only by self-report. The most common adverse events were nausea and sedation. No subjects discontinued because of these side effects, nor were there any reported interactions between the valproic acid (Depakote) and substances of abuse.

Riggs and associates have published three open studies assessing the treatment of multiple comorbid dis-

TABLE 45.2 *Representative Studies of Pharmacotherapy for Adolescent Substance Use Disorders*

Reference	n	Age (years)	Sample Description	Design	Medication	Duration	Daily Dose	Outcome	Comments
Kaminer, 1992	1	16	Males with cocaine dependence, ADHD, and MDD; initial treatment began while hospitalized and then switched to outpatient	Case report	Desipramine	6 month follow-up	200 mg	Mood and craving improved after 3 weeks and was sustained for 6 months	No AEs reported
Kaminer, 1994a	2	Adolescents; exact age N/A	Male adolescents with cocaine abuse; treatment setting N/A	Case report	Desipramine	N/A	N/A	One patient was abstinent for 30 days then became noncompliant; the second discontinued treatment because of adverse event	Letter to the editor AE: postural hypotension
Myers et al., 1994	2	16, 17	Teenage males with alcohol dependence and mood disorder; treatment began on inpatient setting, then switched to outpatient	Case report	Disulfiram	4 months	250 mg	Remained abstinent for up to 4 months; both patients relapsed in follow-up	One case was also receiving fluoxetine for depression; no AEs reported
Donovan et al., 1996	8	14–18	Adolescents with mood lability and marijuana abuse/dependency in outpatient treatment	Open trial	Depakote	5 weeks	1000 mg with serum levels 45–113 μg/mL	Significant decline in amount of marijuana used per week ($p < 0.007$) Significant decrease in mood symptoms ($p < 0.001$)	Unclear diagnostic categorization; no serious AEs SUD measured by self-report and affective symptoms measured by clinical impression
Riggs et al., 1996	15	14–18	Males with CD, ADHD, and SUD in residential program	Open trial	Pemoline	3 weeks	112.5–185.5 mg	ADHD scores decreased significantly ($p < 0.002$) in 13/13 11/13 reported improved rehabilitation	2 patients discontinued because of AEs: insomnia and "feeling spacey"
Lifrak et al., 1997	2	16, 18	Males with alcohol dependence in outpatient treatment	Case report	Naltrexone	26 weeks	50 mg	First case abstinent for entire duration; second case decreased alcohol use; both reported decreased craving	Letter to the Editor No AEs reported
Wold and Kaminer, 1997	1	17	Male with alcohol dependence in partial hospital program	Case report	Naltrexone	1 month follow-up	50 mg	Craving free at time of publication	Letter to the Editor No AEs reported

Study	N	Age	Population	Design	Medication	Duration	Dose	Results	Comments
Riggs et al., 1997	10	14–16	Males with CD, SUD, and MDD who had been in residential treatment for at least 1 month	Open trial	Fluoxetine	7 weeks	20 mg	7/8 showed marked improvement mood ($p < 0.0001$) and 7/8 reported improved rehabilitation with medication	Screened out those with personal or family history of affective disorders; 2 patients discontinued treatment but not because of AEs; medication well tolerated
Geller et al., 1998	25	12–18	Males with bipolar I, II or MDD with "bipolar risk factors" and SUD; all treated on outpatient basis	Double-blind Placebo-controlled	Lithium	6 weeks	Average dose 1700 mg; Average level of 0.9 mEq/L	Significant decrease in number of positive urine tests for lithium group only ($p < 0.042$); No difference in mania scores	4 subjects failed to complete protocol but not because of lithium side effects; 1 had seizure following LSD ingestion; Most common lithium AEs: polyuria and polydipsia
Riggs et al., 1998	13	14–17	Nondepressed males with CD, SUD, and ADHD, all in residential program	Open trial	Buproprion	5 weeks	300 mg	Clinically significant decline in mean Conners scores ($p < 0.02$); 2/13 subjects reported decreased craving; 11/13 wanted to continue on medication	1 subject discontinued medication because of hypomanic symptoms; Unlike fluoxetine study, authors did not exclude those with past or family history of affective disorders; Other common AEs: headache, fatigue
Cornelius et al., 2001	13	15–19	Adolescents with MDD and alcohol abuse or dependence in outpatient treatment	Open trial	Flouxetine	12 weeks	20 mg	Improvement in mood and SUD symptoms	Generally well tolerated with good compliance
Solhkhah, et al., 2001	13	N/A	Adolescents with SUD, ADHD, and mood symptoms in outpatient treatment	Open trial	Buproprion	6 months	Mean daily dose = 315 mg	Improvements in SUD, ADHD, and mood symptoms	Generally well tolerated
Total studies	12	12–17	Majority with comorbid psychiatric illness	Case reports = 5; Open trials = 6; Controlled studies = 1	Multiple agents	3 weeks to 6 months	Standard pediatric dosing	Overall, moderate improvement in SUD symptoms	AEs similar to those expected in non-SUD groups but greater difficulties with compliance

ADHD, attention deficit hyperactivity disorder; AE, adverse event; BPD, bipolar disorder; CD, conduct disorder; MDD, major depressive disorder; SUD, substance use disorder.

orders in adolescents with SUD and delinquent behaviors in a long-term residential program. It is important to note that in all of these studies the subjects were inpatients. Consequently, the limited access to substances of abuse and the effect of inpatient treatment may have confounded the impact of pharmacotherapy.

Pemoline (Cylert), (112.5 to 185.5 mg) was assessed in a 3-week open trial in 15 adolescents with CD, ADHD, and SUD (Riggs et al., 1996). Three of the subjects were receiving other psychotropic medications (clonidine (Catapres) and paroxetine [Paxil]). All subjects had a significant improvement in ADHD symptoms ($p < 0.002$) while 10/13 reported that the pemoline (Cylert) assisted in their substance rehabilitation. No subjects developed a significant elevation in their liver function tests, nor did any subjects test positive for substances of abuse for the duration of the study. No interactions between pemoline (Cylert) and any substances of abuse were reported.

Another study by the same group assessed the use of fluoxetine (Prozac) (20 mg) in a 7-week open trial in 10 adolescents with the commonly occurring triad of SUD, CD, and major depression (Riggs et al., 1997). Seven of the eight subjects had significant improvement in mood ($p < 0.001$), and the majority reported that the fluoxetine (Prozac) assisted in their substance rehabilitation. The medication was well tolerated and no interactions between fluoxetine (Prozac) and any substances of abuse were reported. There were no positive drug tests for the duration for the study.

Cornelius et al., also openly evaluated the efficacy of fluoxetine (Prozac) (20 mg) in 13 adolescents with MDD and alcohol abuse or dependence (Cornelius et al., 2001). The fluoxetine (Prozac) was well tolerated throughout the entire 12 week duration of outpatient treatment and was associated with a significant reduction in MDD symptoms ($p < .001$) for all subjects. Overall, there was a significant reduction drinking days ($p < .08$) and drinks per drinking day ($p < .005$) with 7/13 subjects having their SUD rated as much improved.

More recently, Riggs and associates openly evaluated the use of buproprion (Wellbutrin) (300 mg) in 13 teens with CD, SUD, and ADHD (Riggs et al., 1998). They found a significant decline in both the mean scores on the Conners hyperactivity ($p < 0.01$) and inattention scales ($p < 0.02$), and 11/13 subjects wanted to continue on the medication. However, only 2/13 reported decreased substance craving, while 2 subjects tested positive for drugs during the study. No interactions between the buproprion (Wellbutrin) and any substances of abuse were reported. One subject had to discontinue the study because of the development of hypomania.

Solhkhah et al., also openly evaluated the role of buproprion (Wellbutrin) (mean dose = 315 mg) in 13 adolescents with ADHD and affective illness (Solhkhah et al., unpublished data). Preliminary data after 6 months of outpatient treatment indicate measurable reduction in craving, improvements in mood, and ADHD symptoms with few adverse events. Reduction in SUD symptoms appeared to be related to improvements in mood rather than a direct anti-craving effect of the buproprion.

Agents of Prevention

The fifth class of agents are those that help to prevent the development of future SUD through treatment of existing psychiatric illness. Clinical observation has suggested that treatment of psychiatric illness leads to improved SUD outcome. Conversely, there has been a long-standing concern that the use psychiatric medications for childhood disorders, especially stimulants, may be a risk factor for the future development of SUD (Goldman et al., 1998). Recent research in ADHD has shed light on this important and controversial issue. Biederman et al. (1999) compared the rates of SUD in children and adolescents who had previously received pharmacological treatment with the rates of those who had never had their ADHD symptoms treated. They observed that pharmacotherapy for ADHD was associated with an 85% reduction in the development of SUD (Biederman et al., 1999). Loney et al. (1999) observed that children who received stimulant therapy for their ADHD had lower rates of alcoholism and similar rates of drug abuse when they reached young adulthood, compared to children of equal severity ADHD who did not receive stimulants. Molina and colleagues (1999) also found lower rates of alcohol consumption and of problems related to alcohol and marijuana use in ADHD youth who received stimulant treatment than in those with ADHD who did not receive such treatment. In contrast, Lambert and Hartsough (1998) reported higher rates of substance abuse in young adults who had received ADHD treatment in childhood; however, these findings may have been confounded by the overrepresentation of CD in the treatment group.

TREATMENT OF PEDIATRIC SUBSTANCE USE DISORDER

Despite recent advances, the psychopharmacology of pediatric SUD is still an emerging field with a paucity of empirical data. However, several psychosocial therapies have been found to be effective for the treatment of SUD in adults and adolescents. These include various family therapies, cognitive behavior therapy, and multisystemic therapy. Pharmacological treatments should be considered in the specific addiction states for which research suggests there is clinical efficacy. Youth with SUD who have comorbid psychopathology, particularly those with bipolar disorder, appear to be the group most likely to respond to pharmacological interventions for their SUD. Only a few agents have been found to be effective in SUD youth without comorbid psychopathology. These include naltrexone (ReVia) for alcohol addiction and possibly buproprion (Wellbutrin) for nicotine dependence. Unfortunately, no effective pharmacological treatments have been found for marijuana or ecstasy (MDMA) addictions in youth. Because of the encouraging adult data and the recent increase in opiate use among teens, methadone substitution should also be viewed as a potentially useful treatment despite the lack of existing data on adolescents. Pharmacological interventions should typically be initiated in combination with self-help and psychosocial interventions.

Treatment should begin in the least restrictive setting that ensures personal safety, as it is important to maximize family involvement from the onset. In youth with SUD, family involvement increases compliance with treatment and leads to higher rates of sustained abstinence (Bergmann et al., 1995). It is important to review with the patient and family that medication is one aspect of the treatment plan and is more likely to be effective when used in conjunction with other treatments. In addition, the clinician should also review how the medication will work, the possible side effects, and the time frame in which benefit may be expected. An informed and involved family is more likely to encourage compliance from an adolescent than one that has never met their child's treatment team. An adult caretaker and not the patient should store, administer, and monitor all prescription medications to maximize compliance and minimize the potential for abuse.

Youth with SUD require frequent visits with the treatment team, especially if they have comorbid psychiatric illness. During each visit, the clinician should monitor the patient's SUD and psychiatric symptoms, their social stressors, their compliance with medication and any adverse effects they may have experienced. Random urine "dipstick" testing for substances of abuse during the office visit, with tests such as the Roche "On Trac" system, may be a useful piece of the treatment plan provided that the adolescent is aware

that such testing may be performed. Such tests are sensitive and measure recent use of marijuana, cocaine, amphetamines, phencyclidine and opiates. These tests, which cost approximately $20, do not require laboratory equipment and may be easily completed by clinical staff.

SAFETY AND ADVERSE EVENTS

Patients with SUD are at increased risk for adverse events, as they may combine their medications with drugs of abuse. The combination of tricyclic antidepressants (TCAs) and marijuana has produced delirium in several youth (Wilens et al., 1997b). Any sedating medication such as benzodiazepines should be avoided in patients at risk of using significant amounts of alcohol or opiates. Likewise, monoamine oxidase inhibitors (MAOIs) should be avoided in patients at risk of using sympathomimetic substances such as cocaine or amphetamines. Patients with SUD may also have significant medical illness that can affect drug pharmacokinetics. For example, naltrexone (ReVia), disulfiram (Antabuse), valproic acid (Depakote), and pemoline (Cylert) should be avoided in patients with significant liver dysfunction, as use of these agents has been associated with hepatic impairment.

Many of the pharmacological agents used in SUD are metabolized via the p448 cytochrome system in the liver, and their metabolism can be altered by medications that induce or inhibit this system. For example, agents such as fluoxetine (Prozac), which impair or compete with the hepatic micrsosmoal system, may inhibit the metabolism of methadone. Other agents have very narrow therapeutic windows and minor elevations in blood levels can produce significant adverse events. For these agents, which include the TCAs and lithium, regular blood monitoring and careful titration should be employed when these agents are combined with other prescription medications.

Another major safety concern in the treatment of youth with SUD is abuse of prescribed medications. Particular controversy has arisen around the use of stimulant medication in youth with SUD and ADHD. In one controlled study of adults, the use of methylphenidate (Ritalin) did not increase cocaine use or craving for cocaine (Grabowski et al., 1997), suggesting that the abuse potential of stimulants may be overestimated. Riggs et al. (1996) did not report any difficulties with abuse when administering pemoline (Cylert) to a group of adolescents with SUD and ADHD. While Riggs and associates have observed that youth with SUD do not typically abuse stimulants, they discourage the use of stimulants as first-line treatment for youth with SUD and ADHD (Riggs, 1998). Similarly, we recommend careful consideration before using agents with addiction potential and would consider using alternative agents with minimal addiction potential, such as buproprion (Wellbutrin) or a TCA, for treatment of ADHD. If stimulants are used, we suggest using longer-acting preparations while avoiding short-acting stimulants in abuse-prone youth. Likewise, the selective serotonin reuptake inhibitors (SSRIs) or buspirone (BuSpar) are reasonable initial choices for youth with anxiety and SUD. If agents with abuse potential are used, they should be stored in a secure place and carefully monitored with frequent pill counts.

TREATMENT RECOMMENDATIONS

While research on the pharmacological treatment of pediatric SUD is limited, the following are suggested guidelines for the implementation of pharmacological agents in the treatment of pediatric SUD. These guidelines are based on the existing treatment literature and are organized according to the agents' mechanism of action.

Aversive Agents

In general, the use of aversive therapies in pediatric populations is discouraged (Bukstein, 1997). However, aversive agents, such as disulfiram (Antabuse), may have a potentially useful but narrow role for highly compliant youth at inpatient or day treatment settings whose families are actively involved in their child's treatment. For such youth with alcohol addictions, disulfiram (Antabuse) may be useful to prevent relapses during weekend or extended passes from their treatment setting. Disulfiram (Antabuse) use should be avoided in patients with psychoses or significant liver disease, as it can exacerbate both conditions. Disulfiram (Antabuse) can also affect the metabolism of several psychotropic medications and illicit substances, including the TCAs and marijuana.

Agents of Substitution

There are few empirical data on the use of substitution agents in youth with SUD. However, there is significant evidence supporting the efficacy of opiate substitution therapy for adults with opiate addiction with agents such as methadone, buprenorphine, and LAAM. While heroin use is increasing in adolescents, fewer than 10% of youth diagnosed with opiate addictions in 1997 received methadone substitution treatment (Hopfer et al., 2000). The limited role of methadone is likely due in part to strict federal regulations that require any patient under the age of 18 to have had two documented failures of a methadone-free rehabilitation before they are eligible for methadone substitution. In addition, permission from the youth's guardian must be obtained for therapy (Hopfer et al., 2000). Despite these barriers, opiate substitution therapy is considered a first-line treatment for pregnant adolescents with opiate addictions (Kaminer, 1995). Youth with severe, recalcitrant opiate addiction who have failed traditional treatments may be candidates for opiate substitution therapy; however, the efficacy and safety of such treatments have not been adequately studied in adolescents.

Anticraving Agents

The anticraving agents, such as naltrexone (ReVia) and buproprion (Wellbutrin), have potential use in the treatment of youth with SUD. Naltrexone (ReVia) should be considered an adjunctive treatment for any youth with heavy alcohol use, including repetitive binges, who report persistent craving. The average effective dose for adolescents is 50 mg/day. Because naltrexone (ReVia) can produce liver function test elevations, we recommend baseline liver function tests as well as periodic monitoring for the duration of naltrexone (ReVia) use.

Buproprion (Wellbutrin) has been approved for smoking cessation in adults and is likely to be similarly efficacious in younger populations. Preliminary data suggest that buproprion (Wellbutrin) may have limited efficacy as an anticraving agent for other substances of abuse (Riggs et al., 1998, Wilens, unpublished data). Buproprion (Wellbutrin) should be used with caution in youth with a history of seizures or eating disorders, as it may exacerbate seizures in these groups. In our clinic, buproprion (Wellbutrin) has been observed to be an effective treatment for pediatric depression and ADHD, which suggests that it might be a reasonable choice in youth with SUD and either of these comorbid psychiatric disorders (Solhkhah and Wilens, unpublished data).

Recently, ondansetron (Zofran) was to found to reduce alcohol consumption in adults whose SUD began before age 25 (Johnson et al., 2000). These findings suggest that ondansetron (Zofran) may be potentially effective for craving reduction in youth with SUD. While ondansetron (Zofran) has been prescribed to children as an antiemetic, its anticraving effects have yet to be studied in pediatric populations.

TREATMENT OF COMORBID PSYCHIATRIC ILLNESS

Most of the empirical data on the pharmacological treatment of SUD in youth have been with agents that treat comorbid psychiatric conditions. The following are pharmacotherapy guidelines for youth with SUD and commonly occurring comorbid psychiatric illnesses.

Attention-Deficit Hyperactivity Disorder

The pharmacological treatment of ADHD in individuals who are actively using substances appears to be a difficult task that is often complicated by poor compliance (Levin and Kleber, 1995; Wilens, unpublished data). Current recommendations include a period of abstinence in the range of 2 to 4 weeks before implementing medications for ADHD (Riggs, 1998). Behavioral and psychosocial interventions can be used in the interim for ADHD as well as for the SUD. While the majority of youth with SUD and ADHD do not abuse their ADHD medications (Riggs, 1998), agents with minimal abuse liability should be initially selected. Buproprion (Wellbutrin) is a useful agent as it has very low abuse liability and may improve both the ADHD and substance-craving symptoms simultaneously. Pemoline (Cylert) also has minimal abuse liability, making it a reasonable choice for ADHD in youth with SUD (Riggs et al., 1996). Because of associated hepatic toxicity, it should be avoided in youth with hepatic dysfunction. For any patient receiving pemoline (Cylert), baseline liver function tests as well as regular monitoring should be undertaken. The TCAs have low abuse liability and may be particularly helpful for youth with comorbid ADHD and anxiety. If stimulants are to be used, longer-acting preparations such as Concerta are less likely to be abused than those with shorter duration (Jaffe, 2002).

Anxiety

Pharmacological treatment of anxiety disorders in individuals actively abusing substances is often difficult. Two to four weeks of abstinence is recommended, during which time alternative interventions can be initiated. Agents that have low abuse liability, such as the SSRIs, TCAs, or buspirone (Buspar), are recommended. If benzodiazepines are clinically indicated, it

is reasonable to begin with longer-acting agents such as clonazepam (Klonopin) or chlorazepate (Tranxene) and to carefully monitor their use through methods such as pill counts.

Depression

Although adults with depression and SUD often experience remission of their depressive symptoms after 2 to 4 weeks of abstinence, similar reemission in youth with SUD appears less likely (Bukstein et al., 1992; Riggs et al., 1997). Ideally, 2 to 4 weeks of abstinence should be achieved before initiating pharmacological treatment. In the interim, psychotherapy may be helpful. The literature suggests that antidepressants may effectively reduce SUD and depressive symptoms in adults with both disorders. While there are limited data on youth, fluoxetine (Prozac) and buproprion (Wellbutrin) are considered effective treatments for pediatric depression (Daviss et al., 2001; Emslie et al., 1999), and fluoxetine (Prozac) has been observed to significantly reduce depressive symptoms in youth with SUD (Cornelius et al., 2001; Riggs et al., 1997). What remains unanswered in youth is whether the antidepressants will reduce the SUD symptoms as they have in depressed adults with SUD (Garbutt et al., 1999; Donovan and Nunes, 1998).

Given the current literature, antidepressant therapy should be initiated in youth with SUD and depression if the depressive symptoms persist during a period of abstinence, if such abstinence is unable to be achieved, or early in treatment if there is a history of recurrent depression. The efficacy of buproprion (Wellbutrin) in youth with SUD and depression is currently being explored (Solhkhah and Wilens, unpublished data). The antidepressants have little abuse potential and are generally very safe, although buproprion (Wellbutrin) should be avoided in youth with eating disorders or seizures.

Bipolar Disorder

There is strong evidence that bipolar disorder is associated with SUD in adolescents (Wilens et al., 1999) and that pharmacological interventions are an effective treatment for youth with SUD and bipolar disorder. Two studies, including one randomized controlled study, have reported that mood stabilizers, specifically lithium and valproic acid (Depakote), significantly reduced substance use in bipolar youth (Donovan and Nunes, 1996; Geller et al., 1998). In addition, these agents are considered effective agents for the treatment of bipolar illness (Wozniak and Biederman, 1997). Therefore, a period of abstinence is not necessary before implementing pharmacological interventions, as treatment should be initiated quickly in youth with bipolar disorder and SUD. The mood stabilizers have little abuse potential, but their therapeutic window is narrow. In clinical practice, baseline thyroid and renal function should be checked prior to initiation of lithium and followed periodically thereafter. Prior to starting valproic acid (Depakote), liver and blood chemistries should be drawn and then checked periodically while valproic acid (Depakote) is used. For both agents, monitoring of blood levels is suggested. Other mood-stabilizing agents, such as gabapentin (Neurontin), may also be helpful, but have yet to be studied in youth with SUD.

Psychoses

Psychotic symptoms often require immediate treatment, including hospitalization, to ensure patients' safety. Therefore, antipsychotic medication can be started immediately in youth with psychoses and SUD. Two possible exceptions where it may be reasonable to delay the use of antipsychotic medication, include acutely intoxicated youth with no prior history of psychotic symptoms whose safety can be ensured without antipsychotic medication, and youth with hallucinogen-persisting perception disorder. In hallucinogen-persisting perception disorder, the psychotic symptoms are rarely life threatening, and it has been reported that antipsychotics, particularly risperidone (Risperdal), have exacerbated perceptual symptoms in adults and adolescents (Morehead, 1997; Solhkhah et al., 2000). The atypical neuroleptics appear to have lower rates of neurological side effects, and therefore may be reasonable initial choices when selecting an antipsychotic for youth with SUD.

Prevention

An emerging literature suggests that treatment of psychiatric illness may reduce the risk of developing SUD later in life. The findings are most dramatic for stimulant therapy of ADHD, as several studies have observed decreased SUD rates in children whose ADHD was treated with stimulants, compared to ADHD children who received no such treatment (Biederman et al., 1999; Loney et al., 1999; Molina et al., 1999). There is also preliminary evidence that treatment of bipolar disorder can reduce future substance use (Wilens et al., 2000). While these findings are encouraging, further research is needed to support the initial data and to

determine if they are generalizable to other psychiatric disorders.

CONCLUSION

Even though the pharmacotherapy of adolescent addictions is a relatively new field, it appears to have a role in the treatment of many youth with SUD. Pharmacological agents have been shown to reduce excessive craving, to reduce associated comorbid psychopathology, and to prevent the future development of SUD in certain at-risk youth. Despite the present lack of empirical evidence, opiate substitution therapy should be considered in youth with heroin addiction. As with all treatments, the expectations, risks, and benefits should be reviewed with the patient and their caretakers. For SUD treatment to be successful, the provider should closely monitor and address the patient's SUD and psychiatric symptoms, treatment compliance, and social stressors.

Further research should continue to address the developmental reciprocity across the life span for the treatment of addictions. To this end, trials of promising pharmacological agents for the treatment of SUD, such as acamprosate and ondansetron (Zofran), seem warranted in youth. In addition, future studies should assess whether resolution of psychopathology translates into improvement in SUD in youth, as it does in a subgroup of adults. While preliminary results suggesting that pharmacological treatment of ADHD may reduce the risk for future SUD are encouraging, more studies are needed to support these initial findings and to determine the generalizability to other psychiatric conditions. Research exploring the issues of duration of abstinence prior to pharmacotherapy and the sequencing of the various pharmacological and psychosocial therapies for addictions is necessary. Finally, further research into the pharmacotherapy of marijuana, ecstasy (MDMA), and heroin addiction in youth is needed, given the prevalence of abuse of these agents among adolescents.

REFERENCES

Bergmann, P., Smith, M. and Hoffmann, N. (1995) Adolescent treatment: implications for assessment practice guidelines and outcome management. *Pediatr Clin North Am* 42:453–472.

Biederman, J., Wilens, T., Mick, E., Spencer, T., and Faraone, S. (1999) Pharmacotherapy of attention-deficit/hyperactivity disorder reduces risk for substance use disorder. *Pediatrics* 104:e20 (online).

Bukstein, O., ed. AACAP Official Action: Practice Parameters for the Assessment and Treatment of Children and Adolescents with Substance Use Disorders (1997). *J Am Acad Child Adolesc Psychiatry* 36(10) (Suppl): 140S–155S.

Bukstein, O., Brent, D., and Kaminer, Y. (1989) Comorbidity of substance abuse and other psychiatric disorders in adolescents. *Am J Psychiatry* 146:1131–1141.

Bukstein, O., Lilly, G., and Kaminer, Y. (1992) Patterns of affective comorbidity in a clinical population of dually diagnosed adolescent substance abusers. *J Am Acad Child Adolesc Psychiatry* 31:1041–1045.

Cloninger, R., Bohman, M., and Sigvardsson, S. (1981) Inheritance of alcohol abuse. *Arch Gen Psychiatry* 38:861–868.

Cornelius, J., Bukstein, O., Birmaher, B., Salloum, O., Lynch, K., Pollock, N., Gershon, S., and Clark, D. (2001) Fluoxetine in adolescents with major depression and alcohol use disorder: an open-label trial. *Addict Behav* 26:735–739.

Crum., R., Bucholz, K., Helzer, J., and Anthony, J. (1992) The risk of alcohol abuse and dependence in adulthood: the association with educational level. *Am J of Epidemiology* 135:989–999.

Daviss, W., Bentivoglio, P., Racusin, R., Brown, K., Bostic, J., and Wiley, L. (2001) Buproprion sustained release in adoelcents with comorbid attention-deficit hyperactiivty disorder and depression. *J Am Acad Child Adolesc Psychiatry* 40:307–314.

De Bellis, M., Clark, D., Beers, S., Soloff, P., Boring, A., Hall, J., Kersh, A., and Keshavan, M. (2000) Hippocampal volume in adolescent-onset alcohol use disorders. *Am J Psychiatry* 157:737–744.

DeMilio, L. (1989) Psychiatric syndromes in adolescent substance abusers. *Am J Psychiatry* 146:1212–1214.

DeWit, D., Adlaf, E., Offord, D. and Ogborne, A. (2000) Age at first alcohol use: a risk factor for the development of alcohol disorders. *Am J Psychiatry* 157:745–750.

Donovan, S. and Nunes E. (1998) Treatment of comorbid affective and substance use disorders: therapeutic potential of anticonvulsants. *Am J Addictions* 7:210–220.

Donovan, S., Susser, E., and Nunes E. (1996) Divalproex sodium for use with conduct disordered adolescent marijuana users: letter to the editor. *Am J Addictions* 5:181.

Donovan, S., Susser, E., Nunes, E., Stewart, J., Quitkin, F., and Klein, D. (1997) Divalproex treatment of disruptive adolescents: a report of 10 cases. *J Clin Psychiatry* 58:12–15.

Emslie, G., Walkup, J., Pliska, S., and Ernst, M. (1999) Nontricyclic antidepressants: current trends in children and adolescents. *J Am Acad Child Adolesc Psychiatry* 38:517–528.

Garbutt, J., West, S., Carey, T., Lohr, K., and Crews, F. (1999) Pharmacological treatment of alcohol dependence: a review of the evidence. *JAMA* 281:1318–1325.

Geller, B., Cooper, T., Sun, K., Zimerman, B., Frazier, J., Williams, M., and Heath, J. (1998) Double-blind and placebo-controlled study of lithium for adolescent bipolar disorders with secondary substance dependency. *J Am Acad Child Adolesc Psychiatry* 37:171–178.

Goldman, L., Genel, M., Bezman, R., and Slanetz, P. (1998) Diagnosis and treatment of attention deficit/hyperactivity disorder in children and adolescents. *JAMA* 279:1100–1107.

Grabowski, J., Roache, J., Schmitz, J., Rhoades, H., Creson, D., and Korszun, A. (1997) Replacement medication for cocaine dependence: methylphenidate. *J Clin Psychopharm* 17:485–488.

Henggeler, S., Pickrel, S., and Brondino, M. (1999) Multisystemtic treatment of substance-abusing and dependent delinquents: outcomes, treatment, fidelity and transportability. *Mental Health Services Research* 1:171–184.

Hopfer, C., Mikulich, S., and Crowley, T. (2000) Heroin use among adolescents in treatment for substance use disorders. *J Am Acad Child Adolesc Psychiatry* 39:1316–1323.

Hovens, J., Cantwell, D., and Kiriakos, R. (1994) Psychiatric comorbidity in hospitalized adolescent substance abusers. *J Am Acad Child Adolesc Psychiatry* 33:476–483.

Jaffe, S. (2002) Failed attempts at intranasal abuse of concerta. *J Am Acad Child Adolesc Psychiatry* 41:5.

Johnson, B., Roache, J., Javors, M., DiClemente, C., Cloninger, C., Prihoda, T., Bordnick, P., Ait-Daoud, N., and Hensler J. (2000) Ondansetron for reduction of drinking among biologically predisposed alcoholic patients: a randomized controlled trial. *JAMA* 284:963–971.

Johnston, L., O'Malley, P., and Bachman, J. (2000) Monitoring the Future: National Results on Adolescent Drug Abuse: Overview of Key Findings, 1999. The University of Michigan Institute for Social Research and the National Institute on Drug Abuse. NIH Publication No. 00–4690.

Kaminer, Y. (1992) Case study: desipramine facilitation of cocaine abstinence in an adolescent. *J Am Acad Child Adolesc Psychiatry* 31:312–317.

Kaminer, Y. (1994a) Cocaine craving: letter to the editor. *J. Am. Acad. Child Adolesc. Psychiatry* 33:592.

Kaminer, Y. (1994b) Disulfiram in adolescence?: letter to the editor. *J. Am. Acad. Child Adolesc. Psychiatry* 34:2–3.

Kaminer, Y. (1995) Issues in the pharmacological treatment of adolescent substance abuse. *J Child Adolesc Psychopharm* 5:93–106.

Kaminer, Y. (1999) Addictive disorders in adolescents. *Psychiatr Clin North Am* 22:275–288.

Kaminer, Y. and Burleson, J. (1999) Psychotherapies for adolescent substance abusers: 15-month follow-up of a pilot study. *Am J Addict* 8:114–119.

Kandel, D. (1992) Epidemiological trends and implications for understanding the nature of addiction. In: O'Brien, C. and Jaffe, J. ed. *Addictive States* New York: Raven Press, pp. 23–40.

Kandel, D., Johnson, J., Bird, H., Weissman, M., Goodman, S., Lahey, B., Regier, D., and Schwab-Stone, M. (1999) Psychiatric comorbidity among adolescents with substance use disorders: findings from the MECA study. *J Am Acad Child Adolesc Psychiatry* 38:693–699.

Kessler, R., Crum, R., Warner, L., Nelson, C., and Schulenberg, J. (1997) Lifetime co-occurrence of DSM III-R abuse and dependence with other psychiatric disorders in the national comorbidity survey. *Arch Gen Psychiatry.* 54:313–321.

Kranzler, H., Amin, H., Modesto-Lowe, V., and Oncken, C. (1999) Pharmacologic treatments for drug and alcohol dependence. *Psychiatr Clin North Am* 22:401–423.

Lambert, N. and Hartsough, C. (1998) Prospective study of tobacco smoking and substance dependencies among samples of ADHD and non-ADHD participants. *J Learn Disabil* 31:533–544.

Levin, F., Evans, S., McDowell, D., Brooks, D., Rhum, M., and Kleber, H. (1998) Buproprion treatment for adult ADHD and cocaine use. Abstract Presented at CPPD 1998 Annual Meeting.

Levin, F. and Kleber, H. (1995) Attention deficit hyperactivity disorder and substance abuse: relationships and implications for treatment. *Harv Rev Psychiatry* 2:246–258.

Lifrak, P., Alterman, A., O'Brien, C. and Volpicelli, J. (1997) Naltrexone for alcoholic adolescents: letter to the editor. *Am J Psychiatry* 154:439–440.

Loney, J., Kramer, J., and Salisbury, H. (1999) Medicated versus unmedicated ADHD children: adult involvement with legal and illegal drugs. In: Jensen, P. and Cooper, J. ed. *Diagnosis and Treatment of ADHD*. In Press.

Molina, B., Pelham, W., and Roth, J. (1999) Stimulant medication and substance use by adolescents with a childhood history of ADHD. Poster and Presentation at the Biennial Meeting of the International Society for Child and Adolescent Psychopathology. June 1999.

Morehead, D. (1997) Exacerbation of hallucinogen-persisting perception disorder with risperidone. *J Clin Psychopharm* 17:327–328.

Myers, W., Donahue, J., and Goldstein, M. (1994) Disulfiram for alcohol use disorders in adolescents. *J Am Acad Child Adolesc Psychiatry* 33:484–489.

O'Brien, C. (1996) Recent development in the pharmacotherapy of substance abuse. *J Consult Clin Psychol* 64:677–686.

Ozechowski, T. and Liddle, H. (2000) Family-based therapy for adolescent drug abuse; knows and unknowns. *Clin Child Family Psychol Rev* 3:269–1298.

Riggs, P. (1998) Clinical approach to treatment of ADHD in adolescents with substance use disorders and conduct disorder. *J Am Acad Child Adolesc Psychiatry* 37:331–332.

Riggs, P., Leon, S., Mikulich, S., and Pottle, L. (1998) An open trial of buproprion for ADHD in adolescents with substance use disorders and conduct disorder. *J Am Acad Child Adolesc Psychiatry* 36:1271–1278.

Riggs, P., Mikulich, S., Coffman, L., and Crowley, T. (1997) Fluoxetine in drug-dependent delinquents with major depression: an open trial. *J Child Adolesc Psychopharm* 7:87–95.

Riggs, P., Thompson, L., Mikulich, S., Whitmore, E., and Crowley, T. (1996) An open trial of pemoline in drug-dependent delinquents with attention-deficit hyperactivity disorder. *J Am Acad Child Adolesc Psychiatry* 35:1018–1024.

Rohde, P., Clarke, G., Lewinson, P., Seeley, J., and Kaufman, N. (2001) Impact of comorbidity on a cognitive-behavioral group treatment for adolescent depression. *J Am Acad Child Adolesc Psychiatry* 40:795–802.

Solhkhah, R., Finkel, J., and Hird, S. (2000) Possible risperidone induced-visual hallucinations: letter to the editor. *J Am Acad Child Adolesc Psychiatry* 39:1074–1075.

Stowell, J. and Estroff, T. (1992) Psychiatric disorders in substance abusing adolescent inpatients: a pilot study. *J Am Acad Child Adolesc Psychiatry* 31:1036–1040.

Weinberg, N., Rahdert, E., Colliver, J., and Glantz, M. (1998) Adolescent substance abuse: a review of the past 10 years. *J Am Acad Child Adolesc Psychiatry* 37:252–259.

Wilens, T., Biederman, J., Abrantes, A., and Spencer, T. (1997a) Clinical characteristics of psychiatrically referred adolescent outpatients with substance use disorder. *J Am Acad Child Adolesc Psychiatry* 36: 941–947.

Wilens, T., Biederman, J., and Mick, E. (1998) Does ADHD affect the course of substance abuse? Findings from a sample of adults with and without ADHD. *Am J Addictions* 7:156–163.

Wise, B., Cuffe, S., and Fischer T. (2001) Dual diagnosis and successful participation of adolescents in substance abuse treatment. *Journal of Substance Abuse Treatment* 219:161–165.

Wilens, T., Biederman, J., Millstein, R., Wozniak, J., Hahesy, A., and Spencer, T. (1999) Risk for substance use disorders in youths with child and adolescent-onset bipolar disorder. *J Am Acad Child Adolesc Psychiatry* 38:680–685.

Wilens, T., Biederman, J., and Spencer, T. (1996) Attention deficit hyperactivity disorder and the psychoactive substance use disorders. In: Jaffe, S., ed. *Pediatric Substance Use Disorders: Child Psychiatric Clinics of North America*. Philadelphia: W. B. Saunders, pp. 73–91.

Wilens, T., Biederman, J., and Spencer, T. (1997b) Case study: adverse effects of smoking marijuana while receiving tricyclic antidepressants. *J Am Acad Child Adolesc Psychiatry* 36:45–48.

Wilens, T., Biederman, J., Milberger, S., Hahesy, A., Goldman, S., Wozniak, J. and Spencer, T. (2000) Is bipolar disorder a risk for cigarette smoking in ADHD youth? *Am J Addict* 9:187–195.

Wold, M. and Kaminer, Y. (1997) Naltrexone for alcohol abuse: letter to the editor. *J Am Acad Child Adolesc Psychiatry* 36:6–7.

Wozniak, J. and Biederman, J. (1997) Childhood mania: insights into diagnostic and treatment issues. *J Assoc Acad Minority Physicians* October:78–83.

46 | Individuals with mental retardation

MICHAEL G. AMAN, RONALD L. LINDSAY, PATRICIA L. NASH, AND L. EUGENE ARNOLD

Recent years have witnessed a proliferation in the variety of psychoactive agents that are available. The selective serotonin reuptake inhibitors (SSRIs), atypical antipsychotics, St. John's wort, and the newer antiepileptic drugs are some examples. This has stimulated more widespread treatment and, perhaps, empirical study of psychoactive agents in young people with mental retardation (MR). Much of this work was summarized in a recent text (Reiss and Aman, 1998), which will largely be the source of the discussion that follows. Recently, Rush and Frances (2000) surveyed about 100 expert clinicians and researchers about their views regarding psychosocial issues and appropriate pharmacotherapy in patients with MR. Periodically, we will refer to the *Expert Consensus Guidelines on Mental Retardation* (Rush and Francis, 2000) when trying to place a given treatment or issue in its current context. However, although the *Guidelines* were based on the views of influential figures in the field, it is important to be aware that they reflect the *opinions* of these workers and do not necessarily reflect established scientific fact.

In this chapter, we attempt to review the latest information on drug therapy for psychiatric conditions in children and adolescents with MR. Before doing this, however, it is appropriate to address special considerations in this clinical population that may impinge on the use of psychotropic medicines.

SPECIAL CONSIDERATIONS IN MENTAL RETARDATION

Prevalence of Psychopathology and Behavior Problems in Mental Retardation

Mental retardation is associated with a much higher prevalence of psychopathology than is found in the general population, and this is true of children and adolescents as well as adults. Rutter et al. (1976) found that the rate of behavior problems in children with MR was several times higher (30%–42%) that of normal-IQ children (5.4%). Studies of "dual diagnosis" (presence of both MR and mental illness) typically find prevalences that are three to six times that found in the general population (Bruininks et al., 1988). Of course, this higher rate of psychopathology is likely to translate to a greater use of psychotropic medicines, hopefully in combination with other treatments, in children with MR.

Associated Physical Ailments

Mental retardation tends to be associated with a multitude of medical and neurological conditions that require treatment in their own right. When this treatment is medicinal, this means that the potential for drug–drug interactions will be higher than in the general population. A good example of this is the co-occurrence of epilepsy, the prevalence of which increases with functional handicap. Some experts estimate that the prevalence of epilepsy is as high as 40% among patients with profound MR. As both psychotropic drugs and antiepileptic drugs are active on the central nervous system (CNS), the potential for adverse effects in CNS functioning as well as in metabolism of one of the drugs would seem to be elevated.

Problems Establishing Psychiatric Diagnoses

The practice of psychopharmacology assumes an appropriate fit between the patient's disorder and choice of drug. As the severity of MR increases, the presence of psychiatric conditions may become increasingly difficult to recognize and distinguish. There are several reasons for this. First, the individual may have difficulty introspecting and/or communicating feelings, thoughts, and concerns. Such self-report can be at the very core of some diagnostic formulations, such as depressive disorders, anxiety disorders, and schizophrenia. Many clinicians deal with this by relying in part on physical manifestations of mental illness to help identify the condition e.g., Szymanski et al., 1998). For example, overt tearfulness, altered sleep and eating patterns, psychomotor slowing, and agitation may be important "physical" cues in hypothesizing the presence of major depression. Second, severe intellectual handicap may even preclude the presence of certain psychiatric disorders. For example, can an individual with no expressive or receptive language experience delusions or hallucinations?

A third issue is that the very appearance of mental illness may change or "transmogrify" in patients with MR. For example, several workers have conducted factor analyses of behavior rating scales among patients with MR. It is not uncommon to observe that the factor structure is altered in this population, compared with in typically developing children. In the *Expert Consensus* survey (Rush and Frances, 2000), experienced workers were asked how confident they were that they could diagnose various psychiatric disorders reliably. These workers were confident in diagnosing autistic disorder much of the time. This was followed by obsessive-compulsive disorder (OCD) and major depressive disorder. Somewhat surprisingly, conduct disorder and attention-deficit hyperactivity disorder (ADHD) were not perceived as disorders that could be diagnosed with high reliability. Panic disorder, posttraumatic stress disorder (PTSD), and schizophrenia were seen as among the most difficult disorders to diagnose among patients with MR.

Finally, a fourth issue concerns whether developmental level must be taken into account when diagnosing a disorder in young people with MR. For example, a typically developing 2-year-old child ordinarily would not be diagnosed as having ADHD, even if he or she had marked inattention, impulsiveness, and high activity level. A common recommendation, appearing in parts of the *Diagnostic and Statistical Manual of Mental Disorders* (DSM), is that developmental level should be taken into account when considering certain diagnostic categories. This is intuitively compelling, and it is practiced by many clinicians. It is not necessarily true, however, that some form of developmental adjustment needs to be made when considering significant others' ratings of children with MR. For example, parents and teachers may already make some allowance when rating such children.

Also, one should be aware that mental age is not necessarily a good indicator of what the individual aspires to socially. For example, a 15-year-old with an IQ of 55 usually does not desire to associate with 8-year-olds. The more common experience is that he or she will want to be with other teenagers. At this stage, the astute clinician has to be alert to the possible need to take developmental level into account—e.g., the threshold may have to be elevated somewhat before diagnosing a developmental condition such as ADHD. At the same time, there is virtually no research on this and some kind of automatic adjustment cannot be assumed to be appropriate.

Choice of Appropriate Assessment Instruments

If one accepts the position that the structure of mental illness may differ for young people with MR, then it is also reasonable to choose assessment instruments that are appropriate to that population. There are several tools that have been developed for parent and teacher ratings of patients with MR. Examples are the Aberrant Behavior Checklist, the Developmental Behaviour Checklist, the Nisonger Child Behavior Rating Form, and the Diagnostic Assessment of the Severely Handicapped (see Hurley et al., 1998; Chapter 32, this volume).

These instruments have the advantage of being congruent with different behavioral structures observed in MR. They also contain behaviors ordinarily not seen in typically developing children (e.g., pica, stereotypies, and self-injury), and many of them have the added advantage of normative data for young people who are mentally retarded. Hence, the choice of an appropriate assessment tool assumes some specialist knowledge of the field.

Proneness to Adverse Events

There has been some suggestion that patients with MR may be more prone to develop side effects than patients in the general population (Arnold, 1993). For example, Handen et al. (1991) found that children with ADHD and MR showed high rates of tics, dysphoria, and lack of social responsiveness when treated with moderate doses of methylphenidate. The rates of these side effects appeared substantially to exceed those ordinarily seen in typically developing children. If it is true that there is a higher vulnerability in general to adverse events in this population, it would seem to make sense. By definition, many people with MR have some CNS dysfunction, and this may make them more vulnerable to toxic effects. In the *Expert Consensus* survey, the respondents endorsed the use of lower initial doses, slower dose increases, and slower dose decreases when phasing out medicines, while at the same time endorsing the same maximum doses and maintenance doses as used for the general population (Rush and Frances, 2000). The reasons for slower dosing were not reported, but this would be consistent with concerns over greater sensitivity to adverse events.

PHARMACOTHERAPY OF SPECIFIC PSYCHIATRIC DISORDERS

Attention Deficit Hyperactivity Disorder

More research has been done on pharmacotherapy of ADHD in children and adolescents with MR than for other disorders. Reviews by Aman (1996), Arnold et al. (1998), and Handen (1993) summarize the psychostimulant research (methylphenidate, amphetamine, and magnesium pemoline). Of the 10 or more group studies of methylphenidate or dextroamphetamine in children, adolescents, and adults with ADHD and MR/DD since 1980, all but one were positive and statistically significant. They showed substantial benefit for motor overflow, attention span, and impulsiveness. Improvements were also seen in cognitive performance, some measures of social behavior, and independent play. The sole negative study was of adolescents and adults without ADHD, most of them with profound MR (see Aman, 1996). No studies of mixed amphetamine salts (Adderall) or magnesium pemoline (Cylert) were found for this population (Arnold et al., 1998).

The response rate to psychostimulants in all of the group studies using children or adolescents with diagnosed ADHD was 54% (Aman, 1996). This is below the rate of 57%–69% reported by Arnold (2000) for a single stimulant (87% response if two are tried in succession) in typically developing children, and substantially below the 2/3 to 3/4 response rate often quoted by other authors. Nevertheless, this response rate is good enough that psychostimulants are commonly used in young people having MR and ADHD. Several single-subject studies have also shown beneficial changes with methylphenidate and dextroamphetamine.

Aman (1996) postulated that focus of attention, IQ, and mental age may be useful predictors of psychostimulant response. In his theory, children with narrow attentional focus are generally expected to respond more poorly than those with broader attentional focus, and those with lower IQ and lower mental age are predicted to respond more poorly. Castellanos et al. (1992) reported that in 72 normally developing children, the 13 with IQ above 120 responded better to dextroamphetamine, while those with IQ below 120 responded equally well to either dextroamphetamine or methylphenidate, but they could not replicate this in a prospective study (personal communication).

Tricyclic antidepressants (TCAs) are not as well studied as stimulants for treatment of ADHD even in normally developing children and adolescents, but are well enough studied that they are established as a second-line treatment. There are no controlled studies of TCAs in MR. Two case series reported ADHD symptom improvement, but seizures were a problem in one series (Szymanski, 1998).

Summarizing 22 studies of antipsychotic effects on hyperactivity in patients with MR, Baumeister et al. (1998) found modest reductions in overactivity. As with most psychoactive medications, anticonvulsants have also been used in the past for treatment of ADHD. There are a few controlled studies of carbamazepine showing benefit in treatment of ADHD, but most of the controlled studies (in typically developing children) were negative (Rett, 1968). Although anticonvulsants have thus fallen into disfavor for ADHD, they may have a role in two instances: (1) preventing seizures in a child whose only effective medication causes seizures, and (2) treating children with a pre-existing seizure disorder, in which case titration of the anticonvulsant to a dose slightly higher than that needed for seizure control may also benefit behavior. In contrast, fenfluramine, another previously favored treatment, has fallen into disfavor for a different reason—safety. Although controlled studies of fenfluramine for ADHD in MR were largely positive, reports of valvular dysfunction in adults taking it for weight reduction appear to have effectively ended its use, even though the problem has not been reported in children (Gillberg et al., 1998).

In the *Expert Consensus* survey (Rush and Frances, 2000), the respondents ranked the following most highly for managing ADHD in patients with MR: psychostimulants (first line) followed by α_{-2} agonists, bupropion, and tricyclics. The appearance of α_{-2} agonists in this list is curious, as there is virtually no research on these drugs in children with MR and few studies in normal-IQ ADHD children. When treating a child with MR and ADHD, the standard of care appears to be a trial of one or more psychostimulants, followed, if necessary, by cautious trials of a TCA if not contraindicated by a history of seizure disorder. After that, there are relatively few data to guide the practitioner.

Anxiety Disorders

Diagnosing an anxiety disorder in children can be difficult, because children often are unable to recognize and describe anxiety in themselves. Instead, they may complain of somatic symptoms. Younger children may exhibit behavioral changes such as tearfulness, difficulty separating from a parent, temper tantrums, or defiant behavior. Diagnosing an anxiety disorder in a child or adolescent with MR is even more difficult. Masi and colleagues (1998, 2000) described the clinical features of common psychiatric disorders, including anxiety disorders in persons with MR. Anxiety is often inferred from behavioral symptoms, and this is especially true of the more severely impaired individuals. Symptoms such as aggression, agitation, and self-injury can be interpreted as manifestations of anxiety. Therefore, it can be difficult to separate treatment of anxiety from treatment of these behavioral symptoms. Behavioral treatment programs have been used to treat anxiety in individuals with MR.

Treatment of anxiety disorders in children with psychopharmacologic agents has become much more common in the past decade. There are few studies of the use of these drugs in typically developing children and even fewer in children with MR. Most recommendations are based on experience with adults with a dual diagnosis or with typically developing children. The classes of medications used for the treatment of anxiety disorders include SSRIs, benzodiazepines, TCAs, and buspirone. In the *Expert Consensus Guidelines* (Rush and Frances, 2000), the SSRIs were rated as a first-line treatment for anxiety disorders. Buspirone was also a first-line treatment, with the benzodiazepines considered second line.

Generalized anxiety

Of the SSRIs, fluoxetine has been studied most extensively. Birmaher et al. (1994) and Fairbanks et al. (1997) both found significant improvement in various anxiety disorder symptoms in typically developing children. Fluoxetine was also found to be effective in the treatment of selective mutism (Black and Udhe, 1994; Dummit et al., 1996). Fluoxetine has also been studied in individuals with MR and autistic disorder. In an open trial, Cook et al (1992) found that fluoxetine was associated with significant improvement in the Clinical Global Impression (CGI) severity ratings in 15 of 23 individuals (65%) with autistic disorder and in 10 of 16 individuals (62%) with MR. All of the SSRIs appear to have similar properties and have been approved for panic disorder, phobias, OCD, and anxiety disorder. Sertraline has been approved for treatment of PTSD, and paroxetine, for social phobia.

Buspirone is a relatively new antianxiety medication that acts as an agonist of 5-HT_{1a} receptors. A number of open trials of buspirone in children and adolescents have shown significant improvements in anxiety and

aggression. Buspirone has been suggested as an agent for comorbid conditions of anxiety and ADHD. Ratey et al. (1991) evaluated effects of buspirone on anxiety, aggression, and self-injurious behavior in six adults with MR. While it appears that there was a decrease in aggression and self-injurious behavior, results on anxiety ratings were mixed. Ratey et al. (1989) also reported that 9 of 14 developmentally disabled individuals showed decreases in nervousness, tantrums, agitation, self-injurious behavior, and ritualistic behavior.

Benzodiazepines act by binding to the gamma-aminobutyric acid (GABA) receptors. The shorter-acting agents have been used to treat anxiety at low doses and to induce sedation at higher doses. The longer-acting agents have been used primarily for the treatment of anxiety. Simeon et al. (1987, 1992) found alprazolam to be effective in the treatment of generalized anxiety disorder in typically developing children. Clonazepam was effective in improving anxiety disorders and decreasing the frequency of panic attacks in four adolescents (Kutcher and Mackensie, 1988). Benzodiazepines have had a longer history in psychopharmacology but also have more negative qualities, making their use less attractive. Sedation, cognitive slowing, and paradoxical effects have diminished their use in children generally.

Tricyclic antidepressants have been used for decades to treat depression and anxiety in the general population, and clomipramine has been used to treat OCD. Clomipramine has been studied with respect to treating school phobia or school refusal (Berney et al., 1981). Gittleman-Klein and Klein (1971) found imipramine to be superior to placebo in treating school refusal. As the TCAs may improve other disorders such as nocturnal enuresis, ADHD, and sleep disorders, they may be attractive for children with any of these comorbid conditions and anxiety disorder.

Obsessive-compulsive disorder

In the MR population, OCD can be manifested as adherence to specific routines, performance of rituals, or stereotypies. If the person is not able to fulfill these routines and rituals, he or she may become agitated, upset, and uncooperative. The diagnosis of OCD in children with MR is based more on behavioral observations than on a description of internal factors. Treatment is recommended if these behaviors interfere with the person's ability to function and learn. In the *Expert Consensus* survey (Rush and Frances, 2000) treatment with an SSRI was recommended. Clomipramine, a TCA, may also be considered. Bodfish and Madison

(1993) found that 7 of 10 subjects with MR and compulsive behavior disorder responded favorably to fluoxetine treatment. Sertraline was beneficial in reducing fears and face-rubbing in a case report of a 33-year-old woman with moderate MR (Wiener and Lamberti, 1993). Barak et al. (1995) found a significant reduction in the severity of rituals in 9 of 11 adults with MR (82%) who were treated with 75 mg of sustained-release clomipramine.

Conclusion

It is a curious fact that antianxiety agents have rarely been studied in subjects with MR. When they have, they have often been tried for reducing hostile or aggressive behavior. Sandman and Barron (1992) and Barron and Sandman (1985) have presented data showing that many patients with severe or profound MR have a true paradoxical excitement when given older types of antianxiety drugs. Practitioners have no real option but to rely on data from studies of typically developing children when managing youngsters with MR.

Bipolar Disorder

According to the Expert Consensus Panel for Mental Retardation Rush and Frances, (2000), the mainstays of the pharmacological treatment of acute mania or bipolar disorder in adults are anticonvulsant medications (divalproex, valproic acid, or carbamazepine) or lithium. Both divalproex or valproic acid and lithium were preferred treatments for classic, euphoric manic episodes. Divalproex or valproic acid was preferred over lithium and carbamazepine for mixed or dysphoric manic episodes and rapid-cycling mania. For depressive episodes associated with bipolar disorder, the addition of an antidepressant (SSRI, bupropion, or venlafaxine) was recommended. According to the Expert Consensus Panel, the presence of MR does not affect the choice of medication for these psychiatric disorders in adults.

There has been only one double-blind, placebo-controlled long-term trial of lithium as a treatment for bipolar disorder in adults with MR (Naylor et al., 1974). In this study, 14 adults with borderline to severe MR and bipolar disorder were treated with lithium (with levels between 0.6 and 1.0 mEq/L) for 1 year. The number of weeks of illness was significantly lower in the treatment group. A year-long, single-blind, placebo-controlled trial of lithium in five persons with bipolar mood disorder and MR treatment resulted in re-

mission of symptoms (Rivinus and Harmatz 1979). Mania reemerged after discontinuation of lithium and another lengthy remission was achieved for all subjects when they restarted lithium therapy.

Two commonly used anticonvulsant medications for the treatment and prophylaxis of bipolar mood disorder in adults with MR are carbamazepine and valproic acid. Reid et al. (1981) compared carbamazepine to placebo in a double-blind, crossover fashion in 12 overactive adults with severe MR. Those described as having elevated moods and distractibility responded to treatment, while those without mood disturbance did not. Glue (1989) treated 10 adults with MR and rapid-cycling bipolar mood disorder with lithium alone, lithium and carbamazepine, and carbamazepine alone. None of the patients treated with carbamazepine alone responded, while half of the patients showed partial or complete improvement with lithium alone or in combination with carbamazepine.

Sovner (1989) reported that five individuals with bipolar mood disorder responded to standard treatment with divalproex sodium after failing treatment with neuroleptics and/or carbamazepine. A recent retrospective review of divalproex treatment in 28 adults with MR and severe behavior problems showed improvement (Ruedrich et al., 1999).

Bipolar mood disorder in childhood prior to adolescence is less common than in adolescence, and its occurrence in a child with MR is more likely to be missed (Hucker, 1975). As a result, there are few studies on the treatment of children with bipolar mood disorder and MR, and these are primarily limited to case reports. There are *no* well-designed studies of lithium's effectiveness in treating mania in childhood bipolar disorder (Viesselman, 1999). Dostal and Zvolsky (1970) and Goetzl et al. (1977) reported that lithium therapy was effective in 14 of 17 adolescents and young adults (82%) with MR in inpatient settings. Linter (1987) reported on an adolescent boy with short-cycle manic-depressive psychosis and MR who responded to lithium. There is evidence that lithium may be helpful if the diagnosis is clear-cut and/or when there is a strong family history of bipolar disorder. However, lithium is associated with many side effects in children such as bedwetting, tremor, drowsiness, ataxia, confusion, nausea, vomiting, diarrhea, headache, polyuria, and weight gain. Thus, alternatives to lithium such as anticonvulsant therapy may be preferable (Kastner et al., 1990). Children are more likely than adults to have mixed or rapid-cycling bipolar disorder, which usually responds better to an anticonvulsant than to lithium.

A review of the use of valproic acid (Viesselman,

1999) indicated that there were three open-label studies of the use of this anticonvulsant in adolescent mania. Seventeen of the 22 adolescent subjects in these studies (77%) responded to treatment, which was well tolerated by all. These three studies were limited by their open design, and two of the three studies allowed significant doses of concomitant neuroleptics.

In the absence of sound research on antimanic medicines in young people with MR, clinicians treating such patients have no choice but to extrapolate from the available work with typically developing children and with adults having MR. Given lithium's side effect profile and narrow therapeutic index, it may be wise to give valproate and/or carbamazepine a trial before resorting to lithium.

Conduct Disorder

Because the symptoms are so disruptive to the family and to the child, conduct disorder is one of the most common reasons for referral to a pediatrician or child psychiatrist. In patients with MR, this disorder is seen less as organized, planned illicit activities and more as impulsive, unpredictable acts of violence or destruction. Such individuals may exhibit aggression toward caregivers, teachers, family members, or themselves, and they may be emotionally labile. If behavior therapy has not been effective, pharmacological treatment may be necessary.

Botteron and Geller (1999) listed stimulants as first-line therapies for disruptive disorders in typically developing children, followed by antipsychotics, lithium, and carbamazepine. The psychostimulants have usually been shown to provide some improvement in disruptive behavior, although ADHD symptoms have ordinarily been the main target of treatment (Arnold, 2000). Brown et al. (1991) found methylphenidate to be helpful in adolescents who were hospitalized for conduct disorder but without a diagnosis of ADHD.

Although antipsychotic medications are the treatment of choice for schizophrenia, they are prescribed more often to treat aggression (often in the context of conduct disorder) than for psychosis among children and adolescents (Gracious and Findling, 2001). Haloperidol was found to be effective in treating aggressive, destructive children (Cunningham et al., 1968) and aggressive children with conduct disorder (Campbell et al., 1984). Molindone and thioridazine have also been studied with some success for use in conduct disorder Greenhill et al., 1985).

Lithium, carbamazepine, valproate, and antipsychotics have all been tried, with variable success, as therapy for conduct disorder in typically developing children (Werry and Aman, 1999). Campbell et al. (1984, 1995) found lithium to be effective in reducing aggressive behavior in children hospitalized for conduct disorder. Others (Rifkin et al., 1997) did not regard lithium carbonate as a good choice for such children. Lithium's side effects (tremors, enuresis, ataxia, drowsiness, confusion, nausea, vomiting, diarrhea) make it a less desirable treatment if equally effective agents exist.

Divalproex (Depakote) was found to reduce temper outbursts and emotional lability in 10 adolescents with conduct disorder (Donovan et al., 1997). Studies of carbamazepine have yielded conflicting results. Cueva et al. (1996) did not find carbamazepine to be more effective than placebo in treating children hospitalized for conduct disorder in a double-blind, placebo-controlled study. As in the case of lithium, side effects (rashes, leukopenia, nausea, drowsiness) can be an issue with carbamazepine, offsetting its use.

Whereas some drug studies have been done in children with normal IQ who have conduct disorder, there are very few studies involving children with MR and disruptive behavior problems. We are not aware of any studies of psychostimulants primarily to manage conduct problems in children with MR. However, most studies of children with both MR and ADHD have observed improvements on subscales assessing conduct problems, especially as rated by teachers (Aman et al., 1991, Aman et al., 1993). Given the low toxicity and well-tolerated side effects of the stimulants, they should at least be considered for treating conduct disorder in children and adolescents with MR, especially if they have ADHD.

Kastner et al. (1993) evaluated valproic acid in 18 children and adults (mean age, 19.7 years) with self-injury or aggression, irritability, sleep disorder, and evidence of cycling. Fourteen (78%) responded positively as assessed by the CGI in this uncontrolled study. The authors found that 11 subjects with established or suspected epilepsy responded significantly better than participants with no evidence of epilepsy.

Recently, Janssen Pharmaceutica launched several studies of risperidone in children with borderline IQ or MR and a diagnosis of disruptive behavior disorder (usually oppositional defiant disorder or conduct disorder). To be admissible into the study, subjects needed to be 5 to 12 years old, inclusive, and score above 24 on the Conduct Problem subscale of the Nisonger Child Behavior Rating Form (NCBRF). One 6-week acute trial (*n* = 118) was conducted in the United States (Aman et al., in press), whereas the other (*n* = 110) was based in Canada (Snyder et al., in press). The findings of the two studies were virtually identical, with significant drug-related declines occurring on the Conduct Problem subscale of the NCBRF, significant increases on both NCBRF prosocial subscales, and decreases on several problem behavior subscales (Insecure/Anxious, Hyperactive, Self-injury/Stereotypic). These improvements were obtained with mean doses of 1.23 mg/day (Aman et al., in press) and 0.98 mg/day (Snyder et al., in press). Other drug-related improvements occurred on clinician CGI ratings, parent ratings on the Aberrant Behavior Checklist (Irritability, Lethargy/Social Withdrawal, Hyperactivity/Noncompliance subscales), and parent ratings of the most troublesome symptom. The most common side effects included somnolence, headache, vomiting, dyspepsia, weight increase, and hyperprolactinemia.

The U.S. sample was followed openly on risperidone (0.02–0.06 mg/kg/day) for an additional 48 weeks (Findling et al., 2001). Some 50 children continued to end point, whereas 57 eventually withdrew from the trial for a variety of reasons (11, adverse events; 11, insufficient response; 35 "other" [loss to follow-up, withdrawal of consent, etc]). Subjects who received placebo in the acute trial had significant improvements as rated by parents on the Conduct Problem subscale of the NCBRF as they went on to active medication. Subjects already receiving risperidone in the acute trial continued to show improvement on the Conduct Problem subscale in the open-label continuation. Clinician CGI ratings also indicated improvement for participants who were switched from placebo to risperidone.

The most common adverse events in this trial (Findling et al., 2001) were somnolence (33%), headache (33%), rhinitis (28%), and weight gain (21%). Mean weight gain was 5.5 to 7.0 kg (depending on subgroup), whereas a gain of 4.89 kg would be expected for such children over this duration. Extrapyramidal symptoms were reported in 16% of subjects, but there was no tardive dyskinesia. Mean prolactin levels increased for approximately 4 to 6 weeks and then declined over the remainder of the trial to levels moderately higher than baseline values.

In the *Expert Consensus* survey (Rush and Frances, 2000), respondents were asked to rate which classes of medication may be helpful for treating patients with severe and persistent physical aggression and those who destroyed property. The atypical antipsychotics were rated most highly, followed by "anticonvulsant/mood stabilizer." These were followed (with much lower priority) by antidepressants and beta-blockers. Among the atypical antipsychotics, risperidone was rated most highly, followed by olanzapine; others had much lower ratings. Divalproex or valproic acid and carbamazepine were rated highest of the mood stabi-

lizers, and the SSRIs were rated far higher than all other antidepressants. Whether the experts' views will be substantiated by research remains to be seen.

Major Depressive Disorder

Sovner et al. (1998) have done an excellent job summarizing the data on antidepressants in patients with developmental disabilities. There have been nine reports of antidepressant use in adults with depression and MR and three reports of antidepressant use in children and adolescents. Eight of nine reports in adults were positive. The drugs studied included nialimide (n = 27), fluoxetine (9), imipramine (6), amoxapine (2), and nortriptyline (1) (total n = 45). In addition, Sovner et al. identified four reports of antidepressant use in children. One involved successful treatment with fluoxetine in an adolescent, another indicated efficacy with imipramine and amitriptyline in 9 of 12 children (Dosen, 1982), and a third showed successful management in 3 of 4 children treated with imipramine or tryptophan plus nicotinamide (Dosen, 1990). One study of fluoxetine in depressed children with autism and MR witnessed improvement in depression but not in compulsive symptoms (Ghaziuddin and Tsai, 1991).

Although there are many studies of antidepressants in typically developing children with depression, Viesselman (1999) found only one positive well-controlled outcome study, that being Emslie et al.'s (1997) trial of fluoxetine. It is possible that the CNS develops in such a way that serotonergic antidepressants may be more effective in children than catecholaminergic agents (Viesselman, 1999). Faced with the general lack of evidence with children having depression and MR, it would appear most rational to resort to use of SSRI agents first (supported, if appropriate, with cognitive behavior therapy and monitored with hard data to verify any changes). If the SSRIs are not useful, the clinician can then resort to cyclic antidepressants.

In the *Expert Consensus* survey, the use of the SSRIs was endorsed as the first-line treatment for a major depressive episode (Rush and Frances, 2000). The SSRIs were followed, at some distance, by venlafaxine, nefazodone, bupropion, and tricyclics, in that order. The warning against using bupropion in the presence of epilepsy constitutes a limitation on its use in the developmental disabilities. Clearly, more research is needed on the effects of antidepressants in both children and adolescents with MR and depression, as there are only four studies available thus far and that did not focus on age.

One of the main problems in this area concerns questions about how to diagnose depression in young people who may have limited or nonexistent language skills and extremely poor ability to report on their internal state. Bryan and Herjanic (1980) offered guidelines based on their own clinical experience. They identified 10 signs that may be helpful for diagnosing depression in children with MR, as follows: (1) low mood, as signaled by sadness, tearfulness, or social withdrawal; (2) changes in behavior, such as alterations in mood, hostility, irritability, or loss of interest in previously enjoyed activities; (3) alteration in sleep pattern; (4) alterations in eating habits and/or weight; (5) physical complaints without any apparent physiological basis; (6) change in school behavior and/or academic performance; (7) altered energy level; (8) changes in physical appearance and/or speech; (9) regression to earlier, less developed, behavior patterns; and (10) expressions of grim thoughts.

Eating Disorders

Psychotropic medication use is associated more with causing difficulties with eating rather than as a treatment for eating disorders. None of the medications investigated in the treatment of primary anorexia nervosa have been shown to be efficacious. Pica is defined as the eating of non-food substances. In the *Expert Consensus* survey (Rush and Frances, 2000) 63% of the respondents stated that no medication treatment is indicated for this disorder. Should medication be considered, then SSRI medications were most commonly endorsed. Another alternative is treatment with mineral or nutritional supplements, such as zinc or iron.

Enuresis

The pharmacologic treatment of enuresis in children and adults with MR is a subject that has been more extensively studied than most other diagnoses. Enuresis causes significant anxiety for those experiencing it as well as for those who care for them. Approximately 20% of 5-year-old children wet the bed at least monthly, while by age 6 only 10% wet the bed. There is a 15% remission rate each year after age 6.

Behavioral therapies are the treatment of choice for enuresis in both typically developing children and children with MR. No medical intervention should be undertaken before considering behavioral interventions, such as a star chart for dry nights, evening fluid restriction, bladder-stretching exercises (where children are asked to hold their urine for as long as they can, past the initial bladder spasm), and/or the buzzer-and-pad. However, some MR/DD patients will be unable to cooperate with such strategies and may need medical

help. Two drugs have been studied extensively for treating enuresis: desmopressin acetate (DDAVP) and imipramine hydrochloride.

Desmopressin (the synthetic analog of vasopressin) acts by increasing water retention and urine concentration in the distal tubules of the kidney. This drug is administered intranasally (20–40 µg or one to two sprays) using a unit-dose, spray pump delivery system. The duration of action is 10 to 12 hours. The medication is expensive.

A review of 18 controlled studies in otherwise typically developing children (Moffatt et al., 1993) demonstrated that only about 24% of children were completely dry while on medication and that 94% relapsed after medication was discontinued. In the Swedish Enuresis Trial (SWEET), 399 children aged 6–12 years with primary enuresis participated in an open, multicenter trial of DDAVP (Tullus et al., 1999). Subjects were observed for 4 weeks and had their DDAVP dose titrated over 6 weeks (20–40 µg), followed by a 1-year long-term treatment period. A total of 245 children (61%) experienced a 50% or more reduction in the number of wet nights, with resolution of enuresis in 77 children. The greatest therapeutic effect was observed in children 6–7 years of age. There were no studies on the effectiveness of DDAVP in children with MR.

Imipramine acts directly on the bladder, combining an anticholinergic effect that increases bladder capacity with a noradrenergic effect that decreases bladder detrusor excitability. Treatment with imipramine carries cardiovascular risks, including slowing of cardiac conduction, hypertension, and tachycardia. Overdosage can result in ventricular tachycardia, coma, and seizures. Initial rates of suppression of enuresis in typically developing children ranged from 10% to 60% in eight controlled, double-blind studies, but relapse rates following treatment were more than 90% (Schmitt, 1997). The available data suggest that children with MR have a less favorable response to imipramine (Blackwell and Currah, 1973). Two of three double-blind studies conducted in children with MR reported unfavorable results with imipramine, while one study (Rett, 1968) reported benefit in a heterogeneous group of children, characterized as "brain damaged," with an average IQ below 65.

The Psychoses and Schizophrenia

Turner (1989) surveyed the literature on prevalence of schizophrenia in patients with MR and found an average rate of about 3%. As in the case of most psychiatric disorders, this greatly exceeds rates found in the general population. Turner noted that the reliability of making such a diagnosis in people with MR is hindered because some symptoms commonly encountered (lethargy, vegetative behavior) may be confused with negative symptoms of schizophrenia.

Craft and Schiff (1980) assessed fluphenazine in a mixed group of "mentally ill" (psychotic) and nonpsychotic patients with MR. As determined by global assessments, the behavior of the participants (regardless of presence of "mental illness") improved significantly. Some 22 of the 102 participants (22%) developed extrapyramidal symptoms. Menolascino and colleagues (1985) studied the effects of thiothixene and thioridazine in 31 schizophrenia patients with MR and 30 schizophrenia patients without retardation. Change was assessed with the Global Evaluation Scale, the Katz Rating Scale, and the Brief Psychiatric Rating Scale. Blinded staff members rated both groups as significantly improved following drug therapy. Menolascino et al. reported a significantly faster clinical response with thiothixine (than with thioridazine) for subjects with MR, whereas the opposite occurred for normal-ability participants. Interestingly, the average doses of both drugs were lower for the patients with MR than those of normal IQ, although it was not reported whether these differences were statistically significant.

Two other reports have appeared relating to atypical antipsychotics. Sajatovic et al. (1994) treated five patients (mean IQ = 68) with clozapine (225 to 400 mg/day). All had research diagnostic criteria (RDC) for schizophrenia, schizophreniform, or schizoaffective disorder. Four responded clinically, and ratings on the Brief Psychiatric Rating Scale and Global Assessment Scale indicated statistically significant improvement. Buzan et al. (1998) treated 10 adults having schizoaffective disorder with clozapine (mean dose = 495 mg/day). The CGI severity ratings, Global Assessment of Functioning, and assessments of tardive dyskinesia all improved, but one patient's treatment was suspended because of neutropenia, which developed at 2 weeks.

All of the above trials were conducted in adults and, to the best of our knowledge, there are no trials of antipsychotic medication in children with psychoses and MR. To date there have been two double-blind trials of antipsychotic drugs in normal-IQ children and adolescents with schizophrenia, as well as several open-label trials (Ernst et al., 1999). The majority of these studies and case reports have demonstrated substantial reductions in schizophrenic symptoms. Given the lack of data on children and adolescents having both MR and schizophrenia, it seems that clinicians have little choice but to follow the standard of care applied with normal-IQ schizophrenic children, namely to use antipsychotic medications. In light of the Menolascino et al. (1985) adult study, it is possible that lower doses will prove to be effective.

In the *Expert Consensus* survey (Rush and Frances, 2000) the expert clinicians rated newer atypical antipsychotics highest for treatment of schizophrenic patients who are compliant with medication. Risperidone was rated highest of the atypicals, followed by olanzapine. In the case of patients with numerous failed trials with other antipsychotics, the experts voted for clozapine. For patients noncompliant with oral medication, respondents endorsed long-acting depot antipsychotics. Once again, these were impressions based on personal clinical experiences rather than hard empirical data.

Tics and Movement Disorders

Tourette's syndrome is a well-studied condition, characterized by motor and phonic tics and by behavioral and psychological problems. While many neurotransmitters were implicated in the etiology of this disorder, it is now believed that the dopaminergic system and noradrenergic systems are involved. Two major clinical trials (Shapiro et al., 1989; Sallee et al, 1997) indicated that haloperidol and pimozide reduced the severity of tics by 65%. However, these medications are associated with side effects (including possible cognitive impairment, sedation, dysphoria, and tardive dyskinesia) that may limit their effectiveness in children with MR.

Clonidine can be useful in treating the behavioral and attentional problems in Tourette's syndrome but is only 25% to 35% effective in controlling tics (Leckman et al., 1991). Two recent open trials found botulinum toxin A (BTX) injections effective and well tolerated for treating tics in Tourette's syndrome (Awaad, 1999; Kwak et al., 2000). With no trials of any of these agents in subjects with MR, the clinician has no choice but to extrapolate from studies with typically developing children, while taking a very data-based approach to ensure that any treatments used are, in fact, effective.

Self-Injury

We will rely heavily on a literature review for this section (Aman, 1993). Self-injury may be defined as external trauma resulting from repetitive acts directed against oneself. Within residential institutions, the prevalence of self-injury is typically between 10% and 15%, whereas outside of institutions the prevalence is often reported as being between 1% and 2.5% (Aman, 1993). Factors associated with self-injury include severity of MR, age (higher in adolescence and young adulthood), and male gender (although weakly, because of certain X-linked syndromes such as Lesch-Nyhan syndrome) (Rojahn, 1994).

In the *Expert Consensus* survey (Rush and Frances, 2000), the respondents identified newer atypical antipsychotics and anticonvulsants or mood stabilizers as first-line treatments for self-injury. Antidepressants, naltrexone, and conventional antipsychotics were given ratings at least midway or higher on the scale provided.

Antipsychotics

These agents have been used perhaps more than any others to manage self-injury (Aman, 1993). The data on effectiveness are mixed. In general, evidence for efficacy is strongest for thioridazine, where moderate doses may be helpful; doses as high as those sometimes used to manage schizophrenia may even be harmful (Aman, 1993). Unfortunately, recent evidence of thioridazine QT prolongation indicates that caution should be exercised in its use (Hartigen-Go et al., 1996). Although it is difficult to explain neurochemically, empirical data suggest that chlorpromazine is not particularly helpful for managing self-injury, whereas the evidence for haloperidol is both positive and negative.

There have been numerous trials of use of the atypical antipsychotics in patients with developmental disabilities, but most of these trials were uncontrolled open-labeled studies or case reports (Aman and Madrid, 1999). Findings were reported for 86 adults and 1 child with prominent self-injury. The reports of adults assessed clozapine (1 report) and risperidone (4 reports). Improvement was observed for a majority of participants in all of these trials. The patients presented with a multitude of conditions, ranging from nonspecific MR and associated behavior problems, to pervasive developmental disorders (including autism), to various psychiatric disorders, including schizophrenia and manic disorder. Self-injury appeared to respond to treatment regardless of concomitant condition. In the only clozapine report with a child (who had autistic disorder), a mean dose of 283 mg/day caused a transient reduction in self-injury.

In the *Expert Consensus* survey, the respondents endorsed risperidone, olanzapine, and quetiapine, in that order, followed by high-potency traditional antipsychotics, for managing self-injury. A placebo-controlled study comparing risperidone with a classical antipsychotic, such as haloperidol, could provide valuable data for this field.

Mood stabilizers

Aman's (1993) review of lithium treatment for self-injury revealed that the drug has only inconsistently been shown to suppress such behaviors. The available case reports have been far more positive than the placebo controlled research. Kastner et al.'s (1993) positive but uncontrolled study of lithium in adolescents and adults practicing aggression and self-injury was described earlier (see Conduct Disorder, above). Finally, single-subject studies of carbamazepine have yielded mixed results (Aman, 1993).

In the *Expert Consensus* survey (Rush and Frances, 2000), the respondents endorsed divalproex/valproic acid and carbamazepine as first-line medicines, followed by lithium and gabapentin (second-line interventions). Unfortunately, there are insufficient data on use of any of these—except, perhaps, on lithium—to draw any conclusions at this time.

Antidepressants

In the *Expert Consensus* survey, respondents endorsed the SSRIs as a first-line treatment for self-injury, followed by nefazodone and venlafaxine. Some workers have speculated that repetitive forms of self-injury may reflect underlying depression or OCD. Both of these, in turn, would suggest that serotonergic antidepressants may prove helpful. We were unable to find any empirical data on the use of TCAs or nefazodone and venlafaxine for managing self-injury. There have been at least seven studies or case reports of clomipramine use for treatment of self-injury (Aman et al., 1999). Four of these indicated a decrease in self-injury, one showed no change, and two actually suggested worsening of self-injury. There have also been at least five studies and nine case reports of the effects of SSRIs on self-injury (Aman et al., 1999). Four of the studies were positive (involving fluoxetine and sertraline), whereas one (involving paroxetine) was negative. Eight of nine case reports (involving fluoxetine and paroxetine) were positive, and one report on fluoxetine use was negative. Thus, the preliminary data suggest that the SSRIs (and possibly clomipramine) may be helpful, but their role is by no means defined at this time. There are insufficient data to recommend use of any of the other antidepressants.

Beta blockers

In the 1980s and early 1990s there was a flurry of reports on the use of beta-blockers for a wide variety of "acting-up" conditions (Fraser et al., 1998). Six of these described outcomes in a total of 33 self-injurious patients with MR. In the large majority of cases (88%), the subjects were reported to show at least some decline in self-injury. Aggression was often reduced as well. Most of these reports were flawed methodologically, and several assessed the beta-blocker in conjunction with preexisting antipsychotic medication. As the combination tends to drive up antipsychotic blood concentrations, this makes it difficult to know whether any benefit should be attributed to the beta-blocker, to increased antipsychotic levels, or to both (Fraser et al., 1998). It is also important to note that the doses were far below those commonly reported for controlling aggression in the general population. Children with MR can probably be managed with doses that are the equivalent of 150 mg of propranolol or less.

Naltrexone

Naltrexone was chosen as a possible "rational" treatment for self-injury, based on the notion that these patients either have a lower-than-normal threshold for pain or that self-injury produces surges of endorphins that are reinforcing to the patient. Sandman et al., (1998) have reviewed the literature on naltrexone and concluded that 35% to 70% of patients with self-injury show at least some benefit with the drug. We hold different opinions, but some of us are less enthusiastic. Like other agents used to manage self-injury (e.g., antipsychotics, beta-blockers), naltrexone appears to have some sedative action, which may be more relevant than the drug's opiate-blocking action. There usually is not an all-or-none effect, as the neurochemical-behavioral model might suggest. The Expert Consensus Panel (Rush and Francis, 2000) gave naltrexone an overall rating of 5.5 (on a scale of 0–9), which suggests that the experiences of these experts have been mixed. Theoretically, it should work best where the self-injurious behavior appears to be self-stimulation. Naltrexone is not likely to be effective if self-injury is a response to some undiagnosed physical pain or depressive desperation, and it is variably successful for instrumental self-injurious behavior (e.g., to get attention or vent frustration), depending on how strong the environmental reinforcers for such behavior are.

Sleep Disorders

Sleep problems can cause considerable difficulty in and of themselves and can also exacerbate and be exacerbated by other psychiatric and behavioral problems in individuals with MR. The Expert Consensus Panel (Rush and Frances, 2000) recommended sleep hygiene strategies such as establishing a bedtime routine, regular schedules for bedtime and waking up, reduction of environmental disruptions and stimulation, and restriction of caffeine intake; these are applicable to both adults and children. A patient who has not responded to the above interventions might benefit from trazodone or zolpidem.

Benzodiazepines (such as clonazepam) are used widely to induce sleep, but they disrupt the normal sleep architecture. Children also have a tendency to become more irritable and hyperactive with hypnotics. In severe cases, benzodiazepines could be given for 3–5 days to facilitate a behavioral treatment program. Trazodone, though not specifically studied in children, may be a safer alternative for more chronic sleep problems if over-the-counter (OTC) diphenhydramine does not work.

New-onset sleep problems may be a side effect of psychoactive or other medication, and the first intervention should be consideration of adjusting the dosage or time of day the medication is given. For example, sleep disruption from stimulants can generally be relieved by adjustments based on careful history of the time–action effects.

Antihistamines such as diphenhydramine, a mainstay of OTC sleep preparations, are also used widely by parents for their children at doses of 1 mg/kg. Most of the reports of the use of clonidine for sleep disorders are clinical and anecdotal case reports of use in children with ADHD (Wilens et al., 1994; Prince et al., 1996). There are some safety concerns about using clonidine once a day at bedtime, especially in patients who take a daytime stimulant. Melatonin was studied using a double-blind, placebo-controlled, crossover design (Jan et al., 1994) on a mixed group of 15 children with sleep disturbances, with some improvement reported. However, caution is warranted in using this agent because melatonin is unregulated, and there are concerns about the purity and safety of some commercially available preparations (Werry and Aman, 1999).

Once again, empirical data are generally lacking for children with MR. Clinicians seeing pediatric patients with MR and sleep problems have little recourse but to extrapolate from the literature on typically developing children.

CONCLUSIONS

To summarize, there are many considerations that complicate the use of pharmacotherapy in children with MR. These include (1) a much higher prevalence of psychiatric and psychological problems, (2) the presence of concomitant medical conditions, (3) altered presentation of the disorder, (4) uncertainty over how to handle developmental level, (5) the use of different assessment instruments, and (6)a perhaps greater propensity to side effects.

From what is known about use of psychotropic drugs in children with MR, this is clearly an "orphan" population. We are not aware of any studies indicating that children and adolescents with MR have responded to psychotropic medication in a qualitatively different manner from that of typically developing children. Nevertheless, the only condition for which there is good evidence for a clear-cut diagnosis–drug fit is ADHD. For treatment of virtually all other conditions, practitioners are forced to extrapolate from drug research on adults with MR and on typically developing children.

Our advice to clinicians is to make the best decision that they can, based on the evidence, while opting for agents with the best side effect profiles and that are supported, when possible, with other appropriate therapies. Because of the experimental nature of pharmacotherapy in this population, practitioners should endeavor to confirm the utility of treatment with hard data. Where possible, periodic drug holidays are recommended to determine if continued therapy is needed. Until far more drug research is available on young people with MR, this will continue to be one of the more challenging populations in which to practice psychopharmacology.

REFERENCES

Aman, M.G. (1993) Efficacy of psychotropic drugs for reducing self-injurious behavior in the developmental disabilities. *Ann Clin Psychiatry* 5:171–188.

Aman, M.G. (1996) Stimulant drugs in the developmental disabilities revisited. *J Dev Phys Disabil* 8:347–365.

Aman M.G., Arnold, L.E., and Armstrong S. (1999) Review of serotonergic agents and perseverative behavior in patients with developmental disabilities. *J Child Adolesc Psychopharmacol* 5:279–289.

Aman, M.G., De Smedt, G., Derivan, A., Lyons, B., Findling, R.L., and the Risperidone Disruptive Behavior Study Group (In press). Risperidone treatment of children with disruptive behavior symptoms and subaverage IQ: a double-blind, placebo-controlled study. *Am J Psychiatry*

Aman, M.G., Kern, R.A., McGhee, D.E., and Arnold, L.E. (1993) Fenfluramine and methylphenidate in children with mental retardation and ADHD: clinical and side effects. *J Am Acad Child Adolesc Psychiatry* 32:851–859.

Aman, M.G. and Madrid, A. (1999) Atypical antipsychotics in persons with developmental disabilities. *Ment Retard Dev Disabil Res Rev* 5:253–263.

Aman, M.G., Marks, R.E., Turbott, S.H., Wilsher, C.P., and Merry, S.N. (1991) Clinical effects of methylphenidate and thioridazine

in intellectually subaverage children. *J Am Acad Child Adolesc Psychiatry* 30:816–824.

Arnold, L.E. (1993) Clinical pharmacological issues in treating psychiatric disorders of patients with mental retardation. *Ann Clin Psychiatry* 5:189–198.

Arnold, L.E. (2000) Methylphenidate vs. amphetamine: comparative review.*J Attention Disord* 3:200–211.

Arnold, L.E., Gadow, K., Pearson, D.A., and Varley, C.K. (1998) Stimulants. In: Reiss, S. and Aman, M.C., eds. *Psychotropic Medications and Developmental Disabilities: The International Consensus Handbook*. Columbus, OH: The Ohio State University Nisonger Center, pp. 229–257.

Awaad, Y. (1999) Tics in Tourette syndrome: new treatment options. *J Child Neurol* 14:316–319.

Barak, Y., Ring, A., Levy, D., Granek, I., Szor, H., and Elizur, A. (1995) Disabling compulsions in eleven mentally retarded adults: an open trial of clomipramine SR. *J Clin Psychiatry* 56:459–461.

Barron, J. and Sandman, C.A. (1985) Paradoxical excitement to sedative-hypnotics in mentally retarded clients. *Am J Ment Defic* 90:124–129.

Baumeister, A.A., Sevin, J.A., and King, B.H. (1998) Neuroleptics. In: Reiss, S. and Aman, M.G., eds. *Psychotropic Medications and Developmental Disabilities: The International Consensus Handbook*. Columbus, OH: The Ohio State University Nisonger Center, pp. 133–150.

Berney, T., Kolvin, I., Bhate, R.F., Garside, R.F., Jeans, J., Kay, B., and Scarth, L. (1981) School phobia: a therapeutic trial with clomipramine and short term outcome. *Br J Psychiatry* 138:110–118.

Birmaher, B., Waterman, G.S., Ryan, N.D., Cully, M., Balach, L., Ingram, J., and Brodsky, M. (1994) Fluoxetine for childhood anxiety disorders. *J Am Acad Child Adolesc Psychiatry* 33: 993–999.

Black, B. and Udhe, T.W. (1994) Treatment of elective mutism with fluoxetine: a double-blind, placebo-controlled study. *J Am Acad Child Adolesc Psychiatry* 33:1000–1006.

Blackwell, B. and Currah, J. (1973) The psychopharmacology of nocturnal enuresis. In: Kolvin, I., McKeith, R., and Meadow, S., eds. *Bladder Control and Enuresis*. London: Hineman, pp. 231–257.

Bodfish, J.W. and Madison, J.T. (1993) Diagnosis and fluoxetine treatment of compulsive behavior disorder of adults with mental retardation. *Am J Ment Retard* 98:360–367.

Botteron, K. and Geller, B. (1999) Disorders, symptoms, and their pharmacotherapy. In: Werry, J.S. and Aman, M.G., eds. *Practitioner's Guide to Psychoactive Drugs for Children and Adolescents, 2nd ed.* New York: Plenum Medical, pp. 185–209.

Brown, R.T., Jaffe, S.L., Silverstein, J., and Magee, H. (1991) Methylphenidate and adolescents hospitalized with conduct disorder: dose effects on classroom behavior, academic performance, and impulsivity. *J Clin Child Psychol* 20:282–292.

Bruininks, R.H., Hill, B.K., and Morreau, L.E. (1988) Prevalence and implications of maladaptive behaviors and dual diagnosis in residential and other service programs. In Stark, J.A., Menolascino, F.J., Albarelli, M.H., and Gray, V.C., eds. *Mental Retardation and Mental Health. Classification, Diagnosis, Treatment, Services*. New York: Springer-Verlag, pp. 3–29.

Bryan, D.P. and Herjanic, B. (1980) Depression and suicide among adolescents and young adults with selective handicapping conditions. *Educ Q* 1:57–65.

Buzan, R.D., Dubovsky, S.L., Firestone, D., et al. (1998) Use of clozapine in 10 mentally retarded adults. *J Neuropsychiatry* 10:93–95.

Campbell, M., Adams, P.B., Small, A.M., Kafantaris, V., Silva, R.R., Shell, J., Perry, R., and Overall, J.E. (1995) Lithium in hospitalized aggressive children with conduct disorder: a double-blind and placebo-controlled study. *J Am Acad Child Adolesc Psychiatry* 34:445–453.

Campbell, M., Small, A.M., Green, W.H., Jennings, S.J., Perry, R., Bennett, W.G., and Anderson, L. (1984) Behavioral efficacy of haloperidol and lithium carbonate. A comparison in hospitalized aggressive children with conduct disorder. *Arch Gen Psychiatry* 41:650–656.

Castellanos, F.X., Gulotta, C., and Rapoport, J. (1992) Superior Intellectual functioning and stimulant drug response in ADHD. Poster at May 26–29, 1992 New Clinical Drug Evaluation Unit (NCDEU) meeting, Boca Raton, Florida.

Cook, E.H. Jr., Rowlett, R., Jaselskis, C., and Leventhal, B.L. (1992) Fluoxetine treatment of children and adults with autistic disorder and mental retardation. *J Am Acad Child Adolesc Psychiatry* 31: 739–745.

Craft, M.J. and Schiff, A.A. (1980) Psychiatric disturbance in mentally handicapped patients. *Br J Psychiatry* 137:250–255.

Cueva, J.E., Overall, J.E., Small, A.M., Armenteros, J.L., Perry, R., and Campbell, M. (1996) Carbamazepine in aggressive children with conduct disorder: a double-blind and placebo-controlled study. *J Am Acad Child Adolesc Psychiatry* 35:480–490.

Cunningham, M.A., Pillai, V., and Blanchford-Rogers, W.J. (1968) Haloperidol in the treatment of children with severe behavior disorders. *Br J Psychiatry* 114:845–854.

Donovan, S.J., Susser, E.S., Nunes, E.V., Stewart, J.W., Quitkin, F.M., and Klein, D.F. (1997) Divalproex treatment of disruptive adolescents: a report of 10 cases. *J Clin Psychiatry* 58:12–15.

Dostal, T., and Zvolsky, P. (1970) Antiaggressive effects of lithium salts in severe mentally retarded adolescents. *Int Pharmacopsychiatry* 5:203–207.

Dosen, A. (1982) Ervaringen met psychofarmaca bij zwakzinnige kindern. *Tijschr Kindersgeneesk* 50:10–19.

Dosen, A. (1990) Psychische en gedragsstoornissen bij zwakssinnigen. Amsterdam: *Boom*.

Dummit, E.S., 3rd, Klein, R.G., Tancer, N.K., Asche, B., and Martin, J. (1996) Fluoxetine treatment of children with selective mutism: an open trial. *J Am Acad Child Adolesc Psychiatry* 35:615–621.

Emslie, G.J., Rush, A.J., Weinberg, W.A., Kowatch, R.A., Hughes, C.W., Carmody, T.J., and Rintelmann, J. (1997) A double-blind, randomized, placebo-controlled trial of fluoxetine in children and adolescents with depression. *Arch Gen Psychiatry* 54:1031–1037.

Ernst, M., Malone, R.P., Rowan, A.B., George, R., Gonzalez, N.M., and Silva, R.R. (1999) Antipsychotics (neuroleptics). In Werry, J.S. and Aman, M.G., eds. *Practitioner's Guide to Psychoactive Drugs for Children and Adolescents, 2nd ed.* New York: Plenum, pp. 297–327.

Fairbanks, J., Pine, D.S., Tancer, N.K., Dummit, E.S., Kentgen, L.M., Martin, J., Asche, B.K., and Klein, R.G. (1997) Open fluoxetine treatment of mixed anxiety disorders in children and adolescents. *J Child Adolesc Psychopharmacol* 17:17–29.

Findling, R., Aman, M., and Derivan, A. (2000). Long-term safety and efficacy of risperidone in children with significant conduct problems and borderline IQ or mental retardation. Presented at the 39th Annual American College of Neuropsychopharmacology, San Juan, Puerto Rico, December 2000.

Fraser, W.I., Ruedrich, S., Kerr, M., and Levitas, A. (1998) Beta-adrenergic blockers. In: Reiss, S. and Aman, M.G., eds. *Psychotropic Medications and Developmental Disabilities: The International Consensus Handbook*. Columbus, OH: The Ohio State University Nisonger Center UAP, (pp. 271–289).

Ghaziuddin, M. and Tsai, L. (1991) Fluoxetine in autism with depression. *J Am Acad Child Adolesc Psychiatry* 30:508–509.

Gillberg, C., Aman, M.G., and Reiss, A.L. (1998) Fenfluramine. In: Reiss, S.A. and Aman, M.G., eds. *Psychotropic Drugs and Developmental Disabilities: The International Consensus Handbook*. Columbus, OH: The Ohio State University Nisonger Center, pp. 303–310.

Gittelman-Klein, R. and Klein, D. (1971) Controlled imipramine treatment of school phobia. *Arch Gen Psychiatry* 25:205–207.

Glue, P. (1989) Rapid cycling affective disorders in the mentally retarded. *Biol Psychiatry* 26:250–256.

Goetzl, U., Grunberg, F., and Berkowitz, B. (1977) Lithium carbonate in the management of hyperactive aggressive behavior of the mentally retarded. *Compr Psychiatry* 18:599–606.

Gracious, B.L. and Findling, R.L. (2001) Antipsychotic medications for children and adolescents. *Pediatr Ann* 30:138–145.

Greenhill, L.L., Solomon, M., Pleak, R., and Ambrosini, P. (1985) Molindone hydrochloride treatment of hospitalized children with conduct disorder. *J Clin Psychiatry* 46: 20–25.

Handen, B.L. (1993) Pharmacotherapy in mental retardation and autism. *Sch Psycho Rev* 22:162–183.

Handen, B.L., Feldman, H., Gosling, A., Breaux, A.M., and McAuliffe, S. (1991) Adverse side effects of methylphenidate among mentally retarded children with ADHD. *J Am Acad Child Adolesc Psychiatry* 30:241–245.

Hartigan-Go, K., Bateman, D.N., Nyberg, G., Martensson, E., and Thomas, S.H. (1996) Concentration-related pharmacodynamic effects of thioridazine and its metabolites in humans. *Clin Pharmacol Ther* 60: 543–553.

Hucker, S.J. (1975) Pubertal manic depressive psychosis and mental subnormality—a case report. *Br J Ment Subnormality* 21:34–37.

Hurley, A.D., Reiss, S., Aman, M.G., Salvador-Carulla, L., Demb, H.B., Loschen, E.L., and Einfeld, S.L. (1998) Instruments. In Reiss, S. and Aman, M.G., eds. *Psychotropic Drugs and Developmental Disabilities: The International Consensus Handbook*. Columbus, OH: The Ohio State University Nisonger Center UAP, pp. 85–94.

Jan, J.E., Espezel, H., and Appleton, R.E. (1994) The treatment of sleep disorders with melatonin. *Dev Med Child Neurol* 36:97–107.

Kastner, T., Finesmith, R., and Walsh, K. (1993) Long-term administration of valproic acid in the treatment of affective symptoms in people with mental retardation. *J Clin Psychopharmacol* 13: 448–451.

Kastner, T., Friedman, D.L., and Plummer, A. (1990) Valproic acid for the treatment of children with mental retardation and mood symptomatology. *Pediatrics* 86:467–472.

Kutcher, S. and Mackensie, S. (1988). Successful clonazepam treatment of adolescents with panic disorder. *J Clin Psychopharmacol* 18:299–301.

Kwak, C.H., Hanna, P.A., and Jankovic J. (2000) Botulinum toxin in the treatment of tics. *Arch Neurol* 57: 1190–1193.

Leckman, J.F., Harden, M.T., Riddle, M.A., Stevenson, J., Ort, S., and Cohen, D.J. (1991) Clonidine treatment of Gilles de la Tourette's syndrome. *Arch Gen Psychiatry* 48:324–328.

Linter, C.M. (1987) Short-cycle manic-depressive psychosis in a mentally handicapped child without family history. *Br J Psychiatry* 151:554–555.

Masi, G. (1998). Psychiatric illness in mentally retarded adolescents: clinical features. *Adolescence* 33(130):425–434.

Masi, G., Favilla, L., and Mucci, M. (2000) Generalized anxiety disorder in adolescents and young adults with mild mental retardation. *Psychiatry* 63:54–64.

Menolascino, F.J., Ruedrich, S.L., Golden, C.J., and Wilson, J.E.

(1985) Diagnosis and pharmacotherapy of schizophrenia in the retarded. *Psychopharmacol Bull* 21:316–322.

Moffatt, M.E., Harlos, S., Kirshen, A.J., and Burd, L. (1993) Desmopessin acetate and nocturnal enuresis: how much do we know? *Pediatrics* 92:420–425.

Naylor, G.D., Donald, J.M., LePoidevin, D., and Reid, A.H. (1974) A double-blind trial of long-term lithium therapy in mental defectives. *Br J Psychiatry* 124:52–57.

Prince, J.B., Wilens, T.E., Biederman, J., Spencer, T.J., and Wozniak, J.R. (1996) Clonidine for sleep disturbances associated with attention deficit hyperactivity disorder: a systematic chart review of 62 cases. *J Am Acad Child Adolesc Psychiatry* 35:599–605.

Ratey, J., Sovner, R., Parks, A., and Rogentine, K. (1991) Buspirone treatment of aggression and anxiety in mentally retarded patients: a multiple-baseline, placebo lead-in study. *J Clin Psychiatry* 52: 159–162.

Ratey, J.J., Sovner, R., Mikkelsen, E., and Chmielinski, H.E. (1989) Buspirone therapy for maladaptive behavior and anxiety in developmentally disabled persons. *J Clin Psychiatry* 50:382–384.

Reiss, S. and Aman, M.G. (1998) *Psychotropic Medications and Developmental Disabilities: The International Consensus Handbook*. Columbus, OH: The Ohio State University Nisonger Center UAP.

Reid, A.D., Naylor, G.J., and Ka, D. (1981) A double-blind placebo controlled crossover trial of carbamazepine in overactive severely mentally handicapped patients. *Psychol Med* 11:109–113.

Rett, A. (1968) Der Verwendung von Trimeprimin in der Kinderheikunde. *Medi Welt* 47:2616.

Rifkin, A., Karajgi, B., Dicker, R., Perl, E., Boppana, V., Hassan, N., and Pollack, S. (1997) Lithium treatment of conduct disorders in adolescents. *Am J Psychiatry* 154:554–555.

Rivinus, T.M. and Harmatz, J.S. (1979) Diagnosis and lithium treatment of affective disorders in the retarded: five case studies. *Am J Psychiatry* 136:551–544.

Rojahn, J. (1994) Epidemiology and topographic taxonomy of self-injurious behavior. In: Thompson, T. and Gray, D.B., eds. *Destructive Behavior in Developmental Disabilities: Diagnosis and Treatment*. Thousand Oaks, CA: Sage pp. 49–67.

Ruedrich, S., Swales, T.P., Fossaeeca, C., Toliver, J., and Rutkowski, A. (1999) Effect of divalproex sodium on aggression and self-injurious behavior in adults with intellectual disability: a retrospective review. *J Intellect Disabil Res* 43:105–111.

Rush, A.J. and Frances, A., eds. (2000). The Expert Consensus Guideline Series. Treatment of Psychiatric and Behavioral Problems in Mental Retardation (Issue No. 3, Special Issue). *Am J Ment Retard* 105:159–228.

Rutter, M., Tizard, J., Yule, W., Graham, P., and Whitmore, K. (1976) Isle of Wight studies, 1964–1974. *Psychol Med* 6:313–332.

Sajatovic, M., Ramirez, L.F., Kenny, J.T., and Meltzer, H.Y. (1994) The use of clozapine in borderline-intellectual-functioning and mentally retarded schizophrenic patients. *Compr Psychiatry* 35: 29–33.

Sallee, F.R., Nesbitt, L., and Jackson, C. (1997). Relative efficacy of haloperidol and pimozide in children and adolescents with Tourette's disorders. *Am J Psychiatry* 154:1057–1062.

Sandman, C.A. and Barron, J.L. (1992) Paradoxical response to sedative/hypnotics in patients with self-injurious behavior and stereotypy. *J Dev Phys Disabil* 4:307–316.

Sandman, C.A., Thompson, T., Barrett, R.P., Verhoeven, W.M., McCubbin, J.A., Schroeder, S.R., and Hetrick, W.P. (1998) Opiate blockers. In : Reiss, S. and Aman, M.G., eds. *Psychotropic Drugs and Developmental Disabilities: The International Consensus Handbook*. Columbus, OH: The Ohio State University Nisonger Center UAP, pp. 85–94.

Schmitt, B.D. (1997) Nocturnal enuresis. *Pediatr Rev* 18:183–190.

Shapiro, A.K., Shapiro, E., Fulop, G. Hubbard, M., Mandeli, J., Nordlie, J., and Philips, R.A. (1989) Controlled study of haloperidol, pimozide, and placebo for the treatment of Gilles de la Tourette's syndrome. *Arch Gen Psychiatry* 46:722–730.

Simeon, J. and Ferguson, B. (1987) Alprazolam effects in children with anxiety disorders. *Can J Psychiatry* 32:570–574.

Simeon, J., Ferguson, B., Knott, V., Roberts, N., Ganthier, B., DuBoise, C., and Wiggins, D. (1992) Clinical, cognitive, and neurophysiological effects of alprazolam in children with overanxious and avoidant disorders. *J Am Acad Child Adolesc Psychiatry* 31:29–33.

Snyder, R., Turgay, A., Aman, M.G., Binder, C., Fisman, S., Carroll, A., and The Risperidone Conduct Study Group. (In press) Effects of risperidone on conduct and disruptive behavior disorders in children with subaverage IQs. *J Am Acad Child Adoles Psychiatry*.

Sovner, R. (1989) The use of valproate in the treatment of mentally retarded persons with typical and atypical bipolar disorders. *J Clin Psychiatry* 50:40–43.

Sovner, R., Parry, R.J., Dosen, A., Gedye, A., Barrera, F., Cantwell, D.P., and Huessy, H.R. (1998) Antidepressants. In Reiss, S. and Aman, M.G., eds. *Psychotropic Drugs and Developmental Disabilities: The International Consensus Handbook*. Columbus, OH: The Ohio State University Nisonger Center UAP, pp. 85–94.

Szymanski, L.S., King, B., Goldberg, B., Reid, A.H., Tonge, B.J., and Cain, N. (1998) Diagnosis of mental disorders in people with mental retardation. In: Reiss, S. and Aman, M.G., eds. *Psychotropic Medications and Developmental Disabilities: The International Consensus Handbook*. Columbus, OH: The Ohio State University Nisonger Center, pp. 3–17.

Tullus, K., Bergstron, R., Fosdal, I., Winnergard, I., and Hjalmas, K. (1999) Efficacy and safety during long-term treatment of primary monosymptomatic nocturnal enuresis with desmopressin. *Acta Paediatr*. 88:1274–1278.

Turner, T.H. (1989) Schizophrenia and mental handicap: a historical review, with implications for further research. *Psychol Med* 19: 301–314.

Viesselman, J.O. (1999) Antidepressant and antimanic drugs. In: Werry, J.S. and Aman, M.G., eds. *Practitioner's Guide to Psychoactive Drugs for Children and Adolescents, 2nd ed*. New York: Plenum Medical, pp. 249–296.

Werry, J.S. and Aman, M.G. (1999) Anxiolytics, sedatives, and miscellaneous drugs. In: Werry, J.S. and Aman, M.G., eds. *Practitioner's Guide to Psychoactive Drugs for Children and Adolescents, 2nd ed*. New York: Plenum, pp. 433–469.

Wiener, K, and Lamberti, J.S. (1993) Sertraline and mental retardation with obsessive-compulsive disorder. *Am J Psychiatry* 150: 1270.

Wilens, T., Biederman, J., and Spencer, T. (1994) Clonidine for sleep disturbances associated with attention deficit hyperactivity disorder. *J Am Acad Child Adolesc Psychiatry* 33:424–426.

47 | The medically ill child or adolescent

JONATHAN A. SLATER

Due both to the expansion of the psychopharmacological armamentarium and the advances in the medical treatment of severely ill pediatric patients, child and adolescent psychiatrists are increasingly being called upon to manage these patients adjunctively with psychiatric medication. This need has been tempered with concerns over the potential effects of psychotropic medications on the developing central nervous system (CNS) (Jensen, 1998; Vitiello, 1998). The management of these medically ill children and adolescents falls into several categories:

1. Pediatric patients with comorbid psychiatric disorders requiring continued treatment for their psychiatric symptomatology (e.g., a schizophrenic patient admitted with an asthma exacerbation)

2. Pediatric patients with psychiatric syndromes arising secondary to their medical condition (e.g. a hypoxic patient who becomes agitated secondary to delirium)

3. Pediatric patients with psychiatric symptomatology secondary to medications being used to treat medical conditions (e.g., a transplant patient treated with high-dose corticosteroids for organ rejection who develops irritability)

4. Pediatric patients who develop psychiatric syndromes following acute medical illness or injury or invasive procedures (e.g., a child who develops posttraumatic stress disorder [PTSD] following a motor vehicle accident and trauma; a child who develops PTSD following stem cell transplantation)

5. Pediatric patients who develop psychiatric syndromes in association with chronic illness (e.g., major depression in a patient with cystic fibrosis)

6. Pediatric patients with complex syndromes involving both medical or neurological and somatoform symptoms (e.g., a patient with both seizures and pseudoseizures).

In considering the treatment of such patients, it is essential to employ a model of consultation that takes into account multiple levels of consultation (Lewis, 1996), including the individual dynamics of the child,

and his or her experience of illness; the family dynamics; any psychopathology in a caregiver; the relationship(s) between the child and family and the hospital staff; and dynamics between levels of hospital personnel (e.g., between attending physicians and house staff, between physicians and nursing staff).

Psychotropic medication can only be considered after careful consultation with the child and/or family and liaison with the consultee, culminating in a diagnostic formulation that transcends merely a *Diagnostic and Statistical Manual of Mental Disorders, 4th ed.* (DSM-IV) diagnosis, and after the consideration of other treatment modalities.

Nonpharmacological treatment interventions might include alteration of visitation patterns for the child; behavioral interventions on the unit; involvement of other hospital staff, including Child Life staff or teachers, for example; other efforts to mobilize the child, including physical therapy; cognitive-behavioral interventions (including short-term psychotherapy for anxiety or depressive symptoms, or hypnotic interventions for pain, for example); efforts to help orient a delirious or cognitively impaired patient with a calendar and clock, for example; and efforts to communicate with patients who cannot speak using sign language or letter-boards (e.g., with an intubated but conscious patient). Even in the case of severely ill or debilitated patients, one must never forget that "there is a child in there." Medication is only an adjunctive treatment.

ASSESSMENT AND EVALUATION

Assessment and evaluation of the medically ill child or adolescent is often complicated in various ways by the physical state of the child:

1. The child is too weak to participate in a lengthy interview.
2. Irritability secondary to the effects of being ill and in the hospital affect the receptivity of the patient (or family) to being interviewed.

631

3. Medical illness or medication side effects may directly affect cognition; virtually all classes of medication have been implicated. In adult patients, glucocorticoids can impair memory at relatively low doses (Keenan et al., 1995; Newcomer et al., 1999), as there are postulated effects on hippocampal neurons. Newcomer et al., (1999) have reviewed the literature on illnesses in adults in which memory inversely correlates with cortisol levels, such as in Cushing's disease, Alzheimer's dementia, schizophrenia, and depression. There is no similar literature on the pediatric population. The risk of memory impairment puts chronic steroid treatment, such as that seen in certain pediatric rheumatologic disorders and severe asthmatics, for example, into a different perspective, however. Documentation of memory both before and during chronic steroid treatment might help determine detrimental effects in the pediatric population.

4. Medical illness commonly affects parameters such as sleep, appetite, and energy level that are often used in diagnostic assessment.

For these reasons, the interview of a medically ill pediatric patient is generally briefer than that of a physically healthy child. Because the illness biases psychiatric assessment, the consultant must rely heavily on premorbid history and other informants such as the parents, nurses, and primary care physician in assessing the meaning of current symptoms. Diagnostic criteria as supplied by DSM-IV should also be used.

Neuropsychological testing is generally not useful in the case of an evolving medical or neurological illness, but it can be useful in establishing a baseline assessment of cognitive function, such as in an oncology patient who will undergo intrathecal chemotherapy or CNS irradiation, or in a patient with hepatic encephalopathy who will undergo liver transplantation. Testing can later be repeated to be compare post-treatment results with pretreatment results.

The Mini Mental State Examination (Folstein et al., 1975) has been adapted and studied for use with children (Ouvrier et al., 1993; Besson and Labbe, 1997) and other screening tools to assess cognitive function in children have also been developed (Ouvrier et al., 1999). These tools are invaluable, as so often altered mental status in a child can be related to impaired cognitive function or early delirium.

USE OF PSYCHOPHARMACOLOGIC AGENTS IN MEDICALLY OR NEUROLOGICALLY ILL CHILDREN AND ADOLESCENTS

Principles of rational use of psychopharmacologic agents in this population should follow that of their general use—i.e., when possible, such treatment should be evidence based; the target symptoms cause significant distress and/or impairment; and the criteria for improvement should be objectively measured and documented (Kutcher, 2000). In addition, aspects specific to the medically compromised child should be taken into account—for example, the consequences of anxiety in a patient with severe asthma or cystic fibrosis, who oxygenates more poorly when anxious, or the potential consequences of noncompliance in depressed patients who are being "passively suicidal" through their attitude.

Lack of adherence or compliance is a major factor to consider in treating pediatric patients, especially medially ill adolescents, as has been well documented in treating a variety of conditions, such as diabetes, asthma, and organ transplantation. In pediatric patients, lack of adherence is approximated to be about 50 % (Cohen and Jermain, 1998). Treatment of these patients with psychopharmacologic agents can therefore be quite challenging, because of the lack of consistency of administration of both medical and psychiatric drugs. If possible, concrete methods of measuring compliance (serum drug levels or electronic monitoring) should be used. For example, Bender et al. (2000) electronically measured the extent to which a metered dose inhaler (MDI) was being used by asthmatic children. This monitoring was more accurate than self-report or measuring the weight of the canister for assessing compliance.

A "differential diagnosis" of lack of adherence should be undertaken to ascertain the underlying etiology, which can include lack of understanding of how to administer medication, access to the medication, logistic difficulties (such as the difficulty of administering medicines 3 or 4 times a day), lack of appreciation of the need for a drug if effects are not immediately seen, and side effects. Doses may be skipped, the incorrect dose may be given, or the medication may be discontinued improperly (Cohen and Jermain, 1998), making pill counts, diaries or logs of medication administration by the patient or family, and careful questioning by the treating clinician paramount.

Since medically ill children and adolescents are often taking multiple medications, ways of improving adherence, such as using pill boxes or other prepackaging methods, closer supervision, using simpler regimens (e.g., bid rather than tid dosing), and providing patient education and contracts, can be valuable (Litt, 1992).

Diagnostic Issues in the Medically Ill Pediatric Patient

Differential diagnosis in the medically ill patient involves untangling the effects of appropriate psychological distress in response to physical illness, untreated pain, comorbid psychiatric syndromes, medication side effects, and neuropsychiatric syndromes secondary to illness, such as delirium.

The child psychiatrist is often asked to ascertain the artificial dividing line between medical and psychiatric symptoms. To act effectively, the approach must be collaborative; the model, integrative; and the specific tools, both behavioral, to address adaptation and increasing functionality, and psychopharmacologic, to address specific symptoms, such as decreasing anxiety or improving the patient's energy state or mood.

Such an approach "de-pathologizes" the need for behavioral intervention, by focusing on the negative effects of stress on the course of an illness, using examples such as cardiovascular disease or peptic ulcer disease. This may help reframe pathological emotional response as a normal response to an abnormal situation. Studies on hypnosis, for example, show that children can be taught to increase the level of immunoglobulins in their saliva using hypnosis (Olness et al., 1989).

The pharmacological approach to using psychoactive medication in medically ill pediatric patients is thus predicated on a comprehensive formulation that attempts to tease apart psychiatric syndromes and psychopathology from symptoms of medical illness. In the more seriously medically ill patient, the etiology of altered mental status, or acute changes in mood, anxiety, or behavior should be considered medical in etiology until proven otherwise. In general, treatment of patients with medical conditions predisposing to psychiatric symptomatology should begin with treatment of the underlying medical conditions.

PSYCHOPHARMACOLOGICAL CONSIDERATIONS IN THREE SPECIFIC CLINICAL SYNDROMES

The Patient in Pain

Pain assessment in children and adolescents is a subject unto itself, and one that any clinician working with a child in pain must be familiar with (Franck et al., 2000). Treatment of pain in children and adolescents must include cognitive-behavioral interventions such as preparation and rehearsal, hypnosis, guided imagery, breathing exercises, muscle relaxation, and distraction; consideration of other complementary interventions such as acupuncture or biofeedback is common (Powers, 1999; Chen et al., 2000; Rusy and Weisman, 2000).

Psychopharmacologic treatment of pain in children has been the subject of recent reviews (Green and Ko-

walik, 1994; Leith and Weisman, 1997; Galloway and Yaster, 2000; The Medical Letter, 2000; see Table 47.1. Green and Kowalik (1994) have underscored the intricate relationship between pain and anxiety, and that between pain and depression.

Recently, more attention has been directed toward pain management in the terminal patient. Galloway and Yaster (2000) underscore the important point that pediatric pain is often undertreated, because of unrealistic concerns about addiction or therapeutic diversion, or concerns that pharmacologic treatment of pain somehow either represents "giving up" or may bring death sooner because of respiratory depression, for example. Choice of medication for pain in this population depends on the clinical context (as reviewed in Galloway and Yaster, [2000] pp. 716, 717) ; pediatric HIV patients in particular have specific pain management needs. In general, consideration should be given to topical anesthetics, conscious sedation, specific agents that treat acute pain or chronic pain, adjuvant medication, and agents that treat anxiety (anticipatory anxiety, such as preprocedural, or otherwise), or insomnia that is associated with pain. Galloway and Yaster (2000) advocate an approach to pain management that is multimodal at its onset, with cognitive-behavioral interventions being used along with nonsteroidal anti-inflammatory drugs (NSAIDS), local anesthetics, opioids, and adjuvants to limit pain perception and distress.

Topical anesthetics such as EMLA cream, which is a mixture of lidocaine and prilocaine, can be quite effective in reducing pain associated with venipunture or intravenous line insertion, circumcision, and laser treatment of port wine stains (Wilder, 2000).

Conscious sedation implies that patients have a depressed level of consciousness but nevertheless have intact protective reflexes, the ability to maintain their airway, and the ability to respond appropriately to requests and physical stimulation (Kennedy and Luhmann, 1999). Sedative agents familiar to psychiatrists that are used in this manner for procedures include chloral hydrate, given orally or rectally in a dose of 25 to 100 mg/kg; midazolam, given intramuscularly or intravenously in a dose of 0.05 to 0.15 mg/kg, rectally in a dose of 0.3 to 0.5 mg/kg, or orally in a dose of 0.2 to 0.75 mg/kg; and midazolam, which is felt to be preferable to diazepam for this purpose (Kennedy and Luhmann, 1999). Midazolam is also available in a nasal spray (Ljungman et al., 2000).

Green and Kowalik (1994) reported on the use of midazolam in two studies–in one, prior to laceration repairs, and in the other, in children with acute lymphocytic leukemia (ALL). In the laceration repair study (Hennes et al., 1990), a single 0.2 mg/kg dose of mid-

TABLE 47.1 *Medications Used To Treat Pain and Anxiety in Children and Adolescents*

Disorder	Medication	Dose	Comments	Reference
Cancer pain	Amitriptyline	0.5–1.5 mg/kg hs	Tumor invasion of nerve	Miser and Miser, 1989 (f)
	Amitriptyline	0.5–1.5 mg/kg hs	Cancer pain	Berde et al., 1993
	Doxepin	25–75 mg hs	Cancer pain	Snow et al., 1992
	Imipramine	0.3–0.4 mg/kg hs Every 2–3 days Up to 1–2 mg hs	Tumor invasion of nerve; doxepin and nortriptyline may also be considered	Miser and Miser, 1992
Postoperative pain	Lorazepam	0.25 mg q8h IV	Post-salpingo-oophorectomry Given alernating with small dose of burpenorphine	Richtsmeier et al., 1992
	Diazepam	2 mg po	11-year-old with cerebral palsy, mental retardation, post-hamstring release With concomitant morphine at 0.1 mg/kg q2h	Richtsmeier et al., 1992
Headache	Amitriptyline	25 mg/day for children 50 mg/day for adolsecents	Migraine	Berde et al., 1993
	Amitriptyline	10–20 mg hs Serium levels = 15–21 ng/mL	Migraine in children 5 to 42 months old	Elser and Woody, 1990 (E)
	Valproic acid	10–15 mg kg divided bid	Migraine	Prensky, 2001
Fibromyalgia	Amitriptyline	25 mg hs		Berde et al., 1993
Neuropathy	Amitriptyline	0.1 mg/kg/day 1–2 h before bedtime. Titrate to 0.5–2 mg/kg/day over 2–3 weeks	Diabetic neuropathy	Shannon and Berde, 1989 (G)
	Doxepin	0.1 mg/kg/day 1–2 h before bedtime. Titrate to 0.5–2 mg/kg/day over 2–3 weeks	Instead of amitriptyline if anticho-linergic side effects are not well tolerated	Shannon and Berde, 1989 (G)
	Amitriptyline	50 mg/day	Neuropathy secondary to vincris-tine in 7-year-old boy Resolution in 4 days	Heiligenstein and Steif, 1989 (H)
	Amitriptyline	25–100 mg/day	Neuropathy secondary to VE Pesid (VP-16) and cisplatin	Granowetter, 1993
	Amitriptyline	0.5–1.5 mg/kg hs	Vincristine induced, radiation plex-opathy and tumor invasion of nerve or plexus Works in 3–5 days	Miser and Miser, 1989
	Gabapentin	300–1200 mg tid	Neuropathy secondary to chemoth-erpeutic agents	
Phantom limb	Amitriptyline	5 mg hs	6-year-old patient with osteogenic sarcoma	Rogers, 1989
	Amitriptyline	Start with 25 mg/day Titrate up to maximum of 100 mg/day	Pain diminishes over a few days Need 3–6 months of treatment	Granowetter, 1992 (see Q)
	Gabapentin	14–40 mg/kg	6/7 children/young adults had pain resolve within 2 months	Rusy et al., 2001
Adjuvant pain medication	Lorazepam	25 μm/kg	Acute pain	Golianu, et al., 2000
Chronic pain	Carbamazepine	Begin at 4 mg/kg Tirate to maximum 16 mg/kg divided bid		Berde et al., 1993 Green and Kowalik, 1994

(continued)

TABLE 47.1 *(continued)*

Disorder	Medication	Dose	Comments	Reference
Reflex sympathetic Dystrophy	Gabapentin		11-year-old girl with refractory reflex sympathetic dystrophy	Tong and Nelson, 2000
Conscious sedation for procedures	Chloral hydrate	25–100 mg/kg po or rectally		
	Midazolam	0.05–0.15 mg/kg IM or IV		Kennedy and Luhmann, 1999
		0.3–0.5 mg/kg rectally		
		0.2–0.75 mg/kg po	Also available in a nasal spray	Ljungman et al., 2000
Laceration repairs	Midazolam	0.2 mg/kg	Used as a single dose	Hennes et al., 1990
	Midazolam	0.2 mg/kg	Used as a single dose prior to lumbar puncture or bone marrow aspiration	Friedman et al., 1991
Anticipatory and acute anxiety	Alprazolam	0.005 mg/kg, titrated to 0.003–0.075 mg/kg	In pediatric cancer patients	Pfefferbaum et al., 1987
Anticipatory nausea	Lorazepam	0.04–0.08 mg/kg	Lack of active metabolites	Galloway and Yaster, 2000
Potentiation of opioid analgesics	Methylphenidate Dextroamphetamine	2.5–10 mg bid 2.5–5 mg bid	Diminishes sedative effects of opioids as well	Yee and Berde, 1994

Adapted from Green, W. and Kowalite, S.C. (1997)

azolam was used as part of a placebo-controlled, double-blind study, resulting in 70 % reduction in anxiety in the treatment group. In a study of pediatric cancer patients (Friedman et al., 1991), a single 0.2 mg/kg dose of midazolem was given prior to lumbar puncture or bone marrow aspiration, resulting in a significant reduction in pain and anxiety-related behaviors in the treatment group. Benzodiazepines may also be effective as anxiolytics or hypnotics in the armamentarium for pain management or as premedication for procedures (Pfefferbaum et al., 1987; Pfefferbaum and Hagberg, 1993; Green and Kowalik, 1994). Green Kowalik (1994) noted Pfefferbaum et al., (1987) use of alprazolam for treatment of anticipatory and acute anxiety in pediatric cancer patients, with initial doses of 0.005 mg/kg being titrated to a range of 0.003–0.075 mg/kg. In the author's experience, small doses of lorazepam (0.5 to 1 mg) can be quite effective in these patients.

Acute pain is managed with either nonopioids such as acetaminophen, NSAIDs, or, when severe, opioids such as meperidine, morphine, methadone, hydromorphone, fentanyl, or sufentanil (Golianu et al., 2000). The latter are generally used parenterally, and when the patient is converted to oral analgesics, agents such as codeine, oxycodone, and hydrocodone are often used.

Tramadol is an opioid agonist that also inhibits the reuptake of both norepinephrine and serotonin, and is used to treat moderate pain in the pediatric patient, although there are few published reports on this population (Tobias, 2000). Psychopharmacological agents are most commonly used as adjuvant medication in pediatric patients with acute pain, with drugs such as lorazepam at 25 µg/kg often being effective (Golianu et al., 2000).

Psychostimulant medication can be useful in the treatment of severe, acute pain, such as that seen during a sickle cell crisis (Yaster et al., 2000). Dextroamphetamine and methylphenidate are also effective as adjuvants, as they have independent analgesic effects, and potentiate the effects of opioid analgesics. The increase in alertness afforded by the use of psychostimulants can also allow the use of larger doses of opioids (Yaster et al., 2000). Methylphenidate and dextroamphetamine have been used to diminish the sedative effects of opioid analgesic medication (Yee and Berde, 1991) in adolescent patients with malignancies or sickle crisis, and may also potentiate the effects of analgesics. Doses used by Yee and Berde (1991) were 2.5 to 10 mg bid of methylphenidate, or 2.5 to 5 mg bid of dextroamphetamine.

Antineuropathic agents include tricyclic antidepressants (TCAs), antiepileptic agents (AEDs), and clonidine. Other adjunctive medications include those given for anorexia or nausea, such as antihistamines, steroids, and antiserotonin (5-hydroxytryptamine) agents. Benzodiazepines can be given for anticipatory nausea, with lorazepam (0.04 to 0.08 mg/kg) being perhaps the most efficacious agent because of the absence of active metabolites (Galloway and Yaster, 2000). Although antidopaminergic agents such as chlorpromazine and promethazine may be useful because of their antiemetic, antipruritic, and sedative effects, caution is warranted when using these agents on account of potential dysphoria and extrapyramidal side effects.

More recently, gabapentin has been added to the arsenal of medications used for the treatment of chronic pain, along with other anticonvulsant drugs, such as carbamazepine and clonazepam, as used in the treatment of neuropathies in children (Berde et al., 1993; Green and Kowalik 1994).

The Pediatric Cancer Patient

Psychopharmacology in the pediatric cancer population has recently been reviewed by Spiegel (1998) and Slater (2002). A focus on treating specific symptoms, as opposed to a disorder-specific approach, has been recommended, with attention paid to potential cytochrome P450 drug interactions. Procedural phobias, PTSD, and separation anxiety are not uncommon in the pediatric cancer patient. Procedural phobias can be worsened by insomnia, and anxiety may be a concomitant of incompletely treated pain or represent an exacerbation of a premorbid condition. Anxiety can also be secondary to delirium, medication side effects, or metabolic sequelae of illness. Antihistamines or benzodiazepines may be used to treat insomnia, sedation, or generalized anxiety, although they may worsen mental status in the setting of delirium or cognitive impairment. Alprazolam may be given sublingually; midazolam, diazepam, and lorazepam may be given intramuscularly; diazepam and lorazepam may be given intravenously; and clonazepam is given orally and may be the anxiolytic of choice to be used on a more chronic basis. The selective serotonin reuptake inhibitors (SSRIs) have not been studied systematically in this population, although anecdotally they show promise in treating anxiety and depression in this population. Fluvoxamine in particular has been shown to be quite efficacious in treating anxiety in the nonmedically ill pediatric population (Research Unit on Pediatric Psychopharmacology Anxiety Study Group, 2001). The diagnosis of depression can be quite challenging in the pediatric cancer population because of the effects of illness, medication side effects, and hospitalization on children with cancer, making neurovegetative signs especially less reliable, since these factors can cause depressive symptoms. Sub syndromal PTSD, adjustment disorders, and pain can all be confused with major depressive disorder. Tricyclic antidepressants may be useful for treating mood and anxiety symptomatology in conjunction with insomnia and pain, although an-

ticholinergic (constipation, sedation, dry mouth, urinary retention) or cardiac side effects (orthostatic hypotension, potential effects on cardiac conduction) may make SSRIs the treatment of choice in most cases; the use of low TCA doses makes side effects less likely.

Delirium is not uncommon in the pediatric cancer patient, as it can be due to a number of factors, including primary disease, medication or radiation side effects, metabolic derangement, sepsis, prolonged intensive care unit (ICU) stays, drug withdrawal, or inadequately treated pain. Delirium should be part of the differential diagnosis of any abrupt change in mental status, such as intense anxiety, somnolence, psychosis, confusion, agitation, or aggressive behavior. Treatment must include identification and treatment of the underlying etiology.

Psychopharmacologic treatment is generally most effectively carried out with high-potency neuroleptics such as haloperidol (Lipowski, 1990) or risperidone, which was reported in a case study to be effective in the treatment of delirium in a 14 year old boy (Sipahimalani and Masaud, 1997). Haloperidol can be given parenterally, and clinical lore has it that when given via his route, it has significantly few anticholinergic and hypotensive side effects (Trzepacz, 1996). However, there have been reports of significant QTc prolongation and torsade de pointes as complications of high-dose intravenous haloperidol therapy (DiSalvo and O'Gara, 1995, Hatta et al., 2001); hypotension and extrapyramidal side effects have also been reported (Blitzstein and Brandt, 1997, Franco-Bronson and Gajwani, 1999). The initial intravenous or oral dose of haloperidol for a child 6 to 12 years of age is 0.5 mg for mild agitation, 1.0 mg for moderate agitation, and 2 mg for severe agitation (Williams, 1996). In adolescents, this author would recommend beginning with 1 mg for mild agitation, 2 mg for moderate agitation, and 3–5 mg for severe agitation, depending on the size of the patient, with doses given either orally or intravenously. Risperidone may be used orally, beginning with a dose of 0.25 to 0.5 mg, and repeating this twice daily as needed. The clinician should be vigilant in watching for potential side effects such as parkinsonism, dystonic reactions, akathisia, effects on the QT interval (Welch and Chue, 2000), and neuroleptic malignant syndrome (seen more commonly in patients with CNS disease).

Since pediatric cancer survivors are at greater risk for attentional disorders, mood disorders, and PTSD, the clinician may need to include psychopharmacolgic treatment along with cognitive, behavioral, and milieu interventions. Although most psychiatric medications have not been studied in this population, judicious use of such agents, with close attention to drug interactions and side effects, may be warranted in the setting of significant emotional or behavioral symptoms.

Use of Antidepressants in Unexplained, Idiopathic Syndromes with Physical Symptomatology

O'Malley et al. (1999) have reviewed the adult literature on the use of antidepressant medication in the treatment of etiologically unexplained syndromes, including fibromyalgia, chronic fatigue syndrome, functional gastrointestinal syndromes, idiopathic pain, tinnitus, and headache. Despite there being a clear limitation in controlling for the effects of treating depressive illness associated with these syndromes, pooled data suggest the efficacy of antidepressant agents; patients on antidepressants are, overall, three times more likely to improve compared with patients treated with placebo. Goodnick and Sandoval (1993) reviewed the treatment of chronic fatigue and related disorders with psychotropic agents, noting that doses typically used in these studies (all with adults) were typically lower than those generally used in the treatment of psychiatric disorders. Serotonergic agents (such as clomipramine) seemed more effective in treating pain rather than depression, and adrenergic agents (e.g., bupropion) are more effective for depressive symptoms.

This research has not been replicated in pediatrics. This author has anecdotally found efficacy of antidepressant agents in pediatric patients with chronic fatigue, fibromyalgia, and functional gastrointestinal disorders. Most commonly, SSRIs such as sertraline are used in low doses (12.5–25 mg). While one must use caution in treating patients empirically in a non–evidence-based fashion, unexplained illness carries with it significant morbidity in terms of both disability and potential iatrogenic disorders, because of the multiple invasive tests, pharmacologic interventions, and procedures to which these patients are exposed. In this setting, consideration of empirical antidepressant trials may be warranted.

SUGGESTED TREATMENT ALGORITHM

Figure 47.1 provides a suggested treatment algorithm for use of psychopharmacologic interventions in the medically ill child or adolescent. The use of psychiatric medication in this population must clearly be seen as adjunctive treatment to other nonpharmacologic interventions. Parents are often wary of additional medications to what is often an already complicated medical regimen. In addition, there may be negative stigma associated with using medications directed at mood or behavior. The medical team may either be preferentially receptive to pharmacologic recommendations from the psychiatrist or wary of medications that they may find unfamiliar.

For these reasons, it is essential that a comprehensive evaluation be done, and that an overall intervention "package" be presented to both the family and medical team. Nonpharmacologic interventions should be discussed first, and only then should psychiatric medication be discussed. The latter should be addressed in a fashion that places medication within the broader therapeutic context, with an emphasis on improving the comfort level of the patient, and treating symptoms that are distressing, impairing, or having a negative impact on the medical treatment.

Target symptoms and the means of assessing them, the duration of treatment, and potential side effects should be discussed openly. The potential side effects of *not* treating troubling emotional or behavioral symptoms that might respond to medication should also be discussed. The treatment alliance with both the family and the medical team is essential to psychopharmacologic treatment in this population. In addition, an important job of the psychiatric consultant is to determine which medications can be *removed* or *reduced* in dosage, and which ones may be adversely affecting a patient's mental status.

The following case provides an example of treating a young patient in pain, using elements of the proposed treatment algorithm. A consultation was requested for a 14-year-old male in with ALL in the ICU who seemed lethargic, depressed, and disoriented. The consultant's initial recommendations were to help orient the patient with a large clock and calendar, with frequent verbal reminders, and environmental interventions directed at trying to normalize his disrupted sleep–wake cycle (such as earplugs at night). The pharmacologic recommendations, which were made in conjunction with the pain consultant, were to discontinue the patient's lorazepam and zaleplon, to slowly taper his midazolam and fentanyl, and to begin gabapentin for pain management. Finally, once these changes were made, treatment with low-dose dextroamphetamine was considered. When these recommendations were carried out in sequence, the patient's level of alertness increased dramatically, his confusion abated, and his mood and energy level improved considerably, while maintaining adequate pain control. This was done with careful ex-

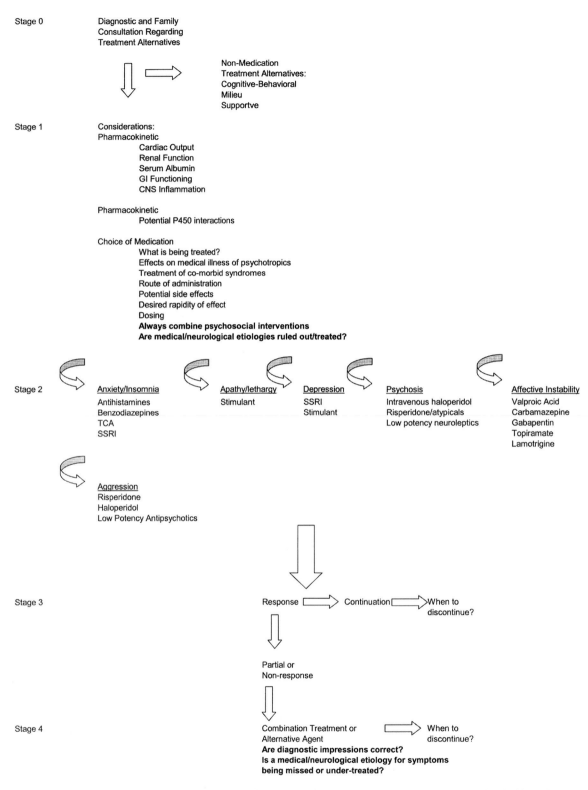

FIGURE 47.1 Suggested algorithm for the use of psychotropic medications in the medically ill child or adolescent. CNS, central nervous system; GI, gastrointestinal; SSRI, selective serotonin reuptake inhibitor; TLA, tricyclic antidepressant.

planation to his parents on a day-to-day basis, who were quite grateful for psychiatry's involvement.

It is very important to choose medications with the least possibility of making an ill pediatric patient suffer additional morbidity from side effects to medication directed at mood or behavior. For these reasons, mood stabilizers such as lamotrigine (which carries with it the risk of a severely toxic rash) should be seen only as third- or fourth-line agents.

Close attention to the QTC interval should be paid whenever an antipsychotic agent is used, as virtually all of these agents have been reported to cause torsades de pointes. Lower-potency antipsychotics carry with them the risk of worsening or precipitating delirium due to anticholinergic side effects, as well as having a greater risk of cardiotoxic effects. Benzodiazepines can cause paradoxical disinhibition or worsen delirium in susceptible patients, and the patient must be closely monitored for potential withdrawal effects if they are discontinued following chronic use.

DISCONTINUATION OF PSYCHOACTIVE MEDICATION

Several factors should be part of the decision-making process regarding the length of time a medically ill child or adolescent should remain on psychoactive medication:

1. What is the relationship of the psychiatric symptoms or syndrome to the underlying medical illness? Were the symptoms premorbid, secondary to, or coincident with the medical illness? Is there a family history of similar syndromes in nonmedically ill family members that might warrant consideration of treating the psychiatric disorder more independently from the medical condition?

2. What is the status of the underlying medical condition? Has the syndrome resolved, such as in the case of a delirium, the anxious anticipatory response to a procedure, or steroid boost for organ rejection; or is the medical illness chronic (e.g., HIV or diabetes mellitus)?

3. How severe was the psychiatric syndrome? For example did the mania in a transplant recipient occur during a steroid boost, or is there psychosis and suicidal ideation in a patient with hyperthyroidism?

4. What is the potential risk of a relapse or recurrence from discontinuing medication. For example, should successful antidepressant treatment of an or-

gan transplant recipient who had previously been noncompliant as part of passive suicidal ideation?

In general, following guidelines established for the treatment of other child psychiatric disorders would seem to be the most prudent initial approach to the question of discontinuation, with the caveats listed above. In the author's experience, continuing treatment for at least 6 months to a year following successful treatment of a psychiatric syndrome (assuming that the symptoms or syndrome was not situational, such as anxiety prior to a procedure or a resolved delirium) would seem to be a reasonable starting point.

SUMMARY AND CONCLUSIONS

Psychopharmacologic treatment of the medically ill child or adolescent often involves little empirical basis for decision making. Clinicians must attempt to extrapolate assistance from the literature on medically ill adults and from literature on use of psychoactive drugs in the medically healthy population, knowing that such extrapolations are not always evidence based. Medically ill children are not immune to psychopathology and emotional symptoms that may benefit or even require psychopharmacologic intervention. In fact, there is a higher incidence of psychopathology in children with chronic illness, especially if there is CNS involvement. Rutter et al. (1970) found an overall prevalence of psychiatric illness in 12% of a chronically ill pediatric population and in 34% of the same group if there was CNS disease. Treating these children involves a synthesis of data on the use of psychiatric medications in children, knowledge of how pharmacokinetics and pharmacodynamics may be altered in medical syndromes or in the presence of complicated medical regimens, and, above all, a multidisciplinary effort of close collaboration of all professionals involved in a child's care.

REFERENCES

Bender, B., Wamboldt, F.S., O'Connor, S.L., Rand, C., Szefler, S., Milgrom, H., and Wamboldt, M.Z. (2000) Measurement of children's asthma medication adherence by self report, mother report, canister weight, and Doser CT. *Ann Allergy Asthma Immunol* 85:416–421.

Berde, C.B., Sethan, N., and Koka, B.V. (1993) Pediatric pain management. In: Warfield, C.A., ed. *Principles and Practice of Pain Management*. New York: McGraw-Hill, pp. 325–346.

Besson, P.S., and Labbe, E.E. (1997) Use of the modified mini-mental state examination with children. *J Child Neurol* 12:455–460.

Blitzstein, S.M. and Brandt, G.T. (1997) Extrapyramidal symptoms from intravenous haloperidol in the treatment of delirium. *Am J Psychiatry* 154:1474–1475.

Chen, E., Joseph, M.H., and Zeltzer, L.K. (2000) Behavioral and cognitive interventions in the treatment of pain in children. *Pediatr Clin North Am* 47:513–525.

Cohen, L.J. and Jermain, D.M. (1998) Neuropsychopharmacology I: basic principles. In: Coffey C.E. and Brumback R.A., eds. *Textbook of Pediatric Neuropsychiatry*. Washington, DC: American Psychiatric Press, pp. 1275–1286.

Di Salvo, T.G. and O'Gara, P.T. (1995) Torsade de pointes caused by high-dose intravenous haloperidol in cardiac patients. *Clin Cardiol* 18:285–290.

Elser, J.M. and Woody, R.C. (1990) Headache in the infant and young child. *Headache* 30:366–368.

Emmanuel, N.P., Lydiard, R.B., and Crawford, M. (1997) Treatment of irritable bowel syndrome with fluvoxamine. *Am J Psychiatry* 154:711–712.

Folstein, M.F., Folstein, S.E., and McHugh, P.R. (1975) "Mini-mental state." A practical method for grading the cognitive state of patients for the clinician. *J Psychiatr Res* 12:189–198.

Franck, L.S., Greenberg, C.S., and Stevens, B. (2000) Pain assessment in infants and children. *Pediatr Clin North Am* 47:487–512.

Franco-Bronson, K., and Gajwani, P. (1999) Hypotension associated with intravenous haloperidol and imipenem. *J Clin Psychopharmacol* 19:480–481.

Friedman, A.G., Mulhern, R.K., Fairclough, D., et al. (1991) Midazolam premedication for pediatric bone marrow aspiration and lumbar puncture. *Med Pediatr Oncol* 19:499–504.

Galloway, K.S., and Yaster, M. (2000) Pain and symptom control in terminally ill children. *Pediatr Clin North Am* 47:711–746.

Gershon, M. *The Second Brain*. New York: HarperCollins, 1998.

Golianu, B., Krane, E.J., Galloway, K.S., et al. (2000) Pediatric acute pain management. *Pediatr Clin North Am* 47:559–587.

Goodnick, P.J. and Sandoval, R. (1993) Psychotropic treatment of chronic fatigue syndrome and related disorders. *J Clin Psychiatry* 54:13–20.

Granowetter, L., Rosenstock, J.G., Packer, R.J. (1992). Enhanced cis-platinum neurotoxicity in pediatric patients with brain tumors. J. Neurooncol 1983; 1:293–297.

Green, W. and Kowalik, S.C. (1994) Psychopharmacologic treatment of pain and anxiety in the pediatric patient. *Child Adolesc Psychiatr Clin North Am* 3:465–484.

Hatta, K., Takahashi, T., Nakamura, H., Yamashiro, H., Asukai, N., Matsuzaki, I., and Yonezawa, Y. (2001) The association between intravenous haloperidol and prolonged QT interval. *J Clin Psychopharmacol* 21:257–261.

Heiligenstein, E. and Steif, B.L. (1989) Tricyclics for pain. *J Am Acad Child Adolesc Psychiatry* 28:804–805.

Hennes, H.M., Wagner, V., Bonadio, W.A., et al. (1990) The effect of oral midazolam on anxiety of preschool children during laceration repair. *Ann Emerg Med* 19:1006–1009.

Jackson, J.L., O'Malley, P.C., Tomkins, G., et al. (2000) Treatment of functional gastrointestinal disorders with antidepressants: a meta-analysis. *Am J Med* 108:65–72.

Jensen, P.S. (1998) Ethical and pragmatic issues in the use of psychotropic agents in young children. *Can J Psychiatry* 43:585–588.

Keenan, P.A., Jacobson, M.W., Soleymani, R.M., and Newcomeer, J.W. (1995) Commonly used therapeutic doses of glucocorticoids impair explicit memory. *Ann N Y Acad Sci* 761:400–402.

Kennedy, R.M., and Luhmann, J.D. (1999) The "ouchless emergency department." Getting closer: advances in decreasing distress during painful procedures in the emergency department. *Pediatr Clin North Am* 46:1215–1247.

Kutcher, S. (2000) Practical clinical issues regarding child and adolescent psychopharmacology. *Child Adolesc Clin North Am Psychopharmacol* 9:245–260.

Leith, P.J. and Weisman, S.J. (1997) Pharmacologic interventions for pain management in children. *Child Adolesc Psychiatr Clin North Am* 6:797–816.

Lewis, M. (1996) The consultation process in child and adolescent psychiatric consultation-liaison in pediatrics. In: Lewis, M., ed. *Child and Adolescent Psychiatry: A Comprehensive Textbook, 2nd ed.* Baltimore: Williams and Wilkins, pp. 935–939.

Lipowski, Z.J. (1990) *Delirium: Acute Confusional States.* New York: Oxford University Press.

Litt, I.F. (1992) Compliance with pediatric medication regimens. In: Yaffe, S.J. and Aranda, J.V., eds. *Pediatric Pharmacology: Therapeutic Principles in Practice, 2nd ed.* Philadelphia: W.B. Saunders., pp. 45–54.

Ljungman, G., Kreuger, A., Andreasson, S., et al. (2000) Midazolam nasal spray reduces procedural anxiety in children. *Pediatrics* 105 (1 Pt 1):73–78.

Miser, A.W. and Miser J.S. (1989). The treatment of cancer pain in children. *Pediatr Clin North Am* 36:979–999.

Miser, A.W. and Miser, J.S. (1993) Management of childhood cancer pain. In: Pizzo, P.A., Poplack, O., eds. *Principles and Practice of Pediatric Oncology, ed 2.* Philadelphia: JB Lippincott, pp. 1039–1050.

Newcomer, J.W., Selke, G., Melson, A.K., Hershey, T., Craft, S., Richards, K., and Alderson, A.L. (1999). Decreased memory performance in healthy humans induced by stress-level cortisol treatment. *Arch Gen Psychiatry* 56:527–533.

O'Malley, P.G., Jackson, J.L., Santoro, J., Tomkins, G., Balden, E., and Kroenke, K. (1999) Antidepressant therapy for unexplained symptoms and symptom syndromes. *J Fam Pract* 48:980–990.

Offord, D.R., Boyle, M.H., Szatmari, P., Rae-Grant, N.I., Links, P.S., Cadman, D.T., Byles, J.A., Crawford, J.W., Blum, H.M., Byrne, C., et al. (1917). Ontario Child Health Study. II. Six-month prevalence of disorder and rates of service utilization. *Arch Gen Psychiatry* 44:832–836.

Olness, K., Culbert, T., and Uden, D. (1989) Self-regulation of salivary immunoglobulin A by children. *Pediatrics* 83:66–71.

Ouvrier, R., Hendy, J., Bornholt, L., and Black, F.H. (1999). SYSTEMS: School-Years Screening Test for the Evaluation of Mental Status. *Child Neurol* 14:772–780.

Ouvrier, R.A., Goldsmith, R.F., Ouvrier, S., and Williams, I.C. (1993) The value of the mini-mental state examination in childhood: a preliminary study. *J Child Neurol* 8:145–148.

Pfefferbaum, B. and Hagberg, C.A. (1993) Pharmacological management of pain in children. *J Am Acad Child Adolesc Psychiatry* 32:235–242.

Pfefferbaum, G., Overall, J.E., Boren, H.A., et al. (1987) Alprazolam in the treatment of anticipatory and acute situational anxiety in children with cancer. *J Am Acad Child Adolesc Psychiatry* 26:532–535.

Powers, S.W. (1999) Empirically supported treatments in pediatric psychology: procedure-related pain. *J Pediatr Psychol* 24:131–145.

Prensky, A. (2001) Childhood migraine headache syndromes. *Curr Treatment Options Neurol* 3:257–270.

Research Unit on Pediatric Psychopharmacology (RUPP) Anxiety Study Group (2001) Fluvoxamine for the treatment of anxiety disorders in children and adolescents. *N Engl J Med* 344:1279–1285.

Rogers, A.G. (1989) Use of amitriptyline (Elavil) for phantom limb pain in younger children. *J Pain Symptom Manage* 4:96.

Richtsmeier, A.J., Barkin, R.L., and Alexander, M. (1992) Benzodiazepines for acute pain in children. *J Pain Sympt Manage* 7:492–495.

Rusy, L.M., Troshynski, T.J., and Weisman, J. (2001) Gabapentin in phantom limb pain management in children and young adults: report of seven cases. *J Pain Symptom Manage* 21:78–82.

Rusy, L.M., and Weisman, S.J. (2000) Complementary therapies for acute pediatric pain management. *Pediatr Clin North Am* 47: 589–599.

Rutter, M., Tizard, J., and Whitmore, K. (1970) *Education, Health and Behavior*. New York: John Wiley and Sons.

Shannon, M. and Berde, C.B. (1989) Pharmacologic management of pain in children and adolescents. *Pediatr Clin North Am* 36:855–871.

Sipahimalani, A. and Masand, P. S. (1997) Use of risperidone in delirium: case reports. *Ann Clin Psychiatry* 9:105–107.

Slater, J. A. (2002) Psychiatric Issues in Pediatric Cancer. In: Lewis, M., ed. *Child and Adolescent Psychiatry: A Comprehensive Textbook, 3rd Edition*. Baltimore: William and Wilkins.

Snow, B.R., Gusmorine, P., and Pinter, I. (1992) Behavioral medicine and cancer: A clinical guide. In: Lewis, M.M., ed. *Musculoskeletal Oncology: A Multidisciplinary Approach*. Philadelphia: WB Saunders, pp. 449–463.

Spiegel, I. (1998) Pediatric psychopharmacology. In: Holland, J., ed. *Psycho-oncology*. New York: Oxford University Press, pp. 954–961.

The Medical Letter, Inc. (2000) Drugs for pain. 42 (1085): 73–78.

Tobias, J.D. (2000) Weak analgesics and nonsteroidal anti-inflammatory agents in the management of children with acute pain. *Pediatr Clin North Am* 47:527–543.

Tong, H.C. and Nelson, V.S. (2000) Recurrent and migratory reflex sympathetic dystrophy in children. *Pediatr Rehabil* 4:87–89.

Trzepacz, P.T. (1996) Delirium. Advances in diagnosis, pathophysiology, and treatment. *Psychiatr Clin North Am* 19:429–448.

Vitiello, B. (1998) Pediatric psychopharmacology and the interaction between drugs and the developing brain. *Can J Psychiatry* 43: 582–584.

Warnock, J.K. (1997) Nefazodone-induced hypoglycemia in a diabetic patient with major depression. *Am J Psychiatry* 154:288–289.

Welch R. and Chue, P. (2000) Antipsychotic agents and QT changes. *J Psychiatry Neurosci* 25:154–160.

Wilder, R.T. (2000) Local anesthetics for the pediatric patient. *Pediatr Clin North Am* 47:545–558.

Williams, D.T. (in press) Neuropsychiatric signs, symptoms, and syndromes. In: Lewis, M., ed. *Child and Adolescent Psychiatry: A Comprehensive Textbook, 3rd ed*. Baltimore: Williams and Wilkins, pp. 344–349.

Williams, D.T. (1996) Neuropsychiatric signs, symptoms, and syndromes. In: Lewis, M., ed. *Child and Adolescent Psychiatry: A Comprehensive Textbook, 2nd ed*. Baltimore: Williams and Wilkins, pp. 636–650.

Yaster, M., Kost-Byerly, S., and Maxwell, L.G. (2000) The management of pain in sickle cell disease. *Pediatr Clin North Am* 47: 699–710.

Yee, J.D. and Berde, C.B. (1994) Dextroamphetamine or methylphenidate as adjuvants to opioid analgesia for adolescents with cancer. *J Pain Symptom Manage* 9:122–125.

48 | Psychopharmacology during pregnancy: infant considerations

ELIZABETH A. WALTER AND C. NEILL EPPERSON

Over 10 million women in the United States will suffer from the symptoms of mental illness during their child-bearing years (Bourdon et al., 1992; U.S. Census Bureau, 2000) and more than 50% of pregnancies are unplanned. These two facts emphasize the importance of educating women's health care providers regarding the risks associated with mental illness and the medications used to treat these disorders.

As all psychoactive medications readily cross the placenta, the impact on the fetus of any medication prescribed to a pregnant woman must be considered and discussed. Documentation that the patient is capable of weighing and understanding the risks and benefits of taking medication during pregnancy should be recorded in the patient's medical record. Adverse effects to the fetus associated with drug exposure in utero can be organized into three general classes: (1) fetal teratogenicity, (2) neonatal toxicity, and (3) behavioral teratogenicity. Medications are considered teratogenic when exposure to the drug during organogenesis (first 12 weeks of gestation) results in an increased incidence of major birth defects compared with the baseline risk in the general population. The incidence of major birth defects in the United States is 2%–4%, with the cause of 65%–70% being unknown (American Medical Association, 1983). *Neonatal toxicity* refers to difficulties in physical and behavioral adjustment shortly after delivery, while *behavioral teratogenicity* refers to long-term neurobehavioral disturbances related to antenatal drug exposure.

The Food and Drug Administration (FDA) classifies medication into five categories—A, B, C, D, and X—which reflect the degree of risk to the fetus, based on available animal and human data (Physicians Desk Reference, 1995). Experts believe that this rating system can be misleading because it does not adequately elucidate the differences between risk categories (Teratology Society, 1994). A FDA subcommittee and the Office of Research on Women's Health of the National Institutes of Health are reviewing these guidelines.

While exposure to psychiatric drugs possibly presents risk to the developing fetus, exposure to the sequelae of maternal mental illness is not without its adverse consequences. Symptoms affecting the unborn child can be as overt as deliberate maternal self-harm, with death or injury to the fetus, or they can be more insidious, revealing themselves in the form of poorer attention to prenatal care issues or participation in unsafe behaviors. When considering whether to continue medications when a woman with mental illness finds she is pregnant or wishing to become pregnant, both she and her clinicians should consider the risk of relapse in someone with her specific disorder and her particular treatment history. Numerous studies have documented high rates of relapse for schizophrenia (Dencker et al., 1986; Carpenter et al., 1990), anxiety (Pollack and Smoller, 1995), and mood disorders (Suppes et al., 1991; Kupfer et al., 1992) when drug therapy is discontinued.

Pregnancy does not protect a woman from mental illness, nor does it ameliorate the symptoms. Affective disturbance is not uncommon during pregnancy; there are high rates of recurrence of both mania and bipolar depression (Krener et al., 1989; Finnerty et al., 1996; Viguera et al., 2000) as well as unipolar depression (Gotlib et al., 1989). The prevalence rate for unipolar depression (10%) is similar in pregnant and nonpregnant women (O'Hara, 1986; Gotlib et al., 1989). A number of studies document an association between pregnancy and the onset of obsessive-compulsive symptoms (Ingram, 1961; Buttolph and Holland, 1990; Neziroglu et al., 1992), while other studies report continued or worsening symptoms of panic disorder (Cohen et al., 1996; Ware and DeVane, 1990; Northcott and Stein, 1994). Furthermore, mounting evidence suggests that untreated symptoms may lead to medically adverse outcomes. For example, placental abruption (Cohen et al., 1989) has been reported as a consequence of panic disorder, and depression and anxiety were associated with an increased risk for developing preeclampsia (Kurki et al., 2000).

This chapter aims to provide a review of the literature summarizing the effects of in utero psychotropic medication exposure on the developing fetus, newborn, and child. Studies of psychotropic medications in pregnancy from 1966 to 1995 were extensively reviewed by Altshulter and colleagues (1996). This chapter will summarize those findings when appropriate, and focus primarily on data not included in their review. On the basis of this information, we will conclude by providing treatment recommendations about the use of frequently prescribed psychotropic medication during pregnancy. Although of substantial and related import, a comprehensive review of the literature regarding the use of psychotropic medications in lactating women could not be included here. The authors refer the interested reader to two recent reviews on the topic (Yoshida et al., 1999; Burt et al., 2001).

EMPIRICAL DATA

Antidepressants

Selective serotonin reuptake inhibitors

Four prospective studies of antidepressant exposure during pregnancy compared with nonteratogen-exposed controls (NTECs) have been conducted since 1993. In the first of these studies, Pastuzsak et al. (1993) compared the pregnancy outcomes of 128 first-trimester fluoxetine-exposed infants with the outcomes of 74 infants with first-trimester exposure to tricyclic antidepressants (TCAs) and NTECs (defined as women exposed to environmental agents or medications that do not increase the baseline teratogenic risk). Their investigation revealed no difference in the rates of major malformations in the antidepressant-exposed groups compared with NTECs.

Chambers and colleagues (1996) followed 228 women who were either exposed early (first or second trimester) or late (third trimester) in their pregnancy to fluoxetine and compared them to NTECs. There was no increase in the rate of major anomalies in the fluoxetine-exposed groups, although there were a number of differences between the groups. First, there was an increased incidence of three or more minor malformations (defined as having no cosmetic or functional importance) in the fluoxetine-exposed infants compared

to controls (15.5% vs. 6.5% controls; $p = 0.03$). Secondly, late-exposed infants had higher rates of premature delivery (before 37 weeks gestation) than the early-exposed or control groups (14.3% vs. 4.1% vs. 5.9%, respectively; $p = 0.03$). Excluding preterm infants, rates of admission to special care nurseries was 23% of infants born to the late-exposed group compared with early-exposed (9.5%) or controls (6.3%) ($p = 0.01$). Full-term, late-exposed infants had lower birth weights and decreased lengths than either the early-exposed or control groups. Maternal weight gain was approximately 3 kg less in the late-exposed group.

Nulman et al. (1997) evaluated women exposed across pregnancy to TCAs, fluoxetine, or NTECs and found no difference in neurodevelopment (global IQ, temperament, mood, arousability, activity level, distractibility, or language, and behavioral development) in preschool children. There were no significant differences in rates of perinatal complications or major malformations between these groups. Finally, Kulin and colleagues (1998) studied pregnancy outcomes in 267 women exposed to either sertraline, paroxetine, or fluvoxamine, primarily in the first trimester. Compared to a healthy control group, exposure to these other Selective serotonin reuptake inhibitors (SSRIs) was not associated with an increase in fetal malformations, miscarriage, still birth, prematurity, or changes in birth weight. A number of other reports have not found an increased rate of major malformations with the use of SSRIs (Rosa, 1994; McElhatton et al., 1996; Goldstein et al., 1997; Ericson et al., 1999). A postmarketing report from the manufacturer (Eli Lilly) shows no increase in perinatal complications after third-trimester exposure to fluoxetine (Goldstein, 1995).

Studies in rats and rabbits demonstrate that in utero exposure to fluoxetine does not produce physical deformities in the offspring or affect fetal viability or litter size, thus suggesting no physical teratogenic effects (Byrd and Markham, 1994). Other reports evaluating chemical teratogenicity have found changes in brain serotonin receptor binding and density (Cabrera and Battaglia, 1994) as well as alterations in the density of serotonin transporters after prenatal exposure to fluoxetine (Cabrera-Vera et al., 1997). The significance of these changes and their clinical implications for humans, however, are unclear. Studies in rats evaluating behavioral teratogenicity after in utero exposure to fluoxetine or paroxetine do not indicate adverse effects on behavioral paradigms (Vorhees et al., 1994; Coleman et al., 1999). Manufacturers' data regarding pregnancy outcomes in their preclinical studies reveal an association between maternal exposure to high doses of some of the SSRIs and decreased maternal weight gain, pup birth weight, increased stillbirths, and pup deaths. Again, the significance of these findings in relationship to human pregnancies is unclear.

Tricyclic antidepressants

Altshuler and colleagues (1996) reviewed 13 studies assessing the risk of congenital malformations after first-trimester exposure to TCAs. In this analysis, first-trimester exposure to these agents was not associated with an increase in congenital defects. Two studies evaluating women with first-trimester exposure to TCAs and comparing this to all births in the population found no increased rates of major malformations (McElhatton et al., 1996; Ericson et al., 1999). Animal studies suggest that fetal exposure to these antidepressants can result in changes in offspring characteristics such as decreased birth weight (Coyle, 1975; Jason et al., 1981), although this is not a consistent finding (Ali et al., 1986).

In rare instances, infants exposed to TCAs through delivery have developed a neonatal withdrawal syndrome. Symptoms can include jitteriness (Eggermont, 1973), transient myoclonus (Bloem et al., 1999), seizure (Cowe et al., 1982), tachypnea, tachycardia, difficulty feeding, diaphoresis, and irritability (Webster, 1973). Anticholinergic effects of TCAs include gastrointestinal stasis and bladder distension (Wisner and Perel, 1988). Two studies have evaluated behavioral teratogenicity. Nulman et al. (1997) found no differences in global IQ, language development, or behavioral development among three groups of preschool children exposed to either fluoxetine, TCAs, or NTEC in utero. Motor and behavioral function after antenatal exposure to TCAs was normal (Misri and Sivertz, 1991).

Behavioral abnormalities in rodent studies include decreased social (File and Tucker, 1984) and environmental interactions (Coyle, 1975; Jason et al., 1981). Neurochemical abnormalities including alterations in adrenergic receptor binding (De Ceballos et al., 1985b; Ali et al., 1986), dopamine receptors (De Ceballos et al., 1985a), and serotonin receptors (De Ceballos et al., 1985b) as well as decreased dopamine levels (Jason et al., 1981) have been documented in animals after fetal exposure to these agents. The significance of these animal findings as it relates to human development is uncertain.

Other antidepressants

The Collaborative Perinatal Project followed the outcome of 21 infants exposed to monoamine oxidase inhibitors (MAOIs) during pregnancy. Three infants had major anomalies (Heinonen et al., 1977). Alternatively, in case reports, two infants exposed to phenelzine across pregnancy did not have any congenital anomalies (Pavy et al., 1995; Gracious and Wisner, 1997). One, albeit dated, animal study with phenelzine showed increased mortality and stillbirths (Werboff et al., 1961), although this finding is not uniform across all agents in this class (Poulson and Robson, 1963). An infant exposed to phenelzine throughout pregnancy did not show any abnormalities in growth or development during a 16-month follow-up period (Gracious and Wisner, 1997).

Scant data exist about the effects of trazodone, nefazodone, venlafaxine, or mirtazapine. Limited animal data do not suggest teratogenicity; however, little or no human data are available. Reports on individual agents have been reviewed by Briggs and colleagues (1998).

Mood-Stabilizing Agents

Lithium

In 1976, a final report from the International Register of Lithium Babies contained information on 225 infants exposed to lithium in the first trimester. Cardiovascular anomalies occurred in 18 (8%) of the newborns, of which 6 (2.7%) had Ebstein's anomaly (Weinstein, 1976). A comprehensive review of this report and the multiple studies that have been conducted since (Cohen et al., 1994) revealed that the risk of congenital defects after in utero exposure to lithium is less than previously anticipated. Currently, the risk for Ebstein's anomaly after first-trimester exposure to lithium is estimated to be 1 in 1000 (0.1%) (Altshuler et al., 1996), or 10–20 times greater than the general population risk of 1 in 20,000 (Weinstein, 1976). Thus, the absolute risk for Ebstein's anomaly is small.

In several case reports and small case series, lithium exposure in the second and third trimester has been associated with "floppy baby" syndrome; characterized by hypotonia and cyanosis. Other perinatal effects that have been reported with near-term maternal lithium treatment are bradycardia, thyroid abnormalities, atrial flutter, electrocardiographic (EKG) abnormalities, enlarged heart and liver, diabetes insipidus, polyhydramnios, seizures, shock, and gastrointestinal bleeding. These effects have been summarized by Briggs et al. (1998) and most have been self-limiting, resolving within 1–2 weeks of delivery. A small study that relied on parental reports to evaluate neurobehavioral development after second-or third-trimester exposure to lithium revealed no significant developmental differences between the lithium-exposed children and their non-exposed siblings (Schou, 1976).

Antiepileptic drugs

Data evaluating the teratogenic effects of in utero exposure to antiepileptic drugs (AEDs) have been obtained from children born to women with epilepsy. The incidence of children with birth defects born to women with seizure disorders is at least two to three times the population average of about 2% (Kelly, 1984). It is uncertain to what extent this increase is caused by genetic factors associated with epilepsy, prenatal exposure to AEDs, or a combination of these factors (Shapiro et al., 1976). Prospective studies, however, suggest that excess teratogenicity is attributable to AEDs rather than to epilepsy (Jäger-Roman et al., 1986; Kaneko et al., 1988). Animal research has demonstrated teratogenic effects for most anticonvulsants (Sullivan and McElhatton, 1975, Nau and Loscher, 1984).

In utero exposure to either valproic acid (VPA) or carbamazepine (CBZ) is associated with a higher incidence of neural tube defects (NTDs), approximately 1%–2% (Lindhout and Schmidt, 1986) and 0.5%–1% (Rosa, 1991) respectively, as compared with rates in the general population of 0.038%–0.096% (Centers for Disease Control, 1995). Studies suggest a dose–response relationship between VPA and NTDs (Samren et al., 1997), with an incidence of up to 5% occuring at higher drug doses (>1500 mg/day) (Omtzigt et al., 1992). Other major congenital defects suspected with VPA exposure are orofacial clefts, urogenital abnormalities, cardiac defects, and skeletal anomalies, although the exact risks are unclear (Briggs et al., 1998). A syndrome of facial dimorphism, nail dysplasia, digital hypoplasia, cleft lip and palate, cardiac defects, and cognitive abnormalities initially identified as fetal hydantoin syndrome is now recognized with other anticonvulsants, including CBZ and VPA (Yerby and Leppik, 1990). In addition to major congenital defects, infants exposed to AEDs in utero tend to have more minor malformations (Yerby et al., 1992) that can occur independently or with syndromes associated with CBZ or VPA exposure.

Although the data are conflicting, numerous studies have suggested that, compared to controls, children of mothers with epilepsy and antenatal exposure to AEDs have developmental delays, lower intelligence, and neurologic dysfunction. Often these studies have failed to control for confounding factors such as socioeconomic status (SES), maternal seizure frequency during pregnancy (Lösche et al., 1994), the type of maternal epilepsy, parental education level (Gaily et al., 1990), or multiple AED exposure in utero (Koch et al., 1999). Of the AEDs studied, CBZ monotherapy has been the most extensively evaluated. A prospective, controlled study (Scolnick et al., 1994) found no differences in global IQ in 36 infants exposed to CBZ monotherapy. Similarly, Van der Pol and colleagues (1991) found no difference in neurologic or cognitive functioning in children antenatally exposed to CBZ compared to unexposed controls.

Antipsychotic Drugs

In a meta-analysis, Altshuler and colleagues (1996) reviewed five studies that evaluated the effects of first-trimester use of low-potency phenothiazines in nonpsychotic women treated for hyperemesis gravidarum. The results suggest that first-trimester exposure to low-potency phenothiazines in women without psychotic disorders increases the baseline risk of congenital anomalies by 0.4%. Studies evaluating the effect of antenatal exposure to high-potency antipsychotic drugs, primarily haloperidol, have often been conducted in nonpsychotic women treated for hyperemesis gravidarum. These studies, as well as animal research, do not support a link between haloperidol and neonatal deformities (Tuchmann-Duplessis and Mercier-Parot, 1971; manufacturer's data McNeil Pharmaceutical, 1993). Experience with other high-potency neuroleptics in the phenothiazine class including perphenazine (Slone et al., 1977), thiothixene, and trifluroperazine (Slone et al., 1977), have not indicated that these medications increase the risk for major malformations (Briggs et al., 1998).

Information about the use of atypical antipsychotic drugs (APDs) during pregnancy is limited to case reports and case series. Over 30 cases of clozapine use during pregnancy have been documented. No major congenital anomalies were noted in 21 of these children (Lieberman and Safferman, 1992; Waldman and Safferman, 1993; Barnas et al., 1994; Tenyi et al., 1994; DiMichele et al., 1996; Stoner et al., 1997; Briggs et al., 1998; Dickson and Hogg, 1998). Nine cases of adverse outcomes were reported to the FDA, but, because of the lack of all known exposures, these abnormalities could be caused by chance and do not suggest that antenatal clozapine exposure increases fetal risk (Briggs et al., 1998).

A preliminary report by the Lilly Worldwide Pharmacovigilance Safety Database found no major or minor malformations in 20 of 23 prospectively identified pregnancies in which olanzapine exposure occurred (Goldstein et al., 2000). There were three (13%) spontaneous abortions, consistent with the rate in control pregnancies (Keily, 1991; McBride, 1991), and no anomalies were noted in these fetuses. There was one stillbirth at 37 weeks, leaving a total of 19 prospectively identified pregnancies. Sixteen normal infants (84%) were born without complications. Six were exposed to olanzapine throughout pregnancy, one during the first and second trimesters, and eight during the first trimester only. A case of a healthy child exposed to olanzapine during the first trimester has also been reported (Littrell et al., 2000). Consistent with these early reports in humans, animal studies have also failed to demonstrate a teratogenic effect associated with olanzapine treatment (Hagopian et al., 1987).

Near-term in utero exposure to APDs has been linked primarily to extrapyramidal side effects (EPS) in neonates (Tamer et al., 1969; O'Connor et al., 1981; Auerbach et al., 1992), although reports of neonatal jaundice (Scokel and Jones, 1962) and functional bowel obstruction (Falterman and Richardson, 1980) have also been attributed to these drugs. Signs of neonatal EPS include hypertonicity, tremulousness, opisthotonus, torticollis, exaggerated deep tendon reflexes, and irritability. The EPS are usually transient, lasting only days, however, there are isolated reports of symptoms occurring for up to 10 months (Tamer et al., 1969, Levy and Wisniewski, 1974). Of the case reports available for clozapine, one infant exposed to clozapine through pregnancy had a seizure of uncertain etiology 8 days after delivery (Stoner et al., 1997).

Data addressing long-term neurobehavioral sequelae after maternal use of APDs during pregnancy are limited. Comments on selected cases of children exposed in utero to phenothiazines did not reveal any behavioral difficulties (Kris, 1965). Slone and colleagues (1977) found no difference in IQ between phenothiazine-exposed and unexposed children tested at 4 years of age.

Administration of APDs can require the use of concomitant agents to help control EPS. Two studies suggest a possible association between benztropine exposure and major malformations (Heinonen et al., 1977; Briggs et al., 1998). One of these studies also suggests a link between first-trimester exposure to trihexyphenidyl and minor malformations (Heinonen et al., 1977). Conflicting reports exist about the teratogenic risk of diphenhydramine. One study supports an association between diphenhydramine use in the first trimester and oral clefts (Saxen, 1974), while other studies do not report an increased risk for major congenital anomalies (Heinonen et al., 1977; Aselton et al., 1985).

Benzodiazepines

Benzodiazepines (BZDs) are commonly prescribed in the psychiatric practice to treat anxiety, insomnia, and unpleasant side effects associated with other psychotropic agents. While early case–control studies found that maternal BZD exposure increased the risk of cleft lip and cleft palate, a recent meta-analysis (Dolovich et al., 1998) examining pooled data from cohort studies published between 1966 and 1998 found no association between antenatal BZD exposure and oral cleft or other major malformations. However, when examining case–control studies published during this period, the authors did find a small, but significant, odds ratio of 1.79 (95% confidence interval, 1.13 to 2.82; $\chi^2 = 11.39$, p = 0.01) suggesting an association between oral clefts and first trimester BZD use. However, other statistical analyses cast doubt on the validity of these marginally significant results (Dolovich et al., 1998; Cates 1999).

With respect to specific BZDs, one case–control study of 1427 malformed newborns and 3001 control infants linked diazepam to congenital defects such as inguinal hernia, cardiac defects, and pyloric stenosis (Bracken and Holford, 1981). Data from Michigan Medicaid collected during 1980–1983 revealed high rates of congenital anomalies in women with heavy BZD use (mainly diazepam) throughout pregnancy (Bergman et al., 1992), however, alcohol and multiple substance abuse were confounders. There have been no reports linking lorazepam, clonazepam, or alprazolam to congenital defects in humans.

With respect to neonatal adjustment, "floppy infant" syndrome has been most frequently associated with heavy use of diazepam throughout pregnancy and/or at the time of delivery (Rementeria and Bhatt, 1977); there has been one case report linking daily use of lorazepam (7.5–12.5 mg/day) to this syndrome (Di Michele et al., 1996). There have been several reports of neonatal withdrawal with restlessness, irritability, and tremors with heavy use of diazepam (Remeteria and Bhatt, 1997) and alprazolam (Oo et al., 1995) around delivery. One case report linked clonazepam (unspecified amount) to apneic episodes over the first 10 weeks of age. The infant had normal neurological development when evaluated at 5 months of age (Fisher et al., 1985). Finally, one study found an association between BZD use during pregnancy and poorer performance on a mental developmental scale at 5, 10, and 18 months of age (Viggegal et al., 1993); no such association has been found by others (Bergman et al., 1992).

Electroconvulsive Therapy

As there are no prospective, controlled trials of electroconvulsive therapy (ECT) administration during pregnancy, experience with this treatment modality is derived from over 300 case reports and case series. Studies have demonstrated efficacious treatment of psychiatric symptoms during pregnancy with ECT (Forssman, 1955; Impastato et al., 1964). In a review of 300 cases, Miller (1994) found 28 reports of ECT-associated pregnancy complications including transient, benign fetal arrythymias, mild vaginal bleeding, abdominal pain, and self-limited uterine contractions. There was no association between ECT and major congenital malformations. Follow-up studies of children who were exposed to ECT in utero, while dated, did not demonstrate any long-term neurobehavioral abnormalities (Forssman, 1955; Impastato et al., 1964).

TREATMENT RECOMMENDATIONS

General Considerations.

Before recommending continuation, alteration, or initiation of medications in preparation for or during pregnancy, the health care provider must evaluate the drug's effects on the fetus, the mother's previous response to treatment, and the potential repercussions of untreated psychiatric illness. It is imperative that the provider and the patient make a collaborative decision regarding treatment(s), and that this decision includes a discussion and documentation of associated risks and benefits to both the mother and unborn child.

Pharmacologic management across pregnancy can be complicated by pharmacokinetic variations in maternal, placental, and fetal drug metabolism. Maternal physiologic changes related to pregnancy include increased plasma volume, enhanced glomerular filtration, and induction of hepatic microsomal mixed function oxidase system. Changes in lithium (Redmond, 1985), TCA (Wisner et al., 1993), SSRI (Hostetter et al., 2000), and anticonvulsant (Kilpatrick and Moulds, 1991) blood levels have been reported and are believed to be secondary to physiologic alterations induced by pregnancy. Psychotropics, therefore, may require periodic monitoring and adjustment when therapeutic response across pregnancy is questionable. However, deterioration in clinical status should be the main indication for making a dose adjustment, rather than decreases in psychotropic drug levels.

Mood disorders

Unipolar depression.

Once the diagnosis of depression is made, treatment will depend on the severity. Mild to moderate depression may respond to nonpharmacologic interventions such as interpersonal therapy (Klerman et al., 1984; Spinelli, 1997) or cognitive therapy (Beck et al., 1979). Chronic, episodic, moderate, or severe depression will require medication in most cases (Frank et al., 1990). Current information suggests that neither SSRIs nor TCAs are associated with teratogenesis and can be used safely during pregnancy. As the bulk of the experience with SSRIs has been with fluoxetine, this is a reasonable medication choice. Given that fluoxetine has been associated in one study (Chambers et al., 1996) with difficulties in neonatal adjustment, some clinicians have suggested tapering medication 10–14 days prior to parturition (Wisner et al., 1999), although this practice is controversial. Others, however, have not observed problems with near-term exposure and believe that the risk of relapse or exacerbation of depression during the postpartum period is greater if medication doses are decreased. A recent study found that SSRIs, similar to TCAs, can require increasing dosages across pregnancy to maintain symptom remission (Hostetter et al., 2000).

The TCAs, with increased maternal side effects and, rarely, neonatal toxicity, are best reserved for women who are asymptomatic with TCA treatment or who have failed to respond to SSRIs. Because of metabolic and pharmacologic changes associated with pregnancy, women in the second half of pregnancy are likely to require 1.3–2 times the amount of medication as in the nonpregnant state or the first trimester to maintain remission of depressive symptoms (Wisner et al., 1993). Medication levels can be evaluated prior to pregnancy and if symptoms recur, a blood level could be checked and medication titrated to a therapeutic response. Because few data exist about the teratogenic risk to the developing fetus and there are significant potential side effects (hypertensive crisis), MAOIs should be reserved for women who have not responded to other medication or for whom the risk of relapse and associated adverse maternal behavior is high. Guidelines for the management of MAOIs during pregnancy have been published and suggest increased obstetric monitoring, genetics counseling, and consultation with the anesthesia service (Gracious and Wisner, 1997).

Electroconvulsive therapy, an effective treatment for depression during pregnancy (Forssman, 1955; Impastato et al., 1964), should be considered when other treatment modalities have failed. Guidelines for ECT during pregnancy are available (Repke and Berger, 1984; Wise et al., 1984, American Psychiatric Association, 1990) and should include a pre-ECT evaluation with pelvic exam, discontinuation of nonessential anticholinergic medication, uterine tocodynamometry, and intravenous hydration. During ECT, elevation of the right hip, intubation, diminishing excessive hyperventilation, and external fetal cardiac monitoring are recommended.

For women who are planning to become pregnant and who have had mild to moderate depression, a trial of medication taper and discontinuation is appropriate. Plans for relapse should be discussed prior to the trial. This strategy may not be appropriate for women who have had severe or multiple episodes of depression, as a recent study reported that pregnant women with a history of recurrent depression were at significant risk for relapse when medication was discontinued (Cohen et al., 1997).

Bipolar Disorder

Studies have documented high rates of relapse in bipolar disorder when medications are stopped during pregnancy (Suppes et al., 1991; Baldessarini et al., 1996) or during the postpartum period (Kendell et al., 1987; Leibenluft, 1996). A recent study (Viguera et al., 2000) demonstrated similar relapse rates for pregnant and nonpregnant women who had discontinued lithium in the preceding 10 months. The risk of recurrence was increased if lithium was discontinued rapidly (1–14 days) instead of more gradually (15–30 days) (Viguera et al., 2000). Of the women who remained stable in the first 40 weeks after discontinuation, postpartum recurrence, particularly of depressive or mixed states, was 2.9 times more common in pregnant women.

For women who have had few episodes of illness or who have been stable on medication for extended periods, an attempt to slowly wean medications prior to pregnancy is reasonable. Gradual tapering of medication is essential, as studies have found that rapid discontinuation of lithium is associated with high relapse rates (Baldessarini et al., 1997; Viguera et al., 2000). Discussion with the patient and family should address the risks associated with lithium, such as cardiac anomalies as well as with anticonvulsants such as NTDs. This should be balanced by a discussion of the risk of relapse and the adverse effects of untreated affective symptoms on neonatal outcomes including premature delivery, low birth weight, and lower Apgar scores (Cohen and Rosenbaum, 1998). Women who have chronic illness, or severe symptoms or those who have not tolerated med-

ication discontinuation in the past should be maintained on medications. If lithium is being used at the time of delivery, blood levels should be closely monitored, as rapid fluid shifts occurring during the first few days after parturition can have a dramatic influence on lithium levels. Some practioners have recommended tapering the lithium dose by 25%–30% just prior to delivery to avoid toxic levels in the puerperium (Altshuler et al., 1996). However, one must consider the fragility of the client when lowering lithium doses below that found to have been previously therapeutic.

Although each mood-stabilizing agent has been associated with some degree of teratogenicity, lithium, with a revised risk for Ebstein's anomaly at 0.1%, appears to have a more favorable liability profile than either VPA or CBZ, which are associated with a higher incidence of NTDs at 1%–2% (Lindhout and Schmidt, 1986) and 0.5%–1% (Rosa, 1991) respectively. Additionally, both of these anticonvulsants are now being associated with specific syndromal anomalies (Yerby and Leppik, 1990) as well as an increased number of minor malformations (Yerby et al., 1992). However, if VPA or CBZ have been most effective in controlling symptoms in the past, 4 daily mg of folate 1 month prior to conception and continuing until the end of the first trimester should be administered (MRC Vitamin Study Research Group, 1991). Women who have taken lithium during the first trimester should have cardiac ultrasonography between 18 and 20 weeks of gestation, and those exposed to anticonvulsants should have maternal serum α-fetoprotein levels measured before the 20th week of gestation, a sonography to screen for NTDs, and amniocentesis to evaluate α-fetoprotein levels (American Academy of Pediatrics, 2000).

Schizophrenia

The consequences of discontinuing medication with subsequent psychotic relapse can be grave. Continuing maintenance medications that have been effective is appropriate. If a medication change is necessary, treatment with haloperidol is recommended because this agent has been used extensively, it has not been associated with teratogenesis, and it possesses only a small risk for EPS in the newborn.

Women who first experience psychotic symptoms in pregnancy should have a thorough evaluation to rule out organic etiologies. Despite common treatment practices of prescribing atypical antipsychotics to people with new-onset psychosis, relatively little is known about their safety during pregnancy, so that haloperidol (or another mid- to high-potency neuroleptic) would be a reasonable first choice. If a typical neuroleptic is not indicated or is poorly tolerated, the growing data available for clozapine and olanzapine suggest that they are not teratogenic and may be reasonable alternatives.

Data regarding the use of adjunctive medications such as anticholinergics or BZDs to alleviate motor side effects, anxiety, and sleep disturbance are limited and somewhat conflicting. However, the most recent data suggest that the association between oral-facial clefts and BZDs is quite small (Dolovich et al., 1998) or even doubtful (Cates, 1999). As with all medications, attempts should be made to use the smallest effective dose of these agents. When high doses of these adjunctive medications are required to control side effects, one could consider switching to olanzapine to decrease the need for these adjunctive agents. Emerging evidence suggests that atypical antipsychotics, with the exception of risperidone and ziprasidone, can alter glucose homeostasis, leading to impaired glucose tolerance and, in some cases, diabetes (Wirshing et al., 1998; Kingsburg et al., 2001). Thus, it may be warranted to perform a glucose tolerance test prior to initiation of treatment and after chronic therapy with one of these agents.

Anxiety

Panic disorder

The effects of pregnancy on the course of panic disorder are variable, with some studies finding improvement of symptoms (George et al., 1987; Cowley and Roy-Byrne, 1989), while others report stable or worsening of symptoms (Northcott and Stein, 1994). Cognitive behavior therapy (CBT) should be offered to all women. For those with mild panic disorder, CBT may lead to remission or significant relief of symptoms, obviating the need for medications. In women with more severe illness, CBT may serve as an augmentative strategy and may decrease symptoms, thus requiring less medication. Either SSRIs or TCAs may be used safely during pregnancy to treat panic disorder. Benzodiazepines can also be used in pregnancy, as the association between first-trimester exposure and orofacial clefts is questionable (Dolovich et al., 1998). In addition, it appears that relatively low doses of lorazepam, alprazolam, and clonazepam may be administered during pregnancy without resulting in significant neonatal adjustment difficulties, although effects of prolonged use of BZDs on long-term development need clarification.

Obsessive-compulsive disorder

It is uncertain how pregnancy may affect the natural history of obsessive-compulsive disorder (OCD). Some studies have reported an association between pregnancy and OCD (Neziroglu et al., 1992; Williams et al., 1997), but this is not a universal finding (Lo, 1967). Treatment of OCD should begin with CBT. If symptoms do not respond to this intervention, a trial of an SSRI can be initiated. For women who do not respond to SSRIs or for whom clomipramine has been helpful in the past, clomipramine therapy may be instituted during pregnancy without increasing the risk of teratogenesis (Briggs et al., 1998). However, clomipramine therapy presents some difficulties, as significant neonatal toxicity can occur. A number of case reports have documented seizures, myoclonus and jitteriness as part of a withdrawal syndrome associated with near term exposure (Briggs et al., 1998).

SUMMARY

Millions of childbearing women face the decision of whether to institute or continue taking a psychotropic medication(s) during pregnancy. Thus, clinicians should become familiar with the risks associated with the agents most frequently encountered in their psychiatric practice. It is vital that clients are involved in the decision making and that documentation of such discussions is recorded in the patient's chart. As the mother's decisions regarding the management of her illness may influence the course of her pregnancy and potentially the infant outcome, input from the infant's father (when appropriate), the other medical professionals involved in the woman's pregnancy and the infant's care should be included whenever possible. Women with active mental illness may require additional support from ancillary and paraprofessionals during the pregnancy and the early postpartum period. Instituting a multidisciplinary team approach will provide the pregnant client and her soon-to-be-born infant the greatest opportunity for a positive outcome.

REFERENCES

Ali, S.F., Buelke-Sam, J., Newport, G.D., and Slikker, W., Jr. (1986) Early neurobehavioral and neurochemical alterations in rats prenatally exposed to imipramine. *Neurotoxicology* 7:365–380.

Altshuler, L.L., Cohen, L., Szuba, M.P., Burt, V.K., Gitlin, M., and Mintz, J. (1996) Pharmacologic management of psychiatric illness during pregnancy: dilemmas and guidelines. *Am J Psychiatry* 153: 592–606.

American Academy of Pediatrics Committee on Drugs (2000) Use of psychoactive medication during pregnancy and possible effects on the fetus and newborn. *Pediatrics* 105:880–887.

American Medical Association (1983) Drug interactions and adverse drug reactions. In: *AMA Drug Evaluations*. Chicago, IL: American Medical Association; pp. 31–44.

American Psychiatric Association (1990) The Practice of Electroconvulsive Therapy: Recommendations for the Treatment, Training and Privileging: A Task Force of the American Psychiatric Association. Washington, DC: American Psychiatric Press, 16:72–73.

Aselton, P., Jick, H., Malunsky, A., Hunter, J.R., and Stergachis, A. (1985) First-trimester drug use and congenital disorders. Obstet Gynecol 65:451–455.

Auerbach, J.G., Hans, S.L., Marcus, J., and Maeir, S. (1992) Maternal psychotropic medication and neonatal behavior. Neurotoxicol Teratol 14:399–406.

Baldessarini, R.J., Tondo, L., Faedda, G.L., Suppes, T.R., Floris, G., and Rudas, N. (1996) Effects of the rate of discontinuing lithium maintenance treatment in bipolar disorders. J Clin Psychiatry 57:441–448.

Baldessarini, R.J., Tondo, L., Floris, G., and Rudas, N. (1997) Reduced morbidity after gradual discontinuation of lithium treatment for bipolar I and II disorders: a replication study. Am J Psychiatry 154:551–553.

Barnas, C., Bergant, A., Hummer, M., Saria, A., and Fleischhaker, W.W. (1994) Clozapine concentrations in maternal and fetal plasma, amniotic fluid and breast milk [letter]. Am J Psychiatry 151:945.

Beck, A.T., Rush, A.J., Shaw, B.F., and Emery, G. (1979) Cognitive Therapy of Depression. New York: Guilford Press.

Bergman, U., Rosa, F.W., Baum, C., Wiholm, B.E., and Faich, G.A. (1992) Effects of exposure to benzodiazepine during fetal life. Lancet 340:694–696.

Bloem, B.R., Lammers, G.J., Roofthooft, D.W.E., De Beaufort, A.J., and Brouwer OF. (1999) Clomipramine withdrawal in newborns [letter]. Arch Dis Child Fetal Neonatal Ed 81:77.

Bourdon, K.H., Rae, D.S., Locke, B.Z., Narrow, W.E., and Reiger, D.A. (1992) Estimating the prevalence of mental disorders in U.S. adults from the Epidemiologic Catchment Area Survey. Public Health Rep 107:663–668.

Bracken, M.B., and Holford, T.R. (1981) Exposure to prescribed drugs in pregnancy and association with congenital malformations. Obstet Gynecol 58:336–44.

Briggs, G.G., Freeman, R.K., and Yaffe, S.J. (1998) Drugs in pregnancy and lactation: A Reference Guide to Fetal and Neonatal Risk, 5th ed. Baltimore: Williams & Wilkins.

Burt, V.K., Suri, R., Altshuler, L., Stowe, Z., Hendrick, V.C., and Muntean, E. (2001): The use of psychotropic medications during breast-feeding. Am J Psychiatry 158:1001–1009.

Buttolph, M.L., and Holland, D.A. (1990) Obsessive-compulsive disorders in pregnancy and childbirth. In: Jenike, M.A., Baer, L., and Minichiello, W.E., eds. Obsessive-Compulsive Disorders: Theory and Management, 2nd ed. Chicago; Year Book Medical, pp. 89–97.

Byrd, R.A., and Markham, J.K. (1994) Developmental toxicology studies of fluoxetine hydrochloride administered orally to rats and rabbits. Fundam Appl Toxicol. 22:511–518.

Cabrera, T.M., and Battaglia, G. (1994) Delayed decreases in brain 5-hydroxytryptamine 2a/2c receptor density and function in male rat progeny following prenatal fluoxetine. J Pharmacol Exp Ther 269:637–645.

Cabrera-Vera, T.M., Garcia, F., Pinto, W., and Battaglia, G. (1997) Effect of prenatal fluoxetine (Prozac) exposure on brain serotonin neurons in prepubescent and adult male rat offspring. J Pharmacol Exp Ther 280:138–145.

Carpenter, W.T., Jr., Hanlon, T.E., Heinrichs, D.W., Summerfelt, A.T., Kirkpatrick, B., and Levine, J., Buchanan, R.W. (1990) Continuous versus targeted medication in schizophrenic outpatients: outcome results. Am J Psychiatry 147:1138–1148.

Cates, C. (1999) Benzodiazepine use in pregnancy and major malformations or oral clefts: pooled results are sensitive to zero transformation used. BMJ 319:918–9.

Centers for Disease Control (1995) Surveillance for anencephaly and spina bifida and the importance of prenatal diagnosis. United States, 1985–1994. MMWR CDC Surveill Summ 44:1–13.

Chambers, C.D., Johnson, K.A., Dick, L.M., Felix, R.J., and Jones, K.J. (1996) Birth outcomes in pregnant women taking fluoxetine. N Engl J Med 335:1010–1015.

Cohen, L.S., Friedman, J.M., Jefferson, J.W., Johnson, E.M., and Weiner, M.L. (1994) A reevaluation of risk of in utero exposure to lithium. JAMA 271:146–150.

Cohen, L.S., Sichel, D.A., Faraone, S.V., Robertson, L.M., Dimmock, J.A., and Rosenbaum, J.F. (1996) Course of panic disorder during pregnancy and the puerperium: a preliminary study. Biol Psychiatry 39:950–954.

Cohen, L.S., Robertson, L.M., Goldstein, J., Sichel, D.A., Grush, L.R., and Weinstock, L.S. (1997) Impact of pregnancy on risk of relapse of MDD. In 1997 Annual Meeting Syllabus and Proceedings Summary. Washington, DC: American Psychiatric Association, pp. 23–24.

Cohen, L.S., and Rosenbaum, J.F. (1998) Psychotropic drug use during pregnancy: weighing the risks. J Clin Psychiatry 59 (Suppl 2): 18–28.

Cohen, L.S., Rosenbaum, J., and Heller, V.L. (1989) Panic attack–associated placental abruption: a case report. J Clin Psychiatry 50:266–267.

Coleman, F.H., Christensen, H.D., Gonzalez, C.L., and Rayburn, W.F. (1999) Behavioral changes in developing mice after prenatal exposure to paroxetine (Paxil). Am J Obstet Gynecol. 181:1166–1171.

Cowe, L., Lloyd, D.J., and Dawling, S. (1982) Neonatal convulsions caused by withdrawal from maternal clomipramine. BMJ 284:1837–1838.

Cowley, D.S. and Roy-Byrne, P.P. (1989) Panic disorder during pregnancy. J Psychosom Obstet Gynaecol 10:193–210.

Coyle, I.R. (1975) Changes in developing behavior following prenatal administration of imipramine. Pharmacol Biochem Behav 3:799–807.

De Ceballos, M.L., Benedi, A., De Felipe, C., and Del Rio, J. (1985a)Prenatal exposure of rats to antidepressants enhances agonist affinity of brain dopamine receptors and dopamine-mediated behavior. Eur J Pharmacol 116:257–262.

De Ceballos, M.L., Benedi, A., Urdin, C., and Del Rio, J. (1985b) Prenatal exposure of rats to antidepressant drugs down-regulates beta-adrenoceptors and 5-HT₂ receptors in cerebral cortex: lack of correlation between 5-HT₂ receptors and serotonin-mediated behavior. Neuropharmacology 24:947–952.

Dencker, S.J., Malm, U., and Lepp, M. (1986) Schizophrenic relapse after drug withdrawal is predictable. Acta Psychiatr Scand 73: 181–185.

Dickson, R.A., and Hogg, L. (1998) Pregnancy of a patient treated with clozapine. Psychiatr Serv 49:1081–1083.

DiMichele, V., Ramenghi, L.A., and Sabatino, G. (1996) Clozapine and lorazepam administration in pregnancy [letter]. Eur Psychiatry 11:214.

Dolovich, L., Addis, A., Vaillancourt, J.M.R., Power, J.D.B., Koren, G., and Einarson, T.R. (1998) Benzodiazepine use in pregnancy and malformations or oral clefts: meta-analysis of cohort and case–control studies. BMJ 317:839–843.

Eggermont, E. (1973) Withdrawal symptoms in neonates associated with maternal imipramine therapy. *Lancet* 2:680.

Ericson, A., Källén, B., and Wiholm, B.-E. (1999) Delivery outcome after the use of antidepressants in early pregnancy. *Eur J Clin Pharmacol* 55:503–508.

Falterman, L.G. and Richardson, D.J. (1980) Small left colon syndrome associated with maternal ingestion of psychotropic drugs. *J Pediatr* 97:300–310.

File, S.E. and Tucker, J.C. (1984) Prenatal treatment with clomipramine: effects on the behavior of male and female adolescent rats. *Psychopharmacology* 82:221–224.

Finnerty, M., Levin, Z., and Miller, L.J. (1996) Acute manic episodes in pregnancy. *Am J Psychiatry* 153:261–263.

Fisher, J.B., Edgren, B.E., Mammel, M.C., and Coleman, J.M. (1985) Neonatal apnea associated with maternal clonazepam therapy: a case report. *Obstet Gynecol* 66(Suppl):34S–35S.

Forssman, H. (1955) Follow-up study of sixteen children whose mothers were given electric convulsive therapy during gestation. *Acta Psychiatr Neurol Scand* 30:437–441.

Frank, E., Kupfer, D.J., Perel, J.M. Cornes, C., Jarrett, D.B., Mallinger, A.G., Thase, M.E., McEarchran, A.B., and Grochocinski, V.J. (1990) Three year outcomes for maintenance therapies in recurrent depression. *Arch Gen Psychiatry* 47;1093–1099.

Gaily, E., Kantola-Sorsa, E., and Granstrom, M.-J. (1990) Specific cognitive dysfunction in children with epileptic mothers. *Dev Med Child Neurol* 32:403–414.

George, D.T., Ladenheim, J.A., and Nutt, D.J. (1987) Effect of pregnancy on panic attacks. *Am J Psychiatry* 144:1078–1079.

Goldstein, D.J. (1995) Effects of third-trimester fluoxetine exposure on the newborn. *J Clin Psychopharmacol* 15:417–420.

Goldstein, D.J., Corbin, L.A., and Fung, M.C. (2000) Olanzapine-exposed pregnancies and lactation: early experience. *J Clin Psychopharmacol* 20:399–403.

Goldstein, D.J., Corbin, L.A., and Sundell, K.L. (1997) Effects of first-trimester fluoxetine exposure on the newborn. *Obstet Gynecol* 89:713–718.

Gotlib, I.H., Whiffen, V.E., Mount, J.H., Milne, K., and Cordy, N.I. (1989) Prevalence rates and demographic characteristics associated with depression in pregnancy and the postpartum. *J Consult Clin Psychol.* 57:269–274.

Gracious, B.L. and Wisner, K.L. (1997) Phenelzine use throughout pregnancy and the puerperium: a case report, review of the literature, and management recommendations. *Depression Anxiety* 6:124–128.

Hagopian, G.S., Meyers, D.B., and Markham, J.K. (1987) Teratology studies of LY170053 in rats and rabbits. *Teratology* 35:60a–61a.

Heinonen, O.P., Slone, D., and Shapiro S. (1977) *Birth Defects and Drugs in Pregnancy.* Littleton, MA: Publishing Services Group.

Hostetter, A., Stowe, Z.N., Strader, J.R., McLaughlin, E., and Llewellyn, A. (2000) Dose of selective serotonin uptake inhibitors across pregnancy: clinical implications. *Depression Anxiety* 11:51–57.

Impastato, D.J., Gabriel, A.R., and Lardaro, H.H. (1964) Electric and insulin shock therapy during pregnancy. *Dis Nerv Syst* 1:542–546.

Ingram, I.M. (1961) Obsessive illness in mental hospital patients. *J Ment Sci* 107:382–402.

Jäger-Roman, E., Deichl, A., Jakob, S., Hartmann, A.M., Koch, S., Rating, D., Steldinger, R., Nau, H., and Helge, H. (1986) Fetal growth, major malformations, and minor anomalies in infants born to women receiving valproic acid. *J Pediatr* 108:997–1004.

Jason, K.M., Cooper, T.B., and Friedman, E. (1981) Prenatal exposure to imipramine alters early behavioral development and beta-adrenergic receptors in rats. *J Pharmacol Exp Ther* 217:461–466.

Kaneko, S., Otani, K., Fukushima, Y., Ogawa, Y., Nomura, Y., Ono, T., Nake, Y., Teranishi, T., and Goto, M. (1988) Teratogenicity of antiepileptic drugs: analysis of possible risk factors. *Epilepsia* 29:459–467.

Keily, M. (1991) *Reproductive and Perinatal Epidemiology.* Boca Raton; FL: CRC Press, p. 69.

Kelly, T.E. (1984) Teratogenicity of anticonvulsant drugs. I: Review of the literature. *Am J Med Genet* 19:413–434.

Kendell, R.E., Chalmers, J.C., and Platz, C. (1987) Epidemiology of puerperal psychoses. *Br J Psychiatry* 150:662–673.

Kilpatrick, C.J., and Moulds, R.F.W. (1991) Anticonvulsants in pregnancy. *Med J Austr* 154:199–202.

Kingsbury, S.J., Fayek, M., Trufasiu, D., Zada, J., Simpson, G.M. (2001) The apparent effects of ziprasidone on plasma lipids and glucose. *J Clin Psychiatry* 62:347–349.

Klerman, G.L., Weissman, M.M., Rounsaville, B.H., and Chevron, E.S. (1984) *Interpersonal Psychotherapy of Depression.* New York; Basic Books.

Koch, S., Titze, K., Zimmermann, R.B., Schröder, M., Lehmkuhl, U., and Rauh, H. (1999) Long-term neuropsychological consequences of maternal epilepsy and anticonvulsant treatment during pregnancy for school-age children and adolescents. *Epilepsia* 40:1237–1246.

Krener, P., Simmons, M.K., Hansen, R.L., and Treat, J.N. (1989) Effect of pregnancy on psychosis: life circumstances and psychiatric symptoms. *Int J Psychiatry Med* 19: 65–84.

Kris, E.B. (1965) Children of mothers maintained on pharmacotherapy during pregnancy and postpartum. *Cur Ther Res* 7:785–789.

Kulin, N.A., Pastuszak, A., Sage, S.R., Schick-Boschetto, B., Spivey, G., Feldkamp, M., Ormond, K., Matsui, D., Stein-Schechman, A.K., Cook, L., Brochu, J., Rieder, M., and Koren, G. (1998) Pregnancy outcome following maternal use of the new selective serotonin reuptake inhibitors: a prospective controlled multicenter study. *JAMA* 279:609–610.

Kupfer, D.J., Frank, E., Perel, J.M., Cornes, C., Mallinger, A.G., Thase, M.E., McEachran, A.B., and Grochocinski, V.J. (1992) Five-year outcome for maintenance therapies in recurrent depression. *Arch Gen Psychiatry* 49:769–773.

Kurki, T., Vilho Hiilesmaa, V., Raitasalo, R., Mattila, H., and Ylikorkala, O. (2000) Depression and anxiety in early pregnancy and risk for preeclampsia. *Obstet Gynecol* 95:487–490.

Leibenluft, E. (1996) Women with bipolar illness: clinical and research issues. *Am J Psychiatry* 153:163–173.

Levy, W., and Wisniewski, K. (1974) Chlorpromazine causing extrapyramidal dysfunction in a newborn infant of a psychotic mother. *NY State J Med* 74:684–685.

Liebermann, J.A. and Safferman, A.Z. (1992) Clinical profile of clozapine: adverse reactions and agranulocytosis. *Psychiat Q* 63:51–70.

Lindhout, D. and Schmidt, D. (1986) In-utero exposure to valproate and neural-tube defects. *Lancet* 2:1392–1393.

Littrell, K.H., Johnson, C.G., Peabody, C.D., and Hilligoss, N. (2000) Antipsychotics during pregnancy. *Am J Psychiatry* 157:342.

Lo, W.H. (1967) A follow-up study of obsessional neurotics in Hong Kong Chinese. *Br J Psychiatry* 113:823–832.

Lösche, G., Steinhausen, H.-C., Koch, S., and Helge, H. (1994) The psychological development of children of epileptic parents. II. The differential impact of intrauterine exposure to anticonvulsant drugs and further influential factors. *Acta Paediatr* 83:961–966.

McBride, W.Z. (1991) Spontaneous abortion. *Am Fam Physician* 43: 175–82.

McElhatton, P.R., Garbis, H.M., Elefant, E., Vial, T., Bellemin, B., Mastroiacovo, P., Arnon, J., Rodriguez-Pinilla, E., Schaefer, C., Pexieder, T., Merlob, P., and Dal Verme, S. (1996) The outcome of pregnancy in 689 women exposed to therapeutic doses of antidepressants. A collaborative study of the European Network of Teratology Information Services (ENTIS). *Reprod Toxicol* 10: 285–294.

Miller, L.J. (1994) Use of electroconvulsive therapy during pregnancy. *Hosp Community Psychiatry* 45:444–450.

Misri, S. and Sivertz, K. (1991) Tricyclic drugs in pregnancy and lactation: a preliminary report. *Int J Psychiatry Med* 21:157–171.

MRC Vitamin Study Research Group (1991) Prevention of neural-tube defects: results of the Medical Research Council Vitamin Study. *Lancet* 338:131–137.

Nau, H. and Loscher, W. (1984) Valproic acid and metabolites: pharmacological and toxicologic studies. *Epilepsia* 25(Suppl 1):S14–S22.

Neziroglu, F., Anemone, R., and Yaryura-Tobias, J.A. (1992) Onset of obsessive-compulsive disorder in pregnancy. *Am J Psychiatry* 149;947–950.

Northcott, C.J. and Stein, M.B. (1994) Panic disorder in pregnancy. *J Clin Psychiatry*. 55:539–542.

Nulman, I., Rovet, J., Stewart, D.E., Wolpin, J., Gardner, H.A., Theis, J.G.W., Kulin, N.A., and Koren, G. (1997) Neurodevelopment of children exposed in utero to antidepressant drugs. *N Engl J Med* 336:258–262.

O'Connor, M., Johnson, G.H., and James, D.I. (1981) Intrauterine effects of phenothiazines. *Med J Aust* 1:416–417.

O'Hara, M.W. (1986) Social support, life events, and depression during pregnancy and the puerperium. *Arch Gen Psychiatry* 43:569–573.

Omtzigt, J.G., Nau, H., Los, F.J., Pijpes, L., and Lindhout, D. (1992) The disposition of valproate and its metabolites in the late first trimester and early second trimester of pregnancy in maternal serum, urine, and amniotic fluid: effect of dose, co-medication, and the presence of spina bifida. *Eur J Clin Pharmacol* 43:381–388.

Oo, C.Y., Kuhn, R.J., Desai, N., Wright, C.E., and McNamara, P.J. (1995) Pharmacokinetics in lactating women: prediction of alprazolam transfer into milk. *Br J Clin Pharmacol* 40:231–236.

Pastuszak, A., Schick-Boschetto, B., Zuber, C., Feldkamp, M., Pinelli, M., Sihn, S., Donnefeld, A., McCormack, M., Leen-Mitchell, M., Woodland, C., Gardner, A., Hom, M., and Koren, G. (1993) Pregnancy outcome following first-trimester exposure to fluoxetine (Prozac). *JAMA* 269:2246–2248.

Pavy, T.J., Kliffer, A.P., and Douglas, M.J. (1995) Anaesthetic management of labour and delivery in a woman taking long-term MAOI. *Can J Anaesth* 42:618–620.

Key to FDA use in pregnancy ratings. *Physicians' Desk Reference, 49th ed.* (1995) Montvale, NJ: Medical Economics Data Production Co., p. 2797.

Pollack, M.H., and Smoller, J.W. (1995) The longitudinal course and outcome of panic disorder. *Psychiatr Clin North Am* 18:785–801.

Poulson, E. and Robson, J.M. (1963) The effect of amine oxidase inhibitors on pregnancy. *J Endocrinol* 27:147–155.

Redmond, G.P. (1985) Physiologic changes during pregnancy and their implications for pharmacological treatment. *Clin Invest Med* 8:317–322.

Rementeria, J.L., and Bhatt, K. (1977) Withdrawal symptoms in ne-

onates from intrauterine exposure to diazepam. *J Pediatr* 90:123–126.

Repke, J.T. and Berger, N.G. (1984) Electroconvulsive therapy in pregnancy. *Obstet Gynecol* 63:39S-41S.

Rosa, F.W. (1991) Spina bifida in infants of women treated with carbamazepine during pregnancy. *N Egl J Med* 324:674–677.

Rosa, F.W. (1994) Medicaid antidepressant pregnancy exposure outcomes. *Reprod Toxicol* 8:444–445.

Samren, E.B., van Duijn, C.M., Koch, S., Hiilesmaa, V.K., Klepel, H., Bardy, A.H., Mannagetta, G.B., Deichl, A.W., Gaily, E., Granström, M.L., Meinadi, H., Grobbee, D.E., Hofman, A., Janz, D., and Lindhout, D. (1997) Maternal use of anti-epileptic drugs and the risk of major congenital malformations: a joint European prospective study of human teratogenesis associated with maternal epilepsy. *Epilepsia* 38:981–990.

Saxen, I. (1974) Cleft palate and maternal diphenhydramine intake. *Lancet* 1:407–408.

Schou, M. (1976) What happened to the lithium babies? A follow-up study of children born without malformations. *Acta Psychiatr Scand* 54:193–197.

Scokel, P.W. and Jones, W.D. (1962) Infant jaundice after phenothiazine drugs for labor: an enigma. *Obstet Gynecol* 20:124–127.

Scolnik, D., Nulman, I., Rovet, J., Gladstone, D., Czuchta, D., Gardner, A., Gladstone, R., Ashby, P., Weksberg, R., Einarson, T., and Koren, G. (1994) Neurodevelopment of children exposed in utero to phenytoin and carbamazepine monotherapy. *JAMA* 271:767–770.

Shapiro, S., Slone, D., Hartz, S.C., Rosenberg, L., Siskind, V., Monson, R.R., Mitchell, A.A., and Heinonen, O.P. (1976) Anticonvulsants and parental epilepsy in the development of birth defects. *Lancet* 1:272–275.

Slone, D., Siskind, V., Heinonen, O.P., Monson, R.R., Kaufman, D.W., and Shapiro, S. (1977) Antenatal exposure to the phenothiazines in relation to congenital malformations, perinatal mortality rate, birth weight, and intelligence quotient score. *Am J Obstet Gynecol* 128:486–488.

Spinelli, M.G. (1997) Interpersonal psychotherapy for depressed antepartum women: A pilot study. *Am J Psychiatry* 154:1028–1030.

Stoner, S.C., Sommi, R.W., Marken, P.A., Anya, I., and Vaughn, J. (1997) Clozapine use in two full-term pregnancies [letter]. *J Clin Psychiatry* 58:364–365.

Sullivan, F.M. and McElhatton, P.R. (1975) Teratogenic activity of the antiepileptic drugs phenobarbital, phenytoin, and primidone in mice. *Toxicol Appl Pharmacol* 24:271–282.

Suppes, T., Baldessarini, R.J., Faedda, G.L., and Tohen, M. (1991) Risk of recurrence following discontinuation of lithium treatment in bipolar disorder. *Arch Gen Psychiatry* 48:1082–1088.

Tamer, A., McKay, R., Arias, D., Worley, L., and Fogel, B.J. (1969) Phenothiazine-induced extrapyramidal dysfunction in the neonate. *J Pediatr* 75:479–480.

Tenyi, T., Trixler, M., Vereczkey, G., and Dorka, A. (1994) [Use of clozapine during pregnancy] Clozapine alkalmazasarol terhessegsoran. *Orv Hetil* 135:1967–1969.

Teratology Society, Public Affairs Committee (1994) FDA classification of drugs for teratogenic risk. *Teratology* 49:446–447.

Tuchmann-Duplessis, H. and and Mercier-Parot, L. (1971) Influence of neuroleptics on prenatal development in mammals. In: Tuchmann-Duplessis, H., Fanconi, G., Burgio, G.R., eds. *Malformations, Tumors and Mental Defects, Pathogenetic Correlation's.* Milan: Carlo Erba Foundation. As cited in Shepard, T.H. *Catalog of Teratogenic Agents, 6th ed.* Baltimore: Johns Hopkins University Press, 1989, pp. 308–309.

U.S. Census Bureau (2000) Resident Population Estimates of the United States by Age and Sex. Washington, DC:

Van der Pol, M.C., Hadders-Algra, M,. Huisjes, H.J., and Touwen, B.C. (1991) Antiepileptic medicaton in pregancy: late effects on the children's central nervous system development. *Am J Obstet Gynecol* 164:121–128.

Van Waes, A. and Van de Velde, E. (1969) Safety evaluation of haloperidol in the treatment of hyperemesis gravidarum. *J Clin Pharmacol* 9:224–237.

Viggegal, G., Hagberg, B.S. and Laegreid, L., and Aronsson, M. (1993) Mental development in late infancy after prenatal exposure to benzodiazepines—a prospective study. *J Child Psychol Psychiatry* 34:295–305.

Viguera, A., Nonacs, R., Cohen, L.S., Tondo, L., Murray, A., and Baldessarini, R.J. (2000) Risk of recurrence of bipolar disorder in pregnant and nonpregnant women after discontinuing lithium maintenance. *Am J Psychiatry* 157:179–184.

Vorhees, C.V., Acuff-Smith, K.D., Schilling, M.A., Fisher, J.E., Moran, M.S., and Buelke-Sam, J. (1994) A developmental neurotoxicity evaluation of the effects of prenatal exposure to fluoxetine in rats. *Fundam Appl Toxicol* 23:194–205.

Waldman, M.D. and Safferman, A.Z. (1993) Pregnancy and clozapine [letter]. *Am J Psychiatry* 150:168–169.

Ware, M.R. and DeVane, C.L. (1990) Imipramine treatment of panic disorder during pregnancy. *J Clin Psychiatry* 51:482–484.

Webster, P.A.C. (1973) Withdrawal symptoms in neonates associated with maternal antidepressant therapy. *Lancet* 2:318–319.

Weinstein, M.R. (1976) The international register of lithium babies. *Drug Information J* 10:94–100.

Werboff, J., Gottlieb, J.S., Dembicki, E.L., and Havlena, J. (1961) Postnatal effect of antidepressant drugs administered during gestation. *Exp Neurol* 3:542–555.

Williams, K.E. and Koran, L.M. (1997) Obsessive-complusive disorder in pregnancy, the puerperium, and the premenstruum. *J Clin Psychiatry* 58:330–334.

Wirshing, D.A., Spellberg, B.J., Erhart, S.M., Marder, S.R., and Wirshing, W.C. (1998) Novel antipsychotics and new onset diabetes. *Biol Psychiatry* 544:778–783.

Wise, M.G., Ward, S.C., Townsend-Parchman, W., Gilstrap, L.C., and Hauth, J.C. (1984) Case report of ECT during high-risk pregnancy. *Am J Psychiatry* 141:99–101.

Wisner, K.L., Gelenberg, A.J., Leonard, H., Zarin, D., and Frank, E. (1999) Pharmacologic treatment of depression during pregnancy. *JAMA* 282:1264–1269.

Wisner, K.L. and Perel, J.M. (1988) Psychopharmacologic agents and electroconvulsive therapy during pregnancy and the puerperium. In: Cohen, R.L., ed. *Psychiatric Consultation in Childbirth Settings*. New York: Plenum, pp. 165–206.

Wisner, K.L., Perel, J.M. and Wheeler, S.B. (1993) Tricyclic dose across pregnancy. *Am J Psychiatry* 150:1541–1542.

Yerby, M.S., Leavitt, A., Erickson, D.M., McCormick, K.B., Loewenson, R.B., Sells, C.J., and Benedetti, T.J. (1992) Antiepileptics and the development of cognitive abnormalities. *Neurology* 42(Suppl 5):132–140.

Yerby, M.S. and Leppik, I. (1990) Epilepsy and the outcomes of pregnancy. *J Epilepsy* 3:193–199.

Yoshida, K., Smith, B., and Kumar, R. (1999) Psychotropic drugs in mothers' milk: a comprehensive review of assay methods, pharmacokinetics and of safety of breast-feeding. *J Psychopharmacol* 13(1):64–80.

49 | Psychopharmacological treatment of preschoolers

SAMUEL L. JUDICE AND LINDA C. MAYES

In recent years, child psychiatrists have developed a special interest and expertise in infancy and early childhood. Concurrently there has been an increase in knowledge about the first years of life from many different disciplines, resulting in a better understanding of the complex interactions among biology, environment, and experience in shaping early development. These advances highlight the critical nature of interventions in the first years of life, as young children may have unique problems that require special developmentally tailored interventions. However, the models of mental health service intervention offered for very young children "vary according to the discipline evaluating and treating the child, the prevailing theoretical emphasis within a discipline or individual practitioner, the explicit goals of the intervention, the diagnostic nosology relied upon, and the characteristics of a particular community or culture vis-à-vis work with young children and families" (Mayes, 1998, p. 219).

One model of treatment being relied upon with increasing frequency with younger children is the prescription of psychotropic medications, a trend that parallels the increasing use and apparent effectiveness of psychotropic agents for behavioral and emotional disorders in other age groups. This trend in the treatment of preschool children has raised many controversial issues. For the child psychiatrist or pediatrician contemplating treating a very young child with a psychotropic medication, several issues warrant consideration above and beyond those concerns about the mental health needs for older children and adolescents in general. In this chapter we will review these special considerations and the data on safety and efficacy of various psychotropic medications in very young children so as to help guide the clinician in weighing the risks and benefits of such an intervention. We will also address a research agenda and highlight the special considerations in studying psychotropic medications in preschool children.

Toward these goals, we reviewed all available studies of psychotropic medication use in preschool children. As appropriate, review papers were also consulted, especially in areas concerning preclinical and animal studies. A Medline and PsycINFO search was conducted using specific search criteria. The search was limited to manuscripts published in the English language in peer-reviewed journals. Studies that were designed for children ≤5 years of age were emphasized. Other studies that contained mixed ages of children were also included if the results were stratified or analyzed in a way that would allow for the extraction of data for preschool children. Because of the paucity of treatment studies of preschool children, the selection of data for this review included both studies with and without nontreated comparison groups as well as case reports and retrospective chart reviews. To help determine the adequacy of research data to inform prescribing practices, studies were divided into one of three categories, as suggested in the International Algorithm Project (Jobson and Potter, 1995; Vitiello, 1997; Jensen 1999). *Level A* denotes adequate data to inform prescribing practices for efficacy and short-term safety with ≥2 randomized controlled trials (RCT). *Level B* indicates 1 RCT or ≥2 RCTs with mixed results. *Level C* indicates that data were only based on informed clinical opinion, case reports, uncontrolled trials, or retrospective chart reviews.

PREVALENCE OF PSYCHOTROPIC MEDICATION USE IN THE PRESCHOOL AGE GROUP

There exists substantial evidence that an increasing number of very young children are being treated with psychotropic medications for a variety of psychiatric and behavioral problems including hyperactivity, impulsivity, tantrums, poor social relatedness, selective mutism, irritability, aggression, and sleep disturbances.

Zito and colleagues (2000), studying the use of psychotropic medications in very young children, reported that 1% to 1.5% of all children aged 2 to 4 years who were enrolled in two Medicaid programs and one managed care organization were receiving stimulants, α_2 agonists, antidepressants, or antipsychotic medications. The investigators also reported that the prevalence of psychopharmacological interventions in this age group had tripled during the last decade. For example, the use of α_2 agonists increased 28-fold during that period—the biggest increase in any one agent.

Several other studies provide evidence that the prescription of psychotropic agents to very young children has increased during the last decade. In a review of information from the Intercontinental Medical Statistics Study, Minde (1998) described a threefold increase in methylphenidate prescriptions in Canada for the treatment of "common general behaviour problems" from 1993 to 1997. Minde also summarized findings from Strasbourg, France, showing that 12% (1367/11595) of all children beginning school were receiving psychotropic medication, primarily phenothiazines for behavioral problems or sleep disturbances. Minde's (1998) summary of findings from Germany indicated that of children aged 2–5 years, 20% were treated (with or without psychotropic interventions) for psychiatric symptoms ($n = 652$). The three most common psychotropic interventions were chlorpromazine for sleep problems 8% (53/652), imipramine for enuresis 6.5% (43/652), and diazepam for hyperactivity 3% (18/652).

In an analysis of Michigan Medicaid claims, Rappley and colleagues (1999) identified 223 children aged 3 years or younger who received the diagnosis of attention-deficit hyperactivity disorder (ADHD), the majority of whom had significant comorbid conditions, including language disorders, mental retardation and developmental disorders, oppositional/conduct disorders, adjustment disorder, emotional disturbance, child maltreatment, and chronic health conditions. While only a quarter of these children received psychological services, 57% (127/223) received psychotropic medications, and almost half of these (69/127) were prescribed two or more psychotropic medications. Taken together, these three studies identify an important change in psychotropic prescribing practices for very young children. Since three of the four study populations from the two studies based on data from the United States were derived from Medicaid populations, it may be that prescribing practices differ for children in poverty from those for children from other socioeconomic strata. However, insufficient data are presently available to address this question.

While it remains unclear from these studies as to *who* is prescribing these psychotropic medications to young children, a panel of experts seems more cautious in its prescribing practices for young children than a general sample of physicians. Surveying the editorial board of the *Journal of Child and Adolescent Psychopharmacology,* Coyle (2000) described the membership as "expert clinicians and researchers [in child psychiatry] who are likely to treat the most difficult cases" (p. 1060). Coyle surveyed the editorial board about their prescribing of stimulants, α_2 agonists, antidepressants, and antipsychotics for 2 to 4 year old children. With 72% responding, most (28/35) of the child psychiatrists reported either no use or very rare use of these medications in this age group. Only three reported prescribing an α_2 agonist (clonidine) on rare occasions. The few positive responses indicated that these psychotropic medications were used for severe, intractable cases such as the management of children with severe, self-injurious behavior. The rarity of psychotropic interventions in very young children as reported in Coyle's survey by experts in pediatric psychopharmacology implies that they may be more reluctant to prescribe psychotropic medications to preschool children than the general group of physicians surveyed in population-based studies of prescribing practices.

THE DILEMMA OF DIAGNOSIS IN PRESCHOOL POPULATIONS

Any therapeutic intervention needs to be guided by a diagnosis: the more refined the criteria for making that diagnosis, the more targeted its intervention. Variations in diagnostic criteria contribute to differences in evaluating the efficacy of any therapeutic intervention. These principles are no different for mental health interventions or for behavioral and psychological impairments and disorders—a refined diagnostic nosology is key. Unfortunately, this requirement poses a serious dilemma for the use of psychotropic medications with young children, since the nosology of developmental and behavioral disorders in this age group is only in the last two decades beginning to be developed. While severe developmental disorders such as autism and mental retardation have been well described and established, the specific criteria for other emotional and behavioral disorders in young children are far less clear. Complex problems such as failure to thrive, sleeping and feeding difficulties, and even language delays are more often symptoms rather than specific diagnoses, and usually reflect interactions between biological vulnerabilities and environmental circumstances. Even disorders that are more specific in older children (e.g., anxiety or conduct disorders) are less well demarcated in the preschool-age children, in whom increased activity, worries, and rituals may be developmentally normative (Mayes, 1998).

Several investigators are concentrating on refining diagnostic criteria in preschool children. The Zero to Three classification system (Zero to three/National Center for Clinical Infant Programs, 1994) is one such effort in which categories such as regulatory disorder may be a more functional description of early difficulties regulating states of arousal. Others are working in the areas of ADHD, oppositional defiant disorder (ODD), early onset-schizophrenia, major depressive disorder, and even bipolar affective disorder (Lahey et al., 1994; Jensen, 1998). However, the validity and reliability of the diagnoses of ADHD, mood disorders, and schizophrenia in very young children have been challenged (Coyle, 2000), and some clinicians may confuse "symptoms" of psychopathology (e.g., increased activity level) for developmentally appropriate behaviors. Conversely, child psychiatrists and other mental health professionals may treat young children with the premise that intervening at a young age offers the opportunity to make a difference in a potentially malleable condition, or with the expectation that mental disorders afflicting children at a young age may have a more severe and pernicious course. Given the problems with diagnostic nosology in young children, most of the work on the epidemiology of childhood disorders has focused on older children. Therefore, not much is known about the prevalence of psychiatric disorders in preschool-age children. Psychiatric disorders of preschool-age children can be categorized by two different approaches: taxonomic and quantitative. A taxonomic approach uses a category diagnosis as found in the *Diagnostic and Statistical Manual of Mental Disorders, 4th ed.* (DSM-IV) and a quantitative approach measures a behavior or developmental function continuously. The Child Behavior Checklist is an example of a quantitative approach. Prevalence studies can also look at prevalence of mental illness in a community sample of preschool aged children, or they can focus on clinic-based populations.

Lavigne and colleagues (1996), using categorical approaches with a community sample of 3860 preschoolers aged 2–5 years in a primary care pediatric sample, found the five most frequent axis I diagnoses (DSM III-R) to be ODD (17%), ADHD (2%), avoidant disorder (0.7%), overanxious disorder (0.7%), simple phobia (0.6%), and functional enuresis (0.7%). Five percent of children also met criteria for parent–child relational

problem. In terms of a quantitative screen, 10% of the study population had rates for behavior problems above the 90th percentile on the Child Behavior Checklist. Keenan and colleagues (1997) studied 104 preschool-age children from low-income families enrolled in the Women, Infants, and Children (WIC) Program. The preschool children ranged in age from 4:6 to 5:8 years. Keenan and colleagues found the following DSM-III-R diagnoses: simple phobia (11.5%), ODD (8%), ADHD (6%), social phobia (5%), conduct disorder (5%), separation anxiety (2%), major depression, and overanxious disorder (1% each). Twenty-three percent of the preschool children were identified as having a clinically significant score on the Child Behavior Checklist. Hooks and colleagues (1988) looked at the prevalence of psychiatric diagnoses among 193 preschoolers (<5 years of age, mean age 40 months) who presented to a psychiatric clinic. They found emotional disorders diagnosed in 32%, no diagnosis in 29%, specific developmental delay in 22%, pervasive developmental disorder in 17%, parent–child problems in 11%, global developmental delay in 6%, and disruptive behavioral problems in 4%. This sample may have been biased as it was based in a university tertiary mental health care setting, which may have elevated the referrals for autism and related disorders. Thus, depending on the population sampled, problems with behavior and/or emotional difficulties (e.g., anxiety) may be sufficiently severe among preschool-age children to warrant consultation with a mental health professional and potential treatment with a psychotropic agent.

The major psychotropic drug classes (stimulants, α_2 agonists, antidepressants and neuroleptics) that have been studied in the preschool population are summarized below.

Stimulants

Methylphenidate, (MPH) the most commonly used psychotropic, is prescribed for 150,000 to 200,000 2- to 4-year-old children (Marshall, 2000), and its use has increased threefold in that age group from 1991 to 1995 (Zito et al., 2000). There are a total of 12 studies and case reports on the use of stimulants in preschool aged children (Tables 49.1 and 49.2). All of the studies involved children with problems with impulsivity, aggression, overactivity, tantrums, and/or poor attention or concentration. These symptoms fall under the rubric of ADHD, although across the preschool years, defining the range of normal for levels of activity and distractability remains a complex nosological issue. While stimulants are the most studied medication in preschool-aged children, there are only eight controlled

TABLE 49.1 *Randomized Controlled Studies of Stimulants in Preschool-Aged Children*

Study	Drug	N	(n)	Age (years)	Diagnosis	Study Design	Medication Dosage	Length of Study	Primary Results	Side Effect or Safety Issues
Schleifer et al., 1975	MPH	26	(26)	3–5	"Hyperactive"	Crossover	MPH 2.5 mg/day to 30 mg/day	28–42 days	Improved on mother, not teacher, report and not on neuropsychiatric measures	Increased dysphoria and social withdrawal
Connors, 1975	MPH	59	(59)	4–5:11	"Minimal brain dysfunction"	Parallel design	MPH 11.8 mg/day (MPH 1.5 mg/kg/d)	42 days	27/29 children improved	Minimal SEs with a trend toward elevated blood pressure
Barkley et al., 1984	MPH	54	(18)	4–5:11	ADHD DSM-II criteria	Crossover	MPH 0.3 mg/kg/day MPH 1 mg/kg/day	21–30 days	"Normalizing" of hyperactive subjects with more positive mother interactions	The higher the dose the more frequent the SEs
Speltz et al., 1988	DEX	1	(1)	4	ADHD DSM-III-R criteria	Time series design	DEX 2.5 mg/bid DEX 5 mg/bid	9 weeks and follow-up at 2 years	Decrease in tantrums and aggressive oppositionality	Increased whining, listlessness, solitary play, and abdominal pain; decreased appetite
Barkley, 1988	MPH	27	(27)	3–5	ADHD DSM-III criteria	Crossover	MPH 0.3 mg/kg/day MPH 1 mg/kg/day	21–30 days	45% decrease in off-task behaviors on higher dose only	Mothers reported more SEs when child was on MPH compared to placebo
Mayes et al., 1994	MPH	69	(14)	3–5	ADHD DSM-III-R criteria with or without DD	ABA design	MPH 0.3 mg/kg/day with increases of 2.5 to 5 mg per dose	24 days	71% of preschool-aged children responded to MPH	51% had SEs: irritability, decreased appetite, lethargy and dysphoria
Monteiro-Musten et al., 1997[a]	MPH	31	(31)	4–5:11	ADHD DSM-III-R criteria	Crossover	MPH 0.3 mg/kg/day MPH 0.5 mg/kg/day	21–30 days	90% of subjects improved	SEs were mild and clinically negligible[a]
Handen et al., 1999	MPH	11	(11)	4–5	ADHD DSM-III-R DD	Crossover	MPH 0.3 mg/kg/dose from qd to tid MPH 0.6 mg/kg/dose from qd to tid	21 days	73% of preschool children with DD and ADHD improved	45% experienced social withdrawal and irritability

ADHD, attention-deficit hyperactivity disorder; DD, developmental disabilities; DEX, dexedrine; MPH, methylphenidate; N, total number of subjects in entire study; n, number of preschool-age subjects in study; SE, side effect.

[a]See also Firestone et al. (1998), which is a re-analysis of the data of Monteiro-Musten et al. (1997).

TABLE 49.2 *Uncontrolled Studies of Stimulants in Preschool-Aged Children*

Study	Drug	N	(n)	Age (years)	Diagnosis	Study Design	Medication Dosage	Length of Study	Primary Results	Side Effect or Safety Issues
Cohen et al., 1981	MPH	24	(24)	Mean age 5.2	"Hyperactive"	Open label	MPH 10–30 mg/day	20 weeks	MPH no better than no treatment	More solitary play
Alessandri and Schramm, 1991	DEX	1	(1)	4	ADHD DSM-III-R criteria	Open label	DEX 5 mg/day	16 weeks	Improved attention and social functioning	More solitary and parallel play
Byrne et al., 1998	MPH DEX	16	(16)	Mean age 5.2	ADHD DSM-IV criteria	Open label	MPH 15–20 mg/day DEX 7.5–15 mg/day	5 months	Improved attention and social relations; decreased problem behaviors	No mention of side effects as this was not a focus of the study
Ghuman et al., 2001	MPH DEX	27	(27)	3–5	ADHD, DD DSM-IV criteria	Chart review	MPH 0.55–1.16 mg/kg DEX 0.43–0.6 mg/kg	24 months	74% improved at 3 months 70% improved at 12 and 24 months	63% had SEs 11% had to stop medication due to SEs: irritability, dysphoria, headache, and dullness

ADHD, attention-deficit hyperactivity disorder; DD, developmental disabilities; DEX, dextroamphetamine; MPH, methylphenidate; N, Total number of subjects in study; n, number of preschool-age subjects in study; SE, side effects.

studies (e.g., those studies utilizing a strategy to compare response across individuals or treatment groups) involving a total of 187 children (Table 49.1; Connors, 1975; Schleifer et al., 1975; Barkley et al., 1984; Speltz et al., 1988; Barkley, 1988; Mayes et al., 1994; Monteiro-Musten et al., 1997; and Handen et al., 1999), and two of these eight studies examined children with developmental disabilities (Mayes et al., 1994; Handen et al., 1999). Of the eight controlled studies, only one evaluated dextroamphetamine (Speltz et al., 1988), while the other seven controlled studies examined MPH. The control studies were all short-term, lasting 14 days to 42 days in length. The mean subject number was approximately 19, with a range of 1 to 31 subjects. While Greenhill et al. (1999) noted that small-subject number, single site controlled trials are able to identify significant stimulant drug effects because of the large placebo-active drug differences, it is likely that the studies contained in Table 49.1 with subject numbers as low as 1, 11, and 14 (Speltz et al., 1988; Mayes et al., 1994; Handen et al., 1999, respectively) were underpowered.

As a group, these studies are difficult to compare, because they used varying definitions of target symptomatogy, dosages of medication, and measures for improvement. The controlled stimulant studies reported a variable response rate. The most positive results included improvements on mother–child interactions and improved behavioral compliance in controlled settings (e.g., very structured classrooms) and during structured test settings (Connors, 1975; Barkley et al., 1984; Barkley, 1988; Monteiro-Musten et al., 1997). One study reported no improvements on objective measures (Schleifer et al., 1975), and another study found no difference in children's spontaneous behavior during play (Barkley et al., 1984). Several studies noted serious side effects, including increased whining, listlessness, dysphoria, solitary play, and irritability (Schleifer et al., 1975; Speltz et al., 1988; Mayes et al., 1994; Handen et al., 1999). The side effects tended to be dose related, but several children had to discontinue stimulant treatment because of persistent severe side effects. Subjects with developmental disabilities were more vulnerable to the serious side effects. Thus, while there is some evidence that stimulants may be helpful for a subset of preschoolers, the sum of published data is presently mixed and no optimal methods for stimulant dosing or monitoring are specified for preschool children. There are also no studies examining the long-term impact of stimulants on children's behavior and development.

Thus, in terms of informing clinical practice, data regarding stimulants are currently at level B (Jobson and Potter, 1995; Vitiello, 1997; Jensen 1999), on account of mixed findings for short-term efficacy. For short-term safety data in pediatric psychopharmacology, Jensen et al. (1999) recommend evidence from a minimum of 300 youths exposed to the active drug in controlled trials. Presently, there are only 187 preschoolers reported in controlled trials of stimulants, an inadequate number for full evaluation of short-term safety. As noted above, commonly reported side effects in four of the controlled studies included irritability, dysphoria, listlessness, and whining. One study reported a side effect rate as high as 50% in preschoolers with or without developmental disabilities (Mayes et al., 1994). Conversely, some studies reported clinically insignificant side effects (Connors, 1975; Barkley, 1988; Monteiro-Musten et al., 1997). Thus, a risk–benefit analysis of stimulant use is difficult to accomplish with these small numbers, with data on short-term safety meeting level B criteria, and long-term safety meeting level C criteria.

Data from preclinical models may help in some considerations of the safety of stimulants in younger children, although extrapolating from preclinical models to humans can be fraught with limitations. Treatment of mice with amphetamines produces cell loss in the substantia nigra (Sonsalla et al., 1996). Dextramphetamine (DEX) (but apparently not MPH [Wagner, et al., 1980]) causes long-lasting alterations of dopaminergic systems in rats with depletions of dopamine and loss of dopamine uptake sites after repeated administration, suggesting a toxic interaction with dopaminergic neurons. In vervet monkey striatum, an acute methamphetamine dose did produce extensive dopamine neurotoxicity (Melega et al., 1997). Sprague-Dawley rats given high-dose (25 mg/kg subcutaneous) injections of DEX, MPH, methamphetamine, and MDMA have shown loss of serotonin uptake sites (Battaglia et al., 1987). Hepatic tumors occur in rodents when the animals are treated with high oral doses of 4 to 47 mg/kg of MPH (Dunnick and Hailey, 1995) although such tumors have not been reported in stimulant-treated preschool-age children (Greenhill et al., 1999). Indeed, failure to demonstrate toxicity findings in humans at therapeutic doses that may parallel those in preclinical models may be a result of differences of species, dose, route of administration, and end point selected (Greenhill et al., 1999).

α_2 Agonists

The data from Zito et al. (2000) indicated that there was a 28-fold change in clonidine prescriptions in preschool-aged children from 1991 to 1995. There are currently no controlled studies looking at α_2 agonists in preschool-age children. However, there are three open label studies examining response in preschool-age children and one studying neonates. These four studies (Table 49.3) examined a total of 12 preschoolers and 7 neonates. At best, the data are at level C in terms of quantity of data to inform prescribing practices. Clonidine or guanfacine has been used in open label reports to treat a variety of symptoms, from neonatal narcotic abstinence syndrome to post-traumatic stress disorder (PTSD) and ADHD (Table 49.3). Clonidine was found to be helpful in treating symptoms of PTSD (aggression, impulsivity, mood liability, insomnia, and hyperarousal) in seven preschool children in a day hospital setting, with only transient reports of sedation (Harmon and Riggs, 1996). Clonidine was also found helpful in a preschool child with hyperactivity and impulsivity believed to be due to HIV-1 encephalopathy, and once again only transient sedation was noted early in treatment (Cesena et al., 1995). Lee (1997), presenting the one published set of findings regarding guanfacine in preschool aged children, re-

ported efficacious effects in the treatment of ADHD in four subjects 2–3 years old. Reported side effects included transient chest pain in one child and transient sedation in another.

Hoder et al. (1984) studied clonidine in seven newborn infants with neonatal narcotic abstinence syndrome and found no significant changes in blood pressure, pulse, or electrocardiograms (EKG) in any of the seven infants. One infant had a transient abnormal eye exam and two infants developed a transient mild metabolic acidosis. On follow up 4–9 months later, four infants were found to be developmentally age appropriate. However, Huisjes et al. (1986) reported that 22 children exposed in utero to clonidine as result of treatment for maternal hypertension had increased sleep disturbances and hyperactivity, compared to a control group at a mean age of 6 years. It is unclear whether these differences were a direct effect of clonidine on prenatal development. More sophisticated preclinical studies need to be done in this area. At best the level of short-term and long-term safety regarding clonidine is level C.

TABLE 49.3 *Studies of α_2 Agonists*

Study	Drug	N	(n)	Age	Diagnosis	Study Design	Medication Dosage	Length of Study	Primary Results	Side Effect or Safety Issues
Hoder et al., 1984	CLD	7	(7)	Neonates	Neonatal narcotic abstinence syndrome	Open label	CLD 3–4μg/kg/day	6–27 days, Mean 13 days	6/7 newborns were effectively treated for narcotic withdrawal	2 infants developed a transient, mild metabolic acidosis; BP, P, and EKG remained normal
Cesena et al., 1995	CLD	1	(1)	4:8 years	Hyperactivity, impulsivity and aggressive behavior due to HIV-1 encephalopathy	Open label	CLD 0.075 mg/day	4 months	Normalization of attention; decreased hyperactivity and impulsivity	Transient sedation early in treatment
Harmon and Riggs, 1996	CLD	7	(7)	3–6 years	PTSD DSM-IV criteria	Open label	CLD 0.1 mg/day to 0.2 mg/day	Not stated	71% significantly improved Decreased aggression, impulsivity, mood liability, hyperarousal, anxiety, and nightmares	Transient sedation; insignificant BP changes; rebound hypertension on abrupt discontinuation
Lee, 1997	GNF	4	(4)	2–3 years	ADHD DSM-IV criteria	Open label	GNF 0.5 mg/day to 1.25 mg/day	2–6 months	Decreased impulsive, hyperactive, and aggressive behaviors; less tantrums; better maternal and child relations	Sedation and transient benign chest pain reported

ADHD, attention-deficit hyperactivity disorder; BP, blood pressure; CLD, clonidine; EKG, electrocardiogram; GNF, guanfacine; *N*, total number of subjects in study; *n*, number of preschool-age subjects in study; PTSD, post-traumatic stress disorder.

Antidepressants

In the Zito et al. study (2000), antidepressants were the second most commonly prescribed psychotropic medication. There are a total of 10 studies or case reports in the literature examining antidepressant use in preschool children (Table 49.4). None of the 10 studies are randomized, double-blind, or placebo-controlled trials. The ten uncontrolled studies looked at a total of 37 preschool children. Six of the studies looked at a total of 29 preschoolers with autism or childhood schizophrenia (Campbell et al., 1971a; Petti and Campbell, 1975; Holttum et al., 1994; Sanchez et al., 1996; DeLong et al., 1998; Hollander et al., 2000). While these six studies are difficult to compare, given the small sample sizes and the different treatment medications, these open-label studies suggest that clomipramine, venlafaxine, and fluoxetine may be helpful to reduce some psychiatric symptoms found in autistic

preschoolers. Tricyclics were reported to have mixed results (Campbell et al., 1971a; Sanchez et al., 1996). Several case reports and case series also reported promising results with fluoxetine in treating selective mutism (Wright et al., 1995; Dummit et al., 1996), ADHD unresponsive to stimulants (Campbell, et al., 1995), and specific phobia with panic attacks (Avci et al., 1998). Nonetheless, there is a paucity of data to guide clinicians in using antidepressants in preschool children, and controlled trials need to confirm initial promising results from case studies and case series. At best, the data are at level C for short-term efficacy.

In terms of toxicology and long-term side effects, data in humans are not available and data from animal studies are informative but not definitive. Prenatal exposure of rats to fluoxetine has yielded mixed findings, as reviewed elsewhere (Emslie et al., 1999). Vorhees et al. (1994) reported reduced litter sizes at high doses, but no significant effects on locomotor activity or per-

TABLE 49.4 *Studies of Antidepressants in Preschool-Aged Children*

Study	Drug	N	(n)	Age (years)	Diagnosis	Study Design	Medication Dosage	Length of Study	Primary Results	Side Effect of Safety Issues
Campbell et al., 1971a	IMP	10	(9)	2–5	Autism, schizophrenia DSM-I criteria	Independent blinded rater	IMP 6–75 mg/day	7–18 weeks	7/9 unchanged or worse IMP was not a useful drug for this population	Worsening of psychosis and disorganized behavior; 1 boy had a grand mal seizure
Petti and Campbell, 1975	IMP	1	(1)	3:2	Schizophrenia, autism DSM-I criteria	Independent blinded rater	IMP 25–125 mg/day	43 days	Marked increases in play and motor initiative as well as language production	Grand mal seizures developed while on IMP
Holttum et al., 1994	CLO	1	(1)	3:9	Autism, Trichotillomania DSM-III R criteria	Open label	CLO 4 mg/kg	3 months	Improvements in spontaneous verbalizations, mood, and social tolerance Trichotillomania reduced with CLO and a behavior plan	No significant SEs
Campbell, et al., 1995	FLX	1	(1)	3	ADHD DSM criteria[a]	Open label	FLX 5–10 mg/day	6 weeks	Improved attention span and more appropriate social interactions	BP, P, and weight remained normal; no SEs reported
Wright et al., 1995	FLX	1	(1)	4:10	Selective mutism DSM-IV criteria	Open label	FLX 8 mg/day	12 months	Resolution of selective mutism by day 20	No adverse medication SEs
Dummit et al., 1996	FLX	21	(5)	5	Selective mutism DSM-IV and III-R criteria	Open label	FLX 10–20 mg/day	9 weeks	4/5 showed improvement and 1/5 was much improved	2/5 had significant SEs: restlessness, disinhibition, and somatic complaints

(continued)

TABLE 49.4 *Studies of Antidepressants in Preschool-Aged Children (continued)*

Study	Drug	N	(n)	Age (years)	Diagnosis	Study Design	Medication Dosage	Length of Study	Primary Results	Side Effect of Safety Issues
Sanchez et al., 1996	CLO	8	(3)	3:5–5:2	Autism DSM-IV and III-R criteria	independent blinded rater	CLO 50–175 mg/day	5 weeks	No improvements noted	Aggravation of stereotypies; 1 boy withdrew due to urinary retention; 2/3 were worse
Avci et al., 1998	FLX	1	(1)	2:5	Specific phobia with panic attacks DSM—IV criteria	Open label	FLX 0.25 mg/kg/day (FLX 5 mg/day)	3 months	Resolutions of symptoms within 1 month	No SEs
DeLong et al., 1998	FLX	37	(1) (3)	2:5–5:11	Autism DSM-IV criteria	Open label	FLX 0.2 mg/kg/day to 1.4 mg/kg/day	13–33 months	9/13 had excellent response with improvements in language, cognition, and social interactions	SEs required cessation of treatment: hyperactivity, agitation, and lethargy
Hollander et al., 2000	VNF	10	(2)	3:6–5:5	Autism or PDD-NOS DSM-IV criteria	Chart review	VNF 12.5–25 mg/day	4.5–6 months	Both children rated as very much improved: more aware, focused, more verbal, less impulsive, and less repetitive	Hyperactivity and more self-stimulation

ADHD, attention-deficit hyperactivity disorder; BP, blood pressure; CLO, clomipramine; FLX, fluoxetine; IMP, imipramine; N, total number of subjects in study; (n), number of preschool-age subjects in study; P, pulse rate; PDD-NOS, pervasive developmental disorder, not otherwise specified; SE, side effect; VNF, venlafaxine.
[a]DSM-III-R or DSM-IV criteria used not specified by authors.

formance. In contrast, Cabrera and Battaglia (1994) reported that prenatal exposure of fluoxetine resulted in biochemical and functional alterations in central serotinergic systems, but this effect was not evident until adulthood. In later developmental periods, long–term fluoxetine treatment has been reported to up-regulate 5-HT uptake sites and 5-HT$_2$ receptors in adult rat brains (McCann et al., 1994). However, the applicability of these findings to developing preschool children remains unknown (Emslie et al., 1999).

Neuroleptics

Some of the earliest studies of psychotropic medications in preschool-age children involved neuroleptics. In autism, antipsychotics are the most frequently used psychoactive agents for the reduction of stereotypies, temper tantrums, aggressiveness against self or others, and hyperactivity (Campbell et al., 1999). There are seven studies with preschoolers with a total subject number of 59. Each of these seven studies involved medication trials with preschool children diagnosed with autism or childhood schizophrenia (Table 49.5). Only one study was a randomized, double-blind, placebo-controlled trial (Campbell et al., 1978), and it examined 21 preschool subjects treated with haloperidol. This study demonstrated that for autistic children less than 4.5 years of age, haloperidol was not significantly effective. There was a correlation between age and dose response: only children older than 4.5 benefited from the active medication, and they also tolerated higher optimum doses. Excessive sedation was the main effect reported. In a secondary analysis of pooled data from three studies with mixed age children (Anderson et al., 1984, 1989; Campbell et al., 1978; *n* = 125), older age was identified again as a variable predictive of a haloperidol response (Locascio et al., 1991). Trifluperidol, thiothixene, and molindone showed some limited improvements by blind raters, although side effects included extrapyramidal symptoms, transient leukopenia, transient rash, periorbital edema, sedation and irritability (Fish et al., 1969, Campbell et al., 1970, 1971b). All side effects were resolved by lowering dosage, and no side effects were seen at therapeutic doses.

In general, the untoward effects of antipsychotics in children are similar to those seen in adults. However, within the therapeutic dose range, parkinsonism is rare in preschool-age children (Campbell et al., 1999). No

TABLE 49.5 *Studies of Neuroleptics in Preschool-Aged Children*

Study	Drug	N	(n)	Age (years)	Diagnosis	Study Design	Medication Dosage	Study Length	Primary Results	Side Effect or Safety Issues
Fish et al., 1969	TFP	10	(10)	2–5	Childhood schizophrenia DSM-II criteria	Independent blinded rater	TFP 0.17–0.67 mg/day	4–15 weeks	8/10 improved with less disorganized speech and behavior Decreased irritability and hyperactivity	5/10 had mild EPS symptoms; 1 child had a transient elevated SGOT; 1/10 got worse
Campbell et al., 1970	THX	10	(9)	3–5	Childhood schizophrenia DSM-II criteria	Independent blinded rater	THX 1–6 mg/day	7–11 weeks	8/10 improved	2/10 got worse; 3/10 had mild EPS; 1/10 had transient leukopenia
Campbell et al., 1971	MLD	10	(10)	3–5	Childhood schizophrenia DSM-II criteria	Independent blinded rater	MLD 1–2.5 mg/ day	6–12 weeks	6/10 improved	No SEs on therapeutic doses
Campbell et al., 1978	HPD	40	(23)	2:6–4:5	Autism DSM-III criteria	RCT	HPD Mean dose, 0.07 mg/ kg/day	10 weeks	Not significantly effective	Excess sedation was main SE; laboratory and vital sign measures were normal
Nicolson et al., 1998	RISP	10	(4)	4:5–5:8	Autism DSM-IV criteria	Open label	RISP 1–1.5 mg/ day	12 weeks	Decreased aggression, tantrums, hyperactivity, and stereotypies	Weight gain and transient sedation
Schwam et al., 1998	RISP	1	(1)	3	Autism DSM-IV criteria	Open label	RISP 0.5 mg/day	5 weeks	Resolution of refusal to eat	None stated
Posey et al., 1999	RISP	2	(2)	1:11–2:5	Autism DSM-IV criteria	Open label	RISP 0.5–1.25 mg/day	12 months	Reduced aggression and improved social relatedness	1/2 patients developed persistent tachycardia and QT prolongation

EPS, extrapyramidal side effects; HPD, haloperidol; MLD, molindone; N, total number of subjects in study; n, number of preschool-age children in study; RCT, randomized, double-blind, controlled trial; RISP, risperidone; SE, side effect; TFP, trifluperidol; THX, thiothixene.

randomized, double-blind, placebo-controlled studies on long-term efficacy or safety of neuroleptics in preschool-age children exist. Three prospective, long-term studies including preschool children in their mixed-age subject population suggest however, that withdrawal dyskinesias may occur in approximately one-third of young children treated with haloperidol, and that in each subsequent treatment episode, dyskinesias may occur earlier and have a longer duration (Malone et al., 1991; Armenteros et al., 1995; Campbell et al., 1997). Of particular note is that the withdrawal dyskinesias have been reported to be reversible (Campbell et al., 1999). Hence, information regarding clinical efficacy and safety of neuroleptics in preschool-age children is at level C.

There are very limited data on the efficacy and safety of atypical neuroleptics in preschool-age children to inform prescribing practices. Only three open label case reports on risperidone exist, containing a total of seven young autistic children (Table 49.5; Nicolson et al., 1998; Schwam et al., 1998; Posey et al., 1999. These three studies suggest that risperidone may be helpful in treating aggression, hyperactivity, stereotypies, tantrums, and refusal to eat, as well as in improving social relatedness in young autistic children. Significant side effects observed with risperidone in these studies include weight gain, transient sedation, and, in one child, tachycardia with QT prolongation. Given that risperidone and other atypical neuroleptics are believed to have a lower risk of dyskinisias than haloperidol and other typical neuroleptics, this perceived advantageous side effect profile will likely ensure the continued use of this medication in young children. According to Campbell et al. (1999), "[s]afety and efficacy studies, including long-term effects on growth, pubertal development, and cognitive performance will be needed for the atypical neuroleptics. . . . Most of the conditions (autism, childhood schizophrenia and severe mental retardation) for which neuroleptics are used are diagnosed in early childhood and require drug treatment over a period of years, often throughout pubertal development" (pp. 542–543). The clinical utility of neuroleptics and atypical neuroleptics remains to be documented in preschool children, as well as their comparative efficacy and safety. Preclinical animal studies relevant to clinical use of neuroleptics in preschool-age children are also needed, as the long-term effects of early exposure have been implied in laboratory animals. For example, Rosengarten and Friedhoff (1979) demonstrated long-lasting increased dopamine receptor sensitivity in rat pups whose mothers were given moderately high doses of haloperidol. Prenatal exposure to haloperidol resulted in a decrease in do-

pamine receptor binding in Wistar rat pups, but in contrast, postnatal exposure to haloperidol through breast milk resulted in an increase in receptor binding (Rosengarten and Friedhoff, 1979). The significance for humans is unclear.

RECOMMENDATIONS FOR CLINICIANS AND A RESEARCH AGENDA

The Zito et al. study (2000) appropriately focused attention on the gap between research and clinical practice in pharmacologically treating preschool-age children with behavioral and psychiatric problems. In response, a national action agenda on children's mental health has been developing through a series of conferences first held at the White House (Marshall, 2000; U.S. Public Health Service, 2000). Recommendations stemming from these meetings included the following:

1. In assessing and diagnosing a child, a skilled professional should consider the symptomatolgy in the context of the child's developmental level, social and physical environment, and reports from parents, teachers, and other caretakers.
2. Psychotropic medications are usually not the first line of treatment for a preschool-age child with a mental disorder, and the first goal should be to understand the factors that may contribute to the illness.
3. If psychotropic interventions are used, they should not be the only treatment strategy or model and the target symptomatolgy should be constantly monitored.
4. More research is needed to determine the effects and benefits of psychotropic interventions in children (National Institutes of Health, 2000).

Admittedly, many clinicians argue that mental disorders, if left untreated in young children, may themselves cause long-term morbidity and deficits in socioemotional and cognitive functioning, and that the "well-documented risks of the illness and the potential risks of treatments (as yet undocumented in humans) must be considered in tandem" (Emslie et al., 1999, p. 525).

Nonetheless, there is considerable cause for concern about the use of psychotropic medication in preschool-age children during a period of continued rapid neural maturation (including synaptic remodeling and construction). The cortical synaptic density reaches its maximum at the age of 3 years and is substantially modified by the pruning process during the next 7 years (Huttenlocher, 1990). At the same time, the cerebral metabolic rate peaks between 3 and 4 years of age (Chugani et al., 1987). Studies in preclinical models indicate that the aminergic systems that are the target of the action of these pharmacological interventions play an important role in neurogenesis, neuronal migration, axonal outgrowth, and synaptognesis (Coyle, 1997). Therefore, it would seem prudent to exert clinical restraint in using psychotropic medications in very young children, while increasing research efforts to elucidate long-term efficacy and safety for those agents in this age group. One such effort currently underway is the Preschool ADHD Treatment Study (PATS), a multicenter trial of Ritalin in 300 children under the age of 6 to address concerns about safety and dosing in this rarely studied age group (Marshall, 2000). Recent attention on the gaps between the prescribing practice of drugs such as Ritalin and lack of research information to inform that practice have helped to emphasize the importance of such a study and aid in securing funding as well as institutional review board approval (Marshall, 2000).

Until data from studies such as the PATS emerge, it would seem prudent to only use these medications in cases where the target symptoms are so severe and persistent that they would have serious negative consequences for the child if left untreated—when the benefits outweigh the risks of psychotropic intervention. Additionally, any consideration of use of medication in this age group should always be accompanied by a full developmental and medical evaluation and family history, as well as information from any participating preschool program. The developmental context of symptoms and the severity of the functional impairment are essential to consider in the work-up of a young child presenting with behavioral or emotional difficulties. In addition to a full assessment, areas of particular relevance for young children include a higher index of suspicion of neglect, abuse, or other adverse environmental factors and of elevated lead levels, and a frequent need for further evaluations, including speech and language assessments, or cognitive and neuropsychological testing (American Academy of Child and Adolescent Psychiatry, 1995; Stubbe and Martin, 2000).

If a decision is made to begin psychotropic medication with a preschool-age child, a close monitoring regimen should be in place that includes regular assessment of cardiovascular function, i.e., periodic EKGs (to assess PR and QT intervals) and blood pressure checks, blood levels (where available), and a detailed evaluation of physical and behavioral side effects. If side effects develop, the dosage should be decreased or the medication discontinued. If the child does not respond to the medication, then the medication should be discontinued before trying a second agent so as to avoid

polypharmacy (Woolston, 1999), a particularly concerning problem with younger children. Clinicians may also consider trials on and off medication in an individual child—a crossover regimen—so as to gather more data on an individual child's response.

In terms of a research agenda, practitioners and professional associations, where feasible and practical, should encourage the enrollment of young children in responsibly conducted, rigorous clinical trials, rather than simply providing the medication in the absence of supporting evidence. Creating these rigorous trials may require collaboration across sites to maximize sample sizes. Additionally, these designs should incorporate both short-term efficacy evaluations and longer-term follow-up. As much as possible, given the state of diagnostic nosology for young children, clinical trials should incorporate recognized diagnostic nosological categorical schemas (e.g., Zero to Three [1994], DSM-IV) as well as measures of psychological and developmental functioning. For example, studies of the impact of stimulants on young children's impulsivity and distractibility should utilize parent and teacher report measures in their assessment of efficacy, as well as measures of reaction time and stimulus processing on and off medication. Finally, it is also important that clinical investigators establish partnerships with neuroscientists studying the impact of commonly prescribed psychotropic agents in preclinical models. Data from preclinical perspectives will inform designs and hypotheses for efficacy and safety trials in humans.

ACKNOWLEDGMENTS

This work was supported by the National Institute on Drug Abuse (RO1 DA-06025), by NICHD P01-HD03008, and by a Research Scientist Development Award to L.C.M. (KO2 DA-00222). S.L.J. was supported by a NIMH research training fellowship (5T32 MH-18268).

REFERENCES

Alessandri, S.M., and Schramm, K. (1991) Effects of dextroamphetamineon the cognitive and social play of a preschooler with ADHD. *J Am Acad Child Adolesc Psychiatry* 30:768–772.

American Academy of Child and Adolescent Psychiatry (1995) Practice Parameters for the Psychiatric Assessment of Children and Adolescents. *J Am Acad Child Adolesc Psychiatry* 34:1386–1402.

Anderson, L.T., Campbell, M., Adams, P., Small, A.M., Perry, R., and Shell, J. (1989) The effects of haloperidol on discrimination learning and behavioral symptoms in autistic children. *J Autism Dev Disord* 19:227–239.

Anderson, L.T., Campbell, M., Grega, D.M., Perry, R., Small, A.M., and Green, W.H. (1984) Haloperidol in infantile autism: effects on learning and behavioral symptoms. *Am J Psychiatry* 141: 1195–1202.

Armenteros, J.L., Adams, P.B., Campbell, M., and Eisenberg, Z.W.

(1995) Haloperidol-related dyskinesias and pre- and perinatal complications in autistic children. *Psychopharmacol Bull* 31:363–369.

Avci, A., Diler, R.S., and Tamam, L. (1998) Fluoxetine treatment in 2.5-year-old girl. *J Am Acad Child Adolesc Psychiatry* 37:901–902.

Barkley, R.A. (1988) The effects of methylphenidate on the interactions of preschool ADHD children with their mothers. *J Am Acad Child Adolesc Psychiatry* 27:336–341.

Barkley, R.A., Karlsson, J., Strzelecki, E., and Murphy, J.V. (1984) Effects of age and Ritalin dosage on the mother–child interactions of hyperactive children. *J Consult Clin Psychol* 52:750–758.

Battaglia, G., Yeh, S.Y., O'Hearn, E., Molliver, M.E., Kuhar, M.J., and De Souza, E.B. (1987) 3,4-Methylenedioxymethamphetamine and 3,4-methylenedioxyamphetamine destroy serotonin terminals in rat brain: qualification of neurodegeneration by measurement of [3-H] paroxetine-labeled serotonin uptake sites. *J Pharmacol Exp Ther* 242:911–916.

Byrne, J.M., Bawden, H.N., DeWolfe, N.A., and Beattie, T.L. (1998) Clinical assessment of psychopharmacological treatment of preschoolers with ADHD. *J Clin Exp Neuropsychol* 20:613–627.

Cabrera, T.M., and Battaglia, G. (1994) Delayed decreases in brain 5-hydroxytryptamine 2A/2C receptor density and function in male rat progeny following prenatal fluoxetine. *J Pharmacol Exp Ther* 269:637–645.

Campbell, M., Armenteros, J.L., Malone, R.P., Adams, P.B., Eisenberg, Z.W., and Overall, J.E. (1997) Neuroleptic-related dyskinesias in autistic children: a prospective, longitudinal study. *J Am Acad Child Adolesc Psychiatry* 36:835–843.

Campbell, M., Anderson, L., Meier, M., Cohen, I., Small, A., Samit, C., and Sachar, E. (1978) A comparison of haloperidol and behavior therapy and their interaction in autistic children. *J Am Acad Child Adolesc Psychiatry* 17:640–655.

Campbell, M., Fish, B., Shapiro, T., and Floyd, A. (1971a), Imipramine in preschool autistic and schizophrenic children. *J Autism Child Schizophrenia* 1:267–282.

Campbell, M., Fish, B., Shapiro, T., Floyd, A. (1971b) Study of molindone in disturbed preschool children. *Curr Ther Res* 13:28–33.

Campbell, M., Fish, B., Shapiro, T., Floyd, A. (1970) Thiothixene in young disturbed children: a pilot study. *Arch Gen Psychiatry* 23:70–72.

Campbell, M., Rapoport, J.L., and Simpson, G.M. (1999) Antipsychotics in children and adolescents. *J Am Acad Child Adolesc Psychiatry* 38:537–545.

Campbell, N.B., Tamburino, M.B., Evans, C.L., and Franco, K.N. (1995) Fluoxetine for ADHD in a young child. *J Am Acad Child Adolesc Psychiatry* 34:1259–1260.

Cesena, M., Lee, D.O., Cebollero, A.M., and Steingard, R.J. (1995) Case study: behavioral symptoms of pediatric HIV-1 encephalopathy successfully treated with clonidine. *J Am Acad Child Adolesc Psychiatry* 34:302–306.

Chugani, H.T., Phelps, M.E., and Mazziotta, J.C. (1987) Positron emission tomography study of human brain functional development. *Ann Neurol* 22:487–497.

Cohen, N.J., Sullivan, J., Minde, K., Novak, C., and Helwig, C. (1981) Evaluation of the relative effectiveness of methylphenidate and cognitive behavior modification in the treatment of kindergarten-aged hyperactive children. *J Aborn Child Psychol* 9:43–54.

Connors, C.K. (1975) Controlled trial of methylphenidate in preschool children with minimal brain dysfunction. *Int J Ment Health* 4:61–74.

Coyle, J.T. (1997) Biochemical development of the brain: neurotransmitters and child psychiatry. In: Popper, C., ed. *Psychiatric Pharmacosciences of Children and Adolescents.* Washington, DC: American Psychiatric Press, pp. 3–25.

Coyle, J.T. (2000) Psychotropic drug use in very young children. *JAMA* 283:1059–1060.

DeLong, G.R., Teague, L.A., and Kamran, M.M. (1998) Effects of fluoxetine treatment in young children with idiopathic autism. *Dev Med Child Neurol* 40:551–562.

Dummit, E.S., Klein, R.G., Tancer, N.K., Asche, B., and Martin, J. (1996) Fluoxetine treatment of children with selective mutism: an open trial. *J Am Acad Child Adolesc Psychiatry* 35:615–621.

Dunnick, J., and Hailey, J. (1995) Experimental studies on the long-term effects of methylphenidate hydrochloride. *Toxicology* 103:77–84.

Emslie, G.J., Walkup, J.T., Pliszka, S.R., and Ernst, M. (1999) Nontricyclic antidepressants: current trends in children and adolescents. *J Am Acad Child Adolesc Psychiatry* 38:517–528.

Firestone, P., Monteiro-Musten, L., Pisterman, S., Mercer, J., and Bennett, S. (1998) Short-term side effects of stimulant medication are increased in preschool children with attention-deficit/hyperactivity disorder: a double-blind placebo-controlled study. *J Child Adolesc Psychopharmacol* 8:13–25.

Fish, B., Campbell, M., Shapiro, T., and Floyd, A. (1969) Comparison of trifluperidol, trifluoperazine and chlorpromazine in preschool schizophrenic children: the value of less sedative antipsychotic agents. *Curr Ther Res* 11:589–595.

Ghuman, J.K., Ginsburg, G.S., Subramaniam, G., Ghuman, H.S., Kau, A.S.M., and Riddle, M.A. (2001) Psychostimulants in preschool children with attention-deficit/hyperactivity disorder: clinical evidence from a developmental disorders institution. *J Am Acad Child Adolesc Psychiatry* 40:516–524.

Greenhill, L.L., Halperin, J.M., and Abikoff, H. (1999) Stimulant medications. *J Am Acad Child Adolesc Psychiatry* 38:503–512.

Handen, B.L., Feldman, H.M., Lurier, A., and Murray, P.J.H. (1999) Efficacy of methylphenidate among preschool children with developmental disabilities and ADHD. *J Am Acad Child Adolesc Psychiatry* 38:805–812.

Harmon, R.J., and Riggs, P.D. (1996) Clonidine for posttraumatic stress disorder in preschool children. *J Am Acad Child Adolesc Psychiatry* 35:1247–1249.

Hoder, E.L., Leckman, J.F., Poulsen, J., Caruso, K.A., Ehrenkranz, R.A., Kleber, H.D., and Cohen, D.J. (1984) Clonidine treatment of neonatal narcotic abstinence syndrome. *Psychiatry Res* 13:243–251.

Hollander, E., Kaplan, A., Cartwright, C., and Reichman, D. (2000) Venlafaxine in children, adolescents, and young adults with autism spectrum disorders: an open retrospective clinical report. *J Child Neural* 15:132–135.

Holttum, J.R., Lubetsky, M.J., and Eastman, L.E. (1994) Comprehensive management of trichotillomania in a young autistic girl. *J Am Acad Child Adolesc Psychiatry* 33:577–581.

Hooks, M.Y., Mayes, L.C., and Volkmar, F.R. (1988) Psychiatric disorders among preschool children. *J Am Acad Child Adolesc Psychiatry* 27:623–627.

Huisjes, H.J., Hadders-Algra, M., and Touwen, B.C.L. (1986) Is clonidine a behavioural teratogen in the human? *Early Hum Dev* 14:43–48.

Huttenlocher, P.R. (1990) Morphometric study of human cerebral cortex development. *Neuropsychologia* 28:517–527.

Jensen, P.S. (1998) Ethical and pragmatic issues in the use of psychotropic agents in young children. *Can J Psychiatry* 43:585–588.

Jensen, P.S., Bhatara, V.S., Vitiello, B., Hoagwood, K., Feil, M., and Burke, L. (1999) Psychoactive medication prescribing practices for U.S. children: gaps between research and clinical practice. *J Am Acad Child Adolesc Psychiatry* 38:557–565.

Jobson, K.O., and Potter, W.Z. (1995) International psychopharmacology algorithm report. *Psychopharmacol Bull* 31:457–459.

Keenan, K., Shaw, D., Walsh, B., Delliquadri, E., and Giovannelli, J. (1997) DSM-III-R disorders in preschool children from low-income families. *J Am Acad Child Adolesc Psychiatry* 36:620–627.

Lahey, B., Applegate, B., McBurnett, K., Biederman, J., Greenhill, L., Hynd, G., et al. (1994) DSM-IV field trials for attention—deficit/hyperactivity disorder in children and adolescents. *Am J Psychiatry* 151:1673–1685.

Lavigne, J.V., Gibbons, R.D., Christoffel, K.K., Arend, R., Rosenbaum, D., Binns, H., et al. (1996) Prevalence rates and correlates of psychiatric disorders among preschool children. *J Am Acad Child Adolesc Psychiatry* 35:204–214.

Lee, B.J. (1997) Clinical experience with guanfacine in 2- and 3-year-old children with attention deficit hyperactivity disorder. *Infant Ment Health J* 18:300–305.

Locascio, J.J., Malone, R.P., Small, A.M. et al. (1991) Factors related to haloperidol response and dyskinesias in autistic children. *Psychopharmacol Bull* 27:119–126.

Malone, R.P., Ernst, M., Godfrey, K.A., Locascio, J.J., and Campbell, M. (1991) Repeated episodes of neuroleptic-related dyskinesias in autistic children. *Psychopharmacol Bull* 27:113–117.

Marshall, E. (2000) Planned Ritalin trial for tots heads into uncharted waters. *Science* 290:1280–1282.

Mayes, L.C. (1998) Mental health services for infants and young children. In: Young, J. and Ferrari, P., eds. *Designing Mental Health Services and Systems for Children and Adolescents: A Shrewd Investment* Philadelphia: Brunner/Mazel, pp. 219–230.

Mayes, S.D., Crites, D.L., Bixler, E.O., Humphrey, F.J., and Mattison, R.E. (1994) Methylphenidate and ADHD: influence of age, IQ, and neurodevelopmental status. *Dev Med Child Neurol* 36:1099–1107.

McCann, U., Hatzidimitriou, G., Ridenow, A., Fischer, C., Yuan, S., Katz, J., and Ricaurte, G. (1994) Dexfenfluramine and serotonin neurotoxicity: further preclinical evidence that clinical caution is indicated. *J Pharmacol Exp Ther* 269:792–798.

Melega, W.P., Raleigh, M.J., Stout, D.B., Lacan, G., Huang, S.C., and Phelps, M.E. (1997) Recovery of striatal dopamine function after acute amphetamine- and methamphetamine—induced neurotoxicity in the vervet monkey. *Brain Res* 766:113–120.

Minde, K. (1998) The use of psychotropic medication in preschoolers: some recent developments. *Can J Psychiatry* 43:571–575.

Monteiro-Musten, L., Firestone, P., Pisterman, S., Bennett, S., and Mercer, J. (1997) Effects of methylphenidate on preschool children with ADHD: cognitive and behavioral functions. *J Am Acad Child Adolesc Psychiatry* 36:1407–1415.

National Institutes of Health (2000) *Treatment of Young Children with Mental Disorders.* NIH Publication No. 00–4702 (September 2000). Washington, DC: U.S. Gov't. Press.

Nicolson, R., Awad, G., and Sloman, L. (1998) An open trial of risperidone in young autistic children. *J Am Acad Child Adolesc Psychiatry* 37:372–376.

Petti, T., and Campbell, M. (1975) Imipramine and seizures. *Am J Psychiatry* 132:538–540.

Posey, D.J., Walsh, K.H., Wilson, G.A., McDougle, C.J. (1999) Risperidone in the treatment of two very young children with autism. *J Child Adolesc Psychopharmacol* 9:273–276.

Rappley, M.D., Mullan, P.B., Alvarez, F.J., Eneli, I.U., Wang, J., and Gardner, J.C. (1999) Diagnosis of attention-deficit/hyperactivity disorder and use of psychotropic medication in very young children. *Arch Pediatr Adolesc Med* 153:1039–1045.

Rosengarten, H., and Friedhoff, A.J. (1979) Enduring changes in dopamine receptor cells of pups from drug administration to pregnant and nursing rats. *Science* 203:1133–1135.

Sanchez, L.E., Campbell, M., Small, A.M., Cueva, J.E., Armenteros, J.L., and Adams, P.B. (1996) A pilot study of clomipramine in young autistic children. *J Am Acad Child Adolesc Psychiatry* 35:537–544.

Schleifer, M., Weiss, G., Cohen, N., Elman, M., Cvejic, H., and Kruger, E. (1975) Hyperactivity in preschoolers and the effect of methylphenidate. *Am J Orthopsychiatry* 45:38–50.

Schwam, J.S., Klass, E., and Alonso, C. (1998) Risperidone and refusal to eat. *J Am Acad Child Adolesc Psychiatry* 37:572–573.

Sonsalla, P.K., Jochnowitz, N.D., Zeevalk, G.D., Oostveen, J.A., and Hall, E.D. (1996) Treatment of mice with methamphetamine produces cell loss in the substantia nigra. *Brain Res* 738:172–175.

Spelz, M.L., Varley, C.K., Peterson, K., and Beilke, R. (1988) Effects of dextroamphetamine and contingency management on a preschooler with ADHD and oppositional defiant disorder. *J Am Acad Child Adolesc Psychiatry* 27:175–178.

Stubbe, D.E., and Martin, A. (2000) The use of psychotropic medications in young children: the facts, the controversy, and the practice. *Conn Med* 64:329–333.

Mental Health (1999) A Report of the Surgeon General. U.S. Department of Health and Human Services. Rockville, MD: U.S. Department of Health and Human Services, Substance Abuse and Mental Health Services Administration, Center for Mental Health Services, National Institutes of Health, National Institute of Mental Health.

Vitiello, B. (1997) Treatment algorithms in child psychopharmacology research. *J Child Adolesc Psychopharmacol* 7:3–8.

Vorhees, C.V., Acuff-Smith, K.D., Schilling, M.A., Fisher, J.E., Moran, M.S., and Buelk-Sam, J. (1994) A developmental neurotoxicity evaluation of the effects of prenatal exposure to fluoxetine in rats. *Fundam Appl Toxicol* 23:194–205.

Wagner, G.C., Ricaurte, G.A., Johanson, C.E., Schuster, C.R., and Seiden, L.S. (1980) Amphetamine induces depletion of dopamine and loss of dopamine uptake sites in caudate. *Neurology* 30:547–550.

Woolston, J.L. (1999) Combined pharmacotherapy: pitfalls of treatment. *J Am Acad Child Adolesc Psychiatry* 38:1455–1457.

Wright, H.H., Cuccaro, M.L., Leonhardt, T.V., Kendall, D.F., and Anderson, J.H. (1995) Case study: fluoxetine in the multimodal treatment of a preschool child with selective mutism. *J Am Acad Child Adolesc Psychiatry* 34:857–862.

Zero to Three/National Center for Clinical Infant Programs (1994) *Zero to Three: Diagnostic Classification of Mental Health and Developmental Disorders of Infancy and Early Childhood.* Washington, DC: National Center for Clinical Infant Programs.

Zito, J.M., Safer, D.J., dosReis, S., Gardner, J.F., Boles, M., and Lynch, F. (2000) Trends in the prescribing of psychotropic medications to preschoolers. *JAMA* 283:1025–1030.

50 | Agitation and aggression

JEAN A. FRAZIER

Violence and aggression are multifactorial in etiology, involving individual (genetic, brain) as well environmental and societal factors (Filley et al., 2001). The treatment of violence requires a multisystems approach, which in children and adolescents with clear neuropsychiatric conditions, may require psychopharmacologic intervention.

DEFINITIONS

In health, aggression is appropriate, as dictated by biological necessity (self-defense) or sanctioned by society (warfare). Aggression does not always result in injury. In sharp contrast, violence, an aggression subtype, is deliberate, unwarranted, avoidable, and leads to physical injury (Filley et al., 2001).

Types of Aggression

Aggression may be acute or chronic, or verbal or physical. The target can be oneself, others, and/or property (see Table 50.1).

An overlap exists between self- and other-directed aggression. For example, impulsive-aggressive youth are at higher risk for destruction of others, property, and self (Apter et al., 1995).

Risk and Protective Factors

For a summary of individual and environmental risk factors and protective factors in aggressive behavior in youth, see Tables 50.02a and 50.2b.

Developmental Considerations

Healthy preschool children have rich fantasy lives and do not have the ability to understand that real people do not bounce back to life like cartoon characters. Healthy adolescents believe nothing bad will happen to them if they engage in risky behaviors.

Vulnerable youths who wish to belong are enticed by organizations such as gangs. Vulnerable teens may engage in copy-cat behaviors, as evidenced in suicide pacts and in the school threats that occurred in the aftermath of the Columbine (Colorado) school shooting.

MENTAL ILLNESS IN YOUTH: PREDISPOSITION TO AGGRESSION?

In the United States, few children suffering from psychiatric disorders actually receive treatment (Satcher, 2001). The impact of untreated psychiatric disorders is costly, with aggression being one important consequence. For example, many of the youths involved in school violence over the past 2 years had emotional difficulties prior to their destructive acts, yet, most did not receive intervention (Vossekeil et al., 2000).

Mood dysregulation and/or thought disturbance increase the probability of aggression. Recent data suggest a link between mental illness and violence; individuals with psychotic or mood disorders are five times more likely to engage in violence than those in the normal population. Substance abuse more than doubles this risk (Swartz et al., 1998).

CHILDHOOD PSYCHIATRIC DISORDERS AND AGGRESSION

Conduct Disorder

Conduct Disorder (CD) is highly correlated with aggression; however, it is not generally considered a medication-responsive disorder (Biederman et al., 1999; Malone et al., 2000). Children with CD have high degrees of psychiatric comorbidity (Zocolillo, 1992; Pliszka et al., 2000) and psychotropic treatment targeting the comorbid disorder(s) may decrease the symptoms of CD (Puig-Antich, 1982; Biederman et al., 1999).

TABLE 50.1 *Subtypes of Aggression and Characteristics*

Subtype	Description	Premeditated	Destruction or Injury	Physical Arousal
Overt/affective/impulsive	Hostile, defiant, defensive, uncontrolled	No	Towards others, self, and property	High arousal; flight-or-fight response
Covert/predatory	Furtive, hidden, goal-directed	Yes	Towards others and others' property; no destruction of self or one's own property	Minimal arousal
Combined	Combination of above two subtypes	Possible	Destruction of property, injury of others; unplanned injury of self and one's own property	Probable
Agitated delirious state	Delirious state altered mental state	No	Nondirected destruction of property; injury to self or others	Probable

TABLE 50.2a *Risk Factors and Protective Factors for Aggressive Behavior in Youth: Individual Factors*

Risk Factors	Protective Factors
Impulsivity	None, or treatment of impulsivity
Loneliness	Sense of belonging
Affective dysregulation	No symptoms or treatment of affective symptoms
Suicidal thoughts or acts	Absence or treatment of psychiatric disorder or stressors leading to suicidal thinking
Low self-esteem	Therapeutic assessment and intervention
Preoccupation with morbid themes or fantasies	No morbid fantasies or treatment of them
Preoccupation with weapons	No preoccupation with weapons or intervention for preoccupations
Intense anger	No anger, or proper interventions for anger
Conduct disorder and oppositional behaviors	No conduct disorder or oppositional behaviors
Fire-setting Cruelty to animals Stealing Bullying Truancy Discipline problem Blaming others for problems	Intervention for those individuals with these difficulties
Lack of coping strategies	Good coping strategies
Deterioration or lack of ability in school performance	Higher intelligence and good school performance
Head trauma/seizures	No head trauma Treatment for head trauma or seizures
Substances	Abstinence from substances
Psychosis	No psychosis

TABLE 50.2b *Risk and Protective Factors for Aggression in Youth: Environmental Factors*

Risk Factors	Protective Factors
Recent loss, rejection, or disappointment	No recent stressors or access to proper supports during times of stress
Peer culture	Healthy peer group and activities
Gangs	No involvement in gangs
Social isolation	Available and engaged in social activities
Access to weapons	No access to weapons, or removal of weapons from home
Overcrowding	No overcrowding
Low socioeconomic status	Middle to upper socioeconomic status
Rejecting parents	Consistent and understanding adult figures
Family difficulties	Family environment with good conflict resolution
Family violence, Abuse, and/or neglect	No family violence, abuse, and/or neglect
Experiences that cause arousal	Minimize experiences causing arousal
Loud noises High temperatures Watching violent movies Agonistic sports	Monitor children's activities Limit access to TV, particularly shows with violent themes Limit access to the Internet Limit exposure to agonistic sports Attend to noise level When high temperatures do occur, provide proper hydration and dress and find shaded areas

Adapted from Vitella and Staff (1997), Singer et al. (1998), and Fassler (2001).

672

AGGRESSION AND MEDICATION RESPONSIVE PSYCHIATRIC DISORDERS

Attention Deficit Hyperactivity Disorder

Children with attention-deficit hyperactivity disorder (ADHD) have high rates of arrests (Satterfield and Schell 1997), comorbid oppositional defiant disorder (ODD), CD, and affective disorders, which increase their risk of aggression (see Fig. 50.1).

Anxiety and Obsessive-Compulsive Disorder

Children with obsessive-compulsive disorder (OCD) have high rates of comorbid mood disorders, ODD, ADHD, CD, psychosis, and tic disorders (Geller et al., 1996). If untreated, these children may act on violent or sexual thoughts.

Post-Traumatic Stress Disorder

Children with histories of maltreatment are at higher risk for aggression, violent crimes, and juvenile arrests (Commission for the Prevention of Youth Violence, 2000).

Affective Disorders

Youth with affective illness are at greater risk for aggression. For example, among juvenile sex offenders, 35%–50% had comorbid mood disorders (Plizka et al., 2000).

Depression

High levels of aggression have been reported in adolescents with major depressive disorder (MDD) (Knox et al., 2000). Delinquent youth and youth with CD have high rates of affective illness (Puig-Antich 1987; Pliszka et al., 2000). Children and adolescents suffering from both MDD and antisocial behavior are at highest risk for suicidal acts (Brent et al., 1993).

Bipolar Disorder and Aggression: Comorbidity with Conduct Disorder

Youths with bipolar disorder (BPD) have high rates of aggression and CD (Kovacs and Pollock, 1995; Wozniak et al., 1995; Geller et al., 1998; Biederman et al.,

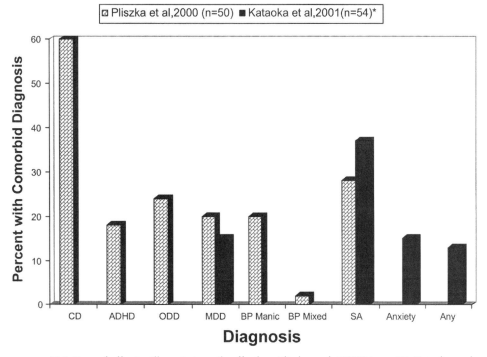

FIGURE 50.1 Rate of affective illness in juvenile offenders. Pliszka et al. (2000) ($n = 50$); Kataoka et al. (2001) ($n = 54$). *The Kataoka article involves female offenders. These youth were assessed only for substance use disorders, depressive symptoms and anxiety using standardized measures. Otherwise, only general information regarding lifetime mental health services was obtained. ADHD, attention-deficit hyperactivity disorder; BP, bipolar; CD, conduct disorder; MDD, major depressive disorder; ODD, opposistional defiant disorder; SA, substance abuse.

1999; Frazier et al., 2001). For example, a recent study found that 60% of juvenile offenders met criteria for CD, and BPD youths had the highest rate of CD (Pliszka et al., 2000).

Bipolar Disorder and Post-Traumatic Stress Disorder

In one study, early BPD was described as an antecedent for trauma and was the most significant predictor of later traumatic events during a 4-year follow-up period (Wozniak et al., 1999).

Psychosis and Aggression

A Finnish birth cohort study found that schizophrenic men were 3.6 times more likely to commit violent crimes than controls, and individuals with other types of psychoses were 7.7 times more likely to commit violent acts (Rasamem et al. 1998).

Substance Abuse

Substance Abuse (SA) disinhibits individuals and exacerbates underlying psychiatric difficulties, leading to increased impulsively and violence. High rates of substance dependence disorders were found in 50 youths in a juvenile detention center and in youths who carry weapons to school (Pliszka et al., 2000; Bell et al., 2001).

Tourette's Syndrome

Sudden explosive outbursts have been described in 25% of patients with Tourette's Syndrome (TS) (Budman et al., 2000). These explosive TS patients had high rates of ADHD (95%), OCD (92%), and ODD (54%).

Developmental Disabilities

Aggression, self-injury, and head-banging are relatively frequent behaviors in this population, which often lead to restrictive programming. In some individuals with developmental disabilities (DD), a coexisting psychiatric condition accounts for aggressive or self-injurious behavior. For example, facial slapping, occurring within the context of a major depressive episode, may represent suicidal gesturing in a mentally retarded individual.

Seizure Disorders

Although violence has long been associated with seizure disorders in the public eye (Marsh and Krauss, 2000), most patients with epilepsy are not violent. Aggressive behavior during the ictal and postictal periods of complex partial seizures is usually nondirected and unintentional, with few serious injurious consequences. For example, only 19 of 5400 patients with epilepsy (0.003%) had aggressive behavior; only 13 (0.002%) were aggressive during the ictal period (Delgado-Escueta et al, 1982).

Incarcerated individuals have a two to four fold greater prevalence of epilepsy, however, a relationship between criminal acts and seizure activity is seldom demonstrated (Marsh and Krauss, 2000). Aggression in seizure-disordered patients is often directed in nature, occurring during the interictal period, in response to a social context, likely related to general brain dysfunction rather than to seizure activity. Therefore, consideration of the social context in which the behavior occurs and of the sociological and biological risk factors is important.

Episodic Dyscontrol Syndrome or Intermittent Explosive Disorder

The *Diagnostic Statistical Manual, of Mental Disorders, 4th ed.* (DSM-IV; American Psychiatric Association, 1994), describes this syndrome as "discrete episodes of a failure to resist aggressive impulses, resulting in serious assault or destruction in the face of limited provocation. These attacks are accompanied by remorse afterwards." This syndrome usually occurs in males with childhood histories of violence, a family history of arrest, poor occupational records, and low socioeconomic status (SES).

Neuropsychological Deficits

Neuropsychological deficits include disinhibition, impulsivity, poor social abilities, inability to anticipate future consequences of one's behavior, inability to learn from one's mistakes, and insufficient self-monitoring. These deficits reduce the number of perceived options that one has in response to situations and result in increased aggression.

Neuropsychological deficits exist in children with Asperger's syndrome, nonverbal learning dysfunction and other learning disabilities, mental retardation (MR), frontal lobe and temporal lobe dysfunction, and traumatic brain injury (Filley et al., 2001).

Delirium or Confusional States

Aggressive behavior can occur during agitated and confusional states in children and adolescents suffering from moderate to severe traumatic brain injury, seizures and delirium. (Joshi et al., 1998; Filley et al., 2001).

TREATMENT OF AGGRESSION

The optimal treatment of aggressive youths requires the involvement of multiple professionals and agencies. Interventions include healthy peer activities, supportive adults, removal of weapons from the home, abstinence from substances, psychoeducation, individual and cognitive behavioral therapy, group and family therapies, school-based interventions, multisystemic therapy, anger management techniques, and psychopharmacology.

Pharmacotherapy

Medical and neurological evaluations of an aggressive youth (to rule out toxins, infections, medical conditions, substance use, seizure disorders, and head trauma) followed by a full psychiatric assessment should be done. An assessment algorithm is presented in Figure 50.2.

Diagnosis-based treatment

Psychopharmacologic treatment of aggression should occur within an individualized multimodal treatment plan and be based on an understanding of the psychiatric disorder, target symptoms, and available pharmacological treatments. Pharmacological intervention requires close monitoring of response over time.

No specific antiaggressive agent exists for children. However, antipsychotics, anticonvulsants, mood stabilizers, antidepressants, sedative-anxiolytics, and beta-blockers are all used to target aggression. Unfortunately, few controlled studies exist that assess these agents.

A review of effective pharmacological treatments for each psychiatric disorder can be found in chapters elsewhere in this volume. Medications that have been evaluated in open and double-blind studies for the behavioral management of aggression in children and adolescents are outlined below (see Table 50.3).

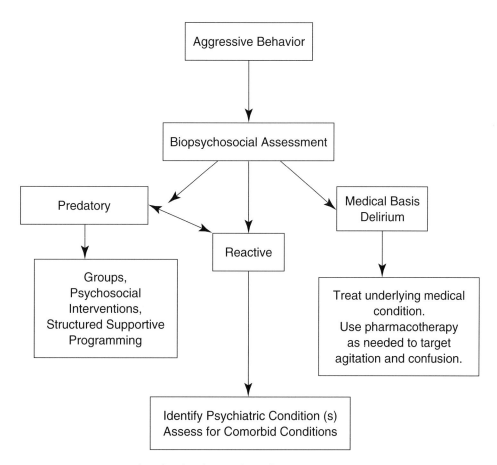

FIGURE 50.2 Assessment algorithm for pharmacologically responsive aggression in youth.

TABLE 50.3 *Psychotropic Medications Found Through Open and Controlled Studies to Be Helpful for Treatment of Agitation or Aggression in Children and Adolescents*

Medication (study design)	Study	Diagnostic Group/Symptoms	Dose and/or Serum Level
Stimulants			
Methylphenidate, dexedrine	Gittelman-Klein et al, 1976 Hinshaw, 1991	ADHD	0.3–1.5 mg/kg/day
Methylphenidate	Buitelaar et al., 1996	ADHD + CD	10 mg bid
Methylphenidate (DB)	Klein et al., 1997	CD + ADHD	Up to 60 mg/day
Methylphenidate	Birmaher et al., 1988 Handen et al., 1999 Aman et al., 1993 Aman et al., 1997 Handen et al., 1999	MR + PDD	0.3–0.6 mg/kg/day
αAgonists			
Clonidine (open)	Comings et al., 1990 Kemph et al., 1993 Schvehla et al., 1994	CD + aggression	0.4–0.6 mg/kg/day
Clonidine (open)	Hunt et al., 1985	ADHD + CD	
Clonidine (open)	Frankhauser et al., 1982	PDD + hyperarousal	0.005 mg/kg/day (transdermal)
Clonidine (DB)	Jaselski et al., 1992	PDD + ODD	0.15–0.2 mg/day
Guanfacine (open)	Hunt et al., 1995	ADHD	Mean dose 3.2 mg/day
Beta-blockers			
Propranolol (open)	Williams et al., 1982	Organic brain dysfunction + aggression	50–1,600 mg/day
Nadolol (open)	Conner et al., 1997	DD	Mean dose 109 mg (30–220 mg/day)
Pindolol (DB)	Buitelaar et al., 1996	ADHD + CD	20 mg bid Side effects prohibitive
Antidepressants			
Imipramine	Puig-Antich, 1982	MDD + CD	Up to 5 mg/kg/day
Clomipramine (DB)	Gordon et al., 1993	PDD + Anger	Mean dose: 152 mg
Fluoxetine (open)	Cook et al., 1992	Mild to profound MR + moodiness + impulse dyscontrol	Range 20–60 mg
Trazodone (open)	Zubieta and Alessi, 1992	Aggression	5 mg/kg/day
Trazodone (open)	Ghazuiddin and Alessi, 1992	Aggression	
Anxiolytics			
Buspirone (open)	Ricketts et al., 1994	DD adults ($n = 5$ and 8)	20–52.5 mg
Buspirone (open)	Verhoeven and Tui-nier, 1996		
Buspirone (open)	Pfeffer et al., 1997	Anxious + Aggression	Up to 50mg/day

(continued)

TABLE 50.3–Continued

Medication (study design)	Study	Diagnostic Group/Symptoms	Dose and/or Serum Level
Mood Stabilizers			
Lithium (DB)	Campbell et al., 1984	CD	500–2000 mg/day
	Campbell et al., 1995		Mean dose 1248 mg/day Mean serum level 1.12 mEq/L
	Malone et al., 2000		900–2100 mg/day (mean level of 1.7)
Anticonvulsants			
Carbamezapine (open)	Kafantaris et al., 1992	CD + aggression	600–800mg/day
Valproate (DB)	Donovan et al., 2000	Explosive temper + mood lability	Range 750–1500 mg/day Mean level 82.2 ± 19.1 ug/mL
Valproate (open)	Kastner et al., 1993	MR + Irritability + Self-injury	Serum levels 64–124 µg/mL
Valproate (retrospective)	Hollander et al., 2000	PDD	Mean dose 892 mg Range 125–2500 mg/day Mean level 75 µg/mL
Neuroleptics			
Molindone	Greenhill et al., 1985	Aggression	
Thioridazine	Gittelman Klein et al., 1976	Aggression	
Haloperidol	Campbell et al., 1984	CD	Range 1–6 mg/day
Haloperidol (open)	Malone et al., 2000	PDD	Mean dose 1.6 ± 0.9 mg/day
Pimozide	Naruse et al., 1982	PDD	Range 2–9 mg/day
Risperidone (retrospective)	Frazier et al., 1999	BPD	Mean dose 1.7 mg ± 1.3 mg
Risperidone (open)	Schreier, 1998	Mood Disorders	Range 0.75–2.5 mg/day
Risperidone (open)	Buitelaar, 2000	Aggression + MR or borderline IQ	Mean dose 2.9 mg Dose range 0.5–4 mg
Risperidone (open)	McDougle et al., 1997	PDD	Mean dose: 1.8 ± 1 mg/day
Risperidone (open)	Horrigan and Barnhill, 1997	Aggression + Explosivity	0.5 mg bid
Risperidone (case Report)	Kramer and Cottingham 1999	Steroid-induced delirium	1 mg
Risperidone (DB)	Findling et al., 2000	CD + Aggression	Mean dose 0.03 ± 0.004 mg/kg/day Range 0.7–1.5mg/day
Olanzapine monotherapy (open)	Frazier et al., 2001	BPD	Mean dose 9.6 ± 4.3 mg/day
Olanzapine (open)	Malone et al., 2000	PDD and MR + Anger	Mean dose 6.5 ± 2.2 mg/day
Droperidol IM	Joshi et al., 1998	Aggression	Mean dose 0.44 ± .22 cc

ADHD, attention-deficit hyperactivity disorder; BPD, bipolar disorder; CD, conduct disorder; DB, double-blind; DD, developmental disability; IM, intramuscular MR, mental retardation; PDD, pervasive developmental disorder

Stimulants

Hundreds of controlled treatment trials of stimulants in children with ADHD have documented efficacy in treating ADHD, as well as improvement of interactions and academic performance. Stimulants have been found to be more effective in ADHD children who are aggressive (Hinshaw, 1991).

Klein et al. (1997) randomized 84 children with CD two-thirds of whom also had ADHD, to placebo or methylphenidate for 5 weeks. Active treatment reduced symptoms of CD; the improvement in CD was unrelated to the severity of ADHD symptomatology.

Recent open and double-blind studies indicate that methylphenidate can help a subset of autistic hyperactive children, particularly those with IQs >45, by decreasing ADHD-like symptomatology without increasing stereotypies, tics, or anxiety (Birmaher et al., 1988; Aman et al., 1993, 1997; Quintana et al. 1995; Handen et al., 1999). While some patients with pervasive developmental disorders (PDD) experienced adverse reactions to stimulants, the majority of them had IQs of <45 (Handen et al., 1999).

Antihypertensives

Antihypertensives typically used in child psychiatry include α agonists (clonidine, guanfacine) and beta-blockers (propranolol, nadolol).

α agonists

Clonidine. An 8-week double-blind study of use of clonidine in children with ADHD showed improvement in hyperactivity and CD in 7/11 (64%) of the children (Hunt et al., 1985).

There are a number of uncontrolled studies that indicate that clonidine may be effective in reducing aggression (Comings et al., 1990; Kemph et al., 1993; Schvehla et al., 1994). Transdermal clonidine decreased hyperarousal in nine children with autism in an uncontrolled study (Frankhauser et al., 1982). In a double-blind study of eight PDD children with ADHD-like symptoms, Jaselski et al. (1992) reported that clonidine had nonsignificant overall effects compared to placebo, however, some of the ratings of aberrant (by teacher) and oppositional (by parent) behavior decreased.

Guanfacine. One 4-week open trial with guanfacine in ADHD children showed improvement in parental ratings of hyperactivity, inattention, and immaturity, but there was no effect on mood problems or aggression (Hunt et al., 1995).

Beta-blockers

Propranolol and nadolol are nonselective beta-blockers acting at β_1 and β_2 receptors.

Propranolol. Williams and colleagues (1982) reported that propranolol, used openly in 30 patients (age range: 7–35 years) with organic brain dysfunction, reduced aggression at high dosages.

Nadolol. An open trial of nadolol in aggressive DD youths decreased aggression. There were no significant effects on inattention or overactivity (Connor et al., 1997).

Pindolol. In a controlled study comparing pindolol with methylphenidate treatment, 32 ADHD children (ages 7–13 years) had modest improvement in CD and ADHD; however, side effects were problematic (Buitelaar et al., 1996).

Antidepressants

Tricyclic Antidepressants. A study of imipramine treatment led to the cessation of CD behaviors in 85% of 13 boys with CD and MDD (Puig-Antich, 1982).

Serotonin reuptake inhibitors and selective serotonin reuptake inhibitors

Clomipramine. Two studies of clomipramine (CMI) treatment in the PDD population have produced conflicting results. Gordon et al., (1993) compared CMI, desipramine, and placebo in a double-blind fashion in children with PDD. Active agents reduced stereotypies, anger, and compulsive behaviors. Side effects included grand mal seizure, prolonged QT interval, and tachycardia. However, an open-label trial of CMI in a younger group of PDD patients (ages 3.5–6.7 years) reported that only one out of seven children improved, while the remaining six worsened on the medication (Sanchez et al., 1996). Behavioral toxicity was severe.

Fluoxetine. An open fluoxetine trial in 17 patients with mild to profound MR showed improvement in 6 of eight children with impulse control problems and moodiness (Cook et al., 1992).

Paroxetine. In an open trial in persons with MR paroxetine reduced the frequency and severity of aggression and self-injury at 1 month, but the improvement was not sustained at 4 months (Davanzo et al, 1998).

Trazodone. Two open studies of trazodone in the treatment of aggressive children led to improvement (Ghazuiddin and Alessi, 1992; Zubieta and Alessi, 1992).

Anxiolytics

Buspirone. At higher doses, buspirone modulates serotonergic activity and acts as a dopamine antagonist. Because of its mechanism, buspirone might be helpful in the autistic population.

Only two open studies with small numbers have been done on adults with DD, while no studies exist on children. The adult studies showed that buspirone reduced self-injury and aggression in the MR population (Ricketts et al., 1994; Verhoeven and Tuinier, 1996). Unfortunately, one open-label study of buspirone in prepubertal children with anxiety and aggression reported improvement in only 3 of the 19 completers (Pfeffer et al., 1997).

Mood stabilizers

Lithium. Three inpatient controlled studies using lithium in aggressive CD youths have been conducted. One double-blind study compared lithium, haloperidol and placebo. Both active agents decreased aggression in youths with CD; however, haloperidol was associated with sedation (Campbell et al., 1984). Two double-blind studies of lithium demonstrated superiority of lithium over placebo in reducing aggression in hospitalized children with CD and aggression (Campbell et al., 1995; Malone et al., 2000). However, a double-blind lithium trial in adolescent inpatients with CD was negative (Rifkin et al., 1997). Two outpatient controlled trials using lithium were also negative (Klein, 1991; Campbell et al., 1995).

Anticonvulsants

Carbamazepine. A pilot study using this agent in 10 youths with CD and aggression showed positive results (Kafantaris et al., 1992). However, a subsequent double-blind study of carbamazepine use in 22 youths with CD, solitary aggressive type, was negative (Cueva et al., 1996).

Valproic acid. A double-blind, placebo-controlled study of valproic acid demonstrated a decrease in explosive temper and mood lability (Donovan et al., 2000).

An open trial of valproic acid in 18 MR patients (8–18 years of age) with irritability and self-injury showed that 12 of 18 (67%) improved (Kastner et al., 1993). Finally, valproic acid was studied in a 10-month retrospective design in PDD spectrum–disordered patients with mood lability, impulsivity, and aggression. Ten of 14 (71%) patients responded to the agent with a decrease in mood lability, impulsivity, aggression, and repetitive behaviors and improvement in social relatedness and language (Hollander et al., 2000).

Neuroleptics

Typical agents Antipsychotics are commonly used to target aggression. Typical agents such as haloperidol, thioridazine, and chlorpromazine are labeled for the treatment of "severe explosive behaviors" in pediatric patients. Several studies have demonstrated the efficacy of typical neuroleptics (haloperidol, molindone, thioridazine) in decreasing aggression in youths (Gittelman-Klein et al., 1976; (Campbell et al., 1984, Greenhill et al., 1985).

Several double-blind studies have demonstrated that typical agents are effective in decreasing problematic behaviors in children with DD. For example, haloperidol reduced anger, hyperactivity, and stereotypies (Campbell et al., 1979) in the dose range of 0.25–4 mg/day. Pimozide reduced problematic behaviors in children with PDD (Naruse et al., 1982). However, the possible long-term side effect of tardive dyskinesia remains a concern when using these agents.

Atypical agents. A number of studies demonstrate that these novel agents may be helpful in decreasing aggression, decreasing fear, and regulating mood in youths.

Risperidone. An outpatient clinic retrospective chart review of risperidone treatment (added to the ongoing medication regimen) in 28 children with BPD (mean age 10.4 ± 3.8 years) found that 57% of the children showed a robust improvement in aggression, mania, and psychosis within the first month of treatment (Frazier et al., 1999). The medication was generally well tolerated. Side effects included sedation, weight gain, drooling, galactorrhea, and hyperprolactinemia.

An open-trial assessing the effectiveness of risperidone in reducing aggression in 11 youths (5.5–16 years old) with concurrent affective symptoms (Schreier, 1998) reported improvement in 8 of 11 (73%) of the children.

There are several open-label trials of risperidone in the treatment of aggressive youths that demonstrate a decrease in aggression (Buitelaar, 2000). Buitelaar (2000) administered risperidone to hospitalized aggressive subjects (age range: 10–18 years old), and all patients had some reduction in aggression, 14 of 26 (54%) had marked reduction and 10 had moderate reduction. In 18 children with PDD spectrum disorders, risperidone open treatment led to improvement in repetitive behavior, aggression, impulsivity, and some elements of social relatedness (McDougle et al., 1997). A large-scale controlled study of risperidone for this indication has been completed, and results are covered in Chapter 42 in this volume (McDougle et al., 2000).

In an open trial in boys suffering from outbursts, risperidone decreased aggression, explosivity, and self-injury (Horrigan and Barnhill, 1997). Sleep and hygiene improved as well. In a 10-week double-blind, placebo-controlled study, Findling et al. (2000) found that risperidone improved conduct symptoms and aggression.

Olanzapine. An open trial of olanzapine monotherapy in youths with BPD showed that treatment improved mania, psychosis, depression, and aggression (Frazier et al., 2001). Olanzapine was well tolerated and medication compliance was excellent. Weight gain was the most significant side effect (mean weight gain of 5 ± 2.3 kg).

An open pilot comparison of olanzapine to haloperidol in 11 children with PDD showed that both agents were effective in reducing problematic behaviors such as social withdrawal, hyperactivity, anger, lability, and stereotypic behaviors. The olanzapine-treated group gained significantly more weight (Malone et al., 2000).

Other

Amantadine. Although this agent showed some initial promise in the treatment of aggression and impulsivity through a case series of children with PDD, a subsequent double-blind amantadine trial (5 mg/kg/day) had mixed results (King et al., 2001a, b). Given the controversial nature of this intervention, amantadine is not a recommended treatment for aggressive PDD children.

Other Pharmacological Approaches

Medications on an as-needed basis

Antihistamines (diphenydramine) and neuroleptics. Vitello et al. (1987) assessed the use of "as needed" medications used to quell fighting and uncooperativeness among patients in a state hospital and found that antihistamines (54%) and neuroleptics (24%) were most commonly used; this form of medication was effective in only 32% of patients. Intramuscular (IM) administration of medications tended to occur when aggression was directed toward staff.

Vitello et al. (1991) later conducted a pilot placebo-controlled study of diphenhydramine for aggressive behavior in 21 boys (ages 5–13 years). Oral or IM administration of diphenhydramine or placebo was used, and pre and post-ratings of aggression were carried out Physical aggression declined significantly, regardless of the agent used or route chosen, and IM injection (regardless of agent) showed a trend toward a greater decline in score.

Aggression or Agitation in Emergency Situations

The etiology of the violent behavior should be ascertained quickly with initiation of the appropriate medical or psychiatric treatment. However, when severe agitation exists, a nonspecific measure may be required emergently to ensure the safety of the patient and those in the immediate environment. Psychopharmacological management in these situations has to occur quickly; relatively safe sedating medications with quick onset of action should be chosen. Although the option of taking medication by mouth should be given, many out-of-control patients refuse oral medication, necessitating IM or intravenous (IV) administration. In many instances, IV access is not practical, because the patient is on a psychiatric unit where IVs are generally not allowed, and/or because the of patient is too agitated. Therefore, IM administration may be required. The benefits of IM administration include (*1*) the medication cannot be "cheeked" or spit out; (*2*) there is no need for IV placement; and (*3*) the onset of action of IM medications is generally more rapid than that oral administration. Safe injection of medication in an agitated youth requires a team of personnel to hold the individual in a reclining position while the IM is being given. An overall suggested approach to the emergency management of the aggressive or agitated youth is presented in Figure 50.3.

Benzodiazepines are generally preferred agents for acute behavioral control because of their safety profile and sedative properties. Violent patients are effectively treated with lorazepam at 1–4 mg, given intravenously over 2 minutes. When medications are given intravenously, respiratory status needs to be closely monitored. The IM administration of lorazepam can be effective in younger patients at doses of 0.5–1 mg and in older youth at 1–2 mg. If a neuroleptic is necessary, haloperidol at 1–5 mg (given with anticholinergics) or chlorpromazine at 25 mg given every 1–2 hours as needed for acute behavioral problems may be necessary. When chlorpromazine is administered intramuscularly, careful attention must be given to vital signs and electrocardiogram (EKG) changes (because of the risk of hypotension and QTc prolongation).

In the case of an intoxicated patient, conservative

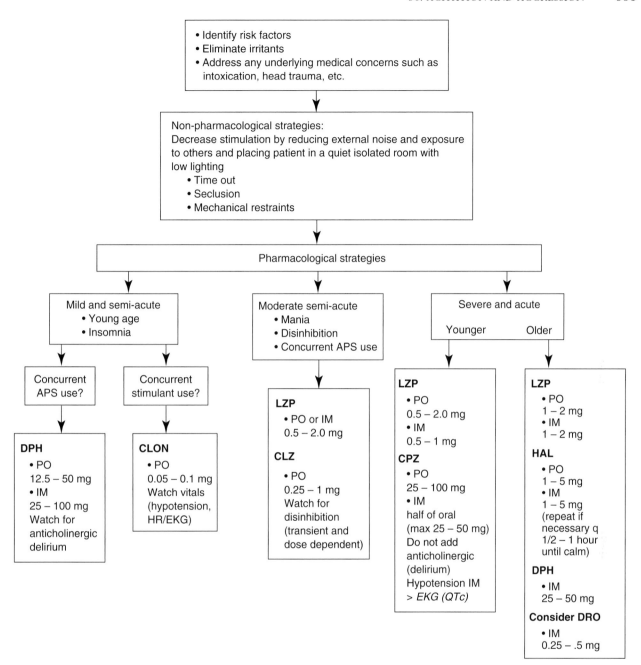

FIGURE 50.3 Childhood aggression or agitation pharmacological approach. **DPH**, diphenhydramine; **CLON**, clonidine; **LZP**, lorazepam; **CLZ**, clonazepam; **HAL**, haloperidol; **DRO**, droperidol.

measures may be adequate. In some instances, medications such as lorazepam are used, instead of or with antipsychotics (IM doses of 1–2 mg can be repeated every hour until the patient is calm; at times doses may need to be repeated every half hour; respiratory suppression should be watched for). Benzodiazepines are preferable to antipsychotics when the recreational drug has strong anticholinergic properties. Antipsychotics

such as haloperidol (Haldol), 1–5 mg every hour, may be required until a patient is stabilized. Clinicians will need to watch closely for extrapyramidal side effects.

If the patient is aggressive and psychotic, continuous medication may need to be given. Small IM or oral (po) doses should be given at 1- to 2-hour intervals (i.e., haloperidol, 1–5 mg [given with anticholinergics] or lorazepam, 0.5–2 mg) until the patient is controlled. At times, doses may be required every ½ hour. Such a dosing strategy, using lower doses at hourly intervals, can be more effective than using large doses initially. This approach can optimize results while avoiding problematic side effects. During the initial treatment, the patient's vital signs should be closely monitored. In patients with head injury, the use of medications is generally contraindicated, as medications can confuse the clinical picture.

The agent droperidol can be helpful in acute emergencies for the management of psychosis and aggression. This ultrashort-acting butyrophenone neuroleptic has onset of action 3–10 minutes after IM or IV administration. Use of droperidol is appealing because of its strong sedative and antiemetic effects, moderate tendency to produce extrapyramidal reactions, and weak anticholinergc and antiadrenergic effects. The sedative effects generally last 2–4 hours, but may persist for up to 12 hours. Usual doses when given IM (2.5 mg/mL) to adults range from 2.5 to 10 mg. The IV doses should not exceed 100 mg twice daily. Droperidol is not intended for long-term use.

A recent report indicated that droperidol (mean dose 0.44 ± 0.22 cc [0.44 ± 0.22 mg]) was effective in 26 aggressive children with externalizing disorders. All children receiving droperidol were able to return to the milieu 2 hours later (Joshi et al., 1998).

Treatment of Agitation that Occurs in Conjunction with a Seizure or in a Delirium

Agitation occurring within the context of a medical or neurological disorder, such as a seizure, requires astute assessment of the underlying disorder and initiation of active treatment for the medical problem. Pharmacologic intervention specifically targeting the agitation and aggression may also be necessary. Pharmacological interventions should be used with caution, while the medical work-up is pursued and treatment initiated.

Low-dose haloperidol was often used in the past within the context of delirium. However, because of concerns regarding the side effects from use of this agent, some of the atypical agents have been used instead. For example, in a recent case report, a 14-year-old girl with a fluctuating psychosis induced by dexamethasone treatment during chemotherapy for pre–B acute lymphocytic leukemia became agitated and aggressive. Her behavior and fluctuating mental status were successfully managed with risperidone, with improvement occurring within 3 weeks (Kramer and Cottingham, 1999).

Developmental Considerations Affecting Treatment

There are discrepant reports regarding the responsivity of aggression in young children to intervention. Treatment outcome may reflect in part the type of aggression that is targeted. Some types of aggression may be more or less responsive to intervention. For example, the covert type of aggression may be less sensitive to treatment (Loeber, 1991), whereas the overt type of aggression (Rebok et al., 1996) is responsive to combined pharmacotherapy and psychotherapeutic interventions.

Adolescents suffering from medication-responsive psychiatric conditions are at high risk for dangerous behaviors. Most teens afflicted with psychiatric disorders struggle to achieve age-appropriate autonomy while trying to accept their illness. As a result, teens are typically noncompliant and resist treatment recommendations that are supported by parents and treators. In addition, adolescents with concerns about side effects, particularly those affecting physical appearance such as weight gain, are prone to noncompliance. Such medication noncompliance in turn leads to an increase in uncomfortable psychiatric symptoms. Often these noncompliant teens turn to illegal substances to self-medicate. The combination of psychiatric symptoms, medication noncompliance, and substance abuse greatly increases the risk of suicidal and homicidal impulsivity.

ASSESSMENT OF RISK FOR VIOLENCE AND LEGAL CONSIDERATIONS

In the assessment of risk for violence one needs to take into consideration the risk factors outlined in Table 50.1. Most aggressive youths are impulsive and noncompliant, often continuing to be at risk despite active treatment.

Providing community support and psychoeducation for the patient and family, as well as involving school personnel, can help in monitoring for signs of dangerousness, relapse, medication noncompliance, and substance abuse. Tight treatment team communication minimizes the likelihood of aggressive behavior.

If a youth is imminently dangerous, health professionals are obligated to protect the individual from acting. Either psychiatric hospitalization or one-to-one close supervision, while optimizing community support, is indicated. All dangerous items (e.g., weapons, medications, etc.) should be removed from the home or locked out of reach. Efforts should be made to decrease stimuli likely to agitate the youth. If a youth is homicidal, psychiatric hospitalization is usually the only course of action. The health professional team has a duty to warn the targeted individual(s) if any are specifically named [Tarasoff Ruling] (Stone, 1976). If the homicidal youth is maintained in the community, increased structure and one-to-one observation are essential, with prohibition of contact with the person(s) toward whom the youth feels homicidal. Access to weapons should be prevented by removing them from the home. Psychopharmacological intervention and psychotherapeutic supports should be optimized. Chronic homicidal or suicidal ideation usually necessitates residential therapeutic placement to provide adequate structure and treatment over a 24-hour period.

In the event that an aggressive act leads to injury or even death, the clinical team should review the event and provide support to each other. In addition, depending on the situation, the clinical team may want to remain available to family members or guardians, as well as to others involved in the child's care, to provide support and education in the aftermath of such an event.

REFERENCES

Aman, M.G., Findling, R.L., Derivan, A., and Merriman, U. (2000) Risperidone versus placebo for severe conduct disorder in children with mental retardation [NCDEU abstract]. *J Child Adolesc Psychopharmacol* 10:253.

Aman, M., Kern, R., McGhee, D., and Arnold, L. (1993) Fenfluramine and methylphenidate in children with mental retardation and ADHD: clinical and side effects. *J Am Acad Child Adolesc Psychiatry* 32: 851–859.

Aman, M.G., Kern, R.A., Osborne, P., Tumuluru R., Rojak, J., and de Medical, V. (1997) Fenfluramine and methylphenidate in children with mental retardation and borderline IQ: clinical effects. *Am J Ment Retard* 101:521–534.

Aman, M. and Langworthy, K.S. (2000) Pharmacotherapy for hyperactivity in children with autism and other pervasive developmental disorder *J Autism Dev Disord* 30:451–459.

American Psychiatric Association (1994) *Diagnostic and Statistical Manual of Mental Disorders, 4th ed.* Washington, DC: American Psychiatric Press.

Apter, A., Gothelf, D., Orbach, I., Wizman, R., Ratzoni, G., Har-Even, D., and Tyano, S. (1995) Correlation of suicidal and violent behavior in different diagnostic categories in hospitalized adolescent patients. *J Am Acad Child Adolesc Psychiatry* 34: 912–918.

Bell, C., Gamm, S., Ballas, P., and Jackson, P. (2001) Strategies for the prevention of youth violence in Chicago public schools. In: Saffi, M., Saffi, S.E., eds. *School Violence: Contributing Factors, Management and Prevention.* Washington DC: American Psychiatric Press.

Biederman, J., Faraone, S.V., Chu, M.P., and Wozniak, J. (1999) Further evidence of a bidirectional overlap between juvenile mania and conduct disorder in children. *J Am Acad Child Adolesc Psychiatry* 38: 468–476.

Birmaher, B., Quintana, H., and Greenhill, L.L. (1988) Methylphenidate treatment of hyperactive autistic children. *J Am Acad Child Adolesc Psychiatry* 27:248–251.

Brent, D.A., Kolko, D.J., Wartella, M.E., Boylan, M.B., Moritz, G., Baughner, M., and Zelerak, J.P. (1993) Adolescent psychiatric in-

patients' risk of suicide attempts at 6 months follow-up. *J Am Acad Child Adolesc Psychiatry* 32:95–105.

Budman, C., Brunn, R.D., Park, K.S., Lesser, M., and Olson, M. (2000) Explosive outbursts in children with Tourette's disorder. *J Am Acad Child Adolesc Psychiatry* 39: 1270–1276.

Buitelaar, J.K. (2000) Open-label treatment with risperidone of 26 psychiatrically hospitalized children and adolescents with mixed diagnoses and aggressive behavior. *J Child Adolesc Psychopharmacol* 10: 19–26.

Buitelaar, J.K., van der Gaag, R.J., Swaab-Barneveld, H., and Kuiper, M. (1996) Pindolol and methylphenidate in children with attention-deficit hyperactivity disorder: clinical efficacy and side-effects. *J Child Psychol Psychiatry* 37: 587–595.

Campbell, M., Adams, P.B., Small, A.M., Kafantaris, V., Silva, R.R., Shell, J., Perry, R., and Overall, J.E. (1995) Lithium in hospitalized aggressive children with conduct disorder: a double-blind and placebo-controlled study. *J Am Acad Child Adolesc Psychiatry* 24:445–453.

Campbell, M., Small A.M., Green W.H., Jennings, S.J., Perry, R., Bennett, W.G., and Anderson, L. (1984) Behavioral efficacy of haloperidol and lithium carbonate. *Arch Gen Psychiatry* 41:650–656.

Campbell, M., Anderson, L.T., and Meier, M. (1979) A comparison of haloperidol, behavior therapy, and their interaction in autistic children. *Psychopharmacol Bull* 15:84–64.

Comings, D.E., Coming, B.F., Tacket, T., and Li, S. (1990) The clonidine patch and behavior problems. *J Am Acad Child Adoles Psychiatry* 29: 667–668.

Commission for the Prevention of Youth Violence (CPYV) (2000) Youth Violence. Medicine, Nursing and Public Health: Connecting the Dots to prevent Violence. Chicago: Commission for the Prevention of Youth Violence, IL pp.1–45.

Connor, D.F., Ozbayrak, K.R., Benjamin, S., Yunshen, and Fletcher, K.E. (1997) A pilot study of nadolol for overt aggression in developmentally delayed individuals. *J Am Acad Child Adolesc Psychiatry* 36:826–834.

Cook, E.H., Rowlett, R., Jaselskis, C., and Leventhal, B.L. (1992) Fluoxetine treatment of children and adults with autistic disorder and mental retardation. *J Am Acad Child Adolesc Psychiatry* 31: 1–7.

Cueva, J.E., Overall, J.E., Small, A.M., Armenteros, J.L., Perry, R., and Campbell, M. (1996) Carbamazepine in aggressive children with conduct disorder: a double-blind and placebo-controlled study. *J Am Acad Child Adolesc Psychiatry* 35:480–490.

Davanzo, P.A., Belin, T.R., Widawski, M.H., and King, B.H. (1998) Paroxetine treatment of aggression and self-injury in persons with mental retardation. *Am J Ment Retard* 102:427–437.

Delgado-Escueta, A.V., Mattson, R.H., King, L., Goldenshon, E.S., Spiegel, L.F., Madsen, J., Crandell, P., Dreifuss, F., and Porter, R.J. (1982) The nature of aggression during epileptic seizure. *N Engl J Med* 305:711–716.

Donovan, S.J., Stewart, J.W., Nunes, E.V., Quitkin, P.M., Parides, M., Daniel, W., Susser, E., and Klein, D.R. (2000) Divalproex treatment for youth with explosive temper and mood lability: a double-blind, placebo-controlled crossover design. *Am J Psychiatry* 157:818–820.

Fassler, D. (2001) A common sense 10 point plan to address the problem of school violence. *Am Acad Child Adolesc Psychiatry* http://www.aacap.org/whatsnew/10point.htm.

Filley, C.M., Price, B.H., Nell, V., Litt, D., Antionette, T., Morgan, A.S., James, F., Bresnahan, S.J., Picus, J.H., Gelbort, M.M., Weissberg, M., and Kelly, J.P. (2001) Toward an understanding of violence: neurobehavioral aspects of unwarranted physical aggression: Aspen Neurobehavioral Conference Consensus Statement. *Neuropsychiatry Neuropsychol Behav Neurol* 14:1–14.

Findling, R.L., McNamara, N.K., Branicky, L.A., Schuluchter, M.D., Lemon, E., and Blumer, J.L. (2000) A double-blind pilot study of risperidone in the treatment of conduct disorder. *J Am Acad Child Adolesc Psychiatry* 39:509–561.

Frankhauser, F.P., Karumanchi, V.C., German, M.L., Yates, A., and Darumanchi, S.D. (1982). A double-blind, placebo-controlled study of the efficacy of transdermal clonidine in autism. *J Clin Psychiatry* 53:77–82.

Frazier, J.A., Biederman, J., Tohen, M., Feldman, P.D., Jacobs, T.G., Toma, V., Rater, M.A., Tarazi, R.A., Kim, G.S., Garfield, S.B., Sohma, M., Gonzalez-Heydrich, J., Risser, R.C., and Nowlin, Z.M.A. (2001) Prospective open-label treatment trial of olanzapine monotherapy in children and adolescents with bipolar disorder. *J Child Adolesc Psychopharmacol* 11:239–250.

Frazier, J.A., Meyer, M.C., Biederman, J., Wozniak, J., Wilens, T., Spencer, T., Kim, G., and Shapiro, S. (1999) Risperidone treatment for juvenile bipolar disorder: a retrospective chart review. *J Am Acad Child Adolesc Psychiatry* 38:960–965.

Geller, D., Biederman, J., Griffin, S., Jones, J., and Lefkowitz, T.R. (1996) Comorbidity of juvenile obsessive-compulsive disorder with disruptive behavior disorders. *J Am Acad Child Adolesc Psychiatry* 35:1637–1646.

Geller, B., Cooper, T., Sun, K., Zimmerman, B., Frazier, J., Williams, M., Heath, J. (1998) Double-blind and placebo-controlled study of lithium for adolescent bipolar disorders with secondary substance dependency. *J Am Acad Child Adolesc Psychiatry* 37:171–178.

Ghazuiddin, N. and Alessi, N.E. (1992) An open clinical trial of trazodone in aggressive children. *J Child Adolesc Psychopharmacol* 2:291–298.

Gittleman-Klein, R., Klein, D.F., Katz, S., Saraf, K., and Pollack, E. (1976) Comparative effects of methylphenidate and thioridazine in hyperkinetic children I: clinical results. *Arch Gen Psychiatry* 33:1217–1231.

Gordon, C.T., State, R.C., Nelson, J.E., Hamburger, S.D., and Rapoport, J.L. (1993) A double-blind comparison of clomipramine, desipramine and placebo in the treatment of autistic disorder. *Arch Gen Psychiatry* 50:441–447.

Greenhill, L.L., Solomon, M., Pleak, R., and Ambrosini, P. (1985) Molindone hydrochloride treatment of hospitalized children with conduct disorder. *J Clin Psychiatry* 46:20–25.

Handen, B.L., Feldman, H.M., Lurier, A., Husaz, R., and Murray, P.J. (1999) Efficacy of methylphenidate among preschool children with developmental disabilities and ADHD. *J Child Adolesc Psychiatry* 38:805–812.

Hinshaw, S.P. (1991). Stimulant medication in the treatment of aggression in children with attentional deficits. *J Clin Child Psychol* 12:301–312.

Hollander, E., Dolgoff-Kaspar, R., Cartwright, C., Rawitt, R., and Novotny, S. (2000) Divalproex sodium in autism spectrum disorders: a pilot trail [NCDEU abstract] *J Child Adolesc Psychopharmacol* 10:251–252.

Horrigan, J.P., and Barnhill, L.J. (1997) Risperidone and explosive aggressive autism. *J Autism Dev Disord* 27: 313–323.

Hunt, R.D., Arnsten, A.F.T., and Asbell, M.D. (1995) An open trial of guanfacine in the treatment of attention-deficit hyperactivity disorder. *J Am Acad Child Adolesc Psychiatry* 34:50–54.

Hunt, R.D., Minderaa, R.B., and Cohen, D.J. (1985) Clonidine benefits children with attention deficit disorder and hyperactivity: report of a double-blind placebo-controlled crossover study. *J Am Acad Child Adolesc Psychiatry* 24:617–629.

Jaselskis, C.A., Cook, E.H., Fletcher, K.E., and Leventhal, B.L. (1992) Clonidine treatment of hyperactive and impulsive children with autistic disorder. *J Clin Psychopharmacol* 12:322–326.

Joshi, P., Hamel, L., Hoshi, A.R.T., and Capozzoli, J.A. (1998) Use of droperidol in hospitalized children. *J Am Acad Child Adolesc Psychiatry* 37:228–230.

Kafantaris, V., Campbell, M., Padron-Gayol, M.V., Small, A.M., Locascio, J.J., and Rosenberg, C.R. (1992) Carbamazepine in hospitalized aggressive conduct disorder children: an open pilot study. *Psychopharmacol Bull* 28:193–199.

Kastner, T., Finesmith, R., and Walsh, K. (1993) Long-term administration of valproic acid in the treatment of affective symptoms in people with mental retardation. *J Clin Psychopharmacol* 13: 448–451.

Kataoka, S.H., Hima, B.T., Dupre, D.A., Moreno, K.A., Yang, X., and McCracken, J.T. (2001) Mental health problems and service use among female juvenile offenders: their relationship to criminal history. *J Am Acad Child Adolesc Psychiatry* 40:549–555.

Kemph, J.P., Devane, C.L., Levin, G.M., Jarecke, R., and Miller, R.L. (1993) Treatment of aggressive children with clonidine: results of an open pilot study. *J Am Acad Child Adolesc Psychiatry* 32:577–581.

King, B.H., Wright, M., Hande, B.L., Sikich, L.M., Zimmerman, A.W., McMahon, W., Cantwell, E., Davanzo, P.A., Dourish, C.T., Dykens, E.M., Hooper, S.R., Jaselskis, C.A., Leventhal, B., Levitt, J., Lord, C., Lubetsky, M.J., Myers, S.M., Ozonoff, S., Shah, B.G., Snape, M., Shernoff, E.W., Williamson, K., and Cook, E.H. (2001a) Double-blind placebo-controlled study of amantadine hydrochloride in the treatment of children with autistic disorder. *J Am Acad Child Adolesc Psychiatry* 40:658–665.

King, B.H., Wright, M., Snape, M., and Dourish, C.T. (2001b) Case series: amantadine open-label treatment of impulsive and aggressive behavior in hospitalized children with developmental disabilities. *J Am Acad Child Adolesc Psychiatry* 40:654–657.

Klein, R.G. (1991) Preliminary results: lithium effects in conduct disorder. In: *CME Syllabus and Proceeding Summary, Symposium 2: The 144th Annual Meeting of the American Psychiatric Association, New Orleans, LA, May 11–16, 1991.* Washington, DC: American Psychiatric Association, pp. 119–120.

Klein, R.G., Abikoff, H., Klass, E., Ganeles, D., Seese, L.M., and Pollack, S. (1997) Clinical efficacy of methylphenidate in conduct disorder with and without attention deficit hyperactivity disorder. *Arch Gen Psychiatry* 54:1073–1080.

Knox, M., King, C., Hanna, G.L., Logan, D., and Ghaziuddin, N. (2000) Aggressive behavior in clinically depressed adolescents. *J Am Acad Child Adolesc Psychiatry* 39:611–617.

Kovacs, M., and Pollock, M. (1995) Bipolar disorder and comorbid conduct disorder in childhood and adolescence. *J Am Acad Child Adolesc Psychiatry* 34:715–723.

Kramer, T.M., and Cottingham, E.M. (1999) Letter to the editor: risperidone in the treatment of steroid-induced psychosis. *J Child Adolesc Psychopharmacol* 9:315–316.

Loeber, R. (1991) Antisocial behavior: more enduring than changeable? *J Am Acad Child Adolesc Psychiatry* 30:393–397.

Malone, R.P., Delaney, M.A., Luebbert, J.F., Cater, J., and Campbell, M. (2000) A double-blind placebo-controlled study of lithium in hospitalized aggressive children and adolescent with conduct disorder. *Arch Gen Psychiatry* 57:649–654.

Marsh, L. and Krauss, G.L. (2000) Review: aggression and violence in patients with epilepsy. *Epilepsy Behav* 1:160–168.

McDougle, C.J., Holmes, J.P., Bronson, M.R., Anderson, G.M., Volkmar, F.R., Price, L.H., and Cohen, D.J. (1997) Risperidone treatment of children and adolescents with pervasive developmental disorders: a prospective, open-label study. *J Am Acad Child Adolesc Psychiatry* 36:685–693.

McDougle, C.J., Scahill, L., McCracken, J.T., Aman, M.G., Tierney, E., Arnold, L.E., Freeman, B.J., Martin, A., McGough, J.J., Cronin, P., Posey, D.J., Riddle, M.A., Ritz, L., Swiezy, N.B., Vitiello, B., Volkmar, F.R., Votolato, N.A., and Walson, P. (2000) Research Units on Pediatric Psychopharmacology (RUPP) Autism Network: background and rationale for an initial controlled study of risperidone. *Child Adolesc Psychiatry Clin North Am* 9: 201–224.

Naruse, H., Naghata, M., Nakane, Y., Shirahashi, K., Takesada, M., and Yamazaki, K. (1982) A multicenter double blind trial of pimozide, haloperidol and placebo in children with behavioral disorder, using a crossover design. *Acta Paediatr Psychiatry* 48:173–184.

Pfeffer, C.R., Jiang, H., and Domeshek, L.J. (1997) Buspirone treatment of psychiatrically hospitalized prepubertal children with symptoms of anxiety and moderately severe aggression. *J Child Adolesc Psychopharmacol* 7:145–155.

Pliszka, S.R., Sherman, J.O., Barrow, M.V., and Irick S. (2000) Affective disorder in juvenile offenders: a preliminary study. *Am J Psychiatry* 157:130–132.

Puig-Antich, J. (1982) Major depression and conduct disorder in prepuberty. *J Am Acad Child Adolesc Psychiatry* 21:118–128.

Puig-Antich, J., Perel, J.M., Lupatkin, W., et al. (1987) Imipramine in prepubertal major depressive disorders. *Arch Gen Psychiatry* 44:81–89.

Quintana, H. and Keshavan, M. (1995) Case study: risperidone in children and adolescents with schizophrenia. *J Am Acad Child Adolesc Psychiatry* 34:1292–1296.

Rasanen, P., Tiihonen, J., Isohanni, M., Rantakallio, P., Lehtonen, J., and Moring, J. (1998) Schizophrenia, alcohol abuse and violent behavior: a 2-year followup study of an unselected birth cohort *Schizophre Bull* 24:437–441.

Rebok, G.W., Hawkins, W.E., Krener, P., Mayer, L.S., and Kellam, S.C. (1996) Effect of concentration problems on the malleability of children's aggressive and shy behaviors. *J Am Acad Child Adolesc Psychiatry* 35:193–203.

Ricketts, R.W., Gota, A.B., Ellis, C.R., Singh, Y.N., Chamber, S., Singh, N.N., and Cooke, J.C. (1994) Clinical effects of buspirone on intractable self-injury in adults with mental retardation. *J Am Acad Child Adolesc Psychiatry* 33:270–276.

Rifkin, A., Karajgi, B., Dicker, R., Perl E., Boppona, V., Hasan, N., Pollack, S. (1997) Lithium treatment of conduct disorders in adolescents. *Am J Psychiatry* 154:554–555.

Sanchez, L.E., Campbell, M., Small, A.M., Cueva, J.E., Armenteros, J.L., and Adams, P.B. (1996) *J Am Acad Child Adolesc Psychiatry* 35:537–544.

Satcher, D. (2001) National Agenda for Children's Mental Health. NIMH Surgeon General National Action Agenda Release. U.S. Dept. of Health and Human Services. Washington, D.C.

Satterfield, J.H., and Schell, a. (1997) A prospective study of hyperactive boys with conduct problems and normal boys: adolescent and adult criminality. *J Am Acad Child Adolesc Psychiatry* 36: 1726–1739.

Schreier, H.A. (1998) Risperidone for young children with mood disorders and aggressive behavior. *J Child Adolesc Psychopharmacol* 8:49–58.

Schvehla, R.J., Mandoki, M.W., and Sumneer, G.S. (1994) Clonidine therapy for comorbid attention deficit hyperactivity disorder and conduct disorder: preliminary findings in children's inpatient unit. *South Med J* 87:692–695.

Singer, M.I., Slovak, K., Frerson, T., York, P. (1998) Viewing preferences, symptoms of psychological trauma, and violent behaviors among children who watch television. *J Child Adolesc Psychiatry* 37:1041–1048.

Stone, A.A. (1976) The Tarasoff decisions: suing psychotherapist to safeguard society. *Harv Law Rev* 90:358–378.

Swartz, M.S., Swanson, J.W., Hiday, V.A., Borum, R., Wagner, R.H., and Burns, B.J. (1998) Violence and severe mental illness: The Effects of substance abuse and nonadherence to medications. *Am J Psychiatry* 15:226–231.

Verhoefen, W.M.A. and Tuinier, S., (1996) The effect of buspirone on challenging behaviour in mentally retarded patients: an open prospective multiple—case study. *J Intell Disability Research* 40: 502–508.

Vitiello, B., Hill, J.L., Elia, J., Cunningham, E., McLevi, S.L., and Gehar, D. (1991) PRN medications in child psychiatric patients: a pilot placebo-controlled study. *J Clin Psychiatry* 52:499–502.

Vitiello, B., Ricciuti, A.J., and Behar, D. (1987) PRN medications in child state hospital inpatients. *J Clin Psychiatry* 48:351–354.

Vitiello, B. and Stoff, D. (1997) Subtypes of aggression and their relevance to child psychiatry. *J Am Acad Child Adolesc Psychiatry* 36:307–315.

Vossekuil, B., Reddy, M., Rein, R. (2000) Safe School Initiative. An interim report on the prevention of targeted violence in schools. Presented at: Awesome Adolescents Conference, McLean Hospital, Boston, MA.

Williams, D.T., Mehl, R., Yudofsky, S., Adams, D., and Roseman, B. (1982) The effect of propranolol on uncontrolled rage outbursts in children and adolescents with organic brain dysfunction. *J Am Acad Child Adolesc Psychiatry* 21:129–135.

Wozniak, J., Biederman, J., Kiely, K., Ablon, J.S., Faraone, S.V., Mundy, E., and Mennin, D. (1995) Mania-like symptoms suggestive of childhood onset bipolar disorder in clinically referred children. *J Am Acad Child Adolesc Psychiatry* 34:867–876.

Wozniak, J., Crawford, M.H., Biederman, J., Faraone, S.V., Spencer, T.J., Taylor, A., and Blier, H. (1999) Antecedents and complications of trauma in boys with ADHD: findings from a longitudinal study. *J Am Acad Child Adolesc Psychiatry* 38:48–55.

Zocolillo, M. (1992) Co-occurrence of conduct disorder and its adult outcomes with depressive and anxiety disorder: a review. *J Am Acad Child Adolesc Psychiatry* 31:547–556.

Zubieta, J.K. and Allessi, N.E. (1992) Acute and chronic administration of trazodone in the treatment of disruptive behavior disorders in children. *J Clin Psychopharmacol* 12:346–351.

51 | Elimination disorders: enuresis and encopresis

WILLIAM REINER

Few somatic regions encompass the variety of emotionally laden physiological and pathophysiological functions as the pelvic cavity, with its associated urinary, defecatory, and sexual structures and functions. Pelvic and perineal considerations, however, have tended to be overshadowed or overlooked and, alternatively, overemphasized or overexplored during the emergence and evolution of theoretical and hypothetical constructs of child development.

Urinary, colorectal, and genital physiological mechanisms are complex and even today incompletely understood. The rather arbitrary diagnostic criteria for psychiatric categorization of disorders of these mechanisms are, then, categorically and neurobiologically rather simplistic. Additionally, genetic components in enuresis (von Gontard et al., 1999) often interact with neurobiology, although at present a strong family history of enuresis primarily implies a greater likelihood of response to vasopressin (AVP) effectors (Hogg and Husmann, 1993; Ornitz et al., 2000) (see Interventions, Nocturnal Enuresis, below). It is fitting to uncover the neurobiological underpinnings of the perineal–pelvic region in order to explicate its pathophysiology. Gleaning clinically relevant data from patients or parents can designate appropriate diagnostic approaches and clinical evaluations as well as therapeutic interventions. This chapter will attempt to provide a brief yet structured approach to both pathophysiology and psychopharmacological interventions for disorders of perineal–pelvic functions in children and adolescents, as well as relevant psychopharmacological effects and side effects on genitourinary, colorectal, and sexual functions.

NEUROANATOMY AND NEUROPHYSIOLOGY OF PELVIC ORGANS

Analogous or neurologically similar mechanisms operate in normal bladder and bowel function, and some of these functions are further integrated with sexual function. However, neurourological data of voiding dysfunctions (that is, urodynamic data from the neurourological clinical laboratory) have greater clinical relevance for psychiatric therapeutic interventions than those from colorectal or sexual dysfunction evaluations. Because of the complexity of the physiology and pathophysiology of the three organ systems, and because of complex interactions among them, focusing on a model of the neurobiology of voiding and the neurourology of voiding dysfunctions will provide insight into all pelvic systems, with specific reference to defecatory or sexual interactions with distinctive physiology that may be clinically relevant. To begin with, typical pelvic organ system functions require the collective integrity of the functional units—that is, appropriate anatomical subunits synchronized with sensory, motor, and autonomic neural contributions. The functional integrity of each pelvic organ system does not require consciousness; that is, bladder, bowel, and sexual functions can be entirely reflexogenic (Elbadawi, 1973; Daniel et al., 1983) and can often, therefore, occur in the absence of cortical integrity. Clinical recognition that these systems may function normally in patients with head injuries, vegetative states, or other cortical insults can itself increase our insight into system dysfunctions.

Normal function, then, requires organ system integrity (Fig. 51.1). Muscular and vascular apparatuses are equally important to sensory and motor innervation (Elbadawi, 1973). In the bladder, for example, muscular function includes storage (distensibility, or compliance) as well as elimination (coordinated muscular contractions) and therefore requires appropriate sphincter tone, contraction, and relaxation. Neurovascular bundles provide critical vascular and neural input and output for all pelvic subunits (Daniel et al., 1983).

The detrusor muscle itself is of complex embryological development, innervation, and function (Hun-

686

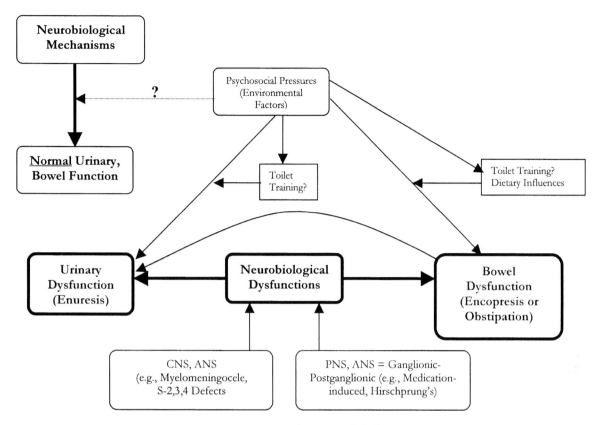

FIGURE 51.1 Mechanisms of urinary and bowel function and dysfunction. ANS, autonomic nervous system; CNS, central nervous system.

ter, 1954). It is composed of irregularly spatially oriented smooth muscle bundles interweaving with each other in equally irregular patterns. Neural innervation has no known myogenic conduction component and thus appears to be neuro*muscular* in conductive origin (Daniel et al., 1983). The *base* of the detrusor is both in continuity with and interlaced by longitudinal smooth muscle bundles from the distal ureters (forming the trigonal muscle) and the urethral smooth muscle at the bladder opening (bladder neck) (Elbadawi and Schenk, 1971). The lissosphincter, or so-called internal urethral sphincter, is thus composed of this bladder neck admixture of smooth muscle units (Elbadawi, 1973, 1982). The rectum, in comparison, has similar anatomical integration of rectal musculature with the internal anal sphincter but with less apparent embryological complexity.

Interestingly, the lissosphincter subunits (the bladder base) have separate pharmacological receptors from the remainder of the detrusor, but without anatomical or histological boundaries, and integrate in micturition. Lissosphincter muscle bundles proceed into the cephalad portion of the prostatic urethra in the male or the urethrovaginal septum in the female (Gil Vernet, 1968; Hutch, 1972). In the male these muscle bundles interlace in complex patterns with the prostatic urethra.

Finally, external urethral sphincter (voluntary sphincter, or rhabdosphincter) is a striated circumscribing structure emanating from the bladder neck and bladder base detrusor through the mid-urethra in the female and intermediate prostatic urethra in the male. While also surrounding Cowper's glands in the male, these rhabdosphincter subunits contract, most likely, only with ejaculation (Hutch, 1972; Elbadawi, 1980), along with simultaneous anal rhabdosphincter, bulbocavernosus muscle, and cremaster muscle contractions.

Lissosphincter and detrusor muscle is innervated by the pelvic plexus, formed from efferent parasympathetic nerves from sacral 2, 3, 4 spinal cord segments and efferent sympathetic nerves from thoracic 10, 11, 12 spinal cord segments to the bladder and urethra (Gil Vernet, 1968; Elbadawi and Schenk, 1971; Elbadawi, 1982). Muscle innervation is from postganglionic parasympathetic cholinergic fibers and postganglionic sympathetic adrenergic fibers, possibly with more cholinergic receptors in the detrusor and adrenergic receptors in the sphincters (Elbadawi and Schenk, 1974; Elbadawi, 1982).

Afferent cholinergic and adrenergic autonomic fibers are similarly present in detrusor and lissosphincter units and include micturition triggers linked with stretch receptors and urinary flow receptors (Gil Vernet, 1968; Hutch, 1972; Elbadawi, 1973, 1982, 1983; Elbadawi and Schenk, 1974; de Groat and Kawatani, 1985). Some of the afferent fibers connect to reflex circuits in the sacral cord for bladder and rectum while connecting in the sacral and thoracic cord for sexual reflex circuits.

External urethral sphincter muscle probably has cholinergic and adrenergic autonomic innervation as well as cholinergic striated muscle innervation (Elbadawi and Schenk, 1974). This rhabdosphincter is unique when compared to other striated muscle in that it has a higher density of neural end-plates as well as blood vessel–independent neural plexuses. Efferent rhabdosphincter innervation is probably via the pudendal nerve while the lissosphincter efferents probably emanate from the pelvic plexus (Elbadawi and Schenk, 1974).

Neurobiological components of colorectal and anal sphincter mechanisms and pathophysiology are similar to the above-mentioned vesical components. In both systems, central, peripheral, and autonomic nervous system reflexes, partly involuntary and partly voluntary, interweave critically for appropriate function. Function and control are mediated through the lower spinal cord, as well as via cortical centers requiring coordinated voluntary (and reflex) relaxation of *external* sphincters, (reflex) relaxation of *internal* sphincters, and simultaneous coordinated contraction of detrusor

muscle in the bladder or peristaltic contraction of colorectal muscularis in the bowel for elimination of stored waste (Elbadawi, 1973, 1980, 1982; Elbadawi and Schenk, 1974; Daniel et al, 1983).

Sensory input is vital, and if filling, stretching, and contracting sensations are misconstrued or absent, elimination will be abnormal (Elbadawi and Schenk, 1974; Curran et al., 2000). Such coordinated functions must in addition be maintained until the respective chambers are emptied completely. Valsalva maneuvers often contribute to efficient emptying in the case of the large bowel; valsalva maneuvers can at times be detrimental to upper and lower urinary tract function and anatomy (Curran et al., 2000). Disruption of any component of sensory or motor function is likely to lead to partial or complete emptying at inappropriate times (incontinence), incomplete or disrupted emptying (withholding), or inability to empty at all (overflow incontinence) (Figs. 51.1 and 51.2).

Thus, normal bladder and urethral physiology is intertwined neurologically, anatomically, and physiopharmacologically to produce effective urinary filling, holding, and release. These functions circumscribe an increasing bladder volume and pressure without involuntary detrusor contractions or sphincter relaxation. A full bladder triggers conscious as well as involuntary recognition, leading at some point to detrusor contraction with sphincter relaxation until the bladder is empty. This must involve, as can be seen, coordinated muscular function with autonomic and voluntary intertwined efferent and afferent signals (Gil Vernet, 1968; Elbadawi, 1973, Elbadawi, 1982, 1983, Elbadawi and Schenk, 1974; Daniel et al., 1983). For

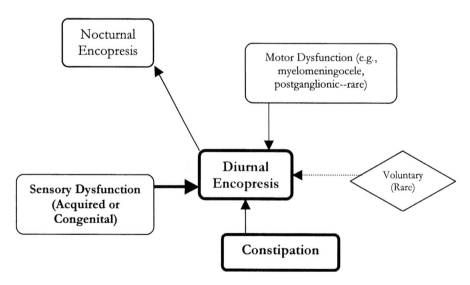

FIGURE 51.2 Mechanisms of encopresis.

proper emptying, muscular contraction must progress smoothly and coherently while sphincter relaxation must be timed accurately and be complete. Cholinergic and adrenergic receptors must then be appropriately stimulated and be normally responsive.

Central versus Peripheral End Organ Failure

There are no data to indicate that purely psychological factors influence elimination functions or dysfunctions directly. Rather, mental states can influence circulating or peripheral neurotransmitters (adrenergic or cholinergic), obfuscating functional subunit sensitivity and responsiveness of the end organs themselves. This alteration in circulating neurotransmitter accentuates pelvic organ dysfunctional states or potential for dysfunction. Simply stated, behavioral interventions for elimination disorders or dysfunction are most useful when targeting central hyperphysiological states and dysfunction such as anxiety, stress disorders, hyperthyroidism, or adrenal dysfunctions. It is neurogenic or myogenic disorder that leads to end organ dysfunction—for example, detrusor-sphincter contraction coupling or detrusor degeneration with sphincter failure. Pharmacological interventions, such as the tricyclic antidepressants (TCAs), can often target end organ dysfunction and central disorders simultaneously.

CLASSIFICATIONS OF ELIMINATION DISORDERS

Pathophysiological Classification of Elimination Disorders

Depending on the timing and the underlying pathophysiology, a child may experience nocturnal enuresis (NE), diurnal enuresis (DE), or both. Incontinence syndromes may in turn be subclassified as (1) intermittent with incomplete emptying (normal detrusor function, closed sphincter); (2) intermittent with slow but complete emptying (absent detrusor function with absent sphincter function); (3) intermittent with bolus emptying (unstable detrusor with normal or abnormal sphincter function); or (4) normal neurobiological urinary function with voiding during sleep (parasomnias, atypical AVP secretion, bladder dysfunctions) (Gil Vernet, 1968; Hutch, 1972; de Groat and Kawatani, 1985; Rerner, 1995; Neveus et al., 1999; von Gontard et al., 1999; Wolfish, 1999; Yeung et al., 1999; Curran et al., 2000; Laberge et al., 2000; Ornitz et al, 2000). Therefore, incontinence can occur while the child is awake or sleeping, attempting voluntary control or voluntary micturition, and recognizing voiding sensation—

voluntary or not—or not recognizing voiding sensation (as in complete neurourological failure).

DSM-IV Classification of Elimination Disorders

The *Diagnostic and Statistical Manual of Mental Disorders, 4th ed.*, (DSM-IV-TR), (American Psychiatric Association, 2000) defines elimination disorders and describes the clinical course, ensuing patient impairment, and associated features. Enuresis, for example, requires either involuntary or intentional voiding into bedding or clothing, a wetting frequency of twice a week for at least three consecutive months, *or* the presence of clinically significant distress in psychosocial functioning, a chronological age of the child of at least 5 years, and the behavior not being exclusively an effect of a substance or of a general medical condition. These criteria are both neurobiologically and clinically irrelevant.

The occurrence of nocturnal enuresis, for example, is inversely proportional to age, with a prevalence of approximately 15% at 5 years of age and a spontaneous rate of remission of about 15% per year thereafter (Forsythe and Redmond, 1974; Klackenberg, 1981). Nearly all children are dry at night by 15 years of age. Additionally, nocturnal enuresis is far more common in males at all ages. Encopresis, as similarly described in the DSM-IV-TR (American Psychiatric Association, 2000), requires repeated passage of feces into inappropriate places, at least one such event a month for at least 3 months, chronological age of the child of at least 4 years, and the behavior not being exclusively due to a substance or general medical condition. Subtypes describe constipation with overflow incontinence or no constipation with overflow incontinence—a contradiction in terms probably referring to neurogenic failure (combined neuromuscular and neurosphincteric dysfunction). A number of psychological, medical, and medication effects are listed as etiologies but correlate poorly with pathophysiological states.

Interestingly, child psychiatric literature and the DSM-IV-TR continue to differentiate primary from secondary enuresis or encopresis (American Psychiatric Association, 2000). Such characterizations are without physiological or pathological basis and have little influence on clinical decision making—they are, in fact, anachronistic in that they are not coherent with neurobiological data accruing over the last 30 years. Additionally, enuresis and encopresis are generally regarded by both patient and parent as well as by social context as impairing without regard to temporal historical data. Incontinence is clinically relevant in and of itself.

Abnormal Urinary Patterns: Classification

A more clinically relevant classification of enuresis divides urinary dysfunction into NE; DE, which in turn can be subdivided into dysfunctional voiding and frequency/dysuria; and NE/DE combined, probably best discussed as a subcategory of DE (Forsythe and Redmond, 1974; Klackenberg, 1981; de Groat and Kawatani, 1985; Hogg and Husmann, 1993; Reiner, 1995; Curran et al., 2000). Such divisions assist the clinician in selecting specific evaluations as well as specific interventions, with goals of prevention or arrest of end organ damage or failure and of improving the child's potential for coping. A careful history from the child and parents or, if necessary, prospective data collection, will generally provide the necessary clinical information pertinent to categorization. It is important to note that encopresis, although tending to occur more during awake periods, can occur during any activity or function.

Nocturnal enuresis

At least 80% of enuretic children wet only while sleeping, although more commonly at night than while napping, and demonstrate no concurrent psychopathology or significant genitourinary pathophysiology (Forsythe and Redmond, 1974; Klackenberg, 1981; Hogg and Husmann, 1993; Reiner, 1995). A normal history, physical examination (including abdominal exam and growth velocity), and a urinalysis are sufficient data through the seventh or eighth years to obviate the need for further urological evaluation. However, constipation is often causally related to all types of enuresis, a connection not frequently made by the clinician, and thus the usefulness of the abdominal exam (Tables 51.1 and 51.2; Yazbeck et al., 1987). The extent of correlation is unclear.

Responders to therapeutic interventions generally need no further evaluation (Koff, 1988; Reiner, 1995). While it is probably wise to refer the remaining enu-

TABLE 51.1 *Bowel Program for Constipation for Children 5–9 Years of Age*[a]

Step	Approach or Intervention	Dose	Administration Technique	Risks or Side Effects
1	History and physical exam			Low to none
2	Oral fiber product, e.g., Metamucil regular flavor (no sugar added), or fiber recommendation of pharmacist	½–¾ level teaspoon, 1–3 times/day	Mix with 1–2 oz. *chilled* juice, water, or liquid of choice, drink *rapidly*; *follow* with 5–6 oz. any liquid over 20 minutes	Low to none
3	USP mineral oil	1 tablespoon daily, for 5 days,[b] then stop	Mix with 3–4 tablespoons milk + 4–5 tablespoons ice cream in a blender for an emulsion with good flavor	Excess oil leads to oil seepage from anus; binds fat-soluble vitamins[b]
4	Sodium docusate (hydrophilic stool softener)	50 mg daily for 1 week, then as needed	Oral	Occasionally, strong urge to defecate ~12 hours after use
5	Mild laxative/stool softener combination (e.g., Senekot + sodium docusate)	As directed for age 1 night per week or less	Oral	Occasional loose stool or urgency to defecate
6	Pediatric Fleets enema or biscodyl suppository	Nightly for first 3 days	Per rectum	Child may experience sense of intrusion; colonic perforation possible (rare)
7	High-fiber foods: unprocessed bran (in cereals, muffins, etc.; dried fruits, prune juice)	10 g of fiber daily	Oral	Low to none
8	Hydration	5–6 6-ounce glasses of water daily	Oral	Low to none
9	Toilet habits	Sit for 10 minutes after breakfast and supper, and as needed	—	Low to none

[a]The aim is passage of at least one large, formed bowel movement every 2 days.
[b]Give evenly other day for 5 days to 5- to 7-year-olds; do not give with meals.

TABLE 51.2 *Bowel Program for Constipation for Larger Children 9–16 Years of Age*

Step	Approach or Intervention	Dose	Administration Technique	Risks or Side Effects
1	Oral fiber product, e.g., Metamucil regular flavor (no sugar added), or fiber recommendation of pharmacist	1 level or rounded teaspoon, 1–3 times/day	Mix with 2–3 oz. *chilled* juice, or liquid of choice, drink *rapidly*; 8 oz additional liquid over 20 minutes	Low to none
2	Sodium docusate (hydrophilic stool softener)	100 mg daily or as directed for age	Oral	Occasionally, strong urge to defecate ~12 hours after use
3	Mild laxative/stool softener combination (e.g., Senekot + softener)	As directed for age, 2 nights per week or less	Oral	Occasional loose stool or urgency to defecate
4	Biscodyl suppository[b]	1 time/week if no bowel movement in 3 days	Per rectum	Child may experience sense of intrusion
6	High-fiber foods: unprocessed bran (in cereals, muffins, etc.; dried fruits, prune juice, pear nectar)	12–16 g of fiber daily	Oral	Low to none
7	Hydration	6–8 6-ounce glasses of water daily	Oral	Low to none
8	Toilet habits	Sit for 10 minutes after breakfast, supper, and as needed	—	Low to none

[a]The aim is passage of at least one large, formed bowel movement every 1–2 days.

[b]Recommended *only* for very severe constipation and only in children over 5 years old.

retic children (after 8 years of age) for urological or urodynamic evaluation, the large majority of even those children will have no pathological findings (Koff, 1988).

Diurnal enuresis

In general, spontaneous diurnal incontinence should be considered pathophysiological (Fig. 51.1). Most commonly, uninhibited detrusor contractions (an unstable detrusor) are the cause alone or in combination with other neuroanatomical subunit dysfunction. Diurnal enuresis demands a urological consultation with diagnostic goals of assessing upper or lower urinary tract damage and of preventing progressive damage. Therapeutic interventions are dictated by the underlying etiology.

Especially in younger children, uninhibited and unpredictable detrusor contractions can be caused by constipation alone, by lower urinary tract infections (UTIs), or by constipation-associated UTIs (Yazbeck et al., 1987; Reiner, 1995). Pediatric pelvic organ structural immaturity prevents complete bladder filling by colorectal obstipation and hyperdistension. By contrast, mature vaginal–uterine or prostatic structural anatomy and associated ligaments provide a fairly rigid barrier between bowel and bladder/bladder neck, protecting the bladder from a hyperdistended colorectum.

Dysfunctional voiding and frequency/dysuria

Dysfunctional voiding is an irregular and unpredictable pattern of detrusor contractions with uncoupled internal and/or external sphincter reflexogenic coordination. Children with these conditions tend to be urinary and fecal withholders and have a muted afferent recognition of filling. Their contractions may be uninhibited because of detrusor instability (high muscle tone, unstable neuromuscular function, or dyscontrol of neural efferent activity) or poor sensory feedback (leading to normal detrusor contraction without the child's realizing that a contraction is about to occur or has already begun). These children tend to have associated fecal soiling (Forsythe and Redmond, 1974; Klackenberg, 1981; Yazbeck et al., 1987; Koff, 1988).

Urinary frequency and dysuria may be caused by high detrusor muscle tone or unstable neuromuscular function, but with good sensation and normal or excessive sphincter control. Extreme bladder sensitivity can also lead to frequency or dysuria. Such sensitivity can be congenital or can be caused by chronic constipation or chronic UTIs. Unfortunately, many children with chronic UTIs do not experience improvement in their symptoms when the infection is controlled. Correcting constipation commonly does, however, lead to some symptomatic improvement (Yazbeck et al., 1987; Koff, 1988). Children with frequency/urgency or dysuria have a presumed neurobiological etiology, including hyperadrenergic states associated with anxiety or stress disorders. Careful history *from the child* about sensory recognition of filling, of being full, of the need or urge to void, and of actual voiding can nearly always delineate abnormal sensory recognition.

INTERVENTIONS FOR ELIMINATION DISORDERS

General Concepts for Enuresis

Historically, interventions for enuresis, as well as encopresis, have often reflected intolerance, seeming harshness, and/or a poor understanding of child development (Glicklich, 1951). The vast majority of children over the age of 6 or 7 years as well as their parents will request treatment. Very occasional parents or children may be interested in intermittent treatment—for example, treatment may be desirable for overnight sleep-overs or for camping. Trials of interventions will be necessary to determine what approaches will work in such children and how much time is required for the intervention to be effective.

In the author's experience, more than half of all children presenting clinically with any form of enuresis, and about 90% with encopresis, will have some aspect of improvement and sometimes even resolution of symptoms with a conservative approach, especially one targeting constipation. The initial step is a "bowel program" or "bowel cocktail" directed towards relative lowering of colonic intraluminal pressure by softening the stool and emptying the colorectal lumen (Yazbeck et al., 1987; Koff, 1988; Reiner, 1995; Neveus et al., 1999; Wolfish, 1999; Yeung et al, 1999; Curran et al., 2000; Laberge et al., 2000). Such a program can utilize a combination of daily high fiber foods and fiber products, the occasional use of a lubricant two or three times per week (mineral oil emulsified with ice cream and milk in a blender), and a stool softener (for example, docusate sodium, 50 mg), possibly with an occasional use of a softener–mild laxative combination (Senekot preparations for children)—see Tables 51.1, 51.2. Maintenance encompasses regular dietary fiber or

fiber supplement plus occasional stool softeners. It is unclear whether lowering intraluminal pressure with such an approach leads to reducing intravesical pressure via neurological overflow (theoretically possible through the sacral 2-3-4 nerve roots) or simply relieves the direct pressure of a hyperdistended colorectum on the bladder, bladder neck, and proximal urethra, while also treating constipation and thus encopresis. Regardless of the mechanism, this intervention is useful and virtually risk-free. Other conservative approaches may include pelvic floor muscle training, biofeedback, or multidisciplinary interventions (Houts, 1991; McKenna et al., 1999; Porena et al., 2000).

Nocturnal Enuresis

For nocturnal enuresis, if a conservative bowel approach is not entirely successful within 3–4 weeks, behavioral approaches may be worthwhile. A conditioning approach (Behrle, 1956; Glazener and Evans, 2001) using commercially available alarm (bell-and-pad) or ultrasound devices, depending upon parental discretion, may suffice. However, the bell often conditions parents more than deep-sleeping children. Indeed, parasomnias and excessively deep sleep (Neveus et al., 1999; Wolfish, 1999; Yeung et al., 1999; Laberge et al., 2000) often preclude the success of alarm systems.

Some additional conditioning may improve results, by having the child take responsibility for washing and changing bedclothes, for example, or by having the parents design a chart program monitoring dry nights and supporting a child's self-esteem (Longstaffe et al., 2000). Unfortunately, while such behavioral programs may occasionally be useful for family dynamics and child and parental self-esteem, few methodologically sound outcome data support these approaches.

A strong family history of NE alone often corresponds to AVP secretion variability (Hogg and Husmann, 1993; Glazener and Evans, 2000). Humans typically secrete higher levels of AVP from the anterior pituitary when *asleep*, regardless of the time of day. However, a substantial percentage of children with NE have a reversed AVP secretion pattern with sleep, perhaps as many as 30% to 75% (Norgaard et al., 1985, 1989; Hogg and Husmann, 1993; Glazener and Evans, 2000). Therefore, such children have *increased* urinary output when sleeping, and a large majority will fail conservative approaches.

Administration of an AVP analog, such as desmopressin acetate (DDAVP), can produce a 30% to 60% reduction in wet nights in general, and about a 50% resolution of enuresis while on the medication (Norgaard et al., 1985; Klauber, 1989; Norgaard et al.,

1989; Sullivan and Abrams, 1999; Glazener and Evans, 2000). When effective, DDAVP response is dose-dependent. Response generally requires dosing of 10 to 40 mg of DDAVP by intranasal spray just at bedtime, or oral dosing with 0.1–0.8 mg in tablet form, divided into twice-daily dosing, with the spray being somewhat more effective than the oral form (Glazener and Evans, 2000). Higher doses increase the side effect potential, particularly for headaches, hypertension, and nasal mucosal bleeding, and may even pose a risk for hyponatremia as well (Klauber, 1989; Glazener and Evans, 2000). A child with enuresis and a *negative* family history of enuresis generally predicts DDAVP failure (Hogg and Husmann, 1993).

Anticholinergics and neuromuscular modulators, such as TCAs and oxybutynin, respectively, can provide some beneficial effects when more conservative approaches are only partly successful, although the complexity of neurobiological interactions implies an equally intricate complex of potential reactions. Agents with the least risk and the most experience should be utilized first. Perhaps the best known and most studied agent is imipramine, which has been shown to be effective in double-blind, placebo-controlled studies, although the serum level must be in the therapeutic antidepressant range (MacLean, 1960; Cole and Fried, 1972; Mikkelsen and Rapoport, 1980; Rapoport et al., 1980; Castleden et al.,1981; Wein et al., 1991; Sullivan & Abrams, 1999). Rapoport et al (Castleden et al., 1981) found that desipramine is as effective as imipramine, but concerns around desipramine cardiotoxicity limit the drug's usefulness. The author's experience is that nortriptyline is effective as well, presumably with lower risk and a more favorable side effect profile. The use of tricyclics, then, should be based on safety, side effect profile, patient response, and partial or complete failure of the previous interventions. Identical parameters should be followed when using TCAs for the treatment of enuresis as those outlined for other indications in Chapter 23. Reports of low-dose effectiveness with TCAs (Norgaard et al., 1985; Glazener and Evans, 2000, albeit without controlled studies, might imply prudence especially in younger children, beginning with a low dose (e.g., nortriptyline or imipramine at 10 mg) and obtaining a serum level after a response is seen or within 2 weeks of a dose change. The TCAs can be added to DDAVP, although the rationale of such an approach can be questioned. Efficacy and safety of other psychopharmacological agents for urinary or bowel dysfunction have not been determined by controlled studies; it might be prudent to avoid such agents at the present time.

Other pharmacological agents can also be useful alone or in combination with the above approaches. Examples of anticholinergic agents that have some efficacy include oxybutynin and tolterodine, which depress detrusor contractility, probably at parasympathetic postganglionic cholinergic receptor sites (Wein et al., 1991; Appel et al., 2000). The long-acting form of oxybutynin was somewhat superior to tolterodine in a double-blind controlled study (Appel et al., 2000). Combination with TCAs may pose unacceptable risks and side effects, especially for younger children, and include sedation, agitation/anxiety, cardiotoxicity, and delirium. Thus, such medication combinations would be best utilized only if more conservative measures and TCAs fail. Figure 51.3 provides an algorithm for NE intervention.

Pediatric urologists tend to be far more experienced and facile in the use of complex neurotransmitter-affecting medication combinations for more complex neurourological conditions—for example, α-adrenergic agonists or antagonists such as clonidine or phentolamine for detrusor–sphincter dyssynergia associated with incomplete emptying, or prostaglandins for increased detrusor muscle-fiber contractility (Wein et al., 1991; Sullivan and Abrams, 1999). It might be prudent, therefore, to consult a pediatric urologist on patients who fail conservative approaches, DDAVP, or TCAs, alone or in combination. However, the child psychiatrist tends to be more aware of the need for medication-appropriate pretreatment evaluations, serum level monitoring, and potential central nervous system (CNS) effects and side effects of drug–drug interactions. Finally, all pharmacological interventions for NE or DE except DDAVP create moderate to severe constipation, which can further accentuate enuresis. A bowel program as described above should probably be initiated at the time of pharmacological intervention in a majority of children.

Diurnal Enuresis, Dysfunctional Voiding, and Frequency/Dysuria

Generally, the approach to DE, dysfunctional voiding, and frequency/dysuria is not excessively different from that to NE. However, even if associated UTIs are absent or successfully treated, these children are very likely to have urological pathology. All interventions are far less likely to be completely effective. Also, the majority of these children also have NE. Probably all of them should be referred for urological or neurourological consultation.

Conservative approaches (as described above) should be utilized first for each of these conditions, al-

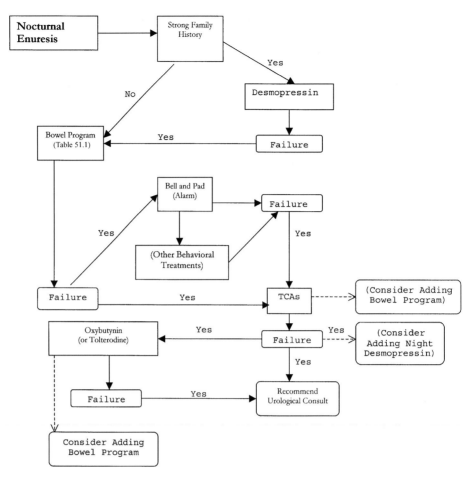

FIGURE 51.3 Paradigm for "pure" nocturnal enuresis intervention. TCAs, tricyclic antidepressants.

though for a very limited time period (perhaps 2–3 weeks). DDAVP is not warranted during the daytime: creating high serum antidiuretic hormone (ADH) environments without a proven ADH deficiency syndrome may be unsafe. The use of TCAs has been reported, but neither with controlled studies nor with reports of serum levels. Clinically, however, TCAs often do appear to be of some benefit even if never "curative" (Castleden et al, 1981; Koff, 1988; Wein et al., 1991; Sullivan and Abrams, 1999).

Oxybutynin and tolterodine (Wein et al., 1991; Appel et al., 2000), can be more effective than other agents in these conditions, probably because of the high prevalence of detrusor instability (Koff, 1988; Wein et al., 1991; Sullivan and Abrams, 1999; Appel et al., 2000; Curran et al., 2000). Diurnal enuresis and dysfunctional voiding in particular, but even urinary frequency and dysuria, can be very distressing to children and are often publicly obvious. Distress may lead

to anxiety and demoralization; stress may lead to increased serum catecholamines. With high concentrations of adrenergic receptors in the bladder and especially in the trigonal muscle and rectal ampulla, anxiety and stress can increase both the sensitivity and motor activity of bladder and rectal function. Therefore, they will accentuate DE and associated dysfunctions and can often effect a nervous bladder or nervous bowel. Nevertheless, even though psychological and psychiatric implications of these conditions are important, the potential seriousness of the urological ramifications demands urological consultation.

Finally, there are children with intermittent minimal incontinence and so-called giggle incontinence (Nirenberg, 1991). Although it is seldom that these conditions require treatment, in such cases where children do request it the standard enuresis approach will generally suffice. Figure 51.4 provides an algorithm for DE interventions.

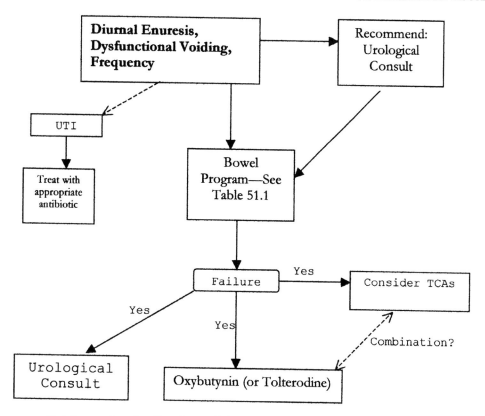

FIGURE 51.4 Interventions for diurnal enuresis intervention. TCAs, tricyclic antidepressants; UTI, urinary tract infection.

PSYCHIATRICALLY INDUCED SEXUAL DYSFUNCTIONS

As in other disorders, knowledge of the neurobiology of normal sexual function and psychosexual development promotes comprehension of dysfunctional states. The reader is referred to more comprehensive treatments of the subject (Bancroft, 1981; Johnson, 1993; Berenbaum, 1998; Meston and Frohlich, 2000; Ryan, 2000). However, it is important to recognize that pathophysiological and physioanatomical sexual dysfunctions and psychosexual developmental obstacles in children are far more prevalent than is generally recognized (Ryan, 2000). An awareness of the phenomenology of sexual dysfunction alone or in concert with psychiatric interventions can benefit patient care as well as compliance. A brief outline of psychiatrically induced or associated sexual dysfunctions will be provided.

Sexual behaviors in children and adolescents are complex and highly variable by individual, by age, and by Tanner stage (Bancroft, 1981; Meston and Frohlich, 2000; Ryan, 2000). Tanner staging, and hormonal effects concurrent with and succeeding puberty,

correlate with a multitude of behavioral phenomena that can be distinct in males and females. Psychopharmacological interventions can at times alter certain sexual behaviors and hormonal effects (Cook et al., 1992; Gitlin, 1994; Piazza et al., 1997; Montejo et al, 2001). Sexual behaviors may be of *parental* or *psychiatric* concern if they put the child at risk (Johnson, 1993). Some areas of *patient* concern may unfold with psychiatric treatment if they include incontinence secondary, for example, to induced constipation—younger children in particular frequently confuse urinary and sexual organs and function; impotence; priapism; anorgasmia; delayed puberty; gynecomastia; and acquired hyposexual or hypersexual states. All have psychosexual as well as potential patient compliance ramifications.

Of particular importance for this discussion, however, is that many sexual behaviors may be inadvertently stimulated, inhibited, or even extinguished by the well-meaning physician, who may fail to recognize the behavioral alterations (Gitlin, 1994; Piazza et al., 1997; Montejo et al., 2001). Specific psychopharmacological agents may have a profound impact on patients' sexual responses or behaviors and may thus affect compliance.

Psychopharmacological interventions can effect specific developmental delays or anomalies. For example, complete pubertal arrest has been associated with valproic acid therapy, with puberty resuming months after discontinuing therapy (Cook et al., 1992) and D_2 blocking agents (in particular, typical neuroleptics) release inhibitory controls in the hypothalamus that can lead to elevated prolactin levels and distressing galactorrhea in girls and boys (Reichlin, 1992).

Psychopharmacological agents are also frequently reported to lead to distinct sexual dysfunctions. Commonly included among these are impotence, decreased libido, and delayed or extinguished orgasm (Gitlin, 1994; Piazza et al., 1997; Michelson et al., 2000; Montejo et al., 2001). Careful review of the methodologies of studies of sexual dysfunctions commonly reveals inadequate phenomenological differentiation among decreased libido, apathy, impotence, and faulty orgasm. In the author's experience in the Psychosexual Disorders Clinic for Children and Adolescents at the Johns Hopkins Children's Center, it would appear that adolescent signs or symptoms typically relegated by many observers to decreased libido or of erectile difficulties often are secondary to apathy or amotivational states secondary to selective serotonin reuptake inhibitor (SSRI) effects (see Chapter 22). Decreasing the SSRI doseage appears to lead to a decrease of apathy and a return of normal libido within 2 to 3 weeks.

Many psychopharmacological agents can, however, decrease and sometimes even extinguish orgasmic response in adolescents. Experience and some data dictate that these include the heterocyclics, monoamine oxidase inhibitors, SSRIs, TCAs, venlafaxine, moclobemide (albeit a low incidence), and neuroleptics (Gitlin, 1994; Plazza et al., 1997; Michelson et al., 2000; Montejo et al., 2001). Trazodone, nefazodone, mirtazapine, bupropion, and benzodiazepines do not appear to affect orgasmic response (Feiger et al., 1996). In the author's experience, adolescent males frequently, and females occasionally, will describe, clinically significant orgasmic delay or anorgasmia, if appropriately questioned after initiation of psychopharmacological treatment. These patients often have already become noncompliant or they may spontaneously request a medication change. Onset of orgasmic difficulties is commonly seen within 1 week of the initial dose and does not appear to be dose related. Tapering the SSRI dosage may have little or no effect.

Treatments recommended for pharmacologically induced anorgasmia have anecdotally included administration of dopamine agonists (most commonly bupropion) or histamine blockade, yet no research has focused on such interventions or combinations of medications. Withdrawal of medication effects return of orgasmic response most commonly within a week or two. Additional interventions that can be useful include (1) switching to nefazodone (Feiger et al., 1996) or mirtazapine if clinically indicated, or (2) teaching pelvic (sexual) relaxation techniques.

Trazodone and the Risk of Priapism

The incidence of spontaneous priapism is not known exactly but is estimated to be about 1 in 100,000 men per year at baseline; however, in prepubertal and pubertal children it is estimated to be about 1 in 5000 to 8000 boys (Merlob and Livne, 1989; Thompson et al., 1990). Trazodone is known from clinical data to increase the incidence of priapism to about 1 in 8000–10,000 men per year, obviously related to the number of men treated (Warner et al., 1987; Azadzoi et al, 1990), and likely more in boys, although no data are available for children treated with trazodone. Trazodone's mechanism of action in priapism appears to be its α-adrenergic blocking potential rather than any smooth muscle relaxation (which could additionally effect venous closure; Warner et al., 1987; Azadzoi et al., 1990; Thompson et al., 1990; Pecknold and Langer, 1996). This is potentially even more serious for the child and adolescent male, for whom α-adrenergic blockade will coincide with the already very high (arterial) flow states. Additionally, seriously accentuated risk is evident because prepubescent and pubescent males have anatomically marked low venous outflow. High-flow states combined with low outflow increases the likelihood of spontaneous erections as well as of priapism. Clitoral priapism is also conceivable, with similar vascular dynamic phenomena, and has been reported rarely in adults (Pescatori et al., 1993).

It is difficult to justify, therefore, any use of trazodone in boys, adolescent males, or young men, especially given its relatively limited usefulness as an antidepressant or even a sedative. Even in girls its use is questionable. Nefazodone would appear to be a far better alternative, especially in that it has no recognized sexual side effects, is well tolerated once the patient adapts to the sedative effect, and is not associated with priapism. That is, risks do not include a known increase in priapism above the background incidence (Thompson et al., 1990; Feiger et al., 1996; Pecknold and Langer, 1996).

REFERENCES

American Psychiatric Association (2000) *Diagnostic and Statistical Manual of Mental Disorders, 4th ed.,* (DSM IV-TR). Washinton, DC: American Psychiatric Association, pp. 116–121.

Appel, R.A., Sand, P., Dmochowski, R., et al., (2000). Prospective randomized controlled trial of extended-release oxybutynin chloride and tolterodine tartrate in the treatment of overactive bladder: results of the Object Study. *Mayo Clin Proc* 78:358–363.

Azadzoi, K.M., Payton, T., Krane, R.J., and Goldstein, I. (1990) Effects of intracavernosal trazodone hydrochloride: animal and human studies. *J Urol* 144:1277–1282.

Bancroft, J. (1981) Hormones and human sexual behaviour. *Br Med Bull* 37:153–158.

Behrle, R.C. (1956) Evaluation of a conditioning device in the treatment of nocturnal enuresis. *Pediatrics* 17:849.

Berenbaum, S. (1998) How hormones affect behavioral and neural development: gonadal hormones and sex differences. *Dev Neuropsychol* 14:175–196.

Castleden, C.M., George, C.F., Renwick, A.G., and Asher, M.J. (1981) Imipramine—a possible alternative to current therapy for urinary incontinence in the elderly. *J Urol* 125:318–320.

Cole, A.T. and Fried, F.A. (1972) Favorable experiences with imipramine in the treatment of neurogenic bladder. *J Urol* 107:44–45.

Cook, J.S., Bale, J.F., Jr., and Hoffman, R.P. (1992) Pubertal arrest associated with valproic acid therapy. *Pediatr Neurol* 8:229–231.

Curran, M.J., Kaefer, M., Peters, C., Logigian, E., and Bauer, S.B. (2000) The overactive bladder in childhood: long-term results with conservative management. *J Urol* 163:574–577.

Daniel, E.E., Cowan, W., and Daniel, V.P. (1983) Structural bases for neural and myogenic control of human detrusor muscle. *Can J Physiol Pharmacol* 61:1247–1273.

de Groat, W.C. and Kawatani, M. (1985) Neural control of the urinary bladder: possible relationship between peptidergic inhibitory mechanisms and detrusor instability. *Neurourol Urodyn* 4:285–300.

Elbadawi, A. (1973) Autonomic innervation of the bladder and urethra. In: *Proceedings of the 16th Congress Société Internationale d'Urologie*, Vol. 2. Paris: Doin, pp. 311–316.

Elbadawi, A. (1980) Autonomic Innervation of Accessory Male Genital Glands. In *Male Accessory Sex Glands* (eds E. Spring-Mills & E.S.E. Hafez), pp. 101–128. Amesterdam: Elsevier.

Elbadawi, A. (1982) Neuromorphological basis of vesicourethral function: 1. Histochemistry, ultrastructure, and fuction of intrinsic nerves of the bladder and urethra. *Neurourol Urodyn* 1:3–50.

Elbadawi, A. (1983) Autonomic muscular innervation of the vesical outlet and its role in micturition. In: F.J., Hinman, ed. *Benign Prostatic Hypertrophy* New York: Springer-Verlag, pp. 330–348.

Elbadawi, A. and Schenk, E.A. (1971) A new theory of the innervation of bladder musculature. 2. The innervation apparatus of the ureterovesical junction. *J Urol* 105:368–371.

Elbadawi, A. and Schenk, E.A. (1974) A new theory of the innervation of bladder musculature. 4. Innervation of the vesicourethral junction and external urethral sphincter. *J Urol* 111:613–615.

Feiger, A., Kiev, A., Shrivastava, R.K., Wisselink, P.G., and Wilcox, C.S. (1996) Nefazodone versus sertraline in outpatients with major depression: focus on efficacy, tolerability, and effects on sexual function and satisfaction. *J Clin Psychiatry* 57:53–62.

Forsythe, W.I. and Redmond, A. (1974) Enuresis and spontaneous cure rate. Study of 1129 enuretis. *Arch Dis Child* 49:259–263.

Gil Vernet, S. (1968) *Morphology and Fuction of Vesicoprostatourethral Musculature.* Tieviso: Canova.

Gitlin, M.J. (1994) Psychotropic medications and their effects on sexual function: diagnosis, biology, and treatment approaches. *J Clin Psychiatry* 55:406–413.

Glazener, C.M. and Evans, J.H. (2000) Desmopressin for nocturnal enuresis in children. *Cochrane Database Syst Rev* 2:

Glazener, C.M. and Evans, J.H. (2001) Alarm interventions for nocturnal enuresis in children (Cochrane Review). *Cochrane Database Syst Rev* 1:CD002911.

Glicklich, L.B. (1951) An historical account of enuresis. *Pediatrics* 8:859.

Hogg, R.J. and Husmann, D. (1993) The role of family history in predicting response to desmopressin in nocturnal enuresis. *J Urol* 150:444–445.

Houts, A.C. (1991) Nocturnal enuresis as a biobehavioral problem. *Behav Ther* 22:133–151.

Hunter, D.T. (1954) A new concept of the urinary bladder musculature. *J Urol* 71:695–704.

Hutch, J.A. (1972) *Anatomy and Physiology of the Bladder, Trigone, and Urethra,* New York: Appleton-Century-Crofts, pp. 1–180.

Johnson, T.C. (1993) Assessment of sexual behavior problems in preschool-aged and latency-aged children. In: A., Yates, ed. *Child and Adolescent Psychiatric Clinics of North America, Sexual and Gender Identity Disorders* Philidelphia: W.B. Saunders, pp. 431–449.

Klackenberg, G. (1981) Nocturnal enuresis in a longitudinal perspective. A primary problem of maturity and/or a secondary environmental reaction? *Acta Paediatr Scand* 70:453–457.

Klauber, G.T. (1989) Clinical efficacy and safety of desmopressin in the treatment of nocturnal enuresis. *J Pediatr* 114:719–722.

Koff, S.A. (1988) Evaluation and management of voiding disorders in children. *Urol Clin North Am* 15:769–775.

Laberge, L., Tremblay, R.E., Vitaro, F., and Montplaisir, J. (2000) Development of parasomnias from childhood to early adolescence. *Pediatrics* 106:67–74.

Longstaffe, S., Moffatt, M.E. and Whalen, J.C. (2000) Behavioral and self-concept changes after six months of enuresis treatment: a randomized, controlled trial. *Pediatrics* 105:935–940.

MacLean, R.E. (1960) Emipramine hydrochloride (Tofranil) and enuresis. *Am J Psychiatry* 117:551.

McKenna, P.H., Herndon, C.D., Connery, S., and Ferrer, F.A. (1999) Pelvic floor muscle retraining for pediatric voiding dysfunction using interactive computer games. *J Urol* 162:1056–1062; discussion 1062–1063.

Merlob, P. and Livne, P.M. (1989) Incidence, possible causes and followup of idiopathic prolonged penile erection in the newborn. *J Urol* 141:1410–1412.

Meston, C.M. and Frohlich, P.F. (2000) The neurobiology of sexual function. *Arch Gen Psychiatry* 57:1012–1030.

Michelson, D., Bancroft, J., Targum, S., Kim, Y., and Tepner, R. (2000) Female sexual dysfunction associated with antidepressant administration: a randomized, placebo-controlled study of pharmacologic intervention. *Am J Psychiatry* 157:239–243.

Mikkelsen, E.J. and Rapoport, J.L. (1980) Enuresis: psychopathology, sleep stage, and drug response. *Urol Clin North Am* 7:361–377.

Montejo, A.L., Llorca, G., Izquierdo, J.A., and Rico-Villademoros, F. (2001) Incidence of sexual dysfunction associated with antidepressant agents: a prospective multicenter study of 1022 outpatients. Spanish Working Group for the Study of Psychotropic-Related Sexual Dysfunction. *J Clin Psychiatry* 62:10–21.

Neveus, T., Hetta, J., Cnattingius, S., Tuvemo, T., Lackgren, G., Olsson, U., and Stenberg, A. (1999) Depth of sleep and sleep habits among enuretic and incontinent children. *Acta Paediatr* 88:748–752.

Nirenberg, S.A. (1991) Normal and pathologic laughter in children. *Clin Pediatr (Phila)* 30:630–632.

Norgaard, J.P., Pedersen, E.B., and Djurhuus, J.C. (1985) Diurnal anti-diuretic-hormone levels in enuretics. *J Urol* 134:1029–1031.

Norgaard, J.P., Rittig, S., and Djurhuus, J.C. (1989) Nocturnal enuresis: an approach to treatment based on pathogenesis. *J Pediatr* 114:705–710.

Ornitz, E.M., Russell, A.T., Gabikian, P., Gehricke, J.G., and Guthrie, D. (2000) Prepulse inhibition of startle, intelligence and familial primary nocturnal enuresis. *Acta Paediatr* 89:475–481.

Pecknold, J.C. and Langer, S.F. (1996) Priapism: trazodone versus nefazodone. *J Clin Psychiatry* 57:547–548.

Pescatori, E.S., Engelman, J.C., Davis, G., and Goldstein, I. (1993) Priapism of the clitoris: a case report following trazodone use. *J Urol* 149:1557–1579.

Piazza, L.A., Markowitz, J.C., Kocsis, J.H., Leon, A.C., Portera, L., Miller, N.L., and Adler, D. (1997) Sexual functioning in chronically depressed patients treated with SSRI antidepressants: a pilot study. *Am J Psychiatry* 154:1757–1759.

Porena, M., Costantini, E., Rociola, W., and Mearini, E. (2000) Biofeedback successfully cures detrusor-sphincter dyssynergia in pediatric patients. *J Urol* 163:1927–1931.

Rapoport, J.L., Mikkelsen, E.J., Zavadil, A., Nee, L., Gruenau, C., Mendelson, W., and Gillin, J.C. (1980) Childhood enuresis. II. Psychopathology, tricyclic concentration in plasma, and antienuretic effect. *Arch Gen Psychiatry* 37:1146–1152.

Reichlin, S. (1992) Hypothalmus and pituitary. In: Foster, D.W. and Williams R.H., eds. *Williams' Textbook of Endocrinology.* Philadelphia: W.B. Saunders, pp. 135–219.

Reiner, W.G. (1995) Enuresis in child psychiatric practice. In: Riddle, M.A., ed *Child and Adolescent Psychiatric Clinics of North America, Pediatric Psychopharmacology II,* Vol. 4. Philidelphia: W.B. Saunders, pp. 453–460.

Ryan, G. (2000) Childhood sexuality: a decade of study. Part II—dissemination and future directions. *Child Abuse Negl* 24:49–61.

Sullivan, J. and Abrams, P. (1999) Pharmacological management of incontinence. *Eur Urol* 36:89–95.

Thompson, J.W., Jr., Ware, M.R. and Blashfield, R.K. (1990) Psychotropic medication and priapism: a comprehensive review. *J Clin Psychiatry* 51:430–433.

von Gontard, A., Eiberg, H., Hollmann, E., Rittig, S., and Lehmkuhl, G. (1999) Molecular genetics of nocturnal enuresis: linkage to a locus on chromosome 22. *Scand J Urol Nephrol Suppl* 202:76–80.

Warner, M.D., Peabody, C.A., Whiteford, H.A., and Hollister, L.E. (1987) Trazodone and priapism. *J Clin Psychiatry* 48:244–245.

Wein, A.J., Van Arsdalen, K., and Levin, R.M. (1991) Pharmacologic therapy. In: Krane, R.J. and Siroky, M.B., eds. *A Clincial Neurourology* Boston: Little, Brown and Company, pp. 523–549.

Wolfish, N. (1999) Sleep arousal function in enuretic males. *Scand J Urol Nephrol Suppl* 202:24–26.

Yazbeck, S., Schick, E., and O'Regan, S. (1987) Relevance of constipation to enuresis, urinary tract infection and reflux. A review. *Eur Urol* 13:318–321.

Yeung, C.K., Chiu, H.N., and Sit, F.K. (1999) Sleep disturbance and bladder dysfunction in enuretic children with treatment failure: fact or fiction? *Scand J Urol Nephrol Suppl* 202:20–23.

IV | EPIDEMIOLOGICAL, RESEARCH, AND METHODOLOGICAL CONSIDERATIONS

The use of drugs in childhood is often considered an "orphan" indication, as if childhood was an anomalous and rare state of being and the diseases of childhood were of secondary importance.

... the fallacy entailed in the assumption that protection of subjects and the research enterprise represent confrontative values.

... research inaction in clinical practice is not an ethically neutral stance; the lack of serious research may, and often does, signify a willingness for society to consign children to chronic suffering.

A. Klin and D.J. Cohen (1994)
The Immorality of Not Knowing: The Ethical Imperative to Conduct Research in Child and Adolescent Psychiatry. Ethics in Child Psychiatry, pp. 2–3

THE volume's fourth and final section consists of five chapters. The first is a comprehensive overview of pharmacoepidemiology that describes the scope of this subfield and its potential clinical, research, and policy implications. The next chapter presents the underlying methodological rationale and action-oriented agenda that clinical trials in pediatric psychopharmacology research call for, with a special emphasis on multisite collaborative efforts. The chapter on regulatory issues addresses the approval and labeling process of psychotropic drugs and underscores the importance of efficient collaboration with federal regulatory agencies. The fourth chapter, at the very core of this volume and of Donald Cohen's lifelong mission, addresses our shared ethical imperative to continue research in pediatric psychopharmacology. This section closes with a chapter on international (non-American) perspectives on the field, taking the European Union and Japan as specific case studies in point.

52 Pediatric psychopharmacoepidemiology: who is prescribing? and for whom, how, and why?

PETER S. JENSEN, ARYEH EDELMAN, AND ROBIN NEMEROFF

Despite the fact that medications are commonly used to treat childhood medical illnesses, concerns are often expressed by the lay public, the media, and health professionals about using medications for children with emotional or behavioral problems. Given the lack of necessary information concerning safety and efficacy of many (but not all) of the commonly used psychotropic agents (Jensen et al., 1999a), the general need for caution concerning the use of medications in treating children's psychiatric disorders is not only understandable but also arguably a core component of ethical clinical practice based on the principle of "do no harm." Nonetheless, some claims about the use of psychotropic medications in children, such as reports about dramatic rates of overprescribing, may have less basis in fact but are instead rooted in misunderstanding, stigma, and/or fear.

Potential misunderstandings about the nature of current prescribing practices turn in part on the central issue of the prevalence of child psychiatric disorders. To the extent that one believes that psychiatric disorders are rare in children, any amount of prescribing of psychotropic agents is likely to be viewed as overprescribing. But in fact, research shows that up to 21% of children between the ages of 9 and 17 have diagnosable mental or addictive disorders (Shaffer et al., 1996). Without awareness of the reality of childhood mental illness and the impact that these conditions exert on children's development, the myth will persist among many persons that psychotropic medications should not be used at all with children. This one-size-fits-all assumption likely does great harm in delaying many parents and professionals in making informed

treatment choices. The accusatory question sometimes heard by parents, "Are you drugging your child?", suggests a double standard for the use of psychotropic medications: although childhood mental illness can be just as devastating as other life-long ailments such as asthma and diabetes, psychotropic agents that have been proven effective are often not even considered. As in treating asthma or diabetes, delaying effective treatments of childhood mental illness also poses significant risks, such as enduring declines in functioning and disturbances in development. In many instances, psychotropic medications constitute an essential tool to assist suffering children and their families.

As will be seen in the course of this review, there are substantial regional, professional, and demographic variations in actual prescribing patterns and practices, such that it is quite possible to make a case for both under- and overprescribing, i.e., appropriate and inappropriate use of psychotropic medications (Jensen, 2000). Thus, in this politicized atmosphere, it is essential for clinicians and prescribers to separate fact from fancy concerning actual prescribing practices. Such information should serve not only to define gaps in research knowledge but also to heighten professionals' awareness about evolving practice trends, so that more informed discussion can take place in professional and public arenas.

This chapter reviews and clarifies what is known and not known about the actual prevalence of psychotropic medication prescribing and use. Because much of the current concern has been galvanized by the recent dramatic upswings in prescribing rates, we first review the actual changes in prescribing practices that have taken place in the last decade, and how these changes have varied across various patient demographic groups (e.g., age, gender, ethnicity) and professional disciplines (e.g., primary care versus speciality mental health providers). Second, we discuss current prescribing rates across the various classes of medication, as well as medication combinations (so-called polypharmacy). Third, we describe what is known about the appropriateness of medication prescribing practices, not just in terms of under- and overprescribing but also in terms of inadequate prescribing. Finally, we describe the implications of our findings for future research and policy initiatives.

TIME TRENDS

The most prominent pattern in pediatric psychopharmacoepidemiology witnessed over the past two decades has been the dramatic increases in stimulant prescriptions, primarily for children with presumptive attention-deficit hyperactivity disorder (ADHD). Recently, Hoagwood and colleagues (2000) analyzed databases from 1989 to 1996 from the National Ambulatory Medical Care Survey (NAMCS). In this survey of office visits to physicians throughout the United States, these authors found that the proportion of visits by children or adolescents ages 0 to 17 years with a diagnosis of ADHD that also resulted in a prescription of psychostimulant medication had increased significantly between 1989 and 1996. In 1989, slightly more than one-half of the visits by children or adolescents with ADHD involved stimulant treatment. But by 1991, 77.8% of visits by children or adolescents with ADHD involved stimulant treatment. Since then, the proportion of visits by children with an ADHD diagnosis that have involved stimulant treatment has remained relatively stable.

Perhaps more tellingly, Safer and colleagues (1996a) estimated that the rate of methylphenidate treatment within pediatric populations in the United States increased twofold from 1990 to 1995—in fact not a new phenomenon, but a long-standing pattern of continued increases. Thus, biennial surveys of the Baltimore County public school students from 1971 to 1987 portrayed a consistent pattern of twofold increases of psychotropic treatment every 4 to 7 years—91% of which was methylphenidate (Safer et al., 1996a)—among students diagnosed with ADHD (Safer et al., 1988). This same trend has continued from the early 1990s to the present. Thus, in 1991, 2.5% of all Baltimore County public school students who were surveyed re-

ceived methylphenidate to treat ADHD. But by 1995, that proportion increased nearly twofold from 1991.

Paralleling these reported increases, the Drug Enforcement Administration, which records the rate of methylphenidate distribution across the United States, notes that the national average of methylphenidate distribution in 1990 was 60 g 10,000 population (Morrow et al., 1998). By 1995, the distribution rate increased more than 2.5-fold. Rates of methylphenidate distribution differed over five-fold among different regions of the country, but even despite these variations, methylphenidate distribution rates increased in every region of the United States during the first half of the 1990s (Morrow et al., 1998). According to Safer et al. (1996a), and based on analysis of multiple data sources, while rates of treatment prevalence have risen, they have not risen as fast as production quotas, in part because children tend to be treated over a longer time period and throughout the school year, compared to earlier periods.

Time Trends in Nonstimulants

Examining medication-prescribing practices more broadly than methylphenidate alone, Kelleher and associates (1989) used the NAMCS data set to estimate the national rate of psychotropic treatment among children and adolescents under the age of 18 years. On the basis of the 1985 NAMCS data, the authors noted that psychotropic drugs (including antidepressant, antianxiety, antipsychotic, or stimulant medications) were ordered or provided in 1.5% of all visits by children and adolescents. Stimulants and antidepressants were the most frequently prescribed psychotropic agents, followed by antipsychotic and antianxiety agents. More recent analyses by Hoagwood and associates (2000) from the 1989–1996 NAMCS and Child Behavior Study (CBS) national databases revealed that the prevalence of psychotropic medication prescribing for ADHD increased from 70.1% in 1989 to 82.9% of children's visits in 1996. Interestingly, from 1991 to the more recent (1996) survey, the prevalence of visits during which nonstimulant psychotropic treatment is prescribed had increased only slightly.

Similar findings have been noted by Pincus and colleagues (1998), who, also using NAMCS databases, found that the number of visits by children younger than age 18 where a medication was prescribed increased between 1985 and 1993–4—from 1.10 million visits to 3.73 million. Relatedly, 3.3% of all primary care pediatric medical visits in 1985 involved a psychotropic prescription, but by 1993–4 this rate had risen to 9.6%, though most of this increase is due to psychostimulants.

Trends in Who Prescribes

Kelleher et al. (1989) examined their NAMCS database in an attempt to discover which medical practitioners were prescribing psychotropic agents for pediatric patients in 1985. They found that psychiatrists prescribed more frequently than any other medical provider among all classes of psychotropic agents. Pediatricians prescribed the least frequently of all practitioners.

These patterns appear to have changed somewhat since then, however, with pediatricians accounting for the most psychotropic medication prescriptions. Pincus and colleagues (1998) compared data from the 1985 NAMCS and the 1994 NAMCS surveys regarding the prevalence of psychotropic treatment for children and adolescents under the age of 18 years prescribed by primary care physicians. They estimated that in comparison to the 0.59 million children in 1985 who received a psychotropic medication from a primary care physician, 2.10 million children in 1994 were treated with psychotropic drugs by primary care physicians. Relatedly, in a survey of children and adolescents ages 0 to 19 years who were treated with methylphenidate in the state of Michigan, Rappley and colleagues (1995) discovered that 59.5% of all children who were medicated were treated by a pediatrician, and only 11.4% were treated by a psychiatrist. Likewise, in a recent survey of toddlers who received psychotropic treatment in Michigan, Rappley and colleagues (1999) found that medicated children were most likely to receive this treatment from pediatricians.

Not only does the absolute total number of prescriptions differ among physician specialities, but also the likelihood that one will receive a prescription from a given specialty varies, once the patient is seen in the provider's office. From the 1996 NAMCS database, Hoagwood et al. (2000) found that prescription prevalence rates vary among different providers: 94.9% of visits by children with ADHD to family practitioners entailed the prescription of stimulants, while only 74.2% of such visits to psychiatrists and 75.4% of visits to pediatricians resulted in a stimulant prescription. Furthermore, while 14.8% of the visits to psychiatrists resulted in a nonstimulant prescription, only 1.9% of visits to family practitioners involved nonstimulant medication prescriptions. When considering the likelihood of any medication being prescribed (stimulants or nonstimulants) for a child with presumed ADHD, 11% of psychiatrist visits resulted in no prescription at all, as opposed to 3.2% of visits to family practitioners. The prescribing practices of pediatricians were similar to that of psychiatrists, except that fewer visits to pediatricians involved the prescription of nonstimulant medications.

Trends in Who Receives Medications: Effects of Age and Gender

Kelleher and colleagues' (1989) study indicated that age was a significant factor in predicting whether a child received a psychotropic medication. At that time, visits by children ages 0–3 comprised 43% of all visits by children or adolescents in which no psychotropic drug was prescribed, and within that age group, only 15% of those visits entailed a medication prescription. Moreover, no children ages 0 to 3 years received a stimulant prescription in that sampled population. During the same time period, visits by adolescents ages 13–17 comprised 18.3% of all child and adolescent visits for stimulant treatment, while the children in the 4- to 8-year age group comprised of 53.3% of stimulant visits.

The population that receives psychotropic medications appears to have changed over the last decade, however. Safer and Krager (1994) note that from the time of their initial survey in the mid-1970s until their 1993 survey, the prevalence of psychotropic treatment for ADHD among secondary school students in Baltimore County public schools had increased substantially. In 1975, the vast majority of children being treated with psychotropics for ADHD were elementary school students, and only 11.3% of all students treated with psychotropics for ADHD were in secondary schools. By 1987, the rate of secondary school students being treated with psychotropics for ADHD had more than doubled. The ratio of secondary school students to all students being treated with psychotropics for ADHD continued to increase during the 1990s.

Furthermore, Safer and Krager (1994) discovered that during the late 1980s and early 1990s, the increases in psychopharmacological treatment for ADHD among female secondary school students was more significant than among male secondary school students. However, among elementary school students, no significant difference between male and female students was found.

The rise in prescribing is also being seen in very young children as well as in older adolescents. Examining the years 1991, 1993, and 1995, Zito and colleagues (2000) analyzed three databases: two Medicaid populations, one in a Midwestern state and the other in a mid-Atlantic state, and a health maintenance organization (HMO) in the northwest. Prevalence was determined by the number of persons per thousand with a Medicaid prescription claim or HMO pharmacy records over 1 year. In 1995, the prevalence of stimulant use among preschoolers (ages 2 to 4) in the Midwestern Medicaid population was 12.3/1000 people. Concerning trends from 1991 to 1995, these authors found that stimulant prescriptions had increased three fold in this youngest age group, and even larger increases were noted in the 15- to 19-year-old group (311%). Among preschoolers, the increase for children 4 years of age was greater than those 2 years old.

Not just stimulants, but the use of other medications also appears to be changing in young children. For example, among younger children in Zito and colleagues' (2000) analysis of three databases, time trends from 1991 to 1995 indicated that the use of clonidine in the preschool population had increased 28.2-fold and antidepressants 3 fold. Within the general category of antidepressants, the use of selective serotonin reuptake inhibitor (SSRIs) had increased more dramatically than other agents.

Trends in Polypharmacy

Over the past decade, the proportion of children and adolescents treated with multiple concurrent psychotropic medications (so-called polypharmacy) also appears to have increased. As recently as 1988, only 9% of 4- to 17-year-old outpatients in Baltimore County community mental health clinics whose files were analyzed by Safer (1997) had been treated with multiple concurrent medications. Yet, the rate of polypharmacy among a sample of outpatients from 1992 to 1994 was as high as 21%.

In this same study, inpatient records of children who had been referred to the community clinics indicated that polypharmacy has become more prevalent among inpatient populations as well. While 26% of the 1988 sample received polypharmaceutical treatment in an inpatient psychiatric unit, as many as 42% of the 1992–4 sample children had been treated with concurrent multiple medications during their inpatient hospital stays.

Rates of polypharmacy appear to vary from setting to setting. For example, Kaplan and associates (1994) surveyed two public, university-affiliated outpatient clinics, one in New York and one in Ohio, discovering that the proportion of children who received multiple concurrent psychotropic medications differed between the two clinics. In Ohio, 22% of all medicated youths (ages 2 to 19 years) were treated with multiple psychotropic medications, while only 11% of those medicated

in the New York clinic received multiple concurrent medications.

One more recent study describing the prevalence of polypharmacy within a specific population was conducted by Zarin and colleages (1998a). These authors surveyed 65 psychiatrists who were treating children or adolescents under the age of 15 years with a diagnosis of ADHD, and found that 37% and 12% of psychiatrists treated their patient with two versus three or more psychotropic medications, respectively, at the time of the index visit. Specifically, 39% of the psychiatrists prescribed a stimulant medication in combination with a nonstimulant medication.

A study by Zima and colleagues (1997) indicates the prevalence of polypharmacy in a population of foster children in Los Angeles. Sixteen percent of the sample, of which 18% had been diagnosed with ADHD, major depression, bipolar disorder, or psychotic disorder, had taken a psychotropic medication during the previous year. Medicated children on average were taking 2.1 medications. Nearly half of the children on medication in the past year had been treated with multiple medications simultaneously. The most common mixture of medications was methylphenidate and clonidine. Not surprisingly, rising rates of polypharmacy have been noted in other intensive service settings as well, such as among children in special education (Mattison, 1997).

It should be noted that polypharmacy per se is not necessarily an inappropriate practice. Most medical disorders, from asthma to AIDS to allergies, are managed with medication combinations. However, it is important to note that the use of multiple concurrent medications appears to rising substantially, suggesting that there is a great need for research data and well-designed studies to inform this practice. In some instances, it may be that the combination, while popular, may be more likely to result in side effects and not particular advantages in treatment efficacy and clinical outcomes (Connor et al., 2000).

CURRENT LEVELS OF PSYCHOTROPIC MEDICATION PRESCRIBING

Jensen and colleagues (1999a) analyzed two national databases (1995 NAMCS and the 1995 National Disease Therapeutic Index [NDTI] to obtain national estimates of the prevalence of psychotropic prescriptions for children younger than 18 years old. Unlike regional surveys, these databases are based on representative samples of physicians in outpatient settings (NDTI) and/or representative samples of children adjusted for age, ethnicity, and region of the county (NAMCS). These data indicated that in 1995 there were over 2 million office visits to physicians that resulted in a pre-scription of a psychostimulant medication, principally for ADHD, and as many as 6 million prescriptions. In addition, levels of prescribing physician visits for other psychotropic agents were quite substantial—over 300,000 visits resulting in the prescription of a SSRI, another 300,000 resulting in a prescription of a mood stabilizer, and over 250,000 visits where a tricyclic an-tidepressant (TCA) was prescribed. The sample sizes for all medications other than stimulants and SSRIs were too small to compute reliable national estimates of prescribing frequency; nonetheless, after stimulants and SSRIs, the most frequently prescribed psychotropic substances (in descending order) were TCAs, central adrenergic agonists, lithium, anticonvulsant mood sta-bilizers, antipsychotics, and benzodiazepines.

Thus, at the national level, the most is known about the stimulants, particularly methylphenidate, rather than other classes of medications. The various data sets, whether based on NAMCS, pharmaceutical in-dustry sources (NDTI), or the several state-level Med-icaid databases, indicate that most of the stimulant medications are currently prescribed by primary care providers. Zarin et al. (1998b), drawing on the NAMCS 1995 data, noted that among primary care, psychiatry, and other specialties (such as neurology), 12.4% of all ADHD medication–related visits in the sample were to a psychiatrist, 75.4% to primary care physicians, and 12.2% to other specialties.

At regional levels and even within providers of a given discipline, there are substantial variations in pre-scribing frequency. For example, Gadow (1997) de-scribed data from a representative sample of 1520 chil-dren ages 5 to 12 across three states, and noted significant differences in treatment prevalence among the 3 surveyed regions. Other investigators have also reported that substantial differences exist in the per-centage of children prescribed methylphenidate within and among states (Rappley et al., 1995; Zito et al., 1997). For example, Rappley and colleagues (1995) found a 10-fold difference in the proportion of pre-scription rates between counties in Michigan, while in Maryland, Zito et al. (1997) found regional methyl-phenidate use rates ranging from 1% to 5%, a fivefold difference.

The reasons for medication and the way in which it tends to be used may also vary as a function of local factors. For example, LeFever et al. (1999) surveyed the prevalence of drug administration by school nurses to public school students with ADHD, grades 2

through 5 in two cities in Virginia (the state with the highest per capita methylphenidate distribution rate in 1995) during the 1995–6 school year. The authors found an interesting discrepancy between the two cit-ies: in city A, 3.7% of children who were "young for their grade," 8.2% of those who were the "expected age," and 12.4% of the "old-for-grade" group were treated with medication in school for ADHD. In con-trast, the respective percentages for city B were 62.7%, 8%, and 10.1%. Furthermore, the stark contrast be-tween the two cities in prevalence of medication for those who were "young for their grade" was consistent across all genders and races. Logistic regression models showed that being male or white in either city, or being young for one's grade in city B predicted drug treat-ment in school for ADHD. In contrast, in city A, being old for one's grade and having an income below the median family income predicted drug administration in school for ADHD.

Gender and Use of Psychotropic Medication

With few exceptions most studies, whether based on clinic settings, state-wide medication databases, or ep-idemiologic samples, have suggested that boys are two to four times more likely to receive a psychotropic medication than girls. For example, in Gadow's study (1997) of children across Missouri, New York, and Wisconsin, 5% of the children in the sample were re-ceiving some psychotropic medication—8% boys and 3% girls. LeFever and colleagues similarly found that male/female stimulant prescription rates differed dra-matically, but also as a function of ethnicity: 17% of white males, 9% of black males, 7% of white girls, and 3% of black girls received medication.

In recent years the psychostimulant male/female ra-tio appears to have narrowed to 1:6, in contrast to the 1:12 ratio in the mid-1980s (Safer, 1994). Similarly, Zito et al. (2000) noted that the male/female ratio for prescription frequency has also narrowed among pre-schoolers in two of three data sets (roughly 4–7:1 to 3–4:1). One interesting exception to this general male female ratio has been noted, however. Zito et al. (1998b) report that for children under the age of 15 years, males are more likely to receive psychotropic treatments (specifically methylphenidate, desipramine, and imipramine) than females. But in youth ages 15 years and older, females received the majority of psy-chotropic prescriptions.

The likelihood of males more frequently being pre-scribed medication, at least for ADHD, is not a simple function of the greater prevalence of the disorder among males. For example, in a longitudinal community survey of over 1000 youth, Angold et al. (2000) found that 72.2% of the children diagnosed with ADHD were medicated with stimulants at some point. However, while 80.4% of the ADHD boys received stimulant medication, only 41.3% of the ADHD girls did, suggesting that even among cases of well-diagnosed ADHD, girls may be less likely to receive medication.

While more studies are needed of medication differences in male and female populations, these differential male/female ratios also appear to apply to speciality mental health settings. For example, Kaplan and Busner (1997) surveyed children and youth across a number of state, county, and private settings, and found that 65%, 63%, and 61% of state, county, and private medicated samples were male (respectively), in comparison to the 30%, 38%, and 33% of the nonmedicated population that was male.

Preschoolers

In the first report of its kind, Rappley et al. (1999) examined the prevalence of psychotropic drug use in children ages 3 years and younger with ADHD, analyzing data from the claims of the Michigan Medicaid system of health care during the 15-month period of October 1, 1995, to December 31, 1996. The authors found 223 children with ADHD 3 years or younger, one-fourth of whom were 2 years or younger. All 223 children had other medical problems; in addition, 28.7% had one comorbid diagnosis, and 14.8% had two or three comorbid diagnoses. Of note, 57% of these children received psychotropic medication. Of those medicated, 54.3% received only one drug, while the rest received two or more. Methylphenidate was the most commonly prescribed drug (33% of all 223 children), followed by clonidine (22%), dextroamphetamine sulfate (14%), imipramine (11%), and thioridazine (8%). Furthermore, providers of the children who received medication were more likely to have a pediatrician as their primary care doctor, and almost half of these children had no contact with psychiatry or neurologist specialists.

As noted above, Zito and colleagues (2000) reported stimulant use in a Medicaid population of 12.3/1000 preschoolers, with rates of stimulants, antidepressants, and other medications such as clonidine increasing dramatically since 1991. Unfortunately, in the absence of efficacy data and details on the actual diagnoses of the children, as well as no documentation of the children's actual functioning or types of care received, this study did not shed light on whether these prescribing practices constituted appropriate or inappropriate care.

Ethnic Differences in Medication Use

Zito and colleagues (1998a) analyzed the Maryland Medicaid prescription reimbursement claims for the fiscal year of 1991, focusing on children ages 5 through 14 years, and found that African Americans made prescription claims less frequently than Caucasians. Interestingly, the greatest disparity existed within stimulant prescriptions, for which Caucasians were 2.5 times more likely to make a reimbursement claim than African Americans. Concerning antidepressant and lithium claims, the disparity was 2.3 to 1, and among antipsychotic and benzodiazepine medications, the disparity was 2.1 to 1 and 2 to 1, respectively. The authors noted that this disparity is significantly greater than the race disparity among reimbursement claims for nonpsychotropic medications in the same population.

Because the representativeness of the above sample was restricted in terms of geographic region and socioeconomic status, the results of this study cannot necessarily be generalized to other populations. To address this problem, Zito and colleagues (1999) authors analyzed the several databases from 1989 through 1996 to determine the prevalence and trends of treatment for children ages 5 through 14 with ADHD. Over the course of the 8 years analyzed, concerning race and ethnicity, the authors found only that the Asian or American Indian groups were represented less frequently in ADHD visits. In contrast, Angold et al. (2000) conducted a longitudinal survey of 1422 students (as well as parents and teachers) who had been randomly selected from public schools in 11 North Carolina counties. Stimulant prevalence was determined at each stage of the study by assessing whether the child or adolescent had received a stimulant medication within the preceding 3 months. Among a group of children with ADHD not otherwise specified, American Indian status predicted increased likelihood of receiving a stimulant prescription.

Prescribing Practices in Specialty Mental Health Settings

One area of increasing interest concerns the use of psychotropic medications in inpatient settings. This issue is of exceptional importance, since the most severely ill children are treated in inpatient units and, arguably, the most powerful and potentially toxic medications are likely to be used in these settings. To examine the extent of medication use in these settings, Zito and colleagues (1994) surveyed the prevalence of psychotropic prescriptions for 501 children and adolescents in one of four inpatient settings operated by the New York State Office of Mental Health during the first 3 months of 1991. Their data revealed that 98% of the initial sample had received a psychotropic medication during the 3-month period that was surveyed. The most frequently prescribed psychotropic medications were neuroleptics, followed by anticholinergic agents. Neuroleptics were prescribed more frequently to patients staying longer than 90 days, with 75% of these patients receiving neuroleptic medication.

Similarly, Kaplan and Busner (1997) assessed the prevalence of psychotropic use during 1991 among inpatient pediatric (< 18 years) populations who were treated by child psychiatrists in a New York suburban area. One state, one county-university, and one private hospital were surveyed. Findings showed that overall, 79% (state), 68% (county-university), and 76% (private) of the child and adolescent patients in the population received a psychotropic treatment during the course of the study. The prevalence of antidepressant treatment in the private hospital was very high (80%) but relatively low in the other hospitals (26% each). Antipsychotics were prescribed to 74% of the county hospital patients, and to 57% and 35% of the patients at the other locations. Stimulants were prescribed only rarely (2%, 3%, and 4% of patients). Lithium was prescribed to 35% and 34% of state and county hospital patients, respectively, and to 16% of private hospital patients. Other mood stabilizers (anticonvulsants) were prescribed frequently to private and county hospital patients (31% and 23%, respectively).

These authors also examined which medications were prescribed to patients with specific diagnoses. The majority of antidepressants were prescribed for patients with major depression, dysthymia, or bipolar disorder. Antipsychotics were prescribed frequently for conduct/oppositional disorder, psychosis, and major depression or dysthymia. In the state hospital, the proportion of nonpsychotic patients who received antipsychotic treatment depended on patients' age: thus, the frequency of children who were not diagnosed with a psychotic disorder but who were treated with antipsychotic medication was greater among children 12 years and younger, in contrast to children ages 13 to 18 years.

The issue of atypical antipsychotic medications may be of special interest, given evidence of their increasing use, and the still largely as yet unknown safety-efficacy profile. Malone and associates (1999) have presented epidemiological data on the prevalence of antipsychotic drug use among children and adolescents under the age of 20 years in a Midwestern Medicaid population. The authors note that from 1990 to 1996, the prevalence of antipsychotic medication use increased 63%, from approximately 0.34% to 0.52%. Furthermore, the prevalence of novel antipsychotics (clozapine and risperidone) increased from nearly 0% in 1990 to 0.2% in 1996, while the prevalence of conventional antipsychotics (such as haloperidol) increased only slightly (although they still are more frequently prescribed than the novel antipsychotics) as of 1996. Clearly, these newer forms of atypical antipsychotic medications, increasingly used with little data to inform their use is very much in need of intensive study in children and adolescents.

Antipsychotic medication use has been examined in outpatient settings as well. Kaplan and colleagues (1994) investigated the prescribing practices of child and adolescent psychiatrists in public, university-affiliated outpatient clinics in New York and in Ohio, in a group of randomly selected patients ages 2 to 19 years (mean age of 11.6 years). The most frequently used medications were antipsychotics (37% in New York and 18% in Ohio), stimulants (35% and 51%), and antidepressant drugs (24% and 26%). Also prescribed were lithium (7% and 10%), clonidine (0% and 8%), carbamazepine (0% and 8%), propranolol (4% and 0%), and antihistamines (2% and 7%). Medicated patients in both populations were more likely to have been hospitalized in the past; furthermore, in the New York sample, patients in the medicated population were more likely to be diagnosed with psychosis or ADHD with concurrent conduct/oppositional disorder than the nonmedicated children.

These authors also found that 65% (New York) and 67% (Ohio) of the sampled medicated patients who received an antipsychotic prescription were not diagnosed with a psychotic disorder. Similarly, 0% and 20% of the sampled medicated patients who received a stimulant medication were not diagnosed with ADHD, and 27% and 42% of the sampled medicated patients who received antidepressants were not diagnosed with major depression, dysthymia, bipolar disorder, or related conditions. In discussing the appropriateness of the medication treatments in the survey, the authors concluded that approximately 10% of the treatments in each sample were deemed inappropriate.

In other outpatient settings, Safer (1997) evaluated case folders of children ages 4 to 17 who had enrolled in one of four community mental health center clinics located in Baltimore County, between 1988 and 1992 and in 1994. All four centers were staffed by board—certified child psychiatrists. Just as seen in primary care settings, findings showed that the prevalence of psychotropic prescriptions for outpatient children (children who were treated in the clinics) had increased from 1988–1992 to 1994 from 40% to 65%. In contrast to earlier studies based mostly on primary care–treated children (e.g., Safer et al., 1996b), the authors found that the prevalence of stimulant treatment had decreased over time, from 58% to 31% of all psychotropic prescriptions for outpatient children, while the prevalence of nonstimulant treatment increased. The SSRI antidepressant prevalence increased from 5% to 21%, the prevalence of any antidepressant treatment increased from 31% to 46%, antimaniac compounds, from 8% to 17%, and prescription of multiple concurrent psychotropics, from 9% to 21%.

OVER-, UNDER-, OR INADEQUATE PRESCRIBING?

The scientific and clinical issues of over- versus undertreatment hinge largely on considerations that have rarely been addressed in most previous studies. In terms of the question of over- versus undertreatment of ADHD, *only community-based epidemiologic sampling methods* with independent determination of diagnostic status can yield meaningful estimates of treated and untreated prevalence rates of ADHD. Unfortunately, most of the public discussion to date of degree of treatment of ADHD has relied on school-based, HMO, or Medicaid medication databases (e.g., see Wolraich et al., 1998; LaFever et al., 1999; Zito et al., 2000). Without rigorous diagnostic approaches of children at the individual case level, it cannot be known whether any single prescription, much less any prescription rate, is in fact appropriate or inappropriate. Likewise, without a systematic diagnostic survey of the larger nonreferred population, we cannot know the extent of underdiagnosis and undertreatment, arguably the larger public health problem (Jensen, 2000).

To address this gap, Jensen et al. (1999b) analyzed data from a survey of 1285 children ages 9 to 17 years in four communities to determine the prevalence of ADHD in this population, as well as the forms of treatment provided to these children. Findings indicated that only 8 (12.1%) of the 66 children with ADHD were given a stimulant medication while 1 child was given a tricyclic medication, suggesting that in these communities, stimulants are underprescribed. In addition, the authors found that eight children without full ADHD diagnoses (four of whom were diagnosed with some other disorder) were treated with stimulants.

However, these children displayed high levels of ADHD symptoms, although not as high as those diagnosed with ADHD. Because the average number of ADHD symptoms among nonmedicated children diagnosed with ADHD was virtually the same as the mean number of ADHD symptoms displayed by medicated, ADHD children, the authors concluded that the children who did not meet full criteria for ADHD yet who were being treated for it may have met criteria for ADHD prior to instituting treatment.

In the only other epidemiologic study to date that can address the issue of over- vs. underprescribing, Angold and colleagues (2000) surveyed 1422 students ages 9, 11, and 13 years in 11 North Carolina counties. Stimulant prescribing prevalence was determined at multiple time points of the study by assessing whether the child or adolescent had received a stimulant medication within the preceding 3 months. The authors report that 57% of the children who were prescribed stimulant medications at any point during the study were not diagnosed with ADHD. Furthermore, they found that 72.2% of the children diagnosed with ADHD were medicated with stimulants at some point. Using logistic regression, the authors found that among the children with full ADHD, being male and younger predicted stimulant use. Among the ADHD–not otherwise specified group, a high level of ADHD symptoms in the parent report, the presence of oppositional defiant disorder, and being an American Indian predicted stimulant treatment.

Unfortunately, findings from the North Carolina study are complicated by the fact that *within the stimulant-treated group* without ADHD, high levels of parent- and teacher-reported ADHD symptoms were found, with these same children also having a higher overactive-distractible rating by interviewers, thus raising important concerns about the validity of the diagnoses (diagnoses were based on parent and child interview only, and not on teacher interview).

If both these studies' findings accurately reflect valid regional levels of over- and underprescribing, their results should be understood to reflect particular geographic regions and should not be considered indicative of rates across the country. For example, various authors estimated in 1995 that only between 1.2 to 1.5 million of the 3 million children with ADHD were on stimulants (Safer et al., 1996; Jensen, 2000). Even treated children have been estimated to receive only an average of five prescriptions per year (Zito et al., 1998b), which is quite different from the lengthy periods of sustained prescribing suggested in this current study.

Hence, prescribing practices appear to vary widely

in different parts of the nation. These studies suggest that there may be pockets of overprescribing in certain communities, but an equally serious public health concern is that many children who need treatment are not receiving it (Jensen, 2000). Even among those that are being treated, treatment is often inadequate, with poor follow-up and poor care. For example, among those families receiving community treatments in the recently completed Multimodal Treatment Study of Children with ADHD (MTA), only two-thirds of these very carefully diagnosed children with ADHD with highly motivated, treatment-seeking families actually obtained medication during a 14-month period. By and large, even among those children receiving medication, most were undertreated—receiving less than adequate doses, intermittent rather than consistent medication, and little follow-up (MTA Cooperative Group, 1999).

These and other findings (e.g., see Sloan et al., 1999) suggest general inadequacy of many assessment, treatment, and prescribing practices, such as failure to use *Diagnostic and Statistical Manual of Mental Disorders* (DSM) criteria to establish the diagnosis, failure to include teacher-based information as a necessary component of the diagnostic assessment, use of stimulant treatment response as a diagnostic indicator, and failure to assess for other comorbid diagnostic conditions. Nonetheless, sufficient details of actual treatment practices (in contrast to those that should constitute state-of-the-art treatment) remain less than fully explicated, and these details will remain elusive without in-depth epidemiologic studies of treated, partially treated, and untreated populations.

RESEARCH AND POLICY IMPLICATIONS

While this review of the literature shows increases in trends in the use of medications across all classes, most questions about the adequacy of treatment practices, and the fit between diagnosis and treatment have not been addressed by most studies to date (with the possible exceptions of Jensen et al., 1999b, and Angold et al., 2000). Consequently, strong conclusions about the meaning of the available findings are not possible, and the extant data leave several major questions unanswered.

First, it is unclear to what extent these changes in medication prescribing patterns reflect good or bad clinical practices, or both. To determine the prevalence of children who might benefit from medication treatments, population-based studies are needed that simultaneously determine the extent of treated and untreated disorder and that also carefully examine whether children without a bona-fide psychiatric disorder are being treated. Second, even among children with a valid disorder, the degree to which a given treatment is the correct treatment cannot be known without a careful case-by-case determination of the diagnosis and a review of the child's history of other treatments tried. Third, determination of appropriate practices must rest on a body of knowledge grounded on controlled clinical trials designed to determine which treatments work for which conditions. And lastly, as that knowledge base grows, such information should also identify which one is the treatment of choice and/or which one should be tried first for which child, i.e., clinical strategies and algorithms should be examined.

For example, if a given psychosocial treatment has been shown to be the safest and most effective choice, use of medication for such a condition in a given child might be considered inappropriate or overprescribing. Likewise, where a given medication has been proven the most effective and safest of available alternatives, an instance in which it can be determined that a given child has not received such treatment might be considered under-prescribing. And in still more complex situations, careful consideration of data that allow the matching of specific patients to specific treatments might suggest that a given treatment is appropriate or inappropriate for a particular child, even though the larger group of children with the same disorder but without a distinguishing characteristic that allows patient-to-treatment matching would warrant an altogether different treatment, or treatment at a different dosage, intensity, or combination. Thus, to truly assess the quality and appropriateness of medication treatments, researchers must study the larger context of a child's treatment experience, rather than merely surveying prescription trends. These considerations suggest the following agenda for future studies to enhance our understanding of data from psychopharmacoepidemiologic studies:

• First, additional studies of the safety and efficacy of various medication treatments are needed. Paralleling these medication efficacy studies, additional research on other treatments, such as various forms of psychotherapy, are needed, as well as studies of treatment combinations (medication and psychotherapy, and medication combinations). Part of this research agenda must address the ordering of treatments and the determination of what to do when an initial treatment results in a partial response or no response altogether, such as the testing of treatment algorithms (e.g., see Plizka et al., 2000).
• If evidence from efficacy studies can be obtained

to support various treatment practices, future pharmacoepidemiologic studies need to probe more deeply than most studies to date into the extent to which evidence-based practices are being employed across practitioners and communities. How do these practices vary by provider specialty, by setting, or by patient characteristics?

• Future, more fully informative pharmacoepidemiologic studies must gather more information about the prevalence of medication use, coupled with the simultaneous determination of the presence or absence of independently determined diagnoses (rather than just what physicians report the diagnosis to be).

• Pharmacoepidemiologic studies must gather more information about the prevalence of medication use in the presence or absence of other types of treatment. To determine the appropriateness of medication practices, the use of medication in conjunction with other types of treatment and the failure of other past treatments that were tried before the current medication choice must be ascertained.

To date, most pharmacoepidemiologic studies have fallen far short of these criteria. In some instances, data have been analyzed without meaningful attendant clinical information, yet have been inappropriately invoked into discussions to address these complex clinical questions. Such interpretive activities stretch far beyond the data, are likely to be misleading, and in fact may do harm in terms of increasing stigma, delaying persons from seeking care, and distracting the field from pursuing a sensible public policy and research agenda.

These caveats noted, there are several areas that deserve special attention, where analyses and social–cultural factors and sources of influence need to be better understood. How are we to understand minority and ethnic differences in decreased medication use, above and beyond their likelihood of use of medications for other conditions? While these analyses have not yet been confirmed across a wide range of data sets, such findings are provocative, and may warrant more systematic studies of attitudes, barriers, and stigma within some minority communities. If such findings are confirmed in other statewide and national medication data bases, more in-depth studies of specific minority populations seem warranted.

Other factors, such as the availability (or lack of availability) of community resources or the ingress of managed care policies that shape clinical behavior, might be invoked to explain possible changes in prescribing and help-seeking behaviors. In addition, studies of physician attitudes as well as parent and family attitudes about medications' use and usefulness are very much needed. These factors should be studied within representative samples of physician prescribers and parents, and examined as a function of other available family, community, and physician resources, to determine the impact of possibly converging forces shaping change in medication practices. More specifically within physicians as a group, the role of training and provider discipline should be explored.

In sum, although the research cited in this chapter represents the best psychopharmacoepidemiology studies available, methodological limitations from all available data sets, including restriction to single settings or limited data sets, call into question the generalizability of many of the findings, given the imprecision of prevalence estimates and variations in treatment practices across communities. Most importantly, they leave unanswered many questions about the interpretation of these findings. For pharmacoepidemiology to rise to the challenge of its promise, it must follow the lead of other more mature fields of epidemiology that have moved past simple forays into simple descriptive statistics of rates of specific phenomena, and pursue better sampling strategies and more in-depth assessments so that it might begin to shed light on the underlying forces and factors that explain the overall findings. Such studies will be expensive, but they must be vigorously pursued for the field to move ahead and for true understanding to emerge.

REFERENCES

Angold, A., Erkanli, A., Egger, H.L., and Costello, E.J. (2000) Stimulant treatment for children: a community perspective. *J Am Acad Child Adolesc Psychiatry* 39:975–984.

Connor, D.F., Barkley, R.A., and Davis, H.T. (2000) A pilot study of methylphenidate, clonidine, or the combination in ADHD comorbid with aggressive oppositional-defiant or conduct disorder. *Clin Pediatr* 39:15–25.

Gadow, K.D. (1997) An overview of three decades of research in pediatric psychopharmacoepidemiology. *J Child Adolesc Psychopharmacol* 7:219–236.

Hoagwood, K., Kelleher, K.J., Feil, M., and Comer, D.M. (2000) Treatment services for children with ADHD: a national perspective. *J Acad Child Adolesc Psychiatry* 39:198–206.

Jensen, P.S. (2000) Stimulant treatment for children: a community perspective: commentary. *J Am Acad Child Adolesc Psychiatry* 39:984–987.

Jensen, P.S., Bhatara, V.S., Vitiello, B., Hoagwood, K., Feil, M., and Burke, L.B. (1999a) Psychoactive medication prescribing practices for U.S. children: gaps between research and clinical practice. *J Am Acad Child Adolesc Psychiatry* 38:557–565.

Jensen, P.S., Kettle, L., Roper, M.S., Sloan, M.T., Dulcan, M.K., Hoven, C., Bird, H.R., Bauermeister, J.J., and Payne, J.D. (1999b) Are stimulants over-prescribed? Treatment of ADHD in four communities. *J Am Acad Child Adolesc Psychiatry* 38:797–804.

Kaplan, S.L. and Busner, J. (1997) Prescribing practices of inpatient child psychiatrists under three auspices of care. *J Child Adolesc Psychopharmacol* 7:275–286.

Kaplan, S.L., Simms, R.M., and Busner, J. (1994) Prescribing practices of outpatient child psychiatrists. *J Acad Child Adolesc Psychiatry* 33:35–44.

Kelleher, K.J., Hohmann, A.A., and Larson, D.B. (1989). Prescription of psychotropics to children in office-based practice. *Am J Dis Child* 143:855–859.

LeFever, G.B., Dawson, K.V., and Morrow, A.L. (1999) The extent of drug therapy for attention deficit-hyperactivity disorder among children in public schools. *Am J Public Health* 89:1359–1364.

Malone, R.P., Sheikh, R., and Zito, J.M. (1999) Novel antipsychotic medications in the treatment of children and adolescents. *Psychiatric Serv* 50:171–174.

Mattison, R.E. (1997) Use of psychotropic medications in special education students with serious emotional disturbance. *J Child Adolesc Psychopharmacol* 7:149–155.

Morrow, R.C., Morrow, A.L., and Haislip, G. (1998) Methylphenidate in the United States, 1990 through 1995. *Am J Public Health* 88:1121.

MTA Cooperative Group (1999) 14-month randomized clinical trial of treatment strategies for attention deficit hyperactivity disorder. *Arch Gen Psychiatry* 56:1073–1086.

Pincus, H.A., Tanielian, T.L., Marcus, S.C., Olfson, M., Zarin, D.A., Thompson, J., and Zito, J.M. (1998) Prescribing trends in psychotropic medications: primary care, psychiatry, and other medical specialties. *JAMA* 279:526–531.

Pliszka, S.R., Greenhill, L.L., Crismon, M.L., Sedillo, A., Carlson, C., Conners, C.K., McCracken, J.T., Swanson, J.M., Hughes, C.W., Llana, M.E., Lopez, M., and Toprac, M.G. (2000) The Texas children's medication algorithm project: report of the Texas Consensus Conference Panel on Medication Treatment of Childhood Attention-Deficit/Hyperactivity Disorder. Part I. attention-deficit/hyperactivity disorder. *J Am Acad Child Adolesc Psychiatry* 39:908–919.

Rappley, M.D., Gardiner, J.C., Jetton, J.R., and Houang, R.T. (1995) The use of methylphenidate in Michigan. *Arch Pediatr Adolesc Med* 149:675–678.

Rappley, M.D., Mullan, P.B., Alvarez, F.J., Eneli, I.U., Wang J., and Gardiner, J.C. (1999) Diagnosis of attention-deficit/hyperactivity disorder and use of psychotropic medication in very young children. *Arch Pediatr Adolesc Medi* 153:1039–1045.

Safer, D.J. (1997) Changing patterns of psychotropic medications prescribed by child psychiatrists in the 1990s. *J Child Adolesc Psychopharmacol,* 7:267–274.

Safer, D.J. and Krager, J.M. (1988) A survey of medication treatment for hyperactive/inattentive students. *JAMA* 260:2256–2258.

Safer, D.J. and Krager, J.M. (1994) The increase rate of stimulant treatment for hyperactive/inattentive students in secondary schools. *Pediatrics* 94:462–464.

Safer, D.J., Zito, J.M., and Fine, E.M. (1996a) Increased methylphenidate use for attention deficit disorder in the 1990s. *Pediatrics* 98:1084–1088.

Safer, D.J., Zito, J.M., and Fine, E.M. (1996b) The case of the missing methylphenidate. *Pediatrics* 98:730–731.

Shaffer, D., Fisher, P., Dulcan, M., Davies, M. and Piacentini, J., Schwab-Stone, M., Lahey, B., Bourdon, K., Jensen, P., Bird, H., Canino, G., and Regier, D., (1996) The second version of the NIMH diagnostic interview schedule for children (DISC-2). *J Am Acad Child Adol Psychiatry* 35:865–877.

Sloan, M., Jensen, P., and Kettle, L. (1999) Assessing services for children with ADHD: gaps and opportunities. *J Attention Disord* 3:13–29.

Wolraich, M.L., Hannah, J.N., Baumgaertel, A., and Feurer, I.D. (1998) Examination of DSM-IV criteria for attention deficit/hyperactivity disorder in a county-wide sample. *J Dev Behav Pediatr* 19:162–168.

Zarin, D.A., Suarez, A.P., Pincus, H.A., Kupersanin, E., and Zito, J.M. (1998a) Clinical and treatment characteristics of children with attention-deficit/hyperactivity disorder in psychiatric practice. *J Am Acad Child Adolesc Psychiatry* 37:1262–1270.

Zarin, D.A., Tanielian, T.L., Suarez, A.P., and Marcus, S.C. (1998b). Treatment of attention-deficit hyperactivity disorder by different physician specialties. *Psychiatr Serv* 49:171.

Zima, B.T., Bussing, R., Crecelius, G.M., Kaufman, A., and Belin, T. (1997) Psychotropic medication treatment patterns among school-aged children in foster care. *J Child Adolesc Psychopharmacol* 7:135–147.

Zito, J.M., Craig, T.J., and Wanderling, J. (1994) Pharmacoepidemiology of 330 child/adolescent psychiatric patients. *J Pharmacoepidemiol* 3:47–62.

Zito, J.M., Safer, D.J., dosReis, S., Gardner, J.F., Boles, M., and Lynch, F. (2000) Trends in the prescribing of psychotropic medications to preschoolers. *JAMA* 283:1025–1030.

Zito, J.M., Safer, D.J., dosReis, S., Magder, L.S., Gardner, J.F., and Zarin, D.A. (1999) Psychotherapeutic medication patterns for youths with attention-deficit/hyperactivity disorder. *Arch Pediatr Adolesc Med* 153:1257–1263.

Zito, J.M., Safer, D.J., dosReis, S., Pharm, B.S., Magder, L.S., and Riddle, M.A. (1997) Methylphenidate patterns among medicated youths. *Psychopharmacol Bull* 33:143–147.

Zito, J.M., Safer, D.J., dosReis, S., and Riddle, M.A. (1998a). Racial disparity in psychotropic medications prescribed for youths with Medicaid insurance in Maryland. *J Am Acad Child Adolesc Psychiatry* 37:179–184.

Zito, J.M., Safer, D.J., Riddle, M.A., Johnson, R.E., Speedie, S.M., and Fox, M. (1998) Prevalence variations in psychotropic treatment of children. *J Child Adolesc Psychopharmacol* 8:99–105.

53 Clinical trials methodology and design issues

BENEDETTO VITIELLO

There is an increasing interest in clinical trials of psychotropic medications in children and adolescents. Several factors contribute to this interest. It is now evident that mental illness often starts in the first two decades of life and both parents and clinicians are more attentive to the presence of psychopathology in youths. New classes of psychotropic medications with a more favorable safety profile than that of older drugs have become available, and are often prescribed to children *off-label*, that is without pediatric indications approved by the Food and Drug Administration (FDA). Efficacy and safety cannot be entirely extrapolated to children from data collected from adults, as development can affect pharmacokinetics, metabolism, therapeutic response, and drug toxicity. Thus, there are currently no reasonable alternatives to conducting well-designed clinical trials in youths with mental illness as a necessary step toward developing effective and safe treatments for this age group.

The general principles of experimental methodology and design of pediatric clinical trials do not differ from those used for adult studies (Chow and Liu, 1998; Friedman et al., 1998). In applying these principles to children, however, certain aspects emerge that deserve special attention and discussion. A comprehensive presentation of clinical trial methodology cannot be accomplished within the limits of this chapter, which will focus on the main elements of clinical trial design relevant to research in pediatric psychopharmacology.

IDENTIFYING THE RESEARCH QUESTIONS

Experimental design and methods depend primarily on the questions to be answered (Kraemer and Telch, 1992). Clinical trials are meant to address clinically relevant questions and generate data that are ultimately relevant to the treatment of patients in usual practice. The importance of clearly identifying the primary experimental question cannot be over-emphasized, as it the foundation for the entire research effort (Table 53.1). A single clinical trial, no matter how large and sophisticated, can be expected to answer only a limited number of questions with some certainty. In fact, in most cases a trial can fully address only one primary research hypothesis, all the others being relegated to a secondary rank by lack of adequate statistical power in subgroup analyses. Clinical trials, in addition to requiring considerable investment of financial resources, often take several years for completion. Thus, in planning a trial, it is essential that the research questions be expected to remain relevant for the foreseeable future. Even so, with the rapid progress of medicine, there is no guarantee that they will not become obsolete before the end of the study.

Clinicians, families, patients, and policy makers can be faced with various questions about the pharmacological treatment of children and adolescents with mental illness. The following are some types of questions that are often formulated into research hypotheses for clinical trials:

- Is a particular treatment effective and safe in relieving specific symptoms?
- Is the treatment effective in reversing functional impairment?
- Is the treatment effective in inducing full recovery from the disorder?
- Is long-term treatment needed to maintain improvement or prevent relapse and recurrence?
- Is the treatment effective across different conditions and clinical settings? Is it effective when implemented in usual clinical practice conditions?
- How does the treatment compare with alternative pharmacological or psychosocial treatments with respect to efficacy, safety, and cost/benefit ratio?

Thus far, only relatively few of the above questions have been systematically addressed for many mental

TABLE 53.1 *Steps in Designing and Conducting a Clinical Trial*

1. Identification of the research questions
   - Are the questions clinically relevant? If *yes*, continue
   - Will addressing these questions advance current knowledge? If *yes*, continue
   - Are these questions formulated as testable hypotheses? If *yes*, continue

2. Definition of the study sample
   - Do the inclusion criteria identify a representative sample of the patients to whom the study results will be relevant?
   - Is the rationale for each exclusion criterion specified (e.g., criterion identifies patients for whom the treatment or the study procedures would not be clinically appropriate)?
   - If this intended to be a NIH-funded study, are the requirements for inclusion of sex/gender and race/ethnicity groups satisfied?
   - Have the potential referral sources been identified? (e.g., clinicians, schools, direct advertisement to families)

3. Choice of the research setting
   - Academic institution versus practice setting, inpatient versus outpatient or residential

4. Structure of the experiment
   - Design (e.g., parallel groups, crossover, discontinuation)
   - Comparison group (e.g., placebo, active medication, psychotherapy, treatment as usual)
   - Assessment instruments to measure efficacy and safety
        Select the primary outcome measure(s)
   - Sample size and power calculation (i.e., study sensitivity)
        Specify the smallest treatment effect that is of clinical interest and that the study should be able to detect with adequate precision
   - Plan for ensuring patient safety
        Safety variables to be measured before and during the study
        Special safety procedures (e.g., contraception for sexually active females)
        Treatment end points (i.e., defining when experimental treatment of individual patients entered into the study will be interrupted)
        Study end points (i.e., defining when the entire study will be interrupted)
        DSMB (required for NIH-defined phase III trials, often needed for other multisite studies)
        If no DSMB, who will monitor safety?
   - Is the proposed experiment scientifically valid? If *yes*, continue
   - Is the proposed experiment ethically acceptable? If *yes*, continue
   - Is the proposed experiment feasible? If *yes*, continue

5. Finalization of protocol and consent forms

6. Securing financial support
   - E.g., grants from public agencies, private foundations, or industry

7. Review of the protocol and informed consent form by IRBs and, if applicable, DSMB
        Approved? If *yes*, continue

8. Preparation of study material
   - Clinical research forms
   - Study medications
   - Manual of operations
   - Treatment manuals
   - Structure of the database

9. Training of research staff
   - Are raters of diagnostic and outcome variables reliable? If *yes*, continue

10. Publication by-laws (for multisite trials)

11. Study implementation
    - Advertisement
    - Patient screening
    - Patient enrollment, treatment, and assessment

12. Monitoring for data quality
    - Ongoing review of accuracy and completeness of data before entry into the database
    - Periodic checks of possible errors (e.g., "box-and-whiskers" plotting)
    - Periodic monitoring of the consistency between database and source documents (e.g., direct comparison for a random sample of the records)

(continued)

TABLE 53.1 *Steps in Designing and Conducting a Clinical Trial (continued)*

13. Monitoring for study safety
    - Periodic review of interim analysis of safety data by DSMB
    - Review of interim analysis of efficacy data (if planned)
14. Completion of data collection and data entry
15. Completion of data cleaning
16. Database is locked
17. Analysis of data according to the protocol statistical plan
18. Study blind is broken
19. Preparation of the primary report and submission for peer review
20. Presentation of results at scientific meetings
21. Publication of results in scientific literature
22. Broad dissemination of results

DSMB, Data and Safety Monitoring Board; IRB, Institutional Review Board; NIH, National Institutes of Health.

health treatments used in children and adolescents. Another set of questions pertains to the possible advantage of choosing a certain treatment strategy (as compared to a single treatment) over an alternative approach, and can be addressed utilizing treatment algorithms. For instance:

- How does pharmacotherapy compare to psychotherapy for efficacy and safety?
- How does the combination of pharmacotherapy and psychotherapy compare with either alone?
- Is it preferable to administer the most intensive (and usually also most expensive) treatments first, or should such treatments be reserved for patients who have failed other less intensive treatments?

Other questions relate to identifying which type of patients benefit most from the treatment, and under which conditions and through which mechanisms treatments work. In clinical trials, these are usually considered secondary questions. For example, in a clinical trial that includes both children and adolescents, it may be important to inquire whether the treatment effects differ among prepubertal as compared to pubertal subjects.

Studies aimed at gathering feasibility and toxicity data on new treatments are usually referred to as *phase I trials*. *Phase II trials* are relatively small studies (typically with sample size less than or about 100 subjects) with the purpose of detecting preliminary evidence of efficacy and safety. *Phase III trials* are larger studies with enough statistical power to test in a conclusive way specific hypotheses about treatment effects. The term *clinical trials* is often broadly used to designate phase III trials.

In recent years, emphasis has been put on the differ-

ences between efficacy and effectiveness of treatment. *Efficacy* is usually defined as the ability of a treatment to decrease relevant symptoms compared to a control under ideal experimental conditions (i.e., homogeneous sample, intense monitoring, good compliance, blinding, placebo as a control, and academic research setting). Effectiveness is the ability to produce clinically meaningful changes, in both symptoms and level of functioning, under usual practice conditions (i.e., a heterogeneous study population with comorbid conditions, in a community setting, and with an ecologically appropriate comparison group). Most of the existing scientific literature in child psychopharmacology belongs more to the efficacy realm. The importance for clinical research to extend beyond ideal experimental conditions to arrive at truly informative conclusions on the effects of treatment interventions has been recently underscored both for adult and child psychiatry (Weisz and Jensen, 1999; Wells, 1999). There are differences in design and methods between efficacy and effectiveness research, the former typically using the randomized double-blind, placebo-controlled trial with stringent inclusion and exclusion criteria, a relatively brief duration of treatment, and symptom scores as outcome measure. In effectiveness research, the inclusion criteria are as broad and diverse as the population likely to receive the treatment in clinical practice. The sample is usually large, and the emphasis is on functional outcomes. Although there is general agreement on the concepts of efficacy and effectiveness, they are often interpreted in different ways. In some contexts, for example, effectiveness research can be a systematic recording of clinical outcomes, without any attempts to control for possible biases through randomization and other experimental methods. In other cases, effectiveness research uses a randomized design and is indeed a clinical trial. Thus, a clear-cut categorization of studies using the dichotomy efficacy versus effectiveness is often difficult to accomplish, as many studies blend characteristics of both. It may be better to cast efficacy and effectiveness as two ideal extremes of a spectrum along which individual studies may have more or less hybrid features. Still, it is important in framing research questions to consider these concepts, as they have implications for study design and methods.

DEFINING THE STUDY SAMPLE

The study sample must be representative of the patient population to whom the results are intended to be relevant. Given the high level of comorbidity usually encountered in child psychiatry, narrow inclusion criteria will identify a homogeneous, but also less common, type of patients. Broader criteria will allow recruitment of a more representative group of patients, but a larger sample size will be needed to account for the greater heterogeneity of the sample. Narrow criteria are typically employed in trials aimed at testing the efficacy of novel treatments, as an initial step toward studying effectiveness in larger, more representative and heterogeneous samples of patients. In any case, it is important to document the source of subject referral to the study and reasons for exclusion as a way of defining the representativeness of the experimental sample and gauging the ecological validity of the study results.

It has become standard to use structured or semistructured diagnostic interviews as a way of arriving at reliable and reproducible diagnosis. For this purpose, the Schedule for Affective Disorders and Schizophrenia for School-age Children (K-SADS; Kaufman et al., 1997), the Diagnostic Interview for Children and Adolescents (DICA; Welner et al., 1987), the Diagnostic Interview Schedule for Children (DISC; Shaffer et al., 2000), and the Autism Diagnostic Interview (ADI; Lord et al., 1994) have been used. In addition to a validated diagnosis, it is important to ensure that study subjects meet certain criteria for severity by requiring a minimum score on the primary outcome measures for entering the study.

In planning federally funded studies, attention must be paid to the current requirements for inclusion of sex/gender and racial/ethnic minorities. According to the National Institutes of Health (NIH) policy, all clinical research must include female subjects and members of racial/ethnic minority groups, unless a clear and compelling rationale is provided indicating that inclusion is inappropriate with respect to the health of the subjects

or the purpose of the research (NIH, 1994). Additional requirements apply to NIH-defined phase III clinical trials. These studies usually involve several hundreds or more human subjects, for the purpose of evaluating an experimental intervention in comparison with a standard or control intervention or comparing two or more existing treatments (NIH, 1994). In situations where previous studies neither support nor negate significant differences in treatment response by sex/gender and/or race/ethnicity, the trial must enroll a sufficient and appropriate number of research subjects of sex/gender and race/ethnic subgroups to allow secondary analyses of the treatment effects in these subgroups to be conducted. However, these secondary analyses are not required to have enough statistical power to test the study primary hypothesis in each subgroup. Rather, they are intended to be exploratory and hypothesis generating. In situations where there is already evidence from previous studies that the treatment effects are different in sex/gender and/or race/ethnicity subgroups, the phase III trial must have enough power to test the study primary hypothesis in these subgroups. Only when previous research has already definitively excluded the presence of clinically significant treatment effects among subgroups can the requirement to enroll adequate gender and ethnic representation be waived. As of October 1, 2000, all research applications or proposals for NIH grants, cooperative agreements, or contracts for phase III clinical trials must include a description of the plans to conduct subgroup analyses as appropriate to the specific research situation described above (NIH, 2000).

SELECTING THE TREATMENT OUTCOMES

Research questions must be quantified and expressed in mathematical terms as hypotheses that can be experimentally tested. To this end, suitable measures of treatment effects must be identified. In the absence of biological markers of psychopathology, the assessment of treatment effects relies on recordings of behavior. The choice of outcome, and therefore also of its measure, depend on the research questions. Thus, if the primary interest is to test the ability of the treatment to improve symptoms, rating scales of proven reliability and validity are adopted to document the presence and severity of symptoms before and during treatment. For instance, clinical trials in attention deficit hyperactivity disorder (ADHD) have used rating scales of the symptoms relevant to this disorder, such as the Conners Teacher and Parent Rating Scales (Conners, 1997) and the Swanson, Nolan, and Pelham Rating Scale (SNAP)

(Swanson, 1992). Likewise, trials in youths with depression have employed instruments such as the Child Depression Rating Scale (Poznanski et al., 1984), Children's Depression Inventory (Kovacs, 1985), and the Beck Depression Inventory (Beck et al., 1988). Symptom scales can be completed by the research clinician (observer) based on information provided by the patient, family, and/or teacher. Whenever possible, observer-completed scales are preferred, as they tend to be more sensitive to treatment effects. Because research observers typically undergo training to achieve acceptable interrater reliability, their scores have usually less variance than those provided by patients or nonresearch raters. In some situations, such as ADHD, the primary outcome variable consists of rating scales completed by parents and teachers, because it would be impractical for researchers to observe the child across the relevant settings and for extended periods of time. It is sometimes possible to count discrete behavioral episodes as the outcome measure. Thus, in studying treatments for children with school refusal, efficacy can be quantified by counting number of days in school (Bernstein et al., 2000). Activity monitors have been used to document the effects of stimulant drugs in ADHD (Porrino et al., 1983). The appeal of this approach is immediately evident, as it uses an objectively quantifiable and easily interpretable outcome measure. Direct observation scales of behavior have also been developed, such as the classroom observation code (Abikoff et al., 1977) and the analog classroom assessment (Swanson et al., 1998) for hyperactive children. Data collected during direct observation of the child can be of value, provided the cross-sectional observation is truly representative of the child behavior and the raters are consistent in recording the variables of interest. Global rating scales such as the Clinical Global Impression (CGI) scales (Guy, 1976) are commonly used in psychiatric trials, both in adults and children. In some cases, these scales have been modified to focus on information relevant to specific disorders such as bipolar disorder (Spearing et al., 1997), depression, and obsessive-compulsive disorder (Hoen-Saric et al., 2000). These types of measurement tend to capture different time periods. Direct observations are cross-sectional recordings of behavior, usually over a period of fractions of an hour, which are expected to be representative of the typical functioning of the child. Symptom rating scales are usually retrospective assessments that gather information on symptom severity over the recent past, such as the past few days or past weeks. When counts of discrete episodes of a behavior are utilized, the time frame is variable and often spans

weeks or months. Global ratings try to integrate all the information on the patient's condition, including retrospective reporting. Their comprehensiveness, joined with the retrospective component of the assessment, tends to increase the sensitivity of global ratings. In medicine, retrospective measures are generally more sensitive to clinically significant changes than cross-sectional ones (Fischer et al., 1999). Symptom rating scales, counts of discrete events, direct observations, and global ratings all offer diverse and potentially valuable perspectives on the possible treatment effects. The selection depends mainly on the type of disorder being studied and the availability of instruments with acceptable psychometric properties. Typically, child psychopharmacology trials have used symptom rating scales based on retrospective reports of behavior (Emslie et al., 1997; MTA Cooperative Group, 1999). Whenever possible, it is advisable to include different types of assessment in a clinical trial as a way of enhancing the resolution of the experiment and thus its capacity of detecting treatment effects.

If measures of symptom change are still the most commonly employed dependent variables in clinical trials, there is increasing awareness of their limitations in capturing truly clinically significant changes. In fact, children are typically referred for treatment because of functional impairment. Symptoms alone are not sufficient for diagnosing most psychiatric disorders, for which evidence of symptom-induced functional impairment is required. The dearth of rating scales that quantify level of functioning and are sensitive to treatment effects is one of the major limitations of the current clinical trial methodology. A few scales exist, such as the Children's Global Adjustment Scale (C-GAS) (Shaffer et al., 1983) and Health of the Nation Outcome Scales (HoNOSCA; Gowers et al., 1999), but their sensitivity in detecting treatment effects in large clinical trials is still unclear. Another set of outcome variables of great interest is those relevant to cost/benefit analyses. A number of such analyses have been conducted in adult psychopharmacology, but it can be expected that they will soon become an integral part of child trials as well. To this end, instruments have been developed to record and quantify use of mental health services (e.g., the Child and Adolescent Services Assessment; Ascher et al., 1996).

The ability of rating scales to detect possible treatment effects is contingent on both the construct validity of the instrument and the reliability of the study raters. The former can be achieved by selecting scales with demonstrated good psychometrics, the latter by carefully training study raters and requiring good interrater reliability before collecting data. Because clinical trials often last years, rater "drifting" from post-training reliability is possible and repeated testing of reliability during the study is advisable.

Child clinical trials often include multiple outcome measures and multiple informants. One major methodological challenge is how to integrate this information in a coherent data analysis. Repeated testing of the same research hypothesis using multiple rating instruments inflates the risk of finding a false-positive result (type I error) and requires protection with adjustments such as the Bonferroni's correction. Multivariate statistics (i.e., MANOVA) can be used in an attempt to capture treatment effects simultaneously on multiple outcomes. This approach is more commonly adopted in psychology research than in psychopharmacology trials, possibly because of statistical and practical drawbacks. In fact, special requirements apply to multivariate analyses, such as the need for adequate sample size for each parameter being tested. Moreover, the handling of missing data can be especially challenging. When the number of outcome measures increases, the likelihood of having incomplete data sets also increases. Data imputation may not be always possible and patients with incomplete sets of outcome measures may have to be dropped from the analyses. Thus, whenever possible, it is preferable to identify one outcome variable that can provide information on the primary outcome of interest, and arrange the other outcome variables in hierarchical order.

The primary outcome variable should be not only sensitive to possible treatment effects but also easily interpretable from a clinical perspective. It is often desirable, in addition to reporting the group mean of the continuous measurement, to report also the rate of responders in each treatment group. This can be accomplished in different ways, most commonly through the use of a global measure of improvement, such as the CGI, or by selecting a priori a cut-off score on a continuous symptom scale to identify patients who improved. If responder status is so defined, it is desirable to show the cumulative distribution curve of the scores of the primary measure for each treatment group as a way to visualize the difference between treatments. An example of such a curve is shown in Figure 53.1, which is taken from a secondary analysis of the Multimodal Treatment Study of Children with of ADHD (Swanson et al., 2001). In this plot, the differences in outcome between treatment groups are evident not only at the a priori designated cut-off defining responders (i.e., SNAP ≤1.0) but also across a range of scores, and without intersections between the curves (which would

have indicated that any group difference in response rate was contingent on the choice of a particular cut-off). These plots are easily interpretable and are an appealing way of presenting the results of a clinical trial.

CHOOSING THE APPROPRIATE COMPARISON GROUP

The presence of a control or comparison group is, together with randomization, an essential feature of controlled clinical trials. It allows discrimination between specific effects of a treatment and effects common to other interventions. Various types of comparison groups can be utilized in controlled trials, such as no treatment, placebo, dose–response, and active control (FDA, 1999). The selection of which comparison to use is primarily dictated by the main purpose of the study. In many cases, the research question is whether the experimental treatment is different from no treatment. To test such a hypothesis in an unbiased fashion, a placebo arm is usually adopted as a control, thus leading to a reformulation of the primary question, which becomes whether the experimental treatment is different from a nonspecific treatment like placebo. This reformulation has implications for the interpretation of the results. In fact, treatment with placebo does not equal absence of treatment, but can be defined as nonspecific therapeutic management that controls for the specific components of the experimental treatment. Because placebo is not usually employed in clinical practice, it can be argued that placebo-controlled studies lack full ecological validity, as they compare a particular treatment with an experimental condition (placebo) that is not a real treatment option. Still, the placebo-controlled design allows several important questions to be answered, and is especially valuable when no treatment has been proven effective for the disorder under study. In these cases, a placebo can be easily justified from both a scientific and an ethical perspective.

More debatable is the use of placebo in conditions when effective treatments already exist. In these situations, ethical objections can be made to assigning patients to an inferior treatment. Moreover, families may refuse enrollment into such studies, thus decreasing the representativeness of the study sample. When testing an experimental medication in situations where effective treatment already exists, different types of questions can arise. We may be interested in testing whether the novel treatment is (1) better than no treatment (or non-specific treatment), (2) comparable to an established treatment of proven efficacy, or (3) superior to

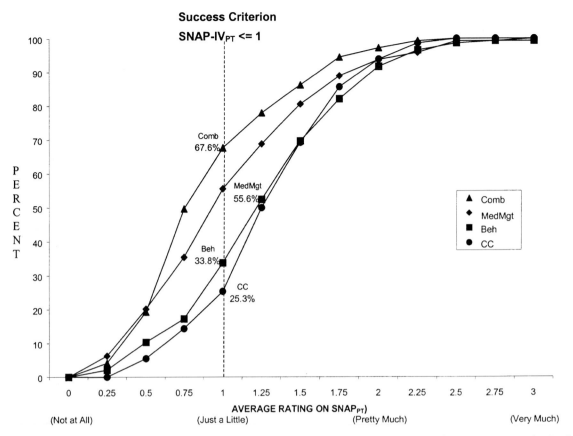

Success Criterion

SNAP-IV_PT <= 1

FIGURE 53.1 Cumulative distribution curves of final ADHD scores by treatment group in the MTA Study. The SNAP rating is average score of the 18 items corresponding to the DSM-IV defining symptoms for attention-deficit-hyperactivity disorder and oppositional defiant disorder (range: 0, not present to 3; very much). Beh, Behavior therapy; CC, community control (treatment as usual); Comb, combined medication management and behavior therapy; MedMgt; medication management; Reproduced with permission from Swanson et al. (2001).

an established treatment of proven efficacy. For statistical reasons, addressing the last two questions requires a substantially larger number of research subjects, as further discussed in this chapter. In some conditions, such as depressive disorder, the placebo response rate can be as high as 70% and highly variable across studies (Birmaher et al., 1998). In these cases, placebo is generally considered an acceptable comparison group, provided its use is limited in time, closely monitored, and not likely to expose patients to harm (Ellenberg and Temple, 2000). If however, the question is whether the novel treatment is as effective as the established one, an active comparison can be considered. Active comparisons can be specific medications or psychotherapies of proven efficacy, or treatment as usual (TAU). If a psychosocial treatment is the comparison group in a psychopharmacology trial, complete blindness of the study is usually impossible, as the participants will know if they have been assigned to psycho-

therapy or not. In this cases, it is important to try to control for possible ascertainment biases by having blind independent raters complete the primary outcome measurements. The TAU is particularly useful as a comparison when the experimental intervention is a novel treatment *strategy* (novel for content of treatment or/and way of implementation) and the aim is to test whether it is superior to usual treatment (MTA Cooperative Group, 1999). If TAU is utilized as a control, it should be defined in the protocol and characterized during the study. In fact, TAU does not usually equal standard treatment and can vary widely both within and between studies. In many cases, TAU consists of assessment and referral to whatever treatment the family can find in the community. Thus, available services in the community, family resources, and barriers to care can all contribute to determining TAU for individual patients. If TAU is found to be inferior to the experimental treatment, it can be difficult to interpret the results without a careful definition of TAU in that particular study.

SUPERIORITY AND NONINFERIORITY STUDIES

Most psychopharmacology trials are aimed at testing whether the experimental treatment is better than a control. In these cases, the null hypothesis is that experimental treatment and control have equal effect on the primary outcome. If enough difference is found between the treatment groups, the null hypothesis is rejected and the treatment considered superior to the control. By convention, *enough difference* is one that could have occurred by chance in no more than 5 cases in 100, or $P \le 0.05$). When previous research supports the efficacy of a treatment for a disorder, it may be of interest to test whether a new treatment is at least as efficacious as one of established efficacy. The current methodology of clinical investigation is based on proving a null hypothesis wrong with sufficient degree of certainty. Proving equality through a clinical trial is, in an epistemological sense, not possible, as the failure to find a difference (i.e., to reject the null hypothesis) does not equal proving absence of a difference. The equality hypothesis can, however, be turned into an inferiority hypothesis, which becomes testable. Under this approach, the null hypothesis is that there is at least a specified difference in outcome between the treatment groups. This specified difference is the clinically acceptable limit, which is the smallest difference in outcome that can be considered clinically important and would make one treatment superior to the other. If the results of the trial fail to demonstrate such a difference, the null hypothesis is rejected and the new treatment is considered non inferior to the standard one. Noninferiority trials are commonly called "active control equivalence studies" (ACES), although the term *noninferiority* is more correct from a methodological point of view (Temple and Ellenberg, 2000). Non-inferiority trials need to reproduce in design, methods, and sample the characteristics of the previously successful superiority trials that support the efficacy of the standard treatment. The non-inferiority trial can be utilized when there is a standard treatment that has been proven consistently effective in previous superiority trials across a variety of studies. Stimulant medications for the treatment of ADHD meet this criterion, and testing of new treatments of ADHD in non-inferiority trials versus methylphenidate or amphetamine would be a reasonable approach. For antidepressants, however, the outcome of placebo-controlled studies is much less consistent and predictable. It is estimated that at

least one-third of industry-sponsored trials of antidepressants are unable to discriminate between active medication and placebo (Temple and Ellenberg, 2000). Thus, there is the possibility that a non-inferiority trial of antidepressants does not have assay sensitivity and incorrect conclusions of clinical equivalence could be drawn. For this reason, the FDA currently requires superiority trials to demonstrate efficacy of antidepressants (FDA, 1999).

COMMON DESIGNS

Like in adults, in children most clinical trials follow a parallel-group design, where patients are randomized to receive one treatment out of a choice of two or more alternatives (Emslie et al., 1997; March et al., 1998; MTA Cooperative Group, 1999). This design has various advantages that derive from its simplicity and reliance on the randomization process to control for possible assignment biases. One disadvantage, however, is that there are differences in treatment response across individual subjects. These differences increase the variance of the outcome measures and this variance needs to be accounted for with an adequate sample size. In some situations, a crossover design can be adopted in child psychopharmacology. In this design, each subject is given sequentially and in random order all the treatments that are being tested, thus controlling for the impact of individual characteristics on treatment effects. The crossover is appealing because it allows a study hypothesis to be tested with equal sensitivity but with substantially smaller sample size than would be needed in a parallel-group design. But the crossover design has also important disadvantages that limit its application to only certain situations. For instance, one of the treatments being tested may have a carryover effect and impact on the next treatment. Conditions that are chronic and stable in time, such as ADHD, and treatments that are have short duration of action, such as methylphenidate, offer a situation that is fitting for a crossover design because symptoms promptly reappear once the treatment is discontinued (Greenhill et al., 2001). On the contrary, crossover designs would not usually be appropriate for clinical trials of antidepressants.

A particular type of parallel design is the *discontinuation design*, where patients who had improved while receiving a certain treatment are randomly and blindly assigned to continue active treatment or switch to placebo. Discontinuation studies aim at testing whether there is therapeutic benefit in continuing treatment beyond a certain point. In this design, worsening of symptoms, relapse, or recurrence of the disorder is the primary outcome variable. Only a few discontinuation studies have been conducted in child psychopharmacology (Gillberg et al., 1997; Emslie et al., 2000). The value of this type of investigation in informing long-term treatment of children is, however, evident. When the short-term efficacy and safety of a treatment are demonstrated, the attention is properly placed on the potential benefit and risks of extended treatment. Childhood psychopathology occurs in the context of development and one cannot always assume that continuous medication treatment is needed for maintaining improvement. Discontinuation studies, however, present various challenges that make them a particular difficult design to implement. Some concerns are ethical. Does the potential benefit of not taking the medication outweigh the risk of relapse? How will the patients be selected? Usually, patients with a history of relapsing upon drug discontinuation will have to be excluded. How careful is the monitoring during the study? How serious can the consequences of relapse be? Can patients who relapse be promptly treated and successfully returned to a remission status? Other challenges are methodological. The power of the study depends on an expected difference in relapse rate between placebo and active treatment. It is probably more difficult to predict relapse rate than treatment response, and long duration of study may be needed to detect differences in relapse rate. If, in an effort to minimize risk to participants, the definition of relapse is too lax, relatively minor fluctuations in symptoms will qualify for relapse, with consequently equally high rates in both arms of the study. The mere knowledge that a patient may have been switched to placebo at a specified point in time leads to a negative expectation in the patient, family, and clinician, and to a tendency to overrate relatively minor symptomatic changes. To obviate this bias, some studies in adults with depression have used a variable discontinuation design with blinding of the time of the possible treatment discontinuation (Rosenbaum et al., 1998).

When two or more different treatments are used concomitantly, it may be of interest to study in the same experiment both the effects due to each treatment (main effects) and the possible interaction between them (interaction effect). *Interaction* here means that the effect of one treatment is modified (e.g., decreased or enhanced) by the coadministration of the other treatment. In these cases, a factorial design can be considered. This design has been used, for instance to study the effects of clomidine and methylphenidate administered separately or in combination to children with ADHD and tic disorders (Tourette's Syndrome Study Group 2002). The simplest form is the 2 × 2 factorial design, where one group of patients is assigned to treatment A, another to treatment B, a third to both A and B, and the fourth to receive neither (placebos for A and B). A potential advantage of this design is that it can test the efficacy of two treatments with about half the sample size required to test them in separate experiments. This potential advantage, however, is only realized if an interaction between the two treatments can be excluded (Keppel 1991). The application of factorial designs to pediatric psychopharmacology trials has thus far been limited, probably because of the difficulties in interpreting the main effect in the presence of interaction effects. In fact, even trials that can be conceptualized according to a factorial in design have been analyzed as conventional parallel-group studies (MTA Cooperative Group, 1999).

HOW MANY STUDY SUBJECTS ARE NEEDED?

In a clinical trial, sample size is one of the critical determinants of the capacity of discriminating between group treatment effects. The other elements that affect experimental sensitivity are variability in treatment response across study subjects, the psychometric properties of the assessment instruments, and the precision with which these instruments are used by the investigators. Assuming that other critical variables remain constant, the larger the sample size, the greater the sensitivity of the trial. Conclusions from a trial are expressed as probability statements and are subject to two sorts of potential errors: incorrectly rejecting the null hypothesis when the observed difference is in fact due to chance (type I error, or α) and failing to reject the null hypothesis when there is a real difference between treatment groups (type II error, or β). It is usual to contain the chances of making a type I error to no more than 5% ($\alpha = 0.05$). It is desirable to keep the chances of making a type II error to no more than 10%, but for many studies a chance of no more than 20% is considered acceptable. The power of the study to detect a certain difference in outcome can be expressed as 1-β. Thus an acceptable power should be at least 80% and a power of 90% or greater is highly desirable. Once the α and β values are established, the other variables needed to calculate the sample size are the difference between treatment groups and the variance of the outcome measure. The *effect size* (ES) expresses that group difference in standard deviation units. Cohen's ES (*d*) is in fact the difference in outcome measure at the end of treatment between the study groups divided by the standard deviation of the control group or the pooled standard deviation. It is usually accepted that ES values of about 0.2 are small, 0.5, mod-

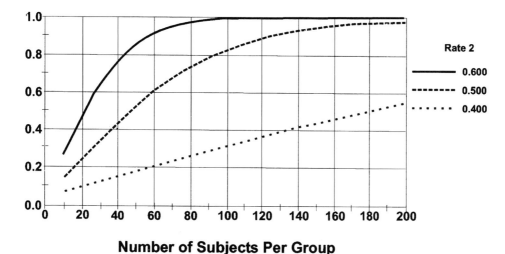

FIGURE 53.2 Statistical power as a function of the difference in response rate between treatment groups (rate 1 vs. rate 2) and of sample size. Reproduced with permission from Borenstein et al. (2000).

erate; and 0.8 or greater, large (Cohen, 1988). When the smallest ES that the study should be expected to detect is specified, the needed sample size can be easily computed using appropriate formulas, tables, or computer programs (Fleiss, 1981, Cohen, 1988, Borenstein et al., 2000). Obviously the larger the ES we are interested in detecting, the smaller the needed sample will be. For example, in order to detect as statistically significant ($\alpha = 0.05$) with acceptable power (1-$\beta = 80\%$) an ES of 1.0, only 17 subjects per group will be needed. This number increases to 33 for an ES of 0.8, to 64 for an ES = 0.5, and to 180 for an ES = 0.3.

When the outcome is expressed categorically (i.e., responder rate), sample size is computed using different formulas based on the same principles. Thus, if the study is expected to have an 80% chance (that is a power of 80%) to find a statistically significant difference ($p \leq 0.05$) *between two treatments* when the response rate is 30% in one group and 60% in the other, a sample size of 40 group is needed. The sample size increases to about 100/group if the rates are 30% versus 50% (Fig. 53.2). Variants on the same theme are used to calculate the sample size needed for other designs, such as crossover and factorial designs, as well as for studies using repeated measurements or 'time to event' as outcome (Friedman et al., 1998).

STATISTICAL SIGNIFICANCE AND CLINICAL SIGNIFICANCE

A difference can be statistically significant but have no clinical relevance. Statistical significance is determined by sample size, and with enough subjects a study can find even clinically irrelevant differences to be statistically significant (Kraemer, 1992). Thus, in designing clinical trials it is essential to determine what is the smallest difference between treatment that would be clinically meaningful, and calculate the sample size based on it. Larger sample sizes would be unnecessary, as they would detect trivial differences of no clinical interest. In recent years, increased attention has been put on effect sizes rather than on statistical significance as a way to focus on clinical relevance of research results (Kraemer, 1992; Borenstein, 1998). Confidence intervals (CI) can be used to estimate the precision of the observed difference. As with statistical power, the precision of the study increases with sample size, with consequent narrowing of the CI (Fig. 53.3). If the 95% CI does not include zero, one can accept the existence of a difference between treatments.

PROTOCOL IMPLEMENTATION

The challenges of intervention research do not end with the preparation of a clinically relevant, scientifically valid, and ethically acceptable protocol. Conduct of the study requires constant attention to both the clinical and experimental components of the trial. Some protocol deviations can be expected in almost every study, but procedures should be in place to minimize both their number and impact, as deviations decrease the assay sensitivity of the experiment and thus the likelihood of detecting treatment effects. A discussion of the monitoring procedures to ensure the quality of the re-

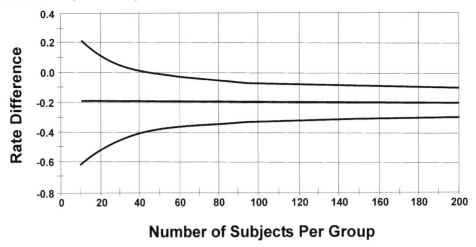

FIGURE 53.3 Two-sided 95% limits for rate diffderence as a function of sample size. Reproduced with permission from Borenstein et al. (2000).

search is beyond the scope of this chapter. The reader interested in the conduct of clinical trials is referred to other sources of information (Meinert, 1986; Friedman et al., 1998). Two aspects, however, are worth mentioning as relevant to the proper planning of treatment studies: ongoing monitoring of study safety and maintenance of the experimental blindness.

Safety must be monitored at two levels: the individual subject level and the study as a whole. The former is accomplished by careful assessment of emerging adverse events and measurement of relevant laboratory parameters; the latter, by periodic review of safety data across treatment groups to detect possible differences or a trend toward differences between groups. Because the interim reviews would unblind the investigators, a separate panel of experts is usually appointed to serve as the Data and Safety Monitoring Board (DSMB). Typically, DSMBs review cumulative study data every 3–6 months, or as needed, based on study characteristics. On the basis of such reviews, the DSMB can modify the study procedures to decrease risk to the participants, require further interim analyses, interrupt the study pending additional analyses, or even terminate the study if the trial has reached a safety or efficacy end point (i.e., the research question has been addressed and further collection of data would not be informative). Since 1998, a DSMB has been required for all phase III clinical trials sponsored by the NIH (NIH, 1998). Phase I and II trials may also need a DSMB if they have multiple clinical sites, are blinded, and/or employ particularly high-risk interventions or

vulnerable populations. Even when DSMB is deemed unnecessary, however, a plan to monitor study safety is required.

In double-blind studies, investigators are usually required to remain blind to treatment assignment of study participants. Breaking individual patient blindness when the participation of each patient has ended but the entire study has not been completed may introduce biases in data collection. In fact, researchers may be given clues to correctly guessing treatment assignment of future study patients. However, trials often last several years, and it is highly impractical and ethically questionable to withhold information about treatment assignment from patients, families, and treating clinicians for long periods of time. One way of providing prompt feedback to individual study participants while still maintaining the investigators blind is to refer patients who have completed all data collection to a clinician who is separate from the investigators and can become unblinded as to the type of treatment received in the study. This strategy has been employed with success in child trials (Research Units in Pediatric Psychopharmacology Anxiety Study Group, 2001).

CONCLUSIONS

Mounting a clinical trial in child psychopharmacology requires the integration of considerable clinical and research expertise. Attention must be paid to multiple design and methodological aspects, and scientific goals must be reconciled with ethical principles. Assessment instruments and outcome measure must be developmentally appropriate. Protocol implementation requires constant monitoring for quality of data gathering and study safety. Ultimately, the success of a trial depends on the contribution from researchers of different backgrounds and expertise, including, among others, child psychiatrists, psychologists, psychiatric nurses, pediatricians, statisticians, and data managers. Involvement of family and patients in the projects from the earlier phases of development is critical. More than any other type of research, clinical trials are team efforts. The presence of excellent single components does not guarantee per se successful performance without extensive overall planning and coordination.

REFERENCES

Abikoff, H., Gittelman-Klein, R., and Klein, D.F. (1977) Validation of a classroom observation code for hyperactive children. *J Consult Clin Psychol* 21:519–533.

Ascher, B., Farmer, E., Burns, B., and Angold, A. (1996) The Child and Adolescent Services Assessment (CASA): description and psychometrics. *J Emotional Behav Disord* 4:12–20.

Beck, A.T., Steer, R.A., and Garbin, M.G. (1988) Psychometric properties of the Beck Depression Inventory: twenty-five years of evaluation. *Clin Psychol Rev* 8:77–100.

Bernstein, G.A., Borchardt, C.M., Perwien, A.R., Crosby, R.D., Kushner, M.G., Thuras, P.D., and Last, C.G. (2000) Imipramine plus cognitive-behavioral therapy in the treatment of school refusal. *J Am Acad Child Adolesc Psychiatry* 39:276–283.

Birmaher, B., Brent, D.A., Kolko, D., Baugher, M., Bridge, J., Holder, D., Iyengar, S., and Ulloa, R.E. (2000) Clinical outcome after short-term psychotherapy for adolescents with major depressive disorder. *Arch Gen Psychiatry* 57:29–36.

Birmaher, B., Waterman, G.S., Ryan, N.D., Perel, J., McNabb, J., Balach, L., Beaudry, M.B., Nasr, F.N., Karambelkar, J., Elterich, G., Quintana, H., Williamson, D.E., and Rao, U. (1998) Randomized, controlled trial of amitriptyline versus placebo for adolescents with "treatment-resistant" major depression. *J Am Acad Child Adolesc Psychiatry* 37:527–535.

Borenstein, M. (1998) The shift from significance testing to effect size estimation. In: Schooler, N., ed. *Research and Methods, Vol. 3* In: Bellack, A.S. and Hersen, M., eds. Comprehensive Clinical Psychology Oxford: Elsevier Science, pp. 314–349.

Borenstein, M., Rothstein, H., and Cohen, J. (2000) Power and precision: a computer program for power analysis and confidence intervals. Biostat, http://www.Power-Analysis.com.

Chow, S.-C. and Liu, J.-P. (1998) *Design and Analysis of Clinical Trials—Concepts and Methodologies.* New York: John Wiley & Sons.

Cohen, J. (1988) *Statistical Power Analysis for the Behavioral Sciences, 2nd ed.* Hillsdale, NJ: Lawrence Erlbaum Associates.

Conners, C.K. (1997) Conners' Rating Scales-Revised. North Tonawanda, NY: Multi-Health Systems.

Ellenberg, S.S. and Temple, R. (2000) Placebo-controlled trials and active-control trials in the evaluation of new treatments. *Ann Intern Med* 133:464–475.

Emslie, G.J., Rush, A.J., Weiberg, W.A., Kowatch, R.A., Hughes,

C.W., Carmody, T., and Rintelmann, J. (1997) A double-blind, randomized, placebo-controlled trial of fluoxetine in children and adolescents with depression. *Arch Gen Psychiatry* 54:1031–1037.

Emslie, G.J., Wagner, K.D., Carpenter, D.J., Riddle, M.A., Birmaher, B., Geller, B., Rosenberg, D., Gallagher, D., and Carpenter, D. (2000) Efficacy and safety of paroxetine in juvenile OCD. Presented at the 47th Annual Meeting of the American Academy of Child and Adolescent Psychiatry, October 24–29, New York, NY.

Fisher, D., Stewart, A.L., Bloch, D.A., Lorig, K., Laurent, D., and Holman, H. (1999) Capturing the patient's view of change as a clinical outcome measure. *JAMA* 282:1157–1162.

Fleiss, J.L. (1981) *Statistical Methods for Rates and Proportions.* New York: John Wiley & Sons.

Food and Drug Administration (FDA) (1999) International Conference on Harmonization: choice of control group in clinical trials. *Fed Register* 64(185):51767–51780.

Friedman, L.M., Furberg, C.D., and DeMets, D.L. (1998) *Fundamentals of Clinical Trials, 3rd ed.* New York: Springer-Verlag.

Gillberg, C., Melander, H., von Knorring, A.L., Janols, L.O., Thernlund, G., Hagglof, B., Eidevall-Wallin, L., Gustafsson, P., and Kopp, S. (1997) Long-term stimulant treatment of children with attention-deficit hyperactivity disorder symptoms. A randomized, double-blind, placebo-controlled trial. *Arch Gen Psychiatry* 54:857–864.

Gowers, S.G., Harrington, R.C., Whitton, A., Lelliott, P., Beevor, A., Wing, J., and Jezzard, R. (1999) Brief scale for measuring the outcomes of emotional and behavioural disorders in children. Health of the Nation Outcome Scales for Children and Adolescents (HoNOSCA). *Br J Psychiatry* 174:413–416.

Greenhill, L.L., Swanson, J.M., Vitiello, B., Davies, M., Clevenger, W., Wu, M., Arnold, L.E., Abikoff, H.B., Bukstein, O.G., Conners, C.K., Elliott, G.R., Hechtman, L., Hinshaw, S.P., Hoza, B., Jensen, P.S., Kraemer, H.C., March, J.S., Newcorn, J.H., Severe, J.B., Wells, K., and Wigal, T. (2001) Impairment and deportment responses to different methylphenidate doses in children with ADHD: the MTA titration trial. *J Am Acad Child Adolesc Psychiatry* 40:180–187.

Guy, W. (1976) ECDEU *Assessment Manual for Psychopharmacology, Revised.* U.S. Dept. of Health and Human Services, Publication No. (ADM) 91–338, Rockville, MD: Government Printing Office.

Hoehn-Saric, R., Ninan, P., Black, D.W., Stahl, S., Greist, J.H., Lydiard, B., McElroy, S., Zajecka, J., Chapman, D., Clary, C., and Harrison, W. (2000) Multicenter double-blind comparison of sertraline and desipramine for concurrent obsessive-compulsive and major depressive disorders. *Arch Gen Psychiatry* 57:76–82.

Kaufman, J., Birmaher, B., Brent, D., Rao, U., Flynn, C., Moreci, P., Williamson, D., and Ryan, N. (1997) Schedule for Affective Disorders and Schizophrenia for School-Age Children–Present and Lifetime Version (K-SADS-PL): initial reliability and validity data. *J Am Acad Child Adolesc Psychiatry* 36:980–988.

Keppel, G. (1991) *Design and Analysis: A Researcher's Handbook, 3rd ed.* Englewood Cliffs, NJ: Prentice Hall.

Kovacs, M. (1985) The Children's Depression Inventory (CDI). *Psychopharmacol Bull* 21:995–998.

Kraemer, H.C. (1992) Reporting the effect size of effects in research studies to facilitate assessment of practical or clinical significance. *Psychoneuroendocrinology* 17:527–536.

Kraemer, H.C., and Telch, C.F. (1992) Selection and utilization of outcome measures in psychiatric clinical trials. *Neuropsychopharmacology* 7:95–94.

Lord, C., Rutter, M., and LeCouteur, A. (1994). Autism Diagnostic

Interview–Revised: a revised version of a diagnostic interview for caregivers of individuals with possible pervasive developmental disorders. *J Autism Dev Disord* 24:659–685.

March, J.S., Biederman, J., Wolkow, R., Safferman, A., Marekian, J., Cook, E.H., Cutler, N.R., Dominguez, R., Ferguson, J., Muller, B., Riesenberg, R., Rosenthal, M., Sallee, F.R., and Wagner, K.D. (1998) Sertraline in children and adolescents with obsessive-compulsive disorder: a multicenter randomized controlled trial. *JAMA* 280:1752–1756.

Meinert, C.L. (1986) *Clinical Trials: Design, Conduct, and Analysis.* New York: Oxford University Press.

MTA Cooperative Group (1999) A 14-month randomized clinical trial of treatment strategies for attention-deficit/hyperactivity disorder. *Arch Gen Psychiatry* 56:1073–1087.

National Institutes of Health (NIH) (1994) NIH guidelines on the inclusion of women and minorities as subjects in clinical research. *NIH Guide,* March 18, 1994 (also available at http://grants.nih.gov/grants/funding/women_min/guidelines_update.htm).

National Institutes of Health (1998) NIH policy for data and safety monitoring. *NIH Guide,* June 10, 1998 (also available at http://grants.nih.gov/grants/guide/notice-files/not98-084.html).

National Institutes of Health (2000) NIH guidelines on the inclusion of women and minorities as subjects in clinical research—updated August 2, 2000. *NIH Guide,* August 2, 2000 (also available at http://grants.nih.gov/grants/guide/notice-files/NOT-OD-00-048.html).

Porrino, L.J., Rapoport, J.L., Behar, D., Sceery, W., Ismond, D.R., and Bunney, W.E. (1983) A naturalistic assessment of the motor activity of hyperactive boys. II. Stimulant drug effects. *Arch Gen Psychiatry* 40:688–693.

Poznanski, E.O., Feeman, L.N., and Mokros, H.B. (1984) Children's Depression Rating Scale–Revised. *Psychopharmacol Bull* 21:979–989.

Research Units in Pediatric Psychopharmacology (RUPP) Anxiety Study Group (2001) Fluvoxamine treatment of anxiety disorders in children and adolescents. *N Engl J Med* 344:1279–1285.

Rosenbaum, J.F., Fava, M., Hoog, S.L., Acroft, R.C., and Krebs, W.B. (1998) Selective serotonin reuptake inhibitor discontinuation syndrome: a randomized clinical trial. *Biol Psychiatry* 44:77–87.

Shaffer, D., Fisher, P., Lucas, C.P., Dulcan, M.K., and Schwab-Stone, M.E. (2000) NIMH Diagnostic Interview Schedule for Children Version IV (NIMH DISC-IV): description, differences from previous versions, and reliability of some common diagnoses. *J Am Acad Child Adolesc Psychiatry* 39:28–38.

Shaffer, D., Gould, M.S., Brasic, J., Ambrosini, P., Fisher, P., Bird, H., and Aluwahlia, S. (1983) A Children's Global Assessment Scale (C-GAS). *Arch Gen Psychiatry* 40:1228–1231.

Spearing, M.K., Post, R.M., Leverich, G.S., Brandt, D., and Nolen, W. (1997) Modification of the Clinical Global Impressions (CGI) Scale for use in bipolar illness (BP): the CGI-BP. *Psychiatry Res* 73:159–171.

Swanson, J.M., (1992) *School-Based Assessments and Interventions for ADD Students.* Irvine, CA: KC Publishing.

Swanson, J.M., Kraemer, H.C., Hinshaw, S.P., Arnold, L.E., Conners, C.K., Abikoff, H.B., Clevenger, W., Davies, M., Elliott, G.R., Greenhill, L.L., Hechtman, L., Hoza, B., Jensen, P.S., March, J.S., Newcorn, J.H., Owens, E.B., Pelham, W.E., Schiller, E., Severe, J.B., Simpson, S., Vitiello, B., Wells, K, Wigal T., and Wu, M. (2001) Clinical relevance of the primary findings of the MTA: success rate based on severity of ADHD and ODD symptoms at the end of treatment. *J Am Acad Child Adolesc Psychiatry* 40:168–179.

Swanson, J.M., Wigal, S., Greenhill, L.L., Browne, R., Waslik, B., Lerner, M., Williams, L., Flynn, D., Agler, D., Crowley, K., Fineberg, E., Baren, M., and Cantwell, D.P. (1998) Analog classroom assessment of Adderall in children with ADHD. *J Am Acad Child Adolesc Psychiatry* 37:519–526.

Temple, R., and Ellenberg, S.S. (2000) Placebo-controlled trials and active-control trials in the evaluation of new treatments. Part 1: ethical and scientific issues. *Ann Intern Med* 133:455–463.

Tourette's Syndrome Study Group (2002) Treatment of ADHD in children with tics. A randomized controlled trial. *Neurology* 58:527–536.

Weisz, J.R., and Jensen, P.S. (1999) Efficacy and effectiveness of psychotherapy and pharmacotherapy with children and adolescents. *Ment Health Servi Res* 1:125–158.

Wells, K.W. (1999) Treatment research at the crossroads: the scientific interface of clinical trials and effectiveness research. *Am J Psychiatry* 156:5–10.

Welner, Z., Reich, W., Herjanic, B., Jung, K.G., and Amado, H. (1987) Reliability, validity, and parent child agreement studies of the Diagnostic Interview for Children and Adolescents (DICA). *J Am Acad Child Adolesc Psychiatry* 26:649–653.

54 | Regulatory issues

THOMAS P. LAUGHREN

Psychiatric illness is recognized in the pediatric population, and there is evidence of substantial use of psychotropic medications in this age group, including in the preschool population (Zito et al., 2000). Unfortunately, the evidence base is inadequate to support the current level of prescribing in this area; neither the efficacy nor the safety of these medications in pediatric patients is well established for most indications. This lack of critical information to support prescribing is reflected in the approved labeling for most of the drug products that are prescribed for pediatric patients with psychiatric illness, which simply states that safety and effectiveness have not been established in pediatric patients. Thus, most prescribing of psychotropic drugs in the pediatric population is off-label, and each child treated is, in a sense, an experiment, but one that is not likely to generate much useful information. There is a critical need for more and better information on the efficacy, safety, dosing, and pharmacokinetics of the psychotropic drugs used to treat psychiatric illness in pediatric patients. There are a number of explanations for the lack of research in pediatric psychopharmacology (Jensen et al, 1994), but this is not the focus of this chapter. Rather, it will review Food and Drug Administration (FDA) initiatives in recent years to stimulate drug research in the pediatric population and the impact of these initiatives on drug development in pediatric psychopharmacology. The chapter will also consider the assessment of safety, the balancing of science and ethics, the preschool population, and other problems that must be addressed for drug development in this area to progress. The chapter will begin with a brief overview of drug development and the regulatory process. In some cases it will be necessary to limit details of the discussion to protect the proprietary rights of individual sponsors who have drug development programs underway in this area.

DRUG DEVELOPMENT AND THE REGULATORY PROCESS

The FDA has regulatory authority over the development and marketing of new drugs, including labeling and advertising for approved drug products. Preclinical testing precedes human testing with a new drug. At least two animal species are exposed to a wide range of doses of the drug for varying durations, and assessments include observation for abnormal signs, routine measurements (laboratory parameters, vital signs, electrocardiograms [EKGs]), and both gross anatomical and histopathological evaluation (Williams, 1990). Plasma is sampled for concentrations of parent drug and metabolites to estimate pharmacokinetic parameters and also to attempt to discover plasma concentration–adverse effect relationships. Findings from early animal studies of a new drug determine both the doses chosen for early human trials and the identification of organ systems selected for careful safety monitoring. In addition, animal models that may be predictive of efficacy in human disease may be utilized to try to identify the concentrations to target in human studies.

Once a pharmaceutical company has done sufficient chemistry and manufacturing work to have a drug substance that is suitable for human testing and has completed enough of the preclinical studies to justify human testing, it submits what is known as an Investigational New Drug (IND) application to initiate such testing. Human testing of a new drug begins with *phase 1 trials* focusing on human pharmacology, pharmacokinetics, and tolerability, generally in normal adults (Posvar and Sedman 1989); (Colburn, 1990). The goal of these early trials is to find a range of tolerable doses. This phase is typically initiated with a single, rising-dose trial in which subjects are exposed to progressively higher single doses of the new drug. The single-dose trial is followed by a multiple, rising-dose trial of several weeks duration, permitting the assessment of steady-state pharmacokinetics. Safety assessments in these early trials include recording of abnormal signs, symptoms, laboratory parameters, vital signs, EKGs, and other special assessments, selected on the basis of the known pharmacology of the drug and findings from animal studies. Plasma samples are evaluated to discover plasma concentration–adverse event relationships.

Patients are generally first exposed to a new drug in

phase 2 trials to evaluate the efficacy of the drug in patients with the disease of interest, and to determine the common short-term adverse events associated with the drug. Although these are sometimes called *dose-ranging trials*, phase 2 trials are almost always too small to provide definitive dose–response information. *Phase 3 trials* are the definitive trials for providing adequate evidence of efficacy for the claimed indications. These trials often include open extensions after the controlled part of a study to provide safety data during longer-term use, and they also extend the drug into more heterogeneous groups, e.g., the elderly, patients with concomitant illnesses, and patients taking concomitant medications. The patients on long-term extended use are sometimes studied in randomized withdrawal studies to demonstrate long-term efficacy. Although safety monitoring tends to be somewhat less intense during this phase than in earlier phases, it may involve more directed approaches to test specific hypotheses. The more heterogeneous populations studied and the longer exposures may permit the discovery of subgroups at particular risk for adverse events through pharmacokinetic screening (Sheiner and Benet., 1985; Temple, 1985).

What is usually missing from the typical drug development scenario is attention to pediatric patients who may suffer from the same disease being studied in adults. The next section will review FDA initiatives that try to stimulate interest in including the pediatric population in the planning of drug development programs. A later section will suggest how even preclinical programs can be modified to include juvenile animals, with the anticipation that adverse effects specific to certain phases of human development might be detected by looking at animals in parallel phases of development.

Once a pharmaceutical company has completed its drug development program, it submits what is known as a New Drug Application (NDA) to gain FDA approval for marketing. For a standard NDA, the FDA has 10 months to make a decision on the application, which can be to approve it, refuse to approve it, or declare it approvable, but with some more information required before final approval. Approval may be accompanied by commitments to conduct phase 4 (post-marketing) studies to follow up on certain questions or concerns. Regardless of whether there are phase 4 commitments, all drugs are subject to post-marketing surveillance. The FDA has a voluntary (spontaneous reporting) system that depends on clinicians and others to report adverse events to the FDA's Medwatch system. As signals emerge in this voluntary reporting system, there may be requirements for additional changes to labeling, additional studies, etc. In addition, the pharmaceutical company may continue with its development program by focusing on new indications (claims), new subgroups in the population, including pediatric patients, new formulations, new schedules of administration, comparisons with other agents, or use in combination with other agents.

FOOD AND DRUG ADMINISTRATION INITIATIVES TO PROMOTE PEDIATRIC DRUG DEVELOPMENT

The FDA's regulatory authority regarding new drugs involves oversight of the development of new drugs under INDs, actions on NDAs submitted after the completion of development programs, drug labeling, and advertising. The FDA does not regulate the practice of medicine, however, so that physicians may prescribe approved drugs in the treatment of any illnesses or any patients for which they consider these drugs appropriate, regardless of whether there are approved indications for those illnesses. As noted, such off-label use is more the rule than the exception in pediatric psychopharmacology. While the FDA does not usually have any direct role in regulating such practices, the agency has long been concerned about the lack of information needed for the safe and effective use of various medications in the pediatric population. Several initiatives have been launched over the years in an attempt to stimulate research interest and activity in pediatric clinical pharmacology. This section will begin with a brief review of initiatives occurring prior to 1997 (Laughren, 1996), and then will discuss the two most recent and important initiatives—i.e., the pediatric provision of the Food and Drug Administration Modernization Act (FDAMA) of 1997, and the 1998 Pediatric Rule.

Pre-1997 Initiatives

The first action intended to improve labeling from the standpoint of pediatric use information was the creation in 1979 (FDA, 1979) of the Pediatric Use subsection under the Precautions section of labeling. The final rule for this labeling change reaffirmed the need for substantial evidence from adequate and well-controlled trials in support of any new pediatric indications, and in the absence of such evidence, it called for the standard disclaimer, i.e., that "safety and effectiveness in children have not been established." Unfortunately, the creation of this subsection by itself did not serve as an effective stimulus to pediatric drug research, and most labeling still contains the standard disclaimer rather than the needed information.

In 1992, the FDA launched a second initiative, again focusing on the Pediatric Use section of labeling (FDA, 1992). This proposed rule emphasized an alternative approach to obtaining "substantial evidence of effectiveness." It was noted that, under certain circumstances, pediatric indications and use information in labeling could be based on adequate and well-controlled studies in adults. In particular, it was noted that, if the agency "concludes that the course of the disease and the drug's effects are sufficiently similar in the pediatric and adult populations," the agency may permit extrapolation from the adult efficacy data to pediatric patients. Supplementary pharmacokinetic data for dosing and additional pediatric safety information would be needed. This proposed rule did still allow for the option of the standard disclaimer in the event it was judged that extrapolation from adult data was not reasonable and other data supporting a pediatric indication were not available. The final rule for this second initiative was published on December 13, 1994, and became effective January 12, 1995 (FDA, 1994). It specifically requested sponsors of already approved drug products to "re-examine existing data to determine whether the Pediatric Use subsection of labeling could be modified based on adequate and well-controlled studies in adults, and other information supporting pediatric use, and, if appropriate, submit a supplemental application to comply" (59FR64240) with this new regulation by December 13, 1996. This new rule did not add a new requirement for sponsors to conduct pediatric studies. However, in line with past Agency views that manufacturers are responsible for providing information on off-label use they know is occurring, this new rule included language from the Food, Drug, and Cosmetic (FD&C) Act and existing regulations suggesting that, under certain circumstances, the agency could actually require new pediatric studies for either an already approved drug being used in pediatric populations or for a drug under development that was very likely to be used in pediatric populations. Such requirements, however, have been very difficult to enforce, and the expectation was that pediatric studies would almost always be a voluntary effort on the part of the pharmaceutical industry. Importantly, this new rule did establish a pediatric subcommittee under the Medical Policy Coordinating Committee in the Center for Drug Evaluation and Research, to oversee the implementation of the rule and to track the response to this rule. Unfortunately, again, the 1994 rule did not have a significant stimulatory effect on pediatric drug research.

Food and Drug Administration Modernization Act (1997)

With exhortation having failed to induce pediatric studies, legislation in 1997 utilized a different approach. The FDAMA was signed into law November 21, 1997 (FDA, 1997). Section 111 of this act provided pharmaceutical sponsors with the possibility of gaining an additional 6 months of market exclusivity (freedom from generic competition) either for new drugs, i.e., not yet approved, or for drugs already approved and marketed, if the existing patent or other exclusivity had not yet lapsed. In either case, it would first be necessary to establish that information relating to the use of the active drug moiety in some pediatric population had the potential for producing health benefits in that population and for the FDA to specifically request such information. For a new drug being developed in adults, this could be a development program for that same indication, but now in the pediatric population, or for a different indication in pediatric patients. A new drug being developed primarily for a pediatric indication would also qualify for exclusivity under the FDAMA. For an already approved drug, this could be a development program (1) for a new indication in pediatric patients not already approved in adults, or (2) for an indication(s) in pediatric patients that is (are) already approved in adults. This is an entirely voluntary program that is intended to provide incentives to sponsors to develop new drugs and/or new indications for pediatric patients.

For any of the situations described for which additional exclusivity might be gained, the FDAMA requires the following to gain that exclusivity: (1) a written request for the pediatric studies must be issued by the FDA; (2) study reports filed as an NDA or supplement by the sponsor must meet the terms of the written request, including conducting the requested studies and submitting the results before the deadline specified in the written request; and (3) the sponsor's drug must have remaining exclusivity or patent protection at the time the data are submitted. Thus, the FDAMA provides no incentives for sponsors of drugs that are available for generic manufacturing. For already marketed drugs, a fourth requirement was that the drug must be on a list of drugs potentially useful in pediatric populations that was required of the FDA by the FDAMA. According to the FDAMA, the FDA was to develop by May 21, 1998, a list of already marketed drugs for which additional pediatric information might be beneficial. The list consists of all drugs approved for use in adults for indications that occur in the pediatric population. The priority list was published on May

20, 1998. It included psychotropics approved for the following indications: generalized anxiety disorder; panic disorder; attention-deficit hyperactivity disorder (ADHD); mania; obsessive-compulsive disorder (OCD); schizophrenia; and insomnia.

Generally, the FDAMA process is initiated by pharmaceutical company sponsors who submit what is referred to as a Proposed Pediatric Study Request (PPSR). If the FDA makes a determination that studying the drug in the pediatric population would provide a public health benefit, it issues a written request, which is a fairly detailed description of what studies a sponsor would need to conduct to address the pediatric questions of interest. The written request may or may not reflect elements in the sponsor's PPSR. Importantly, the new law does not require that the study results be positive to support the additional exclusivity; it requires only that the studies be conducted and reported as requested, including meeting the deadline in the written request. Furthermore, it should be noted that the FDA must be careful to include all the appropriate indications and all the appropriate age ranges for a particular drug at the time of issuing the written request, since exclusivity attaches to any existing exclusivity or patent protection on the entire active moiety belonging to the pharmaceutical sponsor. The second period of exclusivity outlined in the FDAMA is limited to the drug product studied and has not been of interest to sponsors. Thus, it has not acted as an incentive for a sponsor to do additional studies for another pediatric indication not included in the original written request.

The FDA was required to report to Congress by January 1, 2001, on the effectiveness of the program in improving information about important pediatric uses for approved drugs. The pediatric exclusivity provision of the statute expired on January 1, 2002. However, new legislation that provides for a continuation of the authority for FDA to grant extensions to patent exclusivity for pediatric development programs was signed into law January 4, 2002. This law is known as the Best Pharmaceuticals for Children Act (BPCA) of 2001.

Although the pediatric exclusivity provisions of the FDAMA, and the BPCA, represent a voluntary program, they have proved to be the first successful stimulus to the conduct of pediatric studies.

Pediatric Rule of 1998

The 1998 Pediatric Rule was published in final form December 2, 1998 (FDA, 1998), and became effective April 1, 1999. Unlike the pediatric section of the FDAMA, which is voluntary, the Pediatric Rule gives the FDA authority to require pediatric studies for certain new and marketed drug and biological products. Unlike the FDAMA, which focuses only on the drug substance, whether for a new or already approved drug, the Pediatric Rule may be triggered by several different types of development programs that companies might propose. These include programs either for a new drug substance or for any of the following four programs that might be proposed for an already marketed drug substance: (1) a new indication; (2) new dosage form; (3) new dosing regimen; or (4) new route of administration. For any of these situations, it is necessary first to establish that the drug and its indication(s) may provide a "meaningful therapeutic benefit" or there may be "substantial use" in the pediatric population. *Meaningful therapeutic benefit* is defined as either (1) a significant improvement in the treatment, diagnosis, or prevention of a disease, compared to marketed products adequately labeled for that use in the relevant pediatric population, or (2) the drug is in a class of drugs or for an indication for which there is a need for additional therapeutic options. If the drug product already has or is expected to have "substantial use," meaning use in more than 50,000 patients for the labeled indication, then pediatric studies are required. In compelling circumstances, the FDA may require the sponsor of an already marketed drug product to conduct pediatric studies under the Pediatric Rule, even if they are not proposing a new development program. Those circumstances are (1) there is substantial use of the drug product in the pediatric population for the labeled indications, or the drug product represents a meaningful therapeutic benefit over existing treatments for pediatric patients, and (2) the absence of labeling poses significant risks to pediatric patients.

For drug development programs that trigger the Pediatric Rule, pediatric studies are to be completed at the time the NDA or supplement is submitted, unless the studies are waived or deferred. Reasons the FDA may waive the requirement for studies include (1) it is judged that a "meaningful health benefit" would not result from the studies and a case cannot be made for "substantial use"; (2) the sponsor is able to show that studies are either impossible or impractical; (3) the drug product may be anticipated to be unsafe or ineffective in pediatrics; or (4) reasonable efforts to develop a formulation for the pediatric population of interest (if one is needed) have failed. The FDA may defer the submission of studies until after approval of the application. Reasons for deferral of pediatric studies include (1) approval of the new drug product is ready for adult use before the required pediatric studies can be completed, or (2) it is judged that additional safety (including marketing experience) or efficacy information is needed in adults before it would be appropriate to study children. It was not expected that the need for pediatric information would delay approval of drugs appropriately studied in adults.

Goal of All Food and Drug Administration Pediatric Initiatives: Improved Pediatric Labeling

It is important to understand that the goal of all of these pediatric initiatives is to improve labeling with regard to pediatric use of drugs, including, as appropriate, negative information if the result of the pediatric development program. At the present time, labeling of psychotropic drugs has very little information pertinent to the safe and effective use of these products in pediatric patients. The following summarizes current labeling pertinent to indicated uses for psychiatric disorders in pediatric patients:

• There are several drugs, including methylphenidate, amphetamines, and pemoline, approved for the treatment of ADHD, a disorder considered to be primarily pediatric.
• Clomipramine, fluvoxamine, and sertraline labeling all describe positive results of trials of these drugs in pediatric patients with OCD, in effect, granting an indication for these drugs in pediatric OCD.
• The Pediatric Use section of lithium labeling indicates that safety and effectiveness in patients with mania below the age of 12 years have not been established, thereby implying that data are available down to age 12 years.
• Two drugs approved for the treatment of Tourette's disorder have labeling language pertinent to pediatric use. Pimozide labeling indicates that patients with Tourette's disorder down to age 8 years have been studied, although, it also suggests that data for patients under age 12 years are very limited. Haloperidol labeling simply indicates that this drug is indicated for children with Tourette's disorder, without any further specification of age.
• Imipramine is approved for enuresis.
• Doxepin is approved for "psychoneurosis" with labeling suggesting that safety and effectiveness in patients below the age of 12 years have not been established, thereby implying that data are available down to age 12 years.
• Trifluoperazine is approved for "psychotic children," aged 6 to 12.
• Finally, both chlorpromazine and haloperidol are approved for "(1) the treatment of severe behavioral problems in children (1 to 12 years of age) marked by combativeness and/or explosive hyperexcitable behavior (out of proportion to immediate provocations), and (2) in the short-term treatment of hyperactive children who show excessive motor activity with accompanying conduct disorders consisting of some or all of the following symptoms: impulsivity, difficulty sustaining attention, aggressivity, mood lability and poor frustration tolerance."

The use of psychotropic drugs in pediatric patients, however, is far more widespread than is supported by current labeling, and there is clearly a need for better data to guide clinicians in the pharmacological treatment of pediatric patients with psychiatric disorders. Given the regulatory tools now available to the FDA to promote research in pediatric psychopharmacology, it is important to identify those psychiatric indications in the pediatric population that would benefit from study, so that the FDA can encourage and/or require studies in these areas. To fully implement these initiatives, it is critical to develop diagnostic criteria where these do not yet exist. In considering new claims, whether for a specific disease or syndrome or a nonspecific sign or symptom, it is important to understand that similar standards are applied by the FDA in evaluating the proposed claim. Although it would be at least theoretically possible for a sponsor to define an entity not yet well accepted and then study it, in most cases the proposed clinical entity that is the focus of the new claim needs to be already accepted in the relevant clinical or academic community. The newly proposed clinical entity also needs to be operationally definable, and it needs to identify a reasonably homogeneous patient group. The latter two criteria are important to ensure the validity of the clinical trials supporting the claim and to make it possible to inform clinicians in labeling about the use of the proposed treatment. In addition to diagnostic criteria, it will be important to improve assessment methods, and to develop optimal study designs for these programs.

IMPACT OF RECENT FOOD AND DRUG ADMINISTRATION INITIATIVES IN PEDIATRIC PSYCHOPHARMACOLOGY

Written Requests under the Food and Drug Administration Modernization Act

A *written request* is a formal communication from the FDA to the sponsor of a drug product that specifies in detail what pediatric trials are needed for a particular pediatric indication(s) to gain additional exclusivity under the FDAMA. As of March, 2002, the FDA has issued 10 written requests for psychotropic drug products, all focused on one or more of the following five indications: major depressive disorder (MDD), OCD, generalized anxiety disorder (GAD), schizophrenia, and bipolar disorder. Except for one written request that was focused on a need for additional pharmacokinetic and longer-term safety data, these requests have required (*1*) one or more efficacy trials, (*2*) pharmacokinetic data, and (*3*) both short- and longer-term safety data.

Major depressive disorder

Current regulations [21 CFR 201.57(f)(9)(iv)] indicate that a new claim in a pediatric population could be established by extrapolating the efficacy results of adequate and well-controlled studies in adults for the same entity, if it can be established that the disease is the same entity in adults and children and would be expected to respond similarly to the drug. If that conclusion cannot be reached, a single controlled trial might be sufficient to support efficacy in the new population (see Guidance for Industry-Providing Clinical Evidence of Effectiveness for Human Drug and Biological Products, at www.fda.gov/cder/guidance/index. htm). This approach also requires some reason to believe that the course of the disease and the effects of drug treatment are reasonably similar in adult and pediatric populations so that data from the adult efficacy studies appear pertinent to pediatric patients with MDD. Unfortunately, there is reason to question the continuity between adult and pediatric depression and this concern about the extrapolability of adult depression data is more than theoretical. While there are now two published positive reports of selective serotonin reuptake inhibitor (SSRI) treatment of child and adolescent depression with fluoxetine (Emslie et al., 1997) and paroxetine (Keller et al., 2001), there is a preponderance of negative studies of older antidepressants in pediatric patients. It is true that all of the negative studies utilized tricyclic antidepressants, and that, in addition, there were other other possible explanations for the negative outcomes, e.g., sample size, entry criteria, and outcome measures. Nevertheless, these negative trials lead to a substantial concern about the ability to extrapolate positive antidepressant findings from adult to pediatric patients. Consequently, a pediatric depression claim for any antidepressant already approved in adult depression should be supported by two independent, adequate, and well-controlled clinical trials in pediatric depression. The relevant pediatric age groups for study of MDD are children (ages 7 through 11 years) and adolescents (ages 12 through 17 years).

The trials needed have been similar to those in adults: randomized; double-blind; parallel group; placebo-controlled, and 6–8 weeks in duration. The FDA has recommended that at least one of the two studies be a fixed dose–response study, and that randomization should either be stratified by age groups studied, or that some other means is used to ensure adequate representation of both age groups.

Obsessive compulsive disorder

For OCD, a sufficiently strong case has been made for the continuity between adult and pediatric OCD to permit a pediatric claim for a drug already approved in adults to be supported by a single independent, adequate, and well-controlled clinical trial in pediatric OCD. The relevant pediatric age groups for study of OCD are children (ages 7 through 11 years) and adolescents (ages 12 through 17 years).

Generalized anxiety disorder

Except for a recent study suggesting the effectiveness of fluvoxamine in pediatric patients with GAD and/or the commonly comorbid disorders, social phobia or separation anxiety disorder (Research Unit on Pediatric Psychopharmacology (RUPP) Anxiety Study Group, 2001), there have been only rare attempts to systematically study drug treatments in pediatric anxiety disorders. While GAD is defined in the same way for adult and pediatric patients, there are no systematic data upon which to make a judgement about extrapolation of results in adult studies to pediatric patients, and it is not clear that the condition really is the same entity in children. Consequently, a pediatric GAD claim for any anxiolytic already approved in adult GAD should be supported by two independent, adequate, and well-controlled clinical trials in pediatric GAD. The relevant pediatric age groups for study of GAD are children (ages 6 through 11 years) and adolescents (ages 12 through 17 years).

Results of programs initiated on the basis of written requests

As of the date of this chapter (circa March, 2002), labeling changes regarding pediatric use have resulted from only two programs—the study of buspirone in pediatric GAD and a pharmacokinetic study of fluvoxamine in pediatric OCD (fluvoxamine already had a controlled clinical trial in pediatric patients). Two placebo-controlled trials with buspirone in pediatric GAD did not reveal a treatment effect, and this negative outcome is reflected in Buspar labeling. A pharmacokinetic study of fluvoxamine dosed at 100 mg bid in pediatric patients with OCD showed two- to threefold higher steady-state plasma fluvoxamine levels in children (ages 8 through 11 years) compared to adolescents. Female children had significantly higher exposures than male children. On the basis of these findings, Luvox labeling was modified to suggest that (1) a therapeutic effect may be achieved with lower doses in female than in male children, and (2) the dose may need to be increased to the adult maximum of 300 mg/day in adolescents to achieve a therapeutic effect.

Requests Initiated under Pediatric Rule

The 1998 Pediatric Rule gives the FDA authority under certain circumstances to require pharmaceutical sponsors who are developing new adult claims for drugs to conduct studies in pediatric patients having the same disorder.

• In four instances, the agency has invoked this rule at the time of approval of supplements for new indications for psychotropic drugs already approved for other psychiatric indications. It was noted in the approval letters for these supplements that, since the drugs in question would likely be used in children and/or adolescents with the newly approved indications, the FDA required the sponsors of these products to conduct studies that would be pertinent to such use in the pediatric population. Since the products were ready for approval in adults, the FDA deferred the required pediatric studies to a future date. Alternatively, sponsors could make an argument for waiver of the requirement. The drug products and indications for which the FDA has required studies under the Pediatric Rule are as follows: paroxetine for social anxiety disorder; sertraline for post-traumatic stress disorder (PTSD); olanzapine for acute mania in bipolar disorder; and fluoxetine in premenstrual dysphoric disorder (PMDD).

• In another instance (insomnia), the agency has chosen not to require pediatric studies, on the advice of the Pediatric Advisory Subcommittee (see transcript of November 16, 1999, meeting of Pediatric Advisory Subcommittee of the Anti-Infective Drug Products Advisory Committee at www.fda.gov/ohrms/dockets/ac/cder99.htm). Prompted by a question from a pharmaceutical sponsor developing a drug as a hypnotic for the treatment of primary insomnia in adults regarding whether or not they might be required to develop their drug for certain sleep disorders in pediatric patients, the FDA brought the issue to the subcommittee meeting. This subcommittee concluded that there was no basis for the FDA to require or encourage the study of typical adult hypnotics for primary insomnia or any other sleep disorders in pediatric patients, and their only recommendation was for further study of certain sleep disorders in the pediatric population. In particular, they recommended that an entity known generally as sleep phase dysregulation in patients either in neonatal or pediatric intensive care units be further defined so that it might be better studied at some future time. The FDA, therefore, did not invoke the Pediatric Rule at the time of approval of the hypnotic NDA in question.

• In one other instance, i.e., Metadate CD (approved April 3, 2001), a new formulation of methylphenidate for ADHD, the Agency has invoked the Pediatric Rule. It was noted in the approval letter for this NDA that the drug in question would likely be used for treating ADHD in children younger than 6 years and the FDA was deferring the requirement to conduct studies that would be pertinent to use in this population. Alternatively, the sponsor could make an argument for waiver of the requirement and submit justification to the Agency.

RENEWED COMMERCIAL INTEREST IN ATTENTION DEFICIT HYPERACTIVITY DISORDER

Attention-deficit hyperactivity disorder is probably the best studied of the psychiatric disorders found in pediatric patients, at least from the standpoint of pharmacological treatment. Methylphenidate, amphetamines, and pemoline have been approved for the treatment of ADHD for many years. For a period of roughly 15 years subsequent to the approval of the last of these drugs (pemoline), there appeared to be virtually no commercial interest in drug development for ADHD. For a number of reasons, attention has been refocused on drug treatments for ADHD, and a substantial number of commercial INDs are currently active in this area. Several programs are for formulations intended for once-a-day dosing with methylphenidate that either provide a zero-order input or attempt to mimic the bimodal input pattern of typical dosing with immediate-release methylphenidate. One of these programs has resulted in the approval of Concerta, an osmotically controlled-rate–release formulation of methylphenidate for once-a-day dosing, and another program has resulted in the approval of Metadate CD, another formulation of methylphenidate for once-a-day dosing. Other programs are exploring enantiomers of already approved products for ADHD, drugs currently approved for indications other than ADHD, and some entirely new compounds.

This renewed interest in ADHD has been a stimulus for the FDA to rethink its policies regarding what is needed in a development program for a product for

ADHD. As for other psychiatric indications, the expectation would be for placebo-controlled trials. In support of a controlled-release formulation, or an active enantiomer, of an already approved drug, one adequate and well-controlled efficacy trial would suffice. For a new chemical entity, or one not previously approved for ADHD, two adequate and well-controlled efficacy trials would be needed. The usual design for these trials would be a randomized, double-blind, parallel-group study of 2–4 weeks duration with a primary outcome focusing on the defining symptoms of the disease. Laboratory classroom studies are often useful in dose finding and establishing pharmacokinetic–pharmacodynamic relationships. At a minimum, the trials would need to include school-age children, i.e., of ages 6–12 years; ideally, however, they would also include adolescents, and even adults, with ADHD. This disorder is increasingly recognized in preschool children, and a study in this younger population would ordinarily be expected in phase 4. While not needed at this time for approval, longer-term efficacy data should be obtained, since ADHD is a chronic disorder and most patients with this disorder need ongoing treatment. A randomized withdrawal study in responders would establish long-term efficacy and avoid prolonged maintenance on a placebo. Both short-and long-term safety data would be needed, including assessments of growth and development. It is also necessary that any programs for ADHD include the results from juvenile animal studies.

CURRENT REGULATORY CHALLENGES IN PEDIATRIC PSYCHOPHARMACOLOGY

Extending Other Adult Development Programs into Pediatric Populations

At a September 11, 2000, meeting of the FDA's Pediatric Advisory Subcommittee (see transcript of September 11, 2000, meeting of Pediatric Advisory Subcommittee of the Anti-Infective Drug Products Advisory Committee at www.fda.gov/ohrms/dockets/ac/cder00.htm), a question was raised regarding what other adult psychiatric indications might benefit from pediatric studies, i.e., in addition to those already the subject of written requests (MDD, OCD, GAD) or of requirements under the 1998 Pediatric Rule (PTSD, social anxiety disorder, mania, PMDD). The only two disorders for which there was reasonable consensus were schizophrenia and panic disorder. In both cases, the subcommittee recommended that these disorders be studied in adolescence, but not at younger ages. The subcommittee was generally supportive of the age cut-offs the FDA had already proposed for the indications that have been the subject of written requests or requirements for studies under the 1998 Pediatric Rule.

Conduct Disorder

Conduct disorder is of particular interest to the FDA since several pharmaceutical sponsors of antipsychotic drug products have expressed interest in gaining claims for their products for this indication. Conduct disorder is also perhaps the most widely used psychiatric diagnosis in children and adolescents, accounting for 30% to 50% of referrals in some clinics (Kazdin, 1985), and there is reason to believe that the atypical antipsychotics are already fairly widely used for the treatment of conduct disorder. A concern of the FDA and others regarding this diagnosis is the nature of the diagnostic criteria. While it does reside in the *Diagnostic and Statistical Manual of Mental Disorders, 4th ed.* (DSM-IV; American Psychiatric Association, 1994) along with other recognized diagnostic entities—e.g., MDD, schizophrenia, panic disorder, etc.—it is unique in that it consists of a listing of behaviors that either violate the rights of others or in some other way violate societal norms. Thus, it is a disorder that is defined by the distress and dysfunction it causes to others, rather than to the individual with the diagnosis. Indeed, aggression directed against others is a key theme in the defining characteristics of this entity. Obviously, the condition can have adverse consequences for the affected individual as well.

There was some discussion of conduct disorder at the September 11, 2000, meeting of the FDA's Pediatric Advisory Subcommittee, but no agreement regarding whether the FDA should encourage and/or require studies of this entity. One point that was made focused on the nature of the aggression that may be seen in patients diagnosed with conduct disorder. In particular, it was suggested that very different forms of aggression may be seen, in some cases unplanned rage, and in others very well–planned acts of aggression, e.g., stealing a car. The message was that there is considerable heterogeneity in the population labeled with this disorder, making it difficult to characterize the population. As noted above, the fact that others may suffer, perhaps even more than those labeled with this diagnosis, makes it difficult to think of it as a disease entity in the usual sense. Nevertheless, conduct disorder is likely to be the topic of continued discussion as a possible new claim for atypical antipsychotics and perhaps other psychotropics.

Psychopharmacology in Preschool Populations

While psychotropic drugs are being utilized fairly widely in the school-age pediatric population, there is increasing evidence that they are also being prescribed for the preschool population. A recent study (Zito et al., 2000) brought attention to both the absolute extent of prescribing and to the trend for increasing use in this younger age group.

Despite these data showing surprisingly extensive use of psychotropic medications, there are no adequate studies of either the efficacy or safety of these medications in the preschool population. Two important questions raised by Zito et al., were (*1*) what clinical entities are being treated with psychotropics in the 2–4-year-old population, and (*2*) is the absolute use and increase in use justified? The publication of this paper in February 2000, raised sufficient concern to provoke the planning and conduct of several meetings focused at least in part on this topic in the fall of 2000.

• One of these was a session of the FDA's Pediatric Advisory Subcommittee on September 11, 2000, that focused on the question of what clinical entities are in fact being treated in this age group (www.fda.gov/ohrms/dockets/ac/cder00.htm).
• The Surgeon General's Conference on Children's Mental Health was held September 18–19, 2000 (see www.surgeongeneral.gov/cmh/default.htm for a report on this meeting). This meeting was focused more broadly on the mental health of children and the delivery of mental health services, but some attention was paid specifically to the preschool population.
• A joint National Institute of Mental Health (NIMH) FDA workshop (October 2–3, 2000) was organized to examine the current state of knowledge regarding psychotropic medications for young children (Vitiello, 2001).
• Finally, at the Annual Meeting of the American Academy of Child and Adolescent Psychiatry, there was a Research Forum on Developing and Implementing Psychopharmacological Studies in Preschool Children, held on October 25, 2000.

Several views emerged from this series of meetings. First, it seemed to be generally acknowledged that psychiatric diagnosis in the preschool population is at a fairly primitive stage, and that few of the major psychiatric disorders recognized in adults and older pediatric patients have relevance in this younger population. Exceptions include the disorders ADHD and oppositional defiant disorder (ODD). In addition, it was agreed that the pervasive developmental disorders, particularly, autism, were well established in this age group and appropriate clinical targets for drug studies. What also emerged was the view that much of the use of psychotropics in preschool patients may be focused on nonspecific symptoms, e.g., agitation and particularly aggression, rather than on specific disease entities.

It may be useful to point out that there are two reasonably distinct types of clinical entities considered appropriate targets for new claims. Specific diseases or syndromes are the usual focus of a drug claim, e.g., congestive heart failure or rheumatoid arthritis. Nonspecific signs or symptoms not unique to a single disease or syndrome, e.g., pain or fever, may also be the focus for a claim. Antipyretics and analgesics are approved for these nonspecific symptoms on the basis of studies involving different models for each such symptom, e.g., headache pain and dental pain as different pain models. The basis for accepting this nonspecific approach to indications is the view that, while the disease states leading to these nonspecific symptoms may differ markedly, the symptoms themselves are (*1*) universally defined, in whatever disease context they occur; (*2*) readily measured, using commonly accepted assessment methods; and (*3*) respond similarly to drug treatment, whatever the diverse disease state that may lead to the nonspecific symptom. Ideally, we would also understand nonspecific symptoms at a pathophysiologic level, since this would help in establishing such a symptom as really independent of the underlying specific disease state in which it happens to occur. Since we do not fully understand any psychiatric illnesses at a pathophysiological level, this would not be a reasonable requirement for a nonspecific psychiatric symptom.

In psychopharmacology, we have generally not considered potentially nonspecific symptoms (e.g., anxiety, depression, psychosis) separately from the defining disease entity. Psychotropics are now approved for specific syndromes rather than nonspecific symptoms. Approvals are granted for major depressive disorder, and not for depressive symptoms occurring in other settings. Similarly, drugs are approved for specific disorders falling under the "anxiety disorders" umbrella, e.g., panic disorder, OCD, PTSD, social anxiety disorder, and GAD, rather than for anxiety as a nonspecific symptom.

If we were to reach agreement that a particular psychiatric symptom might be reasonably considered a legitimate nonspecific symptom, it would be necessary to consider the possibility of the pseudospecificity of claims focused on such a symptom. Since the essence of such a claim is that the symptom is nonspecific, i.e., it is not limited to any one disease, it seems important to examine efficacy in several different disease models.

To attempt to obtain a claim for a nonspecific symptom in a single disease model would, by definition, be pseudospecific, since such a claim would give the impression that the symptom is specific to that disease. For example, if there were agreement that psychomotor agitation could be considered a nonspecific psychiatric symptom, it would be important to study a drug treatment proposed for this symptom in several different disease models, such as schizophrenia, autism, and mental retardation.

Thus, it will be important to reach agreement on whether or not nonspecific psychiatric symptoms might be considered reasonable clinical targets for drug development programs in the preschool population, or in the pediatric population more generally. There was no such agreement at the series of Fall, 2000 meetings, e.g., with regard to the entity aggression, regarding either how to define it or how to think of it in terms of it being either a specific entity or a nonspecific symptom. Some participants considered aggression a symptom distinct to specific illnesses, while others viewed it as an entity that might be consided nonspecific and occurring in a similar form in association with different disease states. In either case, there were widely varying views on how to define the entity. Clearly, this is a topic in need of much additional discussion, especially given the apparent widespread use of psychotropics for this entity.

Although it was generally agreed that ADHD is a valid diagnosis in the preschool population, it was also acknowledged that this diagnosis requires a careful evaluation to distinguish it from developmentally normal children and those whose symptoms are a result of other psychopathology. Special features are being built into the recent NIMH-funded study of methylphenidate in preschoolers with ADHD, i.e., the Preschoolers with ADHD Treatment Study (PATS), to ensure the validity of the diagnosis and the assessment of change.

Assessing Safety of Psychotropics in Children

The safety of psychotropic drugs used in the pediatric population is a particular concern since the brain is undergoing dramatic changes during this time period, especially at the younger end of this age spectrum. While all of the Fall, 2000 pediatric psychopharmacology meetings addressed safety to some extent, a September 25, 2000, workshop on safety monitoring in pediatric psychopharmacology was specifically focused on this topic—in particular, the need for assessing long-term safety. While there was general agreement that controlled clinical trials are the best approach to ob-

taining information on common adverse events, there was also agreement that more work is needed in designing more sensitive assessment instruments, even for common adverse events. It was generally acknowledged that detecting rare, serious adverse events associated with longer-term use is the more difficult problem. Suggested solutions included cohort or case–control studies, registries, or collecting safety data from practice networks; however, the implementation and funding of such efforts were acknowledged to be difficult barriers. Perhaps most important, none of these methods are suitable for discovering long-term effects on intelligence, personality, and other more subtle aspects of human behavior. The only way to assess these areas for modest effects is long-term controlled studies against placebo or alternative non-drug treatment. Comparisons of different drugs might also be useful.

As noted for ADHD, it is necessary to obtain data from juvenile animal studies in development programs for other psychiatric disorders in pediatric patients. These studies should be designed to examine the safety of a new drug in animals of an age range which is analogous to that of the proposed patient population. In addition to the usual toxicological parameters, such a study would presumably evaluate effects on growth and neurological, behavioral, and reproductive development.

More research into the safety of psychotropic drugs in the pediatric population is needed, including methodology, both in clinical settings and in animal models.

Science and Ethics in Pediatric Psychopharmacology: A Regulatory Perspective

While the issue of the ethical conduct of clinical trials in pediatric psychopharmacology is addressed comprehensively elsewhere in this book, it is important to present an FDA perspective on this important matter. It is also important to have the issue of ethics discussed in the context of the scientific needs for trials presented to the FDA in support of new drug applications. These trials must be adequate and well-controlled (U.S. Department of Health and Human Services, 2001). What this requirement essentially means is that, in order to support an efficacy claim, the trials must be interpretable and must be able to document efficacy. For treatments that are intended to improve symptoms, as is almost always the case for psychotropic drugs, placebo-controlled trials are the usual standard. This is especially true when there is a substantial failure rate in placebo-controlled trials for the drugs known to work in a particular therapeutic area, as again is the case for most psychotropic drugs. Where that is true, the usually proposed alternative, i.e., the active control non-inferiority trial, is problematic because it is not possible to be reasonably certain that such a trial will be able to distinguish effective from ineffective drugs (just as many of the past trials could not tell active drug from placebo). In that case, failure to see a difference between any new drug and control is uninformative (Ellenberg and Temple, 2000; Temple and Ellenberg, 2000). In depression, one of the few cases in pediatric psychopharmacology where there is a substantial history of placebo-controlled trials, there is a particular problem, as most of these trials have been unsuccessful. Thus, from a scientific, regulatory standpoint, the expectation would be for placebo-controlled trials in this area. On the ethical side, the FDA subscribes to the standard provided in the recently published International Conference on Harmonization (ICH) E-10 guidance document regarding when a particular trial design is ethical (FDA, 1999). The standard established in this E-10 document is that a placebo-controlled trial is unaccceptable only if there exist standard drugs that are effective in reducing either mortality or irreversible morbidity. Since that is clearly not the case in pediatric psychopharmacology, the FDA views placebo-controlled trials as acceptably safe, and therefore, ethical. It is, however, particularly important to consider "escape" mechanisms, so that patients doing poorly (e.g., worsening) can be removed from the study promptly. In some cases, it may be possible to use a randomized withdrawal study design (Temple, 1994).

Other Electronic Sources of Information on Regulatory Aspects of Pediatric Drug Development

• The FDA has a pediatric page on its website (www.fda.gov/cder/pediatric) that provides a wealth of information about the implementation of the FDAMA 1997 and the 1998 Pediatric Rule.
• In addition, the International Conference on Harmonization has issued a guidance document pertinent to pediatric drug development: E11, Clinical Investigation of Medicinal Products in the Pediatric Population (www.fda.gov/cder/guidance/index.htm).

SUMMARY

More studies are needed to address the insufficient evidence base for drug treatment of psychiatric disorders in pediatric patients. Recent initiatives, in particular the FDAMA 1997 and the 1998 Pediatric Rule, have provided the FDA with tools for stimulating research in this area. As a result of these initiatives, several clinical development programs in pediatric psychopharmacology are underway and hold promise for improved labeling. However, more work is needed to define clinical targets that might be the focus of additional programs. Improved methodology is needed to address the safety of psychotropic drug use in the pediatric population.

ACKNOWLEDGMENTS
Dr. Laughren is with the Food and Drug Administration, Rockville, MD. However, Dr. Laughren's contribution to this chapter was made in his private capacity. No official support or endorsement by the Food and Drug Administration is intended or should be inferred.

REFERENCES

American Psychiatric Association (1994) *Diagnostic and Statistical Manual of Mental Disorders, 4th ed.* Washington, DC: American Psychiatric Press.

Colburn, W.A. (1990) Controversy V: phase I, first time in man. *J Clin Pharmacol* 30:210–222.

Ellenberg, S.S. and Temple, R. (2000) Placebo-controlled trials and active-control trials in the evaluation of new treatments; Part 2: practical issues and specific cases. *Ann Intern Med* 133: 464–470.

Emslie, G.J., Rush, A.J., Weinberg, W.A., Kowatch, R.A., Hughes, C.W., Carmody, T., and Rintelmann, J. (1997) A double-blind, randomized, placebo-controlled trial of fluoxetine in children and adolescents with depression. *Arch Gen Psychiatry* 54:1031–1037.

Food and Drug Administration (1979) Labeling and prescription drug advertising: content and format for labeling for human prescription drugs. *Fed Register* 44:37434–37467.

Food and Drug Administration (1992) Specific requirements on content and format of labeling for human prescription drugs: proposed revision of "pediatric use" subsection in the labeling. *Fed Register* 57:47423–47428.

Food and Drug Administration (1994) Specific requirements on content and format of labeling for human prescription drugs: revision of "Pediatric Use" subsection in the labeling; final rule. *Fed Register,* 59:64240–64250.

Food and Drug Administration (1997) Section 111 of Title I of the Food and Drug Administration Modernization Act of 1997 [section 505A of the Federal Food, Drug, and Cosmetic Act (21U.S.C.355a).

Food and Drug Administration (1998) Regulations requiring manufacturers to assess the safety and effectiveness of new drugs and biological products in pediatric patients; final rule. *Fed Register* 63:66631–66672.

Food and Drug Administration (1999) International Conference on Harmonization: choice of control group in clinical trials. *Fed Register* 64:51767–51780.

Jensen, P.S., Vitiello, B., Leonard, H., and Laughren, T.P. (1994) Design and methodology issues for clinical treatment trials in children and adolescents. *Psychopharmacol Bull* 30:3–8.

Kazdin, A. (1985) *Treatment of Antisocial Behavior in Children and Adolescents.* Homewood, Il: Dorsey Press, 1985.

Keller, M.B., Ryan, N.D., Strober, M., Klein, R.G., Kutcher, S.P., Birmaher, B., Hagino, O.R., Koplewicz, H., Carlson, G.A., Clarke, G.N., Emslie, G.J., Feinberg, D., Geller, B., Kusumakar, V., Papatheodorou, G., Sack, W.H., Sweeney, M., Wagner, K.D., Weller, E.B., Winters, N.C., Oakes, R., and McCafferty, J.P.

(2001) Efficacy of paroxetine in the treatment of adolescent major depression: a randomized, controlled trial. *J Am Acad Child Adolesc Psychiatry* 40:762–772.

Laughren, T.P. (1996) Regulatory issues in pediatric psychopharmacology. *J Am Acad Child Adolesc Psychiatry* 34:1276–1282.

Posvar, E.L., and Sedman, A.J. (1989) New drugs: first time in man. *J Clin Pharmacol* 29:961–966.

Research Unit on Pediatric Psychopharmacology (RUPP) Anxiety Study Group (2001) Fluvoxamine for the treatment of anxiety disorders in children and adolescents. *N Engl J Med* 344:1279–1285.

Sheiner, L.B., and Benet, L.Z. (1985) Premarketing observational studies of population pharmacokinetics of new drugs. *Clin Pharmacol Ther* 38:481–488.

Temple, R.J. (1985) Food and Drug Administration's guidelines for clinical testing of drugs in the elderly. *Drug Inform J* 19:483–486.

Temple, R.J. (1994) Special study designs: early escape, enrichment, studies in nonresponders. *Commun Statist Theory Meth* 23:499–531.

Temple, R., and Ellenberg, S.S. (2000) Placebo-controlled trials and active-control trials in the evaluation of new treatments; Part 1: ethical and scientific issues. *Ann Intern Med* 133: 455–463.

U.S. Department of Health and Human Services (2001) Adequate and well-controlled trials. Code of Federal Regulations (Revised as of April 1, 2001), Title 21, Part 314.126. Washington, DC: U.S. Government Printing Office.

Vitiello, B., (2001) Psychopharmacology for young children: clinical needs and research opportunities. *Pediatirics* 108:983–989.

Williams, P.D. (1990) The role of pharmacological profiling in safety assessment. *Regul Toxicol Pharmacol* 12:238–252.

Zito, J.M., Safer, D.J., dosReis, S., Gardner, J.F., Boles, M., and Lynch, F. (2000) Trends in the prescribing of psychotropic medications in preschoolers. *JAMA* 283:1025–1030.

55 | Ethical issues in research

KIMBERLY HOAGWOOD

A climate of ambiguity currently surrounds research in pediatric psychopharmacology. This climate has been created by the convergence of disparate beliefs, misunderstandings, and social pressures. This situation creates unique ethical challenges for those embarking on studies of pediatric psychopharmacology. Popular misunderstandings about pediatric mental illnesses abound, including the belief that it does not exist, that it will heal on its own, that it is the mere product of bad parenting. Attitudes about the acceptability or unacceptability of psychotropic medications to treat mental illnesses also are widespread and in some cases deeply held. At the same time, one of the fastest-growing sectors in corporate America is the pharmaceutical industry, and its pediatric arm has experienced especially rapid growth since the advent of federal legislation providing fiscal incentives for pediatric medication development.

Research on detection of child and adolescent mental disorders demonstrates that the problems of under-recognition are pervasive. Since the mid-1980s there have been a series of federal reports indicating that child and adolescent mental health problems are going undetected (U.S. Congress, Office of Technology Assessment, 1991; U.S. Public Health Service, 2000). In recent years, studies have documented that prevalence estimates of mental illnesses, which range from 10% to 20% of all children (Roberts, et al., 1998), are in vast contrast to rates of identification within specific systems. In one of the few studies to carefully assess identification of mental health problems by primary care providers, less than 50% of children with documentable mental illnesses were accurately identified (Horwitz et al, 1992). In analyses of U.S. Department of Education statistics (1998), less than 1% of children are identified as having serious emotional disturbances.

Unfortunately, while these disorders can have a pernicious course (Jensen, 1998), the lack of early recognition, traced in part to poor training of front-line providers and to lack of reimbursement for comprehensive assessments (U.S. Public Health Service, 2000), has cre-

ated a situation in which children's mental health needs often go undetected for years (Duncan et al., 1995).

Several studies on the use of psychotropic medications in children have demonstrated that such use is increasing for children and adolescents, as well as for preschoolers (Jensen et al., 1999b; Zito et al., 2000). Zito and colleagues (2000), for example, found the prevalence of psychotropic medication use in preschool-aged youths to have increased two- to three fold between 1991 and 1995, especially in the use of clonidine, stimulants, antidepressants, and medications with unlabeled indications. Among preschoolers, only one antipsychotic agent (haloperidol) has been labeled by the Federal Drug Administration (FDA) for treatment of mental disorders; methylphenidate has been approved only for children of age 6 years and over. In fact, 80% of all medications, including antibiotics and anesthetics currently available in the U.S. formulary, have not been tested for their safety or efficacy with children (Jensen et al., 1999b), and none of the most common psychotropic medications (methylphenidate, selective serotonin reuptake inhibitors [SSRIs], or clonidine) have been adequately studied in preschool age children. The discrepancy between usage and lack of research support is of concern with regard to all psychotropic medications, as their impact on the developing brain is unknown, and possible long-term effects of exposure to them have not been adequately studied (Cicchetti, 1998; Vitello, 1998).

Research in pediatric psychopharmacology has been justified on the grounds that there is a clear public health need to determine the safety and efficacy of psychotropic medications that may mitigate symptoms of child and adolescent mental illness. Because the impact of these medications cannot be unquestionably inferred from studies of adults (Vitiello and Jensen, 1997), and because of the large number of gaps in knowledge about their safety and efficacy, there has been an increase in the number of pediatric clinical trials targeting basic questions of etiology, course, persistence, and treatment adequacy.

However, the upward trend in the use of psychotropics, combined with lack of an adequate knowledge base on safety and efficacy, and the underrecognition of pediatric mental illnesses, give rise to a range of ethical issues for investigators studying pediatric psychopharmacology. These issues include the complexities of weighing risks and benefits; deciding upon appropriate designs, including discontinuation and placebo-controlled trials; recruiting and retaining appropriate samples; obtaining truly informed consent; ensuring confidentiality; and creating community partnerships. After a brief discussion of the regulations governing the ethical conduct of pediatric investigations, this chapter will discuss each of these ethical issues in turn.

REPORTS, GUIDELINES AND FEDERAL REGULATIONS

While the foundational principles underpinning protection of human subjects in research has remained unchanged since the 1970s, the application of these principles to subpopulations and their interpretation is dynamic and changeable (Hoagwood et al., 1996). Research ethics involving children and adolescents with mental health needs has been the subject of recent federal attention (Arnold et al., 1995; Shore and Hyman, 1999; Charney, 2000). In 1998 the National Bioethics Advisory Commission issued its report, Research Involving Persons with Mental Disorders that May Affect Decision-making Capacity (National Biothics Advisory Commission, 1998). In 1999 the National Institute of Mental Health (NIMH) created a workgroup, the National Advisory Mental Health Council, to provide additional safeguards for and reviews of use of human subjects, in grant applications involving challenging designs, methods, or techniques. In 2000 the National Human Research Protections Advisory Committee (NHRPAC) met to review ethical issues inherent in research involving children, and formed a workgroup to examine the adequacy of the existing regulations in Subpart D (described below). In 2000 the National Institutes of Health (NIH) issued new requirements governing the education of clinical investigators in the protection of research subjects (National Institutes of Health, 2000). The NIMH has also issued program announcements specifically targeting studies of research ethics (National Institutes of Mental Health, 2001). All of these activities reflect the heightened awareness at the federal level of the need to attend carefully to issues of human subjects' protection while ensuring the growth and solidity of the scientific foundation on issues of public health significance.

In addition, a number of professional associations have developed special guidelines governing ethical conduct of research. For example, the American College of Neuropsychopharmacology (ACNP) has established a statement of principles for ethical conduct in neuropsychopharmacologic research involving human beings (American College of Neuropsychopharmacology, 2000). These principles include the expectation that, before conducting such studies, a scientific investigator shall have had adequate training, and shall take all reasonable precautions to preserve the autonomy, rights, and safety of all subjects. The degree of precaution must correspond to the degree of risk expected.

The Belmont Report

The Belmont Report (OPRR, 1979) is generally considered to be one of the critical cornerstones on issues involving ethical principles for studies of human beings. Written in 1979, it identified three ethical principles undergirding human subjects' research: respect for persons, to promote autonomy of research participants; beneficence, to maximize good and minimize harm to individuals or to society; and justice, to ensure that no particular population is bearing the burden for research and that no groups are specifically exploited. All biomedical research must be guided by these three principles.

From a public health scientific standpoint, in addition to these principles, there are several fundamental requirements without which the ethical grounding of a scientific study can be questioned. The first is that the potential yield of the study must be significant in its promise of improving public health. Investigators have been cautioned to focus on scientific issues of genuine significance, rather than questions that may be interesting but trivial or unrelated to general societal benefit (Hyman, 1999). Second, the experimental design must be sound and alternative designs should be considered carefully with respect to both ethical and practical concerns (Vitiello et al., 1999). In addition, the balance between risk and potential benefit should be weighed favorably toward the study participants. Finally, research participants must be fully informed of the risks, benefits, implications, and alternatives to participation.

Federal Regulations

The specific policy that sets the standards for federally funded research was revised in 1991 and includes specific policies for research in children (U.S. Department of Health and Human Services [DHHS], 1991a; b). The main requirements of the policy include the necessity of having research protocols and consent forms approved by Institutional Review Boards (IRBs); of obtaining permission or consent that is fully informed by the parent or other legal guardian for a child's participation in research, and obtaining assent, when possible, from the child; and of ensuring that the risk/benefit ratio is favorable to the child.

In evaluating the concept of risk, several variants are described in the federal code. *Minimal risk* is defined as risk that is not greater than that ordinarily encountered in daily life, or during routine physical or psychological assessments [section 46:102(i) in U.S. Department of Health and Human Services, 1991a]. Minimal risk is not equivalent to no risk and the ways in which it is calibrated and defined differ considerably from one investigation to another and from one IRB to another. Research that involves greater than minimal risk but also includes the prospect of direct benefit is justified if the potential benefit outweighs the potential harm [section 46.405 in U.S. Department of Health and Human Services, 1991b]. According to section 45CFR46, a benefit must be reasonably expected if a study is to be considered to have the prospect of direct benefit. Risks must be presented, however, if they are foreseeable. This definition is much broader and could include possible but unlikely problems. Treatment studies tend to fall into this category. Deliberation of the risks and benefits involves careful consideration of the severity of the child's illness, the availability of alternative treatments, and estimates of the safety and efficacy of the experimental treatment that the child may receive if enrolled in the study. Table 55.1 lists the kinds of research by level of risk and the decisional elements to weigh when considering involvement of children. Consideration of placebo arms within a clinical trial may be weighed against the availability of alternatives to placebo (further discussion of placebo conditions is provided in use of Placebos, below).

Research that does not contain direct benefit to the participant is among the most controversial. Examples of these kinds of studies include invasive medical procedures, exposure to situations that may provoke anxious or upsetting responses, or administration of agents that are potentially toxic. Federal regulations stipulate that this kind of research may be conducted only if, in addition to the other requirements, the following conditions are also met:

1. The study involves only a minor increase over minimal risk.
2. The procedure involves "experiences to the subjects that are commensurate with those inherent in their actual or expected medical, dental, psychological, social or educational situations."

TABLE 55.1 *Elements to Consider in Evaluating the Ethics of Research in Children*

Type of Research	Critical Elements
Research has potential benefit to research subject	Risk/benefit ratio must be favorable to the research subject
Research has no potential benefit to the research subject	No greater than minimal risk is allowed
Research has no potential benefit but relevant knowledge can be gained	No more than a minor increase over minimal risk is allowed Subjects are exposed to experiences reasonably commensurate with those inherent in their lives Research is likely to yield knowledge of vital importance for amelioration of the condition
Research is not otherwise approvable under the above criteria	The Secretary of the Department of Health and Human Services can determine that the proposed research presents a reasonable opportunity to further understanding, prevention, or alleviation of a serious problem affecting health and/or welfare of children

3. The study has the potential to provide knowledge that is of "vital importance" to understanding or treating the pediatric illness.
4. Parental permission and child assent are obtained (section 46.406 in U.S. Department of Health and Human Services, 1991b

The final category of risk involves projects that present greater than a minor increase over minimal risk. These studies are rarely proposed and are considered only if they have the potential to increase scientific knowledge about a serious public health problem affecting children. They require special review and approval by the DHHS.

WEIGHING RISKS AND BENEFITS

The weighing of risks and benefits in research on pediatric psychopharmacology can be among the most complex to address. The primary premise is that risks and benefits should be viewed from the standpoint of the research participant, not that of the investigator or institution. No risk is considered acceptable if the research does not have the potential to benefit the participant or if it will not strengthen knowledge about the condition or treatment for that condition. The scientific validity of the design is one factor that is important for evaluating the potential benefit of a study. The design should reduce risks to the maximum extent possible while preserving the scientific integrity of the design. The design should also maximize benefits to increase the likelihood of benefits for individual participants and for other populations. In addition to design considerations, the potential outcomes need to include both direct and indirect benefits (Fisher, et al. 1996).

Just as there are direct and indirect benefits that must be considered, there are also both direct and indirect risks. The notion of what constitutes a risk needs to be assessed broadly to encompass physical risks, psychological risks, and the social dimensions of risk (Levine, 1981; Roberts, 1998). Risks from medication trials might include dizziness, dry mouth, sleeplessness, or transient discomforts. But in addition to these physiological risks, one should consider the potential risks associated with the withholding of treatment or the dissemination of inaccurate information that may have negative personal consequence.

Because the issues surrounding the weighing of relative risks and benefits vis-a-vis diverse community participation are complex, there are now a growing number of studies establishing formal means of incorporating community perspectives into the research protocol. This can be accomplished by the establishment of advisory boards or the enlistment of special consultants, whose role would be to provide consultation about designs, measures, or involvement of vulnerable populations. High-risk protocols may require special preparation to incorporate into consent forms or other research materials the perspectives of families or other stakeholders. Further discussion of the advantages of establishing formal means of enlisting community stakeholder perspectives is provided in Incentives versus Coercion, below.

Discontinuation Studies

Discontinuation trials, either controlled or open, usually are not likely to have any direct benefit and may well have real risks, such as relapse, suicide, and loss of employment. Such studies need additional scrutiny and safeguards to minimize risk and to strengthen consent procedures. There are some situations in which a discontinuation study may be considered. For example, to determine whether long-term treatment is needed, a study design might randomly assign patients who have responded successfully to a particular treatment to either a continuation or discontinuation of that treatment. Relapse rates across these two conditions could

answer the question as to whether long-term treatment was justified. Discontinuation studies have been conducted for adults with depression and obsessive-compulsive disorders, among other conditions, and they have provided important knowledge about the need for long-term treatment to reduce the risk of relapse (Pato et al., 1988; Kupfer et al., 1992). Such studies in children are only now being undertaken, and most research on the efficacy of psychopharmacology for children involves short-term studies (Vitiello, et al., 1999). Consequently, more research is needed on the effects of long-term exposure to psychopharmacologic treatments.

Justification for discontinuation studies might also include the lack of knowledge about a particular diagnosis or optimal treatments for a particular group of patients; the need to clarify diagnosis; and the need to ascertain whether continuation of medication after a first clinical episode is needed for persons with a certain diagnosis, especially when long-term effects of medication may be of concern. Further reversal of polypharmacy by selective discontinuation of one or more agents may be justification for such a design, with the goal being to simplify the therapeutic regimen

Use of Placebos

The use of placebos in psychopharmacology trials is a controversial issue and one that has been met with considerable confusion, not to say consternation, in the field. The arguments in favor of the use of placebos in clinical trials include the possibility of obtaining clear answers to questions about the relative efficacy of an experimental therapeutic and its side effects, as well as information about whether an established therapeutic is having its intended effects (Roberts et al., 2001). Because placebo response can be high for some mental illnesses in pediatric populations (Emslie et al., 1998), the argument can be made that its use is important for sorting out relative efficacy of therapeutics against belief systems. An additional argument supporting the inclusion of placebo arms in pediatric clinical trials is that these trials can be mounted with relatively small numbers of participants and that the risks are thus mitigated (Roberts et al., 2001). However, strong concerns about the use of placebos have been articulated. Foremost among these is the argument that the ethical duty of clinical investigators is to avoid harm and that placebo arms by definition promote risk by providing no treatment at all for a period of time. This argument is at the core of the World Medical Association's (1997) revision of the Declaration of Helsinki, which argues that clinical research involves an ethical obligation of the investigator to conduct research based upon the therapeutic value for the participant. The revised document states that the risks, benefits, and burdens of a new experimental therapeutic should be tested against those of the currently defined best method and that placebos could be used, but only where no proven prophylactic therapeutic alternative exists (World Medical Association, 1997).

For persons whose symptoms are well managed by current treatments (e.g., children with certain forms of cancer, or children on antirejection medications pursuant to transplants), entry into a placebo design may well be harmful, as it will involve a period of time without medication. The field of pediatric psychopharmacology for children with severe mental illnesses is however, still in its infancy and, unfortunately, with the exception of stimulants for management of ADHD symptoms (MTA Cooperative Group, 1999), the safety and efficacy of most psychotropic agents for pediatric mental illnesses are far from understood. Consequently, arguments can be made that the use of placebos is a necessary first step in establishing baseline data on the efficacy of these agents. Furthermore, for persons identified early in psychiatric illness, including children, entry into a placebo trial may be less risky than the most common alternative, which is, unfortunately, no treatment at all (Charney et al., 2000). Treatment and services for children and adolescents with documented mental health symptoms are currently reaching only one-quarter of these youth, and levels of unmet need are highest among minority populations of children (NIMH Advisory Council, 2001).

Design alternatives have been used to limit the exposure of participants with mental illness to the risks of placebo conditions; these include crossover studies, in which participants receive at different times in the protocol the experimental therapeutic and the placebo. These kinds of designs can enable each participant to receive the experimental agent or compound while also providing a scientifically rigorous approach to the question of interest (Roberts et al., 1998).

In general, the use of placebos in psychopharmacology trials requires additional justification, particularly with very disturbed children. The public health responsibility of publicly funded scientific studies is paramount, and this responsibility implies that only issues of genuine importance be targeted for such studies (Hyman, 1999). There may be times, however, when, for scientific reasons, the use of placebo arms may be ethically justified (Roberts et al., 2001), in part because there are so few psychopharmacology treatments that have been tested to determine their safety or efficacy. Their use should only be pursued after alternative designs or strategies have been considered.

PARTICIPANT RECRUITMENT AND USE OF INCENTIVES

Recruitment for participation involves consideration of several questions in advance. How significant are the study's aims? Why are particular populations, especially if they are vulnerable populations, needed for answering the questions of interest? Can the study be conducted on less vulnerable populations first?

Because children's legal status is limited and because they cannot legally consent to research participation, children are often considered to be a vulnerable population. In addition, children with psychiatric disorders may have (but do not necessarily have) limitations with respect to understanding the conditions under which their participation is being solicited. Therefore, special efforts must be made to ensure that children's assent to participate is voluntary and that they understand fully the risks and benefits of participation. It is often prudent to ask whether a particular study's aims could be directed toward a less vulnerable population first. A clear rationale should be provided for targeting children with psychiatric disorders, as opposed to children or adolescents without these conditions, as the population of interest for a particular study.

Incentives versus Coercion

Incentives offered for research participation need to be considered with respect to two issues: respect for participant's time and compensation for such; and lack of coercion (Macklin, 1986; Roberts, 1998b).

Investigators working with socioeconomically disadvantaged populations have special responsibilities to ensure that access to both research benefits and risks are not unfairly distributed. Once again, the establishment of community advisory boards can be helpful in ascertaining the community's perceptions of risks associated with recruitment and with community perspectives on when recruitment strategies may be viewed as coercive. For example, monetary inducements can be seen as a fair method for compensating research participants for their time. Such compensation can also be viewed as coercive in some communities, as it may be seen as offering inducements that are outside the bounds of convention. These are issues that need to be considered by investigators when developing recruitment procedures that reflect community values, expectations, and beliefs.

In studies involving persons with mental illnesses that may impair their judgment, an investigator should strongly consider using an independent qualified professional to assess the potential participants' capacity to provide informed consent.

A final issue is that ease of access to populations is not considered an acceptable reason for inclusion and can be considered coercive, especially if the population is vulnerable (i.e., foster children). Institutional review boards and review groups are increasingly concerned about the problems of convenience samples and are requiring full explanation of the appropriateness of certain populations for the study in question.

INFORMED CONSENT

Informed consent is in some sense the ethical cornerstone on which human subjects' protection rests. It requires that individuals understand their part in a study and the potential consequences, and are free to choose to participate. As Levine has argued, the consent process should include specific elements: an invitation to participate; a statement of the purpose of the study; the basis of participant selection; and explanation of procedures, risks, and discomforts; how untoward consequences will be handled; the benefits of participation; alternatives to participation; financial consideration; confidentiality; opportunities for continuing disclosure; and measures for ensuring that a person's decision to participate is voluntary (Levine, 1981).

Applebaum and Grisso (1995) identified four central criteria to consider when assessing the adequacy of informed consent procedures:

1. *Capacity.* This involves the ability of the individual to provide consent. Although it is not the same as competence, which is a legal term, it refers to a basic capacity for deciphering linguistic terms and their meanings.

2. *Understanding.* This refers to the ability of the individual to comprehend the terms of the agreement involved in consent. Understanding is sometimes believed to have occurred if the individual can repeat back what has been heard.

3. *Reasoning.* This is the ability of the individual to balance risks and benefits and to foresee risks and anticipated benefits.

4. *Ability to express a choice.* This entails the ability to understand choices and to make decisional preferences.

A variety of features may be included in protocols to improve the process of obtaining informed consent. These include repeated exposure to the information in the protocol; multiple avenues of communication (verbal, written, etc.); language use that is simple, in small units, and comprehensible; use of "patient educators" who can review relevant information with the potential subject, explain the study's purpose and process, and answer any questions; and attention to personal aspects of consent, including motivation, cultural and developmental issues, expectations, and investigator–participant relationship issues (Applebaum and Grisso, 1988; 1995; Sutherland, et al. 1994; Bonnie, 1997; Roberts, 1998a,b).

Impairments in decisional capacity, as can occur with children during development or among psychiatrically impaired individuals, have implications for informed consent procedures. These impairments may be transient, intermittent, or permanent (Roberts, 1998). Clinical syndromes may create distortions of thought, impaired attention or memory, ambivalence, emotional lability, lack of motivation, distractibility, or impulsivity (Dresser, 1996; Bonnie, 1997; Elliott, 1997; Expert Panel Report to the NIH, 1998; Roberts, 1998). Children, by virtue of being children, do not possess full decisional capacity and thus are dependent upon others for providing this. (Munir and Earls, 1992). Another factor that may compromise the ability of individuals to engage in full decisional activities is the nature of the patient–physician relationship. For example, a long-term relationship with a personal physician who then requests that a patient enroll in a protocol may influence the neutrality with which a patient would weigh the advantages and disadvantages of such enrollment (Roberts, 1998b).

CONFIDENTIALITY

Research on pediatric psychopharmacology may involve the divulgence of sensitive information about a child or family that may not have been previously revealed to others or that could produce harm if discovered. Ethical considerations about recruitment and consent can provide important safeguards against the revelation of confidential information, but additional protections are needed to ensure that information remains confidential. Investigators are obligated to ensure that information collected during a research protocol is not divulged to others in a manner inconsistent with the participant's understanding. Procedures for protecting confidentiality must ensure that a participant retains control over what is shared and to whom (Fisher, 1996).

Routine procedures for maintaining confidentiality of data include the use of subject codes rather than identifiers, secure storage, limited access to data, disposal of unnecessary identifying information, and appropriate supervision of research personnel. With newer technologies available for protecting electronic information, but with the additional risks that electronic transmission poses, investigators must be especially cautious to ensure that identifiable information collected during research projects is safeguarded.

The Certificate of Confidentiality is a federally sponsored document that provides immunity to investigators from any governmental or civil order to disclose identifying information from research records. The Certificate is granted under 301(d) of the Public Healthy Service Act. The Certificate provides additional protection against disclosure of confidential information to outside parties. When a Certificate of Confidentiality is granted, both the protections and limitations of it should be explained to the child and caregiver. The application for the Certificate can be obtained at most federal research institutions.

COMMUNITY COLLABORATIONS

As Atkisson, and colleagues have pointed out (1996), research subjects are best seen as active collaborators in the research process. The relationship between investigator and research participant is most respectful when it is structured as a collaborative partnership. This stance requires that participants be fully informed about the risks and benefits of the study, that they understand that the partnership is voluntary, and that they can discontinue participation at any time.

This role of the research participant as being actively engaged in the study, as a collaborator, contrasts with the passive stance that has typically described much medical research in the past. The role of research participant as a collaborator is an ideal that is never fully realized in any study—there are numerous obstacles to it (Atkisson et al., 1996).

Psychopharmacology research in children is designed to generate new knowledge and improve the outcomes for children who suffer from clinical conditions that warrant treatment. Such research relies upon partnerships among investigators, research partnerships, and society. But such research entails risks, so principles must be identified and carefully considered to simultaneously advance knowledge and protect research par-

ticipants by ensuring that investigations are conducted in an ethically informed manner.

At a recent conference, sponsored by Fordham University, the NIMH, and the American Psychiatric Association (APA) (July 2001) a set of key principles was identified for fostering stronger collaborations between researchers and community stakeholders. Among these is the principle that if research is to be conducted in an identifiable community, then prior and ongoing community consultation should be an integral part of the planning, design, conduct, and dissemination of studies of children's mental health. Community consultation should not be seen as a way to obtain acceptance of an already worked out protocol. It must be a true partnership. However, when there is no clearly defined community or when different groups may represent community interests, consultation may be problematic. Yet, the investigator still has the responsibility to accomplish the purposes of community consultation— that is, to identify and understand key stakeholder perspectives, values, and beliefs about the intended study.

These principles of collaboration are especially important in studies involving pediatric psychopharmacology, in part because the misunderstanding of pediatric mental illnesses and the concerns about medications, have created a climate of distrust and confusion. Direct and open communication between stakeholders and researchers is necessary to accomplish the goals of creating an ethical and valid scientific base.

OTHER SPECIAL CONSIDERATIONS AND STRATEGIES

Roberts (1998a) has developed a process for helping investigators develop protocols to ensure that ethically important research elements—design, informed consent, and assurances of confidentiality, for example— explicitly deal with human subjects' protection. The Research Protocol Ethics Assessment Tool is an evaluative checklist for use with participants who may have mental health problems. Although not designed to be used with pediatric populations, it can be useful as an assessment tool by investigators who wish to ensure that key aspects of the research project are holding to the highest ethical standards.

CONCLUSION

Studies of the safety, efficacy, effectiveness, and delivery of pediatric psychopharmacology treatments are among the most important public health issues facing child psychiatry today. Misperceptions about pediatric mental illnesses, about recognition of them, and about whether they are treatable, abound. These misunderstandings have created a climate in which scrutiny over every aspect of a prospective study should be expected. This is as it should be. It is as unethical to conduct studies that have not ensured adequate human subjects' protection as it is to withhold treatments from children who need them or to prescribe treatments for which no evidence of safety or effectiveness exists. Creating an ethically-grounded science base requires more than attention to the jots and tittles within regulations or guidelines. It requires principled commitment to the intrinsic value of science, and to the belief that no harm must ensue from participation in research, and attention to the unique values, histories, and beliefs of the culture or the community into which the researcher enters (Jensen et al., 1999). It is only through establishment of an ethical compact or agreement among investigators, families, and community stakeholders that an ethical and democratized science can be created.

REFERENCES

American College of Neuropsychopharmacology (2000) Statement of Principles of Ethical Conduct for Neuropsychopharmacologic Research in Human Subjects, Nashville, TN.

Applebaum, P.S., and Grisso, T. (1988) Assessing patients' capacities to consent to treatment. N Engl J Med 319:1635–1638.

Applebaum, P.S., and Grisso, T. (1995) The MacArthur Treatment Competence Study I, II, III. Law Hum Behav 19:105–174.

Arnold, L.E., Stoff, D.M., Cook, E., Cohen, D.J., Kruesi, M., Wright, C., Hattab, J., Graham, P., Zametkin, A., Castellanos, F.X., McMahon, W., and Lechman, J.F. (1995) Ethical issues in biological psychiatric research with children and adolescents. J Am Acad Child Adolesc Psychiatry 34:929–939.

Attkisson, C.C., Rosenblatt, A., and Hoagwood, K. (1996) Research ethics and human subjects protection in child mental health services research and community studies. In: Hoagwood, K., Jensen, P.S., and Fisher, C.B., eds. Ethical Issues in Mental Health Research with Children and Adolescents. Mahwah, NJ: Lawrence Erlbaum Associates, pp. 43–58.

Bonnie, R.J. (1997) Research with cognitively impaired subjects. Arch Gen Psychiatry 54:105–111.

Charney, D.S. (2000). The use of placebos in randomized clinical trials of mood disorders: well justified, but improvements in design are indicated. Biol Psychiatry 47:687–688.

Charney, D., Nemeroff, C., Lewis, L., Borenstein, M., Bowden, C., and Caplan, A. (2000) National Depressive and Manic Depressive Consensus Statement on the Use of Placebo in Clinical Trials of Mood Disorders. Chicago, IL

Cicchetti, D. (1998). Early experience, emotion, and brain: illustrations from the developmental psychopathology of child maltreatment. In: Hann, D., Huffman, L.C., Lederhendler, I.I. Meinecke, D. eds., Advancing Research on Developmental Plasticity: Integrating the Behavioral Science and Neuroscience of Mental Health. Bethesda, MD. NIMH.

Dresser, R. (1996). Mentally disabled research subjects: the enduring policy issues. JAMA 276:67–72.

Duncan, B.B., Forness, S.R., and Hartsough, C. (1995) Students identified as seriously emotionally disturbed in day treatment classrooms: cognitive, psychiatric and special education characteristics. Behav Disord 20:238–252.

Elliott, C. (1997) Caring about risks: are severely depressed patients competent to consent to research? Arch Gen Psychiatry 54:113–116.

Emslie, G.J., Rush, A.J., Weinberg, W.A., Kowatch, R.A., Carmody, T., and Mayes, T.L. (1998) Fluoxetine in child and adolescent depression: acute and maintenance treatment in depression and anxiety. Arch Gen Psychiatry 7:32–39.

Expert Panel Report to the National Institutes of Health (NIH) (1998) Research involving individuals with questionable capacity to consent: ethical issues and practical considerations for institutional review boards (IRBs). Presented In Bethesda, MD, February 1998.

Fisher, C.B., Hoagwood, K., and Jensen, P.S. (1996). Casebook on ethical issues in research with children and adolescents with mental disorders. In Hoagwood, K., Jensen P.S., and C.B. Fisher, eds., Ethical Issues in Mental Health Research with Children and Adolescents Mahwah, NJ: Lawrence Erlbaum Associates, pp. 135–257.

Fisher, C., Hoagwood, K., Duster, T., Frank, DA., Grisso, T., Levine, RJ., Macklin, R., Spencer, MB., Takanishi, R., Trimble, JE., Zayas, LH. (in press). Research for mental health science involving ethnic minority children and youth. Am Psychol.

Hoagwood, K., Jensen, P.S., and Fisher, C., eds. (1996) Ethical Issues in Child and Adolescent Mental Health Research. Mahwah, NJ: Lawrence Erlbaum Associates.

Horwitz, S.M., Leaf, P.J., Leventhal, J.M., Forsyth, B., and Speechley, K.N. (1992) Identification and management of psychosocial and developmental problems in community-based, primary care pediatric practices. Pediatrics 89:480–485.

Hyman, S.E. (1999) Protecting patients, preserving progress: ethics in mental health research. Acad Med 74:258–259.

Jensen, P.S. (1998) Ethical and pragmatic issues in the use of psychotropic agents in young children. Can J Psychiatry 43:585–588.

Jensen, P.S., Hoagwood, K., and Trickett, E. (1999a) Ivory tower or earthen trenches? Community collaborations to foster real-world research. J Appl Dev Sci 3:206–212.

Jensen, P.S., Vitiello, B., Bhatara, V., Hoagwood, K., and Feil, M. (1999b) Current trends in psychotropic prescribing practices. Clinical and policy implications. J Am Acad Child Adolesc Psychiatry 5:557–565.

Kupfer, D.J., Frank, E., Perel, J.M., Cornes, C., Mallinger, A.G., Thase, M.E., et al. (1992) Five-year outcome for maintenance therapies in recurrent depression. Arch Gen Psychiatry 49:769–773.

Levine, R.J. (1981) Ethics and Regulation of Clinical Research. Baltimore: Urban & Schwartzenberg.

Macklin, R. (1981). "Due" and "undue" inducements: on paying money to research subjects. IRB: Review of Human Subjects Research. 3:1–6.

MTA Cooperative Group (1999) A 14-month randomized clinical trial of treatment strategies for attention-deficit hyperactivity disorder. Arch Gen Psychiatry, 56:1073–1086.

Munir, K., and Earls, F. (1992) Ethical principles governing research in child and adolescent psychiatry. J Am Acad Child Adolesc Psychiatry 31:408–414.

National Bioethics Advisory Commission (NBAC) (1998) Research involving persons with mental disorders that may affect decision-making capacity. http://www.bioethics.gov

National Institutes of Health (2000) Required education in the protection of human research partaicipants. *NIH Guide:* OD-00–039, June 5, 2000. http://grants.nih.gov/grants/guide/notice-files/NOT-OD-00–039.html.

National Institute of Mental Health Advisory Council (2001) NIMH Advisory Council Workgroup Report: Blueprint for Change: Research on Child and Adolescent Mental Health. Washington, DC: National Institute of Mental Health.

Pato, M.T., Zohar-Kadouch, R., Zohar, J., and Murphy, D.L. (1988) Return of symptoms after discontinuation of clomipramine in patients with obsessive-compulsive disorder. *Am J Psychiatry* 145:1521–1525.

Roberts, L.W. (1998b) Ethics of psychiatric research: conceptual issues and empirical findings. *Compr Psychiatry* 39:99–110.

Roberts, L.W., Lauriello, J., Geppert, C. and Keith, S.J. (2001) Placebos and paradoxes in psychiatric research: an ethics perspective. *Biol Psychiatry* 49:887–893.

Roberts, R.E., Attkisson, C.C., and Rosenblatt, A. (1998) Prevalence of psychopathology among children and adolescents. *Am J Psychiatry* 155:715–725.

Shore, D., and Hyman, S.E. (1999) NIMH symptom challenge and medication discontinuation. *Biol Psychiatry* 46:1009–10.

Sutherland, H.J., Meslin, E.M., and Till, J.E. (1994) What's missing from current clinical trial guidelines? A framework for integrating science, ethics, and the community context. *J Clini Ethics* 4:297–303.

U.S. Congress, Office of Technology Assessment (1991). *Adolescent Health—Volume III: Cross-cutting Issues in the Delivery of Health and Related Services* (OTA-H-467). Washington, DC: U.S. Government Printing Office, June 1991.

U.S. Department of Education (1998) Twentieth Annual Report to Congress on Implementation of the Individuals with Disabilities Education Act. Washington, DC: U.S. Department of Education.

U.S. Department of Health and Human Services (DHHS) (1991a) Protection of Human Subjects. Basic HHS Policy for Protection of Human Research Subjects. Code of Federal Regulations, Title 45, Public Welfare: Part 46, Subpart A: 46.101–46.124, revised June 18, 1991, effective August 19, 1991., Washington, DC; Office of the Federal Register, National Archives and Records Administration, October 1, 1994 (45 CFR Subtitle A), pp. 116–127.

U.S. Department of Health and Human Services (1991b) Protection of Human Subjects, Subpart D: Additional Protections for Children Involved as Subjects in Research, Code of Federal Regulations, Title 45, Public Welfare: Part 46, Subpart D: 46.401–46.409, Revised June 18, 1991, Effective August 19, 1991, Washington, DC: Office of the Federal Register, National Archives and Records Administration, October 1, 1994 (45 CFR Subtitle A), pp. 132–135.

U.S. Public Health Service (2000) Report of the Surgeon General's Conference on Children's Mental Health: A National Action Agenda. Washington, DC:

Vitiello, B. (1998) Pediatric psychopharmacology and the interaction between drugs and the developing brain. *Can J Psychiatry* 43:582–584.

Vitiello, B. in press Ethical issues in pediatric psychopharmacology research. In: Rosenberg, D., Gershon, S., Davanzo P., eds., *Pharmacotherapy for Child and Adolescent Psychiatric Disorders.*

Vitiello, B., Jensen, P.S., and Hoagwood, K. (1999) Integrating science and ethics in child and adolescent psychiatry research. *Biol Psychiatry* 46:1044–1049.

Vitiello, B., and Jensen, P.S. (1997) Medication development and testing in children and adolescents. *Arch Gen Psychiatry* 54:871–876.

World Medical Association (1997) Declaration of Helsinki. Recommendations guiding physicians in biomedical research involving human subjects. *JAMA* 277:925–926.

Zito, J.M., Safer, D.J., DosReis, S., Gardner, J.F., Boles, M., and Lunch, F. (2000) Trends in the prescribing of psychotropic medications to preschoolers. *JAMA* 283:1025–1030.

56 | International perspectives

PER HOVE THOMSEN AND HIROSHI KURITA

This chapter addresses aspects of pediatric psychopharmacology outside of the United States, through the representative examples of the European Union and Japan. In part, the chapter discusses how various classification systems employed for diagnosis are alike and dissimilar. In that connection, areas in which psychopharmacological treatment are indicated are discussed. In addition, the chapter surveys the development of a worldwide order on the use of psychopharmacological treatment for children and adolescents.

THE EUROPEAN UNION

Historical Perspectives of Child Psychiatry in Europe

The discipline of child and adolescent psychiatry is acknowledged as a medical specialty or subspecialty in almost all European countries. The historical development of the discipline of child and adolescent psychiatry varies across Europe. Generally, however, four traditions have made substantial contributions to the current orientation of European child psychiatric institutions: the neuropsychiatric tradition, the remedial clinical tradition, the psychodynamic–psychoanalytical tradition, and the empirical, epidemiological, statistical tradition.

The *neuropsychiatric* tradition goes back to the formerly unified disciplines of psychiatry and neurology. It remains influential in Germany and has been a significant feature in psychiatric research in France, Italy, and many Eastern European countries. This tradition has more recently been extended in some countries to embrace substantial contributions from neuropsychology (Remschmidt and van Engeland, 1999b).

The *remedial clinical* tradition (heilpädagogisch-klinische Tradition) started in Austria and Switzerland, promoted by Hans Asperger in Austria and Paul Moor in Switzerland. The approach was later continued as the so-called psychosomatic tradition in pediatrics and still plays a major role in children's hospitals with departments for child psychosomatics.

The *psychodynamic–psychoanalytical* tradition evolved mainly in Western Europe and was developed from the work of Sigmund Freud, Anna Freud, Melanie Klein, and other pioneers of psychoanalytic work with children (Freud, 1965).

The *empirical, epidemiological, and statistical* tradition has emerged in recent years in a number of European countries and is a strong focus of research in England, Scandinavia, Germany, and Switzerland. It has been strongly influenced by Michael Rutter's work in England and also by research trends from the United States. There has been a swing in recent years toward the empirical approach, particularly focusing on the biological aspects of child and adolescent psychiatry.

The provision of services varies widely across Europe. Using the ratio of child and adolescent psychiatrists to the population under the age of 20 years, the best provision of service is found in Switzerland (1:5300), followed by Finland (1:6600), France (1:7500), and Sweden (1:7700) (Remschmidt and van Engeland, 1999)

Current European Attitudes Toward Medication with Psychotropics

In most European countries in recent years, child and adolescent psychiatry and specifically its medical treatment of children have increasingly been a subject of focus in the media, often presented with a journalistically skeptical, critical approach. The conceptual bases for some of the relevant conditions assumed to be indications for prescriptive treatment (ADHD and depression in particular) have been criticized and posed as problematic by the media, as well as also within the professional circles. The concern in a number of countries has been whether nonspecialists (for example, family physicians) should be authorized to prescribe psychotropic medication to children who have not been evaluated by a specialist in child and adolescent psychiatry.

There is no European consensus, let alone a reference program (such as, for example, that provided by American Psychiatric Association guidelines), for the medical treatment of specific childhood psychiatric conditions (American Academy of Child and Adolescent Psychiatry, 1997). Nonetheless, professional circles in individual countries have held conferences aimed at developing such a consensus and have formulated serviceable guidelines. National Boards of Health in many countries have taken initiatives with similar aims. Finally, the *Journal of the European Association of Child and Adolescent Psychiatry* has published many clinical guidelines in relation to a number of child psychiatric conditions, including attention-deficit hyperactivity disorder (ADHD), depression, and obsessive-compulsive disorder (OCD) (Biederman and Spencer, 2000; Buitelaar and Willemsen-Swinkels 2000; Gillberg, 2000; Kotler and Walsh, 2000; Remschmidt et al., 2000; Robertson and Stern, 2000; Santosh and Taylor, 2000; Thomsen, 2000; Ziervogel, 2000). These guidelines have specified the importance of a thorough and balanced evaluation that includes parental interview, an interview with and observation of the child, and consideration of the developmental history as well as information from different sources. Typically, multimodal interventions are recommended, among which psychoeducational approaches, parental training, and medication are the most important ones.

Since 1971 the so-called Pompidou Group (the cooperation group to combat drug abuse and illicit trafficking of drugs), which is an intergovernmental body, has existed as part of the European Council. This group organized a meeting between the World Health Organization (WHO), 16 European states, and the United States in 1999. A result of the meeting was the recommendation that specialists in ADHD/hyperkinetic disorder (HKD) always evaluate the condition before medication is prescribed. It was further recommended that appropriate standards for clinical care be developed for each European country. Such standards should include guidelines for assessment and diagnosis, medical treatment, types of monitoring and follow-up, dosages of drugs, treatment strategies, and the nature and extent of control in schools. As a guide for future research, it was recommended that there be prevalence studies of ADHD/HKD in different European countries, an exchange of clinical guidelines, and audit systems for the systematic treatment of the disorder, and monitoring and comparison of the use of stimulants in the treatment of ADHD/HKD in European countries (Pompideau Group, 2000).

However, while there seems to be consensus that children with possible ADHD/HKD should be evaluated by specialists in the field, most European countries are confronted with the potential problem of the relative scarcity of child psychiatrists. The lack of specialized child and adolescent psychiatrists to meet the need for specialist treatment may either lead to underdiagnosing and undertreatment of children who are in need of medication for ADHD/HKD, or undermine the sound principle that children who may be treated with psychotropic medication should be evaluated by a specialist in child and adolescent psychiatry.

Trends in the Use of Psychotropics in the European Union

The use of psychotropics for children and adolescents has grown throughout the Western world in the last 10 years. Unfortunately, however, there is no centrally compiled set of statistics that can reliably account for this expanded use. The latest worldwide study was conducted by the WHO in 1985 (World Health Organization, 1985). The study compared data and information from publicly available case registers, obtained for the purpose of studying psychotropic use in children. The prescription rate (i.e., the number of prescriptions for psychotropic drugs that were issued per year per 1000 children in the whole population) was used as an index. The index is far from ideal, but it gives a rough impression of the total use. The study revealed considerable differences in prescription rates. The highest rates were discovered in Scotland, with a rate of 118 prescriptions per 1000 children (Taylor, 1994). Germany (at the time, the existing West Germany) had a rate of 102, whereas Finland had 38 and The Netherlands 2. In Sweden the rate was as low as 8 and in Norway less than 1 prescription per 1000 children. Compared with data from the United States, the European rates were found to be considerably lower.

The results from this worldwide survey showed great differences between countries, which could be interpreted in several ways. It could be that high rates of prescription are associated with high rates of detection of a specific disorder. High rates of prescription might also reflect insufficient availability of alternative treatment strategies, such as psychological treatment or educational treatment. Because prescription practices might have changed considerably during the late 1990s, an updated survey is warranted.

As mentioned in the introduction, the literature on psychopharmacological treatment of representative populations of child and adolescent psychiatric patients is sparse, indeed, almost nonexistent. Nationwide studies are extremely rare, and when there is a lack of a central databank, they are very difficult, if not impossible, to perform. A German study by Elliger and colleagues (1990) analyzed the use of psychotropic drugs in childhood and adolescence based on data from 1985 using the General Drug Classification and Institute of Medical Statistics prescription indices. Judging from the data on prescriptions, psychostimulants were employed on a smaller scale in the late 1980s in Germany than in other countries. The prescription volume of methylphenidate, the leading substance in this therapeutic group, suggested that in 1985 only about 850 and in 1987 almost 750 children were treated with this substance. The authors concluded that historical and irrational factors did cause an extreme underutilization of psychostimulants, and they estimated that the drug prevalence of methylphenidate in the Federal Republic of Germany was no more than 1:10,000 children. Among the psychotropics, the neuroleptics represented the largest group. The main indications for use of neuroleptics was conduct disorder, hyperactivity, and psychotic disorders in adolescent patients; antidepressants were used in children for three main indications: enuresis, attention deficit disorder, and affective disorder.

Simeon et al. (1995) mailed questionnaires to 135 child psychiatrists in 43 countries to obtain more precise information on the views and approaches to the diagnosis and treatment of childhood psychiatric disorders. Of 43 questionnaires returned, data from 38 respondents representing 24 different countries were included. The study indicated that child psychiatrists in Europe and elsewhere outside the United States would use methylphenidate to treat 58% of ADHD patients, with their second choice being imipramine (18%), and 11% would not use medication. The investigators reported that one of the controversies that remained was the diagnosis and treatment of ADHD, as the prescription rates varied extremely from one country to another. In Italy, for example, the diagnosis of ADHD was rarely made and psychostimulants were rarely used. The authors concluded that the choice of medication was frequently restricted by lack of availability as well as by political or social attitudes (Simeon et al., 1995).

A countrywide study based on the national medicinal preparations register in Denmark showed that in 1997, 0.3% of the group aged 0–19 years was under treatment with either antipsychotics, psychostimulants, or antidepressants (Sørensen, 1998). The largest use was found among those aged 16–18 years, for whom selective serotonin reuptake inhibitor (SSRI) preparations comprised 90% of the antidepressants.

The National Health Service in Denmark has a computerized database of all prescription claims issued under the primary health care system one which codes by age and identification (ATC code) and is subdivided by age group (0–15, 16–25, etc.). According to the latest data from the National Health Service (Sørensen, 1998), the number of prescription claims of psychotropic agents issued to children and adolescents has increased during the last decade. This increase seems to be mainly due to an increase in the prescription of SSRIs. The number of patients prescribed SSRIs per 1000 inhabitants in the age group 0–15 years was 0.30 in 1995 and 0.48 in 1999.

In 1995, Bramble published a study on the prescription frequency of antidepressants by British child psychiatrists (Bramble, 1995). A brief postal questionnaire was circulated to 350 members of the British Royal College of Psychiatrists, Child and Adolescent Psychiatry Specialist Sections. There was a 71% response rate, and 85% of the 238 respondents had employed antidepressants, the most popular of these being amitriptyline and imipramine. Nearly one-third of the psychiatrists at that time used neuroagents occasionally, and the SSRIs were used only very rarely. The antidepressant medication was used for a wide range of child and adolescent disorders beyond those of depression and nocturnal enuresis. Approximately 20% of the prescriptions were given for ADHD (hyperkinetic disorder), conduct disorder, and a few cases of autistic disorder. Clomipramine was apparently given for OCD. On the basis of these 1994 data, Bramble concluded that British child psychiatrists tend to use antidepressant medication far less often than American psychiatrists.

A survey on the use of antidepressive agents by an entire country's child and adolescent psychiatric services was recently conducted in Denmark (5 million inhabitants) by sending a questionnaire to all child and adolescent psychiatric departments and specialists with private practices. The response rate from all in- and outpatient clinics as well as from specialists with their own practice was 93.5%. Thirty-two departments and specialists received the survey and 30 were returned. Practitioners were asked to go through their files and report the number of children on medication and the indications for the treatment. Altogether, approximately 5000 children and adolescents were in psychiatric care (out of approximately 1 million children and adolescents in the age group 0–19 years). Of these, 400 (8%) were treated with an antidepressant on the date of the survey (February 8).

In the antipressant group, 92.1% were treated with a SSRI, most commonly citalopram (47.9%) or sertraline (29.3%). The indications for prescribing antidepressants were depression in 59.2%, OCD in 29.8%, anxiety disorder in 10.7%, and eating disorder in 6.3% of those treated with an antidepressant (Sørensen et al. 2002, in press). Of the total population of 0 to 8-year-olds in Denmark, the percentage of children treated with an antidepressant by child and adolescent psychiatry services was 0.03%. The survey provided no information on the amount or number of SSRIs or antidepressants prescribed by general practitioners, which is a subject that has received much attention from the country's public and media.

Under the auspices of the European Council, Sindelaar conducted a study to determine the current trends in the diagnosis and treatment of ADHD/HKD (Sindelar, 2000). Data were gathered by sending questionnaires to all child and adolescent psychiatric centers in 24 European countries. The survey asked practitioners in European countries to estimate by percentage the frequency with which they diagnosed ADHD among their child psychiatric patients, and how often they prescribed medication for ADHD/HKD. A total number of 359 mailed questionnaires were distributed; 119 were returned. The percentage of response differed widely: 85% of the surveys were returned from Iceland, between 10% and 80% from many of the other countries, and 0% from four European countries (Switzerland, Spain, Portugal, and Bulgaria). In total, 33% of the questionnaires were returned.

The aim of the study was to find out how professionals in Europe diagnose and treat children with ADHD/HKD. It was found that the International Classification of Diseases, 10th ed. (ICD-10) was applied much more often than the *Diagnostic and Statistical Manual of Mental Disorders, 4th ed.* (DSM-IV) (76% vs. 29%). Medication was apparently used very seldomly. The study did not indicate the percentage of children in the different countries with a diagnosis of ADHD/HKD who actually received medication. The total number of children or adolescents in psychiatric care was not identified. Practitioners who responded to the survey and who used medication in treating ADHD/HKD most often used stimulants (88.2%) or antidepressant medication as their first or second choice (40.3%), and anticonvulsants (15.1%) or other kinds of medication (20.2%) less frequently. However, most of the respondents noted that they rarely gave medication. The main reasons for not using medication included comorbidity, 38%; noncompliance, 20%, and nonresponse, 8%. Despite the study being cross-sectional, it was interesting to find that 45% of the patients who had been medicated had been treated with medication for more than 2 years and 23% had been treated from 1 to 2 years. As indications for drug treatment, professionals noted severity for 27%, results of examination and investigation for 53%, and a child being nonrespondent to other treatments for 13% of the cases. Only 19% of the professionals stated that drug treatment alone was the most effective form of treatment, while nearly half of those responding reported that the combined treatment of drug plus counseling and/or psychotherapy was the most effective treatment. Twenty percent of the respondents found nondrug treatment to be the most effective form (Pompideau Group, 2000).

We recently surveyed pharmaceutical companies producing antidepressant medication or central nervous system (CNS) stimulants for the European market. Approval for use of such drugs in children and adolescents is limited worldwide. Sertraline, clomipramine, and fluvoxamine have been approved for use in children (for some drugs down to the age of 6 years) for OCD in some European countries (the most wide spread approval being for sertraline in Austria, France, Hungary, Italy, Latvia, Norway, Portugal, Romania, Slovenia, Spain, Sweden, Switzerland, Turkey, United Kingdom, and Denmark) and countries outside Europe. Methylphenidate has been approved for the treatment of children with ADHD in a number of European and non-European countries (Novartis Health care A/S, personal communication).

Several reasons may contribute to these different rates among the European countries. Legislation is one. Cultural preference for nonmedication approaches is another, which might be most predominant in countries more influenced by psychoanalytical reference and theory, such as France, Switzerland, Austria, and Italy. A lack of trained professionals might also explain the difference, as can a lack of professionals to recognize children needing medication will result in a low number of prescriptions. However, the lack of trained professionals in nonmedication treatments (such as psychotherapy) could also contribute to a higher rate of children who are given medication.

The differences in prescribing rates might also reflect the access to alternative treatment options. In Scandinavia, for example, much effort is made to give children with ADHD/HKD special education programs; many schools have special classes for children with ADHD or ADHD-like problems. The general attitude toward the prescription of central stimulants is that educational program and family support must be given and be functioning well, before medication is considered.

Impact of Differing Diagnostic and Assessment Instruments

The ICD-10, which was developed by the WHO as a classification of diseases, was approved in 1990 and implemented in 1993 (World Health Organization,

1993). For mental health there is also a version with research diagnostic criteria, DCR-10, which is similar to the DSM-IV (American Psychiatric Association, 1994). The ICD-10 is used in most European, and Asian, and African countries for clinical purposes; however, most clinical and epidemiological research in Europe is based on the DSM-IV. To date, no pharmacological studies involving antidepressants, antipsychotics, or antianxiety agents have been based on ICD-10 criteria.

One of the most important, general differences between the DSM-IV and the ICD system is that the DSM-IV, like its predecessors, encourages multiple diagnostic codings. The ICD-10, in contrast, generally discourages this practice. The ICD-10 favors a hierarchical structure, so that a lower number (i.e., more severe illness) is recognized as the most important diagnosis. In many cases it excludes the possibility of fulfilling the criteria for another condition. Rather than comorbidity, the ICD-10 operates with mixed categories, such as disturbance of conduct and emotions and hyperkinetic conduct disorder.

The major differences between the two diagnostic systems regarding specific diagnosis are discussed below.

For Anxiety disorders; the ICD-10 delineates special categories of emotional disorders in children in which symptoms of anxiety are considered in relation to age appropriateness, duration, and severity. The DSM-IV focuses on the specific syndrome without considering the influence of development on symptom expression.

The section for emotional disorders in children spans across the following diagnoses: separation anxiety disorder; social anxiety disorder of childhood; phobic anxiety disorder of childhood; generalized anxiety disorder of childhood; other emotional disorders (with onset specific to childhood); and sibling rivalry disorder.

Obsessive-compulsive disorder is a distinct entity in ICD-10 and is not included in anxiety disorders, as it is in the DSM. The ICD-10 delienates subtypes with obsessions or compulsions that are predominant in the condition; however, the subtype that applies to patients with poor insight is not included in the ICD-10. Elective mutism (or selective mutism) is included in the ICD-10 as a disorder of social functioning; however, for both conditions, the main diagnostic criteria are identical.

Attention-deficit hyperactivity disorder is called hyperkinetic disorder in the ICD-10, which does not include the same subtypes as those in the DSM. According to the DSM-IV, ADHD is a broader definition than that given for HKD (hyperkinetic disorder) in the ICD-

10. In both disorders the described behaviors are very similar, but the ICD-10 defines a more severe disorder with a guarded prognosis: (1) all three core problems of attention, hyperactivity, and impulsiveness should be present (whereas the DSM-IV defines three subtypes: predominantly inattentive type, hyperactive impulsive type, and combined type); (2) pervasiveness throughout different situations is determined by more stringent criteria; and (3) the presence of another mental or behavioral disorder is an exclusion criterion.

These criteria result in a much lower prevalence of hyperkinetic disorder, with estimates in the range of 1–5%, as compared to 5–10% in school-aged children for ADHD. In the ICD-10 there is a lower possibility of diagnosing children with attention deficit without hyperactivity. In the ICD-10 another diagnosis of "other specified behavioral and emotional disorders with onset usually occurring in childhood and adolescence" must be used. However, the combined condition of hyperkinetic disorder and conduct disorder is delineated under the diagnosis "hyperkinetic conduct disorder."

The issues of whether depression is underdiagnosed, and more generally, whether the construct of depression is also applicable to children, have been discussed in both Europe (Rutter et al., 1986) and the United States (Beardslee et al., 1985). As in the DSM-IV, the ICD-10 has no specific category for depressive disorder in childhood, so diagnostic criteria developed for adult patients must be applied to children. However, a combination category for depression and conduct disorder is included in the ICD-10, "depressive conduct disorder," for which the child must fulfill criteria for both depression and conduct disorder.

The criteria for conduct disorder (CD) are less strict in the ICD-10 than in the DSM. In a study of the comorbidity of ADHD and conduct disorder, it was found that only 42% of children diagnosed with ADHD also fulfilled the diagnostic criteria for either oppositional defiant disorder (ODD) or CD, according to the DSM-IV, whereas 71% of the same children fulfilled the ICD-10 criteria for CD (Dalsgaard et al., 2001). The ICD-10 retains the distinction socialized/unsocialized, while the DSM-IV has moved to a distinction based on age of onset, childhood/adolescent, for conduct disorders.

Pervasive developmental disorders, including childhood autism, are described in the ICD-10. Asperger's syndrome (ICD-10) and Asperger disorder (DSM-IV) are likewise included in both diagnostic systems.

Three types of eating disorders are included in the ICD-10: anorexia nervosa, bulimia nervosa, and overeating.

There are only minor differences in the diagnostic concepts used in the ICD-10 and DSM-IV. There seem to be no different implications for the use of psychotropics in terms of different use of rating scales or different indications for treatment. For example, the diagnosis of ADHD is based on very similar criteria in the two diagnostic systems. However, the ICD-10, unlike in the DSM, states that the diagnosis must be verified or confirmed by an observation of the child. Certainly, more children in the United States than in Europe are treated with stimulants for ADHD. Furthermore, more children seem to be diagnosed with ADHD in American epidemiological studies than in European ones. While treatment with psychostimulants has reached a frequency of 12%–15% in some areas of the United States, it is considerably lower in Europe—generally less than 1%.

Rating Scales in European Child and Adolescent Psychiatry

In European child and adolescent psychiatry there is increasing use of rating scales in clinical practise. The rating scales most commonly used to cover broad aspects of psychopathology include diagnostic interviews such as the Structured Clinical Interview for DSM-III-R (SCID; Spitzer et al., 1992), and the Kiddie Schedule for Affective Disorders (K-SADS; recently chosen by the Scandinavian countries to be used in research and clinical practice) (Chambers et al., 1985). Most rating scales used in the clinic and in research are either American or from the United Kingdom (the K-SADS, the SCID, the Diagnostic Interview Schedule for Children [DISC], the Children's Interview for Psychiatric Syndromes [CHIPS], or the Children's Assessment Scale [CAS]) or have been derived from these scales.

As for symptom for diagnosis specific interviews or rating scales, the most widely used instruments in the European countries are the Children's Yale-Brown Obsessive-Compulsive Scale (CY-BOCS) for scoring of obsessive-compulsive symptoms (Goodman et al., 1989), the Children's Depression Inventory (CDI) for reporting of depressive symptoms in children (Sherrill and Kovacs, 2000); the Beck Depression Inventory (BDI) for scoring depressive symptoms in adolescents, the Eating Disorder Inventory (EDI) and Eating Attitude Test (EAT), for assessing symptoms of eating disorders; the Connors rating scale, for ADHD; the Structured Clinical Assessment of Neuropsychiatric Disorder Present State Examination (SCAN/PSE), for discerning ICD-10 symptoms of psychopathology, in particular symptoms of psychosis/schizophrenia (World Health Organization, 1993); and the Child Behavior Checklist (CBCL) parent or teacher report of psychopathology (Achenbach, 1993). The CBCL has been standardized according to norms in many European countries (Verhulst et al., 1985; Stanger et al., 1994; Weine et al., 1995; Crunen et al., 1997) the CBCL is used in most epidemiological studies, as well as in many clinical departments, as a clinical test.

JAPAN

Child Psychiatry in Japan: A Historical Perspective

Japanese medicine has long been under the influence of Chinese medicine. This influence gradually faded through the small but steady influx of Dutch medicine between the early 17th and mid-19th centuries, a time during which the Tokugawa Shogun government closed the Japanese border to all except Dutch foreigners. In the period between 1868, when the modern Japanese government headed by the Emperor replaced the Shogun government, ending the international isolation of Japan, and 1945, when World War II ended, Japanese medicine received its major influence from German medicine, although British, French, and American traditions were also visible. Since the end of World War II, American medicine has had the greatest influence on Japanese medicine.

Child psychiatry in Japan has a relatively long history of its own. In the 1950s, several medical schools started child psychiatric services in their departments of psychiatry, primarily through child psychiatrists who had trained in the United States. In 1959, clinical psychiatrists and allied professionals who were interested in mental health and disorders of children first established the Japanese Society of Child Psychiatry. This society published the first issue of the *Japanese Journal of Child Psychiatry and Allied Disciplines* in 1960, the same year as the *Journal of Child Psychology and Psychiatry and Allied Disciplines* in the United Kingdom, a year ahead of the *Journal of the American Academy of Child Psychiatry* in the United States, and well over 30 years before *European Child and Adolescent Psychiatry*.

However, for several reasons, Japanese child psychiatrists, have been less enthusiastic about the psychopharmacological treatment of children than their American colleagues. First, Japanese child psychiatry was strongly psychosocially oriented, possibly because most of its founders came from clinical psychiatry and psychopathology backgrounds. Second, Japanese child psychiatry experienced an intense antipsychiatry movement in the early 1970s, when many Japanese child psychiatrists seem to have fostered a negative attitude toward biological studies in children. Third, there are only a few independent divisions or units of child psychiatry within the 80 medical schools in Japan (Hayashi and Yamazaki, 1998). This is reflected in the poor condition of child psychiatry education in Japan, including of pediatric psychopharmacology. Fourth, almost all of the medications used for child psychiatric disorders are not approved for such use by the Ministry of Health and Welfare of Japan.

For all of those reasons, pediatric psychopharmacology is still an underdeveloped branch of medicine in Japan, and is not comparable to that in the United States. Nevertheless, psychopharmacological treatments have been an important part of therapeutics in Japanese child psychiatry.

In this section, developments over the last four decades and the current status of pediatric psychopharmacology in Japan are reviewed.

Drug Evaluation and Regulatory Affairs

In Japan, the need for scientific drug evaluation was widely recognized after the reports of thalidomide teratogenicity in 1961. According to the recommendation from the World Health Organization in 1963, the Ministry of Health and Welfare of Japan established the monitoring system of side effects of medicines, in collaboration with university medical centers and national hospitals throughout the country. By 1965 it had become mandatory for a pharmaceutical company to report possible side effects of a drug, for at least the 2 years following its approval for commercial distribution. In addition, the system of collecting information on drug side effects from scientific papers throughout the world was set up. Other than governmental efforts, in 1972 the Society for Publishing Clinical Evaluation, a private organization with several prominent child psychiatrists among its founding members, started publishing a journal, *Clinical Evaluation*, to encourage the scientific evaluation of drugs.

In 1970, the Task Force for Evaluation of Children's Behaviors was established. This task force conducted several randomized controlled studies on drugs for children with developmental and behavioral disorders, including mental retardation and autism. The majority of such studies, however, yielded negative results.

The regulatory process

In Japan, all drugs need approval for their clinical use by the Ministry of Health and Welfare, on the basis of their being proven safe and effective through at least one randomized controlled study. Evaluation of a drug for which a pharmaceutical company is seeking approval is conducted by a team of basic and clinical specialists on issues pertaining to drug development and evaluation, as appointed by the Ministry. This specialist team submits an evaluation report on each individual drug to the Central Pharmaceutical Affairs Council, which advises the Ministry of Health and Welfare.

In 1997, the Ministry of Health and Welfare extensively reformed the drug evaluation system and established the Pharmaceuticals and Medical Devices Evaluation Center affiliated with the National Institute of Health Sciences. Under the new system, the Center, through its specialized teams, conducts the evaluation of drugs for which different pharmaceutical companies have sought approval.

Diagnostic and Assessment Issues

Both the DSM-IV (American Psychiatric Association, 1994) and the ICD-10 (World Health Organization, 1993) are used in Japan, with the latter being the official system used to record diseases and the former preferred in research, including for clinical studies on psychotropics. No Japanese version of a structured or semistructured interview scheme based on either the DSM or ICD system for children is yet available.

Rating scales

As compared to the United States and European countries, a much smaller number of reliable and valid rating scales exist to evaluate the efficacy of medications in Japanese youngsters. The development of both Japanese versions of scales developed abroad and original Japanese scales is an ongoing priority area for pediatric psychopharmacology research. To date, representative rating scales originally developed in the United States and Europe that are available in Japanese versions and have demonstrated reliability and validity include the Rutter Scale (Matsuura et al., 1989); the Child Behavior Checklist (CBCL; Nakata et al., 1999); the Childhood Autism Rating Scale (CARS; Kurita et al., 1989); and the Childhood Depression Inventory (CDI; Murata et al., 1992).

The Rating List for Evaluating Abnormal Behaviors in Children, consisting of 258 items rated on a 4-point scale, was the first original Japanese rating scale for children. It showed satisfactory sensitivity and specificity to distinguish between normal and behavior-disordered children (Fujita et al., 1982). This scale was used in several randomized controlled studies of drugs for behavioral problems in children with autism and/

or mental retardation, although most of these studies yielded negative results. Two other original Japanese rating scales are available for the assessment of autism, with proven reliability and validity and potential utility in drug evaluation: the Tokyo Autistic Behavior Scale (TABS; 39 items rated on a 3-point scale by mothers) (Kurita and Miyake 1990; Tachimori et al., 2000), and the Child Behavior Questionnaire (CBQ; 28 items rated on a 4-point scale by mothers) (Osada et al., 2000). These scales are yet to be used in studies evaluating psychotropics for children.

Ethnic Differences

Important biological differences that potentially affect the metabolism of psychotropics have been described between Japanese and non-Asian children. For example, a pharmacogenetic ethnic difference was reported in cytochrome P450 (CYP) 2D6 metabolism of several antipsychotics and antidepressants, and in the CYP 2C19 metabolism of tricyclic agents. In adults, the rate of poor metabolizers of CYP 2D6 substrates is lower in Asians (about 1%) than in Caucasians (about 7%), while that of CYP 2C19 substrates is higher in Asians (15%–30%) than in Caucasians (3%–6%) (Poolsup et al., 2000). Clinicians may need to keep these differences in mind when they use psychotropics in Japanese and other Asian patients, since such differences can lead to different behavioral responses or toxicity.

Two epidemiological differences concerning autism are worth mentioning to highlight other potential biological differences between Japanese and Caucasian children, even if they are not directly related to drug metabolism per se. First, fragile X syndrome exists in a small percentage of male patients with autism in Western countries (Bailey et al., 1993), but is esentially non-existent in Japanese males with autism (Hashimoto et al., 1993). Second, the prevalence of autism is estimated at about 0.1% in Japan (Sugiyama and Abe, 1989), while generally reported at 0.05% in most Western countries (Sponheim and Skjeldal, 1998).

Overcoming Regional Difficulties

Since most psychotropics are not officially approved for use in the treatment of mental disorders in children in Japan, child psychiatrists must prescribe these drugs using their own judgment, including obtaining appropriate informed consent (Yamazaki, 1994). This situation, and the general reluctance of patients (or their guardians) to participate in clinical trials, makes for great difficulty in conducting randomized controlled studies of psychotropics in Japan. There are two avail-

able ways of overcoming such limitations. First, bridging studies can be conducted, in which relevant pharmaceutical data from foreign countries can be supplemented with data from local studies. The International Conference on Harmonization of Technical Requirements for the Registration of Pharmaceuticals for Human Use (ICH), established in 1990 to improve the efficiency of developing pharmaceutical products in Europe, Japan, and the United States, has promoted the concept of such bridging studies. Japanese pharmaceutical companies are now increasingly employing this approach, as it is reasonable to gather data to demonstrate the efficacy and safety of a medication by integrating relevant data from rigorous basic and clinical studies conducted in other countries.

The second approach is to recruit participants, who must provide informed consent to take part in clinical trials of medications, through advertisements in newspapers or other media. This is a reasonable alternative to facilitating clinical trials that meet scientific and ethical standards, but one that has just begun to be used among adults.

Conclusions Regarding Japan

Although the Ministry of Health and Welfare of Japan has improved the evaluation system for psychotropics used in adults since 1997, the system needs further improvement and extension to specifically cover child psychiatric disorders. In this respect, bridging studies that combine data obtained from non-Asian and Asian children will be increasingly important to facilitating the drug evaluation process among Japanese children. More reliable and valid scales, including original Japanese scales and Japanese versions of scales developed abroad for the use of psychotropic studies, need to be broadened and refined.

REFERENCES

Achenbach, T.M. (1993) Manual for the Child Behavior Checklist/ 4–18 and 1991 Profile. Burlington, VT: University of Vermont, Department of Psychiatry.

American Association of Child and Adolescent Psychiatry (1997) Practice Parameters for the Assessment and Treatment of Children, Adolescents, and Adults With Attention-Deficit/Hyperactivity Disorder. J Am Acad Child Adolesc Psychiatry 36:85S–121S.

American Psychiatric Association (1994) Diagnostic and Statistical Manual of Mental Disorders, 4th ed. Washington, DC: American Psychiatric Press.

Bailey, A., Bolton, P., Butler, L., Le Couteur, A., Murphy, M., Scott, S., Webb, T., and Rutter, M. (1993) Prevalence of fragile X anomaly amongst autistic twins and singletons. J Child Psychol Psychiatry 34:673–688.

Beardslee, W., Kleinman, G., Keller, M., Lavori, P., and Podorefsky,

D. (1985) But are they cases? Validity of DSM-III major depression in children identified in a family study. *Am J Psychiatry* 142: 687–691.

Biederman, J. and Spencer, T. (2000) Non-stimulant treatments for ADHD. *Eur Child Adolesc Psychiatry* 9:51–59.

Bramble, D.J. (1995) Antidepressant prescription by British child psychiatrists: practice and safety issues. *J Am Acad Child Adolesc Psychiatry* 34:327–331.

Buitelaar, J.K. and Willemsen-Swinkels, S.H.N. (2000) Medication treatment in subjects with autistic spectrum disorders. *Eur Child Adolesc Psychiatry* 9:85–97.

Chambers, W.J., Puig-Antich, J., Hirsch M., Paez P., Ambrosini, P.J., Tabrizi M.A., and Davies, M. (1985) The assessment of affective disorders in children and adolescents by semistructured interview. Test–retest reliability of the Schedule for Affective Disorders and Schizophrenia for School-Age Children, Present Episode Version. *Arch Gen Psychiatry* 42:696–702.

Crunen, A.A., Achenbach, T.M., and Verhulst, F. (1997) Comparisons of problems reported by parents of children in 12 cultures: total problems, externalizing, and internalizing. *J Am Acad Child Adolesc Psychiatry* 36:1269–1277.

Dalsgaard, S., Hansen, N., Mortensen, P.B., Damm, D., and Thomsen, P.H. (2001) Reassessment of ADHD in a historical cohort of children treated with stimulants in the period 1969–1989. Eur Child Adolesc Psychiatry 10:230–239.

Elliger, T.J., Trott, G.-E., and Nissen, G. (1990) Prevalence of psychotropic medication in childhood and adolescence in the Federal Republic of Germany. *Pharmacopsychiatry* 23:38–44.

Freud, A. (1965) *Normality and Pathology in Childhood*. New York: International University Press.

Fujita, T., Kurisu, E., and Satoh, Y. (1982) A study of extra-normal validity in the Rating List for Evaluating Abnormal Behaviors in Children [in Japanese]. *Clin Eval* 10:201–232.

Gillberg, C. (2000) Typical neuroleptics in child and adolescent psychiatry. *Eur Child Adolesc Psychiatry* 9:2–8.

Goodman, W.K., Price, L.H., Rasmusen, S.A., Mazure, C., Fleischman, R.L., Hill, C.L., Heninger, G.R., and Charney, D.S. (1989) The Yale-Brown Obsessive Compulsive Scale. I. Development, use, and reliability. *Arch Gen Psychiatry* 46:1006–1011.

Hashimoto, O., Shimizu, Y., and Kawasaki, Y. (1993) Low frequency of the fragile X syndrome among Japanese autistic subjects. *J Autism Dev Disord* 23:201–209.

Hayashi, M. and Yamazaki, K. (1998) Surveys on the pregraduate and postgraduate education on child and adolescent psychiatry. *Psychiatry Clini Neurosci* 52 (Suppl): S281–S284.

Kano, Y., Ohta, M., and Nagai, Y. (1998) Tourette syndrome in Japan: a nationwide questionnaire survey of psychiatrists and pediatricians. *Psychiatry Clin Neurosci* 52:407–411.

Kotler, L.A. and Walsh, B.T. (2000) Eating disorders in children and adolescents: pharmacological therapies. *Eur Child Adolesc Psychiatry* 9:108–116.

Kurita, H. and Miyake, Y. (1990) The reliability and validity of the Tokyo Autistic Behavior Scale. *Jpn J Psychiatry Neurol*, 44, 25–32.

Kurita, H., Miyake, Y., and Katsuno, K. (1989) Reliability and validity of the Childhood Autism Rating Scale Tokyo Version (CARS-TV). *J Autism Dev Disord* 19, 389–396.

Matsuura, M., Okubo, Y., Kato, M., Kojima, T., Takahashi, R., Asai, K., Asai, T., Endo, T., Yamada, S., Nakane, A., Kimura, K., and Suzuki, M. (1989) An epidemiological investigation of emotional and behavioral problems in primary school children in Japan: the report of the first phase of a WHO collaborative study in Western Pacific Region. *Soci Psychiatry Psychiatri Epidemio* 24:17–22.

Murata, T., Tsutsumi, T., Sarada, Y., and Nakaniwa, Y. (1992) The validity and reliability of the Japanese version of the CDI [in Japanese]. *Kyushu Neuropsychiatry* 38:42–47.

Nakata, Y., Kanbayashi, Y., Fukui, T., Fujii, H., Kita, M., Okada, A., and Morioka, Y. (1999) A study on the Japanese version of the Child Behavior Checklist for Ages 2 to 3 (CBCL/2–3) [in Japanese]. *Jpn J Psychiatry Neurol Child* 39:305–316.

Osada, H., Kato, S., Naganuma, Y., Setoya, Y., Kubota, Y., Watanabe, Y., Tachimori, H., Kurita, H., and Ohta, M. (2000) The usefulness of Child Behavior Questionnaire (CBQ) as a supplementary scale for diagnosis of pervasive developmental disorders [in Japanese] *Clin Psychiatry* 42:527–534.

Pi, E.H. (1998) Transcultural psychopharmacology: Present and future. *Psychiatry Clin Neurosci* 52(Suppl.): S185–S187.

Pompideau Group (2000) Attention Deficit/ Hyperkinetic Disorders: Their Diagnosis and Treatment with Stimulants. Strasbourg: Council of Europe.

Poolsup, N., Li, Wan Po, A., and Knight, T.L. (2000) Pharmacogenetics and psychopharmacotherapy. *J Clin Pharm Ther* 25:197–220.

Remschmidt, H., Kenninghausen, K., Clement, H.-W., Heiser, P., and Schultz, E. (2000) Atypical neuroleptics in child and adolescent psychiatry. *Eur Child Adolesc Psychiatry* 9:9–19.

Remschmidt, H. and van Engeland, H. (1999) *Child and Adolescent Psychiatry in Europe. Historical Development, Current Situation, Future Perspectives.* Darmstadt, Germany: Steinkopff Verlag.

Robertson, M.M. and Stern, J.S. (2000) Gilles de la Tourette syndrome: symptomatic treatment based on evidence. *Eur Child Adolesc Psychiatry* 9:60–75.

Rutter, M., Izord, C., and Read, P. (1986) Depression in Young People: Clinical and Developmental Perspectives. New York: Guilford Press.

Santosh, P.J. and Taylor, E. (2000) Stimulant drugs. *Eur Child Adolesc Psychiatry* 9:27–43.

Sherrill, J.T. and Kovacs, M. (2000) Interview Schedule for Children and Adolescents (ISCA). *J Am Acad Child Adolesc Psychiatry* 39: 67–75.

Simeon J.G., Wiggins, D.M., and Williams, E. (1995) Worldwide use of psychotropic drugs in child and adolescent psychiatric disorder. *Prog Neuropsychopharmacol Biol Psychiatry* 19:455–465.

Sindelar, B. (2000) Diagnosis and treatment prectices in the field of ADD/ADHD/HD in Europe In: Pompideau Group, eds. *Attention Deficit/Hyperkinetic Disorders: Their Diagnosis and Treatment with Stimulants.* Strasbourg: Council of Europe, pp. 55–101.

Sørensen C.B., Jepsen E.B., Thomsen P.H., and Dalsgaard S. (2002) Indications for and use of antidepressants in a country's child and adolescent psychiatry—a cross-sectional survey in Denmark. Eur Child Adolesc Psychiatry (in press).

Sørensen, L. (1998) Børn og unges forbrug af psykofarmaka, psykostimulantia og antidepressiva. [in Danish] *UfL* 160:7433–7437.

Spitzer, R.L., Williams, J.B., Gibbon, M., and First, M.B. (1992) The Structured Clinical Interview for DSM-III-R (SCID). I: History, rationale and description. *Arch Gen Psychiatry* 49:624–629.

Sponheim, E., and Skjeldal, O. (1998) Autism and related disorders: epidemiological findings in a Norwegian study using ICD-10 diagnostic criteria. *J Autism Dev Disord*, 28:217–227.

Stanger, C., Fombonne, E., and Achenbach, T.M. (1994) Epidemiological comparisons of American and French children: parent report of problems and competencies for ages 6–11. *Eur Child Adolesc Psychiatry* 3:16–28.

Sugiyama, T., and Abe, T. (1989) The prevalence of autism in Nagoya, Japan: a total population study. *J Autism Dev Disord* 19, 87–96.

Tachimori, H., Takahashi, M., Osada, H., Watanabe, Y., Naganuma, Y., Setoya, Y., Kubota, Y., Kato, S., and Kurita, H. (2000) The utility of Tokyo Autistic Behavior Scale (TABS) as a supplementary scale for diagnosis of pervasive developmental disorders. [in Japanese]. *Jpn J Clin Psychiatry* 29:529–536.

Taylor, E. (1994) Physical treatments. In: Rutter, Mi., Taylor, E. and Hersov, L., eds. *Child and Adolescent Psychiatry. Modern Approaches.* Oxford, London, Edinburgh Blackwell Science, pp. 880–899.

Thomsen, P.H. (2000) Obsessive-compulsive disorder: pharmacological treatment. *Eur Child Adolesc Psychiatry* 9:76–84.

Verhulst, F., Akkerhuis, G.W., and Althaus, M. (1985) Mental health in Dutch children: (I) a cross-cultural comparison. *Acta Psychiatr Scand* 323:72–72.

Weine, A.M., Phillips, J.S., and Achenbach, T.M. (1995) Behavioral and emotional problems among Chinese and American children: parent and teacher reports for ages 6 to 13 *J Abnorm Child Psychol* 23:619–639.

World Health Organization (1985) The Prescribing of Psychoactive Drugs for Children. Geneva: World Health Organization.

World Health Organization (1993) *The ICD-10 Classification of Mental and Behavioural Disorders: Diagnostic Criteria for Research.* Geneva: World Health Organization.

Yamazaki, K. (1994) The adaptation and limitation of psychopharmacotherapy for children. [in Japanese]. *Jpn J Dev Disabili,* 16: 1–9.

Ziervogel, C.F. (2000) Selective serotonin reuptake inhibitors for children and adolescents. *Eur Child Adolesc Psychiatry* 9:20–26.

APPENDIX: *Pediatric Psychopharmacogy at a Glance*

STIMULANTS

Drug	Mechanism of Action	Main Indications and Clinical Uses	Dosage (mg/day)	Schedule	Adverse Effects	Comments	Select Brand Names and Preparations Available
Methylphenidate	Dopamine presynaptic release and reuptake blockade	ADHD	15–60 (Ritalin) 18–54 (Concerta)	bid/tid (methylphenidate) qd (Concerta)	Insomnia, decreased appetite, weight loss, dysphoria Possible reduction in growth velocity during long-term use Withdrawal and rebound hyperactivity	Longer-acting preparations may have lower peak and valley effects and less rebound hyperactivity	Ritalin/Methylin: 5, 10, 20 mg t; 20 mg sustained-release t, Concerta: 18, 36, 54 mg Metadate-CD, Ritalin-LA, Focalin, others
Dextroamphetamine	Same as for methylphenidate	ADHD	10–40	bid/tid	Unmasking or induction of tics		Dexedrine: 5 mg t; 5, 10, 15 mg sustained-release spansules
Amphetamine compound	Same as for methylphenidate	ADHD	10–40	qd/bid	Possible induction or acceleration of mania or psychosis		Adderall: 5, 10, 20, 30 mg
Pemoline	Same as for methylphenidate	ADHD	37.5–112.5	qd	Same as other stimulants Abnormal liver function tests and serious hepatotoxity	Liver monitoring necessary Rarely used any more, given hepatotoxic concerns	Cylert: 18.75, 37.5, 75 t; 37.5 mg chewable t

ANTIDEPRESSANTS

Selective serotonin reuptake inhibitors (SSRIs)

Drug	Mechanism of Action	Main Indications and Clinical Uses	Dosage (mg/day)	Schedule	Adverse Effects	Comments	Select Brand Names and Preparations Available
Fluoxetine	Serotonin presynaptic reuptake blockade	OCD, Major depression, other anxiety disorders	2.5–40	qd	Irritability; akathisia; insomnia; appetite decrease (acute use) or increase (chronic) GI symptoms; headaches; dizziness; flu-like symptoms during discontinuation Complex drug interactions	Norfluoxetine metabolite has long half-life All SSRIs have variable degrees of CYP inhibition (see Chapter 5) Higher doses often-needed for OCD	Prozac: 10 mg t/c, 20 mg t; 20 mg/5 mL oral solution
Sertraline	Same as for fluoxetine	OCD, Major depression, other anxiety disorders	25–200	qd			Zoloft: 25, 50, 100 mg t
Paroxetine	Same as for fluoxetine	OCD, Major depression, other anxiety disorders	10–30	qd			Paxil: 10, 20, 30, 40 mg t; 10 mg/5 mL oral suspension
Fluvoxamine	Same as for fluoxetine	OCD, Major depression, other anxiety disorders	12.5–200	bid			Luvox: 25, 50, 100 mg t
Citalopram	Same as for fluoxetine	OCD, Major depression, other anxiety disorders	10–40	qd			Celexa: 20, 40 t; oral suspension

(continued)

APPENDIX: *Pediatric Psychopharmacogy at a Glance (continued)*

Drug	Mechanism of Action	Main Indications and Clinical Uses	Dosage (mg/day)	Schedule	Adverse Effects	Comments	Select Brand Names and Preparations Available
Tricyclic Antidepressants (TCAs)							
Imipramine	Norepinephrine > dopamine presynaptic reuptake blockade	Enuresis, ADHD, ADHD + tic disorders, anxiety disorders, MDD	2.5–5 mg/kg/day	qd/bid	Anticholinergic (dry mouth, constipation, blurred vision) Weight gain Cardiovascular (blood pressure and EKG conduction parameter changes, especially with daily doses > 3.5 mg/kg)	Serum levels can be useful in adjusting dosage, monitoring potential toxicity, and determining metabolizer status	Imipramine hydrochloride: 10, 25, 50 mg t Imipramine pamoate: 75, 100, 125, 150 mg c
Desipramine	Anticholinergic, antihistamine, α_1 postsynaptic effects	Same as for imipramine	2.5–5 mg/kg/day	qd/bid			Desipramine: 10, 25, 50, 75, 100, 150 mg t
Nortriptyline	Same as for imipramine	Same as for imipramine	2–3 mg/kg/day	qd/bid			Nortriptyline: 10, 25, 50, 75 mg
Clomipramine	Same as other TCAs; serotonin presynaptic reuptake blockade	Same as other TCAs, OCD	2–3 mg/kg/day	qd/bid	Treatment requires serum level and EKG monitoring		Clomipramine: 25, 50, 75 t
Other							
Bupropion	Unknown ?Norepinephrine > dopamine presynaptic reuptake blockade	MDD, ADHD	150–450 (single doses ≤ 150 mg)	tid	Irritability; insomnia Drug-induced seizures (in doses > 6 mg/kg) Contraindicated in bulimia	Useful alternative to stimulants in ADHD, but exacerbation of tics has been reported	Wellbutrin: 75, 100 mg t Wellbutrin SR: 100, 150 t
Venlafaxine	Serotonin/norepinephrine presynaptic reuptake blockade	MDD	1–3 mg/kg/day	bid/tid	Similar to SSRIs Nausea, sleepiness, dizziness Dose-dependent sustained diastolic hypertension	Under 150 mg/day, similar to a SSRI Noradrenergic effects at higher doses	Effexor: 25, 37.5, 50, 75, 100 mg t Effexor XR: 37.5, 75, 150 mg c
Trazodone	Serotonin presynaptic reuptake blockade/ 5-HT$_{2a}$ postsynaptic antagonism	Insomnia	25–200	qhs	Nausea, dry mouth, dizziness, constipation; orthostatic hypotension; sedation; priapism (trazodone only)	Nefazodone has less α antagonism than trazodone (i.e., less risk of hypotension and priapism) No pediatric data for trazodone	Trazodone: 50, 100, 150, 300 mg t
Nefazodone	Same as for trazodone	MDD, MDD + anxiety	50–300	bid	mCPP, an anxiogenic metabolite of nefazodone, can accumulate during CYP2D6 inhibition		Serzone: 50, 100, 150, 200, 250 mg t
Mirtazapine	α_2 presynaptic and 5HT$_{2A/3}$ postsynaptic antagonism	MDD	7.5–30	hs	Drowsiness (greater at low doses?) Appetite/weight gain	Useful alternative to SSRIs leading to activation?	Remeron: 7.5, 15 mg

(continued)

Drug	Mechanism	Indications	Dose	Schedule	Side effects	Notes	Preparations
Selegiline	B-selective monoamine oxidase inhibitor (MAOI-B)	ADHD in TS	10–15	bid (A.M., noon)	Hypertensive crisis may occur at higher doses with dietary (tyramine) transgression or with certain drugs; Nausea; dizziness; changes in blood pressure	B-selectivity is maintained at doses ≤ 10 mg/day (in theory allowing for less dietary restrictions)	Eldepryl: 5 mg

MOOD STABILIZERS

Drug	Mechanism	Indications	Dose	Schedule	Side effects	Notes	Preparations
Lithium	Inhibition of phosphatidyl inositol and protein kinase C signaling pathways; Enhancement of serotonergic transmission	Bipolar disorder, manic; prophylaxis of bipolar disorder; MDD; aggressive behavior, conduct disorder; adjunct treatment in refractory MDD	10–30 mg/kg/day Dose adjusted to serum levels in the range of 0.6–1.1 mgEq/L	bid/tid	Polyuria, polydipsia, tremor, ataxia, nausea, diarrhea, weight gain, drowsiness, acne, hair loss; Possible effects on thyroid and renal functioning with long-term administration; Children prone to dehydration are at higher risk for acute lithium toxicity; Lithium levels >2 mEq/L can be life threatening	Therapy requires monitoring of lithium levels, thyroid, and renal function	Lithium carbonate: 150, 300, 600 mg c; Lithium citrate elixir: 8 mEq (300 mg)/5 mL; Sustained-release forms: Lithobid; 300 mg t; Eskalith: 450 mg t
Divalproex	Inhibition of catabolic enzymes of GABA, and of protein kinase C signaling	Bipolar disorder, aggressive behavior, conduct disorder, seizure disorders	15–60 mg/kg/day Dose adjusted to serum levels in the range of 50–125 μg/L	bid/tid	Sedation, nausea, liver toxicity (requires baseline and close monitoring); Thrombocytopenia, pancreatitis	Policystic ovary syndrome has been reported during long term use for seizure control	Depakene (valproic acid): 250 mg; elixir Depakote (divalproex): 125, 250, 500 mg t; sprinkles; 125 mg c
Carbamazepine	Inhibition of glial steroidogenesis; Inhibition of α_2 receptors; Blocks sodium channels; Blocks glial calcium influx	Bipolar disorder, complex partial seizures	10–20 mg/kg/day Dose adjusted to serum levels in the range of 4–14 μg/L	bid	Bone marrow suppression (requires baseline and close monitoring of blood counts); Dizziness, drowsiness, rashes, nausea; Liver toxicity, especially under 10 years of age	Potent inductor of CYP3A4, leading to auto-induction requiring periodic dose adjustment	Tegretol: 100 mg chewable t; 200 mg; elixir, 100 mg/5 mL
Gabapentin	Gabapentin is chemically related to GABA, but its putative GABAergic effects are unclear		100–1000+	tid	Sedation, ataxia at high doses	Broad therapeutic index; Excreted renallly unchanged; No significant drug interactions	Neurontin: 100, 300, 400, 600, 300 mg c

(continued)

APPENDIX: *Pediatric Psychopharmacogy at a Glance (continued)*

Drug	Mechanism of Action	Main Indications and Clinical Uses	Dosage (mg/day)	Schedule	Adverse Effects	Comments	Select Brand Names and Preparations Available
Lamotrigine	Weak 5-HT$_3$ inhibition ?Release of aspartate and glutamate	Bipolar disorder, seizure disorders	75–300	qd	Potentially life-threatening rash Stevens-Johnson syndrome	Slow dose titration (12.5 mg qoWk) may reduce risk of skin reactions	Lamictal: 25, 100, 150, 200 mg t; 5, 25 mg chewable t
Topiramate	Glutamate release antagonist GABA reuptake inhibitor	Bipolar disorder, seizure disorders	50–400	bid	Cognitive difficulties (dulling, word retrieval, attention); dizziness, sedation	Weight loss may be a potentially beneficial side effect	Topamax: 25, 100, 200 mg t

ANTIPSYCHOTICS

Atypical antipsychotics

Drug	Mechanism of Action	Main Indications and Clinical Uses	Dosage (mg/day)	Schedule	Adverse Effects	Comments	Select Brand Names and Preparations Available
Risperidone	Dopamine and 5-HT receptor blockade 5-HT$_{2a}$/D$_2$ affinity ratio: 8:1	Psychosis: positive and negative symptoms; TS; augmentation in OCD; bipolar disorder; autism and PDDs; Aggression and agitation	0.25–4	qd/bid	Sedation; appetite increase; weight gain Low incidence of extrapyramidal adverse effects	—	Risperdal: 0.25, 0.5, 1, 2, 3, 4 mg t; 1 mg/mL elixir
Olanzapine	Dopamine and 5-HT receptor blockade 5-HT$_{2a}$/D$_2$ affinity ratio: 50:1	Same as risperidone	2.5–10	qd/bid	Same as for risperidone		Zyprexa: 2.5, 5, 7.5, 10 mg t
Quetiapine	Dopamine and 5-HT receptor blockade 5-HT$_{2a}$/D$_2$ affinity ratio: 1:1	Same as risperidone	100–600	qd/bid	Same as for risperidone Concerns over potential for cataract formation	—	Seroquel: 25, 100, 200 mg t
Ziprasidone	Dopamine and 5-HT receptor blockade	Same as risperidone	40–160	qd/bid	?Less likely to cause weight gain		Geodon: 20, 40 c
Clozapine	Dopamine and 5-HT receptor blockade 5-HT$_{2a}$/D$_2$ affinity ratio: 30:1	Treatment-refractory psychosis	50–400	bid/tid	Granulocytopenia; agranulocytosis (treatment requires constant monitoring of blood count) Higher risk of seizures (dose-related) Lower incidence of extrapyramidal adverse effects Low risk for tardive dyskinesia	Weekly blood counts (WBC > 3000) mandatory Possibility of going to qoWk monitoring by 6 months Seizure prophylaxis (with valproate or gabapentin) recommended at higher doses	Clozaril: 25, 100 mg t

Typical (Traditional) Antipsychotics

Phenothiazines: low potency

Drug	Mechanism	Indications	Dose range	Frequency	Side effects	Comments	Preparations
Chlorpromazine	D$_2$ receptor blockade	Psychosis, mania, aggressive behavior; agitation; self-injurious behavior; autism	25–400	qd/bid/tid	Anticholinergic (dry mouth, constipation, blurred vision, hypotension—more common with low-potency agents) Weight gain	A warning label from the FDA was introduced for thioridazine in 2000, advising against its use as a first-line drug, given concerns over QTc interval prolongation. Traditional agents are not as effective in treating negative or affective symptoms of psychosis Low-potency agents have high anticholinergic profiles (e.g., sedation, hypotension), whereas high-potency agents are likely to cause extrapyramidal side effects.	Chlorpromazine: 10, 25, 50, 100, 200 mg t; elixir; suppositories; injectable
Thioridazine	D$_2$ receptor blockade 95 mg = 100 mg chlorpromazine	Same as chlorpromazine	25–400	qd/bid/tid	Extrapyramidal reactions (dystonia, rigidity, tremor, akathisia, greater risk with higher potency) Drowsiness		Thioridazine: 10, 15, 25, 50, 100, 150, 200 mg t; elixir
Phenothiazines: medium and high potency							
Perphenazine	D$_2$ receptor blockade 8 mg = 100 mg chlorpromazine	Same as chlorpromazine	4–32	qd/bid/tid	Risk for tardive dyskinesia with long-term administration Withdrawal dyskinesia		Perphenazine: 2, 4, 8, 16 mg t; elixir, injectable
Fluphenazine	D$_2$ receptor blockade 2 mg = 100 mg chlorpromazine	Same as chlorpromazine	5–10	qd/bid/tid	Hypotension, especially when administered IM		Fluphenazine. 1, 2.5, 5, 10 mg; elixir, injectable, long-acting
Other traditional antipsychotics							
Haloperidol (high potency) (butyrophenone)	D$_2$ receptor blockade 2 mg = 100 mg chlorpromazine	Same as chlorpromazine	0.5–10	qd/bid/tid			Haloperidol: 0.5, 1, 2.5, 10, 20 mg t; elixir, injectable, long-acting
Thiothixene (medium potency) (thioxanthene)	D$_2$ receptor blockade 5 mg = 100 chlorpromazine	Same as chlorpromazine	1–20	qd/bid/tid		—	Thiothixene: 1, 2, 5, 10, 20 mg t; elixir, injectable
Molindone (medium potency) (indole derivative)	D$_2$ receptor blockade 10 mg = 100 mg chlorpromazine	Same as chlorpromazine	5–150	qd/bid/tid	Lowest weight gain liability among traditional agents		Molindone: 5, 10, 25, 50, 100 mg t; elixir
Pimozide (high potency)	D$_2$ receptor blockade 1 mg = 100 mg chlorpromazine	Same as other antipsychotics; TS	1–4	qd/bid/tid	Cardiac arrhythmias (EKG: elongated QTc); seizures Extrapyramidal reactions Drowsiness; tardive dyskinesia; withdrawal dyskinesia		Orap: 1, 2 mg t

(continued)

APPENDIX: *Pediatric Psychopharmacogy at a Glance (continued)*

ANTIANXIETY DRUGS

High-potency benzodiazepines

Drug	Mechanism of Action	Main Indications and Clinical Uses	Dosage (mg/day)	Schedule	Adverse Effects	Comments	Select Brand Names and Preparations Available
Clonazepam (long-acting)	Enhancement of GABAergic transmission via binding to a specific benzodiazepine site within the GABA$_a$ receptor	Anxiety disorders; adjunct in treatment-refractory psychosis and in mania; severe agitation; severe insomnia; MDD + anxiety akathisia	0.25–3	qd/bid	Drowsiness, disinhibition, agitation, confusion; depression Withdrawal reactions Potential risk for abuse and dependence Less risk for rebound and withdrawal reactions	—	Klonopin: 0.5, 1, 2 mg t
Alprazolam (short-acting)	Same as for clonazepam	Same as clonazepam	0.25–4	tid	Same as other benzodiazepines Higher risk for rebound and withdrawal reactions	—	Xanax: 0.25, 0.5, 1, 2 mg t
Lorazepam (short-acting)	Same as for clonazepam	Same as clonazepam	0.5–6	tid	Same as for alprazolam	Does not go through phase I reactions; good choice in the context of hepatic insufficiency	Ativan: 0.5, 1, 2 mg t; injectable

Atypical anxiolytic

Drug	Mechanism of Action	Main Indications and Clinical Uses	Dosage (mg/day)	Schedule	Adverse Effects	Comments	Select Brand Names and Preparations Available
Buspirone	5HT$_{1A}$ agonist	Anxiety disorders; adjunct in treatment-refractory OCD	15–60	tid	Drowsiness, disinhibition	No cross-tolerance with benzodiazepines	BuSpar: 5, 10, 15, 30 mg t

NORADERNERGIC AGENTS

Alpha agonists

Drug	Mechanism of Action	Main Indications and Clinical Uses	Dosage (mg/day)	Schedule	Adverse Effects	Comments	Select Brand Names and Preparations Available
Clonidine	Nonspecific α_2 presynaptic agonist	TS; ADHD; aggression/self-abuse; severe agitation; withdrawal symptoms	0.025–0.4	bid/tid/qid	Sedation (very frequent); hypotension (rare); dry mouth; irritability; dysphoria Rebound hypertension Localized irritation with transdermal preparation	Transdermal absorption can be erratic; limited bioavailability	Clonidine: 0.1, 0.2, 0.3 mg t Transdermal patch: Catapres TTS 1, 2, 3 (delivering 0.1, 0.2, 0.3 mg/day/week)
Guanfacine	Selective α_{2a} agonist	ADHD, TS	0.5–4	bid/tid	Same as clonidine Less sedation, hypotension		Tenex: 1, 2 mg t

Beta-blockers

Drug	Action/Class	Dose	Frequency	Adverse Effects/Comments	Formulations
Propranolol	Postsynaptic β blockade	2.0–8.0 mg/kg/d	bid	Akathisia; aggression; self-abuse; agitation	Similar to clonidine. Higher risk for bradycardia (dose dependent) and hypotension (dose dependent) and rebound hypertension	Propranolol: 10, 20, 40, 60, 80 mg t; 60, 80, 120, 160 mg long-acting t
Nadolol		20–200	bid		Bronchospasm (contraindicated in asthmatics). Rebound hypertension on abrupt withdrawal. Contraindicated in diabetics	Nadolol: 20, 40, 80, 120, 160 mg t

ANTIHISTAMINE, ANTICHOLINERGIC

Drug	Action/Class	Dose	Frequency	Adverse Effects/Comments	Formulations
Diphenhydramine	Antihistamine	12.5–100	tid/qid	Sleep disorders; agitation, acute dystonic reactions	Sedation, cognitive impairmaint, anticholergenic (dry mouth, constipation, blurred vision); delirium at high doses	Diphenhydramine: 25, 50 mg t; elixir, injectable
Benztropine	Anticholinergic (muscarinic)	0.5–3	bid/tid	Extrapyramidal reactions (dystonia, rigidity, tremor akathisia)	Same as for diphenhydramine	Benztropine: 0.5, 1, 1 mg; elixir, injectable

ANTIENURETIC

Drug	Action/Class	Dose	Frequency	Adverse Effects/Comments	Formulations
Desmopressin	Antidiuretic hormone analogue	10–40 μg	qhs/bid	Enuresis	Headache; nausea Hyponatremia and water intoxication at toxic doses	Can be useful for acute situations (e.g., sleepaways) or as maintenance treatment	DDAVP: 0.1, 0.2 mg t; nasal spray; 10 μg/spray
Oxybutynin	Antimuscarinic agent	5–15	bid/tid	Enuresis	Anticholinergic side effects	Ditropan: 5 mg t
Tolterodine	Antimuscarinic agent	1–2	bid	Enuresis	Less anticholinergic effects, less sedation	Detrol: 1 mg t

Note: Doses are provided as general guidelines only, and are not meant to be definitive. All doses must be individualized and monitored through appropriate clinical and/or laboratory means. ADHD, attention-deficit hyperactivity disorder; bid, twice daily; c, capsule; CYP, cytochrome P450; EKG, electrocardiogram; FDA, Food and Drug Administration; IM, intramuscular; MDD, major depressive disorder; OCD, obsessive-compulsive disorder; PDD, pervasive developmental disorder; qd, once daily; qhs, each bedtime; qoWk, every other week; t, tablet; tid, three times daily; TS, Tourette's syndrome; WBC, white blood cell count.

Index

Page numbers followed by f and t indicate figures and tables, respectively.

Aberrant Behavior Checklist, 413t, 566
Abnormal Involuntary Movement Scale, 566
Abuse
    child. *See* Child maltreatment
    substance. *See* Substance abuse and dependence disorders
Acetylcholine. *See also* Cholinergic systems
    in attention modulation, 101, 103, 104
    metabolism, 27
Acetylcholine receptors, nicotinic, 241
Acetylcholinesterase, 27
ACh. *See* Acetylcholine
ACTH. *See* Corticotropin
Active control equivalence studies, 719
Acute stress disorder, 580
Adderall. *See* Amphetamine compound
Addiction. *See* Substance abuse and dependence disorders
ADHD. *See* Attention-deficit/ hyperactivity disorder
Adolescents. *See* Children and adolescents
Adoption studies
    aggression, 218
    substance abuse and dependence disorders, 244–45
α_2-Adrenergic agonists, 264–71, 762t. *See also* Clonidine; Guanfacine
    for ADHD, 451t, 455
    for aggression, 678
    for autism and other pervasive developmental disorders, 572
    clinical use, 268–70
    neuropharmacology, 266–68
    for post-traumatic stress disorder, 585
    in preschoolers, 659–60, 660t
    for tic disorders, 168–69, 531–32, 534t
Adrenergic receptors
    α_1-, 28, 29f
    α_2-, 28, 29f
        anatomical distribution, 266
        regulatory properties, 265–66
        in substance abuse and dependence disorders, 243–44
        subtypes, 265, 265f
    antipsychotic drug blockade, 330–31
    ß-, 28, 29f

blockade. *See* Beta blockers
    subtypes, 353–54
    ß$_2$-, internalization, 37–38
    types, 265, 265f
Adrenocorticotropic hormone . *See* Corticotropin
Affect, in mental status examination, 398
Affective disorders. *See* Mood disorders
Affective syndrome, organic, 485
Affiliation, 195–206
    environmental factors, 204
    genetic determinants, 204
    neurobiology relevant to social abnormalities in autism, 204–6
    neurochemistry, 197–204
        dopamine, 203
        gonadal hormones, 201
        nitric oxide, 203–4
        norepinephrine, 203
        opioids and μ-opioid receptors, 201
        oxytocin, 197–99
        oxytocin receptors, 199–200
        prolactin, 200–201
        serotonin, 202–3
        steroids, 201–2
        vasopressin, 200
    neurocircuits and pathology
        amygdala, 196–97
        hippocampus, 197
        hypothalamic medial preoptic areas, 195–96
        limbic areas, 196–97
        other brain regions, 197
        paraventricular nucleus, 196
        ventral bed nucleus of the stria terminalis , 197
Age of onset
    in obsessive-compulsive disorder, 512
    in schizophrenia, childhood-onset, 187–88
Aggression, 210–20, 671–83
    in ADHD, 456, 673
    in adult jail detainees, 210
    in affective disorders, 673, 673f
    affective/impulsive, 212, 672t
    agitated/delirious state subtype, 672t, 674–75
    animal models, 212, 213t, 215, 219–20
    assessment algorithm, 675f

assessment of risk for violence, 682–83
    beta blockers for, 354–55
    in bipolar disorder, 673–74
    Child Behavior Checklist, 217
    in children and adolescents, 211, 671
    comorbid psychiatric disorders, 210, 211t
    in conduct disorder, 671
    definitions, 211–12, 671
    in depression, 673
    in developmental disabilities, 674
    dopamine system in, 216
    electrophysiology, 215–16
    environmental factors, 219–20
    in episodic dyscontrol syndrome, 674
    genetic studies, 217–19
    in inpatient adults, 210–11
    in intermittent explosive disorder, 674
    in intoxicated patient, 680–81
    legal considerations, 682–83
    lithium for, 311
    maternal, 203–4
    measurement, 211
    mental illness and, 671
    neuroanatomical studies, 212, 214
    neurobiology, 210–20
    neuroimaging studies, 214–15
    in neuropsychological deficits, 674
    neurotransmitters in, 216–17
    as nonspecific symptom, 734
    in obsessive-compulsive disorder, 673
    in post-traumatic stress disorder, 673
    predatory, 212, 672t
    prevalence, 210–11
    protective factors, 671, 672t
    psychopharmacotherapy, 675–82, 676t–677t
        α_2-adrenergic agonists, 678
        anticonvulsants, 679
        antidepressants, 678
        antihypertensives, 678
        antipsychotic drugs, 679–80
        anxiolytics, 678–79
        on as-needed (PRN) basis, 680
        beta blockers, 678
        in conjunction with seizures or delirium, 682
        developmental considerations, 682
        in emergency situations, 680–82, 681f

Aggression (*continued*)
  mood stabilizers, 679
  other drugs, 680
  SSRIs, 678
  stimulants, 677–78
  in psychosis, 674, 681–82
  risk factors, 671, 672t
  in schizophrenia, 674
  in seizure disorders, 674
  serotonin system in, 216–17, 218, 219–20
  in substance abuse, 674
  testosterone and gonadal steroids in, 216
  in tic disorders, 674
  treatment, 675
  types, 671, 672t
Agitation
  aggression and, 672t, 674–75
  delirium and, 682
  in seizure disorders, 674, 682
Akathisia, antipsychotic-induced, 334
Alarm system, for nocturnal enuresis, 692
Albumin, in children and adolescents, 50
Alcohol
  acute actions, 241
  chronic effects
    brain morphology, 243
    cerebral blood flow, metabolism, and function, 243
    gender differences, 243
    receptor studies, 243
  deprivation effect, 240
  teratogenic effects, 246
  use
    genetic studies, 244–45
    neuroanatomical substrates of reward, 239–40
    prevalence, 238
Alcoholism, dopamine receptor in, 87
Alertness, in mental status examination, 398
Allelic heterogeneity, 75
Alopecia, divalproex–induced, 318–19
Alprazolam, 343t, 762t
  for pain management, 634
  teratogenicity, 646
Alternative medicine. *See* Complementary and alternative medicine
Amantadine hydrochloride
  for aggression, 680
  for autism and other pervasive developmental disorders, 574–75
American College of Neuropsychopharmacology (ACNP), 738
Amisulpride, for schizophrenia, 553t, 554
Amitriptyline
  for anorexia nervosa, 597
  receptor blockade profile, 287t

Amnesia
  benzodiazepine-induced, 345
  retrograde, after electroconvulsive therapy, 380
AMPA glutamate receptor
  phosphorylation, 40
  receptor, 34
Amphetamine, 757t. *See also* Dextroamphetamine (Dexedrine); Stimulants
  abuse, 239, 260–61
  acute actions, 240
  for ADHD, 448, 449t
    history and overview, 255
    long-acting preparations, 257
    mechanism of action, 256
    pharmacokinetics and drug distribution, 256–57
  long-acting, 453
  neuronal adaptation to, 41
Amygdala
  in affiliative behaviors, 196–97
  in anxiety disorders, 142
  basolateral, 142
  in depression, 125, 128
  extended, in drug reward, 239
  during fear conditioning, 141, 142
  in schizophrenia, childhood-onset, 185–86
  sensitivity to innate fear cues, 143
Anal sphincter, 688
Androgen
  in aggression, 216
  in brain development, 15–16
  modification, for tic disorders, 533
  in tic disorders, 169–70
Anesthesia, in electroconvulsive therapy, 381–82
Animal models
  ADHD, 107
  aggression, 212, 213t, 215, 219–20
  anxiety disorders, 146–47
  drug withdrawal, 240
  early life stress
    primates, 115
    for psychopharmacological research, 119–20
    rodents, 113
  knockout, 77–79, 78f
  mania, 129–30
  schizophrenia, childhood-onset, 185
  substance abuse and dependence disorders, 240
  tic disorders, 171
Animal phobia, 140
Animal studies, in preclinical drug testing, 725
Anorexia nervosa, 224–34. *See also* Eating disorders
  assessment, 594–97, 594t–597t
  behavioral characteristics, 227
  binge eating in, 224, 592–93, 594
  bulimic subtype, 224

clinical phenomenology, 224–25, 592–94
cognitive-behavioral therapy, 599
comorbid psychiatric disorders and traits, 226–27
course of illness, 225
DSM-IV criteria, 592, 593t
etiology, 224
genetic studies, 225–26
hospitalization for, 600, 601
molecular genetics, 233–34
neuroimaging studies, 232–33, 232t
neurotransmitters in, 227–32, 229f
obsessive-compulsive disorder in, 595
outpatient treatment, 601
psychopharmacotherapy, 597–98
restrictor subtype, 224, 592
treatment guidelines, 600–601
Antabuse (disulfiram), for substance use disorders, 606, 612
Antibiotic prophylaxis, for postinfectious OCD and tic disorders, 180
Anticholinergic agents, 763t
  for nocturnal enuresis, 693
  for schizophrenia, during pregnancy, 649
Anticipation, mutation and, 75
Anticonvulsants
  for aggression, 679
  for mood disorders, 312–23
  new (third-generation), 319–23
  for post-traumatic stress disorder, 588
  teratogenicity, 645
Antidepressants, 757t–758t. *See also specific drugs*
  for ADHD, 449t–451t, 453–56
  for aggression, 678
  atypical, 295–306
  for bipolar depression, 472–73
  for bulimia nervosa, 598
  discontinuation, 476
  for etiologically unexplained syndromes, 637
  with lithium, 475
  for major depressive disorder with mental retardation, 623–24
  monoamine oxidase inhibitors as, 295–300. *See also* Monoamine oxidase inhibitors
  neuronal adaptation to, 39–40, 41, 42
  in preschoolers, 661–62, 661t–662t
  for self-injury in mental retardation, 626
  SSRIs as, 274–80. *See also* Selective serotonin reuptake inhibitors
  teratogenicity, 643–44
  tricyclic. *See* Tricyclic antidepressants use of, in Europe, 748–49
Antiepileptic drugs, teratogenicity, 645
Antihistamines, 348–49, 763t
  for anxiety disorders, 349, 502
  central nervous system effects, 348
  in children and adolescents, 349

drug interactions, 348
history, 348
mechanism, 348
pharmacokinetics and drug distribution, 348
pharmacological profile, 348
side effects and toxicity, 348–49
Antihypertensives, for aggression, 678
Antineuronal antibodies, in pathogenesis of OCD and tic disorders, 171, 178
Antipsychotic drugs, 328–37. *See also specific drugs*
α-adrenergic receptor blockade by, 330–31
for ADHD, 456
adverse effects, 331t, 333–36
for aggression, 679–80
for anorexia nervosa, 597
anticholinergic effects, 335
atypical, 328, 329t, 760t
for autism and other pervasive developmental disorders, 567, 568–69
indications, 551
for schizophrenia, 547–48, 550t, 551, 552t–553t
for tic disorders, 528t, 529–30
cardiovascular effects, 335
classification, 547–48
cytochrome P450 metabolism, 332–33, 333t
dermatologic effects, 335
dopamine receptor blockade by, 330
drug interactions, 332–33
endocrine effects, 335
extrapyramidal side effects, 333–34
galactorrhea from, 694
hematological effects, 336
histaminergic receptor blockade by, 331
liver dysfunction from, 334–35
for mania in adults, 489
mechanism of action, 329–32
muscarinic receptor blockade by, 330
ocular effects, 335–36
pediatric use strategy, 336–37
pharmacokinetics, 332
potency, 328, 329t
in preschoolers, 662–64, 663t
response to, dopamine-related alleles in, 87
for schizophrenia, 190, 547–56
decision tree for, 554, 555f
depot, 556
effects and side effects, 549t–550t
guidelines, 556
indications and contraindications, 548
with mental retardation, 625
during pregnancy, 648–49
prevention of relapses, 556
sedation from, 335

seizures from, 334
for self-injury in mental retardation, 626
serotonin receptor blockade by, 330
sexual side effects, 335
for substance use disorders with psychotic symptoms, 614
teratogenicity, 645–46
typical, 328, 329t, 761t
limitations, 328
for schizophrenia, 547–48, 549t–550t
for tic disorders, 527–29, 528t
weight gain from, 334, 336, 530
Anxiety disorders, 497–507
with ADHD, 456–57
animal models, 146–47
antihistamines for, 349
assessment, 409t, 497–500
clinician-rated measures, 498–99
diagnostic interviews, 497–98
observational methods, 499–500
physiological methods, 499–500
questions and answers used in, 498t
self-report rating scales, 499
beta blockers for, 355
brain systems in, 141–47
in cancer patient, 636
cognitive-behavioral therapy
with anxiolytics, 506–7
effectiveness, 504
family-based, 505–6
group, 505
individual, 504–5
limitations, 504
strategies, 504
combination therapy, 506–7
with depression, 476
with depression and school refusal, 432
DSM-IV criteria, 497
early life stress and, 118–19, 145–46
early-onset
clinical characteristics, 138
neurobiology, 138–47
fear systems in, 141–45, 141t
fear conditioning experiments, 141–43
innate fear-producing stimuli, 143–45
pharmacological fear probes, 145
physiological fear probes, 144–45
social fear probes, 143–44
generalized, 139
with mental retardation, 620
pediatric drug development in, 730
hippocampal atrophy and, 146–47
hypothalamic-pituitary-adrenal axis in, 140–41, 145, 146
ICD-10 criteria, 750
informants, 405t
with mental retardation, 619–20

obsessive-compulsive disorder as. *See* Obsessive-compulsive disorder
panic disorder as. *See* Panic disorder
phenomenology, 138–41
phobias as. *See* Phobia
post-traumatic stress disorder as. *See* Post-traumatic stress disorder
during pregnancy, 649
psychopharmacotherapy, 500–503, 507t
benzodiazepines, 502
buspirone, 502
with cognitive-behavioral therapy, 506–7
medication dosing, 500t, 503
other doubtful treatments, 502–3
other potential treatments, 502
SSRIs, 500–501
tricyclic antidepressants, 501–2
psychosocial treatment, 503–6
self-monitoring procedures, 499
separation, 139–40, 291
social, 138–39
with substance abuse and dependence disorders, 613
tic disorders and, 170
treatment options, 506–7, 507t
Anxiety Disorders Interview Schedule for Children, 498
Anxiolytics, 341–50, 762t
for aggression, 678–79
benzodiazepine. *See* Benzodiazepines
with cognitive-behavioral therapy, 506–7
nonbenzodiazepine, 346–50. *See also specific drugs, e.g.,* buspirone
Apathy, from SSRIs, 276
Appearance, in mental status examination, 397
Appetite, increased, divalproex–induced, 318
antipsychotic-induced, 334, 336, 530
Arginine-vasopressin. *See* Vasopressin
Arousal
attention and, 101, 103, 104
emotional, in tic disorders/Tourette's syndrome, 170
Ascending arousal systems, in attention, 101, 103
Asians
CYP2C19 polymorphisms, 62
CYP2D6 polymorphisms, 62
Asperger's syndrome, 564
Assessment for pharmacotherapy, 391–402
clinical interview, 396–97
clinical management, 400, 400t
compliance issues, 401
confidentiality, 401
decision making, 398–99
developmental and family history, 397
developmental history questionnaire, 392f–396f

Assessment for pharmacotherapy (*cont.*)
electrocardiographic, 399
follow-up visits, 401–2
identification of problem hierarchy,
399–400
information sources, 391, 396
informed consent, 401
instruments. *See* Instruments and
scales
laboratory testing, 399
language ability, 399
mental status examination, 397–98
neurological consultation or testing,
399
outcome evaluation, 400–401
therapeutic alliance, 398
treatment plan, 399–400, 400t
Association cortex, 20, 21f
sensory, in attentional processing, 99–
100, 103
Association studies
eating disorders, 233–34
neuropsychiatric disorders
of dopamine-related alleles, 86–87
methodology, 86
of serotonin-related alleles, 88–90
schizophrenia, childhood-onset, 189
tic disorders, 169
Ativan. *See* Lorazepam
Atomoxetine, 294
for ADHD, 455
in children and adolescents, 306
history, 305
mechanism of action, 305
pharmacokinetics and drug
distribution, 305
side effects and toxicity, 305–6
Attachment. *See* Affiliation
Attention
arousal and, 101, 103, 104
brain systems mediating, 99–101,
100f
ascending arousal systems, 101, 103
inferior temporal cortex, 99–100
posterior parietal cortex, 100, 103
prefrontal cortex, 100–101, 103
sensory association cortex, 99–100,
103
subcortical, 101
cortical pathways, 99–101, 100f
deficit
with hyperactivity. *See* Attention-
deficit/hyperactivity disorder
in other neuropsychiatric disorders
of childhood, 107
neuromodulators of
acetylcholine, 101, 103, 104
dopamine, 101, 103
norepinephrine, 101, 103–4
possible mechanisms, 102f
relation to arousal, motivation, and
stress, 104
serotonin, 104

stimulants, 104
subcortical pathways, 101
Attention-deficit/hyperactivity disorder,
447–60
in adults, 447
with aggression, 456, 673
animal models, 107
with anxiety, 456–57
assessment and evaluation, 447–48
assessment instruments, 409t
with bipolar disorder, 457, 493
combination therapy, 432–34, 457
with depression, 457, 475–76
dopamine in
genetic studies, 86–87, 106
imaging studies, 105–6
DSM-IV criteria, 104
in Europe, diagnosis and treatment,
749
genetic studies, 86–87, 106
geographic prevalence, 447
imaging studies
functional, 105
neuroreceptor, 105–6
structural, 105
informants, 404, 405t
mental retardation with, 619
monoamine oxidase inhibitors for,
299, 449t–450t, 454–55
MTA study, 433–34, 458–59
neurobiology, 99–107
pediatric drug development in, 731–32
pindolol for, 354–55
psychopharmacotherapy, 448–56, 449t–
451t
antidepressants, 449t–451t, 453–56
antipsychotics, 456
bupropion, 450t, 454
buspirone, 455–56
cholinergic drugs, 456
controversies in, 459–60
current levels, 705–6
and modulation of attentional
circuits, 102f, 106–7
monoamine oxidase inhibitors, 449t–
450t, 454–55
α₂-noradrenergic agonists, 451t, 455
noradrenergic-specific compounds,
455
over- vs. underprescribing practices,
708–9
psychiatric comorbidity and, 456–57
SSRIs, 450t, 455
stimulants, 255–61, 448, 449t, 450–
53
time trends, 702–4
treatment algorithm, 452t
tricyclic antidepressants, 449t, 453–
54
venlafaxine, 450t, 455
psychosocial treatment, 457–59
cognitive-behavioral approach, 458–
59

operant procedures, 457–58
scales, 448
substance abuse and dependence
disorders with, 613
subtypes, 447
with tic disorders, 165–66
prevalence, 526
stimulants for, 452–53, 535
treatment, 535–37
tricyclic antidepressants for, 454
tricyclic antidepressants for, 291, 449t,
453–54
Attention-Deficit/Hyperactivity Disorder
Rating Scale, 413t
Autism
assessment and evaluation, 565–67
diagnostic instruments, 565
medical work-up, 565–66
psychological work-up, 566
rating scales, 566–67
symptom severity and measurement
of change, 566–67
clinical features, 563–64
comorbid psychiatric disorders, 564
differential diagnosis, 565
in Japanese population, 753
pharmacotherapy, 567–76
α₂-adrenergic agonists, 572
atypical antipsychotics, 568–69
early studies, 567–68
glutamatergic compounds, 574, 576
mirtazapine, 573–74
naltrexone, 357–58
neuroimmune therapies, 576
recent studies, 568–72, 573t–574t
secretin, 572–73
SSRIs, 569–72
stimulants, 572
treatment algorithm for, 575f
tricyclic antidepressants, 291–92
serotonin transporter polymorphism
in, 89
social abnormalities in
opioids in, 206
oxytocin in, 204–5
serotonin in, 205–6
symptoms and criteria, 204
Autism Diagnostic Interview–Revised
(ADI-R), 565
Autoimmune neuropsychiatric disorders,
postinfectious. *See* PANDAS
Autonomic functioning, in
schizophrenia, childhood-onset,
187
Autonomy principle, 380, 738
Axon, 21, 22f
growth and remodeling, 12f, 13
Azapirones, pharmacological profile, 346

Baclofen, for tic disorders, 533–34, 534t
Basal forebrain, cholinergic neurons, 26
Basal ganglia, 20, 21f
functional model, 153–55, 154f

in obsessive-compulsive disorder, 153–55, 154f, 159–60
in postinfectious OCD and tic disorders, 178–79, 179f
striosomes and matrices (matriosomes) in, 155, 156f
in tics and stereotypies, 166, 167f
Basal telencephalon, progenitor cells, 11
Base-state dependency, 408
Bayesian forecasting, in therapeutic drug monitoring, 51–52, 52f
Behavior
activation, from SSRIs, 276, 522
affiliative. See Affiliation
disinhibition, benzodiazepine-induced, 345
in eating disorders, 227
inhibition, social phobia and, 139
maternal. See Maternal behavior
in mental status examination, 398
problems. See also Conduct disorder
in mental retardation, 617
in obsessive-compulsive disorder, 520–21
stereotyped, in obsessive-compulsive disorder, 160–61
suicidal, 476
Behavioral Approach Task (BAT), 499–500
Behavioral teratogenicity, 642
Behavioral therapy. See also Cognitive-behavioral therapy
for ADHD, 457–58
for nocturnal enuresis, 692
for obsessive-compulsive disorder, 514–15
The Belmont Report, 738
Beneficence principle, 380, 738
Benzodiazepines, 341–46
for acute behavioral control of aggression, 680
for anticipatory nausea, 635
for anxiety disorders, 502
in children and adolescents, 345
discontinuation, 346
drug interactions, 344
history, 341
long-term considerations, 345–46
major effects, 341
mechanism of action, 341
for pain management, 634
partial agonists, 344
pharmacokinetics and drug distribution, 342–43, 343t
pharmacological profile, 341–42
for post-traumatic stress disorder, 587–88
premedication workup, 345
for schizophrenia during pregnancy, 649
selection considerations, 343–44
side effects and toxicity, 344–45

structure, 342f
teratogenicity, 646
Benztropine, 763t
teratogenicity, 646
Best Pharmaceuticals for Children Act (BPCA), pediatric exclusivity provisions, 728
Beta blockers, 353–56, 763t
and α₂-adrenergic agonists, 269–70
adult psychiatric indications, 353
for aggression, 678
rage outbursts, and other externalizing behaviors, 354–55
for anxiety disorders, 355
for autism and other pervasive developmental disorders, 568
contraindications, 356
dosage, 355–56
drug interactions, 356
mechanism of action, 353–54
monitoring, 356
overdose, 356
pediatric uses, 354–56
pharmacology, 354
for self-injury in mental retardation, 626–27
side effects and toxicity, 356
Bicoid gene, 4, 5f
Binge drinking, definition, 238
Binge eating
in anorexia nervosa, 224, 592–93, 594
in eating disorders, 224
Binge eating disorder, 592
Bioethics Advisory Commission, 738
Bipolar disorders, 484–94
with ADHD, 457, 493
in adults, neurobiology, 129–30
assessment and evaluation, 486–88
mental status examination, 488
rating scales, 486, 487
screening, 486
structured interviews, 486–87
assessment instruments, 410t
comorbid psychiatric disorders, 484–85
psychopharmacotherapy, 493
definitions, 486
depressive component of, 472–73
diagnostic hospitalization, 493
divalproex for, 319
dopaminergic genes in, 87
DSM-IV criteria, 484, 485t
electroconvulsive therapy, 378
family studies, 485–86
informants, 405t
late-onset, classical presentation, 484
lithium for, 311
maintenance treatment, 493–94
mania in. See Mania
mental retardation with, 621–22
neurobiology, 129–31
neuroimaging studies, 131
neurotrophic factors in, 130

not otherwise specified, 486, 491, 492–93
phenomenology and differential diagnosis, 484–86
and post-traumatic stress disorder, 674
during pregnancy, 648
prevalence, 129
substance abuse and dependence disorders with, 493, 613–14
treatment, 488–94
controlled studies in adults, 488–89
general considerations, 488
inpatient studies, 489–90
outpatient studies, 490–91
utility of preclinical models of mania, 129–30
Bipolarity spectrum, 484, 491
Birth weight, tic disorders and, 170
Bladder
dysfunction. See Enuresis
function, mechanisms, 686–89, 687f
Bleeding complications, from SSRIs, 277
Blood phobia, 140
Body fat, drug distribution and, 49
Body Shape Questionnaire, 596t
Body water, total, drug distribution and, 49–50
Bone morphogenetic protein, 6
Botulinum, for tic disorders, 533, 534t
Bowel
dysfunction. See Encopresis
function, mechanisms, 687f, 689
program, for constipation, 692, 694f
Brain
blood flow. See Cerebral blood flow
development, 3–16
apoptosis, 12
cerebral diversification and expansion, 8, 9f, 10, 10f
critical periods, 14
electroconvulsive therapy and, 380
future applications related to, 16
neuronal and synaptic remodeling, 12–14, 12f
neuronal migration in cerebral cortex, 10–12, 11f
neuronal regeneration in adult, 15
organizer regions, 6, 7f, 8
patterning, 3–4, 5f
regional diversification, 4, 6, 6f
sexual dimorphism, 15–16
imaging studies. See Neuroimaging studies
lesions, obsessive-compulsive disorder and, 151
metabolism. See Cerebral metabolism
neural circuitry, 20–23, 21f–22f
neurotransmitter systems, 23–31
structural abnormalities. See Neuroanatomical studies
Brain-derived neurotrophic factor, tricyclic antidepressants and, 285–86

Brainstem
  cholinergic neurons, 26
  serotonergic neurons, 27
Breast-feeding, SSRIs during, 278
Brief Psychiatric Rating Scale, 413t
Bulimia nervosa, 224–34. *See also*
        Eating disorders
  assessment, 594–97, 594t–597t
  behavioral characteristics, 227
  binge eating in, 224
  clinical phenomenology, 225, 594
  cognitive-behavioral therapy, 599–600
  comorbid psychiatric disorders and
        traits, 226–27
  course of illness, 225
  DSM-IV criteria, 592, 593t
  etiology, 224
  genetic studies, 225–26
  hospitalization for, 600–601
  molecular genetics, 233–34
  neurotransmitters in, 227–32, 229f
  outpatient treatment, 601
  psychopharmacotherapy, 598–99
  purging vs. nonpurging subtypes, 225
  restrictor subtype, 592
  substance abuse in, 595
  treatment guidelines, 600–601
Bupropion, 302–4, 758t
  for ADHD, 450t, 454
    tic disorders and, 536
  in children and adolescents, 303
  history, 302
  for major depressive disorder, 470
  mechanism of action, 302–3
  for post-traumatic stress disorder, 588
  side effects and toxicity, 303
  for substance use disorders, 607, 611,
        612
    with ADHD, 610, 613
    with depression, 613
Buspirone, 762t
  for ADHD, 455–56
  for aggression, 678–79
  for anxiety disorders, 500t, 502
  for autism and other pervasive
        developmental disorders, 568
  in children and adolescents, 347
  discontinuation, 348
  drug interactions, 347
  history, 346
  labeling changes, 730
  for mental retardation with
        generalized anxiety, 620
  pharmacokinetics and drug
        distribution, 347
  pharmacological profile, 346
  for post-traumatic stress disorder, 587
  premedication workup, 348
  side effects and toxicity, 347
  structure, 346f

Calcium, effects on G protein–coupled
        receptors, 36–37

Calcium-calmodulin-dependent kinase II,
        in aggression, 218
Calcium channel blockers, for mania,
        489
Cancer patient, psychopharmacological
        considerations, 636–37
Cannabinoid receptors, 241–42
Cannabis
  acute actions, 241–42
  chronic effects
    brain morphology, 244
    receptor studies, 244
  teratogenic effects, 247
Carbamazepine, 312, 314–17, 759t
  for aggression, 679
  for bipolar disorders, 490
    mental retardation, 621
    during pregnancy, 648
  congenital malformations from, 315
  dermatologic effects, 316
  dosage and administration, 316–17
  hematological effects, 315
  liver toxicity, 316
  for mania, 489, 490
  mechanism of action, 312
  neurological effects, 315
  overdose and toxicity, 316
  pediatric uses, 316
  pharmacokinetics, 312, 314–15
  for post-traumatic stress disorder, 588
  side effects, 315–16
  teratogenicity, 645
  treatment guidelines, 313t
Cardiovascular effects
  antipsychotic drugs, 335
  lithium, 311
  tricyclic antidepressants, 288, 290t,
        291t
Catatonia, electroconvulsive therapy for,
        378
Caucasians, CYP2D6 polymorphisms, 62
Caudate nucleus
  in ADHD, 105
  in postinfectious OCD and tic
        disorders, 178–79, 179f
  in regulation of attention, 101
  in tics and stereotypies, 166
Celexa. *See* Citalopram
Cell adhesion molecules, in neuronal
        remodeling, 13
Cell body, 21, 22f
Cell cycle, cortical neurogenesis, 9f, 10
Central nervous system. *See also* Brain
  alcoholism effects on, gender
        differences, 243
  antihistamine effects on, 348
  development, overview, 3–16
  organizer cells, 6, 7f, 8
  patterning, in vertebrates, 4, 5f
Central serotonin syndrome, 278–79,
        278t
  agents implicated in, 63t, 64, 278t
  manifestations, 63–64, 278t

from monoamine oxidase inhibitors,
        298
Cerebellum
  in ADHD, 105
  glutamatergic neurons, 23
  in regulation of attention, 101
Cerebral blood flow
  in ADHD, 105
  in aggression, 215
  in alcoholism, 243
  in depression, 128
Cerebral cortex
  diversification and expansion, 8, 9f,
        10, 10f
  neuronal and synaptic remodeling, 12–
        14, 12f
  neuronal migration, 10–12, 11f
Cerebral metabolism
  in ADHD, 105
  in alcoholism, 243
Chemical dependency. *See* Substance
        abuse and dependence disorders
Chemical transmission. *See*
        Neurotransmitter(s); Signal
        transduction
Child/Adolescent Impact of Events Scale,
        581
Child and Adolescent Services
        Assessment, 716
Child and Adolescent Trauma Screen,
        581
Child Behavior Checklist, 413t, 751
  in aggression, 217
  in mania, 486
Child maltreatment
  assessment considerations, 120
  definition, 110
  prevalence, 110–11
  relationship to drug use, 245
  relationship to psychopathology, 111
Child Post-Traumatic Stress Disorder
        Checklist, 581
Child psychiatry
  in Europe
    diagnostic and assessment
        instruments, 749–51
    historical perspective, 746
    rating scales, 751
  in Japan
    diagnostic and assessment
        instruments, 752
    historical perspective, 751–52
    rating scales, 752–53
Child Stress Reaction Checklist, 581–82
Child Symptom Inventory, 486
Childhood Anxiety Sensitivity
        Instrument, 413t
Childhood Autism Rating Scale, 435
Childhood disintegrative disorder, 564
Children and Adolescent Psychiatric
        Assessment, 546–47, 546t
Children and adolescents. *See also*
        Preschoolers

abuse of. *See* Child maltreatment
depression in
  early life stress and, 125–26
  neurobiology, 124–29
  neuroimaging studies, 126–29, 127t
drug development in. *See* Pediatric
    drug development; Research in
    children
medically ill. *See* Medically ill child or
    adolescent
pharmacokinetics in, 48–52. *See also*
    Pharmacokinetics
psychiatric disorders in. *See also*
    specific disorders
  prevalence, 701
psychopharmacotherapy for. *See*
    Psychopharmacotherapy,
    pediatric; *specific drugs*
Children's Depression Inventory, 413t
Children's Depression Rating Scale,
    413t, 466
Children's Global Assessment Scale , 466
  in clinical trials, 716
  in schizophrenia, 546t, 547
Children's Interview for Psychiatric
    Syndromes, 412
Children's Psychiatric Rating Scale, 546t,
    547
Children's Yale-Brown Obsessive-
    Compulsive Scale, 413t, 435,
    513–14
  in anxiety disorders, 498
  in autism and other pervasive
    developmental disorders, 566,
    567
Chloral hydrate, for pain management,
    633
Chlordiazepoxide, 343t
Chlorpromazine, 329t, 761t
  for acute behavioral control of
    aggression, 680
  for anorexia nervosa, 597
  for anticipatory nausea, 635–36
Cholecystokinin, in eating disorders, 229–
    30
Cholinergic drugs
  for ADHD, 456
  for tic disorders, 532
Cholinergic interneurons, role of, in
    cortical-striatal-thalamo-cortical
    loops, 155
Cholinergic receptors, 26–27, 26f
Cholinergic systems, 26–27. *See also*
    Acetylcholine
  abnormalities, 27
  anatomy, 26
  function, 27
  synaptic organization, 26–27, 26f
  in tic disorders/Tourette's syndrome,
    168
Chromosome(s). *See also* DNA; Gene(s)
  abnormalities, in schizophrenia,
    childhood-onset, 188–89

structure, 69
  translocation, 75
Cigarette smoking. *See* Tobacco use
Cimetidine, and benzodiazepines, 344
Citalopram, 757t
  adverse effects, 275–79
  cytochrome P450 inhibition by, 277,
    277t
  general properties, 274–75, 275t
  indications, 274, 275t
  for obsessive-compulsive disorder,
    519t
  pharmacokinetic studies in children,
    469
Clinical assessment. *See* Assessment for
    pharmacotherapy
Clinical Global Impression Scale, 412
  in autism and other pervasive
    developmental disorders, 566
  in obsessive-compulsive disorder, 514
Clinical instruments. *See* Instruments
    and scales
Clinical interview, in assessment for
    pharmacotherapy, 396–97
Clinical management, in assessment for
    pharmacotherapy, 400, 400t
Clinical significance, and statistical
    significance, 721, 721f
Clinical trials. *See also* Research in
    children
  common designs, 719–20
  comparison groups, 717–19
  protocol implementation, 721–22
  research questions, 712–15
  safety monitoring, 722
  sample size, 720–21
  statistical significance and clinical
    significance, 721, 721f
  steps, 713t–714t
  study sample, 715
  superiority and noninferiority studies,
    719
  treatment outcomes, 715–17
Clinician-Administered PTSD Scale–
    Child and Adolescent Version,
    582
Clomipramine, 758t
  for aggression, 678
  for anorexia nervosa, 597–98
  for anxiety disorders, 500, 502
  for autism and other pervasive
    developmental disorders, 569–
    70
  electrocardiogram indices for, 520
  for obsessive-compulsive disorder,
    515, 519, 519t, 522
    during pregnancy, 649
    combined with a SSRI, 522
  receptor blockade profile, 287t
  side effects, 522
  for treatment-resistant depression, 475
Clonazepam, 343t, 762t
  in obsessive-compulsive disorder, 522

Clonidine, 264–71, 762t
  for ADHD, 451t, 455
    tic disorders and, 535–36
  adverse effects, 268, 531
  for aggression, 678
  for anxiety disorders, 502
  for autism and other pervasive
    developmental disorders, 572
  binding properties, 266
  cardiovascular safety, 455
  chemical structure, 266, 266f
  clinical use, 268–70
  contraindications, 269
  discontinuation, 269
  dosage and administration, 268
  drug interactions, 269–70
    with methylphenidate, 258, 270
  monitoring, 269
  neuropharmacology, 266–68
  pediatric uses, 264
  pharmacokinetic and
    pharmacodynamic properties,
    266–67
  pharmacological activity, 267–68
  for post-traumatic stress disorder, 585
  premedication workup, 269
  in preschoolers, 659–60, 660t
  for tic disorders, 168–69, 531–32,
    534t
  transdermal, 268, 531–32
Clorgyline, mechanism of action, 297
Clozapine, 329t, 760t
  agranulocytosis from, 336
  for autism and other pervasive
    developmental disorders, 568
  for bipolar disorders, 491
  indications, 328
  for mania, 489
  response to
    dopamine-related alleles in, 87
    serotonin receptor polymorphisms
      in, 90–91, 90t, 91t
  for schizophrenia, 551, 552t
    with mental retardation, 625
  seizures from, 334
  for self-injury in mental retardation,
    626
  teratogenicity, 645, 646
  for tic disorders, 529
Cocaine
  acute actions, 240
  chronic effects
    brain morphology, 242
    cerebral blood flow, metabolism,
      and function, 243
    receptor studies, 242
  neuroanatomical substrates of reward,
    239
  neuronal adaptation to, 41
  teratogenic effects, 247
Codon, 69
Cognitive-behavioral therapy
  for ADHD, 458–59

Cognitive-behavioral therapy (*continued*)
for anxiety disorders
with anxiolytics, 506–7
effectiveness, 504
family-based, 505–6
group, 505
individual, 504–5
limitations, 504
strategies, 504
cognitive strategies, 504
combined with
psychopharmacotherapy. *See*
Combined drug and
psychosocial treatments
for eating disorders, 599–600
in medical context, 428
for obsessive-compulsive disorder, 514–15
for post-traumatic stress disorder, 582–83, 589
for schizophrenia, 556–57
Cognitive deficits
from electroconvulsive therapy, 379–80
in obsessive-compulsive disorder, 153
Cohen's effect size, 720–21
Colorectal sphincter, 688
Columbia Impairment Scale, 412
Combined drug and psychosocial
treatments, 426–41
clinical issues, 434–37
developmental issues, 437
disease management model, 427
dose-response and time-response
issues, 436
evidence-based approach, 428–34
importance of differential therapeutics,
434–35
literature on, 426–27
medical framework for, 427–28
methodological issues, 434
multidisciplinary approach, 428
outcome evaluation, 436–37
practice guidelines, 437–38, 439f–440f
psychoeducation and, 437
rating scales, 435
rationale, 427–28
tailored treatment, 435–36
Communication. *See* Speech and
language
Community collaborations, research in
children and, 743
Comparison group, in clinical trials, 717–19
Complementary and alternative
medicine, 365–74
attitudes of mental health
professionals toward, 366
extent of use, 365–66
Internet sites, 367
liability, 367, 367t
regulatory and ethical issues, 366–67
Compliance issues
in assessment for pharmacotherapy,
401

in medically ill child or adolescent, 632
parental, 421–22
Compulsions. *See also* Obsessive-
compulsive disorder
common, 175
definition, 150
in eating disorders, 225, 227
Concerta. *See* Methylphenidate
Conditional knockouts, 79
Conditioning approaches
for ADHD, 457–58
for nocturnal enuresis, 692
for obsessive-compulsive disorder, 514–15
Conduct disorder
aggression in, 671
comorbidity with bipolar disorder,
673–74
assessment instruments, 409t
depressive, 750
ICD-10 criteria, 750
informants, 405t
lithium for, 311
mental retardation with, 622–23
pediatric drug development in, 732
Confidence intervals, sample size and,
721, 722f
Confidentiality
in assessment for pharmacotherapy,
401
in pediatric research, 742–43
Congenital malformations
carbamazepine-induced, 315
incidence, 642
Conners' Global Index, 413t
Conners-Wells Adolescent Self-Report,
413t
Conscious sedation, 633
Constipation
bowel program for, 692, 694f
relationship to enuresis, 690
Content validity, 407
Contingency management, in cognitive-
behavioral therapy, 504
Contralateral neglect, 100
Control group. *See also* Placebo
in clinical trials, 717–19
Coping Cat program, in anxiety
disorders, 504
Cortical neurons, generation, 8, 9f, 10,
10f
Cortical-striatal-thalamo-cortical loops
in obsessive-compulsive disorder, 152–53, 153–55, 154f, 158f
in tics and stereotypies, 166, 167f
Corticotropin
in anxiety disorders, 118, 146
early life stress and, 113, 115, 116
Corticotropin-releasing factor
in affiliative behaviors, 201–2
in anxiety disorders, 118, 146
in depression, 117–18, 125–26
early life stress and, 113, 115, 116
in eating disorders, 228

ontogeny, 113
in stress response, 111–13, 112f
in substance abuse and dependence
disorders, 242, 246
Corticotropin-releasing factor
antagonists, for prevention or
reversal of early life stress
consequences, 119
Cortisol
in affiliative behaviors, 201–2
in depression, 117–18, 125–26
CREB (*cAMP response element binding*
protein)
phosphorylation
by Protein Kinase A, 35, 36f
regulation, 40
regulation, 40–41
tricyclic antidepressants and, 285–86
up-regulation, by antidepressants, 36
Critical periods, brain development, 14
Crossover study design, 719
Cumulative distribution curve, 717, 718f
Cyclic AMP pathway, G protein–coupled
receptors, 35–36, 36f
Cyclic AMP response element–binding
protein. *See* CREB
Cylert. *See* Pemoline
CYP. *See* Cytochrome P450
Cyproheptadine
for anorexia nervosa, 597
for post-traumatic stress disorder, 587
Cyproterone, for tic disorders, 534
Cytochrome P450
activation, by St. John's wort, 370–71
antipsychotic substrates, 332–33, 333t
developmental aspects, 50–51
drug interactions, 56–65
drug factors, 60
host factors, 60
mechanism, 58
table, 60, 61t–62t
ethnic differences, 753
genetic polymorphisms, 60, 62–63
hepatic, characteristics, 57, 57t
induction, 59–60
inhibition
and clearance of drugs metabolized
by liver, 59
P-glycoprotein and CYP3A as
partners in, 59
by SSRIs, 277, 277t
types, 58–59, 58f
nomenclature, 56
ontogeny, 63
small intestinal, 57
Cytochrome P450 1A2 (CYP1A2),
antipsychotic substrates, 333,
333t
Cytochrome P450 3A (CYP3A)
antipsychotic substrates, 333, 333t
characteristics, 57, 57t
in cytochrome P450 inhibition, 59
developmental aspects, 51
inhibitors, 58

Cytochrome P450 2C19 (CYP2C19),
        genetic polymorphisms, 62
Cytochrome P450 2D6 (CYP2D6)
    antipsychotic substrates, 333, 333t
    developmental aspects, 51
    ethnic differences, 753
    genetic polymorphisms, 60, 62

D8/17 marker, in postinfectious OCD
        and tic disorders, 179–80
DAG (diacylglycerol), 36, 36f
Data analysis, in clinical trial research,
        717, 718f
Data and Safety Monitoring Board
        (DSMB), 722
Death, sudden, desipramine and, 454
Decision making, in assessment for
        pharmacotherapy, 398–99
Deletions, gene, 74
Delirium
    aggression and, 674–75
    agitation and, 682
    in cancer patient, 636
Delusions, in schizophrenia, 191t, 545
Dendrite, 21, 22f
Dendritic spines, 40
Depakote. See Divalproex
Dependence disorders, chemical. See
        Substance abuse and
        dependence disorders
Deprenyl, for ADHD, tic disorders and,
        536–37
Depression, 466–80
    with ADHD, 457, 475–76
    adolescent generalized anxiety
        disorder and, 139
    in adults, neurobiology, 125
    aggression in, 673
    with anxiety, 476
    with anxiety and school refusal, 432
    assessment instruments, 409t
    attention deficit in, 107
    atypical, 472
    bipolar, 472–73
    in children and adolescents
        early life stress and, 125–26
        neurobiology, 124–29
        neuroimaging studies, 126–29, 127t
    classification, 467
    combination therapy, 470, 478, 480
    comorbid psychiatric disorders, 467,
        475–76
    with conduct disorder, 750
    continuation therapy, 476, 477f, 478
    double, 467
    early life stress and, 117–18, 124–26
    electroconvulsive therapy, 378
    ICD-10 criteria, 750
    informants, 405t
    lithium for, 311–12
    maintenance therapy, 478–80, 479f
    mental retardation with, 623–24
    monoamine oxidase inhibitors for,
        299

    with obsessive-compulsive disorder,
        520
    pediatric drug development in, 730
    pharmacotherapy, 467–70
        acute phase, 468–76, 471f
        continuation phase, 476, 477f, 478
        discontinuation, 476
        maintenance phase, 478–80, 479f
        psychoeducation and supportive
            therapy with, 467–68
    during pregnancy, 647–48
    prevalence, 466
    prognosis, 467
    psychotic, 472
    relapse or recurrence
        factors associated with, 478
        management, 476, 478
    SSRIs for, 468–69
    substance abuse and dependence
        disorders with, 613
    subtypes, treatment, 472–75
    suicidal intention and behavior in, 476
    syndrome nosology, 467
    treatment phases, 466
    treatment-resistant, 473–75, 474f
        augmentation or combination
            strategies for, 475
        clomipramine for, 475
        electroconvulsive therapy, 475
        optimizing initial treatment strategy
            for, 473
        reasons for, 473
        switching strategies for, 473, 475
        transcranial magnetic stimulation
            for, 475
    treatment response
        assessment, 466
        definitions, 466, 467t
    tricyclic antidepressants for, 291, 469–
        70
Dermatologic effects
    antipsychotic drugs, 335
    carbamazepine, 316
    lamotrigine, 320–21
Desensitization, 37, 37f
Desipramine, 758t
    for ADHD, 449t, 453
        tic disorders and, 536
    for nocturnal enuresis, 693
    for obsessive-compulsive disorder, 515
    receptor blockade profile, 287t
    stimulants with, 257–58, 457
    for substance use disorders, 607
    sudden death association, 454
Desmopressin, 763t
    for enuresis, 624, 692–93
Detrusor muscle, anatomy and
        physiology, 686–88
Developmental disabilities, aggression in,
        674
Developmental disorders
    pervasive, 563–76. See also specific
        disorder, e.g., autism
        assessment and evaluation, 565–67

    assessment instruments, 410t
    differential diagnosis, 565
    DSM-IV subtypes, 563–76
    ICD-10 criteria, 750
    informants, 405t
    not otherwise specified, 564–65
    in obsessive-compulsive disorder,
        521–22
    pharmacotherapy, 567–76
    in schizophrenia, childhood-onset,
        185
    tricyclic antidepressants for, 291–92
    in tic disorders/Tourette's syndrome,
        166
Developmental history, in assessment for
        pharmacotherapy, 392f–396f,
        397
Dextroamphetamine (Dexedrine), 757t
    for ADHD, 448, 449t. See also
        Amphetamine
    with mental retardation, 619
    for pain management, 635
Diacylglycerol, 36, 36f
Diagnostic and Statistical Manual of
        Mental Disorders-IV (DSM-IV)
    compared to ICD-10, 750–51
    criteria
        ADHD, 104
        anorexia nervosa, 592, 593t
        anxiety disorders, 497
        bipolar disorders, 484, 485t
        bulimia nervosa, 592, 593t
        eating disorders, 592, 593t
        elimination disorders, 689
        manic episode, 484, 485t
        obsessive-compulsive disorder, 150,
            511
        pervasive developmental disorders,
            563–76
        post-traumatic stress disorder, 580
        schizophrenia, 544–45, 544t
Diagnostic Interview for Children and
        Adolescents (DICA)
    in mania, 486
    in post-traumatic stress disorder, 582
    in schizophrenia, 546t, 547
Diagnostic Interview Schedule for
        Children (DISC), 412, 486
Diagnostic interviews, 411–12
    anxiety disorders, 497–98
    bipolar disorders, 486–87
    in clinical trials, 715
    eating disorders, 594–95, 594t, 595t
    in European child psychiatry, 751
    schizophrenia, 546–47, 546t
    semi-structured, 411
    structured, 411–12
Diazepam, 343t
    teratogenicity, 646
Dietary Supplement Health and
        Education Act, 366
Dietary supplements. See
        Complementary and alternative
        medicine

Diphenhydramine, 348, 763t
    for aggression, 680
    for anxiety disorders, 502
    drug interactions, 348
    teratogenicity, 646
Diplopia, carbamazepine-induced, 315
Direct observations, in clinical trials,
        716
Discontinuation studies
    design, 719–20
    risk/benefit analysis, 740
Disruptive behavior disorders, in
        obsessive-compulsive disorder,
        520–21
Distribution curve, cumulative, 717,
        718f
Disulfiram, for substance use disorders,
        606, 612
Divalproex, 317–19, 759t
    alopecia from, 318–19
    appetite increase and weight gain
        from, 318
    for bipolar disorders, 319, 490
        with mental retardation, 621
    dosage, 319
    endocrine and metabolic effects, 318
    gastrointestinal effects, 317–18
    hematological effects, 319
    liver toxicity, 318
    for mania, 489, 490
    mechanism of action, 317
    nervous system effects, 318
    pediatric uses, 319
    pharmacokinetics, 317
    side effects, 317–18
    toxicity, 319
    treatment guidelines, 313t
DNA. See also Chromosome(s); Gene(s)
    cloned, 76–77, 76f, 77f
    histone binding, 70
    methylation, 70–71
    probe, 77
    sense strand, 70
    structure, 69
Donepezil, for tic disorders, 534
Dopamine
    in ADHD, 105–6
    in affiliative behaviors, 203
    in aggression, 216
    in attention modulation, 101, 103
    in drug reward, 239
    in eating disorders, 231
    in obsessive-compulsive disorder, 157,
        158f
    role of, in cortical-striatal-thalamo-
        cortical loops, 155
    in schizophrenia, childhood-onset, 187
    in tic disorders/Tourette's syndrome,
        166–68
Dopamine receptor, 30–31, 30f
    in ADHD, 87, 106
    in alcoholism and substance abuse, 87
    antipsychotic blockade, 330

Dopamine transporter, 31
    in ADHD, 105–6
    in neuropsychiatric disorders, 86–87
    in substance abuse and dependence
        disorders, 242, 243
Dopaminergic agents, for post-traumatic
        stress disorder, 585–86
Dopaminergic genes
    in ADHD, 106
    in neuropsychiatric disorders
        association studies, 86–87
        pharmacogenetic studies, 87–88
    in tic disorders, 87
Dopaminergic neurotransmission, 29–31
    anatomy, 29
    function, 31
    synaptic organization, 30–31, 30f
Double helix, 69
Doxepin, for anxiety disorders, 500
Droperidol, for aggression and
        psychosis, 682
Drosophila, central nervous system
        patterning, 4, 5f
Drugs. See also Medications
    absorption, 45–46, 46f
        in children and adolescents, 48–49
    abuse. See Substance abuse and
        dependence disorders
    bioavailability, 45–46
        in children and adolescents, 48–49
    clearance, 47
    development
        adult, extending to pediatric
            populations, 732
        pediatric. See Pediatric drug
            development
        regulatory process, 725–26
    elimination, 47–48, 47f, 47t
        in children and adolescents, 48, 50
        first-order (linear kinetics), 47
        zero-order or nonlinear (Michaelis-
            Menten) kinetics, 47
    half-life, 47–48, 47f, 47t
    interactions
        cytochrome P450–mediated, 56–65,
            61t–62t
        pharmacokinetic versus
            pharmacodynamic, 54–55, 55f
        preventive strategies, 54, 64–65
        Web sites related to, 64
    maximum concentration, 46, 46f
    metabolism, 55–56, 56f
        in children and adolescents, 50
    protein binding, in children and
        adolescents, 50
    route of administration, 46
    safety monitoring, 402, 722, 734
    steady-state concentration, 47, 47f
    therapeutic monitoring, 51–52, 52f
    volume of distribution, 46–47
        in children and adolescents, 49–50
    withdrawal from, animal models, 240
DSM-IV. See Diagnostic and Statistical

Manual of Mental Disorders-IV
    (DSM-IV)
Duloxetine, 294
Dynorphin, in tic disorders, 168
Dystonic reactions, acute, antipsychotic-
        induced, 333–34
Dysuria, 691–92, 693–94, 695f

Eating Disorder Examination, 596t
Eating Disorder Inventory, 596t
Eating disorders, 224–34. See also
        Anorexia nervosa; Bulimia
        nervosa
    assessment, 494t–497t, 594–97
        diagnostic interviews, 594–95, 594t,
            595t
        laboratory abnormalities, 596–97,
            597t
        physical examination abnormalities,
            595–96, 596t
        self-rating and semistructured
            interview scales, 595, 596t
    assessment instruments, 410t
    behavioral characteristics, 227
    binge eating in, 224
    clinical phenomenology, 224–25, 592–
        94
    cognitive-behavioral therapy, 599–600
    comorbid psychiatric disorders and
        traits, 226–27
    course of illness, 225
    DSM-IV criteria, 592, 593t
    etiology, 224, 592
    genetic studies, 225–26
    ICD-10 criteria, 750
    informants, 405t
    mental retardation with, 624
    molecular genetics, 233–34
    neurobiology, 224–34
    neuroimaging studies, 232–33, 232t
    neurotransmitters in, 227–32, 229f
        cholecystokinin, 229–30
        corticotropin-releasing hormone,
            228
        dopamine, 231
        leptin, 230
        neuropeptide Y and peptide YY,
            228–29
        opioid peptides, 228
        relationship to symptoms, 229f, 230–
            31
        serotonin, 231–32
    not otherwise specified, 592
    psychopharmacotherapy, 597–99
    treatment guidelines, 600–601
Ebstein's anomaly, lithium-induced, 644
Education. See Psychoeducation
Effect size, 720–21
Effectiveness
    definition, 714
    research, 714–15
Effexor. See Venlafaxine
Efficacy, definition, 714

Eldepryl. *See* Selegiline
Electrocardiography
  in assessment for pharmacotherapy,
    399
  in eating disorders, 597
  monitoring
    during clonidine therapy, 269
    during tricyclic antidepressant
      therapy, 288, 291t
Electroconvulsive therapy, 377–84
  administration, 382
  adverse effects, 379–80
  anesthesia, 381–82
  assessment of progress and side
    effects, 382–83
  brain development and, 380
  clinical uses, 378–79
  cognitive impairment after, 379–80
  concurrent medications, 381
  effectiveness, 378, 378t
  electrode placement, 382
  history, 377–78
  lay attitudes, 383
  legal and ethical aspects, 380–81
  for mania, 490
  during pregnancy, 647–48
  procedure, 380–83
  prolonged seizures in, 379
  psychiatric and medical assessment
    prior to, 381
  stimulus pulse characteristics, 382
  teratogenicity, 647
  transcranial magnetic stimulation vs.,
    383–84
  for treatment-resistant depression, 475
  views of health professionals, patients
    and parents, 383
Electroencephalogram
  in aggression, 215–16
  worsening, carbamazepine-induced,
    315
Electrolyte abnormalities, in eating
    disorders, 596–97
Electrophysiology, in aggression, 215–16
Elimination disorders. *See also*
    Encopresis; Enuresis
  central vs. peripheral, 689
  classification
    DSM-IV, 689
    pathophysiological, 689
    by urinary pattern, 689–92
  interventions for, 692–94
  and neurobiology of pelvic organs,
    686–89, 687f
Elimination half-life, 47, 47f, 48
Emotional abuse, definition, 110
Emotional arousal, in tic disorders/
    Tourette's syndrome, 170
Emotional disorders
  ICD-10 criteria, 750
  in schizophrenia, 545
Emotional management therapy, for
    schizophrenia, 557

Empirical/epidemiological tradition, in
    European child psychiatry, 746
Emx genes, 6
Encephalopathy, Wernicke's, 243
Encopresis
  definition, 689
  mechanisms, 688f
Endocrine effects
  antipsychotic drugs, 335
  divalproex, 318
  lithium, 311
Endocrine factors, in tic disorders/
    Tourette's syndrome, 169–70
Endorphins, in social abnormalities of
    autism, 206
Enhancers, gene, 70
Enuresis
  assessment instruments, 410t
  classification, 690
  definition, 689
  diurnal, 691, 693–94, 695f
  informants, 405t
  interventions, 690t, 691t, 692–94
  in mental retardation, 624
  nocturnal, 292, 689, 690–91, 692–93,
    694f
  tricyclic antidepressants for, 292
Environmental factors
  affiliation, 204
  aggression, 219–20
  maternal behavior, 204
  schizophrenia, childhood-onset, 189
  substance abuse and dependence
    disorders, 245–46
  tic disorders/Tourette's syndrome, 169–
    71
Environmental-situational phobia, 140
Epidemiology of
    psychopharmacotherapy. *See*
    Psychotropic drugs, use of
Epidermal growth factor, in cortical
    neurogenesis, 10
Episodic dyscontrol syndrome,
    aggression in, 674
Epoxide hydrolases, in phase 1
    metabolism, 56
Erythromycin, and benzodiazepines,
    344
Essential fatty acids, 372–73
Esterases, plasma, in phase 1
    metabolism, 56
Estrogen, in maternal behavior, 201
Ethanol. *See* Alcohol; Alcoholism
Ethical issues
  in complementary and alternative
    medicine, 366–67
  in electroconvulsive therapy, 380–81
  in research, 734–35, 737–44. *See also*
    Research in children
Ethiopians, CYP2D6 polymorphisms, 62
Ethnic differences
  cytochrome P450, 62, 753
  psychotropic drug use, 706

Ethnicity requirements, in clinical trials,
    715
The European Union, 746–51
  child psychiatry in
    diagnostic and assessment
      instruments, 749–51
    historical perspective, 746
    rating scales, 751
  psychotropic drugs in
    attitudes toward, 746–47
    trends in use of, 747–49
Evening primrose oil, 372–73
Event-related potentials, in aggression,
    216
Evidence-based medicine (EBM), 428–34
  description of framework, 428–29
  evaluation of treatment question, 429,
    429t
  evaluation of treatment studies, 429–
    32, 430t
  Internet resources, 429
  number needed to treat (NNT)
    concept, 431, 431t, 432t
  PECO mnemonic, 429, 429t
  reference sources, 427
Exons, gene, 71
*Expert Consensus Guidelines on Mental
    Retardation*, 617
Exposure, in cognitive-behavioral
    therapy, 504
Exposure and response prevention
  in cognitive-behavioral therapy, 504
  for obsessive-compulsive disorder, 514
External validity, 428
Extrapyramidal side effects
  from antipsychotic drugs, 333–34,
    646
  neonatal, 646
  from SSRIs, 276
  treatment, 334
Eye movements, smooth pursuit, in
    schizophrenia, childhood-onset,
    187, 188

Face validity, 407
Facial processing, as social fear probe,
    143–44
Family history, in assessment for
    pharmacotherapy, 397
Family-oriented therapy
  for anxiety disorders, 505–6
  for schizophrenia, 558
Family practitioners, psychotropic drug
    prescribing by, 703, 705
Family studies
  bipolar disorders, 485–86
  obsessive-compulsive disorder, 152
  PANDAS, 177
  schizophrenia, childhood-onset, 187–
    88, 188t
  tic disorders, 169
Fat, body, drug distribution and, 49
Fatigue, chronic, antidepressants for, 637

Fatty acids, essential, 372–73
FDA. See Food and Drug Administration (FDA)
Fear conditioning
    in anxiety disorders, 142–43
    in children and adolescents, 142–43
    contextual, 142
    cued, 142
    phenomenology and neuroanatomy, 142
Fear probes
    pharmacological, 145
    physiological, 144–45
    social, 143–44
Federal regulations
    pediatric drug development, 725–26, 735. See also Pediatric drug development
    research in children, 738–39, 739t
Females. See Gender differences
Fenfluramine
    for autism and other pervasive developmental disorders, 567
    for bulimia nervosa, 598–99
Fertraline, for post-traumatic stress disorder, 586
Fetal teratogenicity, 642. See also Teratogenicity
Fibroblast growth factor 2, in cortical neurogenesis, 10, 10f
Fibroblast growth factor 8, 8
Fibromyalgia, antidepressants for, 637
Fish oil, 372–73
Flavin-containing monooxygenases, in phase 1 metabolism, 56
Flax seed oil, 372–73
Floppy baby syndrome
    diazepam-induced, 646
    lithium-induced, 644
Fluoxetine, 757t
    adverse effects, 275–79
    for aggression, 678
    for anorexia nervosa, 598
    for anxiety disorders, 500, 500t, 501
    for autism and other pervasive developmental disorders, 571
    and benzodiazepines, 344
    for bulimia nervosa, 598, 599
    central serotonin syndrome from, 64
    cytochrome P450 inhibition by, 277, 277t
    general properties, 274–75, 275t
    indications, 274, 275t
    for major depressive disorder, 468
    for mental retardation with generalized anxiety, 620
    for obsessive-compulsive disorder, 515, 519, 519t
    pharmacokinetic studies in children, 279
    for substance use disorders with depression, 610, 613
    teratogenicity, 643
Fluphenazine, 329t, 761t

    for schizophrenia with mental retardation, 625
    for tic disorders, 528
Flutamide, for tic disorders, 533
Fluvoxamine, 757t
    adverse effects, 275–79
    for anxiety disorders, 145, 500–501, 500t
    for autism and other pervasive developmental disorders, 570–71
    central serotonin syndrome from, 64
    cytochrome P450 inhibition by, 277, 277t
    general properties, 274–75, 275t
    indications, 274, 275t
    labeling changes, 730–31
    for obsessive-compulsive disorder, 515, 519, 519t
    response to, serotonin transporter gene and, 90t, 91, 91t
FMR1 gene, in fragile X syndrome, 75
Focalin. See Mathylphenidate
Follow-up visits, in assessment for pharmacotherapy, 401–2
Food and Drug Administration
    Modernization Act (FDAMA), 44
        pediatric exclusivity provisions, 727–28
        requests initiated under, 729–31
    Pediatric Advisory Subcommittee, 732, 733
    pediatric drug development initiatives, 726–31
    Pediatric Rule, 44
    website, 735
Food interactions, monoamine oxidase inhibitors, 297–98
Forebrain, basal, cholinergic neurons, 26
Founder cells, cortical, 8, 10
Fragile X syndrome, FMR1 gene in, 75
Frontal lobe-like syndromes, from SSRIs, 276
Frontal lobe volume, in depression, 128
Frontotemporal regions, in bipolar disorders, 131

G protein–coupled receptor(s), 21, 22f, 34–38
    activation cycle, 34–35, 35f
    calcium effects on, 36–37
    cyclic AMP pathway, 35–36, 36f
    desensitization, 37, 37f
    down-regulation, 37f, 38
    GABA$_B$, 25, 25f
    glutamate, 23, 24f
    internalization, 37–38, 37f
    in ion channel modulation, 37
    phosphoinositol pathway, 36
    phosphorylation, 37, 40
    regulation
        at receptor level, 37–38, 37f
        by RGS proteins, 35
    second messenger pathways, 35–36

    serotonergic, 27, 28f
G protein–coupled receptor kinase, desensitization by, 37, 37f
GABA receptors, 24–25, 25f
    benzodiazepine binding to, 341–42
    ionotropic, 34
GABAergic agents, for post-traumatic stress disorder, 587–88
GABAergic interneurons
    anatomy, 24
    deficits, 11–12
    progenitor cells, 11
GABAergic projection neurons, 24
GABAergic system, 24–26
    abnormalities, 25–26
    anatomy, 24
    function, 25–26
    synaptic organization, 24–25, 25f
    in tic disorders/Tourette's syndrome, 168
Gabapentin, 321–22, 759t
    for bipolar disorders, 491
    mechanism of action, 321
    for pain management, 636
    pediatric uses, 321–22
    pharmacokinetics, 321
    side effects, 321
    treatment guidelines, 314t
Galactorrhea, from antipsychotic drugs, 694
Gamma aminobutyric acid. See GABA entries
Gap genes, 4, 5f
Gastric emptying, in children and adolescents, 48–49
Gastrointestinal disorders, functional, antidepressants for, 637
Gastrointestinal effects
    divalproex, 317–18
    lamotrigine, 321
    lithium, 310
Gbx2 gene, 8
GDP, in G protein cycle, 34–35, 35f
Gender differences
    alcohol-related central nervous system damage, 243
    brain development, 15–16
    obsessive-compulsive disorder, 512
    psychotropic drug use, 703
    tic disorders, 169–70
Gender requirements, in clinical trials, 715
Gene(s). See also Chromosome(s); DNA
    elements, 70
    enhancers, 70
    exons, 71
    imprinting, 71
    introns, 71
    isolation, 75–77, 76f, 77f
    mutations, 74–75
    promoters, 70
    structure, 69
    transcription, 70–71
Gene arrays, 79–80

Gene expression
  morphogens and, 3–4, 5f
  regulation, 40–41
Gene knockout, 77–79, 78f
Generalized anxiety disorder, 139
  with mental retardation, 620
  pediatric drug development in, 730
Genetic studies. *See also*
        Pharmacogenetics
  ADHD, 86–87, 106
  aggression, 217–19
  alcohol use, 244–45
  anorexia nervosa, 225–26
  bulimia nervosa, 225–26
  obsessive-compulsive disorder, 152
  schizophrenia, childhood-onset, 187–
        89, 188t
  substance abuse and dependence
        disorders, 244–45
  tobacco use, 244
Genetics, reverse, 76
Genome scans, in tic disorders, 169
Genomics, functional, 79–80
Geodon. *See* Ziprasidone.
Giggle incontinence, 694
Glare sensitivity, carbamazepine-induced,
        315
Glial cells, in cortical cell migration, 10–
        11
Global Assessment of Functioning
        (GAF), 412–13, 466
  in obsessive-compulsive disorder, 514
Global instruments and scales, 412–14
Global ratings, in clinical trials, 716
Globus pallidus
  in cortical-striatal-thalamo-cortical
        loops, 153, 154f
  in postinfectious OCD and tic
        disorders, 178
  in tics and stereotypies, 166
Glucocorticoids
  in anxiety disorders, 118, 146
  in depression, 117–18, 125–26
  in stress response, 111–13, 112f
Glutamate receptors, 23, 24f, 34
Glutamate system, 23–24
  abnormalities, 24
  anatomy, 23
  function, 23–24
  in obsessive-compulsive disorder, 159
  in schizophrenia, childhood-onset,
        187
  synaptic organization, 23, 24f
  in tic disorders/Tourette's syndrome,
        168
Glutamatergic compounds, for autism
        and other pervasive
        developmental disorders, 574,
        576
Glycine receptors, ionotropic, 34
Gonadal steroids
  in affiliative behaviors, 201
  in aggression, 216
  in brain development, 15–16

Gray matter
  development, 14
  in schizophrenia, childhood-onset,
        185, 186
Group A beta hemolytic streptococci
        (GABHS) infection
  host immune response, 177–78
  in pathogenesis of OCD and tic
        disorders, 170, 171, 178. *See
        also* PANDAS
Group therapy
  for anxiety disorders, 505
  for schizophrenia, 557–58
Growth factors, signal transduction and,
        73, 73f
Growth hormone, in anxiety disorders,
        145, 146
GTP, in G protein cycle, 34–35, 35f
Guanfacine, 264–71, 762t
  for ADHD, 451t, 455
  adverse effects, 268–69
  for aggression, 678
  for autism and other pervasive
        developmental disorders, 572
  binding properties, 266
  chemical structure, 266, 266f
  clinical use, 268–70
  contraindications, 269
  discontinuation, 269
  dosage and administration, 268
  drug interactions, 269–70
  monitoring, 269
  neuropharmacology, 266–68
  pediatric uses, 264
  pharmacokinetic and
        pharmacodynamic properties,
        266–67
  pharmacological activity, 267–68
  for post-traumatic stress disorder, 585
  premedication workup, 269
  in preschoolers, 660, 660t
  for tic disorders, 532, 534t

Habits, neural substrates, 166–69, 167f
Half-life, drug, 47–48, 47f, 47t
Hallucinations, in schizophrenia, 545
  childhood-onset, 191t
Haloperidol, 329t, 761t
  for acute behavioral control of
        aggression, 680
  for delirium in cancer patient, 636
  in obsessive-compulsive disorder, 522
  in preschoolers, 662
  for schizophrenia during pregnancy,
        648–49
  teratogenicity, 645
  for tic disorders, 527–28, 528t, 529
Hamilton Anxiety Rating Scale, 498
Hamilton Depression Rating Scale, 466
Handbook of Psychiatric Measures,
        404
Health of the Nation Outcome Scales,
        716
Heart rate, in aggression, 216

Hematological effects
  antipsychotic drugs, 336
  carbamazepine, 315
  divalproex, 319
  lithium, 311
Hepatic. *See* Liver
Herbal remedies. *See* Complementary
        and alternative medicine
Heterologous desensitization, 37
Hippocampus
  adult neurogenesis, 15
  in affiliative behaviors, 197
  atrophy
        in anxiety disorders, 146–47
        in depression, 118, 125, 126
        in post-traumatic stress disorder,
              118
  glutamatergic neurons, 23
  lesions, and social behavior in rhesus
        monkeys, 197
  marijuana toxicity, 244
  neurogenesis, 41–42
  in schizophrenia, childhood-onset, 185–
        86
Histaminergic receptor blockade, by
        antipsychotics, 331
Holoprosencephaly, *Otx* genes in, 6
Homeobox *(Hox)* genes, 70
Homeodomain selector genes, 4, 6, 6f
Homicidal patient, management, 682–83
Homologous desensitization, 37
Hox genes, 4
5-Hydroxyindolacetic acid, in eating
        disorders, 229f, 231–32
Hyperactivity, attention deficit with. *See*
        Attention-deficit/hyperactivity
        disorder
Hypericum perforatum, 368. *See also* St.
        John's wort
Hyperkinetic disorder, 750. *See also*
        Attention-deficit/hyperactivity
        disorder
Hyperprolactinemia, antipsychotic-
        induced, 335
Hypertensive-adrenergic crisis, from
        monoamine oxidase inhibitors,
        297–98
Hypomagnesemia, in eating disorders,
        596
Hypomania, in obsessive-compulsive
        disorder, 520
Hypophosphatemia, in eating disorders,
        596–97
Hypothalamic medial preoptic areas, in
        affiliative behaviors, 195–96
Hypothalamic-pituitary-adrenal axis, in
        anxiety disorders, 140–41, 145,
        146

ICD-10 *(International Classification of
        Diseases, 10th Edition)*, 749–
        51
Imaging studies. *See* Neuroimaging
        studies

Imipramine, 758t
    for ADHD, 449t, 453
    for anxiety disorders, 500t, 501–2, 503
    for enuresis with mental retardation, 624
    for major depressive disorder, 470
    for nocturnal enuresis, 292, 693
    receptor blockade profile, 287t
Immediate early genes, in maternal behavior, 204
Immune-mediated neuropsychiatric disorders, neurobiology, 175–81
Immunoglobulin
    for autism and other pervasive developmental disorders, 576
    in neuronal remodeling, 13
    for postinfectious OCD and tic disorders, 180
Immunomodulatory therapy, for postinfectious OCD and tic disorders, 180
Imprinting, gene, 71
Impulse-control disorders, lithium for, 311
Inclusion criteria, clinical trials, 715
Incontinence
    classification of syndromes, 689
    giggle, 694
    intermittent minimal, 694
Inferior temporal cortex, stimulus processing in, 99–100
Informants, 404, 405t
Information sources, in assessment for pharmacotherapy, 391, 396
Informed consent
    in assessment for pharmacotherapy, 401
    for electroconvulsive therapy, 380
    for research in children, 742
Inhalant use, prevalence, 238–39
Inositol-1,4,5-triphosphate, 36, 36f
Inpatients
    adult, aggression in, 210–11
    bipolar disorders in, 489–90
    mania in, 489–90
    psychotropic drug use in, 706–7
Insertions, gene, 74
Institutional Review Board (IRB), 739
Instruments and scales, 404–14
    analyzing and interpreting scores, 408, 411
    for anxiety disorders, 497–500, 498t
    for attention-deficit/hyperactivity disorder, 448
    for autism, 566–67
    baseline data, 404, 406
    for bipolar disorders, 486, 487
    categorical vs. dimensional measures, 408
    clinical tempering of scores, 407–8
    for clinical trials, 715–17
    for combination therapy, 435

content validity, 407
    diagnostic, 411–12
    disorder-specific, 409t–411t, 414
    ease of data collection and usage, 406
    for eating disorders, 595, 596t
    in European child psychiatry, 751
    face validity, 407
    general principles, 404–11
    global, 412–14
    informants, 404, 405t
    in Japanese child psychiatry, 752–53
    low base-rate phenomenon, 407
    multiple informants, 404
    predictive power, 407
    rating attenuation effect, 406
    reliability, 406
    scale sums, composites, and averages, 413–14
    for schizophrenia, 545–47, 546t
    selection considerations, 408
    self-report, 435
    sensitivity, 406–7
    sources, 413t
    specificity, 406–7
    target symptom quantification, 414
    validity, 406–7
Intellectual ability, in mental status examination, 398
Intelligence tests, in autism and other pervasive developmental disorders, 566
Interaction effects, 720
Intermittent explosive disorder, aggression in, 674
Internal validity, 428–29
Internalization, G protein–coupled receptors, 37–38, 37f
International Classification of Diseases-10th edition (ICD-10), 749–51
International Conference on Harmonization (ICH), 735, 753
Internet sites
    complementary and alternative medicine, 367
    drug interactions, 64
    FDA, 735
Interview
    clinical, in assessment for pharmacotherapy, 396–97
    diagnostic. See Diagnostic interviews
Interview for Childhood Disorders and Schizophrenia, 546–47, 546t
Intoxicated patient, aggression in, 680–81
Introns, gene, 71
Investigational New Drug (IND) application, 725
Ionotropic receptors, 21, 22f, 34
Iowa Conners' Rating Scale, 413t
Iproniazid, structure, 297
Irritability, assessment, 487
Isocarboxazid

indications, 296
    mechanism of action, 296
Japan
    biological differences
        autism, 753
        psychotropic drug metabolism, 753
    child psychiatry in
        diagnostic and assessment instruments, 752
        historical perspective, 751–52
        rating scales, 752–53
    drug evaluation and regulatory affairs, 752
    drug regulatory process, 752
    overcoming regional difficulties, 753
Justice principle, in research in children, 738
Kainate receptor, 34
Kava, 373–74
Kiddie-Formal Thought Disorder Story Game and Scale (K-FTDS), 546t, 547
Kiddie Positive and Negative Syndrome Scale for Children and Adolescents (K-PANSS), 546t, 547
Kiddie Schedule for Affective Disorders and Schizophrenia (K-SADS)
    in anxiety disorders, 498
    in mania, 486
    in schizophrenia, 546–47, 546t
Kindling, bipolar disorders and, 130
Klonopin. See Clonazepam
Knockout animals, 77–79, 78f
Korsakoff's psychosis, 243
Labeling, pediatric, for psychotropic drugs, 726–27, 729
Laboratory testing, in assessment for pharmacotherapy, 399
Lactation, psychopharmacotherapy during, 643
Lamotrigine, 320–21, 759t
    for autism and other pervasive developmental disorders, 574
    dermatologic effects and sensitivity reactions, 320–21
    gastrointestinal effects, 321
    mechanism of action, 320
    neurological effects, 320
    pediatric uses, 321
    pharmacokinetics, 320
    side effects, 320
    treatment guidelines, 314t
Language. See Speech and language
Lateral ventricle enlargement, in depression, 128
Law of initial values, 408
Learning, synaptic plasticity in, 14
Lecithin, for bipolar disorders, 491

Legal considerations
    in aggression, 682–83
    in electroconvulsive therapy, 380–81
Leiter International Test of Intelligence–
        Revised, 566
Leptin, in eating disorders, 230
Leukopenia, carbamazepine-induced,
        315
Levodopa, for tic disorders, 534
Liability, in complementary and
        alternative medicine, 367, 367t
Library, cDNA, 76–77, 76f, 77f
Librium, 343t
Light therapy, for seasonal affective
        disorder, 472
Limbic areas
    in affiliative behaviors, 196–97
    in drug reward, 239
Linkage studies
    eating disorders, 233–34
    schizophrenia, childhood-onset, 189
    tic disorders, 169
Lissosphincter, 687–88
Lithium, 309–12, 759t
    for aggression, 679
    antidepressants with, 475
    for bipolar disorders, 490–91
        with mental retardation, 621
        during pregnancy, 648
    for bulimia nervosa, 598
    cardiac effects, 311
    discontinuation, 493
    dosage and administration, 312
    endocrine effects, 311
    gastrointestinal effects, 310
    hematological effects, 311
    for impulse-control disorders, 311
    for mania
        in adults, 488–89, 488t
        in children and adolescents, 489,
            490–91
    mechanism of action, 309
    for mood disorders, 311–12
    neurological effects, 310
    overdose and toxicity, 311
    pediatric uses, 311–12
    pharmacokinetics, 309–10
    predictors of response, 488–89, 488t
    renal effects, 311
    for self-injury in mental retardation,
        626
    side effects, 310–11
    for substance use disorders with
        affective dysregulation, 607
    teratogenicity, 644–45
    therapeutic drug monitoring, 52, 52f
    treatment guidelines, 313t
Liver
    cytochrome P450 enzymes in, 57, 57t,
        59
    hypersensitivity reaction, to pemoline,
        452
    toxicity

antipsychotic drugs, 334–35
carbamazepine, 316
divalproex, 318
nefazodone, 300–301
pemoline, 259
Liver failure, divalproex-induced, 318
Locus ceruleus, noradrenergic neurons,
        28
Locus heterogeneity, 75
Locus of control, medication and, 418
Long-term depression, in learning, 14
Long-term potentiation, in learning, 14
Lorazepam, 343t, 762t
    for acute behavioral control of
        aggression, 680
    for anticipatory nausea, 635
    for pain management, 634
    teratogenicity, 646
Loss, parental
    prevalence, 110–11
    relationship to psychopathology, 111
Loxapine, 329t
Luvox. See Fluvoxamine

Magnetic resonance imaging (MRI)
    in bipolar disorders, 131
    in depression, 128–29
    in schizophrenia, childhood-onset, 185–
        86, 186t
Magnetic resonance spectroscopy (MRS)
    in bipolar disorders, 131
    in schizophrenia, childhood-onset, 186
Major depressive disorder, syndrome
        nosology, 467. See also
        Depression
Males. See Gender differences
Maltreatment, child. See Child
        maltreatment
Managed care, prescribing influence of,
        423
Mania
    acute
        controlled treatment studies in
            adults, 488–89
        diagnostic hospitalization for, 493
        inpatient treatment studies, 489–90
        outpatient treatment studies, 490–
            91
        treatment approach, 491–94, 492f
    assessment instruments, 410t
    attention deficit in, 107
    chronic, 492–93
    comorbid psychiatric disorders,
        psychopharmacotherapy, 493
    euphoric, 491
    informants, 405t
    maintenance treatment, 493–94
    mixed, 491
    neuroimaging studies, 131
    preclinical models, 129–30
    prevalence, 129
    from SSRIs, 276
Mania Rating Scale, 413t

Manic episode, DSM-IV criteria, 484,
        485t
MAPK, activation, 38–39, 39f
Marijuana use, prevalence, 238
Marplan. See Isocarboxazid
Maternal aggression
    definition, 203
    nitric oxide and, 203–4
Maternal behavior. See also Affiliation
    amygdala in, 196–97
    environmental factors, 204
    estrogen in, 201
    hypothalamic medial preoptic areas in,
        195–96
    immediate early genes in, 204
    norepinephrine in, 203
    opioids and μ-opioid receptors in, 201
    oxytocin in, 198
    paraventricular nucleus in, 196
    progesterone in, 201
    prolactin in, 200–201
    serotonin in, 202–3
    steroids in, 201–2
    ventral bed nucleus of the stria
        terminalis in, 197
Maternal separation, as early life stress
        model, 113, 114t, 115, 119
Matrices and striosomes
    in obsessive-compulsive disorder, 155,
        156f
    stereotypies and, 160
Matrix-assisted laser desorption/
        ionization, 80
Measures
    categorical vs. dimensional
        (continuous), 408
    of treatment effect, 715–17
Mecamylamine, for tic disorders, 532–
        33
Meclobemide, mechanism of action, 297
Medial preoptic areas, in maternal
        behavior, 195–96
Medial temporal lobe, 20, 21f
Medically ill child or adolescent, 631–40
    assessment and evaluation, 631–32
    diagnostic issues, 632–33
    nonpharmacological management, 631
    psychopharmacotherapy, 632–40
        in cancer patient, 636–37
        discontinuation of psychoactive
            medications, 638–39
        in etiologically unexplained
            syndromes, 637
        management categories, 631
        for pain, 633–36, 634t–635t
        principles of use, 632
        treatment algorithm, 637–38, 638f
Medications. See also Drugs
    children's thinking about, 419–20,
        419t
    context, meaning of, 421–22
    education points, 400
    follow-up visits, 401–2

Medications (*continued*)
  and locus of control, 418
  meaning of, 418–20, 419t
  noncompliance in taking, reasons, 401
  parental attitudes toward, 421
  parental compliance considerations,
    421–22
  placebo vs., meaning of, 420–21
  process, meaning of, 420–21
  resistance to, causes, 400
  school context, 421
  side effects
    identification, 400–401
    monitoring, 402
  timing considerations, 418
Melatonin, for bipolar disorders, 491
Membrane bound receptors, 21, 22f
Mental health services, use of,
    assessment, 716
Mental retardation, 617–28
  with ADHD, 619
  with anxiety disorders, 619–20
  with bipolar disorders, 621–22
  with conduct disorder, 622–23
  with eating disorders, 624
  with enuresis, 624
  Expert Consensus Guidelines, 617
  with generalized anxiety, 620
  with major depressive disorder, 623–24
  with obsessive-compulsive disorder,
    620–21
  physical ailments associated with, 617
  with psychiatric disorders, 617
    assessment instruments, 411t, 618
    pharmacotherapy, 619–27
    problems establishing psychiatric
      diagnoses, 617–18
    proneness to adverse events, 618–19
  with psychotic disorders, 624–25
  with schizophrenia, 624–25
  with self-injury, 625–27
  with sleep disorders, 627
  with tic disorders and Tourette's
    syndrome, 625
Mental status examination
  in assessment for pharmacotherapy,
    397–98
  in bipolar disorders, 488
  elements, 397–98
Meprobamate, for anxiety disorders,
    500
Mesocorticolimbic dopamine system, in
    drug reward, 239
Mesoridazine, 329t
Metabolic effects, divalproex, 318
Metabotropic receptors. *See* G protein–
    coupled receptor(s)
Metadate. *See* Methylphenidate
Methadone, for substance use disorders,
    606, 612
Methylin. *See* Methylphenidate
Methylphenidate, 757t. *See also*
    Stimulants

for ADHD, 448, 449t, 453
  dosage, 260
  drug interactions, 257–58
  history and overview, 255–56
  long-acting preparations, 257
  long-term use considerations, 260–
    61
  mechanism of action, 256
  with mental retardation, 619
  pharmacokinetics and drug
    distribution, 256–57
  time trends in use of, 702
for aggression, 677–78
for autism and other pervasive
    developmental disorders, 572
with clonidine, 258, 270
and desipramine, 457
long-acting, 453
for pain management, 635
in preschoolers, 655–59, 657t–658t
purified d, threo-, 453
response to, dopamine-related alleles
    in, 87
Midazolam, for pain management, 633–
    34
Mini Mental State Examination, in
    medically ill child or
    adolescent, 632
Mirtazapine
  for autism and other pervasive
    developmental disorders, 573–
    74
  in children and adolescents, 304
  for major depressive disorder, 470
  mechanism of action, 303
  pharmacokinetics and drug
    distribution, 303–4
Modeling, in cognitive-behavioral
    therapy, 504
Molecular genetics, 69–81. *See also*
    Genetic studies;
    Pharmacogenetics
  DNA structure, 69
  functional genomics, 79–80
  gene knockout, 77–79, 78f
  isolation of genes, 75–77, 76f, 77f
  mutations, 74–75
  protein synthesis, 71–72, 72f
  proteomics, 80–81
  RNA, 70–71
  signal transduction, 72–74, 73f
Molindone, 329t, 336, 761t
Monoamine oxidase
  functions, 296
  knockout mouse, 218
  types, 296
Monoamine oxidase inhibitors, 295–300
  for ADHD, 299, 449t–450t, 454–55
  in children and adolescents, 299–300
  for depression, 299
  discontinuation, 299
  food and drug interactions, 297–98
  history, 295–96

indications, 296
limitations, 296, 455
mechanism of action, 296–97
with methylphenidate, 258
monitoring, 299–300
nonselective and irreversible, 296
pharmacokinetics and drug
    distribution, 297
during pregnancy, 647
premedication workup, 299
selective and irreversible, 296–97
selective and reversible, 297
side effects and toxicity, 298–99
structure, 297
teratogenicity, 644
for treatment-resistant depression,
    475
Monoamine systems, in eating disorders,
    229f, 231–32
Mood disorders. *See also* Bipolar
    disorders; Depression
  aggression in, 673, 673f
  eating disorders and, 226
  in juvenile offenders, 673f
  neurobiology, 124–32
  during pregnancy, 647–48
  in schizophrenia, childhood-onset,
    188, 188t
  seasonal, 472
Mood stabilizers, 309–23, 759t. *See also*
    specific drugs, e.g., Lithium
  for aggression, 679
  for autism and other pervasive
    developmental disorders, 568
  for bipolar depression, 472
  mechanism of action, 130
  for self-injury in mental retardation,
    626
  for substance use disorders with
    bipolar disorders, 613–14
  teratogenicity, 644–45
  treatment guidelines, 313t–314t
Mood symptoms, electroconvulsive
    therapy, 378
Morphine, neuronal adaptation to, 41
Morphogens
  brain patterning, 3–4, 5f
  as organizers, 6, 7f, 8
Motor disturbances, in schizophrenia,
    545
Motor tic, 164, 175
Movement disorders, postinfectious
    subtype, 176–81. *See also*
    PANDAS
MTA study, of combination therapy for
    ADHD, 433–34, 458–59
Mullen Scale of Early Development, in
    autism and other pervasive
    developmental disorders, 566
Multidimensional Anxiety Scale for
    Children (MASC), 413t, 499
Muscarinic receptors, 26, 26f
  antipsychotic drug blockade, 330

Mutations, 74–75
Mutism, ICD-10 criteria, 750

Nadolol, 763t
    for aggression, 678
    dosage, 356
    pharmacology, 354
Naloxone, 357
    for tic disorders, 534
Naltrexone
    for autism, 206, 357–58, 567–68
    conditions tested, 359–60
    dosage, 359
    overdose, 360
    for pervasive developmental disorders,
        567–68
    pharmacology, 357
    for post-traumatic stress disorder, 588
    for self-injury, 358–59, 627
    side effects, 359
    for substance use disorders, 607, 611,
        612
Nardil. See Phenelzine
National Advisory Mental Health
        Council, 738
National Bioethics Advisory
        Commission, 738
National Institute of Mental Health
        Diagnostic Interview Schedule
        for Children (NIMH-DISC),
        546t, 547
National Institutes of Health (NIH),
        Office of Dietary Supplements,
        366
Nefazodone, 758t
    for anxiety disorders, 500t, 502
    and benzodiazepines, 344
    central serotonin syndrome from, 64
    in children and adolescents, 301
    drug interactions, 300
    mechanism of action, 300
    pharmacokinetics and drug
        distribution, 300
    for post-traumatic stress disorder, 587
    side effects and toxicity, 300–301
Negative predictive power, 407
Neglect
    contralateral, 100
    definition, 110
Neonatal teratogenicity, 642. See also
        Teratogenicity
Neonatal withdrawal syndrome, tricyclic
        antidepressant-induced, 644
Neonates
    CYP2D6 activity, 51
    extrapyramidal side effects in, 646
Nerve terminal, 21, 22f
Netrins, in neuronal remodeling, 13
Neural circuitry, 20–23, 21f–22f
Neural maturation, in preschoolers, 664–
        65
Neuroanatomical studies
    aggression, 212, 214

obsessive-compulsive disorder, 153–57
schizophrenia, childhood-onset, 185–
        86, 186t
substance abuse and dependence
        disorders, 239–40
Neuroanatomical systems, 20–23, 21f
Neurobiology
    of affiliation, 195–206
    of aggression, 210–20
    of anxiety disorders, 138–47
    of attention-deficit/hyperactivity
        disorder, 99–107
    of childhood schizophrenia, 184–91
    of depression, 124–29
    of eating disorders, 224–34
    of elimination disorders, 686–89, 687f
    of immune-mediated neuropsychiatric
        disorders, 175–81
    of mood disorders, 124–32
    of social abnormalities in autism, 206
    of stress, 111–13, 582
    of substance abuse and dependence
        disorders, 238–48
    of tic disorders/Tourette's syndrome,
        164–72
Neurodevelopmental instability, signs
        and symptoms, 397
Neurogenesis
    cortical, 8, 9f, 10, 10f
    pluripotent cells, 15
Neuroimaging studies
    ADHD, 105–6
    aggression, 214–15
    bipolar disorders, 131
    depression, 126–29, 127t
    eating disorders, 232–33, 232t
    mania, 131
    obsessive-compulsive disorder, 152–53
    schizophrenia, childhood-onset, 186
Neuroimmune therapies, for autism and
        other pervasive developmental
        disorders, 576
Neuroleptic malignant syndrome
    antipsychotic-induced, 334
    electroconvulsive therapy, 378
    vs. serotonin syndrome, 278
Neuroleptics. See Antipsychotic drugs
Neurological consultation or testing, in
        assessment for
        pharmacotherapy, 399
Neurological effects
    carbamazepine, 315
    divalproex, 318
    lamotrigine, 320
    lithium, 310
    SSRIs, 276
Neurons
    adaptation, mechanisms, 39–41
    anatomy, 21, 22f
    migration, cerebral cortex, 10–12, 11f
    regeneration, adult brain, 15
    remodeling, 12–14, 12f
Neurontin. See Gabapentin

Neuropeptide(s), in eating disorders, 227–
        31, 229f
Neuropeptide Y, in eating disorders, 228–
        29
Neuropsychiatric disorders
    association studies
        of dopamine-related alleles, 86–87
        of serotonin-related alleles, 88–90
    in children and adolescents,
        prevalence, 701
    immune-mediated, 175–81. See also
        PANDAS
    pharmacokinetic studies
        of dopamine-related alleles, 87–88
        of serotonin-related alleles, 90–91,
        90t, 91t
Neuropsychiatric Rating Schedule, in
        mania, 487
Neuropsychiatric tradition, in European
        child psychiatry, 746
Neuropsychological deficits, aggression
        in, 674
Neuroticism, serotonin transporter
        polymorphism in, 89
Neurotransmitter(s), 23–31
    in aggression, 216–17
    anatomical systems and, 20–23, 21f
    atypical, 21
    cholinergic, 26–27, 26f
    dopaminergic, 29–31, 30f
    GABAergic, 24–26, 25f
    glutamatergic, 23–24, 24f
    noradrenergic, 28–29, 29f
    in schizophrenia, childhood-onset, 187
    serotonergic, 27–28, 28f
Neurotransmitter receptors. See
        Receptor(s)
Neurotrophin receptors, signaling
        pathways, 38–39, 39f
Neutrophilia, lithium-induced, 311
New Drug Application (NDA), 726
New York Teacher Rating Scale, 413t
Nicotine. See also Tobacco use
    acute actions, 241
    for ADHD, 456
    for tic disorders, 532
Nicotinic acetylcholine receptors, 241
Nicotinic receptors, 26–27, 26f
Nimodipine
    for bipolar disorders, 491
    for mania, 489
Nisonger Child Behavior Rating Form,
        413t
Nitric oxide
    in affiliative behaviors, 203–4
    role of, in cortical-striatal-thalamo-
        cortical loops, 155
Nitric oxide synthetase, in aggression,
        218–19
NMDA receptors, 34
    glutamate, 23, 24f
    hippocampal, function, 23–24
    phosphorylation, regulation, 40

Noninferiority studies, clinical trials, 719
Noradrenergic agents, 762t
Noradrenergic reuptake inhibitors, 294
Noradrenergic-specific compounds, for
      ADHD, 455
Noradrenergic systems, 28–29. *See also*
      Adrenergic *entries*
   anatomy, 28
   in anxiety disorders, 118
   function, 29
   synaptic organization, 28–29, 29f
   in tic disorders/Tourette's syndrome,
      168–69
   tricyclic antidepressant effects on, 284
Nordiazepam, 343
Norepinephrine, 28. *See also*
      Noradrenergic systems
   in affiliative behaviors, 203
   in anxiety disorders, 145
   in attention modulation, 101, 103–4
   in tic disorders, 169
Norepinephrine transporter, 28–29
Nortriptyline, 758t
   for ADHD, 449t, 453–54
   for nocturnal enuresis, 693
   receptor blockade profile, 287t
Nucleus accumbens, in obsessive-
      compulsive disorder, 155–56
Null hypothesis, 719
Number needed to treat (NNT), 431,
      431t, 432t

Observational methods
   anxiety disorders, 499–500
   in clinical trials, 716
Observer Rating Scale of Anxiety, 499
Obsessions
   common, 151, 175
   definition, 150, 511
   in eating disorders, 225, 227
Obsessive-compulsive disorder, 150–61,
      511–23
   age at onset, 512
   aggression in, 673
   in anorexia nervosa, 595
   assessment and evaluation, 513–14
   assessment instruments, 410t
   basal ganglia dysfunction in, 153–55,
      154f, 159–60
   childhood-onset, 150
   clinical course, 150, 175
   clinical features, 511–13, 512t
   cognitive-behavioral therapy, 514–15
   combination therapy, 441
   comorbid psychiatric disorders, 152,
      175, 513, 513f
      treatment, 520–22
      and treatment response, 519
   cortical-striatal-thalamo-cortical
      dysfunction in, 152–53, 153–
      55, 154f, 158f
   definition and nosology, 511
   differential diagnosis, 514
   dopamine system in, 157, 158f

DSM-IV criteria, 150, 511
   eating disorders and, 227
   etiological factors, 151–52
   evolutionary perspective, 151
   Expert Consensus Guidelines, 438,
      439f–440f
   gender differences, 512
   genetic studies, 152
   glutamate system in, 159
   ICD-10 criteria, 750
   informants, 405t
   mental retardation with, 620–21
   neuroanatomical features, 153–57
      basal ganglia, 153–55, 154f
      striatum microstructure, 156–57
      striosome and matrix
         compartments, 155, 156f
      ventral striatum, 153, 155–56
   neurobehavioral characteristics, 151t
   neurobiology, 150–61
   neuroimaging studies, 152–53
   neuropsychological studies, 153
   pediatric drug development in, 730
   phenotypic presentation, 511–12,
      512t
   postinfectious subtype, 176–81. *See
      also* PANDAS
      age at onset, 512
      treatment, 523
   during pregnancy, 649
   prevalence, 150, 175, 511
   right hemisphere involvement in, 153
   serotonin system in, 157–59
   serotonin transporter polymorphism
      in, 89
   stereotypies and, 160–61
   in Sydenham's chorea, 176
   themes, 151
   with tic disorders, 152, 165, 176
   treatment, 180–81, 514–23
      adverse events, 522
      algorithm, 521f, 523
      behavioral, 514–15
      with comorbid psychiatric disorders,
         520–22
      duration, 522
      general principles, 514–15
      guidelines, 519–22
      novel agents, 523
      outcome studies, 522–23
      published studies, 515–19, 516t–
         518t
      resistance, augmentation strategies,
         522
      response
         assessment, 515
         predictors, 519
      selection of initial agent, 519–20
      tricyclic antidepressants for, 291
      unique characteristics, 160
OCD. *See* Obsessive-compulsive disorder
Ocular effects
   antipsychotic drugs, 335–36
   quetiapine, 336

Olanzapine, 329t, 760t
   for aggression, 680
   for autism and other pervasive
      developmental disorders, 568–
      69
   for bipolar disorders, 491
   for mania, 489
   for obsessive-compulsive disorder, 522
   for schizophrenia, 551, 552t–553t,
      554
   teratogenicity, 645–46
   for tic disorders, 529, 530
Omega-3 and omega-6 fatty acids, 372–
      73
Ondansetron
   for substance use disorders, 607, 612–
      13
   for tic disorders, 534
Opiate antagonists, 356–60
   for autism, 357–58
   contraindications, 359–60
   dosage, 359
   mechanism of action, 357
   overdose, 360
   pharmacology, 357
   for post-traumatic stress disorder,
      588
   for self-injury, 358–59
   side effects, 359
Opioid(s)
   acute actions, 241
   chronic effects
      brain morphology, 244
      receptor studies, 243–44
   endogenous
      in eating disorders, 228
      in tic disorders/Tourette's syndrome,
         168
   neuronal adaptation to, 39, 41, 42
   precursor proteins, 357
   in social abnormalities of autism,
      206
   teratogenic effects, 247
Opioid receptors, 241, 357
   in affiliative behaviors, 201
Oppositional defiant disorder
   assessment instruments, 410t
   informants, 405t
Orbitofrontal cortex, in obsessive-
      compulsive disorder, 159
Organic affective syndrome, 485
Organizer cells, central nervous system,
      6, 7f, 8
Orgasmic dysfunction, psychiatrically
      induced, 696
Otx1 gene, 4, 6, 6f
Otx2 gene, 8
Outcome evaluation
   in assessment for pharmacotherapy,
      400–401
   clinical trials, 715–17
   combination therapy, 436–37
Ovaries, polycystic, divalproex-induced,
      318

Overprescribing of psychotropic drugs, 708–9
Overt Aggression Scale (OAS), in mania, 487
Oxazepam, 343t
Oxybutynin, 763t
    for diurnal enuresis, 694
    for nocturnal enuresis, 693
Oxytocin
    in affiliative behaviors, 197–99
    in induction of maternal behavior, 196
    knockout mouse, 198–99
    in social abnormalities of autism, 204–5
    in social memory, 199
Oxytocin receptors
    in affiliative behaviors, 199–200
    distribution, species-specificity, 199–200

P-glycoprotein
    in cytochrome P450 inhibition, 59
    substrates, enhancers, and inducers, 55, 55t
P13 kinase, activation, 39, 39f
Pain, in medically ill child or adolescent, psychopharmacological considerations, 633–36, 634t–635t
PANDAS, 170–71, 176–81
    biological basis, 177–80
    brain systems implicated, 178–79
    comorbid psychiatric disorders, 177
    criteria for, 176–77, 177t
    evidence for, 176
    family studies, 177
    genetic susceptibility and biologic markers, 179–80
    treatment modalities, 180–81
Panic disorder
    childhood separation anxiety and, 139–40
    in children and adolescents, 140
    physiological fear probes, 144–45
    during pregnancy, 649
    respiratory abnormalities, 140
Paranoid personality disorder, in schizophrenia, 188, 188t
Paraventricular nucleus, in affiliative behaviors, 196
Parent
    attitudes toward medications, 421
    loss of
        prevalence, 110–11
        relationship to psychopathology, 111
    medication compliance considerations, 421–22
Parietal cortex, posterior, attentional processing, 100, 103
Parkinsonism, antipsychotic-induced, 334
Parnate. See Tranylcypromine

Paroxetine, 757t
    adverse effects, 275–79
    for aggression, 678
    for anxiety disorders, 500, 500t
    for autism and other pervasive developmental disorders, 571
    central serotonin syndrome from, 64
    cytochrome P450 inhibition by, 277, 277t
    general properties, 274–75, 275t
    indications, 274, 275t
    for major depressive disorder, 468–69
    for obsessive-compulsive disorder, 515, 519, 519t
    pharmacokinetic studies in children, 279, 469
    for post-traumatic stress disorder, 586
Patient education. See Psychoeducation
Paxil. See Paroxetine
Pediatric Anxiety Rating Scale (PARS), 498–99
Pediatric Autoimmune Neuropsychiatric Disorder Associated with Streptococcus (PANDAS), xx
Pediatric drug development. See also Research in children
    in ADHD, 731–32
    in conduct disorder, 732
    ethical considerations, 734–35, 737–44
    FDA initiatives promoting, 726–31
        FDAMA, 727–28
        goal, 729
        impact, 729–31
        Pediatric Rule of 1998, 728–29
        pre-1997, 726–27
    in generalized anxiety disorders, 730
    information sources on regulatory aspects, 735
    in major depressive disorder, 730
    in obsessive-compulsive disorder, 730
    in preschool populations, 733–34
    regulatory challenges, 732–35
    regulatory process, 725–26
    safety considerations, 734
Pediatric OCD Treatment Study, 441
Pediatric psychopharmacotherapy. See Psychopharmacotherapy, pediatric
Pediatric Rule of 1998, 728–29, 731
Pediatricians, psychotropic drug prescribing by, 703, 705
Pelvic organs, neuroanatomy and neurophysiology, 686–89, 687f
Pemoline, 757t
    for ADHD, 448, 449t
        pharmacokinetics and drug distribution, 257
        with substance use disorders, 610, 613
    hepatic hypersensitivity reaction, 452
    liver damage from, 259
Peptide YY, in eating disorders, 228–29

Pergolide, for tic disorders, 530, 534
Perinatal complications
    schizophrenia and, 189
    tic disorders/Tourette's syndrome and, 170
Perphenazine, 329t, 761t
    teratogenicity, 645
Personality disorders
    in eating disorders, 595
    paranoid, in schizophrenia, 188, 188t
    schizotypal, 545
        in schizophrenia, 188, 188t
Pervasive developmental disorders. See Developmental disorders, pervasive
Pharmaceutical industry, prescribing influence of, 422–23
Pharmacodynamics
    in central serotonin syndrome, 63–64
    in pharmacogenetics, 85
Pharmacogenetics, 84–92. See also Genetic studies; Molecular genetics
    in neuropsychiatric disorders
        dopaminergic genes, 87–88
        future applications, 92
        methodology, 86
        serotonergic genes, 90–91, 90t, 91t
    overview of clinical applications, 84
    pharmacodynamic aspects, 85
    pharmacokinetic aspects, 84–85
    relevance to understanding pathogenesis, 85–86
    terminology, 84
Pharmacogenomics, 84
Pharmacokinetics, 44–52
    in central serotonin syndrome, 63–64
    cytochrome P450 and
        developmental aspects, 50–51
        drug interactions, 54–65
    definition, 44
    development principles, 48–52
    of dopamine-related alleles, 87–88
    interrelationships, 44, 45f
    in pharmacogenetics, 84–85
    principles, 45–48
    of serotonin-related alleles, 90–91, 90t, 91t
    target concentration strategy and, 44–45
    therapeutic drug monitoring and, 45, 51–52, 52f
Pharmacological fear probes, 145
Phase I metabolism, 50, 55–56, 56f
Phase I trials, 713, 725–26
Phase II metabolism, 50, 55–56, 56f
Phase II trials, 713, 725–26
Phase III trials. See Clinical trials
Phase IV (post-marketing) studies, 726
Phenelzine
    indications, 296
    mechanism of action, 296
    teratogenicity, 644

Phenothiazines, 761t
    teratogenicity, 645
Philadelphia chromosome, 75
Philopodia, 13
Phobia, 140
    animal, 140
    blood, 140
    environmental-situational, 140
    procedural, in cancer patient, 636
    school, tricyclic antidepressants for,
        291
    social, 138–39
Phonic tic, 164
Phosphodiesterases, 36
Phosphoinositol pathway, G protein–
    coupled receptors, 36
Phosphorylation, protein, 71–72
    regulation, 40
    signal transduction and, 73–74, 73f
Photosensitivity, St. John's wort and,
        370
Physical abuse of child
    definition, 110
    prevalence, 111
    relationship to psychopathology,
        111
Physical illness. See Medically ill child or
        adolescent
Physiological fear probes, 144–45
Pica, 624
Pimozide, 329t, 761t
    side effects, 528
    for tic disorders, 527–28, 528t, 529
Pindolol
    for ADHD, 354–55
        tic disorders and, 536
    for aggression, 678
Placebo, 717–18, 734–35
    risk/benefit analysis, 740–41
    vs. medication, meaning of, 420–21
Plasmapheresis, for postinfectious OCD
        and tic disorders, 180
Platelet dysfunction, divalproex–induced,
        318
PLC-γ, activation, 38–39, 39f
Point mutations, 74
Polycystic ovaries, divalproex–induced,
        318
Polyuria, lithium-induced, 311
Positive predictive power, 407
Positron emission tomography (PET), in
        aggression, 214–15
Post-traumatic stress disorder, 580–89
    aggression in, 673
    assessment, 581–82
    assessment instruments, 410t
    attention deficit in, 107
    bipolar disorder and, 674
    clinical presentation, 580
    cognitive-behavioral therapy, 582–83,
        589
    comorbid psychiatric disorders, 581
    DSM-IV criteria, 580

hypothalamic-pituitary-adrenal axis in,
        140–41
    informants, 405t
    neurobiological systems involved in,
        585t
    pharmacotherapy, 582–88
        adrenergergic agents, 585
        algorithm for, 583–84, 583f
        anticonvulsants, 588
        buproprion, 588
        carbamazepine, 588
        dopaminergic agents, 585–86
        GABAergic and benzodiazepines,
            587–88
        general approach, 588–89
        opioid antagonists, 588
        published studies, 584–85, 584t
        roles of, 584
        serotonergic agents, 586–87
        stimulants, 588
        tricyclic antidepressants, 587
        valproic acid, 588
        venlafaxine, 587
    prevalence, 580
    psychoeducation in, 582
    relationship to drug use, 245
    symptoms, pharmacological actions
        associated with, 586t
Post-Traumatic Stress Disorder Reaction
        Index, 413t, 581
Posterior parietal cortex, attentional
        processing, 100, 103
Postinfectious autoimmune
        neuropsychiatric disorders. See
        PANDAS
Postsynaptic neurons, 21, 22f
Practice guidelines, combination therapy,
        437–38, 439f–440f
Preclinical drug testing, 725
Predictive power, 407
Prefrontal cortex
    in ADHD, 105
    in aggression, 212, 214
    attentional processing, 100–101,
        103
    in depression, 125
    modulation of, 103–4
        by acetylcholine, 104
        by dopamine, 103
        by norepinephrine, 103–4
        by serotonin, 104
        by stimulants, 104
    in obsessive-compulsive disorder, 153
    in tics and stereotypies, 166
Pregnancy
    anxiety disorders during, 649
    bipolar disorders during, 648
    complications
        schizophrenia and, 189
        tic disorders and, 170
    maternal physiologic changes related
        to, 648
    mood disorders during, 647–48

psychopharmacotherapy during, 642–
        50
        anticonvulsants, 645
        antidepressants, 643–44
        antipsychotic drugs, 645–46
        benzodiazepines, 646
        electroconvulsive therapy, 647
        empirical data, 643–47
        mood stabilizers, 644–45
        treatment recommendations, 647–49
    schizophrenia during, 648–49
    testing, in assessment for
        pharmacotherapy, 399
Prenatal stress
    prevalence, 110–11
    relationship to psychopathology, 111
Preschool Behavior Questionnaire, 413t
Preschool Observation Scale of Anxiety,
        499
Preschoolers
    assessment instruments, 411t
    psychiatric disorders in
        diagnostic dilemma, 655–66
        prevalence, 666
    psychotropic drug development in,
        733–34
    psychotropic drug use in, 654–65
        α₂-adrenergic agonists, 659–60,
            660t
        antidepressants, 661–62, 661t–662t
        antipsychotic drugs, 662–64, 663t
        prevalence, 654–55, 706, 737
        recommendations for clinicians and
            research agenda, 664–65
        stimulants, 259, 655–59, 657t–
            658t
Presynaptic neurons, 21, 22f
Priapism, trazodone-induced, 696
Primate models, of mania, 129–30
Pro-dynorphin, 357
Pro-enkephalin, 357
Pro-opiomelanocortin, 357
Problem identification, in assessment for
        pharmacotherapy, 399–400
Procedural phobias, in cancer patient,
        636
Progesterone, in maternal behavior,
        201
Prolactin
    in affiliative behaviors, 200–201
    knockout mouse, 201
Promethazine, for anticipatory nausea,
        635–36
Promoters, gene, 70
Proposed Pediatric Study Request
        (PPSR), 728
Propranolol, 763t
    for aggression, 678
    for anxiety disorders, 355
    dosage, 355–56
    pharmacology, 354
Prosencephalon, homeodomain selector
        genes, 4, 6, 6f

Protein
    acetylation, 71
    binding, in children and adolescents,
        drug distribution and, 50
    glycosylation, 71
    mass spectrometric identification, 80
    methylation, 71
    phosphorylation, 71–72
        regulation, 40
        signal transduction and, 73–74, 73f
    synthesis, 71–72, 72f
Protein chip approach, 80
Protein kinase A (PKA)
    G protein–coupled receptor
        desensitization by, 37, 37f
    phosphorylation targets, 35
Protein kinase C (PKC)
    G protein–coupled receptor
        desensitization by, 37, 37f
    phosphorylation targets, 36
Protein-protein interactions, 80–81
Proteomics, 80–81
Prozac. See Fluoxetine
Pseudostratified ventricular epithelium,
    8, 9f
Psychiatric disorders. See
    Neuropsychiatric disorders
Psychiatrists, psychotropic drug
    prescribing by, 703, 705
Psychodynamic-psychoanalytical
    tradition, in European child
    psychiatry, 746
Psychoeducation
    anxiety disorders, 504–5
    combination therapy, 437
    depression, 467–68
    medications, 400
    post-traumatic stress disorder, 582
Psychopharmacotherapy, pediatric
    assessment for, 391–402. See also
        Assessment for
        pharmacotherapy
    combination therapy, 426–41. See also
        Combined drug and
        psychosocial treatments
    definition, 417
    developmental principles, 1–16
    genetic studies, 84–92. See also
        Pharmacogenetics
    instruments and scales, 404–14. See
        also Instruments and scales
    prescribing practices, 701–10. See also
        Psychotropic drugs, use of
    psychology of, 417–24
        influences on prescribing, 422–23
        meaning of medication, 418–20,
            419t
        meaning of medication context, 421–
            22
        meaning of medication process, 420–
            21
        split treatment prescribing, 423–24
    regulatory challenges, 732–35

and therapeutic alliance, 417
Psychosis
    aggression in, 674
    assessment instruments, 410t
    informants, 405t
    Korsakoff's, 243
    substance abuse and dependence
        disorders with, 614
Psychosocial treatment. See also
        Cognitive-behavioral therapy
    for ADHD, 457–59
    for anxiety disorders, 503–6
    with psychopharmacotherapy. See
        Combined drug and
        psychosocial treatments
    for substance abuse and dependence
        disorders, 605, 611
Psychosomatic tradition, in European
    child psychiatry, 746
Psychotherapy, for schizophrenia, 556–
    58
Psychotic depression, electroconvulsive
    therapy, 378
Psychotic disorders
    with mental retardation, 624–25
    in obsessive-compulsive disorder,
        521
Psychotropic drugs. See also specific
        type, e.g., Antipsychotic drugs
    clinical trials, 712–23. See also
        Clinical trials
    neuronal adaptation to, 39–42
    nonspecific indications, 733–34
    pediatric exclusivity provisions related
        to, 727–28
    pediatric labeling
        current, 729
        regulations, 726–27
    pharmacokinetics, 44–52. See also
        Pharmacokinetics
    in preschoolers. See under
        Preschoolers
    regulatory issues, 725–35. See also
        Pediatric drug development
    safety monitoring, 402, 722, 734
    signal transduction mechanisms, 33–
        39
    summary table, 757t–763t
    therapeutic drug monitoring, 51, 51t
    use of, 701–10
        age differences, 703–4
        current levels, 704–8
        ethnic differences, 706
        in Europe, 746–51
        gender differences, 703, 705–6
        inpatient settings, 706–7
        in Japan, 751–53
        local factors, 705
        misunderstandings about, 701
        outpatient settings, 707–8
        over- vs. underprescribing practices,
            708–9
        polypharmacy trends, 704

regional factors, 705
    research and policy implications,
        709–10
    specialty differences, 703, 705
    time trends, 702–4
    trends in who receives medications,
        703–4
Pubertal arrest, from valproic acid, 694
Putamen
    in postinfectious OCD and tic
        disorders, 178
    in regulation of attention, 101
    in tics and stereotypies, 166
Pynoos Stress Reaction Index, 582
Pyrilamine maleate, 348

Q fraction, cortical neurogenesis, 9f, 10
QTc prolongation, antipsychotic-
    induced, 335
Quantitative trait loci (QTL) mapping,
    in substance abuse and
    dependence disorders, 244–45
Quetiapine, 329t, 760t
    for autism and other pervasive
        developmental disorders, 569
    for bipolar disorders, 491
    ocular effects, 336
    for schizophrenia, 553t, 554
    for tic disorders, 529

Race requirements, in clinical trials,
    715
Rage, beta blockers for, 354–55
Ras gene, activation, 38, 39f
Rate dependency, 408
Rating attenuation effect, 406
Rating scales. See Instruments and scales
Reboxetine, 294
    in children and adolescents, 304
    history, 304
    mechanism of action, 304
    pharmacokinetics, 304
    side effects and toxicity, 304
Receiver/Response Operating
    Characteristic (ROC) curves, in
    schizophrenia, 547
Receptor(s)
    cholinergic, 26–27, 26f
    dopamine, 30–31, 30f
    G protein–coupled (slow-acting, class
        II), 21, 22f, 34–38
    $GABA_A$, 24–25, 25f
    $GABA_B$, 25, 25f
    glutamate, 23, 24f
    ionotropic, 34
    ionotropic (fast-acting, class I), 21,
        22f, 34
    membrane bound, 21, 22f
    muscarinic, 26, 26f
    neurotrophin, 38–39, 39f
    nicotinic, 26–27, 26f
    noradrenergic, 28, 29f
    serotonergic, 27, 28f

Receptor tyrosine kinases
  in neuronal remodeling, 13
  phosphorylation, regulation, 40
  signaling pathways, 38–39, 39f
Reeler gene, in cortical cell migration,
     11
Regression to the mean, 406
Regulatory issues
  in complementary and alternative
     medicine, 366–67
  in drug development, 725–35. *See also*
     Pediatric drug development
Rehabilitation, in schizophrenia, 558–
     59
Reliability, measurement instruments,
     406
Remedial clinical tradition, in European
     child psychiatry, 746
Renal effects, lithium, 311
Repetition suppression, 99
Research in children, 737–44. *See also*
     Clinical trials
  The Belmont Report, 738
  community collaborations, 743
  confidentiality, 742–43
  ethics assessment tool, 743
  federal regulations, 738–39, 739t
  guidelines, 738
  incentives vs. coercion, 741–42
  informed consent, 742
  participant recruitment, 741–42
  risk/benefit analysis, 739–41
     in discontinuation studies, 740
     in placebo group, 740–41
  risk evaluation, 739, 739t
Research Protocol Ethics Assessment
     Tool, 743
Research questions, identifying, 712–15
Respiratory disturbances
  in panic disorder, 140
  as physiological fear probe, 144–45
Retrograde amnesia, after
     electroconvulsive therapy, 380
Rett's disorder, 564
Reverse genetics, 76
Revised Children's Manifest Anxiety
     Scale, 413t
RGS proteins, regulation of G protein
     signaling by, 35
Rhabdosphincter, 687, 688
Rheumatic fever
  with chorea, 176
  tic disorders and, 170
Ribosomes, 71
Risk
  evaluation, research in children, 739,
     739t
  minimal, definition, 739
Risk/benefit analysis
  research in children, 739–41
  SSRIs, 279
Risperidone, 329t, 760t
  for aggression, 679–80

for autism and other pervasive
     developmental disorders, 568
for bipolar disorders, 491
for conduct disorder with mental
     retardation, 622–23
for delirium in cancer patient, 636
for mania, 489
for obsessive-compulsive disorder, 522
in preschoolers, 664
for schizophrenia, 553t, 554
for self-injury in mental retardation,
     626
for tic disorders, 529
weight gain from, 334
Ritalin. *See* Methylphenidate
RNA
  messenger
     transcription, 70–71
     translation and posttranslational
        processing, 71–72, 72f
  splicing, 71
  transfer, 71
Rodent models, of mania, 129

Safety monitoring, 402
  in clinical trials, 722
  research needs, 734
St. John's wort, 368–72
  active constituents and mechanism of
     action, 368
  botany, 368
  in children and adolescents, 371
  for depression, effectiveness, 368–69
  dosage and administration, 371–72
  drug interactions, 370–71, 370t
  pharmacokinetics and drug
     distribution, 369
  preparations, 371
  safety, 369
  serotonin syndrome from, 64, 278–79
  side effects, 369–70
  for uses other than depression, 372
Sample size
  clinical trials, 720–21
  confidence intervals and, 721, 722f
  statistical power and, 720–21
Schedule for Affective Disorders and
     Schizophrenia, Kiddie version–
     Present & Lifetime version (K-
     SADS-PL), 411
  in post-traumatic stress disorder, 582
Schizencephaly, *Emx* genes in, 6
Schizoaffective disorder, 188, 188t
Schizophrenia
  aberrant synaptic pruning hypothesis,
     190
  aggression in, 674
  childhood-onset, 184–91, 543–59
     animal models, 185
     assessment instruments, 545–47,
        546t
     autonomic functioning in, 187
     classification, 184–91, 543–59

clinical phenotype, 184–85
clinical presentation, 545
comorbid psychiatric disorders, 185
conceptual models, 190
differential diagnosis, 547, 548t
environmental factors, 189
epidemiology, 543–44
genetic studies, 187–89, 188t
neuroanatomical studies, 185–86,
     186t
neurobiology, 184–91
neurophysiological studies, 187–89
neurotransmitters in, 187
pharmacotherapy, 190, 547–56
  amisulpride, 553t, 554
  atypical antipsychotics, 547–48,
     550t, 551, 552t–553t
  clozapine, 551, 552t
  decision tree for, 554, 555f
  guidelines, 556
  indications and contraindications,
     548
  olanzapine, 551, 552t–553t, 554
  quetiapine, 553t, 554
  risperidone, 553t, 554
  typical antipsychotics, 547–48,
     549t–550t
premorbid development, 189–90
prevalence, 184
prevention of relapses, 556
psychotherapy
  cognitive and behavioral
     approaches, 556–57
  emotional management therapy,
     557
  family-oriented measures, 558
  group therapy, 557–58
  social skills training, 556–57
rehabilitation, 558–59
risk factors, 191t
smooth pursuit eye movements in,
     187, 188
treatment, 547–58
very early–onset vs. early-onset,
     544
diagnostic criteria, 544–45, 544t
electroconvulsive therapy, 378
mental retardation with, 624–25
neurodevelopmental hypothesis, 190
during pregnancy, 648–49
simple, 545
subtypes, 544t, 545
Schizophrenia spectrum disorders, 188,
     188t
Schizophreniform disorder, 545
Schizotypal personality disorder, 188,
     188t, 545
School context, medications, 421
School phobia, tricyclic antidepressants
     for, 291
School refusal, anxiety disorders with
     depression and, combination
     therapy, 432

Scrambler gene, in cortical cell
    migration, 11
Screen for Anxiety-Related Emotional
    Disorders (SCARED), 499
Seasonal affective disorder, 472
Second messenger pathways, G protein–
    coupled receptors, 35–36
Secretin, for autism and other pervasive
    developmental disorders, 572–
    73
Sedation
    from antipsychotics, 335
    from benzodiazepines, 344
    conscious, 633
Sedative hypnotics, acute actions, 241
Seizures
    aggression/agitation during, 674, 682
    from antipsychotics, 334
    from bupropion, 303
    prolonged, in electroconvulsive
        therapy, 379
    from tricyclic antidepressants, 290
Selective noradrenergic reuptake
    inhibitors, 294
Selective serotonin reuptake inhibitors,
    274–80, 757t
    for ADHD, 450t, 455
    adverse effects, 275–79
        in children and adolescents, 275
        general, 275–76
    for aggression, 678
    for anorexia nervosa, 598
    for anxiety disorders, 500–501, 500t,
        503
    for autism and other pervasive
        developmental disorders, 569–
        72
    for bulimia nervosa, 598
    discontinuation, 469
    discontinuation syndrome, 277
    drug interactions, 277–78, 277t, 469
    future directions, 279
    general properties, 274–75, 275t
    indications, 274, 275t
    for major depressive disorder, 468–69
        with mental retardation, 623
    neurological effects, 276
    neuropsychiatric and behavioral
        effects, 276–77
    for obsessive-compulsive disorder, 158–
        59, 515, 519–20, 519t, 522
        number needed to treat, 431, 431t,
            432t
        tic disorders and, 537
    overdose, 277
    pharmacokinetic studies in children,
        279, 469
    for post-traumatic stress disorder, 586–
        87
    during pregnancy, 647
    for prevention or reversal of early life
        stress consequences, 119
    risk/benefit considerations, 279

selectivity differences, 274–75
    for self-injury in mental retardation,
        626
    serotonin syndrome from, 278–79,
        278t
    side effects, 469, 522
    with stimulants, 457
    teratogenicity, 643–44
Selegiline, 758t
    for ADHD, 450t, 454–55
    indications, 296
    mechanism of action, 296–97
Self-injury
    mental retardation with, 625–27
    naltrexone for, 358–59
Self-report instruments and scales, 435
Sensitivity, measurement instruments,
    406–7
Sensory association cortex, attentional
    processing, 99–100, 103
Separation anxiety, 139–40, 291
Sepsis, vs. serotonin syndrome, 278
Serotonergic genes, in neuropsychiatric
    disorders
    association studies, 88–90
    genetic studies, 90–91, 90t, 91t
Serotonergic neurotransmission, 27–28
    anatomy, 27
    function, 27–28
    synaptic organization, 27, 28f
Serotonin
    in affiliative behaviors, 202–3
    in aggression, 216–17, 218, 219–20
    in anxiety disorders, 145
    in attention modulation, 104
    in autism, 205–6
    in depression, 128
    in eating disorders, 231–32
    knockout mouse, 202–3
    in obsessive-compulsive disorder, 157–
        59
    in tic disorders/Tourette's syndrome,
        169
    tricyclic antidepressant effects on, 284–
        85
Serotonin receptors, 27, 28f
    antipsychotic drug blockade, 330
    polymorphisms
        in clozapine response, 90–91, 90t,
            91t
        disease associations, 89–90
Serotonin reuptake inhibitors
    noradrenergic and, 294
    selective. *See* Selective serotonin
        reuptake inhibitors
Serotonin syndrome, 278–79, 278t
    agents implicated in, 63t, 64, 278t
    manifestations, 63–64, 278t
    from monoamine oxidase inhibitors,
        298
Serotonin transporter, 27, 28f
    in depression, 128
    polymorphisms, 88–89

in substance abuse and dependence
    disorders, 242, 243
Sertraline, 757t
    adverse effects, 275–79
    for anxiety disorders, 500, 500t
    for autism and other pervasive
        developmental disorders, 571
    cytochrome P450 inhibition by, 277,
        277t
    general properties, 274–75, 275t
    indications, 274, 275t
    for obsessive-compulsive disorder,
        515, 519t
    pharmacokinetic studies in children,
        279, 469
    for post-traumatic stress disorder, 587
Serzone. *See* Nefazodone
Set-shifting, prefrontal cortex in, 101
Sex differences. *See* Gender differences
Sexual abuse of child
    definition, 110
    prevalence, 110–11
    relationship to psychopathology, 111
Sexual dimorphism, brain development,
    15–16
Sexual dysfunction
    from antipsychotics, 335
    psychiatrically induced, 695–96
Sheep, oxytocin receptors in, 199–200
Signal transduction
    mechanisms, 33–39
    molecular genetics, 72–74, 73f
Single photon emission computed
    tomography (SPECT)
    in aggression, 214
    in depression, 128
Skin conductance, in aggression, 216
Skin rash
    antipsychotic-induced, 335
    carbamazepine-induced, 316
    lamotrigine-induced, 320–21
Sleep disorders
    benzodiazepine-induced, 344
    mental retardation with, 627
    from SSRIs, 276–77
Small intestine, cytochrome P450
    enzymes in, 57
Smoking. *See* Tobacco use
Smooth pursuit eye movements, in
    schizophrenia, childhood-onset,
    187, 188
SNAP-IV, 413t
Social anxiety, 138–39
Social Effectiveness Training for
    Children, for anxiety disorders,
    505
Social fear probes, 143–44
Social relatedness, in mental status
    examination, 398
Social scrutiny, hypersensitivity to, 139
Social Skills Rating System, 413t
Social skills training, for schizophrenia,
    556–57

Sonic hedgehog (Shh), 6, 7f, 8
Spatial attentional orienting, cholinergic
    sensitivity, 103
Specificity, measurement instruments,
    406–7
Speech and language
    in assessment for pharmacotherapy,
        399
    disturbances
        in mental status examination, 398,
            488
        in schizophrenia, 545
        premorbid development, in
            schizophrenia, childhood-onset,
            190
SSRIs. See Selective serotonin reuptake
    inhibitors
Startle regulation, anxiety disorders and,
    143
Statistical power
    response rate and, 721, 721f
    sample size and, 720–21
Statistical significance, and clinical
    significance, 721, 721f
Stem cells, pluripotent, 15
Stereotypies
    neural substrates, 167f
    obsessive-compulsive disorder and,
        160–61
Steroids
    in affiliative behaviors, 201–2
    gonadal
        in affiliative behaviors, 201
        in aggression, 216
        in brain development, 15–16
Stevens-Johnson syndrome, lamotrigine-
    induced, 320–21
Stimulants, 757t
    acute actions, 240
    for ADHD, 255–61, 448, 449t, 450–
        53
        with clonidine, 258
        with desipramine, 257–58, 457
        discontinuation, 261
        drug interactions, 257–58
        growth deficits associated with, 452
        history and overview, 255–56
        long-acting preparations, 257, 453
        long-term use considerations, 260–
            61
        mechanism of action, 102f, 104,
            256
        with mental retardation, 619
        monitoring, 260
        pharmacokinetics and drug
            distribution, 256–57
        in preschool-age children, 259, 655–
            59, 657t–658t
        selection and dosage considerations,
            259–60
        side effects and toxicity, 255–59
        with SSRIs, 457
        sustained-release formulations, 260

tic disorders and, 452–53, 535
for aggression, 677–78
in attention modulation, 104
for autism and other pervasive
    developmental disorders, 572
chronic effects
    brain morphology, 242
    cerebral blood flow, metabolism,
        and function, 243
    receptor studies, 242
for conduct disorder with mental
    retardation, 622
neuronal adaptation to, 41
for pain management, 635
for post-traumatic stress disorder,
    588
in preschoolers, 259, 655–59, 657t–
    658t
side effects, 452
for substance use disorders, safety
    concerns, 611–12
use of
    in Europe, 748
    time trends, 702
Streptococcal infection, pediatric
    autoimmune neuropsychiatric
    disorders associated with. See
    PANDAS
Stress
    acute, 580
    attention and, 104
    early life, 110–20
        animal models, 113, 115, 119–20
        anxiety disorders and, 118–19, 145–
            46
        clinical research considerations, 120
        definition, 110
        depression and, 117–18, 124–26
        disorders related to, 117–19
        genetic vulnerability, 117
        neurobiological consequences, 113–
            17, 114t
            clinical studies in adults, 116–17
            clinical studies in children, 115–
                16
            primate studies, 115
            rodent studies, 113
        pharmacological prevention or
            reversal of consequences, 119
        prevalence, 110–11
        relationship to psychopathology,
            111
    neurobiology, 111–13, 582
    post-traumatic. See Post-traumatic
        stress disorder
    prenatal, 110–11
    substance abuse and dependence
        disorders and, 245–46
    tic disorders and, 170
Stress response
    corticotropin-releasing factor systems
        in, 111–13, 112f
    ontogeny, 112–13

Striatum
    medium spiny neurons
        in obsessive-compulsive disorder,
            156
        in tic disorders, 168
    microstructure, 156–57
    in obsessive-compulsive disorder, 153,
        155–56, 160
Striosomes and matrices
    in obsessive-compulsive disorder, 155,
        156f
    stereotypies and, 160
Study design, clinical trials, 719–20
Study sample, defining, 715
Substance abuse and dependence
    disorders, 238–48, 605–14
    acute actions of drugs of abuse, 240–
        42
    with ADHD, 613
    aggression in, 674
    animal models, 240
    animal studies, 239
    with anxiety, 613
    assessment instruments, 410t
    with bipolar disorders, 493, 613–14
    chronic effects, 242–44
    comorbid psychiatric disorders, 605–6
        treatment, 607, 610, 613–14
    definitions, 238
    with depression, 613
    dopamine receptor in, 87
    early onset, 605
    with eating disorders, 226–27, 595
    environmental factors, 245–46
    genetic studies, 244–45
    informants, 405t
    neuroanatomical substrates of reward
        in, 239–40
    neurobiology, 238–48
    pharmacotherapy
        adverse effects, 611
        agents of prevention, 610
        agents of substitution, 606–7, 612
        agents that treat comorbid
            psychopathology, 607, 610
        anticraving agents, 607, 612–13
        aversive agents, 606, 612
        classification of agents, 606t
        with comorbid psychiatric disorders,
            607, 610, 613–14
        published studies, 606–10, 608t–
            609t
        recommendations, 612–13
        safety concerns, 611–12
        without comorbid psychopathology,
            611
    prenatal exposure studies, 246–47
    prevalence and patterns of use, 238–
        39
    prevention, 614
    with psychoses, 614
    psychosocial treatment, 605, 611, 614
    risk factors, 244–46

stress and
    in initiation of use, 245
    in progression to dependence, 245–46
    in relapse, 246
    treatment, 610–11
    withdrawal in, animal models, 240
Substantia nigra
    in cortical-striatal-thalamo-cortical loops, 153, 154f
    dopaminergic neurons, 29, 30f
Suicidal intention and behavior, in depression, 476
Sulpiride, for tic disorders, 530
Superiority studies, clinical trials, 719
Surgeon General's Conference on Children's Mental Health, 733
SWAN, 413t
Sydenham's chorea
    neuropsychiatric manifestations, 176
    tic disorders and, 170–71
Symptom scales, in clinical trials, 715–16
Synapse, 21, 22f
    cholinergic, 26–27, 26f
    dopaminergic, 30–31, 30f
    GABAergic, 24–25, 25f
    glutamatergic, 23, 24f
    noradrenergic, 28–29, 29f
    serotonergic, 27, 28f
Synaptic plasticity
    in learning, 14
    visual cortex, 14
Synaptic remodeling, 12–14, 12f

Tardive dyskinesia, antipsychotic-induced, 334
Teacher Report Form, 413t
Telencephalon, basal, progenitor cells, 11
Temporal cortex, inferior, stimulus processing in, 99–100
Temporal lobe
    in aggression, 214
    medial, 20, 21f
Teratogenicity
    alcohol, 246
    anticonvulsants, 645
    antidepressants, 643–44
    antipsychotic drugs, 645–46
    benzodiazepines, 646
    cannabis, 247
    cocaine, 247
    electroconvulsive therapy, 647
    empirical data, 643–47
    FDA rating system, 642
    mood stabilizers, 644–45
    opiates, 247
    tobacco use, 246–47
    types, 642
Terminal illness, pain management, 633
Testbusters, for anxiety disorders, 505
Testosterone
    in aggression, 216
    in tic disorders, 169–70

Tetrabenazine, for tic disorders, 530
Thalamus, 20, 21f
Therapeutic alliance, in assessment for pharmacotherapy, 398
Therapeutic drug monitoring
    Bayesian forecasting in, 51–52, 52f
    indications, 51, 51t
    timing, 51
Thioridazine, 329t, 761t
    QTc prolongation from, 335
    for schizophrenia with mental retardation, 625
    for self-injury in mental retardation, 626
Thiothixene, 329t, 761t
    for schizophrenia with mental retardation, 625
    teratogenicity, 645
Thought content, in mental status examination, 398
Thought Disorder Index, 546t, 547
Thought disorders, in schizophrenia, 545
Thought process, in mental status examination, 398
Three Factor Eating Questionnaire, 596t
Thrombocytopenia, carbamazepine-induced, 315
Thyroid dysfunction, lithium-induced, 311
Tiapride, for tic disorders, 530
Tic(s)
    clinical characteristics, 164–65
    complex, 175–76
    definition, 164
    motor, 164, 175
    phonic or vocal, 164
    premonitory urges, 164
Tic disorders/Tourette's syndrome, 526–38
    with ADHD, 165–66
        prevalence, 526
        stimulants for, 452–53, 535
        treatment, 535–37
        tricyclic antidepressants for, 454
    aggression in, 674
    animal models, 171
    assessment instruments, 411t
    cholinergic systems in, 168
    coexisting conditions, 165–66
    with developmental disorders, 166
    diagnosis, 176
    diagnostic categories, 165
    dopamine-related alleles in, 87
    dopamine system in, 166–68
    endogenous opioid peptides in, 168
    environmental influences, 169–71
        gender-specific endocrine factors, 169–70
        perinatal risk factors, 170
        postinfectious autoimmune mechanisms, 170–71

    psychological stress and emotional arousal, 170
    future prospects, 171–72
    GABAergic system in, 168
    general treatment approach, 534–35
    genetic susceptibility, 169
    glutamate system in, 168
    informants, 405t
    with mental retardation, 625
    natural history, 526–27
    neural substrates, 166–69, 167f
    neurobiology, 164–72
    noradrenergic systems in, 168–69
    with obsessive-compulsive disorder, 152, 165, 176, 520
        prevalence, 526
        treatment, 520, 537
    pharmacotherapy
        androgen modification, 533
        antipsychotic drugs, 527–30, 528t
        baclofen, 533–34, 534t
        botulinum, 533, 534t
        clonidine, 168–69, 531–32, 534t
        with comorbid psychiatric disorders, 535–37
        guanfacine, 532
        indications, 526–27
        mecamylamine, 532–33
        nicotine, 532
        other agents, 534
        pergolide, 530
        risks and benefits, 527
        tetrabenazine, 530
        tiapride and sulpiride, 530
    postinfectious subtype (PANDAS), 170–71, 176–81
        biological basis, 177–80
        brain systems implicated, 178–79
        comorbid psychiatric disorders, 177
        criteria for, 176–77, 177t
        evidence for, 176
        family studies, 177
        genetic susceptibility and biologic markers, 179–80
        treatment modalities, 180–81
    prevalence, 165, 176
    psychotherapy, 535
    serotonin systems in, 169
    treatment, 180–81
Tobacco use. See also Nicotine
    acute actions, 241
    genetic studies, 244
    neuroanatomical substrates of reward, 239
    prevalence, 238
    teratogenic effects, 246–47
Tolterodine, 763t
    for enuresis, 693, 694
Topiramate, 759t
    mechanism of action, 322
    pediatric uses, 322
    pharmacokinetics, 322
    side effects, 322

Topiramate (*continued*)
  for tic disorders, 534
  treatment guidelines, 314t
Tourette's syndrome. *See* Tic disorders/
    Tourette's syndrome
Tramadol, for pain management, 634–
    35
Transcranial magnetic stimulation, 383–
    84
  for treatment-resistant depression, 475
Transcription, gene, 70–71
Transcription factors, 40–41, 70
Translocation, chromosomal, 75
Transmission disequilibrium test (TDT),
    86
Tranylcypromine
  for ADHD, 449t, 454
  indications, 296
  mechanism of action, 296
  structure, 297
Trauma
  neurobiology of, 582
  stress disorder after. *See* Post-
    traumatic stress disorder
Trazodone, 758t
  for aggression, 678
  in children and adolescents, 302
  drug interactions, 301–2
  for major depressive disorder, 470
  mechanism of action, 301
  pharmacokinetics and drug
    distribution, 301
  and risk of priapism, 696
  side effects and toxicity, 302
Treatment as usual, as control group in
    clinical trials, 718–19
Treatment of Adolescents with
    Depression Study (TADS), 441
Treatment Outcome PTSD scale, 582
Treatment outcomes, for clinical trials,
    715–17
Treatment plan, in assessment for
    pharmacotherapy, 399–400,
    400t
Treatment studies, evidence-based
    medicine applied to, 429–32,
    430t
Tremor, hand, lithium-induced, 310
Triazolam, 343t
Tricyclic antidepressants, 284–93, 758t
  absorption, 286–87
  for ADHD, 291, 449t, 453–54
    with mental retardation, 619
  and α₂-adrenergic agonists, 270
  for aggression, 678
  for autism and pervasive
    developmental disorders, 291–
    92
  cardiovascular effects, 288, 290t,
    291t
  in children and adolescents, 290–93
  discontinuation, 293
  distribution, 287

dosages, 292
drug interactions, 288, 289t
effects on noradrenergic system, 284
effects on serotonin system, 284–85
excretion, 287
for major depressive disorder, 291,
    469–70
mechanism of action, 284–86, 286f
metabolism, 287
monitoring, 292–93
for nocturnal enuresis, 292, 693
for obsessive-compulsive disorder, 291
pharmacokinetics, 286–88
for post-traumatic stress disorder, 587
postsynaptic effects, 285–86
during pregnancy, 647
premedication workup, 291t, 292
receptor blockade profile, 287t
for school phobia and separation
    anxiety, 291
side effects, 288, 290, 290t
with stimulants, 258
structure, 284, 285f
teratogenicity, 644
toxicity and overdose, 288, 290
Trifluoperazine, 329t
  teratogenicity, 645
Trihexyphenidyl, teratogenicity, 646
Trinucleotide repeat expansion, 70–71
Tripelennamine, 348
Tryptophan hydroxylase gene, 90
Twin studies
  aggression, 217–18
  obsessive-compulsive disorder, 152
  substance abuse and dependence
    disorders, 244
  tic disorders, 169
Type I error, 720
Type II error, 720
Tyramine, monoamine oxidase inhibitors
    and, 297–98

Underprescribing of psychotropic drugs,
    708–9
Urethral sphincter
  external, 687, 688
  internal, 687–88
Uridine diphosphate glucuronyl
    transferases
  classification, 57–58
  in phase 2 metabolism, 56
Urinary frequency, 691–92, 693–94,
    695f

Valerian, 373
Validity
  external, 428
  instruments and scales, 406–7
  internal, 428–29
Valium. *See* Diazepam
Valproic acid
  for aggression, 679
  for bipolar disorders

with mental retardation, 621–22
during pregnancy, 648
for conduct disorder with mental
    retardation, 622
for post-traumatic stress disorder, 588
pubertal arrest from, 694
for substance use disorders with
    explosive mood disorders, 607
teratogenicity, 645
and valproate sodium. *See* Divalproex
Vancomycin, for autism and other
    pervasive developmental
    disorders, 576
Vasopressin
  in affiliative behaviors, 197, 200
  in nocturnal enuresis, 692
Venlafaxine, 758t
  for ADHD, 450t, 455
  for anxiety disorders, 500t, 502, 503
  in children and adolescents, 305
  history, 304
  for major depressive disorder, 470
  mechanism of action, 304–5
  monitoring, 305
  pharmacokinetics and drug
    distribution, 305
  for post-traumatic stress disorder, 587
  side effects and toxicity, 305
Ventilatory disturbances
  in panic disorder, 140
  as physiological fear probe, 144–45
Ventral bed nucleus of the stria
    terminalis, in affiliative
    behaviors, 197
Ventral striatum, in obsessive-compulsive
    disorder, 153, 155–56
Ventral tegmental area, dopaminergic
    neurons, 29, 30f
Ventricle, lateral, in depression, 128
Ventricular epithelium, pseudostratified,
    8, 9f
Ventricular volume, in schizophrenia,
    childhood-onset, 185, 186
Verapamil
  for bipolar disorders, 491
  for mania, 489
Verbal tic, 164
Vertebrate, central nervous system
    patterning, 4, 5f
Violence. *See also* Aggression
  assessment of risk for, 682–83
  definition, 671
  mental illness and, 671
  weather and, 219
Visual cortex
  critical period, 14
  stimulus processing in, 99–100
Visuospatial attention, posterior parietal
    cortex in, 100
Voiding
  dysfunctional, 691–92, 693–94, 695f
  neurobiology, 686–89, 687f
Voles, oxytocin receptors in, 199, 200

Weather, violence and, 219
Wechsler-III Intelligence scale for
        Children (WISC-III), 566
Weight gain
    from antipsychotics, 334, 336
    from divalproex, 318
Wellbutrin. *See* Bupropion
Wernicke's encephalopathy, 243
White matter
    in ADHD, 105
    development, 14

Withdrawal, drug, animal models, 240
Wnt-1 gene, 8

Xanax. *See* Alprazolam

Yale-Brown-Cornell Eating Disorder
        Scale, 596t
Yale-Brown Obsessive-Compulsive Scale.
        See Children's Yale-Brown
        Obsessive-Compulsive Scale
Yale Global Tic Severity Scale, 413t

Yotari gene, in cortical cell migration, 11
Young-Mania Rating Scale, 487

Zaleplon, 350
Ziprasidone, 336, 760t
    for autism and other pervasive
        developmental disorders, 569
    for tic disorders, 529–30
Zofran. *See* Ondansetron
Zoloft. *See* Sertraline
Zolpidem, for anxiety disorders, 349–50